Health Information Management

Concepts, Principles, and Practice

Second Edition

Kathleen M. LaTour, MA, RHIA, FAHIMA
Shirley Eichenwald Maki, MBA, RHIA, FAHIMA

Editors

AHiMA

American Health Information
Management Association®

The Web sites listed in this book were current and valid as of the date of publication. However, Web page addresses and the information on them may change or disappear at any time and for any number of reasons. The user is encouraged to perform his or her own general Web searches to locate any site addresses listed here that are no longer valid.

ISBN 1-58426-142-0
AHIMA Product Number AB103306

AHIMA Staff:

Claire Blondeau, MBA, Project Editor
June E. Bronnert, RHIA, CCS, CCS-P
Jill Burrington-Brown, MS, RHIA
Michelle L. Dougherty, RHIA, CHP
Melanie A. Endicott, MBA/HCM, RHIA, CCS
Susan Fenton, MBA, RHIA
Kathy Giannangelo, RHIA, CCS
Beth Hjort, RHIA, CHPS
Susan Hull, MPH, RHIA, CCS, CCS-P
Karen Kostick, RHIT, CCS, CCS-P
Elizabeth Lund, Assistant Editor
Donald T. Mon, PhD, FHIMSS
Carol Ann Quinsey, RHIA, CHPS
Harry Rhodes, MBA, RHIA, CHPS
Dan Rode, MBA, FHFMA
Rita A. Scichilone, MHSA, RHIA, CCS, CCS-P, CHC
Mary H. Stanfill, RHIA, CCS, CCS-P
Melissa Ulbricht, Editorial/Production Coordinator
Maggie Williams, MA
Ann Zeisset, RHIT, CCS-P, CCS
Ken Zielske, Director of Publications

American Health Information Management Association
233 North Michigan Avenue, Suite 2150
Chicago, Illinois 60601-5800

ahima.org

Contents

About the Editors and Authors

Kathleen M. LaTour, MA, RHIA, FAHIMA is an assistant professor and chair of the department of healthcare informatics and information management (HIIM) at the College of St. Scholastica in Duluth, Minnesota. She is an active member of the Minnesota Health Information Management Association, where she was selected as the Distinguished Member in 1992. She has served as chair and member of many AHIMA councils and as a member of AHIMA's Board of Directors from 1993 to 1997. She participated in the development of the AHIMA Model Curricula for both bachelor's- and master's-level programs. She has authored several articles and recently contributed a chapter to *Health Information Management Technology: An Applied Approach,* second edition, a textbook published by AHIMA in 2006. She was awarded fellowship in AHIMA in recognition of sustained contributions to the field of HIM and, in 2004, was corecipient of AHIMA's Legacy Award.

Shirley Eichenwald Maki, MBA, RHIA, FAHIMA, is an assistant professor in the department of healthcare informatics and information management at the College of St. Scholastica in Duluth, Minnesota. She also serves as project director for The ATHENS Project (css.edu/programs/athens), a health sciences EHR curriculum model project funded by a grant from the U.S. Department of Education, Title III program. She is the 2001 recipient of the College of St. Scholastica's Max H. Lavine Award for Teaching Excellence. A former president of AHIMA, she was awarded the association's Distinguished Member Award in 1998. In addition, she coauthored with Merida L. Johns, PhD, RHIA, AHIMA's White Paper on the Health and Well-being of HIM Education. She has held the position of director of education and accreditation at AHIMA and has served as an HIM consultant with Pyramid Health Solutions and Quadramed's HIM Division. Finally, she was awarded fellowship in AHIMA in recognition of sustained contributions to the field of HIM and, in 2004, was corecipient of AHIMA's Legacy Award.

Margret K. Amatayakul, MBA, RHIA, CHPS, FHIMSS, is president of Margret\A Consulting, LLC, in Schaumburg, Illinois, a consulting firm specializing in computer-based patient records and associated HIM standards and regulations, such as HIPAA. She has more than 30 years of experience in national and international HIM. A leading authority on electronic health record (EHR) strategies for healthcare organizations, she has extensive experience in EHR selection and project management, and she formed and served as executive director of the Computer-based Patient Record Institute (CPRI). Other positions held include associate executive director of AHIMA, associate professor at the University of Illinois, and director of medical record services at the Illinois Eye and Ear Infirmary. She is a much-sought-after speaker, has published extensively, and has earned several professional service awards. Amatayakul also serves as an adjunct faculty member of the College of St. Scholastica and the University of Illinois at Chicago.

Rita K. Bowen, MA, RHIA, CHPS, has nearly 30 years of experience in healthcare information management. She is currently the privacy officer for the Erlanger Health System in Chattanooga, Tennessee, and has previously held positions as director of health information services, director of medical records, marketing director, and medical records consultant at various hospitals and medical services companies throughout the United States. Bowen has an MA in health information management technology from the College of Saint Scholastica and earned her bachelor's degree in medical science from Emory University in Atlanta. She has a continuous history of activities with AHIMA and the Tennessee HIMA.

Elizabeth Bowman, MPA, RHIA, is a professor in the HIM program at the University of Tennessee Health Science Center in Memphis. She has been an HIM educator for more than 25 years. She received a bachelor's degree from

Millsaps College and a master's degree in public administration with a concentration in healthcare administration from the University of Memphis. She has served as chair of the AHIMA Assembly on Education and received the AHIMA Educator Award in 1999. Additionally, she was awarded the Tennessee Health Information Management Association's Distinguished Member Award in 1998.

Bonnie S. Cassidy, MPA, RHIA, FAHIMA, FHIMSS, CPHQ, received a BS degree in medical record administration from Daemen College in Amherst, New York, and a master's degree from Cleveland State University. A member of the AHIMA Board of Directors, she recently chaired the AHIMA Fellowship Review Committee and was a member of the EHR Transformation Workgroup, the Panel of Accreditation Surveyors for The Commission on Accreditation for Health Informatics and Information Management Education (CAHIIM), and the Clinical Terminology and Classification Practice Council. In addition, she has served as chair of the AHIMA Nominating and Professional Development committees; HIM Steering; QMS Roles and Functions committees; and the Data Quality, E-Health and Corporate Communications and Marketing Task Forces of AHIMA. Her achievements include the AHIMA 2000 Legacy Award, AHIMA's 1995 Professional Achievement Award, and the Distinguished Member Award from the Ohio Health Information Management Association (OHIMA), where she is a past president. In 2005, she was appointed to the Certification Commission for Health Information Technology Work Group on the Certification Process. She has represented the HIM profession on many levels, including as a frequent contributor to the *Journal of AHIMA* and as a presenter at AHIMA educational sessions and annual conventions. Her career has included working as a practitioner for two major teaching hospitals, a consultant for three professional service companies, adjunct faculty for two HIT programs, and vice-president of business development for an HIM-focused consulting company. Currently, she is president of Cassidy & Associates Consulting.

Nadinia Davis, MBA, CIA, CPA, RHIA, FAHIMA, is an assistant professor of HIM at the College of Natural, Applied, and Health Sciences at Kean University in Union, New Jersey. She has worked as a coding consultant and auditor in acute settings and as director of medical records at a rehabilitation institute. Prior to her HIM career, Davis worked in the financial services industry, most recently as an internal auditor. She is former president and a Distinguished Member of NJHIMA, as well as a former member of the AHIMA Board of Directors. She was a coauthor of *Introduction to Health Information Technology,* a contributor to *Effective Management of Coding Services,* and editor and contributor to *Workbook to Accompany Essentials of Health Care Finance.*

Mehnaz Farishta, MS, is manager for marketing and communications at The Shams Group, Inc., an award-winning knowledge management IT software and consulting company in the health information systems marketplace. She has authored and coauthored several articles on the role of information technology in healthcare, especially in the areas of data warehousing, patient safety, and process automation. These articles have been published in noted healthcare publications, including *Journal of AHIMA* and *Topics in Health Information Management.* Prior to joining TSG, Farishta worked as an insurance analyst and consultant.

Susan H. Fenton, MBA, RHIA, works part-time as a manager in practice leadership for the American Health Information Management Association. She is project leader for the National Library of Medicine SNOMED:ICD-9-CM map validation project. Presently, she is pursuing a PhD in health services research at the Texas A&M School of Rural Public Health. She has authored numerous articles and several book chapters.

Sandra R. Fuller, MA, RHIA, is executive vice-president and chief operating officer at AHIMA. Her responsibilities include oversight of the *Journal of AHIMA,* development of HIM practice tools, the annual convention, continuing education and training, certification, publications, accreditation and education, membership, and marketing and sales. A former director of patient data services at the University of Washington Medical Center in Seattle, Fuller completed her term as a member of AHIMA's Board of Directors at the end of 1996. She also has served on AHIMA's Council on Education and its Alliance and Program committees. A former president of the Washington State Health Information Management Association, she received both a bachelor's degree in health information management and a master's degree in management from the College of St. Scholastica in Duluth, Minnesota.

Matthew J. Greene, RHIA, CCS, is functional analyst/HIM specialist and data content team leader for the Department of Veterans Affairs Health Data Repository project. Prior to this position, he was a coder and HIM manager at the Buffalo, New York, and Salt Lake City VA healthcare systems. He received a BS in medical record administration from Daemen College in Amherst, New York. He was awarded the 2004 Distinguished Member Award from the Utah Health Information Management Association (UHIMA). Currently, Greene is serving his second year as director of acute care for UHIMA. In addition, he has volunteered for several AHIMA initiatives, including the eHIM workgroup and the ICD-10-CM Field Test, and he is an active member of the Health Level Seven (HL7) Medical Record/Information Management, Structured Documents, and EHR Technical committees. He has also been a workgroup volunteer for the eGov Consolidated Health Informatics (CHI) initiative.

J. Michael Hardin, PhD, is professor of statistics in the Department of Information Systems, Statistics, and Management Science at the University of Alabama in Tuscaloosa. In addition, he is adjunct professor of health informatics in the Department of Health Services Administration at the University of Alabama at Birmingham (UAB). Prior to these positions, Hardin served for 13 years as professor of health informatics, biostatistics, computer science, and preventive medicine at UAB and was selected as scholar in residence at Loyola University of Chicago. Moreover, he has been a visiting scholar at Trinity College, University of Dublin. A frequent speaker at AHIMA national meetings in the areas of database design, data modeling, and data mining, he has given more than 30 presentations on various topics related to data mining and data warehousing and has taught decision support in health informatics for the past seven years. He has authored or coauthored more than 90 publications and has served as a consultant to several major companies in the area of Medicare program integrity and utilization review.

Laurinda B. Harman, PhD, RHIA, is an associate professor and chair of the Department of Health Information Management at the College of Health Professions at Temple University in Philadelphia. She has been an HIM professional and educator for more than 35 years and has directed HIM baccalaureate programs at George Washington University in Washington, DC, and The Ohio State University in Columbus. She was a faculty member in the health information technology program at Northern Virginia Community College and served as director of education and human resource development for the Department of Health Care Sciences at George Washington University. She edited *Ethical Challenges in the Management of Health Information* and received the AHIMA 2001 Triumph Legacy Award for this important health information resource. The second edition was published in 2006.

Anita C. Hazelwood, MLS, RHIA, FAHIMA, is a professor in the HIM department at the University of Louisiana at Lafayette and has been an HIM professional for nearly 30 years. She is actively involved with AHIMA's Assembly on Education (AOE), has served on several other AHIMA committees, and is currently on the Board of Directors. She also is a member of the Society for Clinical Coding, where she has held several leadership positions. Hazelwood has held numerous positions with the Louisiana Health Information management Association, including past president and delegate, and was selected as its 1997 Distinguished Member. She consults in many types of healthcare facilities and educational institutions and conducts coding workshops for hospitals and physician offices. Moreover, she has written, coauthored, and edited numerous publications, including AHIMA's *Basic ICD-9-CM for Physician Office Coding* and *ICD-10-CM Preview,* for which she received AHIMA's Legacy Award in 2003. She frequently serves as a reviewer for publishers of HIM-related textbooks and electronic materials.

Linda L. Kloss, MA, RHIA, CAE, is AHIMA's executive vice-president and chief executive officer, a position she has held since 1995. Before joining the AHIMA staff, she served from 1976 to 1995 as senior manager for Massachusetts-based MediQual Systems, Inc., and Chicago-based InterQual, Inc., where she participated in the design of computer-based tools for healthcare outcomes evaluation and consulted and lectured widely on quality improvement concepts and methods. Moreover, she has held academic and HIM practice positions in Minneapolis and San Francisco. She served on the AHIMA Board of Directors from 1980 to 1986 and was president in 1985. In addition to AHIMA, Kloss has served on the boards of directors of several not-for-profit organizations in healthcare and higher education. She holds a bachelor's degree in medical record science from the College of St. Scholastica in Duluth, Minnesota, and an MA in organizational development with a concentration in change leadership from DePaul University in Chicago.

Deborah Kohn, MPH, RHIA, CHE, CPHIMS, FHIMSS, is the principal consultant at Dak Systems Consulting in San Mateo, California, a national healthcare information technology advisory consultancy specializing in the analysis, planning, and design of electronic patient record component technologies and systems. She has more than 20 years of experience in healthcare management and information systems. Kohn holds an undergraduate degree from The Ohio State University at Columbus and a graduate degree from UCLA in health services and hospital administration. She is certified in healthcare information and management systems and is a fellow of the Healthcare Information Management Systems Society. Moreover, she is board certified in healthcare management and a diplomate of the American College of Healthcare Executives. An active member of AHIMA and the Association for Information and Image Management International (AIIM), she was awarded AHIMA's prestigious Computer-based Patient Record Advancement Award in 1995 for her efforts in promoting and implementing components of computer-based patient record systems. She also is a recipient of AIIM's Master and Laureate of Information Technology designations, which recognize achievement in the area of document and Web content management.

Elizabeth Layman, PhD, RHIA, CCS, FAHIMA, is a professor and chair in the Department of Health Services and Information Management at East Carolina University, located in Greenville, North Carolina. Previously, she worked at Hennepin County Medical Center and the University of Minnesota Hospitals, both in Minneapolis, from 1974 to 1990. She earned her postbaccalaureate certificate in health information administration from St. Scholastica. She has been involved in healthcare information management for more than 30 years. After earning a master's degree in organizational leadership from the College of St. Catherine, she joined the faculty of the Medical College of Georgia in Augusta, Georgia. She also consulted for the Physicians' Practice Group. In 1995, she earned a doctorate in higher education from Georgia State University. In 2001, she was one of the first two individuals in the country to be awarded the designation of Fellow of the American Health Information Management Association.

Madonna LeBlanc, MA, RHIA, is an assistant professor in the health informatics and information management program at the College of St. Scholastica in Duluth, Minnesota. Prior to her teaching role, she managed health information services at St. Mary's/Duluth Clinic Health System in Superior, Wisconsin. Her responsibilities included a broad spectrum of acute care HIM functions, from physician education to JCAHO survey coordination. Her field experience also includes cancer registry and physician peer administration. She is a graduate of the College of St. Scholastica's MA program in health information management.

Frances Wickham Lee, DBA, RHIA, is an associate professor in the Department of Health Administration and Policy at the Medical University of South Carolina. She received an MBA from Western Carolina University and a doctorate in business administration from the University of Sarasota. An active member of AHIMA, she was awarded the Distinguished Member Award from the Mental Health Section of AHIMA in 1995.

Mary Cole McCain, MPA, RHIA, is a professor of health information management and chair of the health information management department at the University of Tennessee Health Science Center in Memphis. She has held this position since 1973. She also serves as assistant dean in the College of Allied Health Sciences. McCain chaired AHIMA's Assembly on Education and cochaired the Model Curriculum Project for AHIMA. She is a recipient of the Tennessee Health Information Management Association's Distinguished Member Award.

Pamela Oachs, MA, RHIA, is an assistant professor and coordinator of the HIM graduate programs in the College of St. Scholastica's healthcare informatics and information management department. She has more than 15 years of healthcare experience. Her career has included a variety of positions, both managerial and professional, in the areas of utilization management, quality improvement, medical staff credentialing, JCAHO coordination, information technology, project management, and patient access. She has served on the board of the Minnesota Health Information Management Association and is currently serving as president of the Northeastern Minnesota Health Information Management Association.

Carol E. Osborn, PhD, RHIA, is assistant director of coding and compliance at The Ohio State University Medical Center in Columbus. She has been an HIM professional for more than 30 years and is a former faculty member at both the University of Illinois at Chicago and The Ohio State University. Osborn has served AHIMA at both the state and national levels, participating as president of AHIMA's Illinois education task force and as a member of both the AHIMA Council on Education and Item Writing Committee. She authored *Statistical Applications for Health Information Management,* as well as many articles in the *Journal of AHIMA* and *Topics in Health Information Management.* She is former president of the AHIMA Assembly on Education.

Karen R. Patena, MBA, RHIA, is a clinical assistant professor and undergraduate program coordinator in the HIM program, School of Biomedical and Health Information Sciences, at the University of Illinois at Chicago (UIC). She earned an MBA from DePaul University and is currently pursuing a doctorate degree at UIC. She is an alumnus of the University of Illinois health information management program. Previously, Patena was director of the independent study division of AHIMA and a faculty member at Indiana University and Prairie State College. She also has extensive experience in hospital medical record department management, including computer systems planning and implementation. Her areas of expertise include management, quality improvement and TQM, and the use of computers in healthcare and systems analysis. She has presented numerous tutorials at local, state, and national levels on the use of the Internet in HIM. She currently serves on the panel of surveyors for the AHIMA Council on Accreditation.

Lynda A. Russell, EdD, JD, RHIA, CHP, is privacy manager at Cedars-Sinai Medical Center in Los Angeles. She holds a baccalaureate degree in medical record science from the Medical College of Georgia, a master's and doctorate in educational administration and supervision from the University of Central Florida, and a JD from the University of Florida. A member of the California Bar, she is licensed to practice before the Superior Court of California and the Federal Court of the Central District of California. She maintains a Florida license as a risk manager and is certified in healthcare privacy. Russell has been an HIM professional for more than 30 years and has been active professionally on the national, state, and local levels. She served as president of the Florida Health Information Management Association and as a member of the Board of Directors of the California Health Information Association (CHIA). Furthermore, she has held numerous local, state, and national committee appointments, including chair of AHIMA's Educational Strategy Committee and chair of CHIA's Editorial Board, and was the CHIA president for 2004–2005. She serves as a frequent speaker and has published widely on a variety of health information and related topics and on HIPAA.

Patricia B. Seidl, RHIA, CCDM, has more than nine years of project management experience and is currently working in clinical research data management for Astellas Pharma, Inc. She has 18 years of experience in information technology as a systems analyst and project manager. Seidl is currently serving as an adjunct professor for the project management certificate program at the College of St. Scholastica and was a contributing author to *Special Edition: Using Microsoft Project 2000.* She received a bachelor's degree from the College of St. Scholastica and an associate of applied science degree in computer science from the University of Southern Colorado.

Kam Shams, MA, is chairman of The Shams Group, Inc., an award-winning knowledge management IT software and consulting company in the health information systems marketplace. He has been a visionary and innovator in the IT industry for more than 30 years. He started his career in information technology in the early 1970s and has been in healthcare since 1981. Prior to establishing The Shams Group, Inc., he served as vice-president and chief information officer of noted healthcare integrated delivery networks. In the past, he has served on numerous IT user boards and coached CEOs on IT-related issues. He also is a visiting professor at the College of St. Scholastica in Duluth, Minnesota, for the Department of Healthcare Informatics and Information Management, as well as at the University of Tennessee Health Sciences Center in Memphis. Shams has written extensively on how to leverage information technology to enhance healthcare processes for increased quality and best outcomes. He is a regular contributor to several healthcare periodicals and speaks frequently at conferences around the country.

David X. Swenson, PhD, is an associate professor in the management department at the College of St. Scholastica, where he teaches strategic management, organizational development, leadership, and principles of management. He is also clinical associate professor of behavioral sciences at the University of Minnesota Medical School and a forensic psychologist in private practice. He has worked in the field of psychology for more than 35 years. In addition, he has served as director of student development at the College of St. Scholastica, director of clinical services at the Human Resource Center of Douglas County, Wisconsin, and codirector of a training and consulting partnership. He has authored more than 80 publications, including *Stress Management for*

Law Enforcement. A doctoral graduate of the University of Missouri at Columbia in counseling and personnel services, Swenson also has master's degrees in management and educational media and technology and is a diplomate in forensic psychology.

Carol A. Venable, MPH, RHIA, FAHIMA, is a professor and department head of HIM at the University of Louisiana at Lafayette and has been an HIM professional for nearly 30 years. She is actively involved with AHIMA's Assembly on Education (AOE), Panel of Accreditation Surveyors, and several other committees, as well as the Louisiana Health Information Management Association, where she has held many leadership positions and was selected as Distinguished Member in 1991. In addition, she is a member of the Society for Clinical Coding (SCC). Previously, she was director of medical records at Lafayette General Medical Center, has consulted in a variety of healthcare facilities and educational institutions, and conducts coding workshops for hospitals and physician offices. Venable has written, coauthored, and edited numerous publications, including AHIMA's *ICD-9-CM Diagnostic Coding and Reimbursement for Physician Services* and *ICD-10-CM Preview,* for which she was awarded AHIMA's Legacy Award in 2003. She frequently serves as a reviewer for publishers of HIM-related textbooks, certification exams, and electronic materials.

Karen A. Wager, DBA, RHIA, is an associate professor in the Department of Health Administration and Policy at the Medical University of South Carolina in Charleston, where she received a master's degree in health information administration and finance. In 1998, she received a doctorate of business administration from the University of Sarasota. She is a member of AHIMA and has served on various association committees. She was president of the South Carolina Health Information Management Association (SCHIMA) from 1991 to 1992.

Vicki L. Zeman, MA, RHIA, is academic coordinator of professional practice experience for the Department of Health Information Management at the College of St. Scholastica in Duluth, Minnesota. An HIM professional for 30 years, she practiced in a variety of settings for 13 years before becoming an educator. Her last six years in practice were focused on the area of hospitalwide quality improvement. While serving as an instructor in the HIM program for 17 years, she has provided administrative support as coordinator of the RHIT progression program.

Preface

Health information management (HIM) professionals play a critical role in the delivery of healthcare in the United States. They manage patient information systems in a variety of care settings, including hospitals, ambulatory care facilities, nursing homes, home care facilities, hospices, behavioral health facilities, correctional facilities, and so on. As managers of patient information systems, HIM professionals collaborate with other members of the healthcare team to ensure that an individual's health information is accurate, accessible, confidential, and secure. In recent years, health information managers have been playing increasingly diverse roles in other health-related industries, such as insurance companies, managed care, vendor settings, service organizations, and health-related consulting organizations. The dynamic nature of the HIM profession reflects the continuous change that characterizes the healthcare delivery system as a whole. The expansion of career opportunities has demanded new skill sets and competencies for HIM professionals.

Although expansion of the HIM profession is a positive and rewarding trend, it poses unique challenges in preparing students in educational programs, especially at the baccalaureate level, to assume a variety of positions within the healthcare industry. The need to respond to change has driven the efforts of the American Health Information Management Association (AHIMA) to develop model curricula for associate-, baccalaureate-, and master's-level education. The model curricula create clear boundaries between the various levels of HIM education in terms of content, program outcomes, and professional competencies. The accreditation process for HIM programs and the certification examinations for RHIAs and RHITs support these deliberate differences between HIM credentials and educational programs. Over the past several years, HIM programs have revised and developed their curricula to better reflect the AHIMA models.

This text is directed specifically toward health information management at the baccalaureate degree level. Like the companion text for associate degree programs, *Health Infor-* *mation Management: An Applied Approach,* it is the result of AHIMA's ongoing efforts to provide rich resources for the education and training of students in HIA programs. It also offers a reference for current practitioners in the field. This textbook is designed to reflect HIM practice at the baccalaureate level with emphasis on the core set of skills and knowledge set forth in the model curriculum. Its topics reflect the recommended content as defined in the Model Curriculum for Baccalaureate Degree Programs in Health Information Management. The content and organization of the text allow for the effective integration of dynamic concepts into an existing HIM curriculum.

All the content areas of the AHIMA Model Curriculum for Baccalaureate Programs are covered in this text with the exception of those related to the biomedical sciences (anatomy, physiology, pathophysiology/disease processes, medical terminology, pharmacology, and so on), basic human resources management principles, and the skill-development aspects of classification systems. The editors recognize that in some content areas, specialized content-specific textbooks may be required as additional resources, especially for developing competence in coding, the use of basic computer systems, and human resources management.

Central to the organization of this text is the information management model used by the Joint Commission on Accreditation of Healthcare Organizations (JCAHO), shown in figure 5.2. This model presents health information management as an incremental process that begins with the collection of patient-specific data, is followed by the aggregation of data to generate information, the development of comparative data, and, finally, the utilization of such data and derived information to increase knowledge and support decision making.

Use of the model curriculum and the information management model as the foundations of this textbook ensures that the content is covered in a logical and systematic way.

A systems approach to the content is utilized in this text because the audience will be expected to develop skills in problem solving, decision making, systems thinking, and professional leadership. The structure used throughout this text is designed to help students apply concepts and principles in practice in an organized and systematic way. The features used to accomplish this goal include the following:

- Examples and case studies used throughout the text reflect the contemporary spectrum of HIM practice environments.
- Each chapter begins with a section titled Theory into Practice, which includes a case study. The case study gives the learner an appreciation of how the major concepts and principles in the chapter are applied in a real practice-based situation.
- Each chapter contains sections called Check Your Understanding, which allow learners to verify their command of the information presented in the chapter. The sections also provide formative feedback as students proceed through the material.
- Each chapter contains a Real-World Case developed from today's top stories in healthcare delivery.

The text is presented in six parts. Part I introduces the concepts of informatics and information management as they apply to the healthcare industry. It also introduces the profession of health information management.

Chapter 1 introduces the concept of health information management, discusses the overall characteristics and challenges of today's modern healthcare environment, and provides a short history of AHIMA.

Chapter 2 provides an overview of the organizations that deliver, finance, and regulate healthcare services in the United States. It focuses on the impact of accreditation, licensure, regulation, reimbursement systems, and legal and ethical issues in creating the environment for managing and delivering healthcare services. This chapter provides a context for the concepts and applications presented in the remainder of the text.

Chapter 3 introduces the field of informatics as it is applied in healthcare. The chapter surveys the emerging technologies in the clinical environment (for example, imaging, natural language processing, artificial intelligence, and Web technologies). It explores the major issues associated with computerizing clinical data and presents an overview of the types of computer applications used to support clinical decision making. It also identifies the barriers and limitations associated with computerized clinical decision support.

Chapter 4 introduces the body of knowledge, competencies, and ethical principles that constitute the core of the HIM profession's contributions to the healthcare industry. The education, certifications, and associations that are identified with the HIM profession are discussed, as are the functions and roles of HIM professionals.

Chapter 5 introduces the concept of information as an organizational asset that must be managed effectively to provide and sustain its value. The chapter discusses the components of the JCAHO information management model. It presents the principles, tools, and techniques used to develop data, to create a database infrastructure, and to establish reporting capabilities that meet the needs of the various types and levels of information systems users within an organization. The essential characteristics of quality data as well as the principles, regulations, and techniques associated with ensuring data security are presented as the primary concerns of information managers.

The final chapter in this part, chapter 6, introduces the process of information systems development. It begins with a discussion of information systems planning as a component of an organization's strategic planning effort. This chapter focuses on the information systems life cycle: its phases, the activities within each phase, and the unique and complementary roles of information technology staff, information management professionals, and information users in the information systems development effort.

Part II focuses on the development of health information systems from the perspective of individual patients. It addresses the development of personally identifiable health information and the basic concepts of managing health records in both a manual and a computerized environment in today's healthcare facilities.

Chapter 7 addresses healthcare information standards, including the concept of converting data into information in the healthcare environment. It also explores the development of uniform standards that guide data collection in healthcare. It discusses healthcare data sets, including the history, purpose, and use of each. It also introduces emerging healthcare informatics standards that support the transition from paper-based to computer-based health records.

Chapter 8 focuses on the content and structure of patient-specific data and personally identifiable data and information, as collected in individual health records. It addresses data sources, capture of data in a health record, and documentation requirements. This chapter also addresses management issues related to paper-based record systems, including clinical documentation issues, medical word processing as a tool for documentation, forms design, storage and retrieval systems, and chart tracking.

Chapter 9 focuses on the development of health records in a computerized format, including issues related to the transition from paper-based records to electronic or computer-based records. Data capture, imaging, security, and user needs are among the topics addressed. Issues related to the creation and maintenance of computer-based patient records also are discussed.

Chapters 10 and 11 focus on the legal and ethical concepts and issues related to healthcare information systems and HIM practice. Current legal and regulatory issues are explored, including issues related to privacy, confidentiality, security, and access to healthcare data. Work processes related to release of information policies and procedures are addressed. Ethical issues such as those related to computerization of clinical information, the coding–reimbursement connection, and vendor–organization relationships are among those discussed in chapter 11.

Part III focuses on the conversion of patient-specific data and information into aggregate data used for analysis, statistics, and research, as well as clinical and administrative decision making.

Chapter 12 focuses on impersonal uses of healthcare data, that is, data that have been abstracted from individual health records and captured in healthcare databases. Included in this chapter are secondary records such as indexes, registers, and registries, as well as exploration of data sources, data capture, and the healthcare information infrastructure. Information management concepts are applied to healthcare database development.

Chapter 13 provides an introduction to classification systems for healthcare data including ICD-9-CM, CPT, and SNOMED. Emerging clinical vocabularies are introduced, and the concept of data representation in computer-based systems is explored, as is medical linguistics as a basis for clinical classifications and vocabularies.

Chapter 14 provides an overview of the uses of coded data and health information in reimbursement systems. Included in this chapter are issues related to coding management, case-mix management, billing procedures, and severity-of-illness classifications. Methods for managing the quality of coded data are addressed.

Part IV introduces the development and use of comparative data in healthcare and focuses on the development of statistical and research methodologies. It addresses professional competencies put forth in the AHIMA Model Curriculum for HIA programs.

Chapter 15 emphasizes the collection, use, presentation, and verification of statistical healthcare data. Fundamentals of descriptive and inferential statistics are covered, as are standard formulae for facility-based statistics. This chapter focuses on the practical application of descriptive and inferential statistics in a healthcare environment and the application of information management concepts in developing comparative data.

Chapter 16 addresses basic research methods as they are applied to healthcare information. The chapter focuses on the steps in developing a research project, including defining a research problem, performing a literature review, determining research design and methodology, selecting measurement instruments, analyzing data, and presenting study results. Library research techniques and data search and access also are addressed.

Chapter 17 addresses the collection and use of aggregate data in the analysis and evaluation of healthcare services. Topics such as clinical quality assessment, clinical outcomes management, critical pathways and case management, utilization review, and risk management systems are explored. The chapter focuses on healthcare data as a resource in clinical decision making.

Part V explores knowledge-based healthcare data and information and applies the concepts of knowledge management to the use of healthcare information for biomedical and research support as well as for expert systems and decision support. The process of converting knowledge assets into wisdom to create a learning organization is explored.

Chapter 18 presents concepts associated with acquiring clinical knowledge-based data. This chapter addresses national research policy development, medical/health research and investigation, and research protocol data management. The role of HIM professionals in a research environment is explored.

Chapter 19 addresses the application of artificial intelligence concepts to support administrative, executive, and clinical decision making. Specifically, the chapter focuses on the various types and classes of decision support systems being used in healthcare and how they are being used. The concepts of data warehousing and data mining, as they apply to decision support systems, are discussed. Emerging career opportunities for HIM professionals in decision support areas are explored.

Chapter 20 describes the process of transforming information into knowledge within an organization through a knowledge management program. It addresses the human factors that are key to using knowledge assets for the real benefit of an organization and explores the impact of corporate culture and values on the ability to translate knowledge assets into wise actions. Key knowledge management applications in healthcare (online analytical processing, customer relationship management, and so on) are explored. The emerging role of a chief knowledge officer to ensure the availability of, as well as the wise and ethical use of, knowledge resources is explored.

Part VI addresses the tools, techniques, and strategies utilized in managing health information services. It provides an overview of human resources management and focuses on applications of both operational and human resources management principles in the healthcare setting.

Chapter 21 introduces the management discipline, the evolution of management thought, and the functions of management. It presents the principles and basic tools associated with each management function. The relationship between management functions and skills with the various levels of management in an organization is discussed. Communications and problem-solving models and techniques are explored.

Chapter 22 addresses leadership theory and functions, traits related to leadership effectiveness, and key differences between the concepts of managing and leading. The role of a leader in positively facilitating the transition of people through organizational change is explored.

Chapter 23 focuses on the systems nature of work processes in organizations. It introduces the concepts, tools, and techniques associated with designing (and redesigning) effective and efficient work processes, as well as those associated with implementing new or revised work processes. Performance measurement and performance improvement in terms of productivity, quality measurement, benchmarking, and work process redesign are presented as major topics.

Chapter 24 discusses the implementation of appropriate policies, procedures, and practices in each of the seven human resources (HR) activity areas: HR planning and analysis; equal employment opportunity; staffing; HR development; compensation and benefits; health, safety, and security; and employee and labor/management relations. Effective recruitment, selection, and hiring practices also are discussed, as well as job orientation and performance review.

Chapter 25 focuses on training and retaining employees in a highly competitive labor environment and with a rapidly diversifying workforce pool. Topics include orientation programs, staff development programs, continuing education needs identification, and employee retention strategies. A departmental training and development model is presented. Trends in staffing are explored, including flexible scheduling, job sharing, home-based work, and outsourcing.

Chapter 26 focuses on the concepts and tools associated with planning and controlling the financial resources required to operate a department or work unit within a healthcare organization. Basic financial and managerial accounting principles, concepts, and reporting are explained. Operations, labor, and capital budgeting processes and techniques are presented. Organizational and departmental financial performance measures are reviewed, with a special emphasis on accounts receivable management. The role(s) that HIM professionals play in the financial management of the organization is explored.

Chapter 27 addresses project management. The focus is on the various aspects of a project that must be integrated to effectively move it from an idea to a functioning reality. The organization and processes that must be put in place to effectively manage a project are defined. The requisite skill set of project managers as well as the tools and techniques used by effective project managers are explored. The impact that the project context, stakeholder needs and expectations, and competing demands have on the project manager's work is highlighted.

Chapter 28, the final chapter of the text, focuses on the role of the health information professional and manager as a visionary leader and strategist for a department and/or an organization. The principles of strategic management are presented. Models for strategic planning and techniques for implementing a strategic management philosophy into a department or organization are explored.

Six appendixes follow Part VI. Appendix A features sample health record documentation forms. Appendix B presents the list of sample position descriptions developed by AHIMA for HIM positions (available online at ahima. org) such as risk manager, quality improvement director, director of HIM academic program, coder, clinical data specialist, and several others. Appendix C provides a sample notice of health information practices. Appendix D lists Web resources. Appendix E features the 2004 AHIMA Code of Ethics. And finally, appendix F provides a key to the student self-study Check Your Understanding exercises within each chapter.

A complete glossary of HIM terms is included at the end of the book. Throughout the text chapters, boldface type is used to indicate the first substantial reference to key terms included in the glossary. A detailed content index is included at the end of the text. Frequently used abbreviations and acronyms, and initialisms are spelled out on the inside covers of the book for easy reference.

Acknowledgments

The editors and publications staff would like to express appreciation to the many authors who contributed chapters to this textbook. They willingly shared their expertise, met tight deadlines, accepted feedback, and contributed to building the body of knowledge related to health information management. Writing a chapter is a time-consuming and demanding task, and we are grateful for the authors' contributions.

We also would like to thank the following reviewers who lent a critical eye to this endeavor:

Donna Bowers, JD, RHIA, CHP
June E. Bronnert, RHIA, CCS, CCS-P
Jill Burrington-Brown, MS, RHIA
Christopher G. Chute, MD, DrPH
Michelle L. Dougherty, RHIA, CHP
Melanie A. Endicott, MBA/HCM, RHIA, CCS
Susan Fenton, MBA, RHIA
Leslie A. Fox, MA, RHIA, FAHIMA
Jennifer Garvin, PhD, RHIA, CPHQ, CCS, FAHIMA
Kathy Giannangelo, RHIA, CCS
Barry S. Herrin, CHE, Esq.
Beth Hjort, RHIA, CHPS
Susan Hull, MPH, RHIA, CCS, CCS-P
Lolita M. Jones, RHIA, CCS
Karen Kostick, RHIT, CCS, CCS-P
Donald T. Mon, PhD, FHIMSS
Carol Ann Quinsey, RHIA, CHPS
Harry Rhodes, MBA, RHIA, CHPS
Dan Rode, MBA, FHFMA
Rita A. Scichilone, MHSA, RHIA, CCS, CCS-P, CHC
Mary H. Stanfill, RHIA, CCS, CCS-P
Valerie Watzlaf, PhD, RHIA, FAHIMA
Maggie Williams, MA
Ann Zeisset, RHIT, CCS-P, CCS

Finally the editors wish to acknowledge the guidance, patience, and expertise of Claire Blondeau, MBA, AHIMA Project Editor. She is the glue that held the entire project together.

Foreword

To Tomorrow's Health Information Leaders:

In the four years since the first edition of *Health Information Management Concepts, Principles, and Practice* was published, health information has become a top-line issue for the healthcare industry. In January 2004, President George W. Bush called for widespread adoption of interoperable electronic health records (EHRs) within 10 years and appointed a national coordinator for health information technology. Federal leadership, combined with substantial private-sector leadership, has made this the decade of health information transformation. The world's most information intensive industry is finally coming into the information age—and not a moment too soon. Before this decade is over, EHRs will be a reality for nearly all healthcare organizations, decision support will guide caregivers, and citizens will be knowledgeable partners in their health and wellness. Unencumbered by the physical limitations of a paper file, digital data and images will be accessible to support patient care wherever and whenever it is needed. Individuals and families will be as diligent about their health information as they are about their financial and other critical information. Public health and public policy will be based on accurate and timely information. The results of clinical research will be available to aid sound clinical decision making. And, most important, patient care will be safer and more economical and the outcomes of that care will be improved. These are very big goals, but the potential for these and other benefits are now well documented.

Health information management professionals will be on the front lines in delivering the benefits of electronic records and health information computing to patients, to purchasers, and to the health and well-being of our society. In the 78 years since the field was created, the role of the health information management professional has never been more expansive or more relevant. Research shows that HIM professionals practice in 40 work settings and more than a hundred job titles.

Health Information Management: Concepts, Principles, and Practice is a compendium of the knowledge, skills, and competencies needed to succeed as an HIM professional. Editors Shirley Eichenwald Maki, MBA, RHIA, FAHIMA, and Kathleen M. LaTour, MA, RHIA, FAHIMA, designed this text to provide comprehensive coverage of the "science" of health information management and then added the "art" through a rich variety of case studies and exercises. They assembled content experts representing the breadth of information management in healthcare as reflected in AHIMA's Model Curriculum for Baccalaureate Health Information Administration Programs.

The context within which information is managed—the healthcare system; concepts of informatics, information, and information systems management; and the profession of health information management—is expertly covered by contributors Bonnie S. Cassidy, MPA, RHIA, FAHIMA, FHIMSS; Deborah Kohn, MPH, RHIA, CHE, CPHIMS, FHIMSS, and Pamela Oachs, MA, RHIA; Sandra R. Fuller, MA, RHIA; Frances Wickham Lee, DBA, RHIA; and Karen A. Wager, DBA, RHIA. The content of health information and patient records—the laws, standards, and ethical values that affect how it is managed—is presented by Kathleen M. LaTour, MA, RHIA, FAHIMA; Mary Cole McCain, MPA, RHIA; Margret Amatayakul, MBA, RHIA, CHPS, FHIMSS; Lynda A. Russell, EdD, JD, RHIA, CHP, and Rita K. Bowen, MA, RHIA, CHPS; Laurinda B. Harman, PhD, RHIA; and Elizabeth Bowman, MPA, RHIA; Susan H. Fenton, MBA, RHIA, and Matthew Greene, RHIA, CCS; and Anita Hazelwood, MLS, RHIA, FAHIMA, and Carol A. Venable, MPH, RHIA, FAHIMA address the development and use of coded and aggregate information for healthcare management and reimbursement. Authors Carol E. Osborn, PhD, RHIA; Elizabeth Layman, PhD, RHIA, CCS, FAHIMA; Vicki L. Zeman, MA, RHIA; J. Michael Hardin, PhD; Kam Shams, MA; and Mehnaz Farishta, MS, cover the development and use of statistical data to enable meaningful comparisons, support clinical and policy research, and improve the quality of health-care. Finally, concepts and processes for managing health information services are explored by David X. Swenson, PhD; Madonna LeBlanc, MA, RHIA; Shirley Eichenwald Maki, MBA, RHIA, FAHIMA; Karen R. Patena, MBA, RHIA; Nadinia Davis, MBA, CPA, RHIA, FAHIMA; Patricia B. Seidl, RHIA, CCDM; Linda L. Kloss, MA, RHIA, CAE.

HIM professionals are highly specialized knowledge work-ers. The information revolution has expanded the breadth of the knowledge and skills required to be an effective HIM professional. It also has exploded the opportunities for further specialization into any number of information management subspecialty areas such as health statistics, leadership and management, compliance, informatics, and technology. This text is dedicated to you, the health information management student. You are tomorrow's professional leaders, and your efforts will ensure that information technology and informatics science are used fully and effectively to improve health and the quality of healthcare. This text also is dedicated to those who built and nurtured this profession and its legacy of service. As we complete the transition from a paper- to a computer-based healthcare information system, we will be fulfilling the dream of our profession's leaders: high-quality healthcare through high-quality information.

Linda L. Kloss, MA, RHIA, CAE
Chief Executive Officer
American Health Information
Management Association

Part I

Informatics and Health Information Management

Chapter 1
Introduction

*Shirley Eichenwald Maki, MBA, RHIA, FAHIMA,
and Kathleen M. LaTour, MA, RHIA, FAHIMA*

The field of health information management (HIM) has been a recognized field of study for more than 70 years. It was originally called medical record science and members of the profession were originally called medical record librarians. From its inception, the mission of the profession was to elevate the standards of clinical recordkeeping in hospitals, dispensaries, and other healthcare facilities. Since its founding, the professional association, now known as the American Health Information Management Association (AHIMA), and the professionals affiliated with it, have been advocates for the effective management of clinical records to ensure their accuracy, confidentiality and accessibility in every type of healthcare setting. HIM professionals serve the healthcare industry and the public by managing, analyzing, and utilizing the information vital for patient care and making it accessible to healthcare providers when and where it is needed (Johns 2006).

Beginning with the managed care movement in the 1980s, effective information management began to emerge as a top priority for healthcare institutions. Subsequently, events affecting healthcare delivery and the management of healthcare delivery services have placed even greater pressure on healthcare organizations to improve their information-handling capacity and functionality. Johns (2006) emphasizes that the healthcare industry now fully recognizes the importance of information flow across departmental boundaries and the necessity of broad dissemination throughout the organization. Currently, there are significant government and industry initiatives focused on the goal of improving the delivery of healthcare by "bringing timely health information to, and aiding communication among, those making health decisions for themselves, their families, their patients, and their communities" (NCVHS 2001). A series of Institute of Medicine reports, the Department of Health and Human Services recommendations for creating a National Health Information Infrastructure, the Markle Foundation's Connecting for Health, and public/private partnerships for standards development have focused attention on the critical elements needed to achieve this goal.

This chapter provides a brief introduction to the HIM profession and focuses on the changing nature of its core domain of practice. It sets the stage for the remaining chapters in this textbook by providing a context for the broad range of topics that must be addressed in a textbook whose purpose is to describe the concepts, principles, and practices associated with the HIM profession in its current state of transformation. (A full discussion of the HIM profession and related professional associations is presented in chapter 4.)

The Modern Healthcare Environment

In the 1990s, several forces at work in the American healthcare industry had a transformational effect on the HIM profession. During that decade, competition among healthcare providers was stimulated by major changes in the reimbursement system used by Medicare and Medicaid (two federally mandated healthcare programs). Integrated healthcare delivery systems also began to emerge as significant organizational models, and managed care delivery systems continued to expand. As a result of these developments, the availability of timely and accurate clinical information has become critical to the viability of healthcare organizations. Medical and administrative staffs recognize that the information gathered from clinical records is an invaluable organizational asset. They also understand that this information represents an important quality indicator and a vital tool for efficiently managing the business of healthcare in an increasingly tight financial environment.

The wise application of increasingly sophisticated computer technology also has received increased attention among healthcare professionals and organizations. Technology is the obvious solution to the industry's need for greater efficiency in managing the ever-increasing volume of healthcare data. In addition, as diverse healthcare decision makers look for flexibility in how to access and analyze vast electronic repositories of clinical data, advanced decision support technology is critical to meeting that demand.

Today, these trends continue to affect the practice of health information management and healthcare in general as:

- The federal government sets a strategic vision that includes every American having an electronic health record (EHR) by the year 2010 and the creation of regional health information organizations that facilitate the transfer of health information among authorized parties to enhance the quality of care and reduce the cost of healthcare services.
- Payers pilot healthcare reimbursement systems that provide incentives for healthcare organizations to implement computer-based information systems to support quality of care programs.
- Regulators and accreditation agencies focus on the use of computer-based information technologies to reduce the number of medical errors.
- Workforce shortages place greater emphasis on technological systems for improving productivity.
- Integrated information system solutions as well as clinician-friendly hardware and applications are continuing to evolve.
- The Internet and its derived technologies make connectivity across otherwise disparate information systems accessible and affordable for healthcare organizations.

Contemporary Health Information Management

The HIM profession is the only profession that has as its core professional mission the quality of the data collected and maintained in the course of delivering healthcare services. Although clinical and allied healthcare professionals depend on the availability of high-quality data to perform clinical decision making, their primary concern is providing diagnostic and therapeutic services, not managing clinical information. The administrators and managers of healthcare organizations also use collected clinical information to plan and manage healthcare services, but managing the quality of the data they use is not their major concern. Similarly, computer scientists and technicians are concerned primarily with the performance of software and hardware configurations; researchers are concerned primarily with the development of scientific solutions to important questions; third-party payers are concerned primarily with the control of financial resources; and policy makers are concerned primarily with incentives for cost-effectiveness, social justice, and ethical practice. Although they all rely on high-quality data, only the HIM profession is charged with ensuring the availability of high-quality data for a variety of uses and users.

In an information-intensive environment embedded within a technology-supported framework, HIM professionals must build and market their unique knowledge base and competencies in the following areas:

- Practice standards, laws, and regulations related to ensuring the accuracy, completeness, integrity, and security of healthcare information
- Healthcare data standards
- Healthcare data analytics and reporting methods
- Clinical coding, classification, and reimbursement systems
- Health record and information systems design, functions, and maintenance
- Organizational and cross-disciplinary modes of functioning

Once applied in a world of paper-based records and manual systems, the HIM knowledge base and competencies are now needed to effectively transition vital clinical data resources into electronic clinical repositories and EHR systems. These modern technological systems support both the operational and strategic needs of the organization's workforce and decision makers. (Chapter 4 presents an expanded discussion of emerging roles for HIM professionals.)

The HIM profession today remains committed to its original mission to elevate health record standards and practices. It does so, however, in a healthcare environment that is becoming more and more technology driven in both its work processes and information flow, as well as more and more dependent on the quality and accessibility of the information contained within clinical records. HIM professionals work to ensure that their communities and customers are provided high-quality and cost-effective healthcare information services.

HIM skills and competencies are needed by all organizations that use person-specific or aggregate patient data. The national push to adopt health information technology will accelerate the demand for a qualified HIM workforce (Kloss 2005).

Working in strong collaborative partnerships with specialists in information technologies and with specialized healthcare data and information users (physicians, nurses, pharmacists, therapists, administrators, researchers, policy makers, and others), health information managers have become key players within the emerging discipline of healthcare informatics. Healthcare informatics focuses on designing and implementing technology-based information systems to support the specialized activities associated with each type of healthcare worker. For example, nursing informatics focuses on systems that support the work of nurses, and medical informatics focuses on systems that support the work of physicians. Similarly, consumer informatics systems support the activities of patients, long-term care residents, and healthcare clients (Shortliffe et al. 2000).

Thus, to carry on the important legacy of their predecessors, today's HIM professionals support an adapted vision of their unique contribution. They build and maintain an accompanying set of strengthened competencies for the healthcare industry they serve. They envision how the concepts, principles, and practices at the core of the HIM knowledge base and competencies continue to apply in their changing work environment and settings. In addition, they assess their adaptive strengths and weaknesses relative to that vision and, most important, they take action to position themselves appropriately to contribute their unique expertise to the organizations they serve.

Summary

The health information management profession began with the founding of the Association of Record Librarians of North America in 1928. The association's original goal was to improve clinical recordkeeping in healthcare facilities. The association, now known as the American Health Information Management Association, and a new generation of HIM professionals have inherited a powerful legacy from those original medical records pioneers. They also have an extraordinary opportunity and obligation to build on that legacy by elevating the standards for clinical data and information systems in a healthcare environment that demands integrated, computer-based, user-focused data repositories and warehouses. The viability and vitality of the HIM pro-fession in years to come depends on the commitment of current and future professionals to think and act strategically in order to address the data and information needs of an evolving healthcare industry. To meet that challenge, HIM professionals must continually update their knowledge base and competencies through self-assessment and commitment to lifelong learning, and they must actively take part in their professional organizations' activities at the local, regional, state, and national levels.

References

Blum, B.I. 1986. *Clinical Information Systems.* New York: Springer-Verlag.

Johns, M.L. 2006. Introduction. Ch. 1 in *Health Information Management Technology: An Applied Approach,* 2nd ed. Chicago: AHIMA.

Kloss, L. 2005. Supply and demand: A challenge for healthcare and HIM. *Journal of American Health Information Management Association* 76(5):23.

NCVHS. November 1, 2001. *A Strategy for Building the National Health Information Infrastructure.* Washington, DC.

Protti, D.J. 1984. Knowledge and skills expected of health information scientists: A sample survey of prospective employers. *Methods of Information in Medicine* 23(4):204–8.

Shortliffe, E.H., L.E. Perreault, G. Wiederhold, and L.M. Fagan. 2000. *Medical Informatics: Computer Applications in Health Care and Biomedicine.* New York: Springer-Verlag.

Chapter 2
Healthcare Delivery Systems

Bonnie S. Cassidy, MPA, RHIA, FAHIMA, FHIMSS

Learning Objectives

- To understand the history of the healthcare delivery system from ancient times until the present
- To understand the basic organization of the various types of hospitals and healthcare organizations
- To recognize the impact of managed care on healthcare providers
- To recognize the impact of external forces on the healthcare industry
- To identify the various functional components of an integrated delivery system
- To describe the systems used for reimbursement of healthcare services
- To recognize the role of government in healthcare services

Key Terms

Accreditation
Acute care
Ambulatory care
American Association of Medical Colleges (AAMC)
American College of Healthcare Executives (ACHE)
American College of Surgeons
American Health Information Management Association (AHIMA)
American Hospital Association (AHA)
American Medical Association (AMA)
American Nurses Association (ANA)
Average length of stay (ALOS)
Behavioral healthcare
Blue Cross and Blue Shield Association
Case management
Centers for Medicare and Medicaid Services (CMS)
Chief executive officer (CEO)
Chief financial officer (CFO)
Chief information officer (CIO)
Chief nursing officer (CNO)
Chief operating officer (COO)
Clinical privileges
Commission on Accreditation of Health Informatics and Information Management Education (CAHIIM)
Conditions of Participation
Continuous quality improvement (CQI)
Continuum of care
Deemed status
Evidence-based medicine
Extended care facility
Health savings accounts
Health systems agency
Hill-Burton Act
Home healthcare

Hospice care
Integrated delivery network (IDN)
Integrated delivery system (IDS)
Investor-owned hospital chain
Joint Commission on Accreditation of Healthcare Organizations (JCAHO)
Long-term care
Malpractice
Managed care
Managed care organization (MCO)
Medicaid
Medical staff bylaws
Medical staff classifications
Medicare
Mission (statement)
National Committee on Quality Assurance (NCQA)
National Institutes of Health (NIH)
National Practitioner Data Bank (NPBD)
Peer review
Peer review organization (PRO)
Physician assistant (PA)
Postacute care
Prospective payment system (PPS)
Public Health Service (PHS)
Quality improvement organization (QIO)
Reengineering
Rehabilitation services
Skilled nursing facility (SNF)
Subacute care
Tax Equity and Fiscal Responsibility Act (TEFRA)
Telehealth
TRICARE
Utilization Review Act
Workers' compensation

Introduction

A broad array of healthcare services is available in the United States today, ranging from simple preventive measures such as vaccinations to complex lifesaving procedures such as heart transplants. An individual's contact with the healthcare delivery system often begins before she or he is born with family planning and prenatal care and continues through end-of-life planning and hospice care.

Healthcare services are provided by physicians, nurses, and other clinical providers who work in ambulatory care, **acute care,** rehabilitative and psychiatric care, and long-term care facilities. Healthcare services also are provided in the homes of hospice and home care patients. Assisted living centers, industrial medical clinics, and public health department clinics also provide services to many Americans.

Integrated delivery systems (IDSs) provide a full range of healthcare services along a **continuum of care** to ensure that patients get the right care at the right time from the right provider. The continuum extends from primary care providers to specialist and ancillary providers. The goal of IDSs is to deliver high-quality and cost-effective care in the most appropriate setting (Sloane, Sloane, and Harder 1999, p. 9). Most hospitals are integrated into their communities through ties with area physicians and other healthcare providers, clinics and outpatient facilities, and other practitioners. Almost half the nation's hospitals are tied to larger organizational entities, such as multihospital and integrated healthcare systems (IHCSs), **integrated delivery networks** (IDNs), and alliances. A network or IDN is a group of hospitals, physicians, other providers, insurers, and/or community agencies that work together to deliver health services (AHA 2004).

In 2002, there were 1,343 acute care hospitals (27 percent of the total) in networks (AHA 2004). Multihospital systems include two or more hospitals owned, leased, sponsored, or contract managed by a central organization. In 1985, 27.5 percent of hospitals were system members; by 2002, this figure had risen to 46 percent (AHA 2004). Within the context of healthcare, an alliance is a formal organization, usually owned by shareholders/members, that works on behalf of its individual members to provide services and products and to promote activities and ventures (AHA 1999). In 2000, there were 3,344 hospitals in group-purchasing organizations (the dominant kind of alliance). The same hospitals can be registered in more than one category (AHA 2000).

In 2002, there were 321 multihospital or integrated healthcare systems in the United States. The majority were not-for-profit, including religious (56) and secular (209) systems. Fifty-one systems were investor owned, and five were operated by the federal government (Jonas and Kovner 2005, p. 232). This chapter discusses the origin of the healthcare industry in the United States and examines the history from 1800s to the 21st century. Included in this history is the impact of external forces that have shaped the healthcare system of today.

Theory into Practice

In the 1990s, hospitals in the United States faced continued pressure to contain costs, improve quality, and demonstrate their contributions to the health of the communities they served. They adapted to these pressures in various ways. Some hospitals merged with or bought out other hospitals and healthcare organizations. Others created IDSs to provide a full range of healthcare services along the continuum of care, from ambulatory care to inpatient care to long-term care. Still others concentrated on improving the care they provided by focusing on patients as customers. Many hospitals responded to local competition by quickly entering into affiliations and other risk-sharing agreements with acute and nonacute care providers, physicians' groups, and **managed care organizations.**

History of Western Medicine

Modern Western medicine is rooted in antiquity. The ancient Greeks developed surgical procedures, documented clinical cases, and created medical books. Before modern times, European, African, and native American cultures all had traditions of folk medicine based on spiritual healing and herbal cures. The first hospitals were created by religious orders in medieval Europe to provide care and respite to religious pilgrims traveling back and forth from the Holy Land. However, it was not until the late 1800s that medicine became a scientific discipline. More progress and change occurred during the 20th century than over the preceding 2,000 years. The past few decades have seen dramatic developments in the way diseases are diagnosed and treated and in the way healthcare is delivered.

Before the advent of modern Western medicine, epidemics and plagues were common. Epidemics of smallpox, measles, yellow fever, influenza, scarlet fever, and diphtheria killed millions of people. Bubonic plague spread periodically through Europe and killed millions more. Disease was carried by rodents and insects as well as by the travelers who moved along intercontinental trade routes.

The medical knowledge that had been gained by ancient Greek scholars such as Hippocrates was lost during the Middle Ages. The European Renaissance, a historical period beginning in the 14th century, revived interest in the classical arts, literature, and philosophy as well as in the scientific study of nature. This period also was characterized by economic growth and concern for the welfare of workers at all levels of society. With this concept came a growing awareness that a healthy population promoted economic growth.

North America's First Hospitals

Early settlers in the British colonies of North America appointed commissions to care for the sick, to provide for orphans, and to bury the dead. During the mid-1700s, the citizens of Philadelphia recognized the need for a place to provide relief to the sick and injured. They also recognized the need to isolate newly arrived immigrants who had caught communicable diseases on the long voyage from Europe.

In Philadelphia, Benjamin Franklin and other colonists persuaded the legislature to develop a hospital for the community. It was the first hospital in the British colonies of North America. The Pennsylvania Hospital was established in Philadelphia in 1752. (Almost 200 years earlier, Hernando Cortez established the first hospital in Mexico and it still serves patients today.)

Over its first 150 years, the Pennsylvania Hospital served as a model for the organization of hospitals in other communities. The New York Hospital opened in 1771 and started its first register of patients in 1791. Boston's Massachusetts General Hospital opened in 1821.

Standardization of Medical Practice

Human anatomy and physiology and the causes of disease were not well understood before the 20th century. At one time, it was believed that four basic fluids, called humors, determined a person's temperament and health and that imbalances in the proportion of humors in the body caused disease. The therapeutic bleeding of patients was practiced until the early 20th century. Early physicians also treated patients by administering a variety of substances with no scientific basis for their effectiveness.

An individual's early medical education consisted of serving as an apprentice to an established practitioner. Just about anyone could hang out a shingle and call himself a physician. The medical profession recognized that some of its members achieved better results than others, and leaders in the profession attempted to regulate the practice of medicine in the late 1700s. The first attempts at regulation took the form of licensure. The first licenses to practice medicine were issued in New York in 1760. By the mid-1800s, however, efforts to license physicians were denounced as being undemocratic and penalties for practicing medicine without a license were removed in most states.

As the population of the United States grew and settlers moved westward, the demand for medical practitioners far exceeded the supply. To staff new hospitals and serve a growing population, many private medical schools appeared almost overnight. By 1869, there were 72 medical schools in the United States. However, these schools did not follow an established course of study and some graduated students with as little as six months of training. The result was an oversupply of poorly trained physicians.

The **American Medical Association** (AMA) was established in 1847 to represent the interests of physicians across the United States. However, the AMA was dominated by members who had strong ties to the medical schools and the status quo. Its ability to lead a reform of the profession was limited until it broke its ties with the medical schools in 1874. At that time, the association encouraged the creation of independent state licensing boards.

In 1876, the **American Association of Medical Colleges** (AAMC) was established. The AAMC was dedicated to standardizing the curriculum for U.S. medical schools and to developing the public's understanding of the need to license physicians.

Together, the AMA and the AAMC campaigned for medical licensing. By the 1890s, 35 states had established or reestablished a system of licensure for physicians. At that time, 14 states decided to grant licenses only to graduates of reputable medical schools. The state licensing boards discouraged the worst medical schools, but the criteria for licensing continued to vary from state to state and were not fully enforced.

By the early 20th century, it had become apparent that improving the quality of American medicine required regulation through curriculum reform as well as licensure. However, the members of the AMA were divided on this issue. Conservative members continued to believe that the association should stay out of the area of regulation. Progressive members supported the continued development of state licensure systems and the creation of a standardized model for medical education.

The situation attracted the attention of the Carnegie Foundation for the Advancement of Teaching. The president of the foundation offered to sponsor and fund an independent review of the medical colleges then operating in the United States. Abraham Flexner, an educator from Louisville, Kentucky, undertook the review in 1906.

Over the following four years, Flexner visited every medical college in the country and carefully documented his findings. In his 1910 report to the Carnegie Foundation, the AMA, and the AAMC, he described the poor quality of the training being provided in the colleges. He noted that medical school applicants often lacked knowledge of the basic sciences. Flexner also reported how the absence of hospital-based training limited the clinical skills of medical school graduates. Perhaps most important, he reported that huge numbers of graduates were being produced every year and that most of them had unacceptable levels of medical skill. He recommended closing most of the existing medical schools to address the problem of oversupply.

Several reform initiatives grew out of Flexner's report and from recommendations made by the AMA's Committee on Medical Education. One of the reforms required medical school applicants to hold a college degree. Another required that medical training be founded in the basic sciences. Reforms also required that medical students receive practical, hospital-based training in addition to classroom work. These reforms were carried out in the decade following Flexner's report, but only about half the medical schools actually closed. By 1920, most of the medical colleges in the United States had met rigorous academic standards and were approved by the AAMC.

Today, medical school graduates must pass a test before they can obtain a license to practice medicine. The licensure tests are administered by state medical boards. Many states now use a standardized licensure test developed in 1968 by the Federation of State Medical Boards of the United States. However, passing scores for the test vary by state. Most physicians also complete several years of residency training in addition to medical school.

Specialty physicians also complete extensive postgraduate medical education. Board certification for the various specialties requires the completion of postgraduate training as well as a passing score on a standardized examination. The most common medical specialties include the following:

- Internal medicine
- Pediatrics
- Family practice
- Cardiology
- Psychiatry
- Neurology
- Oncology
- Radiology

The most common surgical specialties include:

- Anesthesiology
- Cardiovascular surgery
- Obstetrics/gynecology
- Orthopedics
- Urology
- Ophthalmology
- Otorhinolaryngology
- Plastic and reconstructive surgery
- Neurosurgery

Some medical and surgical specialists undergo further graduate training to qualify to practice subspecialties. For example, the subspecialties of internal medicine include endocrinology, pulmonary medicine, rheumatology, geriatrics, and hematology. Physicians also may limit their practices to the treatment of specific illnesses. For example, an endocrinologist may limit his or her practice to the treatment of diabetes. Surgeons can work as general surgeons or as specialists or subspecialists. For example, an orthopedic surgeon may limit his practice to surgery of the hand, surgery of the knee, surgery of the ankle, or surgery of the spine.

Some physicians and healthcare organizations employ **physician assistants** (PAs) and/or surgeon assistants (SAs) to help them carry out their clinical responsibilities. Such assistants may perform routine clinical assessments, provide patient education and counseling, and perform simple therapeutic procedures. Most PAs work in primary care settings, and most SAs work in hospitals and ambulatory surgery clinics. PAs and SAs always work under the supervision of licensed physicians and surgeons.

Standardization of Nursing Practice

In the 19th century and the first part of the 20th century, religious organizations sponsored more than half the hospitals in the United States. Members of religious orders often provided nursing care in these organizations. As the U.S. population grew and more towns and cities were established, new hospitals were built. Older cities also grew, and city hospitals became more and more crowded.

In the late 1800s, nurses received no formal education and little training. Nursing staff for the hospitals was often recruited from the surrounding community, and many poor women who had no other skills became nurses. The nature of nursing care at that time was unsophisticated. Indeed, the lack of basic hygiene often promoted disease. Many patients died from infections contracted while hospitalized for surgery, maternity care, and other illnesses.

In 1868, the AMA called the medical profession's attention to the need for trained nurses. During the years that followed, the public also began to call for better nursing care in hospitals.

The first general training school for nurses was opened at the New England Hospital for Women and Children in 1872. It became a model for other institutions throughout the country. As hospital after hospital struggled to find competent nursing staff, many institutions and their medical staffs developed their own nurse training programs.

The responsibilities of nurses in the late 19th and early 20th centuries included housekeeping duties. Nurses also cooked meals for patients in kitchens attached to each ward. Direct patient care duties included giving baths, changing dressings, monitoring vital signs, administering medications, and assisting physicians. During this time, nurses were not required to hold a license to practice.

In 1897, a group of nurses attending the annual meeting of the American Society of Superintendents of Training Schools for Nursing founded the Nurses Associated Alumnae of the United States and Canada. In 1911, the organization was renamed the **American Nurses Association** (ANA). During the early meetings of the association, members established a nursing code of ethics and discussed the need for nursing licensure and for publications devoted to the practice of nursing.

At the turn of the 20th century, nurses also began to organize state nursing associations to advocate for the registration of nurses. Their goal was to increase the level of competence among nurses nationwide. Despite opposition from many physicians who believed that nurses did not need formal education or licensure, North Carolina passed legislation requiring the registration of nurses in 1903. Today, all 50 states have laws that spell out the requirements for the registration and licensure of nursing professionals.

Modern registered nurses must have either a two-year associate's degree or a four-year bachelor's degree from a state-approved nursing school. Nurse practitioners, researchers, educators, and administrators generally have a four-year degree in nursing and additional postgraduate education in nursing. The postgraduate degree may be a master's of science or a doctorate in nursing. Nurses who graduate from nonacademic training programs are called licensed practical nurses (LPNs) or licensed vocational nurses (LVNs). Nondegreed nursing personnel work under the direct supervision of registered nurses. Nurses in all 50 states must pass an exam to obtain a license to practice.

Today's registered nurses are highly trained clinical professionals. Many specialize in specific areas of practice such as surgery, psychiatry, and intensive care. Nurse-midwives complete advanced training and are certified by the American College of Nurse-Midwives. Similarly, nurse-anesthetists are certified by the Council on Certification/Council on Recertification of Nurse Anesthetists. Nurse practitioners also receive advanced training at the master's level that qualifies them to provide primary care services to patients. They are certified by several organizations (for example, the National Board of Pediatric Nurse Practitioners) to practice in the area of their specialty.

Standardization of Hospital Care

In 1910, Dr. Franklin H. Martin suggested that the surgical area of medical practice needed to become more concerned with patient outcomes. He had been introduced to this concept in discussions with Dr. Ernest Codman. Codman was a British physician who believed that hospital practitioners should track their patients for a significant amount of time after treatment so that they could determine whether the end result had been positive or negative. Codman also supported the use of outcome information to identify the practices that led to the best results for patients.

At that time, Martin and other American physicians were concerned about the conditions in U.S. hospitals. Many observers felt that part of the problem was related to the lack of organization in medical staffs and to lax professional standards. In the early 20th century, before the development of antibiotics and other pharmaceuticals, hospitals were used mainly by physicians who needed facilities in which to perform surgery. Most nonsurgical medical care was still provided in the home. It was natural, then, for the force behind improved hospital care to come from surgeons.

The push for hospital reforms eventually led to the formation of the **American College of Surgeons** in 1913. The organization faced a difficult task. In 1917, the leaders of the college asked the Carnegie Foundation for funding to plan and develop a hospital standardization program. The college then formed a committee to develop a set of minimum standards for hospital care. It published the formal standards under the title of the Minimum Standards.

During 1918 and part of 1919, the college examined the hospitals in the United States and Canada just as Flexner had reviewed the medical colleges a decade earlier. The performance of 692 hospitals was compared to the college's Minimum Standards. Only 89 of the hospitals fully met the college's standards, and some of the best-known hospitals in the country failed to meet them.

Adoption of the Minimum Standards was the basis of the Hospital Standardization Program and marked the beginning

of the modern **accreditation** process for healthcare organizations. Basically, accreditation standards are developed to reflect reasonable quality standards. The performance of each participating organization is evaluated annually against the standards. The accreditation process is voluntary. Healthcare organizations choose to participate in order to improve the care they provide to their patients.

The American College of Surgeons continued to sponsor the hospital accreditation program until the early 1950s. At that time, four professional associations from the United States and Canada decided to join forces with the college to create a new accreditation organization. This organization was called the Joint Commission on Accreditation of Hospitals. The associations were the American College of Physicians, the AMA, the **American Hospital Association** (AHA), and the Canadian Medical Association. The new organization was formally incorporated in 1952 and began to perform accreditation surveys in 1953.

The Joint Commission, under the name **Joint Commission on Accreditation of Healthcare Organizations** (JCAHO), continues to survey several different types of healthcare organizations today, including:

- Acute care hospitals
- Long-term care facilities
- Ambulatory care facilities
- Psychiatric facilities
- Home health agencies

Several other organizations also perform accreditation of healthcare organizations. These include the American Osteopathic Association (AOA), the Commission on Accreditation of Rehabilitation Facilities (CARF), and the Accreditation Association for Ambulatory Healthcare (AAAHC).

Professionalization of the Allied Health Professions

After the First World War, many of the roles previously played by nurses and nonclinical personnel began to change. With the advent of modern diagnostic and therapeutic technology in the middle of the 20th century, the complex skills needed by ancillary medical personnel fostered the growth of specialized training programs and professional accreditation and licensure.

According to the AMA's definition, *allied health* incorporates the healthcare-related professions that function to assist, facilitate, and/or complement the work of physicians and other clinical specialists. The Health Professions Education Amendment of 1991 describes allied health professionals as health professionals (other than registered nurses, physicians, and PAs) who have received either a certificate, an associate's degree, a bachelor's degree, a master's degree, a doctorate, or postdoctoral training in a healthcare-related science. Such individuals share responsibility for the delivery of healthcare services with clinicians (physicians, nurses, and PAs).

Allied health occupations are among the fastest growing in healthcare. The number of allied health professionals is difficult to estimate and depends on the definition of allied health. Unlike medicine, women dominate most of the allied health professions, representing between 75 and 95 percent in most of the occupations. All 50 states require licensure for some allied health professions (physical therapy, for example). Practitioners in other allied health professions (occupational therapy, for example) may be licensed in some states, but not in others.

The following list briefly describes some of the major occupations usually considered to be allied health professions (Jonas and Kovner 2005, pp. 446–48):

- *Clinical laboratory science:* Originally referred to as medical laboratory technology, this field is now referred to more appropriately as clinical laboratory science. Clinical laboratory technicians perform a wide array of tests on body fluids, tissues, and cells to assist in the detection, diagnosis, and treatment of diseases and illnesses.
- *Diagnostic imaging technology:* Originally referred to as x-ray technology and then radiologic technology, this field is now more appropriately referred to as diagnostic imaging. The field continues to expand to include nuclear medicine technologists, radiation therapists, sonographers (ultrasound technologists), and magnetic resonance technologists.
- *Dietetics:* Dietitians (sometimes called clinical nutritionists) are trained in nutrition. They are responsible for providing nutritional care to individuals and for overseeing nutrition and food services in a variety of settings, ranging from hospitals to schools.
- *Emergency medical technology:* Emergency medical technicians (EMTs) are responsible for providing a wide range of services on an emergency basis for cases of traumatic injury and other emergency situations and in the transport of emergency patients.
- *Health information management:* Health information management (HIM) professionals (formerly called medical record managers) oversee health record systems and manage health-related information to ensure that it meets relevant medical, administrative, and legal requirements. Health records are the responsibility of registered health information administrators (RHIAs) and registered health information technicians (RHITs).
- *Occupational therapy:* Occupational therapists (OTs) evaluate and treat patients whose illnesses or injuries have resulted in significant psychological, physical, or work-related impairment.
- *Physical therapy:* Physical therapists (PTs) evaluate and treat patients to improve functional mobility, reduce pain, maintain cardiopulmonary function, and limit disability. PTs treat movement dysfunction resulting from accidents, trauma, stroke, fractures, multiple sclerosis, cerebral palsy, arthritis, and heart and respira-

tory illness. Physical therapy assistants work under the direction of PTs and help carry out the treatment plans developed by PTs.
- *Respiratory therapy:* Respiratory therapists evaluate, treat, and care for patients with breathing disorders. They work under the direction of qualified physicians and provide services such as emergency care for stroke, heart failure, and shock and treat patients with emphysema and asthma.
- *Speech-language pathology and audiology:* Speech-language pathologists and audiologists identify, assess, and provide treatment for individuals with speech, language, or hearing problems.

Check Your Understanding 2.1

Instructions: On a separate piece of paper, write down the word or term that correctly completes each of the sentences below.

1. The ancient ___ developed surgical procedures, documented clinical cases, and created medical books.
   a. Egyptians
   b. Greeks
   c. Phoenicians
   d. Chinese

2. The ___ was established in 1847 to represent the interests of physicians across the United States.
   a. American Association of Medical Colleges
   b. American College of Surgeons
   c. Committee on Medical Education
   d. American Medical Association

3. Today, medical school students must pass a test before they can obtain a ___ to practice medicine.
   a. Degree
   b. Residency
   c. Specialty
   d. License

4. The first general training school for ___ was opened at the New England Hospital for Women and Children in 1872.
   a. Nurses
   b. Physician assistants
   c. Surgical specialists
   d. Surgeons

5. Modern ___ must have either a two-year associate's degree or a four-year bachelor's degree from a state-approved nursing school.
   a. Nurse practitioners
   b. Licensed vocational nurses
   c. Registered nurses
   d. Licensed practical nurses

6. In 1910, Dr. Franklin H. Martin suggested that the surgical area of medical practice needed to become more concerned with ___.
   a. Patient care
   b. Professional standards
   c. Patient outcomes
   d. Nonsurgical medical care

7. Adoption of the Minimum Standards marked the beginning of the modern ___ process for healthcare organizations.
   a. Accreditation
   b. Licensing
   c. Reform
   d. Educational

8. According to the AMA's definition, ___ incorporates the healthcare-related professions that function to assist, facilitate, and/or complement the work of physicians and other clinical specialists.
   a. Home health
   b. Nursing care
   c. Ambulatory care
   d. Allied health

Modern Healthcare Delivery in the United States

Until the Second World War, most healthcare was provided in the home. Quality in healthcare services was considered a product of appropriate medical practice and oversight by physicians and surgeons. Even the Minimum Standards used to evaluate the performance of hospitals were based on factors directly related to the composition and skills of the hospital medical staff.

The 20th century was a period of tremendous change in American society. Advances in medical science promised better outcomes and increased the demand for healthcare services. But medical care has never been free. Even in the best economic times, many Americans have been unable to take full advantage of what medicine has to offer because they cannot afford it.

Concern over access to healthcare was especially evident during the Great Depression of the 1930s. During the Depression, America's leaders were forced to consider how the poor and disadvantaged could receive the care they needed. Before the Depression, medical care for the poor and elderly had been handled as a function of social welfare agencies. During the 1930s, however, few people were able to pay for medical care. The problem of how to pay for the healthcare needs of millions of Americans became a public and governmental concern. Working Americans turned to prepaid health plans to help them pay for healthcare, but the unemployed and the unemployable needed help from a different source.

Effects of the Great Depression

The concept of prepaid healthcare, or health insurance, began with the financial problems of one hospital, Baylor University Hospital in Dallas, Texas (AHA 1999, p. 14). In 1929, the administrator of the hospital arranged to provide hospital services to Dallas's schoolteachers for 50 cents per person per month. Before that time, a few large employers had set up company clinics and hired company physicians to care for their workers, but the idea of a prepaid health plan that could be purchased by individuals had never been tried before.

The idea caught on quickly, and new prepaid plans appeared across the country. Eventually, these plans became known as Blue Cross plans when the blue cross symbol used by some of the new plans was adopted officially as the trademark for all the plans in 1939.

Another type of prepaid plan, called the Blue Shield plan, was subsequently developed to cover the cost of physicians' services. The idea for the Blue Shield plans grew out of the medical service bureaus created by large lumber and mining companies in the Northwest. In 1939, the first formal Blue Shield plan was founded in California.

Growth in the number of Blue Cross/Blue Shield plans continued through the Depression and boomed during the Second World War. During the war-related labor shortages, employers began to pay for their employees' memberships in the "Blues" as a way to attract and keep scarce workers.

The idea of public funding for healthcare services also goes back to the Great Depression. The decline in family income during the 1930s curtailed the use of medical services by the poor. In 10 working-class communities studied between 1929 and 1933, the proportion of families with incomes under $150 per capita had increased from 10 to 43 percent. A 1938 Gallup poll asked people whether they had put off seeing a physician because of the cost. The results showed that 68 percent of lower-income respondents had put off medical care, compared with 24 percent of respondents in upper-income brackets (Starr 1982, p. 271).

The decreased use of medical services and the inability of many patients to pay meant lower incomes for physicians. Hospitals were in similar trouble. Beds were empty, bills went unpaid, and contributions to hospital fund-raising efforts tumbled. As a result, private physicians and charities could no longer meet the demand for free services. For the first time, physicians and hospitals asked state welfare departments to pay for the treatment of people on relief.

The Depression posed a severe test for the AMA. It was no easy matter to maintain a common front against government intervention when physicians themselves were facing economic difficulties. Because of the economic hardships, many physicians were willing to accept government-sponsored health insurance. In 1935, the California Medical Association endorsed the concept of compulsory health insurance because health insurance promised to stimulate the use of physicians' services and help patients pay their bills.

The AMA's response to the economic crisis emphasized restricting the supply of physicians, rather than increasing the demand for their services, by instituting mandatory health insurance. The AMA reacted by pushing for the closure of medical schools and reductions in the number of new medical students.

By the mid-1930s, however, the AMA began to adjust its position on health insurance. Instead of opposing all insurance, voluntary or compulsory, it began to define the terms on which voluntary programs might be acceptable. Although accepting health insurance plans in principle, the AMA did nothing to support or encourage their development.

The push for government-sponsored health insurance continued in the late 1930s during the administration of President Franklin D. Roosevelt. However, compulsory health insurance stood on the margins of national politics throughout the New Deal era. It was not made part of the new Social Security program, and it was never fully supported by President Roosevelt.

Postwar Efforts toward Improving Healthcare Access

After the Second World War, the issue of healthcare access finally moved to the center of national politics. In the late 1940s, President Harry Truman expressed unreserved support for a national health insurance program. However, the issue of compulsory health insurance became entangled with America's fear of communism. Opponents of Truman's healthcare program labeled it "socialized medicine," and the program failed to win legislative support.

The idea of national health insurance did not resurface until the administration of Lyndon Johnson and the Great Society legislation of the 1960s. The **Medicare** and **Medicaid** programs were legislated in 1965 to pay the cost of providing healthcare services to the elderly and the poor. The issues of healthcare reform and national health insurance were again given priority during the first four years of President Bill Clinton's administration in the 1990s. However, the complexity of American healthcare issues at the end of the 20th century doomed reform efforts.

Influence of Federal Legislation

During the 20th century, Congress passed many pieces of legislation that had a significant impact on the delivery of healthcare services in the United States. Many of these legislative efforts are described in the following subsections.

Biologics Control Act of 1902

Direct federal sponsorship of medical research began with early research on methods for controlling epidemics of infectious disease. The Marine Hospital Service performed the first research. In 1887, a young physician named Joseph Kinyoun set up a bacteriological laboratory in the Marine Hospital at Staten Island, New York. Four years later, the Hygienic Laboratory was moved to Washington, D.C. It was given authority to test and improve biological products in 1902 when Congress passed the Biologics Control Act. This act regulated the vaccines and sera sold via interstate commerce. That same year, the Hygienic Laboratory added divisions in chemistry, pharmacology, and zoology.

In 1912, the service, by then called the U.S. Public Health Service, was authorized to study chronic as well as infectious diseases. In 1930, reorganized under the Randsdell Act, the Hygienic Laboratory became the **National Institutes of Health** (NIH). In 1938, the NIH moved to a large, privately donated estate in Bethesda, Maryland (Starr 1982, p. 340).

Today, the mission of the NIH is to uncover new medical knowledge that can lead to health improvements for everyone. The NIH accomplishes its mission by conducting and supporting medical research, fostering communication of up-to-date medical information, and training research investigators. The organization has played a vital role in recent clinical research on treatment of the following diseases:

- Heart disease and stroke
- Cancer
- Depression and schizophrenia
- Spinal cord injuries

Social Security Act of 1935

The Great Depression revived the dormant social reform movement in the United States as well as more radical currents in American politics. Unionization increased, and the American Federation of Labor abandoned its long-standing opposition to social insurance programs. The Depression also brought to power a Democratic administration. The administration of Franklin D. Roosevelt was more willing than any previous administration to involve the federal government in the management of economic and social welfare.

Even before Roosevelt took office in 1933, a steady movement toward some sort of social insurance program had been growing. By 1931, nine states had passed legislation creating old-age pension programs. As governor of New York, Roosevelt endorsed unemployment insurance in 1930. Wisconsin became the first state to adopt such a measure early in 1932.

Although old-age pension and unemployment insurance bills were introduced into Congress soon after his election, Roosevelt refused to give them his strong support. Instead, he created a program of his own. On June 8, 1934, he announced that he would appoint a committee on economic security to study the issue comprehensively and report to Congress in January 1935. The committee consisted of four members of the cabinet and the federal relief administrator and was headed by the secretary of labor, Frances Perkins.

Although Roosevelt indicated in his June message that he was especially interested in old-age and unemployment programs, the committee included medical care and health insurance in its research. From the outset, the prevailing sentiment on the committee was that health insurance would have to wait. Abraham Epstein was the founder of the American Association for Social Security and a leading figure in the social insurance movement. In an article published in October 1934, he warned the administration that opposition to health insurance was strong. He advised the administration to be politically realistic and cautious on health insurance.

Sentiment in favor of health insurance was strong among members of the Committee on Economic Security. However, many members of the committee were convinced that adding a health insurance amendment would spell defeat for the entire Social Security legislation. Ultimately, the Social Security bill included only one reference to health insurance as a subject that the new Social Security Board might study. The Social Security Act was passed in 1935.

The omission of health insurance from the legislation was by no means the act's only conservative feature. It relied on a regressive tax and gave no coverage to some of the nation's poorest people, such as farmers and domestic workers. However, the act did extend the federal government's role in public health through several provisions unrelated to social insurance. It gave the states funds on a matching basis for maternal and infant care, rehabilitation of crippled children, general public health work, and aid for dependent children under the age of 16.

Hospital Survey and Construction Act of 1946
Passage of the **Hill-Burton Act** was another important development in American healthcare delivery. Enacted in 1946 as the Hospital Survey and Construction Act, this legislation authorized grants for states to construct new hospitals and, later, to modernize old ones. The fund expansion of the hospital system was to achieve a goal of 4.5 beds per 1,000 persons. The availability of federal financing created a boom in hospital construction during the 1950s. The hospital system grew from 6,000 hospitals in 1946 to a high of approximately 7,200 acute care hospitals.

Growth in Number of Hospitals
The number of hospitals in the United States increased from 178 in 1873 to 4,300 in 1909. In 1946, at the close of the Second World War, there were 6,000 American hospitals, with 3.2 beds available for every 1,000 persons.

In 2002, there were 4,927 hospitals in the United States, with a total of 821,000 beds. Of the $1.4 trillion spent on healthcare in 2001, hospital costs totaled $415 billion or 32 percent. The majority of the hospitals in the U.S. are nonprofit or owned by local, state, or federal governments (Jonas and Kovner, 2005, p. 224).

Decline in Number of Hospitals
During the 1980s, medical advances and cost-containment measures caused many procedures that once required inpatient hospitalization to be performed on an outpatient basis. Outpatient hospital visits increased by 40 percent with a resultant decrease in hospital admissions. Fewer patient admissions and shortened lengths of stay (LOS) resulted in a significant reduction in the number of hospitals and hospital beds. Healthcare reform efforts and the acceptance of **managed care** as the major medical practice style of U.S. healthcare resulted in enough hospital closings and mergers to reduce the number of government and community-based hospitals in the United States to approximately 5,000 (Sultz and Young 2004, p. 68).

Public Law 89-97 of 1965
In 1965, passage of a number of amendments to the Social Security Act brought Medicare and Medicaid into existence. These two programs have greatly changed how healthcare organizations are reimbursed. Recent attempts to curtail Medicare/Medicaid spending continue to affect healthcare organizations.

Medicare (Title XVIII of the Social Security Act) is a federal program that provides healthcare benefits for people 65 years old and older who are covered by Social Security. The program was inaugurated on July 1, 1966. Over the years, amendments have extended coverage to individuals who are not covered by Social Security, but who are willing to pay a premium for coverage, to the disabled, and to those suffering from chronic kidney disease.

The companion program, Medicaid (Title XIX of the Social Security Act, was established at the same time to support medical and hospital care for persons classified as medically indigent. Originally targeted to recipients of public assistance (primarily single parent families and the aged, blind, and disabled), Medicaid has expanded to additional groups so that it now targets poor children, disabled, pregnant women, and very poor adults (including those 65 years of age and over). The only exception to these expansions was passage of the Personal Responsibility and Work Opportunity Reconciliation Act of 1996 (PRWORA, P.L. 104-193, 1996), which changed eligibility for legal/illegal immigrants (Jonas and Kovner 2005, p. 56). Medicaid today is a federally mandated program that provides healthcare benefits to low-income people and their children. Medicaid programs are administered and partially paid for by individual states. Medicaid is an umbrella for 50 different state programs designed specifically to serve the poor. Beginning in January 1967, Medicaid provided federal funds to states on a cost-sharing basis to ensure that welfare recipients would be guaranteed medical services. Coverage of four types of care was required: inpatient and outpatient services, other laboratory and x-ray services, physician services, and nursing facility care for persons over 21 years of age.

Many enhancements have been made in the years since Medicaid was enacted. Services now include family planning and 31 other optional services such as prescription drugs and dental services. With few exceptions, recipients of cash assistance are automatically eligible for Medicaid. Medicaid also pays the Medicare premium, deductible, and coinsurance costs for some low-income Medicare beneficiaries.

Four million individuals were enrolled in Medicaid during 1966, its first year of implementation. By December 2002, 39.7 million people were enrolled in Medicaid programs. In 2002, the states and the federal government expended $250.4 billion on Medicaid, most of which was directed toward the elderly, the blind, or the disabled. Elderly and disabled participants comprised about one-quarter of the Medicaid rolls, yet the program expends almost three-quarters of all funds on this group (Jonas and Kovner 2005, pp. 56–57).

Public Law 92-603 of 1972
Utilization review (UR) was a mandatory component of the original Medicare legislation. Medicare required hospitals and **extended care facilities** to establish a plan for UR as well as a permanent UR committee. The goal of the UR process was to ensure that the services provided to Medicare beneficiaries were medically necessary.

In an effort to curtail Medicare and Medicaid spending, additional amendments to the Social Security Act were instituted in 1972. Public Law 92-603 required concurrent review for Medicare and Medicaid patients. It also established the professional standards review organization (PSRO) program to implement concurrent review. PSROs performed professional review and evaluated patient care services for necessity, quality, and cost-effectiveness.

Three major eras occurred in health care policy from 1975 to 2000. Like an archeological site, these eras have mostly accumulated on top of one another, rather than fully replacing what has come before. The three health policy eras can be identified as the following (Etheredge 2001):

- Age of Traditional Insurance (1965–1982), which began with the enactment of Medicare and Medicaid and which was based on open-ended, fee-for-service health insurance;
- Age of Regulated Prices for Government Programs (1983–1992), which was launched with the enactment of the Medicare DRG system; and
- Age of Markets, Purchasing and Managed Care (1993–2000), the era that has seen the population move to managed care plans in both the private and public coverage programs.

Health Systems Agency
The Health Planning and Resources Development Act of 1974 called for a new local organization, the **health systems agency** (HSA), to have broad representation of healthcare providers and consumers on governing boards and committees. Although the governance structure required participation by consumers, interested parties from the provider groups dominated the discussions. HSAs were fundamentally unsuccessful in materially influencing decisions about service or technology expansion. Their decisions became undeniably political, and attempts to achieve consensus based on real service needs were counterbalanced by community interests in economic and employment expansions. Concurrent with attempts to slow cost increases through a planning approach, a number of other legislative initiatives took shape that were directly related to concerns over Medicare costs and service quality (Sultz and Young 2004, pp. 39, 242). The legislation that created the HSAs or nationwide system of local health planning agencies was repealed in 1986.

Utilization Review Act of 1977
In 1977, the **Utilization Review Act** of 1977 made it a requirement that hospitals conduct continued-stay reviews for Medicare and Medicaid patients. Continued-stay reviews determine whether it is medically necessary for a patient to remain hospitalized. This legislation also included fraud and abuse regulations.

Peer Review Improvement Act of 1982
In 1982, the Peer Review Improvement Act of 1982 redesigned the PSRO program and renamed the agencies **peer review organizations** (PROs). At this time, hospitals began to review the medical necessity and appropriateness of certain admissions even before patients were admitted. PROs were given a new name in 2002 and are now called **quality improvement organizations** (QIOs). They currently emphasize quality improvement processes. Every state and territory, as well as the District of Columbia, now has its own QIO. The mission of the QIO is to ensure the quality, efficiency, and cost-effectiveness of the healthcare services provided to Medicare beneficiaries in its locale.

Tax Equity and Fiscal Responsibility Act of 1982
In 1982, Congress passed the **Tax Equity and Fiscal Responsibility Act** (TEFRA). TEFRA required extensive changes in the Medicare program. Its purpose was to control the rising cost of providing healthcare services to Medicare beneficiaries. Before this legislation was passed, healthcare services provided to Medicare beneficiaries were reimbursed on a retrospective, or fee-based, payment system. TEFRA required the gradual implementation of a **prospective payment system** (PPS) for Medicare reimbursement.

In a retrospective payment system, a service is provided, a claim for payment for the service is made, and the healthcare provider is reimbursed for the cost of delivering the service. In a PPS, a predetermined level of reimbursement is established before the service is provided.

Prospective Payment Act (1982)/ Public Law 98-21 of 1983
The PPS for acute hospital care (inpatient) services was implemented on October 1, 1983, according to Public Law 98-21. Under the inpatient PPS, reimbursement for hospital care provided to Medicare patients is based on diagnosis-related groups (DRGs). Each case is assigned to a DRG on the basis of the patient's diagnosis at the time of discharge. For example, under inpatient PPS, all the cases of viral pneumonia would be reimbursed at the same predetermined level of reimbursement no matter how long the patients stayed in the hospital or how many services they received.

Prospective payment systems for other healthcare services provided to Medicare beneficiaries have been gradually implemented in the years since 1983. Implementation of the ambulatory payment classification system for hospital outpatient services, for example, began in the year 2000.

Consolidated Omnibus Budget Reconciliation Act of 1985
The Consolidated Omnibus Budget Reconciliation Act of 1985 made it possible for the Healthcare Financing Administration (HCFA) to deny reimbursement for substandard healthcare services provided to Medicare and Medicaid beneficiaries. (HCFA's name was changed to the **Centers for Medicare and Medicaid Services** [CMS] in June 2001.)

Omnibus Budget Reconciliation Act of 1986
The Omnibus Budget Reconciliation Act of 1986 requires PROs to report instances of substandard care to relevant licensing and certification agencies.

Healthcare Quality Improvement Act of 1986
The Healthcare Quality Improvement Act established the **National Practitioner Data Bank** (NPDB). The purpose of the NPDB is to provide a clearinghouse for information about medical practitioners who have a history of malpractice suits and other quality problems. Hospitals are required

to consult the NPDB before granting medical staff privileges to healthcare practitioners. The legislation also established immunity from legal actions for practitioners involved in some peer review activities.

Omnibus Budget Reconciliation Act of 1989

The Omnibus Budget Reconciliation Act of 1989 instituted the Agency for Healthcare Policy and Research. The mission of this agency is to develop outcome measures to evaluate the quality of healthcare services.

Omnibus Budget Reconciliation Act of 1990

The Omnibus Budget Reconciliation Act of 1990 requires PROs to report actions taken against physicians to state medical boards and licensing agencies.

Health Insurance Portability and Accountability Act of 1996

The Health Insurance Portability and Accountability Act (HIPAA) of 1996 addresses issues related to the portability of health insurance after leaving employment, as well as administrative simplification. One of HIPAA's provisions was the creation of the Healthcare Integrity and Protection Data Bank (HIPDB). Its mission is to inform federal and state agencies about potential quality problems with clinicians and with suppliers and providers of healthcare services.

Biomedical and Technological Advances in Medicine

Rapid progress in medical science and technology during the late 19th and 20th centuries revolutionized the way healthcare was provided. The most important scientific advancement was the discovery of bacteria as the cause of infectious disease. The most important technological development was the use of anesthesia for surgical procedures. These 19th century advances formed the basis for the development of antibiotics and other pharmaceuticals and the application of sophisticated surgical procedures in the 20th century.

To further medical advances in the 21st century, the National Institutes of Health (NIH) sought the input of more than 300 recognized leaders in academia, industry, government, and the public to create a "Roadmap" program to accelerate biomedical advances, create effective prevention strategies and new treatments, and bridge knowledge gaps. The program, which involves a plethora of NIH Institutes and Centers, has three main strategic initiatives (NIH 2005):

1) New Pathways to Discovery, which includes a comprehensive understanding of building blocks of the body's cells and tissues and how complex biological systems operate; structural biology; molecular libraries and imaging; nanotechnology; bioinformatics and computational biology;

2) Research Teams of the Future, including interdisciplinary research, high-risk research, and public-private partnerships; and

3) Re-engineering the Clinical Research Enterprise.

Through these efforts, NIH will boost the resources and technologies needed for 21st century biomedical science.

Figure 2.1 offers a timeline of key biological and technological advances at a glance.

Although surgical procedures were performed before the development of anesthesia, surgeons had to work quickly on conscious patients to minimize risk and pain. The availability of anesthesia made it possible for surgeons to develop more advanced surgical techniques. The use of ether as an anesthetic was first recorded in 1842. At about the same time, nitrous oxide was introduced for use during dental procedures and chloroform was used to reduce the pain of labor. By the 1860s, the physicians who treated the casualties of the American Civil War on both sides had access to anesthetic and pain-killing drugs.

In the 1860s, Louis Pasteur began studying a condition in wine that made it sour and unpalatable. He discovered that the wine was being spoiled by parasitic growths. His research proved that tiny, living organisms (called bacteria) increase through reproduction and cause infectious disease. Pasteur also demonstrated that bacteria could be destroyed by the application of heat and certain chemicals (for example, alcohol). In doing so, he laid the foundation for modern bacteriology. After 20 years of research into the biology of microorganisms, Pasteur began studying human diseases. In 1885, he developed a vaccine that prevented rabies.

Figure 2.1.   Key biological and technological advances in medicine

Time	Event
1842	First recorded use of ether as an anesthetic
1860s	Louis Pasteur laid the foundation for modern bacteriology
1865	Joseph Lister was the first to apply Pasteur's research to the treatment of infected wounds
1880s–1890s	Steam first used in physical sterilization
1898	Introduction of rubber surgical gloves, sterilization, and antisepsis
1895	Wilhelm Roentgen made observations that led to the development of x-ray technology
1940	Studies of prothrombin time first made available
1941–1946	Studies of electrolytes; development of major pharmaceuticals
1957	Studies of blood gas
1961	Studies of creatine phosphokinase
1970s	Surgical advances in cardiac bypass surgery, surgery for joint replacements, and organ transplantation
1971	Computed tomography first used in England
1974	Introduction of whole-body scanners
1980s	Introduction of magnetic resonance imaging
1990s	Further technological advances in pharmaceuticals and genetics; Human Genome Project
2000s	NIH creates roadmap to accelerate biomedical advances, create effective prevention strategies and new treatments, and bridge knowledge gaps in the 21st century

Although the importance of cleanliness had been known since early times, the role that microorganisms played in disease was not understood until Pasteur conducted his research. In 1865, Joseph Lister was the first to apply Pasteur's research to the treatment of infected wounds. Lister began by protecting open fractures from infection by treating the wounds with carbolic acid (a disinfectant). His discovery was called the antiseptic principle. Antisepsis reduced the mortality rate in Lister's hospital after 1865 from 45 to 12 percent. He published his results in 1868, and soon carbolic acid was being used to prevent bacterial contamination during surgery.

During the 1880s and 1890s, physical sterilization using steam was developed. This technological advance had a major impact on surgery and in other areas throughout the hospital. The sterile operative technique was further advanced through the introduction of rubber surgical gloves in 1898. Other advances included the use of sterile gowns, masks, and antibiotics and other drugs.

In 1895, the well-known physicist Wilhelm Roentgen made observations that led to the development of x-ray technology. He found that he could create images of the bones in his hand by passing x-rays through his hand and onto a photographic plate. Radiographic technology is used extensively today to diagnose illnesses and injuries.

Many advances in laboratory testing occurred during the 20th century. Equipment that allows the rapid laboratory processing of diagnostic and prognostic examinations was developed, and the number of diagnostic laboratory procedures increased dramatically. For example, studies of prothrombin time were first made available in 1940, electrolytes in 1941 through 1946, blood gas in 1957, creatine phosphokinase in 1961, serum hepatitis in 1970, and carcinoembryonic antigen (the first cancer-screening test) in 1974.

Diagnostic radiology and radiation therapy have undergone huge advances in the past 50 years. An enormous advance first used in 1971 in England was an imaging modality called computed tomography (CT). The first CT scanners were used to create images of the skull. Whole-body scanners were introduced in 1974. In the 1980s, another powerful diagnostic tool was added, magnetic resonance imaging (MRI). MRI is a noninvasive technique that uses magnetic and radio-frequency fields to record images of soft tissues.

Surgical advances have been remarkable as well. Cardiac bypass surgery was developed in the 1970s, as were the techniques for joint replacement. Organs are now successfully transplanted, and artificial organs are being tested. New surgical techniques have included the use of lasers in ophthalmology, gynecology, and urology. Microsurgery is now a common tool in the reconstruction of damaged nerves and blood vessels. The use of robotics in surgery holds great promise for the future (Sloane, Sloane, and Harder 1999, pp. 6–7).

Check Your Understanding 2.2

Instructions: On a separate piece of paper, match the descriptions with the appropriate legislation.

1. ___ Hill-Burton Act
2. ___ Tax Equity and Fiscal Responsibility Act
3. ___ Public Law 89-79 of 1965
4. ___ Utilization Review Act
5. ___ Omnibus Budget Reconciliation Act of 1989
6. ___ Public Law 92-603 of 1972
7. ___ Healthcare Quality Improvement Act of 1986
8. ___ Omnibus Budget Reconciliation Act of 1990

a. Amendments to the Social Security Act that brought Medicare and Medicaid into existence

b. Authorized grants for states to construct new hospitals

c. Required concurrent review for Medicare and Medicaid patients

d. Required hospitals to conduct continued-stay reviews for Medicare and Medicaid patients

e. Established the National Practitioner Data Bank

f. Required peer review organizations to report actions taken against physicians to state medical boards and licensing agencies

g. Required extensive changes in the Medicare program to control the rising cost of providing healthcare services to Medicare beneficiaries (PPS general implementation)

h. Instituted the Agency for Healthcare Policy

Professional and Trade Associations Related to Healthcare

A number of trade and professional associations currently influence the practice of medicine and the delivery of healthcare services in the United States. Descriptions of a few of the numerous healthcare-related professional and trade associations that currently influence healthcare issues are provided below.

American Medical Association

The AMA was founded in 1847 as a national voluntary service organization. Today, its membership totals approximately 300,000 physicians from every area of medicine. The organization is headquartered in Chicago. Its mission is to promote the science and art of medicine and to improve public health. Its key objectives are:

- To become the world leader in obtaining, synthesizing, integrating, and disseminating information on health and medical practice
- To remain the acknowledged leader in promoting professionalism in medicine and setting standards for medical ethics, practice, and education
- To continue to be an authoritative voice and influential advocate for patients and physicians
- To continue to be a sound organization that provides value to members, related organizations, and employees

In addition, the AMA acts as an accreditation body for medical schools and residency programs. It also maintains and publishes the Current Procedural Terminology (CPT) coding system. CPT codes are used as the basis of reimbursement systems for physician services and other types of healthcare services provided on an ambulatory basis.

American Hospital Association

The AHA was founded in 1899. At its first meeting, eight hospital superintendents gathered in Cleveland, Ohio, to exchange ideas, compare methods of hospital management, discuss economics, and explore common interests and new trends. The original group was called the Association of Hospital Superintendents. Its mission was "to facilitate the interchange of ideas, comparing and contrasting methods of management, the discussion of hospital economics, the inspection of hospitals, suggestions of better plans for operating them, and such other matters as may affect the general interest of the membership" (AHA 1999, p. 110).

The Association of Hospital Superintendents adopted a new constitution in 1906 and a new name, the American Hospital Association. At that time, it had 234 members. Its major concerns were developing hospital standards and building the management skills of it members.

Today, the mission of the AHA is to advance the health of individuals and communities. The association has a current membership of approximately 5,000 hospitals and healthcare institutions, 600 associate member organizations, and 40,000 individual executives active in the healthcare field. Its headquarters are located in Chicago.

The AHA publishes *Coding Clinic,* which provides official ICD-9-CM coding advice.

Joint Commission on Accreditation of Healthcare Organizations

Since its beginning in 1952, the Joint Commission has continually evolved to meet the changing needs of healthcare organizations. The organization changed its name from the Joint Commission on Accreditation of Hospitals (JCAH) to the Joint Commission on Accreditation of Healthcare Organizations (JCAHO) in the late 1980s in recognition of changes in the U.S. health delivery system. Today, the JCAHO is the largest healthcare standards-setting body in the world. It conducts accreditation surveys in more than 19,500 facilities, including ambulatory care facilities, long-term care facilities, behavioral health facilities, healthcare networks, and managed care organizations as well as acute care hospitals (JCAHO 2005).

In the late 1990s, the JCAHO moved away from traditional quality assessment processes and began emphasizing performance and quality improvement. Its ORYX initiative reflected the new approach. The goal of the ORYX initiative was to incorporate the ongoing collection of quality and performance data into the accreditation process.

Today, the JCAHO's standards give organizations substantial leeway in selecting performance measures and improvement projects. Outcome measures document the results of care for individual patients as well as for specific types of patients grouped by diagnostic category. For example, an acute care hospital's overall rate of postsurgical infection would be considered an outcome measure. The outcome measures must be reported to the JCAHO via software from vendors that have been approved by the JCAHO for this purpose.

Blue Cross and Blue Shield Association

The forerunner of the **Blue Cross and Blue Shield Association** was a commission instituted by the AHA in 1929. In 1960, the commission was replaced by the Blue Cross Association and ties to the AHA were broken. In 1982, the Blue Cross Association merged with the National Association of Blue Shield Plans to become the Blue Cross and Blue Shield Association, often referred to as "the Blues."

Blue Cross and Blue Shield coordinate the activities of local plans throughout the United States. The vast majority of hospitals (more than 80 percent) and physicians (nearly 90 percent) contract directly with the Blues (3Dquote.com 2000).

American College of Healthcare Executives

The **American College of Healthcare Executives** (ACHE) is an organization for healthcare administrators. Like most of the organizations already discussed, it is headquartered in Chicago. Its mission is to serve as "the professional membership society for healthcare executives; to meet members' professional, educational, and leadership needs; to promote high ethical standards and conduct; and to enhance healthcare leadership and management excellence."

ACHE has nearly 30,000 members internationally. It also publishes books and textbooks on healthcare services management.

American Nurses Association

The ANA was founded in 1897. Headquartered in Washington, D.C., the ANA is a professional association as well as the strongest labor union active in the nursing profession. It represents the interests of the nation's 2.6 million registered nurses. The ANA's mission is to work for the improvement of health standards and the availability of healthcare services, to foster high professional standards for nurses, to stimulate and promote the professional development of nurses, and to advance the economic and general welfare of its members.

American Health Information Management Association

The **American Health Information Management Association** (AHIMA) is the professional membership organization for managers of health record services and healthcare information. It was founded in 1928 under the name of the Association of Record Librarians of North America. In 1929, the association adopted a constitution and bylaws. Its name was changed to the American Medical Record Association in 1970 and then to AHIMA in 1991.

Today, with headquarters in Chicago, the association has nearly 50,000 members. Its mission is to be a "community of professionals engaged in health information management, providing support to members and strengthening the industry and profession." The association's vision is of "a world in which the public values the contribution of health information management professionals and the American Health Information Management Association, in the advancement of health through quality information."

The association is the sponsoring organization for the **Commission on Accreditation of Health Informatics and Information Management Education** (CAHIIM), which accredits two- and four-year programs in health information management. AHIMA also offers an approval program for master's programs in HIM and coding specialist programs. Additionally, it certifies health information professionals as registered health information technologists (RHITs) for graduates of two-year programs and registered health information administrators (RHIAs) for graduates of baccalaureate programs. Finally, AHIMA offers credentialing examinations for coding professionals as certified coding specialists (CCSs), certified coding specialists for physicians' services (CCS-Ps), and certified coding associates (CCAs).

Other Healthcare-Related Associations

Many other healthcare-related associations in the United States serve their professional members by providing educational, certification, and accreditation services. The best known include the following:

- The American Osteopathic Association
- The American Dental Association
- The American College of Surgeons
- The American League for Nursing
- The American Society of Clinical Pathologists
- The American Dietetic Association
- The Commission on Accreditation of Rehabilitation Facilities
- The American Association of Nurse Anesthetists

Check Your Understanding 2.3

Instructions: On a separate piece of paper, match each organization with the appropriate description.

1. ____ American College of Healthcare Executives
2. ____ American Hospital Association
3. ____ American Medical Association
4. ____ American Nurses Association
5. ____ American Health Information Management Association
6. ____ Blue Cross and Blue Shield Association

a. Part of this organization's mission is to "enhance healthcare leadership and management excellence."
b. This organization was originally called the Association of Hospital Superintendents.
c. This organization was originally a commission instituted by the AHA in 1929.
d. This association was founded in 1928 under the name of the Association of Record Librarians of North America.
e. Part of this organization's mission is to work for the improvement of health standards and the availability of healthcare services.
f. This organization's mission is to promote the art and science of medicine and to improve public health.

Organization and Operation of Modern Hospitals

The term *hospital* can be applied to any healthcare facility that has the following four characteristics:

- An organized medical staff
- Permanent inpatient beds
- Around-the-clock nursing services
- Diagnostic and therapeutic services

Most hospitals provide acute care services to inpatients. Acute care is the short-term care provided to diagnose and/or treat an illness or injury. The individuals who receive acute care services in hospitals are considered inpatients. Inpatients receive room-and-board services in addition to continuous nursing services. Generally, patients who spend more than 24 hours in a hospital are considered inpatients.

The **average length of stay** (ALOS) in an acute care hospital is 30 days or less. (Hospitals that have ALOSs longer than 30 days are considered long-term care facilities. Long-term care is discussed in detail later in this chapter.) With recent advances in surgical technology, anesthesia, and pharmacology, the ALOS in an acute care hospital is much shorter today than it was only a few years ago. In addition, many diagnostic and therapeutic procedures that once required inpatient care can now be performed on an outpatient basis.

For example, before the development of laparoscopic surgical techniques, a patient might be hospitalized for 10 days after a routine appendectomy (surgical removal of the appendix). Today, a patient undergoing a laparoscopic appendectomy might spend only a few hours in the hospital's outpatient surgery department and go home the same day. The influence of managed care and the emphasis on cost control in the Medicare/Medicaid programs also have resulted in shorter hospital stays.

In large acute care hospitals, hundreds of clinicians, administrators, managers, and support staff must work closely together to provide effective and efficient diagnostic and therapeutic services. Most hospitals provide services to both inpatients and outpatients. A hospital outpatient is a patient who receives hospital services without being admitted for inpatient (overnight) clinical care. Outpatient care is considered a kind of ambulatory care. (Ambulatory care is discussed later in this chapter.)

Modern hospitals are extremely complex organizations. Much of the clinical training for physicians, nurses, and allied health professionals is conducted in hospitals. Medical research is another activity carried out in hospitals.

Types of Hospitals

Hospitals can be classified in many different ways according to the:

- Number of beds
- Type of services provided
- Type of patients served
- For-profit or not-for-profit status
- Type of ownership

Number of Beds

A hospital's number of beds is based on the number of beds that it has equipped and staffed for patient care. The term *bed capacity* is sometimes used to reflect the maximum number of inpatients the hospital can care for. Hospitals with fewer than a hundred beds are usually considered small. Most of the hospitals in the United States fall into this category. Some large, urban hospitals have more than 500 beds. The number of beds is usually broken down by adult beds and pediatric beds. The number of maternity beds and other special categories may be listed separately. Hospitals also can be categorized on the basis of the number of outpatient visits per year.

Type of Services Provided

Some hospitals specialize in certain types of service and treat specific illnesses. For example:

- *Rehabilitation hospitals* generally provide long-term care services to patients recuperating from debilitating or chronic illnesses and injuries such as strokes, head and spine injuries, and gunshot wounds. Patients often stay in rehabilitation hospitals for several months.
- *Psychiatric hospitals* provide inpatient care for patients with mental and developmental disorders. In the past, the ALOS for psychiatric inpatients was longer than it is today. Rather than months or years, most patients now spend only a few days or weeks per stay. However, many patients require repeated hospitalization for chronic psychiatric illnesses. (Behavioral healthcare is discussed in more detail later in this chapter.)
- *General hospitals* provide a wide range of medical and surgical services to diagnose and treat most illnesses and injuries.
- *Specialty hospitals* provide diagnostic and therapeutic services for a limited range of conditions (for example, burns, cancer, tuberculosis, or obstetrics/gynecology).

Type of Patients Served

Some hospitals specialize in serving specific types of patients. For example, children's hospitals provide specialized pediatric services in a number of medical specialties.

For-Profit or Not-for-Profit Status

Hospitals also can be classified on the basis of their ownership and profitability status. Not-for profit healthcare organizations use excess funds to improve their services and to finance educational programs and community services. For-profit healthcare organizations are privately owned. Excess funds are paid back to the managers, owners, and investors in the form of bonuses and dividends.

Type of Ownership

The most common ownership types for hospitals and other kinds of healthcare organizations in the United States include the following:

- *Government-owned hospitals* are operated by a specific branch of federal, state, or local government as not-for-profit organizations. (Government-owned hospitals are sometimes called public hospitals.) They are supported, at least in part, by tax dollars. Examples of federally owned and operated hospitals include those operated by the Department of Veterans Affairs to serve retired military personnel. The Department of Defense operates facilities for active military personnel and their dependents. Many states own and operate psychiatric hospitals. County and city governments often operate public hospitals to serve the healthcare needs of their communities, especially those residents who are unable to pay for their care.
- *Proprietary hospitals* may be owned by private foundations, partnerships, or investor-owned corporations. Large corporations may own a number of for-profit hospitals, and the stock of several large U.S. hospital chains is publicly traded.
- *Voluntary hospitals* are not-for-profit hospitals owned by universities, churches, charities, religious orders, unions, and other not-for-profit entities. They often provide free care to patients who otherwise would not have access to healthcare services.

Organization of Hospital Services

The organizational structure of every hospital is designed to meet its specific needs. For example, most acute care hospitals are made up of a board of directors, a professional medical staff, an executive administrative staff, medical and surgical services, patient care (nursing) services, diagnostic and laboratory services, and support services (for example, nutritional services, environmental safety, and HIM services).

Board of Directors

The board of directors has primary responsibility for setting the overall direction of the hospital. (In some hospitals, the board of directors is called the governing board or board of trustees.) The board works with the **chief executive officer** (CEO) and the leaders of the organization's medical staff to develop the hospital's strategic direction as well as its mission, vision, and values:

- *Mission:* A statement of the organization's purpose and the customers it serves
- *Vision:* A description of the organization's ideal future
- *Values:* A descriptive list of the organization's fundamental principles or beliefs

Other specific responsibilities of the board of directors include the following:

- Establishing bylaws in accordance with the organization's legal and licensing requirements
- Selecting qualified administrators
- Approving the organization and makeup of the clinical staff
- Monitoring the quality of care

The board's members are elected for specific terms of service (for example, five years). Most boards also elect officers, commonly a chairman, vice-chairman, president, secretary, and treasurer. The size of the board varies considerably. Individual board members are called directors, board members, or trustees. Individuals serve on one or more standing committees such as the executive committee, joint conference committee, finance committee, strategic planning committee, and building committee.

The makeup of the board depends on the type of hospital and the form of ownership. For example, the board of a community hospital is likely to include local business leaders, representatives of community organizations, and other people interested in the welfare of the community. The board of a teaching hospital, on the other hand, is likely to include medical school alumni and university administrators, among others.

Increased competition among healthcare providers and limits on managed care and Medicare/Medicaid reimbursement have made the governing of hospitals especially difficult during the past two decades. In the future, boards of directors will continue to face strict accountability in terms of cost containment, performance management, and integration of services to maintain fiscal stability and to ensure the delivery of high-quality patient care.

Medical Staff

The medical staff consists of physicians who have received extensive training in various medical disciplines (for example, internal medicine, pediatrics, cardiology, gynecology/obstetrics, orthopedics, and surgery). The medical staff's primary objective is to provide high-quality care to the patients who come to the hospital. The physicians on the hospital's medical staff diagnose illnesses and develop patient-centered treatment regimens. Moreover, physicians on the medical staff may serve on the hospital's governing board, where they provide critical insight relevant to strategic and operational planning and policy making.

The medical staff is the aggregate of physicians who have been granted permission to provide clinical services in the hospital. This permission is called **clinical privileges.** An individual physician's privileges are limited to a specific scope of practice. For example, an internal medicine physician would be permitted to diagnose and treat a patient with pneumonia, but not to perform a surgical procedure. Most members of the medical staff are not actually employees of the hospital. However, many hospitals do directly employ radiologists, anesthesiologists, and critical care specialists.

Medical staff classification refers to the organization of physicians according to clinical assignment. Depending on the size of the hospital and on the credentials and clinical privileges of its physicians, the medical staff may be separated into departments such as medicine, surgery, obstetrics, pediatrics, and other specialty services. Typical medical staff classifications include active, provisional, honorary, consulting, courtesy, and medical resident assignments.

Officers of the medical staff usually include a president or chief of staff, a vice-president or chief of staff-elect, and a secretary. These offices are authorized by vote of the entire active medical staff. The president presides at all regular meetings of the medical staff and is an ex officio member of all medical staff committees. The secretary ensures that accurate and complete minutes of medical staff meetings are maintained and that correspondence is handled appropriately.

The medical staff operates according to a predetermined set of policies. These policies are called the **medical staff bylaws.** The bylaws spell out the specific qualifications that physicians must demonstrate before they can practice medicine in the hospital. The bylaws are considered legally binding. Any changes to the bylaws must be approved by a vote of the medical staff and the hospital's governing body.

Administrative Staff

The leader of the administrative staff is the CEO or chief administrator. The CEO is responsible for implementing the policies and strategic direction set by the hospital's board of directors. He or she also is responsible for building an effective executive management team and coordinating the hospital's services. Today's healthcare organizations commonly designate a **chief financial officer** (CFO), a **chief operating officer** (COO), and a **chief information officer** (CIO) as members of the executive management team.

The executive management team is responsible for managing the hospital's finances and ensuring that the hospital complies with the federal, state, and local regulations, standards, and laws that govern the delivery of healthcare services. Depending on the size of the hospital, the CEO's staff may include healthcare administrators with job titles such as vice-president, associate administrator, department director or manager, or administrative assistant. Department-level administrators manage and coordinate the activities of the highly specialized and multidisciplinary units that perform clinical, administrative, and support services in the hospital.

Healthcare administrators may hold advanced degrees in healthcare administration, nursing, public health, or business management. A growing number of hospitals are hiring physician executives to lead their executive management teams. Many healthcare administrators are fellows of the American College of Healthcare Executives.

Patient Care Services

Most of the direct patient care delivered in hospitals is provided by professional nurses. Modern nursing requires a diverse skill set, advanced clinical competencies, and postgraduate education. In almost every hospital, patient care services constitute the largest clinical department in terms of staffing, budget, specialized services offered, and clinical expertise required.

Nurses are responsible for providing continuous, around-the-clock treatment and support for hospital inpatients. The quantity and quality of nursing care available to patients are influenced by a number of factors, including the nursing staff's educational preparation and specialization, experience, and skill level. The level of patient care staffing is also a critical component of quality.

Traditionally, physicians alone determined the type of treatment each patient received. However, today's nurses are playing a wider role in treatment planning and **case management.** They identify timely and effective interventions in response to a wide range of problems related to the patients' treatment, comfort, and safety. Their responsibilities include performing patient assessments, creating care plans, evaluating the appropriateness of treatment, and evaluating the effectiveness of care. At the same time that they provide technical care, effective nursing professionals also offer personal caring that recognizes the patients' concerns and the emotional needs of patients and their families.

A registered nurse qualified by advanced education and clinical and management experience usually administers patient care services. Although the title may vary, this role is usually referred to as the **chief nursing officer** (CNO) or vice-president of nursing or patient care. The CNO is a member of the hospital's executive management team and usually reports directly to the CEO.

In any nursing organizational structure, several types of relationships can be identified, including the following:

- *Line relationships* identify the positions of superiors and subordinates and indicate the levels of authority and responsibility vested with each position. For example, a supervisor in a postop surgical unit would have authority to direct the work of several nurses.
- *Lateral relationships* define the connections among various positions in which a hierarchy of authority is not involved. For example, the supervisors of preop and postop surgical units would have parallel positions in the structure and would need to coordinate the work they perform.
- *Functional relationships* refer to duties that are divided according to function. In such arrangements, individuals exercise authority in one particular area by virtue of their special knowledge and expertise.

Diagnostic and Therapeutic Services

The services provided to patients in hospitals go beyond the clinical services provided directly by the medical and nursing staff. Many diagnostic and therapeutic services involve the work of allied health professionals. Allied health professionals receive specialized education and training, and their qualifications are registered or certified by a number of specialty organizations.

Diagnostic and therapeutic services are critical to the success of every patient care delivery system. Diagnostic services include clinical laboratory, radiology, and nuclear medicine. Therapeutic services include radiation therapy, occupational therapy, and physical therapy.

Clinical Laboratory Services

The clinical laboratory is divided into two sections: anatomic pathology and clinical pathology. Anatomic pathology deals with human tissues and provides surgical pathology, autopsy, and cytology services. Clinical pathology deals mainly with the analysis of body fluids, principally blood, but also urine, gastric contents, and cerebrospinal fluid.

Physicians who specialize in performing and interpreting the results of pathology tests are called pathologists. Laboratory technicians are allied health professionals trained to operate laboratory equipment and perform laboratory tests under the supervision of a pathologist.

Radiology

Radiology involves the use of radioactive isotopes, fluoroscopic and radiographic equipment, and CT and MRI equipment to diagnose disease. Physicians who specialize in radiology are called radiologists. They are experts in the medical use of radiant energy, radioactive isotopes, radium, cesium, and cobalt as well as x-rays, and radioactive materials. They also are expert in interpreting x-ray, MRI, and CT diagnostic images.

Radiology technicians are allied health professionals trained to operate radiological equipment and perform radiological tests under the supervision of a radiologist.

Nuclear Medicine and Radiation Therapy

Radiologists also may specialize in nuclear medicine and radiation therapy. Nuclear medicine involves the use of ionizing radiation and small amounts of short-lived radioactive tracers to treat disease, specifically neoplastic disease (that is, nonmalignant tumors and malignant cancers). Based on the mathematics and physics of tracer methodology, nuclear medicine is widely applied in clinical medicine. However, most authorities agree that medical science has only scratched the surface in terms of nuclear medicine's potential capabilities.

Radiation therapy uses high-energy x-rays, cobalt, electrons, and other sources of radiation to treat human disease. In current practice, radiation therapy is used alone or in combination with surgery or chemotherapy (drugs) to treat many types of cancer. In addition to external beam therapy, radioactive implants, as well as therapy performed with heat (hyperthermia), are available.

Occupational Therapy

Occupational therapy is the medically directed use of work and play activities to improve patients' independent functioning, enhance their development, and prevent or decrease their level of disability. The individuals who perform occupational therapy are credentialed allied health professionals called occupational therapists. They work under the direction of physicians. Occupational therapy is made available in acute care hospitals, clinics, and rehabilitation centers.

Providing occupational therapy services begins with an evaluation of the patient and the selection of therapeutic goals. Occupational therapy activities may involve the adaptation of tasks or the environment to achieve maximum independence and to enhance the patient's quality of life. An occupational therapist may treat developmental deficits, birth defects, learning disabilities, traumatic injuries, burns, neurological conditions, orthopedic conditions, mental deficiencies, and psychiatric disorders. Within the healthcare system, occupational therapy plays various roles. These roles include promoting health, preventing disability, developing or restoring functional capacity, guiding adaptation within physical and mental parameters, and teaching creative problem solving to increase independent function.

Physical Therapy and Rehabilitation

Physical therapy and rehabilitation have expanded into many medical specialties. Physical therapy can be applied in most disciplines of medicine, especially in neurology, neurosurgery, orthopedics, geriatrics, rheumatology, internal medicine, cardiovascular medicine, cardiopulmonary medicine, psychiatry, sports medicine, burn and wound care, and chronic pain management. It also plays a role in community health education. Credentialed allied health professionals administer physical therapy under the direction of physicians.

Medical **rehabilitation services** involve the entire healthcare team: physicians, nurses, social workers, occupational therapists, physical therapists, and other healthcare personnel. The objective is to either eliminate the patients' disability or alleviate it as fully as possible. Physical therapy can be used to improve the cognitive, social, and physical abilities of patients impaired by chronic disease or injury.

The primary purpose of physical therapy in rehabilitation is to promote optimal health and function by applying scientific principles. Treatment modalities include therapeutic exercise, therapeutic massage, biofeedback, and applications of heat, low-energy lasers, cold, water, electricity, and ultrasound.

Respiratory Therapy

Respiratory therapy involves the diagnosis and treatment of patients who have acute and/or chronic lung disorders. Respiratory therapists work under the direction of qualified physicians and surgeons. The therapists provide such services as emergency care for stroke, heart failure, and shock patients. They also treat patients with chronic respiratory diseases such as emphysema and asthma.

Respiratory treatments include the administration of oxygen and inhalants such as bronchodilators. They set up and monitor ventilatory equipment and provide physiotherapy to improve breathing.

Ancillary Support Services

The ancillary units of the hospital provide vital clinical and administrative support services to patients, medical staff, visitors, and employees.

Clinical Support Services

The clinical support units provide the following services:

- Pharmaceutical services
- Food and nutrition services
- HIM (health record) services
- Social work and social services
- Patient advocacy services
- Environmental (housekeeping) services
- Purchasing, central supply, and materials management services
- Engineering and plant operations

HIM services are managed by registered health information administrators (RHIAs) and registered health information technicians (RHITs). The pharmacy is staffed by registered pharmacists and pharmacy technologists. Food and nutrition services are managed by registered dietitians, who develop general menus, special-diet menus, and nutritional plans for individual patients. Social work services are provided by licensed social workers and licensed clinical social workers. Patient advocacy services may be provided by several types of healthcare professionals, most commonly, registered nurses and licensed social workers.

Administrative Support Services

In addition to clinical support services, hospitals need administrative support services to operate effectively. Administrative support services provide business management and clerical services in several key areas, including:

- Admissions and central registration
- Claims and billing (business office)
- Accounting
- Information services
- Human resources
- Public relations
- Fund development
- Marketing

Check Your Understanding 2.4

Instructions: On a separate piece of paper, indicate whether the statements below are true or false (T or F).

1. ____ Ambulatory care is the short-term care provided to diagnose and/or treat an illness or injury.

2. ____ The influence of managed care and the emphasis on cost control in the Medicare/Medicaid programs have resulted in shorter hospital stays.

3. ___ Hospitals can be classified on the basis of their type of ownership.

4. ___ Government hospitals are operated by a specific branch of federal, state, or local government as for-profit organizations.

5. ___ The board of directors has primary responsibility for setting the overall direction of the hospital.

6. ___ Medical staff classification refers to the organization of physicians according to clinical assignment.

7. ___ A registered nurse qualified by advanced education and clinical and management experience usually administers patient care services.

8. ___ Physicians who specialize in radiology are called radiology technicians.

9. ___ Occupational therapy is made available in acute care hospitals, clinics, and rehab centers.

10. ___ The ancillary units of the hospital provide vital clinical and administrative support services to patients, medical staff, visitors, and employees.

Forces Affecting Hospitals

A number of recent developments in healthcare delivery have had far-reaching effects on the operation of hospitals in the United States.

Subacute Care

Subacute care represents a new movement in healthcare. In the past, the term was used in reference to the services provided to hospitalized patients who did not meet the medical criteria for needing acute care. Today, it refers to the level of skilled care needed by patients with complex medical conditions, typically Medicare patients who have multiple medical problems.

Traditionally, nursing homes, home care providers, and rehabilitation facilities have provided subacute care. Now some hospitals are developing subacute units in response to changing demographics that make it a cost-effective alternative to inpatient acute care.

Development of Peer Review and Quality Improvement Programs

The goal of high-quality patient care is to promote, preserve, and restore health. High-quality care is delivered in an appropriate setting in a manner that is satisfying to patients. It is achieved when the patient's health status is improved as much as possible. Quality has several components, including the following:

- Appropriateness (the right care is provided at the right time)
- Technical excellence (the right care is provided in the right manner)
- Accessibility (the right care can be obtained when it is needed)
- Acceptability (the patients are satisfied)

Peer Review

In **peer review,** a member of a profession assesses the work of colleagues within that same profession. Peer review has traditionally been at the center of quality assessment and assurance efforts. The medical profession's peer review efforts have emphasized the scientific aspects of quality. Appropriate use of pharmaceuticals, postoperative infection rates, and accuracy of diagnosis are among the measures of quality that have been used. Peer review is a requirement of both CMS and the JCAHO.

Quality Improvement

Quality improvement (QI) programs have been in place in hospitals for years and have been required by the Medicare/Medicaid programs and accreditation standards. QI programs have covered medical staff as well as nursing and other departments or processes.

Efforts to encourage the delivery of high-quality care take place at the local and national levels. Such efforts are geared toward assessing the efforts of both individuals and institutions. Currently, professional associations, healthcare organizations, government agencies, private external quality review associations, consumer groups, managed care organizations, and group purchasers of care all play a role in trying to promote high-quality care.

Growth of Managed Care

Managed care is a generic term for a healthcare reimbursement system that manages cost, quality, and access to services. Most managed care plans do not provide healthcare directly. Instead, they enter into service contracts with the physicians, hospitals, and other healthcare providers who provide medical services to enrollees in the plans.

Managed care systems control costs primarily by presetting payment amounts and restricting patient access to healthcare services through precertification and UR processes. (Managed care is discussed in more detail in chapter 14.) Managed care delivery systems also attempt to manage cost and quality by:

- Implementing various forms of financial incentives for providers
- Promoting healthy lifestyles
- Identifying risk factors and illnesses early in the disease process
- Providing patient education

Although the most recent studies suggest that managed care results in lower costs with equal or better quality, most are limited because they have focused on short-term health outcomes (Weinerman et al. 1966, p. 1037). Very little is known about the long-term effects of specific reimbursement or organizational arrangements on quality of care. Further, recent evidence indicates that the quality of care provided under managed care systems may differ across population groups.

Efforts at Healthcare Reengineering

During the 1980s, healthcare organizations adopted **continuous quality improvement** (CQI) processes. Lessons learned from other areas of business were applied to healthcare settings. **Reengineering** came in many varieties, such as focused process improvement, major business process improvement and business process innovation, total quality management (TQM), and CQI. Regardless of its approach, every healthcare organization attempted to look inside and think "process" as opposed to traditional "department" thinking. Healthcare organizations formed cross-functional teams that collaborated to solve organizational problems. At the same time, the JCAHO reengineered the accreditation process to increase its focus on process and systems analysis. Gone were the days of thinking in a "silo." All those silos were turned over, and healthcare teams learned from each other. The drivers of reengineering included cost reduction, staff shortages, and implementation of technology.

Emphasis on Patient-Focused Care

Patient-focused care is a concept developed to contain hospital inpatient costs and improve quality by restructuring services so that more of them take place in the nursing units (patient floors) and not in specialized units in dispersed hospital locations. The emphasis is on cross-training staff in the nursing units to perform a variety of functions for a small group of patients rather than one set of functions for a large number of patients. Some organizations have achieved patient-focused care by assigning multiskilled workers to serve food, clean patients' rooms, and assist in nursing care. However, some organizations have experienced low patient satisfaction with this type of worker because the patients are confused and do not know who to ask to do what.

Hospital staff spend most of their time performing activities in the following nine categories:

- Medical, technical, and clinical procedures
- Hotel and patient services
- Medical documentation
- Institutional documentation
- Scheduling and coordination
- Patient transportation
- Staff transportation
- Management and supervision
- Ready-for-action activities

A study at Lakeland Regional Medical Center, a 750-bed hospital in central Florida, found that medical, technical, and clinical activity consumed one-sixth of the center's personnel-related costs. The study also showed that almost twice that amount of time was spent writing things down. Scheduling and coordination took as much time as medical activity, and ready-for-action activities consumed even more.

The study suggested that restructuring services at Lakeland would reduce the number of staff required for patient care activities from 2,200 to 1,200 and improve care. The amount of physical space allotted to each unit would be sufficient to contain a minilab, diagnostic radiology rooms, linen and general supply, stockrooms, and so on. If such changes were carried out, medical documentation could be reduced by almost two-thirds, scheduling and coordination service by more than two-thirds, and ready-for-action time by two-thirds.

Hospitals have had difficulty in fully and rapidly implementing patient-focused care for the following reasons: the high cost of conversion; the extensive physical renovations required; resistance from functional departments; and other priorities for management, such as mergers and considering potential mergers.

Development of Integrated Healthcare Delivery Systems

Managed care and healthcare organization integration have placed enormous pressure on information systems. The need for cost data, as well as the integration of data from the various components of integrated systems, has placed many demands on systems technology and personnel. A healthcare provider that cannot completely analyze the cost of delivery when dealing with an insurer is at a distinct disadvantage. Similarly, an inability to integrate patient data across a system can produce increased costs, inefficiencies, and even medical errors.

The role of computers has changed rapidly in healthcare organizations, just as it has in many service organizations. The more advanced systems, once called data-processing centers, became management information systems. As computer operations became more powerful and complex, it became possible to think about creating new services or greatly improving existing ones. Innovations were considered strategic uses of information systems because they helped an organization to compete or achieve its goals. Hospitals and integrated health systems have begun to use computers to serve in new functions. For example, a hospital can offer physicians the opportunity to connect to its computer system. Thanks to virtual private networks, a physician can connect to an integrated health system's intranet and work within the system in a private and secure environment without worrying about the downtime often experienced on the Internet.

Check Your Understanding 2.5

Instructions: On a separate piece of paper, write the best terms to complete the following sentences.

1. Today, ___ refers to the level of skilled care needed by patients with complex medical conditions, typically Medicare patients who have multiple medical problems.
   a. Acute care
   b. Ambulatory care
   c. Subacute care
   d. High-quality care

2. Quality has several components, including appropriateness, technical excellence, ___, and acceptability.
   a. Accuracy of diagnosis
   b. Continuous improvement
   c. Connectivity
   d. Accessibility

3. ___ programs have been in place in hospitals for years and have been required by the Medicare/Medicaid programs and accreditation standards.
   a. Quality assurance
   b. Peer review
   c. Managed care
   d. Quality improvement

4. ___ is a generic term for a healthcare reimbursement system that manages cost, quality, and access to services.
   a. Quality improvement
   b. Subacute care
   c. Managed care
   d. Patient-focused care

5. Recent evidence indicates that the quality of care provided under managed care systems may differ across ___.
   a. Population groups
   b. Healthcare settings
   c. Medical facilities
   d. Integrated delivery systems

6. ___ attempts to contain hospital inpatient costs and improve quality by restructuring services.
   a. Continuous quality improvement
   b. Patient-focused care
   c. Managed care
   d. Acute care

7. Managed care and healthcare organization integration have placed enormous pressure on ___.
   a. Integrated delivery systems
   b. Acute care facilities
   c. Rehabilitation facilities
   d. Information systems

8. The role of ___ has changed rapidly in healthcare organizations, just as it has in many service organizations.
   a. Reengineering
   b. Computers
   c. Quality improvement programs
   d. Peer review efforts

Other Types of Healthcare Services

Thus far, this chapter has focused primarily on acute care services delivered for the most part in the hospital setting. However, healthcare delivery is more than hospital-related care. It can be viewed as a continuum of services that cuts across services delivered in ambulatory, acute, subacute, long-term, residential, and other care environments. This section describes several of the alternatives for healthcare delivery along this continuum.

Ambulatory Care

Ambulatory care can be defined as:

> The preventive and/or corrective healthcare provided in a practitioner's office, a clinic, or a hospital on a nonresident (outpatient) basis. The term usually implies that patients go to locations outside their homes to obtain healthcare services and return the same day.

Ambulatory care encompasses all the health services provided to individual patients who are not residents in a healthcare facility. Such services include the educational services provided by community health clinics and public health departments. Primary care, emergency care, and ambulatory specialty care (which includes ambulatory surgery) can all be considered ambulatory care. Ambulatory care services are provided in a variety of settings, including urgent care centers, school-based clinics, public health clinics, and neighborhood and community health centers.

Current medical practice emphasizes performing healthcare services in the least costly setting possible. This change in thinking has led to decreased utilization of emergency services, increased utilization of nonemergency ambulatory facilities, decreased hospital admissions, and shorter hospital stays. The need to reduce the cost of healthcare also has led primary care physicians to treat conditions they once would have referred to specialists.

Physicians who provide ambulatory care services fall into two major categories: physicians working in private practice and physicians working for ambulatory care organizations. Physicians in private practice are self-employed. They work in solo, partnership, and group practices set up as for-profit organizations.

Alternatively, physicians who work for ambulatory care organizations are employees of those organizations. Ambulatory care organizations include health maintenance organizations, hospital-based ambulatory clinics, walk-in and emergency clinics, hospital-owned group practices and health promotion centers, freestanding surgery centers, freestanding urgent care centers, freestanding emergency care centers, health department clinics, neighborhood clinics, home care agencies, community mental health centers, school and workplace health services, and prison health services.

Ambulatory care organizations also employ other healthcare providers, including nurses, laboratory technicians, podiatrists, chiropractors, physical therapists, radiology technicians, psychologists, and social workers.

Private Medical Practice
Private medical practices are physician-owned entities that provide primary care or medical/surgical specialty care services in a freestanding office setting. The physicians have medical privileges at local hospitals and surgical centers but are not employees of those healthcare entities.

Hospital-Based Ambulatory Care Services
In addition to providing inpatient services, many acute care hospitals also provide various ambulatory care services.

Emergency Services and Trauma Care
More than 90 percent of community hospitals in the United States provide emergency services. Hospital-based emergency departments provide specialized care for victims of traumatic accidents and life-threatening illnesses. In urban areas, many also provide walk-in services for patients with

minor illnesses and injuries who do not have access to regular primary care physicians.

Many physicians on the hospital staff also use the emergency care department as a setting to assess patients with problems that may either lead to an inpatient admission or require equipment or diagnostic imaging facilities not available in a private office or nursing home. Emergency services function as a major source of unscheduled admissions to the hospital.

Outpatient Surgical Services

Generally, ambulatory surgery refers to any surgical procedure that does not require an overnight stay in a hospital. It can be performed in the outpatient surgery department of a hospital or in a freestanding ambulatory surgery center. During the 1980s and 1990s, the percentage of surgeries done on an outpatient basis rose dramatically and this trend continues today. The increased number of procedures performed in an ambulatory setting can be attributed to improvements in surgical technology and anesthesia and the utilization management demands of third-party payers.

Outpatient Diagnostic and Therapeutic Services

Outpatient diagnostic and therapeutic services are provided in a hospital or one of its satellite facilities. Diagnostic services are those services performed by a physician to identify the disease or condition from which the patient is suffering. Therapeutic services are those services performed by a physician to treat the disease or condition that has been identified.

Hospital outpatients fall into different classifications according to the type of service they receive and the location of the service. For example, emergency outpatients are treated in the hospital's emergency or trauma care department for conditions that require immediate care. Clinic outpatients are treated in one of the hospital's clinical departments on an ambulatory basis. And referral outpatients receive special diagnostic or therapeutic services in the hospital on an ambulatory basis, but responsibility for their care remains with the referring physician.

Community-Based Ambulatory Care Services

Community-based ambulatory care services refer to those services provided in freestanding facilities that are not owned by or affiliated with a hospital. Such facilities can range in size from a small medical practice with a single physician to a large clinic with an organized medical staff.

Among the organizations that provide ambulatory care services are specialized treatment facilities. Examples of these facilities include birthing centers, cancer treatment centers, renal dialysis centers, rehabilitation centers, and so on.

Freestanding Ambulatory Care Centers

Freestanding ambulatory care facilities provide emergency services and urgent care for walk-in patients. Urgent care centers (sometimes called emergicenters) provide diagnostic and therapeutic care for patients with minor illnesses and injuries. They do not serve seriously ill patients, and most do not accept ambulance cases.

Two groups of patients find these centers attractive. The first group consists of patients seeking the convenience and access of emergency services without the delays and other forms of negative feedback associated with using hospital services for nonurgent problems. The second group consists of patients whose insurance treats urgent care centers preferentially compared with physicians' offices.

As they have increased in number and become familiar to more patients, many of these centers now offer a combination of walk-in and appointment services.

Freestanding Ambulatory Surgery Centers

Generally, freestanding ambulatory surgery centers provide surgical procedures that take anywhere from 5 to 90 minutes to perform and that require less than a four-hour recovery period. Patients must schedule their surgeries in advance and be prepared to return home on the same day. Patients who experience surgical complications are sent to an inpatient facility for care.

Most ambulatory surgery centers are for-profit entities. They may be owned by individual physicians, managed care organizations, or entrepreneurs. Generally, ambulatory care centers can provide surgical services at lower cost than hospitals can because their overhead expenses are lower.

Public Health Services

Although the states have constitutional authority to implement public health, a wide variety of federal programs and laws assist them. The U.S. Department of Health and Human Services (HHS) is the principal federal agency for ensuring health and providing essential human services. All its agencies have some responsibility for prevention. Through its 10 regional offices, HHS coordinates closely with state and local government agencies and many HHS-funded services are provided by these agencies as well as by private-sector and nonprofit organizations.

The Office of the secretary of HHS has two units important to public health: the Office of the Surgeon General of the United States and the Office of Disease Prevention and Health Promotion (ODPHP). ODPHP has an analysis and leadership role for health promotion and disease prevention.

The surgeon general is appointed by the president of the United States and provides leadership and authoritative, science-based recommendations about the public's health. The surgeon general has responsibility for the **Public Health Service** (PHS) workforce (Jonas and Kovner 2005, pp. 108–9).

Home Care Services

Home healthcare is the fastest-growing sector to offer services for Medicare recipients. The primary reason for this is increased economic pressure from third-party payers. In other words, third-party payers want patients released from the hospital more quickly than they were in the past. Moreover, patients generally prefer to be cared for in their own homes. In fact, most patients prefer home care, no matter how complex their medical problems. Research indicates that the medical outcomes of home care patients are similar to those of patients treated in **skilled nursing facilities** (SNFs) for similar conditions.

In 1989, Medicare rules for home care services were clarified to make it easier for Medicare beneficiaries to receive such services. Patients are eligible to receive home health services from a qualified Medicare provider when they are homebound, when they are under the care of a specified physician who will establish a home health plan, and when they need physical or occupational therapy, speech therapy, or intermittent skilled nursing care.

Skilled nursing care is defined as both technical procedures, such as tube feedings and catheter care, and skilled nursing observations. Intermittent is defined as up to 28 hours per week for nursing care and 35 hours per week for home health aide care. Many hospitals have formed their own home healthcare agencies to increase revenues and at the same time allow them to discharge patients from the hospital earlier.

Voluntary Agencies

Voluntary agencies provide healthcare and healthcare planning services, usually at the local level and to low-income patients. Their services range from giving free immunizations to offering family planning counseling. Funds to operate such agencies come from a variety of sources, including local or state health departments, private grants, and different federal bureaus.

One common example of a voluntary agency is the community health center. Sometimes called neighborhood health centers, community health centers offer comprehensive, primary healthcare services to patients who otherwise would not have access to them. Often patients pay for these services on a sliding scale based on income or according to a flat rate, discounted fee schedule supplemented by public funding.

Some voluntary agencies offer specialized services such as counseling for battered and abused women. Typically, these are set up within local communities. An example of a voluntary agency that offers services on a much larger scale is the Red Cross.

Long-Term Care

Generally speaking, **long-term care** is the healthcare rendered in a nonacute care facility to patients who require inpatient nursing and related services for more than 30 consecutive days. SNFs, nursing homes, and rehabilitation hospitals are the principal facilities that provide long-term care. Rehabilitation hospitals provide recuperative services for patients who have suffered strokes and traumatic injuries as well as other serious illnesses. Specialized long-term care facilities serve patients with chronic respiratory disease, permanent cognitive impairment, and other incapacitating conditions.

Long-term care encompasses a range of health, personal care, social, and housing services provided to people of all ages with health conditions that limit their ability to carry out normal daily activities without assistance. People who need long-term care have many different types of physical and mental disabilities. Moreover, their need for the mix and intensity of long-term care services can change over time.

Long-term care is mainly rehabilitative and supportive rather than curative. Moreover, healthcare workers other than physicians can provide long-term care in the home or in residential or institutional settings. For the most part, long-term care requires little or no technology.

Long-Term Care and the Continuum of Care

The availability of long-term care is one of the most important health issues in the United States today. There are two principal reasons for this. First, thanks to advances in medicine and healthcare practices, people are living longer today than they did in the past. The number of people who survive previously fatal conditions has been growing, and more and more people with chronic medical problems are able to live reasonably normal lives. Second, there was an explosion in birth rate following the Second World War. Children born during that period, the so-called baby-boomer generation, are today in or entering their 50s. These factors combined mean that the need for long-term care can only increase in the years to come.

As discussed earlier, healthcare is now viewed as a continuum of care. That is, patients are provided care by different caregivers at several different levels of the healthcare system. In the case of long-term care, the patient's continuum of care may have begun with a primary provider in a hospital and then continued with home care and eventually care in an SNF. That patient's care is coordinated from one care setting to the next.

Moreover, the roles of the different care providers along the patient's continuum of care are continuing to evolve. Health information managers play a key part in providing consultation services to long-term care facilities with regard to developing systems to manage information from a diverse number of healthcare providers.

Delivery of Long-Term Care Services

Long-term care services are delivered in a variety of settings. Among these settings are SNFs /nursing homes, residential care facilities, hospice programs, and adult day-care programs.

Skilled Nursing Facilities/Nursing Homes

The most important providers of formal, long-term care services are nursing homes. SNFs, or nursing homes, provide medical, nursing, and/or rehabilitative care, in some cases, around the clock. The majority of SNF residents are over age 65 and quite often are classified as the frail elderly.

Many nursing homes are owned by for-profit organizations. However, SNFs also may be owned by not-for-profit groups as well as local, state, and federal governments. In recent years, there has been a decline in the total number of nursing homes in the United States, but an increase in the number of nursing home beds.

Nursing homes are no longer the only option for patients needing long-term care. Various factors play a role in determining which type of long-term care facility is best for a particular patient, including cost, access to services, and individual needs.

Residential Care Facilities

New living environments that are more homelike and less institutional are the focus of much attention in the current long-term care market. Residential care facilities now play a growing role in the continuum of long-term care services. Having affordable and appropriate housing available for elderly and disabled people can reduce the level of need for institutional long-term care services in the community. Institutionalization can be postponed or prevented when the elderly and disabled live in safe and accessible settings where assistance with daily activities is available.

Hospice Programs

Hospice care is provided mainly in the home to the terminally ill and their families. Hospice is based on a philosophy of care imported from England and Canada that holds that during the course of terminal illness, the patient should be able to live life as fully and as comfortably as possible but without artificial or mechanical efforts to prolong life.

In the hospice approach, the family is the unit of treatment. An interdisciplinary team provides medical, nursing, psychological, therapeutic, pharmacological, and spiritual support during the final stages of illness, at the time of death, and during bereavement. The main goals are to control pain, maintain independence, and minimize the stress and trauma of death.

Hospice services have gained acceptance as an alternative to hospital care for the terminally ill. The number of hospices is likely to continue to grow because this philosophy of care for people at the end of life has become a model for the nation.

Adult Day-Care Programs

Adult day-care programs offer a wide range of health and social services to elderly persons during the daytime hours. Adult day-care services are usually targeted to elderly members of families in which the regular caregivers work during the day. Many elderly people who live alone also benefit from leaving their homes every day to participate in programs designed to keep them active. The goals of adult day-care programs are to delay the need for institutionalization and to provide respite for the caregivers.

Data on adult day-care programs are still limited, but there were about 3,000 programs in 2000. Most adult day-care programs offer social services, crafts, current events discussions, family counseling, reminiscence therapy, nursing assessment, physical exercise, activities of daily living, rehabilitation, psychiatric assessment, and medical care.

Behavioral Health Services

From the mid-19th century to the mid-20th century, psychiatric services in the United States were based primarily in long-stay institutions supported by state governments and patterns of practice were relatively stable. Over the past 45 years, however, remarkable changes have occurred. These changes include a reversal of the balance between institutional and community care, inpatient and outpatient services, and individual and group practice.

Today, the number of long-stay residents in state mental hospitals is estimated to be well below 80,000. In 1955, it was more than 500,000. The shift to community-based settings began in the public sector and community settings remain dominant. The private sector's bed capacity increased in the 1970s and 1980s, including psychiatric units in nonfederal general hospitals, private psychiatric hospitals, and residential treatment centers for children. Substance abuse centers and child and adolescent inpatient psychiatric units grew particularly quickly in the 1980s, as investors recognized their profitability. In the 1990s, the growth of inpatient private mental health facilities leveled off, and the number of outpatient and partial treatment settings increased sharply.

Some patients with treatment-resistant schizophrenia, severe mood disorders, or chronic cognitive impairment may be dangerous to themselves or others. State and county hospitals may be returning to their traditional role by providing asylum to disabled patients who are unable function in their communities.

Residential treatment centers for emotionally or behaviorally disturbed children provide inpatient services to children under 18 years of age. The programs and physical facilities of residential treatment centers are designed to meet patients' daily living, schooling, recreational, socialization, and routine medical care needs.

Day-hospital or day-treatment programs occupy one niche in the spectrum of **behavioral healthcare** settings. Although some provide services seven days per week, many programs provide services only during business hours, Monday through Friday. Day-treatment patients spend most of the day at the treatment facility in a program of structured therapeutic activities and then return to their homes until the next day. Day-treatment services include psychotherapy, pharmacology, occupational therapy, and other types of rehabilitation services. These programs provide alternatives to inpatient care or serve as transitions from inpatient to outpatient care or discharge. They also may provide respite for family caregivers and a place for rehabilitating or maintaining chronically ill patients. The number of day-treatment programs has increased in response to pressures to decrease the length of hospital stays.

Insurance coverage for behavioral healthcare has always lagged behind coverage for other medical care. Although treatments and treatment settings have changed, rising health-care costs, the absence of strong consumer demand for behavioral health coverage, and insurers' continuing fear of the potential cost of this coverage have maintained the differences between medical and behavioral healthcare benefits.

Although the majority of individuals who are covered by health insurance have some outpatient psychiatric coverage, the coverage is often quite restricted. Typical restrictions include limits on the number of outpatient visits, higher copayment charges, and higher deductibles.

Behavioral healthcare has grown and diversified, particularly over the past 40 years, as psychopharmacologic treatment has made possible the shift away from long-term custodial treatment. Psychosocial treatments continue the process of care and rehabilitation in community settings. Large state hospitals have been supplemented, and in many cases replaced, by psychiatric units in general hospitals, new outpatient clinics, community mental health centers, day-treatment centers, and halfway houses. Treatment has become more effective and specific, based on our growing understanding of the brain and behavior. Recent advances in the biological and behavioral sciences continue to improve opportunities for diagnosing, treating, and preventing psychiatric disorders (Jonas and Kovner 1999, pp. 243–73).

Check Your Understanding 2.6

Instructions: On a separate piece of paper, match the descriptions provided with the terms to which they apply.

1. ___ Behavioral health service
2. ___ Public health service
3. ___ Home care service
4. ___ Hospice program
5. ___ Skilled nursing facility
6. ___ Voluntary agency
7. ___ Residential care facility
8. ___ Day-treatment program
9. ___ Continuum of care
10. ___ Freestanding ambulatory care center

a. Fastest-growing sector of Medicare
b. Provides emergency services and urgent care for walk-in patients
c. Represents a reversal in the balance between institutional and community care
d. Are designed to meet patients' daily living, schooling, recreational, socialization, and routine medical care needs
e. Has an analysis and leadership role for health promotion and disease prevention.
f. Provides healthcare and healthcare planning services usually at the local level and to low-income patients
g. Provides alternatives to inpatient care or serves as transition from inpatient to outpatient care or discharge
h. Care provided mainly in the home to the terminally ill and their families
i. Care provided by different caregivers at several different levels of the healthcare system
j. Healthcare rendered in a nonacute care facility to patients who require inpatient nursing and related services for more than 30 consecutive days

---

Integrated Delivery Systems

Many hospitals have responded to local pressures by rapidly merging, acquiring, and entering into affiliations and other risk-sharing reimbursement agreements with other acute and nonacute providers, hospital-based healthcare systems, physicians and physician group practices, and managed care organizations. Transactions have included mergers of nonprofit organizations into either investor-owned or other nonprofit entities.

The goal of integrated delivery systems (IDSs) or integrated delivery networks (IDNs) is to organize the entire continuum of care, from health promotion and disease prevention to primary and secondary acute, tertiary care, long-term care and hospice care, to maximize its effectiveness across episodes of illness and pathways of wellness. A premium is placed on integration and holistic care, not fragmentation and specialist care.

Strengths and Weaknesses of IDSs

It takes many years to truly integrate these new, often hospital-sponsored aggregations of facilities and services into integrated systems for the delivery of healthcare. Barriers to doing so include:

- The failure to understand the new core business
- An inability to overcome the hospital paradigm, as it may not be consistent with system priorities
- Ambiguous roles and responsibilities throughout the system
- The inability to "manage" managed care
- The inability to execute the strategy
- A lack of alignment or match between various components, such as orientation toward the market versus managerial control of strategy.

The success of a strength is highly dependent on system investments in information technology, managerial leadership, and empowerment and shared-system ownership with physicians (Jonas and Kovner 1999, pp. 173–75).

Information Needs of IDSs

The emergence of IDSs has placed enormous pressure on the need for integrated information systems. The need for financial information, as well as the integration of data from the various components of integrated systems, has placed many demands on systems technology and personnel. A healthcare provider that cannot completely analyze the cost of delivery when dealing with an insurer is at a distinct disadvantage. An IDS must be able to integrate patient data across a system in an effort to analyze ways to reduce costs and inefficiencies.

The Future of IDSs

U.S. hospitals will most likely continue to affiliate with others in large local systems; and there may be enhanced identification of hospitals as part of regional and national chains, depending on financial incentives and other messages in the environment, including antitrust regulation (that is, on how far hospitals are allowed to combine, by law, into monopolies or oligopolies). There probably will be a variety of models in the future together with a reaffirmation by hospitals of their functions in local communities, regardless of ownership or membership in larger systems. The history of hospitals suggests that they will continue to expand wherever possible rather than contract and that they will continue to be controlled by shifting coalitions of community interests, business interests, physicians, third-party payers, trustees, administrators, politicians, and lobbyists. One of the key issues is the availability and channeling of hospital income. Without adequate income, hospital bankruptcies, mergers, and closures will be as commonplace as they were during the Depression in the 1930s.

There is no single or obvious direction for the future. As in the past, the hospital system is what we make it, for good or ill, as charity and business. The quality of American medical care is, indeed, an index of American civilization (Stevens 1999, pp. 364–65).

Licensure, Certification, and Accreditation of Healthcare Facilities

Under the Tenth Amendment of the U.S. Constitution, states have the primary responsibility for public health, which include disease and injury prevention, sanitation, water and air pollution, vaccination, isolation and quarantine, inspection of commercial and residential premises, food and drinking water standards, extermination of vermin, fluoridation of municipal water supplies, and licensure of physicians and other healthcare professionals. Each state has a division or agency that is dedicated to promoting high-quality patient care and safety in healthcare facilities and outpatient services by conducting regular on-site surveys. State and federal licensing/certification programs require that high-performance standards be met in the provision of medical care and in the construction and maintenance of the healthcare facility.

State Licensure

Licensure gives legal approval for a facility to operate or for a person to practice within his or her profession. Virtually every state requires that hospitals, sanatoria, nursing homes, and pharmacies be licensed to operate, although the requirements and standards for licensure may differ from state to state. State licensure is mandatory. Federal facilities such as those of the Department of Veterans Affairs (VA) do not require licensure.

Although licensure requirements vary, healthcare facilities must meet certain basic criteria that are determined by state regulatory agencies. These standards address such concerns as adequacy of staffing, personnel employed to provide services, physical aspects of the facility (equipment, buildings), and services provided, including health records. Licensure

typically is performed annually, and facilities must usually meet the minimum acceptable standards for operation.

Certification for Medicare Participation

In 1965, the Social Security Act established both Medicare and Medicaid. Medicare was the responsibility of the Social Security Administration (SSA), but federal assistance to the state Medicaid programs was administered by the Social and Rehabilitation Service (SRS). SSA and SRS were agencies in the Department of Health, Education, and Welfare (HEW). In 1977, the Health Care Financing Administration (HCFA) was created under HEW to effectively coordinate Medicare and Medicaid. In 1980, HEW was divided into the Department of Education and HHS. In 2001, HCFA was renamed the Centers for Medicare and Medicaid Services (CMS), an agency of HHS.

CMS maintains oversight of the survey and certification of nursing homes and continuing care providers (including hospitals, nursing homes, home health agencies, end-stage renal disease facilities, hospices, and other facilities serving Medicare and Medicaid beneficiaries) and makes available to beneficiaries, providers/suppliers, researchers, and state surveyors information about these activities. In November 2002, CMS began a national Nursing Home Quality Initiative (NHQI). The goals of the initiative are essentially twofold: to provide consumers with an additional source of information about the quality of nursing home care by providing a set of MDS-based quality measures on Medicare's Nursing Home Compare Web site, and to help providers improve the quality of care for their residents by providing them with complementary clinical resources, quality improvement materials, and assistance from the QIOs in every state.

Many nursing homes have already made significant improvements in the care being provided to residents by taking advantage of these materials and the support of QIO staff (CMS 2005).

To be eligible for Medicare and Medicaid reimbursement, providers must demonstrate compliance with the **Conditions of Participation,** which is the process of certification. Certification is the process by which government and nongovernment organizations evaluate educational programs, healthcare facilities, and individuals as having met predetermined standards. The certification of healthcare facilities is the responsibility of the states. However, Title XVIII of the Medicare Act specifies that facilities accredited by the JCAHO and AOA must be deemed in compliance with the Medicare Conditions of Participation for Hospitals; those accredited are said to have deemed status.

Voluntary Accreditation

Accreditation is a voluntary system of institutional or organizational review that an independent body created for the purpose of evaluating the work quality of the subject agencies, using written criteria (Jonas and Kovner 1999, p. 527).

JCAHO operates voluntary accreditation programs for hospitals and other healthcare services. It certifies hospitals as having met the Conditions of Participation required for reimbursement under the federal Medicare program. The definition of Federal **Deemed Status** is as follows:

> In order for healthcare organizations to participate in and receive payment from the Medicare and Medicaid programs, [they] must be certified as complying with the Conditions of Participation, or standards, set forth in federal regulations (JCAHO 2005).

A majority of state governments recognize JCAHO accreditation as a condition of licensure and receiving Medicaid reimbursement. Inspections are typically triannual with accreditation and survey findings made publicly available. The standards are based on the premise that healthcare organizations exist to maximize the health of the people they serve while using resources efficiently. When an organization is found to be in substantial compliance with the JCAHO standards, accreditation may be awarded for up to three years. Hospitals must undergo a full survey at least every three years.

JCAHO publishes accreditation manuals with standards for hospitals, nonhospital-based psychiatric and substance abuse organizations, long-term care organizations, home care organizations, ambulatory care organizations, and organization-based pathology and clinical laboratory services.

Much like JCAHO, the American Osteopathic Association (AOA) Hospital Accreditation Program accreditation is a voluntary program that accredits osteopathic hospitals. Those hospitals that are accredited are recognized by the HHS as having deemed status and thus are eligible to receive Medicare funds (www.cms.hhs.gov 2006). AOA has been accrediting healthcare facilities for more than 30 years under Medicare. It is one of only two voluntary accreditation programs in the United States authorized by CMS to survey hospitals under Medicare. In addition, the program is a cost-effective, user-friendly means to validate the quality of care provided by a facility.

The AOA accreditation program was developed in 1943 and 1944 and implemented in 1945. Under this program hospitals were surveyed each year. In this manner, the AOA was able to ensure that osteopathic students received their training through rotating internships and residencies in facilities that provided high-quality patient care. In 1995, the AOA applied for and received deeming authority to accredit laboratories within AOA-accredited hospitals under the Clinical Laboratory Improvement Amendments of 1988. AOA also has developed accreditation requirements for ambulatory care/surgery, mental health, substance abuse, and physical rehabilitation medicine facilities (AOA 2005).

Reimbursement of Healthcare Expenditures

Together, the Medicare and Medicaid programs and the managed care insurance industry have virtually eliminated fee-for-service reimbursement arrangements.

Evolution of Third-Party Reimbursement

The evolution of third-party reimbursement systems for healthcare services began more than 60 years ago. The evolution created a need for systematic and accurate communications between healthcare providers and third-party payers. Commercial health insurance companies (for example, Aetna) offer medical plans similar to Blue Cross/Blue Shield plans. Traditionally, Blue Cross organizations covered hospital services and Blue Shield covered inpatient physician services and a limited amount of office-based care. Today, Blue Cross plans and commercial insurance providers cover a full range of healthcare services, including ambulatory care services and drug benefits. (Healthcare reimbursement systems are discussed in more detail in chapter 14.)

Most commercial health insurance is provided in the form of group policies offered by employers as part of their fringe benefit packages for employees. Unions also negotiate health insurance coverage during contract negotiations. In most cases, employees pay a share of the cost and employers pay a share.

Individual health insurance plans can be purchased but usually are expensive or have limited coverage and high deductibles. Individuals with preexisting medical conditions often find it almost impossible to get individual coverage.

Commercial insurers also sell major medical and cash payment policies. Major medical plans are directed primarily at catastrophic illness and cover all or part of treatment costs beyond those covered by basic plans. Major medical plans are sold as both group and individual policies. Cash payment plans provide monetary benefits and are not based on actual charges from healthcare providers. For example, a cash payment plan might pay the beneficiary $150 for every day he or she is hospitalized or $500 for every ambulatory surgical procedure. Cash payment plans are often offered as a benefit of membership in large associations such as the American Association of Retired Persons (AARP).

Like the Blues, the commercial insurance companies are subject to supervision by state insurance commissioners. However, such supervision does not include rate regulation. One general requirement is that commercial plans establish premium rates high enough to cover all potential claims made under the insurance they provide.

Government-Sponsored Reimbursement Systems

Until 1965, most of the poor and many of the elderly in the United States could not afford private healthcare services. As a result of public pressure calling for attention to this growing problem, Congress passed Public Law 89-97 as an Amendment to the Social Security Act. The amendments created Medicare (Title XVIII) and Medicaid (Title XIX).

Medicare

Medicare was first offered to retired Americans in July 1966. Today, retired and disabled Americans who are eligible for Social Security benefits automatically qualify for Medicare coverage without regard to income. Coverage is offered under two coordinated programs: hospital insurance (Medicare Part A) and medical insurance (Medicare Part B).

Medicare Part A is financed through payroll taxes. Initially, coverage applied only to hospitalization and home healthcare. Subsequently, coverage for extended care in nursing homes was added. Coverage for individuals eligible for Social Security disability payments for over two years and those who need kidney transplantation or dialysis for end-stage renal disease also was added.

Medical insurance under Medicare Part B is optional. It is financed through monthly premiums paid by eligible beneficiaries to supplement federal funding. Part B helps pay for physician's services, outpatient hospital care, medical services and supplies, and certain other medical costs not covered by Part A. At the present time, Medicare Part B does not provide coverage of prescription drugs. (Medicare Parts A and B are discussed in greater detail in chapter 14.) In January 2006, Medicare Part D was implemented to provide prescription drug coverage for Medicare beneficiaries who select this option.

Medicaid

Medicaid is a medical assistance program for low-income Americans. The program is funded partially by the federal government and partially by state and local governments. The federal government requires that certain services be provided and sets specific eligibility requirements.

Medicaid covers the following benefits:

- Inpatient hospital care
- Outpatient hospital care
- Laboratory and x-ray services
- SNF and home health services for persons over 21 years old
- Physician's services
- Family planning services
- Rural health clinic services
- Early and periodic screening, diagnosis, and treatment services

Individual states sometimes cover services in addition to those required by the federal government.

Services Provided by Government Agencies

Federal health insurance programs cover health services for several additional specified populations.

TRICARE, which was originally referred to as the Civilian Health and Medical Program for the Uniformed Services (CHAMPUS), pays for care delivered by civilian health providers to retired members of the military and the dependents of active and retired members of the seven uniformed services. The Department of Defense administers the TRICARE program. The program also provides medical services to active members of the military.

The VA provides healthcare services to eligible veterans of military service. The VA hospital system was established in 1930 to provide hospital, nursing home, residential, and outpatient medical and dental care to veterans of the First World War. Today, the VA operates more than 950 medical centers throughout the United States. The medical centers are currently being organized into 22 Veterans Integrated Service Networks (VISNs) to increase the efficiency of their services.

Through the Indian Health Service, the HHS also finances the healthcare services provided to Native Americans living on reservations across the country.

State governments often operate healthcare facilities to serve citizens with special needs, such as the developmentally disabled and mentally ill. Some states also offer health insurance programs to those who cannot qualify for private healthcare insurance. Many county and local governments also operate public hospitals to fulfill the medical needs of their communities. Public hospitals provide services without regard to the patient's ability to pay.

Workers' Compensation

Workers' compensation is an insurance system operated by the individual states. Each state has its own law and program to provide covered workers with some protection against the costs of medical care and the loss of income resulting from work-related injuries and, in some cases, illnesses. The first workers' compensation law was enacted in New York in 1910. By 1948, every state had enacted such laws. The theory underlying workers' compensation is that all accidents that occur at work, regardless of fault, must be regarded as risks of industry and that employer and employee should share the burden of loss (Jonas and Kovner 1999, p. 41).

Managed Care

The growth of managed care in the United States has had a tremendous impact on healthcare organizations and healthcare professionals. Managed care is a broad term used to describe several types of prepaid healthcare plans. Common types of managed care plans include health maintenance organizations (HMOs), preferred provider organizations (PPOs), and point-of-service (POS) plans.

Members of HMOs pay a set premium and are entitled to receive a specific range of healthcare services. In most cases, employers and employees share the cost of the plan. Coverage can be provided for an individual employee or his or her whole family. HMOs control costs by requiring members of the plan to seek services only from a preapproved list of providers, who are reimbursed at discounted rates. The plans also control access to medical specialists, expensive diagnostic and treatment procedures, and high-cost pharmaceuticals. They generally require preapproval for specialty consultations, inpatient care, and surgical procedures.

The development of managed care was an indirect result of the federal government's enactment of the Medicare and Medicaid laws in 1965. Medicare and Medicaid legislation prompted the development of **investor-owned hospital chains** and stimulated the growth of university medical centers. Both of these furthered the corporate practice of medicine by increasing the number of management personnel and physicians employed by hospitals and medical schools (Kongstevdt 1993, pp. 3–5).

The new healthcare programs for the elderly and poor laid the groundwork for increased corporate control of medical care delivery by third-party payers. This was done through the government-mandated regulation of fee-for-service and indemnity payments for healthcare services. After years of unchecked healthcare inflation, the government authorized corporate cost controls on hospitals, physicians, and patients, such as diagnosis-related groups (DRGs), prospective payment systems, and the resource-based relative value scale.

Further federal support for the corporate practice of medicine resulted from passage of the HMO Act of 1973. Amendments to the act enabled managed care plans to increase in numbers and expand enrollments through healthcare programs financed by grants, contracts, and loans. After passage of the HMO Act, strong support for the HMO concept came from business; the executive, legislative, and judicial branches of government; and several states where managed care proliferated, such as California, some northeastern states, and particularly Minneapolis-St. Paul, Minnesota.

Bipartisan support for managed care was based on the concept that HMOs can decrease costs and encourage free-market competition in the medical care arena with only limited government intervention. One measure of success of this policy can be found in the virtual disappearance of some 17 national health insurance bills introduced into Congress in the early 1970s (Kongstevdt 1993, pp. 3–5).

Impact of Managed Care Organizations

With more and more Americans receiving their health insurance through managed care organizations (MCOs), the responsibilities of primary care providers have changed. In the fee-for-service model, the primary care provider is responsible only for the patients actually seen in his or her office and a practice is viewed as being made up of individual patients. In a fully capitated managed care setting, however, particularly when the provider is paid through a capitation system rather than by a modified fee-for-service system, he or she is responsible for providing care to a defined population of patients assigned by the MCO. The MCO may audit the provider's practice to determine whether standards of care are being met. In the capitated MCO setting, providers are often held responsible for each patient on their panels, whether or not the patient ever comes to the office to be seen. Thus, if the standard of care set by the MCO for a pediatric practice requires that 90 percent of children receive all their immunizations by two years of age, the denominator used in assessing compliance with this goal is the total number of children two years of age and older in the provider's panel, not just the children actually seen in the provider's office. Standards of care, benchmarks against which the adequacy of care provided by the primary care practitioner is judged, exist for preventive services. Although quality assurance

measures have been required in hospital settings for a long time, it has only been since 1991, with the advent of standards of accreditation for MCOs set by the **National Committee on Quality Assurance** (NCQA), the accrediting body for MCOs, that widespread monitoring of standards of care in ambulatory settings has begun to gain acceptance (Jonas and Kovner 2005, p. 240).

The advent of managed care appeared to tame healthcare cost inflation during the early and mid-1990s, but costs are once again rising very rapidly. In particular, the total cost of pharmaceuticals is skyrocketing. The managed care industry faces continued financial challenges. At the same time, it remains under intense public scrutiny and is facing continued attempts at increased government legislation and regulation. In addition, for many years costs increased faster than premiums could rise to cover them. Thus, escalating costs have forced employers to ask workers to pay for a larger share of healthcare. Political and market forces and the weakness of any stabilizing influences are eroding the ability of managed care firms to control underlying healthcare costs. Moreover, significant increases in the cost of coverage are anticipated through 2006.

From 1960 to 2002, national healthcare spending rose from $27 billion to $1.6 trillion. Within that time period, the population of the United States rose from 186 million to 285 million and the gross domestic product (GDP) rose from $527 billion to $10.4 trillion. One thing that stands out from these numbers is the fact that healthcare spending outgrew the population. According to the statistics, per capita spending on healthcare during that same time period increased from $143 per person to $5,440 per person (Jonas and Kovner 2005, p. 630). Today, healthcare costs are staggering, and total U.S. healthcare expenditures are projected to increase from $1.66 trillion in 2003 to $2.7 trillion in 2010, with annual increases averaging 6.8 percent. Indeed, healthcare spending accounts for a larger share of the GDP (15 percent) in the United States than in any other major industrialized country. Moreover, despite the incredible investment America continues to make in healthcare, an astounding 15 percent of Americans lack healthcare coverage altogether.

Although managed care deserves much of the credit for taming the rampant, double-digit healthcare inflation of the 1980s and early 1990s, the relief from rising medical bills that Americans enjoyed for several years is over and increases in premiums have both HMOs and employers, especially smaller ones, scrambling for countermeasures. The shift to managed care seems to have run out of magic in terms of lowering healthcare costs. Although employers saw health coverage premiums increase only about 2 to 4 percent annually from 1994 through 1997, thanks to widespread implementation of managed care contracts, costs have been soaring ever since. In 2002, small employers saw cost increases of as much as 15 to 20 percent, while larger firms suffered health benefit cost increases of about 16 percent (and some employers of all sizes endured much higher increases). Healthcare costs are escalating in part because of rising drug costs.

Consumer-Driven Health Care

An emerging issue in the private insurance market is that of consumer-driven health care. This strategy seems to be gaining momentum in an effort to both allow employees more choice in their healthcare decisions and to stabilize healthcare costs. The design of consumer-driven plans varies, but, essentially, employers provide employees with a "personal care account," which is a fixed amount and offered in the form of a voucher, refundable tax credit, higher wages, or some other transfer of funds. Employees may choose their own services and providers as well as manage their annual spending. If an employee uses up all the funds in his or her personal care account, he or she is responsible for expenses up to a deductible, at which point wraparound or catastrophic coverage starts. A deductible places a minimum amount at which major medical expenses will be covered (Jonas and Kovner 2005, p. 69).

Health Savings Accounts (HSA)

Health savings accounts, or HSAs (also called medical savings accounts), offer participants the opportunity to control how their healthcare dollars are spent. HSAs combine high-deductible health insurance with a tax-sheltered savings account. President Bush signed the health savings account legislation into law on December 8, 2003.

The benefit of an HSA is that the member pays for the deductible with pretax dollars, which allows a member to save the money that ordinarily would have gone to pay taxes. When members pay off the deductible, the insurance company begins to pay. The money in the HSA earns interest and is owned by the member who holds the account (Health Insurance Carriers 2005).

Continued Rise in Healthcare Costs

For the fifth consecutive year, 2004 saw a double-digit increase in healthcare costs. Specifically, American employers saw a 12 percent increase in premiums paid to insurers. Although the increase was devastating to many employers, they took small comfort in the fact that costs increased at a slightly slower rate. According to a survey conducted by Towers Perrin, a benefits consulting firm, in 2003, employers saw an increase of 16 percent over the previous year. The reasons for the slowdown included fewer hospital stays and the use of generic drugs. The good news is that the slowing trend is expected to continue, but projections for healthcare cost growth still exceed those for overall economic growth. Healthcare cost increases are expected to slow to 6.7 percent per year by 2012 and are predicted to reach 18 percent of the GDP.

On average, employers' annual cost for healthcare coverage per active employee totaled $7,308 in 2004, which was $742 more than in the previous year. (The cost of insuring each "active" employee includes the cost of covering both eligible retired and current employees.) The catalysts for these repeated rises included the cost of prescription drugs, medical innovation, and a growing acceptance of higher-premium health plans that offer greater flexibility in choice of providers. One way that employers attempted to control costs was to implement monitoring and preventive care plans for conditions such as diabetes and heart disease. Blue Cross and Blue Shield of Minnesota offers such a program and has posted annual employer savings as high as $36 million.

The United States continues to spend more on healthcare than any other developed nation, spending 15 percent of the GDP or $5,650 per person (2003 estimate based on a U.S. population of 293 million). The average per capita healthcare spending among 30 member nations of the Organization for Economic Cooperation and Development is less than half as much.

Moreover, the United States is seeing greater growth in spending from one year to the next than other developed nations. Despite the higher costs, however, Americans have a much higher incidence of obesity and their average life expectancy is slightly lower than that of people in Japan, Iceland, Sweden, and Canada.

Healthcare prices in the United States are influenced by many factors. Supply and demand is greatly influenced by insurance companies and health plans. Patients' bargaining power is greatly decreased because providers can negotiate different charges depending on the payer. Many cash-strapped Americans abandon their expensive private healthcare plans and choose not to be insured at all. Unfortunately, patients who are not covered by MCOs are typically charged much higher rates for care. For example, a hospital might charge a set price of $1,900 for a CT scan procedure when billing an individual not covered by a managed care contract but discount the cost to $1,200 for someone who is covered. This is because managed care companies insist on negotiated rates for care (Plunkett Research 2003).

Cost and Quality Controls

The federal government became involved in the quality of care/malpractice issue through the establishment of the National Practitioner Data Bank (NPDB) under the Healthcare Quality Improvement Act of 1986. Congress enacted this legislation to:

- Moderate the incidence of malpractice
- Allow the medical community to demonstrate new willingness to weed out incompetents
- Improve the base of timely and accurate information on medical malpractice

The act required hospitals to request information from the data bank whenever they hire, grant privileges, or conduct periodic reviews of a practitioner. (See chapter 10 for additional discussion of malpractice and other legal issues affecting health information management.)

Major Challenges Affecting the Healthcare Industry

The American healthcare industry is at a crossroads today as a result of several significant factors, including:

- The commercial health insurance and managed care industry face continued challenges, both financially and in terms of public perception.
- Medicare and Medicaid programs are in need of reform to deal with a rapidly aging population.
- The subacute and post-acute care services segments continue to grow and present new challenges to the industry.
- The healthcare industry is entering what will long be remembered as the beginning of the Biotech Era.
- The development of evidence-based medicine calls for greater integration of all professions associated with healthcare, including purchasing and management.
- Malpractice insurance costs for physicians are spiraling out of control.

Commercial Health Insurance Industry

One major challenge facing the healthcare industry is the questionable image of managed care companies in general. Supporters of managed care contend that its structure offers higher-quality care at a lower cost. On the other hand, critics of managed care argue that the system risks lives by allowing plan managers to question—and sometimes reverse—the decisions made by medical professionals while emphasizing cost control at the expense of quality, thus sabotaging the bond of trust that should exist between doctor and patient. Additionally, many detractors of managed care are concerned about the trend of mergers creating huge managed care com-

panies. Some metropolitan markets are dominated by as few as two major health plans. Critics are equally concerned about the lack of autonomy of physicians who are forced to deal with the growing power of managed care giants.

While both supporters and critics make valid arguments, sweeping generalizations about the state of managed care are inherently flawed because no two managed care plans are exactly alike. Neither society nor consumers can afford to turn back the clock to the considerably more expensive, traditional fee-for-service system in which high-quality preventive care was largely nonexistent and patient care was generally provided without regard to cost.

Medicare and Medicaid Programs and an Aging Population

The future obligations of Medicare and Medicaid are significant enough to cause vast problems for the federal budget. Reforms are vital. Meanwhile, the number of seniors covered by Medicare will continue to grow at an exceedingly high rate and new prescription coverage costs will add to the government's financial problems.

Millions of dollars in potential profits are lost as hospitals and health systems write off record amounts of revenues to bad debt. Costs also are being forced upward by legislation passed in response to the overall public mistrust of managed care firms. Moreover, total healthcare expenditures are driven up by the aging baby-boomer generation and the scope and total amount of available healthcare.

In the wake of the tremendous growth of all aspects of the healthcare industry from 1945 onward, efficiency, competition, and productivity were, regretfully, largely overlooked. Much of this occurred because such a large portion of the healthcare bill is paid by federal and state governments. According to CMS, total Medicare and Medicaid program outlays in 2002 reached $377.2 billion, or 18 percent of the federal budget.

Growth of Subacute Care Services

Spending for home healthcare, hospital-based and freestanding nursing facilities has been growing rapidly. Subacute care providers have been growing in number and capacity (President's Advisory Commission 1998).

Postacute Care

Postacute care, also called **subacute care** or transitional care, is a type of short-term care provided by many long-term care and rehabilitation facilities and hospitals. Subacute care is often referred to as care that falls between acute care and traditional skilled nursing home care. It is needed immediately after, or instead of, hospitalization and includes medical services such as short-term rehabilitation, ventilator care/respirator care, intravenous therapy, wound management, and cardiac rehabilitation. This may include rehabilitation services, specialized care for certain conditions (such as stroke and diabetes), and/or postsurgical care and other services associated with the transition between the hospital and the home.

Residents of these units often have been hospitalized recently and typically have more complicated medical needs.

The goal of subacute care is to discharge residents to their homes or to a lower level of care. Subacute care usually lasts between 15 and 100 days, and is covered by Medicare. Some nursing homes have been providing short-term rehabilitation services and ventilator/respirator care for years. However, there recently has been a significant increase in the number of facilities offering these and other subacute services (CDC 2004).

The Biotech Era

Biotechnology is shifting the U.S. healthcare paradigm from a society "struggling to meet the escalating health problems of an aging population to one that focuses on wellness by preventing or delaying the onset of disease" (Burrill 2005). Almost 80 percent of the nation's healthcare spending is for chronic care. With advances in systems biology, this is shifting toward more personalized medicine focused on prevention, and eventually could lead to "a future in which an individual's genetic makeup can be determined to help tailor safer, more effective, cost-efficient treatments" (Burrill 2005).

New tools and a better understanding of how biological systems work is expected to create new treatments for everything from obesity, memory loss, and aging to cancer and cardiovascular illnesses. However, "safety issues in the pharmaceutical industry will continue to dominate the headlines" (Burrill 2005).

Overall, an outcome of the improvements made to the U.S. Healthcare system in the 20th century is a much longer, healthier life. Increased healthcare costs are typically incurred at the end of life. (See figure 2.2.) Much of the focus of biotechnology is directed at improving the care for chronic diseases of the elderly (Lynn and Adamson 2003).

Development of Evidenced-Based Best Practices and Outcomes

Physicians are caught between the desire for high-quality care and the desire for cost control on the part of payers,

Figure 2.2.   Americans' current healthcare expenditures are concentrated in the final part of the life span

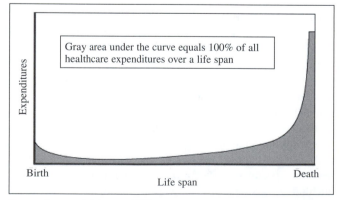

Gray area under the curve equals 100% of all healthcare expenditures over a life span

Source: Lynn and Adamson 2003.

including HMOs, Medicare, and Medicaid. The cost-versus-care debate has spawned an energetic movement to improve the quality of healthcare in the United States, much of it centered around patients' rights.

Evidence-based medicine is the conscientious, explicit, and judicious use of current best evidence in making decisions about the care of individual patients. The practice of evidence-based medicine means integrating individual clinical expertise with the best available external clinical evidence from systematic research. Evidence-based healthcare extends the application of the principles of evidence-based medicine to all professions associated with healthcare, including purchasing and management (Centre for Evidence-based Medicine 2005).

The importance of measuring and monitoring healthcare quality is essential, yet quantifying healthcare quality is complex. The entire process of quality assessment requires judgment and choices that should be influenced by physicians' clinical realities of medical care. It is assumed as well as essential that healthcare providers possess the knowledge to participate actively in the assessment of healthcare quality. Assessing quality requires the development and application of performance measures that are explicit standards of care against which actual clinical care is judged. Given the availability of evidenced-based guidelines for the management of patients, there is a natural inclination to use these consensus statements as a basis for developing performance measures for the evaluation of healthcare quality. Guidelines are not performance measures. Rather, they are written to suggest diagnostic or therapeutic interventions for most patients in most circumstances. The use of guideline recommendations in diagnosing and treating individual patients is left to the discretion of the physician. In contrast, performance measures are standards of care that imply that physicians are in error if they do not care for patients according to these standards. Therefore, in addition to stating an explicit diagnostic or therapeutic action to be performed, performance measures must define how to practically identify those patients for whom a specific action should be taken (American Heart Association 2000).

The Agency for Healthcare Research and Quality (AHRQ) promotes evidence-based practice in everyday care through establishment of 12 evidence-based practice centers (EPCs), which develop evidence reports and assess healthcare technology. Because of the EPC program, AHRQ became a "science partner" with private and public organizations (AHRQ 2004).

Malpractice insurance costs for physicians

Malpractice is the improper or negligent treatment of a patient, as by a physician, resulting in injury, damage, or loss. Garner (1990, p. 959) defines malpractice as

> the failure of rendering professional services to exercise that degree of skill and learning commonly applied under all the circumstances in the community by the average prudent reputable member of the profession with the result of injury, loss or damage to the recipient of those services or to those entitled to rely upon them.

Medical malpractice liability insurance premiums have increased in recent years, with a trend toward increasingly large plaintiffs' awards and higher losses for insurers. Premiums have risen both because insurance companies face increased costs to pay claims (from growth in malpractice awards) and because of reduced income from the insurance companies' investments and other short-term factors. Rapidly rising malpractice premiums may influence physicians, especially those in high-risk fields, to stop practicing medicine, thus reducing the availability of health care in some parts of the country (Beider and Hagen 2004)."

New Models of Healthcare Delivery

Telehealth is a new platform on which healthcare provision can be reshaped to meet the challenges of an aging population and more demanding and discerning patients/citizens. It involves automating all routine healthcare processes, from monitoring blood sugar levels to administering drugs, and extending the distribution of more complex and expert medical expertise by using videoconferencing to deliver consultations or surgical support. Following both these paths delivers benefits to healthcare provisioning, enabling medical staff to work more effectively, whatever their level of expertise or responsibility. Telehealth provides medical staff with a tool to eradicate mundane and low-value healthcare processes and to maximize their core skills and expertise. The same level of automation that is routine among financial and retail verticals, for example, is not as prevalent within the healthcare community. Changes under way have the potential to fundamentally change the delivery of healthcare in the near and long term (HBS Consulting 2003).

The evolution of telehealth is not only expected to reshape the delivery of consultations, monitoring, and treatments, but it also is expected to reshape healthcare providers' and patient/citizens' access to healthcare services. Healthcare delivery is no longer controlled—and will be less and less controlled—by secondary and primary healthcare providers.

Payer Changes in 2000–2010

Escalating costs have forced employers to ask workers to pay for a larger share of their healthcare. Political and market forces and the weakness of any stabilizing influences are eroding the ability of managed care firms to control underlying healthcare costs.

Employers are fighting back, partly by establishing new benefits methods that can accomplish much more than simply raising workers' copayments. For example, many major firms are showing their employees how to use the Internet to obtain better information about diseases and prevention. Insurance providers are using the Internet as a resource as well. For example, Humana's Web-based Emphesys benefits system puts everything from monthly payments to participating physicians to claims on the Internet at a substantial decrease in cost. Some employers are even hiring in-house physicians and nurses to provide primary care in the workplace.

Patients and insurance companies also are dealing with sticker shock as the nation's prescription drug bill soars. Prescription drug costs have increased more than 10 percent every year since 1995, surging 14 percent in 2002. Other factors edging costs upward are exuberance over new medical technology and patients' demand for greater plan flexibility in choosing doctors and specialists at their will.

As mentioned in earlier sections, healthcare costs are staggering and health spending in the United States today accounts for a larger share of the GDP than in any other major industrialized country.

Real-World Case

Community Hospital (CH) was a 250-bed, nonprofit community hospital in a suburb of a major midwestern city. Although it had generated an operating profit in 1998, in 2001, it had to file for protection under Chapter 11 of the Bankruptcy Code. CH had provided general acute care services to residents in the middle-income neighborhoods. Many independent hospitals in the U.S. market had begun joining integrated healthcare networks (IDNs), but CH chose to stay independent because its operations had shown continued modest profits. CH's cash position, however, was deteriorating. In the late 1990s, CH management initiated a cost-cutting program to restore financial health and made leadership changes in the finance area with the objective of improving the collection of accounts receivables. By 1999, CH reported a significant improvement in financial results.

CH management attributed its eventual financial demise to two factors: the Balanced Budget Act (BBA) of 1997 and Year 2000 (Y2K) compliance. Although these factors were important, other internal and avoidable factors led to the demise of CH's financial position.

BBA was plaguing providers everywhere, not just CH. Many hospital leaders sustained the ability to successfully manage their organizations using an approach based on one financial management tool: the income statement. With this approach, periodic reports show a few facts from the balance sheet such as days in accounts receivable, amount of debt, and cash, but attention is really on controlling expenses within available revenue as shown on the income statement.

CH had embarked on a major information technology (IT) upgrade. The hospital had been using a 20-year-old information system (IS). Because of its age, the IT vendor no longer provided system support. Recognizing the need to improve its management ISs and become Y2K compliant, CH leadership decided to install a new clinical and financial IT system.

CH experienced a $20 million reversal in earnings, net patient revenues decreased significantly, and at the same time expenses rose by $18 million. The hospital could no longer manage revenue weakness by reducing expenses. CH faced a series of events that used up cash, and by late FY1999, the

IT project was not going well. Installation expenses were high and patient bills did not go out for months. When patient cash went down and expenses went up, it did not take long for CH to use up its cash. This is when CH began postponing payments to creditors and looking for alternative sources of cash.

Changes in leadership decisions, board oversight, and medical staff partnering can bring some financial turnaround to troubled hospitals. If actions are not undertaken immediately in a hospital whose operations and financial performance are deteriorating, a bankruptcy may be unavoidable.

However, hospitals do not have to spiral downward to bankruptcy. To avoid bankruptcy, CH needed to find ways to recognize its problems more quickly and to take action early enough to avoid insolvency or restructuring. Unfortunately, no one wanted to face tough decisions and make necessary changes. It is hard to make difficult changes when the organizational team does not perceive itself as having a crisis. But, difficult as it may be, earlier effective actions could have made a difference. Finally, in 2001, the hospital filed for bankruptcy.

BBA was just an excuse. The act had a significant impact on the revenues of many hospitals. In CH's case, management estimated that the legislation caused a 5 percent decline in annual revenues. An expense cut to make up lost revenue would have been painful but almost certainly achievable. Nevertheless, CH's patient revenue problems went far beyond the BBA. Patient volume went down, the weakness in collections continued, and bad debt expense increased during this time period.

CH did not have accurate reporting systems and cash monitoring systems that would lead to controlling expenses as the revenue weakened. Upgrading its IT systems also proved difficult. The hospital undertook a process to replace its entire clinical, billing, and collection system with a new software package. The hospital's IT project focused on replacing a 20-year-old system that if, done well, could have positioned CH to meet future needs for compliance with Y2K and Health Insurance Portability and Accountability Act of 1996 (HIPAA) requirements. The original plan called for a six-month installation for a go-live, with numerous postponed deadline dates, all of which were missed. Many of the customizations were cancelled, and shortcuts were made to complete testing of the system controls. As problems mounted, management added more resources to solve the problem. At one point, the CH IT department had 65 people. Unfortunately, the billing and accounts receivable collection systems did not function after go-live. Accounting controls such as balancing reports that would ensure accurate tracking of revenue from the accounts receivable system to the general ledger had not been tested prior to go-live and did not function.

New patient services after go-live could not be billed. Concerns over meeting Y2K time frames had led management to go forward with the IT implementation in May 1999 before the complicated issues of billing from an integrated hospital system and testing of the system's billing capabilities had been worked through. Patient cash for services billed under the old system was collected in June 1999, but there was little cash was collected throughout the rest of the year. Management began piecing together work-around solutions. Although the hospital was able to generate bills again within a few months by feeding information into a separate billing system, collection of accounts receivable required extensive manual intervention and a very long receivables cycle. This work-around solution did not provide robust tools for collecting appropriate payments from managed care payers and following up on denials. In 2000, cash collections from patient activities slowed to a trickle. By mid-2000, the cash-flow difficulties began to create organizational distress.

Concurrent with the BBA, and IS issues, CH experienced a decline in its core operations. The medical staff expressed frustration with a management team it believed was more determined to hire administrative assistants than to bring on medical professionals and more concerned about cosmetic improvements than upgrading patient care floors.

Summary

Throughout history, humans have attempted to diagnose and treat illness and disease. As populations settled into towns and cities, early folk medicine traditions eventually led to the establishment of formalized entities specifically designed to care for the sick.

In the American colonies, enlightened thinkers such as Benjamin Franklin soon saw the need to establish hospitals and to regulate the practice of medicine. The 19th century saw the growth of organizations dedicated to standardizing medical practice and ensuring consistency in the quality of healthcare delivery. Organizations such as the American Medical Association and the American Nurses Association were created to represent the interests of their members and to further ensure the quality of their services.

The 20th century ushered in a completely new concept in the provision of healthcare: prepaid health plans. For the first time, Americans could buy health insurance. However, during the Great Depression of the 1930s and the Second World War, it became obvious that millions of Americans could not afford to pay for healthcare. After the war, the federal government began to study the problem of healthcare access for all Americans. Finally, during the Johnson administration in the 1960s, Congress passed amendments to the Social Security Act of 1935 that created the Medicare and Medicaid programs. These programs were designed to pay for the cost of healthcare services to the elderly and the poor.

As the healthcare industry has grown, so have efforts to regulate it. Some regulation has come from professional and trade associations that are associated with the industry. However, much regulation has come from the federal government, particularly with regard to the Medicaid and Medicare programs. Moreover, the types and variety of healthcare services that are available today have increased dramatically. Every new type of service, and every new way to provide it, brings complex issues that must be addressed in order to ensure that Americans receive the highest-quality healthcare possible at the most affordable price.

Passage of the Medicare and Medicaid programs and establishment of the managed care industry have had a tremendous impact on the way that healthcare in the United States is delivered and paid for. The ramifications of these changes on the American healthcare industry have yet to be fully appreciated. The only thing that is certain is that the American healthcare system continues to be a work in progress.

References

Agency for Healthcare Research and Quality. 2004 (Sept.). *Evidence-based practice centers overview.* Rockville, MD: AHRQ. Available online from ahrq.gov/clinic/epc/.

American Heart Association. 2000. Measuring and improving quality of care: A report from the American Heart Association/American College of Cardiology first scientific forum on assessment of healthcare quality in cardiovascular disease and stroke. Stroke 31(4):1002-12. Available online from circ.ahajournals.org/cgi/content/full/101/12/1483.

American Hospital Association. 2004 (Oct. 25). Fast Facts on U.S. Hospitals from *AHA Hospital Statistics.* Available online from aha.org/aha/resource_center/fastfacts/fast_facts_US_hospitals.html.

American Hospital Association. 1999. *100 Faces of Healthcare.* Chicago: Health Forum.

American Osteopathic Association. 2005. Available online from do-online. osteotech.org/index.cfm

Beider, P. and S. Hagen. 2004 (Jan. 8). Limiting tort liability for medical malpractice. Washington, D.C.: Congressional Budget Office. Available online from cbo.gov.

Burrill, G.S. 2005 (June 20). Healthcare in transition: Biotech drives major changes. Paper presented at BIO 2005, Philadelphia. Available online from sev.prnewswire.com/biotechnology/20050619/NYSU00419062005-1.html.

Centers for Disease Control. 2004. Health care in America: Trends in utilization. Available online from cdc.gov/nchs/datawh/nchsdefs/postacutecare.htm.

Centers for Medicare and Medicaid Services. 2005 (March 4). U.S. Department of Health and Human Services. Available online from Origins of Medicare. cms.hhs.gov/medicare/.

Centre for Evidence-Based Medicine. 2005. Glossary of terms in evidence-based medicine. Oxford: Institute of Health Sciences. Available online from cebm.net/glossary.asp.

Etheredge, L. 2001. *On the Archeology of Health Care Policy: Periods and Paradigms, 1975-2000.* Washington, D.C.: The National Academies Press. Available online from nap.edu/books/NI000569/html/1.html.

Garner, B.A., ed. 1990. *Black's Law Dictionary,* 6th ed. St. Paul, MN: West Group.

Health Insurance Carriers. 2005. Health Savings Accounts. health-insurance-carriers.com/hsa.html.

Joint Commission on Accreditation of Healthcare Organizations. 2005. *Comprehensive Accreditation Manual for Hospitals.* Oakbrook Terrace, IL: JCAHO.

Jonas, S., and A.R. Kovner. 2005. *Healthcare Delivery in the United States,* 8th ed. New York: Springer.

Jonas, S., and A.R. Kovner. 1999. *Healthcare Delivery in the United States,* 6th ed. New York: Springer.

Kongstevdt, P. 1993. *The Managed Care Handbook.* Gaithersburg, MD: Aspen.

Lynn, J. and D.M. Adamson. 2003. White paper: Living well at the end of life: Adapting health care to serious chronic illness in old age. Santa Monica, CA: RAND. Available online from rand.org/pubs/white_papers/2005/WP137.pdf.

National Institutes of Health. 2005. NIH Roadmap: Accelerating medical discovery to improve health. Frequently asked questions. Available online from nihroadmap.nih.gov/faq.asp.

Plunkett Research. 2003 (December). *Plunkett's Health Care Industry Almanac,* 2004 ed. Houston, TX: Plunkett Research, Ltd.

President's Advisory Commission on Protection and Quality in the Health Care Industry. 1998 (March 12). Improving health care quality in an industry in transition. In *Quality First: Better Health Care for All Americans.* Available online from hcqualitycommission.gov/final/

Sloane, R.M., B.L. Sloane, and R. Harder. 1999. *Introduction to Healthcare Delivery Organization: Functions and Management,* 4th ed. Chicago: Health Administration Press.

Starr, P. 1982. *The Social Transformation of American Medicine.* New York: Basic Books.

Stevens, R. 1999. *In Sickness and in Wealth.* Baltimore: Johns Hopkins University Press.

Sultz, H.A., and K.M. Young. 2004. *Healthcare USA—Understanding its Organization and Delivery,* 4th ed. Sudbury, MA: Jones and Bartlett.

3DQuote.com. 2000. Blue Cross national. Available online from 3dquote.com/blue-cross-national-info.htm.

Weinerman, E.R., R.S. Ratner, A. Robbins, and M.A. Lavenbar. 1966 (July). Determinants of use of hospital emergency services. Section 5 in Yale studies in ambulatory medical care. *Am J Public Health Nations Health* 56(7):1037–56.

Chapter 3
Informatics in Healthcare

Deborah Kohn, MPH, RHIA, CHE, CPHIMS, FHIMSS,
and Pamela Oachs, MA, RHIA

Learning Objectives

- To understand the field of informatics as it is being applied in healthcare
- To identify the major issues associated with computerizing health data and information
- To learn the types of computer applications and technologies being used to support the delivery of healthcare and the management of health data and information
- To identify the barriers/limitations associated with computerized health data and information

- To develop a working knowledge of the emerging technologies that support the creation and maintenance of electronic health record (EHR) systems
- To prepare for assuming a leadership role in the development of improved healthcare information systems, integrated patient information systems, and decision support tools

Key Terms

Analog
Application programming interface (API)
Application service provider (ASP)
Applied healthcare informatics
Artificial intelligence (AI)
Autocoding
Automated forms-processing (e-forms) technology
Bar-coding technology
Bit-mapped data
Care Maps®
Clinical care plans
Clinical informatics
Clinical information system (CIS)
Clinical/medical decision support system
Clinical messaging system
Clinical pathways
Clinical practice guidelines
Clinical workstation
Clinician/physician Web portals
Computer-assisted coding
Computer output laser disk/ enterprise report management (COLD/ERM) technology
Consumer informatics
Content
Continuous speech input
Data
Data marts
Data mining
Data repositories
Data types
Data warehouses

Decision support systems
Dental informatics
Diagnostic image data
Digital
Digital signature management technology
Discrete data
Document
Document image data
Document-imaging technology
Document management technology
e-commerce
e-health
Electronic data interchange (EDI)
Electronic document/content management system
Electronic records management technology
Encryption
Enterprise master patient index (EMPI)
Evidence-based medicine
Executive information system (EIS)
Expert decision support system
eXtensible Markup Language (XML)
Extranet
Free-text data
Geographic information system (GIS)
Gesture recognition technology
Healthcare informatics
Health information management (HIM)

Healthcare or health information technology (HIT)
HyperText Markup Language (HTML)
Identity management
Informatics
Information
Information management
Information science
Information systems (IS)
Intelligent character recognition (ICR) technology
Intelligent document recognition (IDR) technology
Interoperable
Interoperability
Interoperate
Intranets
Logical (or conceptual) repository
Management information system (MIS)
Mark sense technology
Master patient index (MPI)
Medical informatics
Metadata
Motion or streaming video/ frame data
Multimedia
Natural language processing technology
Neural networks
Nursing informatics
Object-oriented database
Online/real-time analytical processing (OLAP)
Online/real-time transaction processing (OLTP)

Optical character recognition (OCR) technology
Outcomes management
Par level
Patient/member Web portals
Personal digital assistants (PDAs)
Personal health record (PHR)
Pixel
Physical data repository
Physiological signal processing systems
Point-of-care information systems
Protocol
Public key infrastructure (PKI)
Radio frequency identification (RFID)
Raster image
Real audio data
Relational database
Secure messaging systems
Speech recognition technology
Structured data
Taxonomy
Text mining
Unstructured data
Vector graphic (or signal tracing) data
Web-based systems and applications
Web browser-based or Web native architectures
Web content management systems
Web portal
Web services
Wireless technology
Workflow technology

Introduction

The relatively recent introduction and rapid evolution of the use of computer technology to manage **data** and **information** continues to spearhead healthcare delivery systems and services in the new millennium. This means that well-trained and skilled individuals with knowledge about both healthcare and computerized information technologies will be needed to design, develop, select, and maintain tomorrow's **health information management** (HIM) systems.

This chapter introduces the field of **informatics** as it is currently being applied in the healthcare industry. Also, it describes the current and emerging technologies used to support the delivery of healthcare and the management and communication of patient information. Finally, the chapter discusses health information management as a component of the health informatics infrastructure and the partnerships that HIM professionals will forge with information technology and health informatics professionals in the future.

Theory into Practice

A large, nonprofit, acute care organization in New Jersey currently employs Daryl, an HIM professional, as a systems analyst in its information technology (IT; a.k.a. **information systems** [IS]) department. Daryl supports all the HIM department's applications from an IT perspective. This includes the organization's patient financial (patient billing/accounts receivable; a.k.a. revenue cycle management [RCM]) systems' HIM applications, such as the encoder, and the organization's patient administrative systems' HIM applications, such as the **master patient index** (MPI). Additionally, this includes the organization's patient clinical systems' HIM applications, such as the HIM department's dictation/transcription (a.k.a. voice/text) system and electronic document management system (EDMS).

As such, Daryl plays a key liaison role between IT and HIM. She represents the HIM department's systems at all IT department meetings and chairs the organization's RCM and EDMS technical users groups.

In general, Daryl identifies the HIM department's current and future information system (IS) needs, recommends and facilitates all system changes, implements and customizes new applications, and troubleshoots/resolves application system issues in both installation and production environments. She defines project plans and coordinates the resources to accomplish project plan objectives. Also, she improves and enhances the HIM department's application software by participating in the direction, selection, conversion, and routine management of these applications.

To accomplish this, Daryl's typical day includes researching answers to problems, setting up meetings and appointments with HIM department users, coordinating demonstrations and training sessions, following up on tasks assigned at meetings, testing applications and interfaces, and working with vendors to make enhancements to existing products. She uses the following, important skills:

- Attention to detail
- Knowledge of HIM department fundamentals to understand how technology can be used and modified
- Knowledge of the department's business rules
- Knowledge of the flow of information throughout the organization
- Knowledge of the department's workflow
- Organizational skills
- Project management skills

Recently, Daryl took the lead in identifying HIM requirements for the organization's new **clinical information system** (CIS). Such requirements included providing interface specifications to and from the HIM department's transcription system and setting up the HIM department's security profiles.

Having implemented a transcription system at a former place of employment, Daryl learned how to work with people and analyze both manual and automated systems. The prior experience also gave Daryl more exposure to the fundamentals of project management and taught her how to develop a request for proposal (RFP), complete the steps required to evaluate software, and perform system administration functions.

Therefore, Daryl began the project by assembling an ad hoc committee of transcription users throughout the organization, whether or not these users would be required to interface with the CIS. After the first meeting, the committee determined that not only would all these users be required to interface with the CIS, but also there were other transcription users "hiding" in the organization who needed to be a part of the committee.

After performing a thorough inventory of every transcription system, the committee accounted for six disparate word-processing systems that were used for organizational transcription. The HIM department's word-processing system was used to transcribe the majority of the organization's medical report dictation. However, the other five systems were used to transcribe at least 30 percent of the organization's dictation. These systems included two proprietary systems and three systems each with different versions of Microsoft Word™.

Therefore, the analysis persuaded the committee to recommend to the organization's IT steering committee that, at this time, standardizing on one transcription system (the system used by the HIM department) would be the most appropriate, strategic solution for the organization, its CIS, and its CIS transcription interface requirements.

This recommendation was made after discussion and dissension. For example, all the committee members realized that the recommendation would be difficult to implement because the users of the five remaining transcription systems involved care providers who were unaccustomed to change. Further, it would be expensive in the short term because it would require a significant amount of retraining, additional hardware and server capacity, and the potential consolidation of all transcription positions under the HIM department.

However, in the long term, the benefits of standardizing on one system would allow IS to develop one set of interface instructions as opposed to six. The five remaining systems needed to be upgraded anyway because some of the interfaces could not proceed unless more current operating systems and software versions were installed. In addition, because interfaces are extremely costly to develop and maintain, the long-term advantages of standardizing on one transcription system throughout the organization outweighed the short-term disadvantages of interfacing and maintaining six, disparate systems.

As lead, Daryl realized that the short-term challenges had to be addressed immediately. These challenges included changing provider behavior, retraining various transcriptionists and dictators, and reorganizing HIM department positions with job descriptions and salaries. In other words, solutions to these challenges needed to be designed—and even implemented—before the committee could begin to determine the systems' interface rules and HIM department security profiles for the CIS.

Based on her previous management and healthcare informatics experiences, Daryl knew that responsibilities for several tasks had to be delegated, including the required retraining, marketing of the recommendation, and working with the HIM director and transcription system vendor to expand the department's existing transcription area. Also, the tasks included amending the existing transcription system contract to add software licenses. The delegation took place primarily using existing ad hoc committee members. In addition, Daryl incorporated "outside" clinical champions as well as clinical troublemakers so that the tasks could be accomplished in tandem and any roadblocks could be dismantled along the way.

The Field of Informatics

Informatics is the science of **information management.** It uses a variety of techniques to automate, or use, computers for the management of data and information to support decision-making activities. The management of data and information includes the generation, collection, organization, validation, analysis, storage, and integration of data, as well as the dissemination, communication, presentation, utilization, transmission, and safeguarding of information.

Healthcare informatics is the field of **information science** concerned with the management of all aspects of health data and information through the application of computers and computer technologies. The healthcare industry is information intensive. One needs to spend only a day with a healthcare provider/clinician to realize that the largest percentage of healthcare professional activities relates to managing massive amounts of data and information. This includes obtaining and documenting information about patients, consulting with colleagues, staying abreast of the current literature, determining strategies for patient care, interpreting laboratory data and test results, and conducting research.

The influence of healthcare informatics is broad. **Healthcare or health information technology** (HIT) is having a huge impact not only on the complex financial and administrative aspects of healthcare, but also on its unique clinical practices. For example, CISs, which provide computerized communication and information management for such functions as order entry, results retrieval, care planning, and charting, are installed in every kind of healthcare organization—from major academic teaching hospitals and integrated delivery networks/systems to post–acute care facilities, physician practices, and managed care organizations. In addition, healthcare informatics is changing at the speed of thought.

Historically, the healthcare industry did not value healthcare informatics to the same degree that other vertical market industries do. The healthcare industry has been perceived as slow to understand computerized information management and to incorporate it effectively into the work environment. Perhaps this is because the requirements of the healthcare industry are more demanding than those of other industries in a number of areas. These areas include implications of violations of privacy, support for personal values, responsibility for public health, complexity of the knowledge base and terminology, perception of high risk and pressure to make critical decisions rapidly, poorly defined outcomes, and support for the diffusion of power (Stead and Lorenzi 1999, p. 343).

Recently, the concept of **applied healthcare informatics** has emerged, which emphasizes the use of the computer-based applications in delivering and documenting healthcare services. Therefore, for HIM, applied healthcare informatics is the application of healthcare information technology to HIM. As this concept evolves, the healthcare industry will continue to take note of HIM's contribution to this growing field. In addition, HIM's position within the broad healthcare informatics domain will continue to be reinforced. For more information about the development of healthcare informatics, visit the Web site for the American Medical Informatics Association at amia.com.

The Informatics Revolution in Healthcare

Revolution is an overused word, but when applied to the effect of all that is digital, automated, or electronic in the healthcare industry, it is entirely accurate. Over the past several decades, established relationships, value chains, and strategies have been radically altered or swept away by computer technology.

Evolution of Healthcare Informatics

The term *informatics* was adopted in the early 1970s when European universities and research institutions offered programs to keep up with the introduction and application of computers and computer systems. Likewise, the term *healthcare informatics* as we know it today—the intersection of information and technology and healthcare—was based on an idea born in Europe. However, since the mid-1980s, some of the most original and creative minds in the healthcare professions in the United States have engaged healthcare informatics, giving rise to a discipline in its own right.

Today, the goal of the discipline is to understand the structure, dynamics, design, implementation, and ongoing maintenance of ISs that are composed of people, technology, and organizational factors. This allows the appropriate flow and use of information to be individually optimized for every task in every context for every user in any organization (Turley et al. 2001, p. 48). Thus, the discipline's focus today is on the development, implementation, and use of computer-based applications that support ever-changing business/workflow processes that, in turn, support specific types of users in performing their work or meeting their needs.

For example, some users of the applied healthcare informatics discipline (for example, physicians) work in clinical medicine or medical research, where the term *medical informatics* is used. Other users work in nursing, where *nursing informatics* is a more commonly recognized term. Some users work in dentistry, where the profession is taking new steps toward *dental informatics.* And still other users, including pharmacists and therapists, work in the allied healthcare professions, where the term *clinical informatics* has gained acceptance. Even *consumer informatics* is beginning to be represented as new relationships emerge

between people and the health system. Consequently, the generic term *healthcare informatics* is seen as the broad domain, stressing the interdisciplinary nature of the field and underscoring the need to involve all healthcare professionals and patients.

The value proposition of healthcare informatics can be explained as the study, creation, and implementation of healthcare business/workflow processes designed to improve the communication and understanding of healthcare data and information, as well as to improve the management of the data and information. Thus, the value proposition covers the clinical, technical, public, and commercial aspects of healthcare.

As such, applied healthcare informatics can make it possible to achieve better outcomes for the healthcare delivery and IT industries. Its structures and communication methods allow information to be linked to healthcare work processes and managed as an asset outside the systems that automate those processes. Its data-mining techniques and filters locate information and limit reports to the immediate context. Its presentation metaphors can enhance healthcare users' exploration techniques and adapt to individual learning styles. Its education and training programs are beginning to produce people who know how to develop effective information-enabled work processes.

Health information managers are well positioned to play key roles in ensuring acceptance of healthcare informatics within the healthcare industry. They have the skills needed to exploit the computerized systems and technologies for their unique practical and strategic functionalities. Therefore, they can leverage chief information officers, the health information technology industry, and the field of healthcare informatics as partners to enable people to use information to improve health. In addition, they can provide the leadership needed to develop a better model for the healthcare delivery system.

Examples of Calls to Action and Informatics Successes

Calls to action for the use of information technologies to improve the healthcare delivery system are not new. The 1990s began with the Institute of Medicine's (IOM) report, which was based on the findings of its Committee on Improving the Patient Record, which championed the computer-based patient record (CPR) (Dick and Steen 1991). (CPRs, with its more current term, electronic health records [EHRs], are discussed in detail in chapter 9.) The second portion (Title II) of Public Law 104-191, the Health Insurance Portability and Accountability Act of 1996 (HIPAA), addressed the requirements to support electronic information exchange with goals of administrative efficiency and process improvement. It also mandated the protection of health information.

The millennium began with two additional IOM reports based on the findings of its Committee on Quality of Health

Care in America. The first report shocked the nation with its estimated number of deaths each year resulting from preventable medical errors (Kohn, Corrigan, and Donaldson 1999). The second, follow-up report called for transforming America's "failing" healthcare industry (IOM 2001). Each of these calls to action identified IT needs and the potential for IT benefits.

The IOM's third report in as many years argued that the federal government should lead the development of clinical standards for measuring care and proposed financial incentives for organizations that improve quality (IOM 2002). As such, this report called for five "demonstration" projects, including IT development, to help coordinate the exchange of healthcare information across the industry. The fourth report (IOM 2003) called for the *Consolidated Health Informatics* (CHI) initiative of the Department of Health and Human Services (HHS), the Department of Defense (DoD) and the Veterans Health Administration (VA) to work with the National Committee on Vital and Health Statistics (NCVHS) to identify appropriate clinical data standards that will make health information uniform and understandable to all. In addition, this report mandated that EHRs "operate seamlessly as part of a national network of health information that is accessible by all healthcare organizations" (NCVHS 2001).

Additionally, examples of healthcare informatics successes are steadily growing. Charge collection and billing, automated laboratory testing and reporting, clinical documentation, computerized provider order entry (CPOE), patient and provider scheduling, diagnostic imaging, and secondary data use make up a distinguished healthcare informatics "success" list, proving what is doable and supporting further investment.

Still, many of the healthcare informatics calls to action and successes have not produced compelling outcomes, especially those outcomes that communicate the feasibility of a better health system for more individuals at an affordable cost. Therefore, today's task for informatics is to design, develop, and implement the ISs that enable healthcare organizations to accomplish visions for providing the highest-quality care in the most effective way. To do so, the visions must make the benefits of the proposed systems clearer. In addition, they must establish explicit links between the promised benefits and the key enablers of the benefits—the information technologies.

The National Health Information Network

The National Health Information Network (NHIN; formerly known as the National Health Information Infrastructure [NHII]) is a relatively recent government-sponsored initiative designed to improve the effectiveness, efficiency, and overall quality of health and healthcare in the United States. This will be accomplished by providing a comprehensive view of a patient's health information at the point of care through the development of a comprehensive, interconnected, knowledge-based network of **interoperable** ISs from all sectors of the healthcare industry. Also referred to as the Medical Internet,

providers of care will be able to electronically exchange the information between all electronic health records so that a complete, electronic health record can be assembled whenever and wherever a patient presents for care.

The NHIN was mentioned first by the IOM in its seminal report, *The Computer-based Patient Record: An Essential Technology for Health Care* (Dick and Steen 1991). A decade later, the NHIN was defined further by the NCVHS in its report, *Information for Health: A Strategy for Building the NHII* (NCVHS 2001). Following September 11, 2001, and the anthrax attacks, the NHIN gained national attention in both public and private sectors when the need for enhanced public health surveillance and response became more visible and immediate. Consequently, the IOM's fourth quality report additionally asserted that an NHIN "should be the highest priority for all healthcare stakeholders" (IOM 2003).

HHS provided initial guiding principles and requirements for this network. Based on these and other requirements, in 2004, the Center of Information Technology Leadership determined that over the next 10 years, building a national system of healthcare information exchange would cost a hefty $276 billion, with operating costs another $16.5 billion per year (2004). However, a fully implemented (assuming this 10-year technology rollout and usage schedule) and standardized NHIN, consisting of machine-interpretable data (that is, structured messages, standardized content/data) would deliver national savings of $77.8 billion per year (Walker et al 2005, p. 16). (See table 3.1.)

However, significant barriers exist to achieving the NHIN within the next ten years. Such barriers include a current lack of standards allowing for **interoperability** and data sharing, insufficient funding, a lack of ongoing economic incentives needed to sustain infrastructure operations, and public concern over privacy. Consequently, in late 2004, the HHS Office of the National Coordinator for Health Information Technology (ONC) published a request for information (RFI) to seek public comment about how to develop the NHIN. Over 500 responses were received. A summary report was released in 2005.

Table 3.1.   Annual savings with a NHIN

Provider Type	Net Value, Starting at Year 11
Hospitals/Clinician Offices	$33.5 billion
Payers	$21.6 billion
Laboratories	$13.1 billion
Imaging Centers	$ 8.2 billion
Pharmacies	$ 1.3 billion
Public Health	$ 0.1 billion
TOTAL	**$77.8 billion**

© 2005 Deborah Kohn.

The interoperability and data-sharing strategies available to support an NHIN are fundamentally no different from those available to individual healthcare provider organizations. However, regarding the approach used to develop the NHIN, healthcare organizations must carefully weigh public concerns over privacy and cross, multi-organizational concerns over the continued ownership, control, and advantage their existing data provide them.

Consequently, also in late 2004, HHS stipulated that the NHIN must be built incrementally from collaborative, local, and regional efforts in the public and private sectors. As a result, today's NHIN focus is to begin with a network of connected, public and private regional health information organizations (RHIOs; formerly known as local health information infrastructures [LHIIs]), each facilitating exchange of health information in a "region." And, NHIN activities on the national level most likely will focus on the development and/or adoption of standards and economic incentives that will promote the growth of these regional health information exchange infrastructures.

Regional Health Information Organizations

RHIOs are healthcare provider, payer, and patient collaboratives that regionally exchange healthcare information. They serve anywhere from approximately 500,000 to 1,000,000 plus lives. Typically, an RHIO is made up of diverse healthcare stakeholders providing and receiving services in a medical referral area or, for all intents and purposes, an area served by a regional emergency medical services organization. As such, RHIOs are bigger and fewer than the earlier LHIIs. However, RHIOs typically are no larger than a state.

Many developing RHIOs favor a decentralized or "federated" approach to their technical architectures for regional healthcare information exchange. This model is not the fully integrated, monolithic, centralized database model of most healthcare provider organizations. Instead, it consists of distinct, distributed, disparate, and decentralized databases. Centralization only occurs with an **enterprise-type master patient index** (EMPI) for demographic data, and, perhaps, with **application programming interfaces** (APIs). As such, this model allows information sharing to occur without requiring a unique, national patient identifier and allows contributing organizations to retain ownership and control of their data.

The federated model has other advantages. For example, data ownership is managed by defining business policies and access rules. In addition, new computer systems typically are not required, allowing for an easier transition to regional EHRs. Unfortunately, the drawbacks of this approach remain. Because there is yet no unified data model and standardized codification, decision support and many reporting capabilities are limited. In addition, this approach typically requires more coordination to implement. For example, RHIO stakeholders often have to accept diverse, regional infrastructures and workflows.

Check Your Understanding 3.2

Instructions: Answer the following questions on a separate piece of paper.

1. What is the goal of healthcare informatics? How does healthcare informatics benefit a healthcare organization?
2. Describe at least two major reports published by the Institute of Medicine (IOM) that have each served as a call to action in healthcare informatics.
3. What initiative is referred to as the Medical Internet, and what is its purpose?
4. What barriers exist to achieving the NHIN within the next 10 years?
5. Describe the federated approach that many RHIOs are taking to develop their technical architectures for regional healthcare information exchange. What are the advantages and disadvantages of this approach?

Current and Emerging Information Technologies in Healthcare

To examine the information resources and systems that enable healthcare organizations to accomplish their visions in the most effective way, HIM professionals must possess fundamental knowledge of computer-based information systems' components, regardless of industry. This includes knowledge of system hardware, software, and service components; communication and networking components; the Internet and its derived technologies; and system architectures. For the purposes of this book, it is assumed that students have acquired this knowledge through other, generic computer system courses and related textbooks.

Next, it is appropriate that HIM professionals review some of the current and emerging information technologies used to support the delivery of healthcare as well as the management and communication of health data and information within the healthcare setting. To do this, five categories of current and emerging technologies in healthcare have been defined. These categories support:

- Different types of data and formats
- Efficient access to, and flow of, data and information
- Managerial and clinical decision making
- The diagnosis, treatment, and care of patients
- The security of data and information

Supporting Different Types of Data and Formats

The information technologies currently in use for healthcare applications as well as the new technologies being developed consist of different data types and formats, all used to support the creation, storage, dissemination, and analysis of information in every healthcare setting. Specific examples include emerging **speech recognition technology** and **natural language processing technology.**

Different Data Types and Formats

Healthcare informatics professionals have agreed that an EHR system is not one or even two or more "products." Rather, it is a concept that consists of a plethora of integrated, component information systems and technologies. The automated files that make up the EHR system's component information systems and technologies consist of different **data types,** and the data in the files consist of different data formats.

Some data formats are structured and some are unstructured. For example, the data elements in a patient's automated laboratory order, result, or demographic/financial information system are coded and alphanumeric. Their fields are predefined and limited. In other words, the type of data is discrete, and the format of these data is structured. Consequently, when a healthcare professional searches a database for one or more coded, **discrete data** elements based on the search parameters, the engine can easily find, retrieve, and manipulate the element.

However, the format of the data contained in a patient's transcribed radiology or pathology result, history and physical (H&P), or clinical note system using word-processing technology is unstructured. **Free-text data,** as opposed to discrete, **structured data,** are generated by word processors, and their fields are not predefined and limited. Consequently, when a healthcare professional searches unstructured text, the search engine cannot easily find, retrieve, and manipulate one or more data elements embedded in the text.

Likewise, the format of the data contained in a patient's dictated radiology or pathology result, H&P, or clinical note system using speech recognition technology (real-time speech in, text out) is unstructured. However, the speech recognition technology's engine takes the unstructured, free-text-based speech data and codifies them, often with the help of templates. Hence, the format of the outputted text data becomes structured, with predefined and limited fields. Search engines then easily can find, retrieve, and manipulate one or more data elements embedded in the text.

Diagnostic image data, such as a digitized chest x-ray or a computed tomography (CT) scan stored in a diagnostic image management system, represent a different type of data called **bit-mapped data.** However, the format of bit-mapped data also is unstructured. Saving each bit of the original image creates the image file. In other words, the image is a **raster image,** the smallest unit of which is a picture element or **pixel.** Together, hundreds of pixels simulate the image.

Some diagnostic image data are based on **analog,** photographic films, such as an analog chest x-ray. These analog films must be digitally scanned, using film digitizers, to digitize the data. Other diagnostic image data are based on **digital** modalities, such as computed radiography (CR), CT, magnetic resonance (MR), or nuclear medicine.

Document image data are yet another type of data that are also bit mapped, and the format of which is unstructured. These data are based on analog paper documents or on analog photographic film documents. Most often, analog paper-based documents contain handwritten notes, marks, or signatures. However, such documents can include preprinted documents (such as forms), photocopies of original documents, or computer-generated documents available only in hard copy. Analog photographic film based documents (that is, photographs) are processed using an analog camera and film, similar to analog chest x-rays. Therefore, both the analog paper-based and the photographic film-based documents must be digitally scanned, using scanning devices that are similar to facsimile machines.

The EHR system's component ISs and ITs consist of additional data types, the formats of which also are unstructured. **Real audio data** consist of sound bytes, such as digital heart sounds. **Motion or streaming video/frame data,** such as cardiac catheterizations, consist of digitized film attributes, such as fast forwarding. The files that consist of **vector graphic (or signal-tracing) data,** are created by saving lines plotted between a series of points, accounting for the familiar ECGs, EEGs, and fetal traces.

When more than one **unstructured data** type is present in an IS, the data and system they represent are referred to as **multimedia.** Clearly, the EHR system is multimedia.

Figure 3.1 (p. 50) shows the different types of data and their sources found in EHR system component ISs and ITs.

Speech Recognition Technology

For more than 20 years, the concept of generating an immediately available, legible, final, signed note or report based on computer speech input has been the catalyst for the development and application of different forms of speech recognition technology in healthcare. Unfortunately, the technology remains inaccurate. Systems offering greater than 95 percent accuracy are not acceptable for efficient and often lengthy clinical dictation purposes. Consequently, many still consider speech recognition an emerging technology.

Today, the most common form of speech recognition technology is speaker independent with continuous speech input. Speaker independence does not require extensive training. The software is already trained to recognize generic speech and speech patterns. **Continuous speech input** does not require the user to pause between words to let the computer distinguish between the beginning and ending of words. However, the user still is required to be careful in the enunciation of words.

Although speech recognition vocabularies are expanding due to faster and more powerful computer hardware, only limited vocabularies have been developed. Limited vocabulary-based speech recognition systems require the user to say words that are known or taught to the system. In healthcare, limited vocabulary-based specialties such as radiology, emergency medicine, and psychiatry have realized benefits for dictation from the technology.

Recent data indicate that speech recognition technology may be an acceptable alternative for producing outpatient notes. Although it takes longer to dictate and edit the outpatient notes on the computer compared with dictating and editing the notes for human transcription, decreased delays and costs associated with producing transcribed documents have been realized (Borowitz 2001, p. 102).

Figure 3.1. CPR data types and their sources

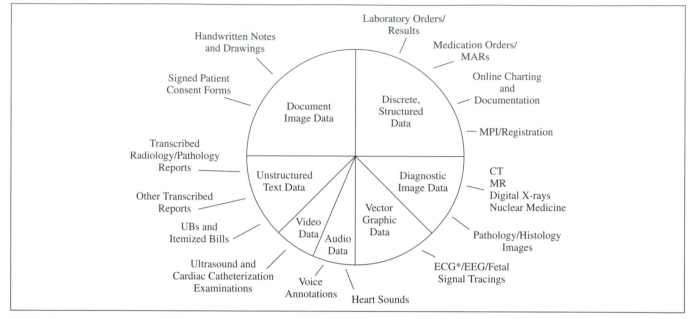

*ECG is the more correct term, but EKG is more widely used.
©2001 Deborah Kohn.

Other areas in healthcare have realized significant benefits from this input technology for specific programs. These programs include data-entry systems, navigating through pathways, pulling down menus, editing text, autodialing phone numbers, and completing multiple-choice-based forms. This usually requires exchanging data with the other applications through seamless, but complex, interfaces.

The ultimate goal in speech recognition technology is to be able to talk to a computer's central processor and rapidly create vocabularies for applications without collecting any speech samples (in other words, without training). It includes being able to talk at natural speed and intonation and in no specific manner. Additionally, it includes having the computer understand what the user wants to say (the context of the word or words) and then apply the correct commands or words as coded data in a structured format. Finally, it includes identifying a user's voice and encrypting the voice-print. Over the next years and decades, clinical vocabularies and algorithms will continue to improve, true speaker independence will be achieved, and natural language understanding will ultimately make structured dictation a reality.

Natural Language Processing Technology

One could argue that natural language processing technology is another name for speech recognition technology. When one talks at natural speed without pausing between words, the *natural language* voice bytes are, indeed, *processed* by this technology. However, natural language processing technology is more than speech recognition technology.

Natural language processing technology considers sentence structure (syntax), meaning (semantics), and context to accurately process and/or extract free-text data, including speech data for application purposes. As such, it differs from simple Boolean word search programs that often complement speech recognition technology-based systems. For example, the narratives "no shortness of breath, chest pain aggravated by exercise" and "no chest pain, shortness of breath aggravated by exercise" look the same to a Boolean word search engine when looking for occurrences of "chest" and "pain" in the same sentence. This Boolean word search approach retrieves approximately 20 percent of the answer 20 percent of the time. It is rife with false positives and false negatives.

On the other hand, natural language processing technology knows the difference in the narratives' meanings. For example, for health record coding applications, it teaches computers to understand English well enough to "read" transcribed reports/notes and then find certain key concepts (not merely words) by identifying the many different phrasings of the concept. By "normalizing" these concepts, different phrases of the same content can all be compared with one another for statistical purposes. For example, "the patient thinks s/he has angina" and "the doctor thinks the patient has angina" have different meanings from a coding perspective (Schnitzer 2000, p. 96). By employing statistical or rules-based algorithms, natural language processing technology can then compare and code these similar expressions accurately and quickly.

Autocoding and **computer-assisted coding** are the terms commonly used to describe natural language processing technology's method of extracting and then translating dictated and then transcribed free-text data, or dictated and then computer-generated discrete data, into ICD and/or CPT codes for clinical and financial applications such as patient billing and health record coding. **Text mining** and **data mining** are the terms commonly used to describe the process of extracting and then quantifying and filtering free-text data and discrete data, respectively.

Early results of several formative studies suggest that natural language processing technology improves health record coding productivity and consistency without sacrificing quality (Warner 2000, p. 78). More recent studies suggest that quality remains in question (AHIMA 2004). Despite the studies' outcomes, vendors continue to integrate natural language processing technology within health record coding reference tools, coding clinic guidelines, drug databases, and legacy information systems to provide complete patient billing, health record coding, and other applications with little or no human intervention.

Check Your Understanding 3.3

Instructions: Answer the following questions on a separate piece of paper.

1. Give an example of structured and unstructured data formats and an example of discrete and free-text data types.
2. What is a key advantage to structured data when searching a database?
3. What are the similarities and differences between a diagnostic image and a document image?
4. Give a healthcare example for each of the following data types: real audio data, motion or streaming data, signal or vector graphic data.
5. What is the difference between (a) speech recognition technology and natural language processing technology and (b) natural language processing searching and Boolean searching?

Supporting Efficient Access to, and Flow of, Data and Information

A plethora of current and emerging information technologies are used to support the efficient access to, and flow of, healthcare data and information. For purposes of this book, the following technologies are highlighted:

- Automatic recognition technologies
- **Electronic data interchange** (EDI) and **e-commerce**
- Enterprise master patient indexes/identity management
- **Data repositories**
- **Electronic document/content management systems**
- **Secure messaging systems**
- Web-derived technologies and applications
- **Application service providers** (ASPs)

Automatic Recognition Technologies

Several technologies are used in healthcare to recognize analog items automatically, such as tangible materials or documents, or to recognize characters/symbols from analog items. Character/symbol recognition technologies recognize electronically scanned characters or symbols from analog items, enabling the identified data to be quickly, accurately, and automatically entered into digital systems. Other recognition technologies identify the actual items.

Character/Symbol Recognition Technologies

Character/symbol recognition technologies include **barcoding, optical character recognition** (OCR), and **gesture recognition technologies.**

Bar-Coding Technology

More than two decades ago, the bar code symbol was standardized for the healthcare industry, making it easier to adopt bar-coding technology and to realize its potential. Since then, bar-coding applications have been adopted for labels, patient wristbands, specimen containers, business/employee/patient records, library reference materials, medication packages, dietary items, paper documents, and more. Benefits have been realized by the uniform consistency in the development of commercially available software systems, fewer procedural variations in healthcare organizations using the technology, and the flexibility to adopt standard specifications for functions while retaining current systems. Because virtually every tangible item in the clinical setting, including the patient, can be assigned a bar code with an associated meaning, it is not surprising to find bar coding as the primary tracking, identification, inventory data-capture, and even patient safety medium in healthcare organizations.

With bar-coding technology, an individual's computer data-entry rate can be increased by eight- to twelvefold in applications such as patient/medication tracking, supply requisitioning, or chart/film tracking. For example, a function such as hand-keying paper chart/film locations into a computer that once took a healthcare professional eight hours to perform now can be done in 30 to 45 minutes with bar-coding technology.

In addition to eliminating time, bar-coding technology eliminates most of the mounds of paperwork (worksheets, count sheets, identification sheets, and the like) that are still associated with traditional computer keyboard entry. When bar-coding systems are interfaced to these types of healthcare information systems, the bar code can be used to enter the data, especially repetitive data, saving additional processing time and paper generation.

More important, the data input error rates with bar coding are as close to zero as most IT professionals think is possible. For all intents and purposes, bar-coded data, with an error rate of approximately three transactions in 1 million, can be considered error free. Thus, it is a most effective remedy for medication errors when used to make sure that the right medication dose is administered to the right patient.

Optical Character Recognition Technology

Like bar coding, OCR technology was invented to reduce manual data input, or hand-keying. OCR technology recognizes machine-generated characters (for example, preprinted numbers and letters) by interpreting the scanned, bit-mapped shapes of the characters' images and then converting the characters into computer-processable codes. OCR technology was initially used to automatically identify financial accounts consisting of preprinted Arabic numbers and Roman letters using the E13B font on thousands of paper-based documents, such as bank checks.

OCR has since been perfected to recognize the full set of preprinted/typeset fonts as well as point sizes. Moreover, it performs well with different Germanic and Romance languages. The best OCR systems compensate for imperfectly formed characters and scanned pages by employing characteristics such as de-skewing, broken character repair, and redaction. De-skewing "straightens" oblique characters, broken character repair "fixes" incomplete characters, and redaction "hides" superfluous characters. OCR is used to perform everything from indexing scanned documents to digitizing full text. Its ability to dramatically reduce manual data input, or hand-keying, and at the same time increase input speed represents the best aspect of this technology.

Unfortunately, like other technologies, OCR has been perfected but is not perfect. The 90 to 95 percent recognition rate realized by most OCR systems may not be sufficient for the kind of text recognition applications OCR software is designed to perform. In addition, after an analog document is scanned by OCR technology, the data become unstructured, free-text data. As with all unstructured text data, when a healthcare professional needs to search the text, the search engine cannot easily find, retrieve, and manipulate one or more data elements embedded in text.

Gesture Recognition Technology

The recognition of constrained or unconstrained, handwritten, English language free text (print and/or cursive, upper- and/or lower-case, characters and/or symbols) typically stored on paper-based, analog documents is known as **intelligent character recognition** (ICR) **technology.** The recognition of hand-marked characters in defined areas of, typically, paper-based, analog documents is known as **mark sense technology.** Collectively, these technologies are referred to as gesture recognition technologies.

Mark sense technology detects the presence or absence of hand-marked characters on analog documents. Consequently, it is used for processing analog questionnaires, surveys, and tests, such as filled-in circles by Number 2 pencils on SAT exam forms.

ICR technology is quite an elaborate information-processing technique. An operation such as the detection of lines or the beginnings of words in sections of handwritten text can be accomplished with relative ease in the normal case. However, subsequent tasks turn out to be extraordinarily complicated. These include segmentation of the words into individual characters and assignment of the individual characters to a definite class of characters, such as words. Consequently, ICR error rates remain high. As such, ICR technology is being adopted slowly, primarily into the data-entry activities of certain types of pen-based computer devices, such as hand-held devices.

Neural networks remain the leading ICR technology. These networks are modeled on the way synapses work in the brain: processing information by recognizing patterns of signals. As such, they adapt themselves into shifting configurations based on what they encounter. In other words, they change as they grow and learn.

Consequently, for each handwritten character or symbol recognized by ICR technology, a confidence level is expressed internally as a percentage and a user picks the threshold below which he or she wants to flag uncertain characters or symbols. Like speech recognition technology, a training or setup period is required for this emerging technology.

Other Recognition Technologies

Automatic recognition technologies that identify actual items include **radio frequency identification** (RFID) and **intelligent document recognition** (IDR) **technologies.**

Radio Frequency Identification Technology

RFID technology allows cars to zip through toll plazas without stopping to tender cash and is the alert buzzer that sounds if someone tries to leave a department store before a salesperson removes the plastic tags. The technology is rapidly evolving, primarily in the consumer products industry. In fact, this industry is moving to adopt standards around RFID so that various industries can "talk to each other."

RFID technology works in the following manner: Chips that emit radio signals are embedded in analog items/products. The signals are read and captured by receivers installed in ceilings or toll booths. The receivers act as data collectors and send the signals to PCs on a network, allowing the items/products to be tracked.

RFID's applicability in the healthcare industry is limited only by the imagination. Like bar codes, it is being used to track moveable patients, clinicians, medications, and equipment. As such, in a wireless environment, conceivably, RFID could replace bar codes for these applications.

However, today, the question surrounding RFID is its business value. First, healthcare organizations must install wireless networks with the required access points. However, this is occurring at a rapid rate, despite RFID. Second, today, passive RFID tags—those that become activated when they are in close proximity to a "reader," similar to a bar code reader—cost around 10 to 20 cents each. In comparison, bar code stickers cost around 1 cent. Therefore, today, if, for example, every medication dose in a healthcare organization were to be RFID tagged, the costs remain substantial when compared to bar code tags. On the other hand, RFID users only have to go to the nearest computer and click on an icon to locate patients, clinicians, or equipment.

Intelligent Document Recognition Technology

Recently, an automatic recognition technology has been developed to recognize types of analog documents or forms, eliminating the need for bar codes or other characters/symbols that identify the documents/forms. IDR trains itself to identify document or form types and to sort the information accordingly for subsequent data entry. This training process requires a period of continuously scanning each type of document/form. As such, the pattern of document/form layouts and information locations educates the system to recognize the document/form for future recognition situations.

Electronic Data Interchange and E-Commerce

EDI allows the transfer (incoming/outgoing) of information directly from one computer to another by using flexible, standard formats. These formats function as a common language among many different healthcare "trading" or "business" partners (payers, government agencies, financial institutions, employer groups, healthcare providers, suppliers, and claims processors) who have agreed to exchange the information electronically but use a wide variety of application software with incompatible native formats. In the healthcare industry, with its traditionally strong reliance on paper-intensive processes, the goal of EDI is to eliminate the administrative nightmares of transferring paper documents back and forth between these partners and then hand-keying the information into the partners' disparate computer systems.

No EDI story has been told more often than that of the former American Hospital Supply Corporation (AHSC) in the late 1970s. AHSC pioneered an electronic connection with its customer hospitals that reinforced its position as the country's largest distributor of hospital supplies. Beginning as a "dumb terminal"–based utility for transmitting electronic purchase orders, over time this proprietary system evolved into a PC-based information system that served as the gateway for what became Baxter Healthcare's purchase orders and confirmations.

By the late 1980s, the healthcare industry's business partners expanded their EDI linkages beyond purchase orders to electronic invoices and payments. At the same time, the American National Standards Institute (ANSI) chartered the Accredited Standards Committee (ASC) X12 to create standard, electronic formats for all business transactions. ASC X12's Insurance Subcommittee (X12 N) Healthcare Task Group developed many standard healthcare transactions, including healthcare claims (837), healthcare payments and remittance advices (835), and healthcare claim status requests (276).

However, acceptance by the healthcare industry to use these standards as the tools for conducting business electronically was atrociously slow. The unfortunate outcome of the industry's self-imposed obstacles to the adoption of standards-based EDI increased the need for paper-based and telephone callback business processes, resulting in even higher costs and less efficiencies than the older, manual systems.

In 1991, the Workgroup for Electronic Data Interchange (WEDI), a public/private task force, was established by HHS to develop an action plan for healthcare standards-based EDI: standardizing and implementing electronic data exchange to reduce the healthcare industry's inefficient administrative processes and increasing costs. WEDI's 1993 report underscored the need to establish uniform content and coding so that healthcare data could be exchanged quickly, easily, and inexpensively via interconnecting networks. Also, the report recommended industrywide, standards-based EDI implementation guidelines. Such guidelines included establishing unique identification numbers for patients, providers, and payers; ensuring security to protect confidential medical and financial information; and enabling eligibility checking, verification of claim status and copayments, and referral information. The then HHS Secretary Louis Sullivan proposed that standards-based EDI would decrease paperwork and result in savings of $4 to $10 billion annually (HHS 1993). These WEDI/HHS recommendations and proposals became the drivers that forced the enactment of Title II, Administrative Simplification, of HIPAA.

HIPAA's proposed rule on the EDI/coding standard transaction set was published in August 2000. Its original compliance date was extended to October 16, 2003, on which date the regulation was officially implemented. The rule mandates that healthcare "covered entities"/"business partners" implement a common standard (ASC X12 N) for the transfer of information and accept the standard-based electronic transaction. This regulation does not apply to the transfer of data and information within a healthcare organization, but it does apply to the transfer of data and information external to and between healthcare organizations.

By the new millennium, the term *EDI* (but not the concept) had become somewhat dated. With the mid- to late 1990s lightning-effect introduction and widespread acceptance of the Internet and its derived technologies, such as the Web, the term *e-commerce* began to replace the term *EDI*. Today, e-commerce is used to describe the integration of all aspects of business-to-business (B2B) and business-to-consumer (B2C) activities, processes, and communications, *including* EDI.

In addition, the term *e-health* is now used to describe the application of e-commerce in the healthcare industry. Several principles and concepts of e-health directly relate to EDI principles and concepts. These include the links among the healthcare trading/business partners; the links to healthcare equipment and supply vendors, providers, and health plans; and the transactions for exchanging data on healthcare eligibility, referrals, claims, and so forth.

Enterprise Master Patient Indexes/ Identity Management

Too often, breakdowns in patient identification cause patient record errors that threaten data integrity. The most common error occurs when healthcare provider organization registration personnel fail to locate existing patient information in the organization's MPI, including the patient's unique identification number. The patient is then assigned another record (in other words, a duplicate record) and a new file is created in the database. When this error occurs, it is unclear into which database file the patient's data should be entered. This often results in unnecessary duplicate tests, billing problems, and increased legal exposure in the case of adverse treatment outcomes.

Another common error occurs when registration personnel incorrectly register a patient under another person's existing, unique identification number. This error of overlay results in the merging of two different patients' data into one file. The clinical risks are obvious.

As healthcare organizations continue to come together into integrated delivery networks (IDNs), the probability increases that information about a patient is spread across multiple databases and in multiple formats. In addition, the information is updated and accessed by multiple transaction processing systems and personnel. This causes problems when the IDN begins to assemble information about a patient in order to deliver care across diverse systems and encounters. Longitudinal applications, such as the EHR system, cannot be successful.

Consequently, healthcare provider organizations are developing strategic initiatives for EMPIs. In the broad sense, this involves the increasingly important service referred to as **identity management.**

EMPIs provide access to multiple repositories of information from overlapping patient populations that are maintained in separate systems and databases. The approach is through an indexing scheme to all unique patient identification numbers and information in all the organizations' databases. As such, EMPIs become the cornerstones of healthcare system integration projects.

EMPIs work in two ways. In the back end, EMPIs coordinate recordkeeping. The indexes receive information from multiple systems that need no modification. The receiving is often performed through an integration gateway or engine. The enterprise index tests to see whether the patient is identified in all of the systems; if not, it may assign a unique identification number or other, related identifier as well as correlate records throughout the enterprise.

In the front end, EMPIs receive requests from existing registration systems to send data to these systems. Usually, these existing registration systems need some reprogramming to enable them to request and receive data from the EMPI. Currently, there is no consistent, accepted trigger event and standard data format to do this.

EMPI building is complex. Variations in ISs, data capture, and organizational goals and objectives present multiple challenges to integrating patient data. For example, EMPI building involves a multitude of decision points. These include deciding whether to employ centralized or distributed data storage; whether to maintain limited, additional information such as allergies and encounter histories or robust information such as problem lists; and whether to establish batch processing or real-time communication between the registration system and the EMPI.

In addition, EMPIs include complex capabilities. These capabilities include merging records pertaining to the same person using probabilistic matching/algorithms, maintaining source systems' pointers, removing duplicate records, and providing a common user interface. Finally, after technical and organizational issues are overcome, the purely operational tasks of linking patients across multiple entities and episodes of care and maintaining these linkages are difficult and can be costly.

Data Repositories

Data repositories are powerful databases that exist in every industry and are designed to store large amounts of data. Typically, these databases are organized into data fields, data records, and data files.

Typically, the model of these databases is relational. In other words, the data are stored physically in the database using two-dimensional tables that create a relation. The format of the data is usually structured, and the type of data is discrete. Therefore, this model forces the database architect to predict how many data fields, records, and files will be stored about a particular event.

Some **relational databases** contain binary large objects (BLOBs) in their tables that consist of unstructured data, such as free-text data, bit-mapped data, real audio data, streaming video data, or vector graphic data. More commonly, relational databases contain pointers in their tables that indicate other, physical data repositories containing the unstructured data.

Another model of these databases is the **object-oriented database.** An object can contain several types of unstructured data. Typically, these data types are stored in the database tables with specific behavior rules or procedures. For example, streaming video data are stored in the database tables with "fast-forward" or "rewind" behavior rules. This model cannot force the database architect to predict how many data fields, records, and files will be stored about a particular event.

Typically, in healthcare provider organizations, the term *data repository* is used to refer to databases that are relational and store structured, discrete, patient clinical, administrative, and financial data. As such, the repositories storing patient clinical data are often called clinical data repositories (CDRs), the repositories storing patient financial data are often called financial data repositories (FDRs), and so on. Sometimes one data repository physically stores all the organization's structured and discrete clinical, administrative, and financial data related to patients.

To provide continuous, high-quality care for patients, all the physical data repositories in healthcare provider organizations must be linked logically. These repositories include the relational databases that store structured, discrete, patient clinical, administrative, and financial data as well as the object-oriented databases that store unstructured, patient free-text, bit-mapped, real audio, streaming video, or vector graphic data. The EMPI primary index keys, the patients' unique identification numbers, are the links.

In addition, the organizations' logically linked, physical data repositories must be designed to allow **online/real-time transaction processing** (OLTP) of the data stored in the repositories. In other words, the data are entered into the repositories by the organizations' various "feeder" applications, and the users must be able to manipulate, update, retrieve, and otherwise act on the data in real time while the data are stored in the repositories. This requires data repositories to include tools designed to perform intricate data searches and retrievals.

For example, a healthcare provider organization's CDR typically incorporates powerful, centralized, relational database management technology. In an online/real-time mode, the CDR allows providers of care to access and manipulate patient-structured and discrete, administrative, and clinical data, such as patient demographic data, physician orders, nursing care plans, and laboratory/radiology/pathology results. It also allows providers to access and manipulate patient-unstructured, free-text data, such as transcribed clinical report data.

Electronic Document/Content Management Systems (ED/CM)

A **document** is any analog or digital, formatted, and preserved "container" of data or information, collectively referred to as **content.** The document is a well-worn and very useful human construct. It really has not changed much in 5,000 years. People like doing some very basic things using documents, things that do not change just because document data/information were once contained on stone tablets and, today, are electronic and contained in spreadsheets, e-mail messages, and laboratory test result reports.

For example, people like to be able to exchange documents, read documents, and know what the documents mean. One reason why many healthcare professionals still resist using data/information systems to accomplish their daily work functions and processes is that viewing or reading an IS's "data" (informational representations of the system's transactions) is, plainly, unaccommodating to the human eye. Unless the data are formatted, accompanied by printlike qualities, such as headings or bolding, and contained in documents, "data" are difficult to interpret.

It is for this reason that documents, and not data, are required for evidentiary discovery purposes. To settle legal disputes, the transaction *presentation, not representation,* is required for all business record documents. In healthcare organizations, this involves the retrieval of the bill "document," the consultation report "document," the photograph "document," the image "document," and so on.

An ED/CM system is any electronic system that manages an organization's analog and digital documents/content (that is, not just the "data") to realize significant improvements in business work processes. Like most ISs, an ED/CM system consists of a number of component technologies that support both digital and analog document/content management.

These component technologies are discussed in the following sections.

Document-Imaging Technology

Document-imaging technology is one, and only one, of the many ED/CM system component technologies. This technology electronically captures, stores, identifies, retrieves, and distributes documents that are not generated digitally and/or are generated digitally but are stored on paper for distribution purposes. Currently, in healthcare provider organizations, documents that typically are not generated in a digital format, are stored on paper, and are candidates for this technology include handwritten physician problem lists/notes; "fill-in-the-blank," typeset nursing forms; preprinted Conditions of Treatment forms; and external documents (documents from the outside).

By digitally scanning (faxing) the documents, the technology converts the analog data on the document into digital, bit-mapped, document images, discussed in a previous section of this chapter. As more and more documents are created, distributed, and stored digitally, the dependence on, and use of, this technology decreases.

Document Management Technology

For every type of document as well as for every section or part of a document, **document management technology** automatically organizes/assembles, secures, and shares documents. Some of the more common document management technology functions include document version control, check in-check out control, document access control, and text/word searches.

Electronic Records Management Technology

Business records are bound by legal and regulatory requirements. Consequently, formats for long-term preservation, storage media for long-term viability, and strategies for record migration and accessibility are required **electronic records management technology** components that must ensure the authenticity, security, and reliability of an organization's electronic records. For example, mass storage is required for the massive amounts of structured and unstructured data as well as the large number and kind of documents stored in ED/CM systems. The major, mass storage medium used in ED/CM systems is magnetic, including disk (for example, Redundant Array of Independent Disks [RAID], Network Attached Storage [NAS], Content Addressable Storage [CAS]) or tape options. For extraordinarily large amounts of data and lengthy document archive requirements, the optical medium might be used, including Compact Disk-Read Only Memory (CD-ROM), CD-Recordable, Digital Versatile Disk (DVD; read only or recordable), or magneto-optical-based Write Once Read Many (WORM) options.

In addition, ED/CM system records must be properly classified under appropriate categories so that appropriate legal and regulatory retention rules can be applied. Users must determine how to identify and declare these records so that the records and/or record documents can be deleted/ purged/destroyed at a defined point in their life cycle.

Workflow/Business Process Management (BPM) Technology

BTM technology allows computers to add and extract value from document content as the documents move throughout an organization. The documents can be assigned, routed, activated, and managed through system-controlled rules that mirror business operations and decision processes. For example, in healthcare organizations, **workflow technology** automatically routes electronic documents into electronic in-baskets of its department clerks or supervisors for disposition decisions.

Computer Output Laser Disk/ Enterprise Report Management Technology

Computer output laser disk (COLD)/enterprise report management (ERM) technology electronically stores, manages, and distributes documents that are generated in a digital format and whose output data are report-formatted/print-stream originated. Unfortunately, documents that are candidates for this technology too often are printed to paper or microform for distribution and storage purposes. COLD/ERM technology not only electronically stores the report-formatted documents but also distributes them with fax, e-mail, Web, and traditional hard-copy print processes. One of the more recent trends for ERM is to store the coded, report-formatted output data natively and convert the data to **eXtensible Markup Language** (XML) or **HyperText Markup Language** (HTML) when needed. In healthcare provider organizations, such documents generated by COLD/ERM technology typically include "green bar" financial system reports, Uniform Bills (UBs)/CMS (formerly known as HCFA) 1500s, laboratory cumulative result summary reports, and transcribed, word-processed medical reports.

Automated Forms-Processing Technology

Automated forms-processing (e-forms) technology allows users to electronically enter data into "online forms" and electronically extract the data from the online forms for various data-manipulation purposes. Powerful contextual verification processes have made such operations highly accurate. In addition, the form document is stored in a form *format,* as the user sees it on the screen, for ease of interpretation.

Digital Signature Management Technology

Digital signature management technology offers both signer and document authentication for analog or digital documents. Signer authentication is the ability to identify the person who digitally signed the document. Implementation of the technology is such that any unauthorized person will not be able to use the digital signature. Document authentication ensures that the document and the signature cannot be altered (unless both the original document and the change document are shown). As such, document authentication prevents the document signer from repudiating that fact.

Secure Messaging Systems

Messaging systems electronically deliver data/information to users. As such, e-mail systems are messaging systems. However, secure messaging systems eliminate the security concerns that surround e-mail but retain the benefits of pro-active, traceable, and personalized messaging. These systems are not transaction (data) processing systems. Also known as secure notification delivery systems, these systems store and forward content to users in an asynchronous, "anytime" mode.

In healthcare, secure messaging systems often are referred to as **clinical messaging systems** because these systems are important, pervasive tools that are included in a broad set of contextual collaboration tools for clinicians. Other clinical collaboration tools include synchronous, real-time tools, such as instant messaging, chat servers, and Web/media conferencing. However, secure clinical messaging is the most heavily used because it crosses time zones, can be done in each clinical user's own time frame, and gives clinical recipients time to think over and then respond to issues, such as notifications of abnormal laboratory test results. In addition, clinical messaging does not require all participants to be available at the same time and eliminates the scheduling problems associated with the real-time tools.

Secure clinical messaging systems work in the following manner: When a CIS generates a patient alert regarding a possible drug interaction or an anomalous test result, the secure clinical messaging system immediately routes the alert, along with patient data, to a caregiver's designated pager number, fax machine number, telephone number, or e-mail address. In turn, clinicians can securely send these alerts to other, related clinicians. Also, messages can be automatically escalated to the next available caregiver if the original caregiver does not respond within a predefined time frame. In addition, messages can be tracked throughout the care delivery network.

Most of today's secure clinical messaging systems fall into one of four architectures: peer-to-peer networking, a message staging server installed inside the network's firewall, a staging server installed outside the firewall (usually hosted), and a wholly outsourced service. A message staging server installed on an organization's virtual private network (VPN) works best for larger organizations that collaborate regularly with the same business partners. A hosted staging server works best for smaller organizations that benefit from a premessage payment plan. When a secure clinical messaging system's staging server is installed inside the network's firewall, the server can act as a "will call" window for authenticated viewing (Tabar 2003).

Web-Derived Technologies and Applications

It is an understatement that the Internet has transformed the healthcare industry and its stakeholders. Likewise, it is an understatement that the Internet will continue to grow, change, and influence everything in the 21st century. Because of this relatively new phenomenon, having only made its impact beginning in the late 1990s, the full range of social, economic, political, cultural, and historical perspectives regarding what we today know as healthcare and information management will continue to be drastically transformed in less than a tenth of the time it took to change over the last half century and in ways that, today, are unimaginable.

Consequently, for HIM professionals to take advantage of the opportunities afforded by the Internet phenomenon, it is important to review some of the many, current technologies and applications that have been developed only because of the Internet and its two dominant applications/**protocols:** e-mail (Simple Mail Transfer Protocol [SMTP]) and the World Wide Web (HyperText Transfer Protocol [HTTP]). For the purposes of this book, the following Web-derived technologies and applications are highlighted: Web-based information systems, Web portals, Web-based **intranets/extranets, Web content management systems,** and **Web services.**

Web-Based Information Systems and Applications

In past decades, healthcare information system (HIS) vendors were forced to migrate their existing systems and products from proprietary, centralized processing-based architectures running on mainframe computers, minicomputers, and microcomputers to open, client/server-based architectures. This required a lot of time and money in terms of company research and development (R&D). In many cases, it involved a total rewrite of the systems' code. For those HIS companies that designed their systems based on client/server architectures, they, too, were required to expend a lot of R&D time and money. This was because such firms typically had to transition from 16-bit to 32-bit hardware and software components, which also involved a total rewrite of the systems' code.

Ironically, at the same time that thousands of computer components were being "thickened" to 32 bits, maintaining thick client workstations and their multitude of corresponding servers became an IT department's worst nightmare. Also, during this time, the Internet and its derived technologies began to be introduced, offering a simpler and more cost-effective alternative to computer system development and maintenance.

However, the mass introduction and acceptance of the Internet and its derived technologies once again forced HIS companies to make another transition: to **Web browser-based or Web native architectures.** This, again, required a lot of R&D. In all cases, it involved a total rewrite of the systems' code.

Unfortunately, many HIS companies with legacy and/or client/server-based systems no longer could afford to make the next transition to Web browser–based/Web native architectures. Consequently, many of these companies began to transition their existing systems and products to Web browser–based/Web native architectures by Web-enabling the systems.

With Web enabling, the HIS companies did not rewrite their systems' code in the newer, Web native programming languages, such as HTML, SGML, XML, or Java and its derivatives. Instead, when an authorized user logs onto the system, he or she is presented with a Web page. From the Web page, the companies' systems applications (for example, applications written in Microsoft's 32-bit Visual Basic) are launched.

Web browser–based or Web native systems are more complex. These are systems where companies have either written or rewritten their systems' code using one or more of the above-mentioned, Web native programming languages. In Web browser–based/Web native systems, the Web browser acts as the primary desktop interface for access to a healthcare organization's repositories. The Web browser is used to display and query (for example, to drill down via hypertext) information stored in databases as quickly as client/server-based systems. (For comparison purposes, in Web browser–based/Web native systems, the retrieval application typically resides on the server. In client/server-based systems, the retrieval application typically is loaded on standard, thick client workstations.)

Web browser–based/Web native systems accept data inputs from other systems and send them to other databases over the network using plug-ins or display controls, such as Active X or CORBA. These systems are OLTP systems and have been proven to reduce network administration and workstation maintenance costs.

Web Portals

No one IS can provide all the applications, data types, and data formats needed by all of the healthcare industry's diverse healthcare organizations and users. Consequently, healthcare provider organizations maintain multiple, disparate "feeder" applications for their data repositories. Depending on their size and systems acquisition philosophies, some healthcare provider organizations maintain and often integrate large numbers of disparate feeder applications, and others maintain and integrate at least two or three.

Each disparate feeder application for the repository has a unique user interface, uses different data nomenclature, and takes limited advantage of data standards. Therefore, it is not only difficult to integrate the information from the disparate systems into the repositories, but it is also difficult for the organizations' users to learn and interact with the different systems.

Consequently, the concept of the **clinical workstation** evolved during the early 1990s so that one single point of access to the data in the repositories and to the applications "feeding" the data into the repositories would be deployed at the clinician's workstation or desktop. This single point of access would include a common user interface to view the information from the disparate applications as well as to launch the applications.

During this time, Microsoft's Windows® operating system products became ubiquitous for PC client workstations. Consequently, the Windows-based graphical user interface (GUI) was originally deployed at the clinical workstation.

However, with the mid- to late-1990s introduction and widespread acceptance of the Internet and its derived technologies, the Web browser began to be deployed as the user interface of choice.

Today, the term *clinical workstation* is still used to describe the presentation of healthcare data and the launching of applications in the most effective way for healthcare providers. However, for all intents and purposes, the concept of Web-based, clinician/physician portals has replaced the concept of the clinical workstation.

A **Web portal** is a single point of personalized access (an entryway) through which to find and deliver information (content), applications, and services. Web portals began in the consumer market as an integration strategy rather than a solution. Portals offered users of the large, public, online Internet service provider Web sites, such as AOL, fast, centralized access (via a Web browser) to an array of Internet services and information found on those Web sites.

Consequently, like clinical workstations, **clinician/physician Web portals** first were seen as a way for clinicians to easily access (via a Web browser) the healthcare provider organizations' multiple sources of structured and unstructured data from any network-connected device. Like clinical workstations, clinician/physician Web portals evolved into an effective medium for providing access to multiple applications as well as the data. And because clinician/physician portals are based on Internet technologies, they became the access points to sources of data and applications both internal and external to the organization.

In short, clinician/physician Web portals have become, and can be considered analogous to, internal, private Webs. As such, the portals provide centralized security both internal and external to the organization. This is accomplished by restricting access to data and applications contained within the portal to authorized users. Examples of authorized users for healthcare provider organizations include a role (for example, physician), an individual (for example, Chris Jones, MD), a group of individuals (for example, all the physicians in the organization), a department (for example, internal medicine), or a group of departments (for example, surgical subspecialties).

In addition, clinician/physician Web portals provide simplified, automated methods of creating **taxonomy,** or classifying data. Consumer portals, such as Yahoo.com, provide good examples of this, whereby files and data corresponding to food, fashion, and travel are organized for easy access. Finally, true clinician/physician Web portals have at least one search engine and allow customization at the role and individual level. As such, search engines must be able to search e-mails, file servers, Web servers, and databases; and customization must allow users to create individual, relevant views. The clinical benefits of these portal features and functions are obvious.

With the success of clinician/physician Web portals, a growing number of healthcare provider and payer organizations have established Web portals for their patients/members.

Each participant receives an account on the Web portal with a unique log-in and password. Typical payer-based portal uses include accessing membership information and choosing a primary care physician. Typical provider-based portal uses include requesting prescription renewals, scheduling appointments, and asking questions of providers via secure messaging. Increasingly, **patient/member Web portals** are allowing patients to pay their bills online and to securely view all or portions of their provider-based, electronic medical record, such as current medical conditions, medications, allergies, and test results.

Although patients/members access the portals over the Internet, all the information, including the secure messaging applications, resides on the provider's/payer's secured servers. As such, these portals dovetail well with HIPAA, which empowers patients/members with the authority to determine who can have access to their healthcare information. Also, patients can use the portal to notify providers if their EHR is incorrect. As consumers seek to take a larger role in their healthcare, such patient/member "entryways" to information (content), applications, and services are expected to become more common.

Intranets/Extranets

Web-based information systems and applications cannot continue to proliferate without creating Web-based intranets designed to enhance communication among an organization's internal employees and facilities and Web-based extranets designed to enhance communication among an organization's external business partners. This is because intranets link every employee within an organization via an easy-to-navigate, comprehensive network devoted to internal business operations and extranets link an organization's external business partners with the same, comprehensive network, but one that is devoted to external business operations.

Just as Web portals are analogous to internal, private Webs, Web-based intranets are analogous to internal, private Internets. Access to data and applications contained within the intranet is restricted to authorized users. This is so that the general Internet public cannot access this private, secure network. However, through its intranet, a healthcare organization can access the Internet's servers for general Internet mail and messaging.

Like Web portals, Web-based intranets are growing at an astounding rate. They offer better security than use of the "public" Internet. Moreover, they are less expensive to implement and easier to use than most private networks of proprietary mail and messaging software products. In fact, today, intranets have become so important that almost every healthcare provider organization uses them as some form of development platform.

For example, these private, secure networks provide every healthcare organization employee basic information, such as message boards, employee handbooks, manuals, mail, cafeteria menus, newsletters, directories, and contact lists.

Also, they are used for the development of the organization's EHR. Here, the challenge is to evolve from the intranet's "static," informational, and brochureware-based Web pages to "dynamic" Web pages where authorized intranet users can access the private network's Web-based applications from anywhere and at anytime. This requires a powerful, stable infrastructure that can handle the transmission of larger amounts of data and support dynamic applications during times of peak use. It also requires continuous management of all the information and content on the intranet so that its users can find what they need to do their jobs better and so that the intranet information is kept current.

Extranets connect intranets that exist outside an organization's firewall. For example, typically, an IDN's autonomous care facilities (for example, acute care, long-term care, home health care), each with its own intranet, need to communicate between and among themselves via secure e-mail or other collaboration tools. As such, the facilities connect the various intranets and form an extranet.

Another example is when organizations connect to their external suppliers of equipment or trading partners so that they can exchange information. In a hospital, the companies that supply medical equipment for the hospital can, with an extranet, "peer into" the **par levels** (the accepted, standard inventory levels for all supplies and equipment in an organization) of the hospital's supply inventory to determine when the various supply par levels are getting lower and it is time to reorder. Thus, forming an extranet prevents a hospital employee from having to check inventory and write a reorder. In this example, the hospital's supplier or trade partner can "peer into" only this portion of the hospital's intranet and automatically send the supplies when needed.

Web Content Management Systems

Publishing a few static or dynamic pages on an organization's intranet- or extranet-based Web site is relatively easy. However, getting a group of people to do this effectively is challenging. Getting many groups of people to create the pages, track the revisions, set up the workflow, and scale and secure the intranet/extranet's framework is quite difficult from an organizational perspective.

Web content management systems label and track the exponential increase in and variety of information that is placed on a Web site so that the information can be easily located, modified, and reused. These systems are a critical component in personalizing an organization's Web-based intranet/extranet, Web portal, and page content for site users and visitors. They also provide crucial versioning and globalization capabilities. *Versioning* enables each of the Web site's content components to be tracked individually. Then, as the content changes, each iteration of the content can be identified and the overall Web site can be recreated as it existed at any specific point in time. *Globalization* enables the look and feel of an organization's Web site to be managed centrally, while specific content is managed for local require-

ments, such as regional healthcare language or procedure differences.

Web Services

Web services technology is a platform for software applications (or services) whose basic communication mechanism is XML, the universal language of the Web and the accepted format for data exchange over the Internet. In addition, Web services utilizes Web-based infrastructure protocols, such as HTTP and transmission control protocol/Internet protocol (TCP/IP). As such, Web services allows programs written in different languages and on different operating systems to communicate with each other in a standards-based way. In other words, Web services is an open, standardized way of integrating disparate, Web browser–based and other applications.

By using XML messages to format/tag data, Web services technology allows for data interchange without the need for translation. In addition, the messages use system-independent vocabularies and protocols, such as Simple Object Access Protocols (SOAP), to transfer the data; Universal Description, Discovery, and Integration (UDDI) to list what services are available; and Web Services Description Language (WSDL) to describe the services available.

Unlike traditional Web-based client/server architecture, such as a Web server/Web page system, Web services technology does not provide the user with a GUI, such as the browser. Instead, it shares business logic, data, and processes through a programmatic interface across a network.

Healthcare organizations have been gradually installing Web services to ease integration of disparate Web-based and legacy applications, often written in incompatible languages. This ensures that the organizations' applications **interoperate** and that healthcare organizations can more easily choose tools for important interorganizational and regional data sharing. (See figure 3.2, p. 60.)

Like other, traditional technologies and systems, Web-derived technologies and applications have inherent benefits. Similarly, the issues surrounding the successful deployment of the technologies and applications in healthcare provider organizations are complex. For example, technical hurdles that must be overcome in using intranets, portals, and Web content management systems are found at every point of the compass; some are obvious, and some are hidden. More important, implementation of the business processes that breathe new life into healthcare organizations via these technologies and systems is difficult. Developing and using Web-derived technologies and applications takes time and commitment, usually without obvious, upfront, hard-dollar benefits.

Application Service Providers

ASPs are service firms that deliver, manage, and remotely host standardized (prepackaged) applications software through centralized servers via a network, not exclusively, but more commonly, the Internet. The software is provided

Figure 3.2. Web services

©2005 Deborah Kohn.

through an outsourcing contract. As such, the ASP is viewed as a type of outsourcing. The contract is based on fixed, monthly usage, "rental-like" fees (for example, flat rate and per registered user fees) or transaction-based fees (for example, per transaction or percentage of revenue). The emphasis of this arrangement is on the functional use, rather than on the ownership, of a system (Nussbaum 2001, p. 3).

ASPs share many characteristics with the other types of outsourcing. The former service bureaus of the 1980s and 1990s, which provided remote time-sharing services, existed during a time when hardware costs and knowledge to operate the hardware were expensive and not widely available. Service bureaus were a type of outsourcing that allowed healthcare provider organizations to concentrate management attention on its core business of patient care and not become distracted or diverted into IT challenges.

Times changed, and the high connectivity costs plus substantial monthly fees associated with service bureaus became less attractive than smaller, more robust and flexible systems that could be operated locally. But the concept of outsourcing did not dissipate. The remote computing option became an extension of the service bureau concept. Currently, this type

of outsourcing is offered by many of the major HIS vendors. The difference is that remote computing outsourcing requires a substantial cadre of healthcare organization–employed and local IT professionals to operate the organization's software while the system's hardware and software reside in the vendor's data center.

The appeal of the ASP to both IT buyers and sellers is based on its position as a type of outsourcing somewhere between remote computing and full-asset outsourcing, which involves the transfer of all staff, long-term relationships, and accountability from internal IT management to a contracted third party. For example, major capital IT expenditures are the responsibility of the ASP. Consequently, healthcare organizations no longer need to fund large, upfront IT expenditures. Traditionally, chief financial officers crafted leases or similar arrangements to help mitigate some of the cash flow impact of IT purchases. However, the ASP is also responsible for all the systems' maintenance and upgrades, which, under a leasing arrangement, are the responsibility of the healthcare organization. In addition, the ASP offers various payment methods, such as fixed monthly fees or transaction-based fees. Consequently, the ASP outsourcing model permits a more predictable monthly cost, potentially over a shorter duration.

Although the ASP model offers many benefits, a number of issues must be understood as detracting from its appeal. Perhaps the least favorable aspect of the ASP outsourcing model is the likelihood that the healthcare organization must accept a standard, off-the-shelf product. For the ASP to maintain its system efficiently and effectively for all its customers, often users are not allowed the level of customization or tailoring to which they are accustomed. Often healthcare organizations lose control on the time of system upgrades as well as the response time for changes to the software. The ASP may be faced with conflicting priorities among its customers in terms of demand for specific features and functions.

Given the need for integration and interfacing between and among a healthcare organization's disparate ISs, it is not a trivial exercise to consider how to integrate and interface ASP offerings into healthcare organizations' existing or future IT environments. Virtually all ASPs in healthcare limit their deliveries to their owned applications. Where multiple source applications are delivered and customer owned, virtually none is provided with a common user interface.

It is also not trivial to change an ASP in the event it files for bankruptcy or no longer participates with its customers in a partner-based relationship. Last but not least, security is a major concern, with the healthcare organization still maintaining full responsibility for firewalls and HIPAA compliance.

Many ASP delivery models reflect the application breadth, source, level of integration, interfaces, customer risks, and associated services. Thus, the delivery of the ASP model varies based on the organization's current environment and value. Currently, the most significant targets for ASP consideration appear to be healthcare provider organizations with smaller investments in IT and/or that have difficulty retaining technical expertise and resources. This includes physician practices, small acute or specialty care facilities, and stand-alone clinics.

Check Your Understanding 3.4

Instructions: Answer the following questions on a separate piece of paper.

1. Give a healthcare example for each of the following automatic recognition technologies: bar coding, OCR, ICR, RFID, and IDR.

2. How are the concepts of EDI, e-commerce, and e-health interrelated?

3. What is driving the heightened interest in EMPI technology within the healthcare industry?

4. What types of data are commonly maintained in an object-oriented database associated with a clinical data repository?

5. What is an ED/CM system? Explain the value of the following technologies: document-imaging technology, Workflow/BPM technology, COLD/ERM technology, automated forms technology, and digital signature management technology.

6. Explain why secure clinical messaging is often preferred over real-time tools such as instant messaging or chats?

7. How are Web browser–based systems different from Web-enabled systems?

8. What is the primary purpose of the clinical workstation and the clinician/physician portal?

9. How do Web portals established by providers/payers assist consumers in taking a larger role in their healthcare?

10. What is the difference between an intranet and an extranet? Give an example of how each can be used in healthcare.

11. What are the benefits and drawbacks of choosing to use the application service provider (ASP) model for providing IT applications to a healthcare organization?

Supporting Managerial and Clinical Decision Making

Many current and emerging information technologies are used to support managerial and clinical decision making. For the purposes of this book, the following technologies and systems are highlighted:

- **Data warehouses** and **data marts**
- **Decision support systems**
- **Artificial intelligence**

Data Warehouses and Data Marts

Data warehouses are large, centralized, enterprise-wide collections of all the historical, demographic, and transactional data and information about businesses that are used to support managerial or, in the case of healthcare provider organizations, clinical decision-making processes. Data warehousing is the acquisition of all the business data and information from potentially multiple, cross-platform sources, such as legacy databases, departmental databases, and online transaction–based databases, and then the warehouse storage of all the data in one consistent format. Data mining is the probing and extracting of all the business data and information from the warehouse and then the quantifying and filtering of the data for analysis purposes.

Like data repositories, data warehouses are powerful databases. And, like data repositories, typically the format of the data in the warehouse is structured and the type of data is discrete.

However, the model of the data warehouse database is typically subject oriented. In other words, the data within the data warehouse are organized along subject lines (customer, product, patient, clinician) rather than along operational lines (accounting, management, medicine, surgery) in order to be accessible and useful across the enterprise. For example, healthcare provider organizations use data warehouses to centrally organize patient information, to establish wellness plans supporting community medicine, and to reduce costs.

In addition, the data are stored in the warehouse database using multidimensional tables rather than two-dimensional tables that create a relation as in relational databases. For example, if a surgeon performs a certain procedure several times during a period of time, the data query also may need to include the average length of stay (ALOS) for the procedure.

Therefore, the warehouse data must be structured so that the identifying data (such as a procedure, time period, or ALOS) reside in the database dimension headers (which are comparable to the row and column headers of a spreadsheet) rather than being repeated for each record as in relational databases. This multidimensional model, sometimes referred to as a physical cube, lends itself to trend analysis and forecasting.

Generally, for day-to-day operations, a healthcare organization needs relatively current data and each operational unit needs only its own data. That is why relational and object-oriented database models for data repositories are well suited for OLTP. But for large-scale, retrospective data analysis, for which **online/real-time analytical processing** (OLAP) is designed, a healthcare organization generally needs not just its current status, but also a historical record over time or time variance, encompassing all the organizational operating units by subject for comparison purposes.

In addition, for large-scale data analysis, a healthcare organization generally requires summary data, not detail data. Using the above surgeon and procedure example, the data query may need to know only the summary figure for the ALOS.

Finally, warehouse data, when correctly recorded, cannot be updated like repository data. Generally, only two kinds of operations occur in a data warehouse: data warehousing and data mining. This is referred to as the nonvolatility of warehouse data.

In healthcare, data warehouses have been used primarily for the following applications (Henchey 1998, p. 68):

- *Clinical management:* For example, every day, patient clinical data are fed into the warehouse from multiple sources to contribute to enterprise-wide best practices and to identify areas of excessive variation from best practices.
- *Operations management*: For example, sophisticated analytical tools, such as cost accounting, case-based budgeting, and variance analysis tools, are included with the warehouse to determine new healthcare market opportunities.
- *Outcomes management:* For example, data mining is conducted to study patient health status or other factors, such as satisfaction, that contribute to clinical outcomes.
- *Population management:* For example, to proactively manage the health of plan members, data mining helps the organization to predict utilization or identify at-risk members requiring case management.
- *Revenue management:* For example, the data warehouse assists healthcare financial analysts in addressing all the different contractual and regulatory reimbursement formulas. With revenue based on a mix of several dimensions, such as fee-for-service, capitation, and risk pooling, only the data warehouse can provide a complete picture of the enterprise's revenue stream and the factors controlling it.

A data warehouse cannot simply be bought and installed. Its implementation requires the integration of many products within its architecture. For example, often data warehouses require advanced data warehousing and mining techniques and tools. The software must be able to locate data that often are stored on multiple servers that may include any type of machine or operating system. The software must be able to maintain **metadata** (indexed data about the data), such as what indexes the acquired data uses. Further, the software must be able to recognize data duplication and exceptions as well as issue alerts when data are not present or have been corrupted.

Data marts can be thought of as miniaturized data warehouses. Data marts are usually geared to the needs of a specific department, group, or business operational unit. Because data marts are considerably smaller in both size and complexity than data warehouses, some healthcare organizations build data marts as a way of testing data warehouses on smaller, more focused scales. What many are finding, though, is that data marts can easily proliferate into a collection of incompatible data stores with accessibility or utility limited to the department or operational unit that designed the mart.

Decision Support Systems

Decision support systems (DSSs) are interactive computer systems that intend to help decision makers use data and models to identify and solve problems and make decisions. A great deal of innovation is occurring related to DSSs, and the technologies that make them up are changing rapidly.

Generally, DSSs are based on either a data repository model or a data warehouse model. Both transfer data from an operational environment (either in real time or retrospectively, in batches at fixed intervals) to a decision-making environment, and both organize the data in a form suitable to decision support applications.

Power (1997) suggests that DSSs can be classified based on one or more of the following five categories:

- *Communications-driven DSSs* emphasize communications, collaboration, and shared decision-making support. A simple Internet bulletin board or threaded e-mail is the most elementary level of functionality in this type of DSS.
- *Data-driven DSSs* emphasize access to and manipulation of internal, and sometimes external, structured business data. Simple file systems accessed by query and retrieval tools provide the most elementary level of functionality in this type of DSS.
- *Document- or graphics-driven DSSs* focus on the retrieval and management of unstructured business data. Basic document- or graphics-driven DSSs exist in the form of Web-based search engines.
- *Knowledge-driven DSSs* can suggest or recommend actions to decision makers. These DSSs are person-

to-computer systems with specialized problem-solving expertise. The expertise consists of knowledge about a particular domain, understanding of problems within that domain, and skill at solving some of those problems.

- *Model-driven DSSs* emphasize access to and manipulation of a model, for example, statistical, financial, optimization, and/or simulation models. Simple statistical and analytical tools provide the most elementary level of functionality in this type of DSS.

A wide variety of DSSs and related tools and technologies exist in healthcare, most of which can be classified as hybrids of the above categories. These systems include, but are not limited to, **clinical/medical decision support systems, management information systems** (MISs), **executive information systems** (EISs), **geographic information systems** (GISs), and **expert decision support systems.**

Clinical/Medical Decision Support Systems

Typically, clinical/medical decision support systems are data driven. They assist clinicians in applying new information to patient care through the analysis of patient-specific clinical/medical variables. Clinical/medical decision support systems can be characterized simply by providing reminders and alerts, clinical guideline advice, therapy critiquing, or benchmarking tools. However, many of these systems are used to enhance diagnostic efforts and, thus, quality of care, by including computer programs that provide extensive differential diagnoses based on the clinical/medical data and information entered by the clinician (Barnett et al. 1987). Many systems streamline workflow processes and enhance efficiencies. Other forms of clinical/medical decision support systems seek to prevent medical errors and improve patient safety. These DSSs include tools such as antibiotic management programs and anticoagulation dosing calculators (Hunt et al. 1998).

For years, clinical/medical decision support systems have been the subject of industry criticism. Clinicians complain that the system tools often are populated with general, textbook-type information that is not actionable or that the tools contain too much information that distracts the clinicians. Also, some systems simply do not blend well into care processes and are perceived as a source of additional work by already busy clinicians. In some instances, the tools are so complicated that clinicians cannot use them effectively. In addition, often the systems have been architected and executed only partially, resulting in limited functionality and unmet expectations (Krohn 2004).

Management Information Systems

Typically, MISs refer to the broad range of data-, document-, or knowledge-driven DSSs that provide information concerned with an organization's administrative functions (in other words, those functions that are associated with the provision and utilization of services). In addition, DSS-based MISs enable management to interrogate the computer on an ad hoc basis for various kinds of information within the organization so as to predict the effect of potential decisions. As such, DSS-based MISs provide information to people who must query these systems to make disposition decisions about valuable resources in a timely, accurate, and complete manner. Such systems are crucial for the effective administration of any organization and include, but are not limited to, general accounting and financial systems, customer relationship management (CRM) systems, enterprise resource planning (ERP) systems, and operations/plant management systems.

Executive Information Systems

EISs are DSSs that support the decision making of senior managers. As such, they provide direct online access to timely, accurate, and actionable information about aspects of a business that are of particular interest to a senior healthcare manager. Typically, this information is provided in a useful and navigable format so that managers can identify broad strategic issues and then explore the information to find the root causes of those issues. According to Kelly (2001), the following EIS features and functions are essential:

- The system must be specifically tailored to executives' information needs.
- The system must be able to access data about specific issues and problems.
- The system must be able to aggregate data into meaningful reports.
- The system must provide extensive online analysis tools, including trend analysis, exception reporting, and drill-down or data-mining capabilities.
- The system must be able to access a broad range of internal and external data.
- The system must be easy to use (typically mouse or touch screen driven).
- The system must be able to be used directly by executives without assistance.
- The system must be able to present information in a graphical form.

Geographic Information Systems

In the strictest sense, GISs are DSSs capable of assembling, storing, manipulating, and displaying geographically referenced data and information. In other words, GISs identify data according to their locations. The applications of GIS in healthcare extend from practical community-based services to sophisticated studies on a global scale. For example, pediatricians consult community-based GISs to observe neighborhoods with high concentrations of lead and decide whether lead screenings would be appropriate for certain patients.

Expert Decision Support Systems

Expert decision support systems (also referred to as systems that use principles of artificial intelligence) use a set of rules or encoded concepts to construct a reasoning process. Such rules or concepts are based on knowledge developed from consultation with experts on a problem and the processing and/or formalizing of this knowledge in such a manner that the problem can be solved. In other words, expert DSSs provide the kind of problem analysis and advice that an expert might provide if he or she were present as a consultant.

Some of the various rules-based processing techniques used by expert DSSs are neural networks and data mining, defined earlier in this chapter. Other techniques include (Siwicki 1996, p. 47):

- *Fuzzy logic:* A rules-based system that mimics human thought and enables a computer to "think" in inexact terms rather than in a definitive, either-or manner
- *Genetic algorithms:* Tools that examine data and determine by programmed stipulations which data best match a stated goal and which data do not
- *Symbolic reasoning:* A method of deduction that follows an explicit line of inferences

Expert systems "learn" based on the continual addition of data to the system. Therefore, in its simplest model, the technologies of speech recognition or ICR can be considered expert. These technologies adapt themselves into shifting configurations based on what they encounter, and they change as they grow and learn.

Artificial Intelligence

In other disciplines and industries, the term *artificial intelligence* is often used synonymously with the term *expert decision support systems.* Because expert decision support systems, especially those using neural network techniques, "learn" as humans do by processing information through recognizing patterns of signals, there are only a few differentiators.

The field of artificial intelligence (AI) is the branch of computer science concerned with endowing computers with the ability to simulate human intelligence and behavior. As such, AI attempts to understand intelligence and intelligent entities and then design computer systems to perform functions normally associated with language, learning, reasoning, and problem solving.

This involves developing systems that think and act like humans. This human-centered approach to AI involves empirical science, which, in turn, involves hypothesis creation and experimental confirmation. This also involves developing systems that think and act rationally. A rationalist approach to AI involves a combination of mathematics and engineering.

Exploring and furthering the application of AI to clinical situations is lofty because of the vital and crucial nature of medical science as well as the need for accurate and timely data and information to support clinical decisions. Consequently, AI to support clinical decision making focuses on the gathering, availability, security, and use of medical information throughout the human life cycle and beyond.

Check Your Understanding 3.5

Instructions: Answer the following questions on a separate piece of paper.

1. What features differentiate a data warehouse from a data repository?
2. What is the primary difference between expert decision support systems and, more common in healthcare, clinical decision support systems?
3. What functional capabilities are associated with applications that use artificial intelligence technology?

Supporting the Diagnosis, Treatment, and Care of Patients

Many current and emerging information technologies are used to support the diagnosis, treatment, and care of patients. For the purposes of this book, the following technologies are highlighted:

- **Physiological signal processing systems**
- **Point-of-care information systems**
- Mobile/wireless technology and devices
- Automated care plans, **clinical practice guidelines, clinical pathways,** and protocols
- Telemedicine/telehealth
- Electronic health record systems
- Computer-based patient information and education

Physiological Signal Processing Systems

The human body is a rich source of signals that carry vital information about underlying physiological processes. Traditionally, such signals have been used in clinical diagnosis as well as in the study of the functional behavior of internal organs.

Earlier in this chapter, physiological signal processing systems, such as ECG, EEG, EMG, and fetal trace systems, were mentioned because these systems store data based on the body's signals and create output based on the lines plotted between the signals' points. The data type used by these systems is referred to as signal tracing or vector graphic data.

Physiological signal processing systems measure biological signals. Also, they help to integrate the medical science of analyzing the signals with such disciplines as biomedical engineering, computer graphics, mathematics, diagnostic image processing, computer vision, and pattern recognition. The integration of these disciplines allows these systems to electronically compile measurement equations, estimate the signals' parameters, and characterize the feedback elements. For example, the computer-based analysis of the neuromuscular system, the definition of cardiovascular system models, the control of cardiac pacemakers, the regulation of blood sugar levels, and the development of artificial organs not only serve patient diagnostic and care purposes, but they also support the development and simulation of instrumentation for physiological research and clinical investigation.

Point-of-Care Information Systems

Computer systems that allow healthcare providers to capture and retrieve data and information at the location where the healthcare service is performed have come a long way since hard-wired computer terminals with green screens were first placed at the patient's bedside more than 25 years ago. Functionally, almost every type of patient clinical and administrative application has been introduced to provide care services at the bedside, in the exam room, at the home, or even on the patient, as in medical monitoring. Technologically, massive changes have occurred in these systems' platforms, footprints, and networking capabilities.

For example, many acute care facilities have installed clinical point-of-care information systems that, among other services, provide online medication order entry, profiles, administration schedules, and records. The records include information about medications not given (with reasons) as well as related information such as fluid balances, physical assessments, laboratory test results, and vital signs. All medications, including unit doses, are bar coded and scanned at or near the patient's bedside along with the patient's wristband and the caregiver's identification badge. This prompts a safety edit, documents administration of the medication, and generates the charge. Other acute care facilities have installed administrative point-of-care (or service) systems that have eliminated admitting areas. Inpatients are greeted at the door with their room assignments, and roving admissions representatives visit patients in the assigned rooms to complete all the admission procedures.

Typically, point-of-care information systems use portable, handheld, wireless devices to enable entry of the data by a bar code scanner, keypad, or touch screen. Also, the devices are used to upload and download information to and from hard-wired workstations. Retrieval of the data occurs at the wireless device or on wall-mounted or portable, cart-based computers. The data also can be entered and retrieved on hard-wired workstations located in areas outside the point of care, such as central areas at patient care units, back offices, central or satellite pharmacies, and physician lounges/homes/offices.

Mobile/Wireless Technology and Devices

Perhaps the biggest influence on, as well as challenge for, point-of-care information systems and their use comes from recent, significant advances in **wireless technology** and smaller, mobile devices. For the healthcare industry, the successful integration of wireless technology and smaller, mobile devices with point-of-care software supports and enhances the clinician's decision-making processes.

True wireless systems use wireless networks and wireless devices to access and transmit data in real time. At the basic level, wireless technology is based on the use of radio waves. For the purposes of this chapter, the technology is divided into two categories: (1) regulated and unregulated, and (2) wide area and in-building.

For the general benefit of the country, Congress has charged the Federal Communications Commission (FCC) with regulation of the radio spectrum. This regulation encompasses licenses for the use of the radio frequencies for commercial radio, television, walkie-talkies, and mobile telephones. Specific portions of the radio spectrum may be assigned to specific users, such as individual radio stations, or set aside for general and usually low power use, such as Citizens Band (CB) radio.

For years, healthcare organizations have used in-building wireless point-of-care information systems, such as telemetry systems. These systems were based on existing technologies and use a portion of the radio spectrum reserved for industrial, scientific, and medical purposes (ISM band). Individual licenses are not required for these types of systems.

Also, provider organizations have long used wide-area wireless technology to support ISs, such as point-of-care systems. This technology involves microwave systems that are based on fixed, point-to-point wireless technology used to connect buildings in a campus network. Microwave systems are regulated and require licenses and compliance with FCC procedures.

Until recently, most in-building wireless systems were proprietary. However, adoption of the IEEE 802.11 wireless technology standard has begun to provide a reasonable level of standardization. The IEEE 802.11 standard allows data transmission speeds up to 11 megabits per second, is relatively low power, and does not require licenses for installation and use. The IEEE 802.11b is an international standard that provides a method for wireless connectivity to fixed and portable devices within a local area. As such, this standard allows interoperability among multiple vendor products.

But it is the widespread adoption of cellular telephone technology that has significantly advanced the development of wireless technology and, consequently, its support for point-of-care systems. A brief look at most healthcare organizations today turns up mobile phones, two-way pagers, Internet-enabled telephones, and **personal digital assistants** (PDAs).

Currently, the majority of these mobile devices are used to meet personal, individual needs. For wireless technology and the smaller mobile devices to be integrated into larger corporate projects such as point-of-care information systems, they must significantly enhance the function and use of existing ISs. Ironically, existing, healthcare provider organization ISs, including point-of-care information systems, were not designed to support clinician workflow but, instead, were developed to automate specific functions, as described above. As a result, often clinicians must access multiple systems to retrieve the information they need and spend 10 minutes each day simply logging on.

On the other hand, mobile devices improve this paradigm by allowing clinicians to use a device personalized to their individual workflows, such as clinical (for example, e-prescribing), dictation, and billing workflows, not functions. In addition, mobile devices provide clinicians the information they need anytime, anywhere, and on any network-addressable device.

Therefore, increasingly, healthcare organizations are taking advantage of wireless technology and mobile devices. Impediments that have prevented a more widespread use of the technology and devices for point-of-care systems and other workflows include:

- Impediments preventing widespread use of wireless technology
  - Vendor difficulty in packaging wireless technology with specific clinical software applications that demonstrate a significant return on investment and add value to the clinician
  - The use of proprietary wireless technology
  - Inconsistent technology deployment
  - The need to make a large investment for the deployment of wireless technology on a wide scale
  - The need to make a large investment for the underlying network infrastructure to support wireless technology
- Impediments preventing widespread use of smaller, portable, point-of-care devices
  - Battery life, including how and when batteries will be recharged
  - Device weight and where the devices will be stored when not in use
  - Screen real estate
  - Application functionality (for example, how the data are delivered in bits and are not presented in a page-oriented fashion, how the processing of the data must be transactional, and how an abundance of frivolous graphics or poor-quality content cannot be tolerated)

Automated Clinical Care Plans, Practice Guidelines, Pathways, and Protocols

The terms used to describe practice mandates, care process guides and documents, disease management (a.k.a. chronic care improvement) decision algorithms, and quality improvement tools are not well standardized. They tend to be used informally and interchangeably, resulting in miscommunication among healthcare professionals.

Consequently, when **clinical care plans,** practice guidelines, pathways, and protocols are automated and used by multidisciplinary teams, patient care can be affected unless the definitions are uniformly applied. For example:

- Healthcare providers create clinical care plans for individual patients for a specific time period. Typically, clinical care plans are based on provider training.
- Clinical practice guidelines are recommendations based on systematic statements or clinical algorithms of proven care options. Often professional organizations and associations, health plans, and government agencies such as the Agency for Health Care Policy and Research develop these guidelines.
- For a specific time period, clinical (or critical) pathways or **Care Maps**® delineate standardized, day-to-day courses of care for a group of patients with the same diagnosis or procedure to achieve consistent outcomes. Typically, pathways or Care Maps are developed by the local healthcare organization or health plan.
- Clinicians often use the term *protocol* to refer to the written documents that guide or specify a practice, including clinical practice guidelines and pathways. Strictly speaking, however, protocols are more detailed care plans for individual patients based on investigations performed by professional societies, drug companies, or individual researchers (Bufton 1999, p. 258).

Providers now recognize the enormous variation in how they diagnose, treat, and care for patients. Consequently, there is a trend to adopt **evidence-based medicine** and **outcomes management** based on more use of guidelines, formalized pathways, and protocols. Automating these guidelines, pathways, and protocols for easier access and use is the first step. Also, there is a trend to incorporate care plans into providers' notes. This is being recognized as automated clinical documentation systems are being introduced into and used by more healthcare organizations.

In short, care plans, guidelines, pathways, and protocols, as well as formularies and other knowledge bases, are becoming automated for easier access and use and for easier maintenance. In particular, practice guidelines and knowledge bases that are available through subscriptions from agencies, societies, and research companies can be kept more current because users can incorporate periodic downloads into their transaction-based or analytic systems.

The challenge for automated care plans, practice guidelines, pathways, and protocols is that, like clinical workstations and Web portals, no one form of clinical documentation or one view of the information suits everyone or all situations. For example, the wide variability of clinical documentation is obvious in H&Ps versus consultations. Such documentation suits some providers, but not others, or some situations, but not all. Similarly, views of data are requested in page, narrative, table, flowchart, or graphic formats. Therefore, automated plans, guidelines, pathways, and protocols require customization capabilities to help individuals and groups better share knowledge to reach similar decisions about patient care. Automated drawing tools and anatomical diagrams are other documentation options.

Another challenge is that it is difficult to convert intricate clinical care processes and guideline, pathway, and protocol content into computer architecture. An even higher level of complexity occurs when the content is merged with reengineered processes, instead of just automating the existing or status quo processes. This is because these actions represent a translation of specific and conceptual clinical information and interpretations into data fields. Therefore, it is recommended that clinicians work with IS analysts, such as health information managers, to ensure that the integrity of the clinical content is preserved during the conversion.

In addition, the task of seamlessly embedding reminders or alerts or defaulted, guideline-based clinical orders into ISs as well as the care processes is challenging. According to Bufton (1999, p. 266), this requires in-depth knowledge of the following:

- The computer system's capabilities and limitations, such as data dictionaries, field lengths, screen builders, data retrieval/analysis/reporting capabilities
- The processes of care, local caseloads, and local practice environments
- The many diverse guidelines, pathways, and protocols

Telemedicine/Telehealth

Interactive, patient–provider consultations across gulfs of time and space represent what is often referred to as classic telemedicine or telehealth. However, the field has always encompassed a plethora of strategies for moving clinical knowledge and expertise instead of moving people. As such, telemedicine/telehealth systems, like EHR systems, are concepts made up of several cost-effective technologies used to bridge geographic gaps between patients and providers.

In other words, telemedicine/telehealth is not video-conferencing technology. Rather, it is clinically adequate, interactive, media conferencing (for example, video conferencing) integrated with other technologies. It can be dynamic and include interactive (or real-time processing) technology, or it can be static and include store-and-forward (or batch processing) technology. It includes telecommunications and remote control–based biomedical technologies. It utilizes in-room systems, roll-abouts, desktop systems, and/or handheld units. Often it is integrated with component technologies of the EHR system and/or derived technologies of the Internet. The access and ability to transmit patient records and the integration with reference databases on the Internet all play into the telemedicine/telehealth model.

Telemedicine/telehealth is not a new way to deliver healthcare. It takes existing ways of delivering healthcare and enhances them, such as enhancing patient–provider consultations via "electronic house calls." It extends care to underserved populations, whether they are located in rural or urban areas, and redefines the healthcare organization's community. It transfers clinical information between places of lesser and greater medical capability and expertise.

Like medicine in general, telemedicine/telehealth technology is made up of a number of specialties and subspecialties. Some examples include:

- Telecardiology
- Teledermatology
- Telehome healthcare
- Teleneurology
- Telenursing healthcare
- Teleophthalmology
- Telepathology
- Telepsychiatry
- Teleradiology
- Telesurgery

The telemedicine/telehealth specialty that has been around for the longest time and, perhaps, is the most notable is teleradiology. Even today, spurred by a rising demand for sophisticated imaging tests as well as a smaller pool of radiologists from which to recruit, teleradiology is taking advantage of the speedy Internet transfer of medical data to outsourced, foreign radiologists who provide preliminary interpretations of scans during their normal business hours. In addition, since the early 1990s, the University of Pittsburgh Medical Center, the Mayo Clinic, and other prestigious provider organizations have employed dynamic telepathology interactions. Teleradiology and telepathology specialties are considered first-generation telemedicine/telehealth systems and services because they do not rely on patient interaction.

The second-generation telemedicine/telehealth systems and services involve those specialties relying on patient interaction and consultations. These include teleophthalmology, telepsychiatry, telehome healthcare, and so on.

The latest generation of telemedicine/telehealth systems and services involves patient interaction beyond the consultation. For example, in October 2001, telesurgeons in New York City performed the world's first complete (that is, from start to finish) telesurgery by successfully operating on the gallbladder of a patient in France. This was accomplished by sending high-speed signals through fiber-optic cables across the Atlantic Ocean to robots in a Strasbourg clinic.

As both a clinical and technological endeavor, telemedicine/telehealth plays a key role in the integration of managing patient care and in the more efficient management of the information systems that support it. However, overcoming multiple technical challenges remains a concern. These challenges include the lack of systems interoperability and network integration as well as metropolitan broad bandwidth limitations. Physician resistance; lack of consistent, proven cost-effectiveness; lack of consistent, proven medical effectiveness; and concerns for safety are other challenges that require overcoming complex behavioral, economic, and ethical constraints.

Electronic Health Record Systems

In 1991, the Institute of Medicine (IOM) defined the computer-based patient record (CPR) as "an electronic patient record that resides in a system specifically designed to support users by providing accessibility to complete and accurate data, alerts, reminders, clinical decision support systems, links to medical knowledge, and other aids" (Dick and Steen 1991, p. 11). Fortunately, by the end of the millennium, a common definition of the CPR was under way by various groups: a system consisting of "electronically stored information about an individual's lifetime health status and health care. It replaces the paper medical record as the primary record of care, meeting all clinical, legal and administrative requirements. . . . [It] provides reminders and alerts, linkages with knowledge sources for decision support, and data for outcomes research and improved management of health care delivery" (Dick, Steen, and Detmer 1997, p. 11).

Fortunately, there also was agreement that the CPR system was not one or even two or more products. According to Dick and Steen, the CPR system is a "set of components that form the mechanism by which patient records are created, used, stored and retrieved. . . . It includes people, data, rules and procedures, processing and storage devices, and communication and support facilities" (1991, p. 12). According to Dick, Steen, and Detmer, the CPR system is "an evolving concept that responds to the dynamic nature of the healthcare environment and takes advantages of technological advances" (1997, p. 11). In other words, the CPR system is a concept consisting of an array of integrated, component information systems and technologies.

However, only within the last years did a universal understanding of the CPR system's components emerge, and, along with that, a new, universal term for the CPR system: the electronic health record (EHR) system. During summer 2003, the Bush administration, through HHS, commissioned the IOM to provide an EHR System (EHR-S) Functional Needs and Priority by Care Settings model for a standardized EHR. In addition, HHS enlisted the Health Level-7 (HL-7) standards development organization to create an EHR-S Functional Model and Standard based on the findings of the IOM and to ballot the Functional Model and Standard by 2004. (HL-7 is the organization that develops, by a voluntary consensus process, standards for patient *clinical* electronic data interchange. Founded in 1987, HL-7 consists of a large, broad healthcare IT membership. In addition, HL-7 was accredited in 1994 by the International Standards Organization's [ISO] American National Standards Institute [ANSI].) During spring 2004, HL-7's second Draft Standard for Trial Use on the EHR-S Functional Model and Standard was passed by its members. After a period of two years,

when the draft standard will be tested, it will be balloted as a fully accredited standard.

The significance of this achievement cannot be understated. The EHR-S Functional Model and Standard laid the foundation for the first-generation, standards-based EHR and defined the system's components as elements of an IT infrastructure by which the patient's EHR is created and managed. This infrastructure represents an aggregation of information from multiple, often disparate, databases and systems within and across the healthcare enterprise. It incorporates a messaging standard for common representation of all pertinent patient data. Stored data are indexed with sufficient detail to support retrieval for patient care delivery, management, and analysis. It includes hardware, application software, system software, user interfaces, networks, communications protocols, and so on.

EHR System Infrastructure

Technically, the EHR system infrastructure consists of multiple **physical data repositories.** Typically, these repositories are organized into data fields, data records, and data files. They store structured, discrete, clinical, administrative, and financial data as well as unstructured, patient free-text, bitmapped, real audio, streaming video, or vector graphic data. They must be linked to form one **logical (or conceptual) repository.** Typically, the EMPI primary index keys constitute these links. (See figure 3.3.)

Technically, the EHR system infrastructure also consists of multiple data types, information systems, software applications, and technologies. Examples of multiple data types were given earlier in this chapter. Examples of multiple ISs include most of those discussed in this chapter, such as clinical information systems, HISs, ambulatory care information systems, electronic document/content management systems, picture archive and communication systems, telemedicine systems, patient appointment and resource scheduling systems, physiological signal processing systems, registration/eligibility/enrollment systems, and DSSs. Examples of mul-

Figure 3.3.   Physical and logical data repositories for CPR systems

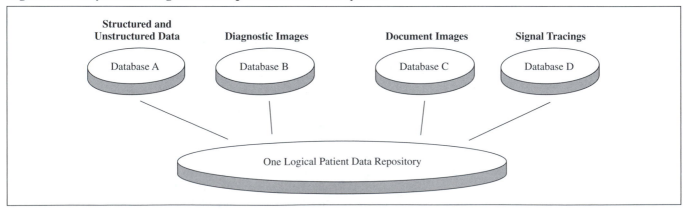

tiple software applications and technologies also include most of those discussed in this chapter, such as workflow and secure messaging software, security/access to ITs, single log-on software, Web-derived technologies, and digital/electronic signature software.

Today, most healthcare organizations have installed at least one or more EHR system infrastructure component technologies or systems. However, unfortunately, the existing components may not be integrated or interfaced.

Typically, several EHR system infrastructure components are implemented in healthcare organizations in parallel. Solely technical attributes of EHR system infrastructure component systems and technologies must not be considered when determining whether and when to implement the various components. Instead, the value of the component to improve the quality of patient care, the fiscal priorities of the organization, the available technical and organizational resources, and the unique business motives and strategies of the organization must be considered.

EHR System Attributes/EHR System Functionality Standards

The 1991 IOM report identified 12 attributes for the CPR system. These attributes represented the elements essential to provide the required functionality that would support healthcare providers with a robust CPR system.

Since then, the attributes have been revised and expanded, most notably those included in the EHR-S Functional Model and Standard. (The EHR-S Functional Model and Standard is discussed in detail in chapter 9.) However, for historical context, it is important to review the original CPR system attributes so that HIM professionals can ensure their completeness as tools with enhanced utility for providing high-quality patient care in light of the ever-changing healthcare environment and technological advances.

Following are the 1991 IOM report's 12 attributes for the CPR system (Dick and Steen 1991):

1. The CPR system offers a problem list.
2. The CPR system measures health status and functional levels (in other words, it measures clinical outcomes).
3. The CPR system documents clinical reasoning and the rationale for patient care decisions.
4. The CPR system provides longitudinal and timely linkages with other patient records.
5. The CPR system protects the privacy of the individual by guaranteeing that the information is confidential (in other words, indicating that the information is sensitive) and the confidential information is secure (for example, by providing audit trail capabilities).
6. The CPR system provides continuous, authorized user access.
7. The CPR system supports simultaneous, multiple user views into the CPR.
8. The CPR system supports timely access to local and remote information resources.
9. The CPR system facilitates clinical problem solving, using specific rule sets or decision support systems.
10. The CPR system supports direct data entry by providers of care, especially physicians.
11. The CPR system supports practitioners in measuring or managing costs and improving quality.
12. The CPR system is flexible to support existing and evolving clinical specialty needs.

According to Dick and Andrews (1995, pp. 66, 78), revised and expanded CPR system attributes were considered crucial to the establishment of robust CPR (and now, EHR) systems. If any one of the attributes were ignored or inadequately addressed in the design and development of the CPR system, the CPR might be jeopardized. Some of these subattributes include:

- The CPR system includes a substantial, flexible, and extensible clinical data dictionary.
- The CPR system supports a well-designed CDR so that the CDR is capable of supporting the extensive and diverse needs of all healthcare practitioners.
- The CPR system includes an array of powerful input capabilities to allow for the direct data entry of caregivers at the point of care.
- The CPR system supports a user-friendly, ergonomically designed presentation of the information for all intended users, including a presentation tailored to the type of individual and to personal preferences.
- The CPR system includes automated, intelligent support that anticipates and facilitates all clinical processes and thinking.

Current Status of Electronic Health Record Systems

No one disputes the fact that EHR systems have the potential to improve care quality and patient safety at lower costs. Furthermore, technologically, the chances of realizing the EHR vision are better today than ever before, primarily thanks to the advent of the Internet and its derived technologies model. As such, much can be done today to prepare and continue to implement the EHR system's component systems and technologies.

However, today, several years after the original IOM report, EHR systems remain far from the various standards for patient medical records. In addition, it is anticipated that still more years will pass before most healthcare organizations fully install EHR systems and, therefore, fully realize the systems' potential.

Some health information technology (HIT) professionals argue that, as originally defined and agreed to, a CPR/EHR system is not what is needed and that the system's objective should not be a theoretical ideal or concept but, rather, a focus on all the patient care processes and related systems and technologies that produce immediate, clear benefits and value (Drazen 2001). For example, implementing clinical DSSs, CPOE systems, medication administration systems, and patient registry systems can provide huge advantages in patient care and safety.

On the other hand, most HIT professionals agree that the biggest challenge in implementing all the processes and related systems and technologies is the inability to seamlessly share information between the various systems and technologies, even with well-established messaging and other standards. This lack of systems interoperability has been caused by the standards' lack of information models for the management of the data, leading to enormous standards flexibility. As such, this flexibility has led most healthcare IS developers to interpret and implement the standards in a conflicting, nonuniform, and proprietary manner. Therefore, despite significant standards development and compliance efforts, healthcare organizations have been left with thwarted attempts for reliable, quick, and cost-effective EHR systems.

Along these lines, some HIT professionals argue that interoperability must precede any EHR use. They view the risk of implementing processes and systems as an opportunity that might lead irreversibly to treatment of health information as a proprietary asset of delivery systems. They believe that if standards are not solidified and built into EHR systems now, a generation of investment will be wasted (Brailer 2005).

Another challenge is that EHR system quantitative returns on investment have not been consistently demonstrated. Consequently, there remains a bewildering array of EHR initiatives, activities, and debates, with only a few proving to be good assessment vehicles. For example, provider organizations continue to buy huge, difficult-to-implement systems from one large vendor for millions of dollars, which does little to restore the confidence that there will be a future market for other, more focused products, especially those products that must focus on smaller provider organizations, such as physician offices.

As long as the healthcare industry continues to do this and as long as interoperability remains elusive, EHR systems will advance, but not quickly or cost-effectively.

Computer-Based Patient Information and Education

During the past decade, the use of e-commerce (in other words, the use of the Internet and its derived technologies to integrate all aspects of business-to-business and business-to-consumer activities, processes, and communications) has transformed every vertical market industry. In the healthcare industry, the following examples illustrate this transformation:

- Increasing numbers of patients access the Internet for information about healthcare providers, treatment options, and personal health information (PHI).
- Health Web sites provide patients with tools to develop and maintain personal, online health records independent of providers.
- Healthcare providers and patients correspond via e-mail, with each viewing and contributing information to the health record.

- Health plans, disease-specific groups, and professional associations use Web sites to provide education and interact with patients.

As a result, plausible scenarios regarding a patient's health information include the following:

- Personal patient information might be obtained and used inappropriately by unauthorized individuals or organizations. Unfortunately, several examples of targeted marketing based on unauthorized use of individually identifiable health information have been cited.
- A patient's information might be accessed fraudulently and altered without detection. Also, the accessed information might be incomplete, incorrect, out-of-date, or misinterpreted, potentially resulting in financial or health-related harm to the patient.
- A patient might inadvertently enter the wrong medication in an allergy portion of a **personal health record** (PHR). In a subsequent episode of care, this information might be accessed and used to make prescribing decisions. The patient might have an allergic reaction and file suit.
- A hacker might break into the records of a provider and make entries in numerous records indicating a serious, chronic disease. The patient's credit rating, employment, or ability to get health insurance might be affected.

Contrary to popular belief, the information patients share with their care providers has never been completely private and protected. A national survey released in January 1999 found that one in five people believes that his or her PHI has been used inappropriately, without his or her knowledge or consent. More striking, one in six Americans engages in some form of privacy-protective behavior to shield themselves from what they consider to be harmful and intrusive uses of their PHI (California HealthCare Foundation 1999).

But because of the Internet and its e-commerce transformation, the situation has become more acute. For example, traditional, organizational HIM processes have become inadequate. Centrally controlled processes such as release of information in accordance with a valid authorization are not easily administered in cyberspace. Authentication of health record entries to verify responsibility and accuracy is more complex when managing an Internet-connected longitudinal, rather than episodic, health record. Safeguarding against misinterpretation of treatment findings is more difficult when patients have online access to information, potentially even seeing test results before the provider.

Computer technology can offer suitable solutions to traditional HIM problems. However, technology without effective policy will neither meet patients' requirements nor be adequate for providers who remain legally responsible for much of the information. According to Goldman and Hudson, without ubiquitous and strong privacy rules and their enforcement, the promise of the Internet and e-commerce to transform the quality of healthcare people receive might become just another failed venture that further disempowers people (2000, pp. 140–48).

Consequently, the quality of care that people receive as well as the integrity of information needed to improve the health of the larger community are at stake. Therefore, more than ever, promoting health through education and protecting patient information are values that must go hand in hand.

E-Health

Simply stated, e-health is the application of e-commerce to the healthcare industry. E-health offers businesses and consumers the opportunity to provide or engage in a number of services, including:

- Personal health records
- Patient appointment scheduling
- Patient registration
- Previsit health screening, evaluations, and assessments
- Postvisit patient education
- Information on health conditions, diseases, wellness, or new healthcare developments
- Support for handheld, point-of-care devices

E-health offers businesses and consumers clear, potential benefits, including:

- Enabling patients and staff to do more with less support
- Streamlining managed care contract administration, EDI, and claims processing
- Building relationships and brand equity with patients, physicians, and affiliated providers
- Improving access to vital patient information
- Reducing care costs
- Improving care delivery
- Building market image and position
- Improving employee productivity and morale
- Facilitating pharmaceutical research, clinical trials, and regulatory submission
- Promoting direct contact with patients

Healthcare organizations must be able to provide high-quality services through e-health to realize the above benefits. Although most organizations have the necessary technology to provide these services, e-health initiatives are often hindered by an organization's culture to accept the profound changes that e-health can bring about.

Following are key qualities required of an e-health culture:

- *Quick:* The growth of e-health requires that organizations respond more quickly to communications from patients and customers. Because of e-health technologies' speed and ease of use, the people served by healthcare organizations have come to expect equally fast replies. To promote this level of speed within the organization's culture, healthcare professionals must support and encourage quick decision making, helping the organization to become accustomed to a faster pace of operation.

- *Patient focused and service oriented:* Although all healthcare organizations are in the business of serving people, many ISs still are not truly patient focused and thus not e-compatible. As e-health technologies continue to allow patients to seek help through a wider variety of sources, organizations that, in the past, did not provide high-quality service through patient-centered systems are going to fall behind. To promote greater patient focus and service orientation in the organization's culture, healthcare professionals must determine where the service shortcomings lie and then make the necessary improvements. For example, a new e-health-based patient appointment and resource scheduling system will not enhance patient service if patients still have to wait an hour to be seen by a provider after they arrive at the point of service.

- *Partnership-friendly:* To implement many of the e-health technologies and systems to support the delivery of healthcare and the management and communication of health data within the healthcare organization, many partnerships and outsourcing relationships with vendors have developed. To promote better relationships with these partners, healthcare organizations must develop other partnerships for purposes other than technology. As such, an organization that is comfortable working with all kinds of partners has a much broader range of tools available because it employs high-tech means to improve service to patients.

As the wave of e-health continues, the challenge to HIM professionals is clear. They can understand the potential of e-health in the industry and can control and direct its power to the benefit of their customers, health plan members, and patients. Or they can allow the technologies to roll uncontrolled through and around their organizations (for example, not establishing strict policies and procedures for PHI included in e-mail messages). If they choose the latter, they will effectively hand over their rich knowledge base and expert skills to faster-moving, better-focused professionals, some of whom may not even exist yet.

Personal Health Records

Personal health records (PHRs) electronically populate elements or subsets of PHI from provider organization databases into the electronic records of authorized patients, their families, other providers, and sometimes health payers and employers. A range of people and groups maintain the records, including the patients, their families, and other providers. The development of PHRs parallels the consumer-centrism long evident in other vertical market industries, such as banking, where consumers maintain and examine their activities 24 hours a day in a secure electronic environment.

PHRs come in a variety of forms and formats, with no standard design or model yet to emerge. In recent years, the American Health Information Management Association

(AHIMA) has vigorously promoted the use of PHRs and has provided definitions and attributes for standardization.

For example, AHIMA defines the PHR as "an electronic, lifelong resource of health information needed by individuals to make health decisions. Individuals own and manage the information in the PHR, which comes from healthcare providers and the individual. The PHR is maintained in a secure and private environment, with the individual determining rights of access. The PHR does not replace the legal record of any provider" (AHIMA 2005).

In addition, AHIMA suggests that the following attributes describe more completely the "ideal" PHR:

Functionality
- Aids the transition from paper to electronic record-keeping
- Allows the individual to refill prescriptions electronically
- Addresses the major issues of health literacy skills (reading and writing) in the context of culture and language
- Allows selective retrieval and formatting of information by individuals or agents
- Is portable (remains with the individual)
- Helps the individual organize personal health information
- Educates the individual about personal health information
- Assists the individual with decision making and health management and wellness (for example, reminders of health activities, health risk assessments, and public health and patient safety alerts)
- Is flexible and expandable to support evolving health needs of the individual and family

Format and Content
- Dynamic record that is continuously updated
- Standard format is electronic
- Incorporates paper documents and other media formats
- Linked with, or contains copies of, provider's legal or electronic records
- Original and immediate source of information is identifiable
- Includes dates of entry and occurrence of all information
- Contains lifelong health information
- Not considered a complete record
- Not restricted by any one format
- Not the legal record or electronic health record of a provider
- Not restricted by culture or language
- Providers use their professional judgment, as they do with any patient-supplied history, for clinical decision support or health management of the individual

Privacy Access and Control
- Private and secure
- Controlled by the individual

- Accessible any place and time by individual
- Accessible in an emergency
- Individual has primary responsibility for the information

Maintenance and Security
- Audit trail shows what information was viewed, by whom, and when
- Amendable by original source as a means of maintaining record integrity
- Individual decides what is incorporated into his or her record

Interoperability
- Achieves easy, accurate, and consistent exchange with others by using communication and health vocabulary standards
- Standard-driven to support evolving health information technology
- Supports structured data collection from individual and stores information using a defined vocabulary
- Links to supportive educational, management, productivity, and quality knowledge bases (AHIMA 2005)

Currently, the most common PHR variations and models include:

- *Shared data record:* The shared data record model consumes the largest number of PHRs and is the most effective. Here, both provider (or employer or health plan) and patient maintain the record. In addition, the provider (or employer or health plan) supports the record. As such, the patient receives and adds information over time. The focus of this model is to keep track of health events, medications, or specific physiological indicators, such as exercise and nutrition.
- *EHR extensions:* The EHR extensions model extends the EHR into cyberspace so that an authorized patient can access the provider's record and check on the record's content. Often this model also allows an authorized patient to extract data from the healthcare provider's record. The record is still maintained by the provider but is available to the patient in an online format.
- *Provider-sponsored information management:* The provider-sponsored information management model represents provider-sponsored information management by creating communication vehicles between patient and provider. Such vehicles can include reminders for immunizations or flu shots, appointment scheduling or prescription refill capabilities, and monitoring tools for disease management in which regular collection of data from the patient is required.

Several issues are at stake. The first is whether a provider organization will be willing to work with a PHR. For example, increasing consumer demand for useful PHRs will make it mandatory that an EHR system be capable of sending and receiving data from a PHR. Another issue is whether a patient can trust the network that is transmitting his or her information. Currently, large-scale deployment and adoption of Internet-based PHRs remains slow because of ongoing privacy and security challenges.

In 2002, the American Society for Testing and Materials (ASTM) Committee E31 (Healthcare Informatics), Subcommittee 26 established a standard for PHRs on the Internet. Content for the standard was based on the e-health tenets developed by AHIMA in 2000.

PHRs have tremendous implications for the future of HIM professionals. HIM professionals will become the custodians of the online dimension of PHRs and their information on top of the organization's EHR system and paper records. Consequently, HIM professionals must answer a number of questions as they begin to create PHRs for consumers/patients, link PHRs to education and the healthcare community, and integrate the PHRs with other patient or health plan member information. For example (Hagland 2001):

- Who will be the stakeholders who will be developing and implementing PHRs?
- How will the PHRs fit into the organization's existing culture and processes for patient information access?
- If the organization has installed component technologies of the EHR system, how will PHRs integrate with those existing components?
- How will PHRs fit into the organization's strategic IT plan?
- What will be the privacy, security, and confidentiality dimensions of the PHRs?
- What will be the budgetary implications?
- What will be the organization's marketing and public relations implications?
- What will be the medicolegal implications?
- If an outsourcing partner maintains the PHRs at least partly or fully, what will be the practical and strategic implications of that decision?

Check Your Understanding 3.6

Instructions: Answer the following questions on a separate piece of paper.

1. Give at least five distinct examples of diagnostic tests that involve physiological signal processing.

2. What patient data are typically collected and viewed (accessed) by care providers using point-of-care systems?

3. What is driving the increased use of computerized care protocols in healthcare?

4. Describe how second- and third-generation telehealth applications differ in functionality from first-generation applications such as teleradiology.

5. Why is it that an electronic medical record created by scanning/faxing analog paper documents into digitized, bit-mapped images does not fit the description of a CPR as defined in the 1991 and 1997 IOM reports?

6. Why is HL-7's Draft Standard for Trial Use on the EHR-S Functional Model and Standard significant?

7. Give at least five examples of services healthcare organizations are offering their customers utilizing e-health technology?

8. What are the characteristics of an e-health culture in a healthcare organization?

9. Describe the differences among the following three common models for the PHR: shared data record, EHR extensions, and provider-sponsored information management.

Supporting the Security of Data and Information

Many current and emerging information technologies are used to support the security of healthcare data and information. They are the same technologies used to support the security of data and information in most vertical market industries. What sets the healthcare vertical market industry apart is the application of the technologies according to the second portion (Title II) of HIPAA, which mandates the protection of health information.

For the purposes of this book, the following technologies are highlighted:

- Encryption/cryptography
- Biometrics technology
- Firewall systems
- Audit trails

Encryption/Cryptography

Computer technology's greatest strengths also are its greatest weaknesses. For example, computer technology, especially the Internet and its derived technologies, easily allows anyone to send and receive information. However, it also easily allows anyone to intercept a transmission.

Cryptography is an applied science in which mathematics transforms intelligible data and information into unintelligible strings of characters and back again. **Encryption** technology uses cryptography to code digital data and information. This is so that the information can be transmitted over communications media and the sender of the information can be sure that only a recipient who has an authorized decoding "key" can make sense of the information.

There are two broad categories of encryption. The first category is symmetric or single-key encryption. Here, each computer uses software that assigns a secret key or code. One computer uses the key to code the message, and the other computer uses the same key to decode the message before the recipient can read it. This form of encryption requires both computers to have the same key.

The second category is asymmetric or **public key infrastructure** (PKI) encryption. PKI does not require that both computers have the same key to decode messages. A private key is known to one computer, which gives a public key to the other computer with which it wants to exchange encrypted data. The public key can be stored anywhere it is convenient, such as on a Web site or with an e-mail. The second computer decodes the encrypted message by using the public key and its own private key.

To prevent abuse, some type of authority is needed to serve as a trusted third party. A certification authority (CA) is an independent licensing agency that vouches for the individual's identity and relationship to the individual's public key. Acting as a type of electronic notary public, a CA verifies and stores a sender's public and private encryption keys and issues a digital certificate or "seal of authenticity" to the recipient.

These keys come in various strengths or levels of security. The strengths vary not only according to the algorithm that codes the data, but also on how well the encoding and decoding keys are maintained. The more bits a key has, the harder it is to break the code without massive computer assistance.

For Internet sites, the use of private and public keys is handled behind the scenes by users' computer browsers and the Web servers for the sites. For example, when a healthcare Internet user performs an online, interactive business transaction, a secure socket layer (SSL) PKI is used to exchange sensitive healthcare data and information.

PKI is becoming the de facto encryption technology for secure data transfers and online authentication. As such, its use will enable healthcare organizations to meet HIPAA's regulations concerning the security of data and electronic signatures.

Biometrics Technology

Biometrics technology verifies a person's identity by measuring (comparing different mathematical representations of) biological and physical features or traits unique to the individual. For example, in signature verification technology, the biometrics of a handwritten signature are measured to confirm the identity of an individual. In data access technology, the biometrics of a hand (hand geometry), fingerprint (fingerprint matching), eye (iris or retinal scanning), voice (voice verification), or facial feature (facial image recognition) are measured to confirm the individual's identity.

Unique, positive identification or verification without the fear of replication or duplication for access to confidential health information is critical. As such, HIPAA requires a mechanism to ensure the authentication of the user and to restrict the user only to those systems that he or she is authorized to access. But because positive identification is so reliable as a personal identifier, individuals might feel that their privacy is threatened or compromised.

Fingerprint matching is the oldest and most popular type of biometrics technology. Everyone has unique, immutable fingerprints made of a series of ridges, furrows, and minute points or contours on the surface of the finger that form a pattern. Retinal scanning is quite accurate because it involves analyzing the layer of blood vessels at the back of the eye. But it is not as popular an identification technology because of the close contact users must make with a scanning device and thus is unfriendly for users wearing eyeglasses or contact lenses. Iris scanning is less intrusive than retinal scanning but is considered clumsy to use.

Facial image recognition requires an unobtrusive, digital camera to develop a dynamic, facial image of the user.

Unfortunately, matching dynamic images is not as easy as matching static images, such as two or more fingerprints or iris scans. Therefore, positive identification based on multiple biometrics technologies currently has the most promising potential for authentication purposes.

Firewall Systems

Firewalls are hardware and software security devices situated between the routers of a private and public network. They are designed to protect computer networks from unauthorized outsiders. However, they also can be used to protect entities within a single network, for example, to block laboratory technicians from getting into payroll records. Without firewalls, IT departments would have to deploy multiple-enterprise security programs that would soon become difficult to manage and maintain.

Firewalls originated during the 1980s and were used to screen a network's incoming data from unwanted, outside addresses. At that time, networks were not large and complicated. Consequently, firewalls were not foolproof and were easy to circumvent.

By contrast, today's massive and complex networks demand firewall systems fortified with software applications that, for example, authenticate users, encrypt messages, scan for viruses and spyware, and produce audit trails. Technically, most firewalls are made up of proxy and filtering services. Proxy services are special-purpose programs allowing network administrators to permit or deny specific applications or features of applications. They screen user names and all information that attempts to enter or leave the private network. Filtering allows the routers to permit or deny decisions for each piece of information that attempts to enter or leave the private network.

Firewalls are based on preestablished rules that allow or deny access to the network or exchange of information between the networks. As such, firewalls enforce security policies so that everything not explicitly permitted is denied. For example, firewall systems determine which inside services may be accessed from the outside, which outsiders are permitted access to the permitted inside services, and which outside services may be accessed by insiders. For a firewall to be effective, all traffic to and from the networks must pass through the firewall, where it can be inspected.

The firewall itself must be immune to penetration. Unfortunately, a firewall cannot offer protection after an attacker has gotten through or around it.

Audit Trails

Audit trails are chronological sets of records that provide evidence of computer system utilization. Data are collected about every system event, such as log-ins, log-outs, file accesses, and data extractions. As such, audit trails are used to facilitate the determination of security violations and to identify areas for improvement. Their usefulness is enhanced when they include trigger flags for automatic, intensified review.

Today, audit trails serve as strong impediments to computer data abuse. For example, the presence of these tools promotes awareness that people who access confidential information can be tracked and held accountable.

Care must be taken to determine which audited data elements are required by law or which ones are exceptions. Following are some suggested data elements to track activity in healthcare information system audit trails:

- Date and time of event
- Patient identification
- User identification
- Access device used
- Type of action (view/read, print, update/add)
- Identification of patient data access by a category of content
- Source of access and software application used
- Reason for access by category (patient care, research, billing)

Practical issues concerning the use of audit trails involve trust. For example, healthcare organizations must be able to distinguish between users who access patient records for patient care and those who access them for unauthorized purposes. Frequent sampling by organizational managers or "tiger teams" is one way to determine system usage within an environment of trust. Delegating to users the responsibility to examine their own audit histories is another way to determine this. It is recommended that the results of audit trails be published and included in employee performance reviews.

Check Your Understanding 3.7

Instructions: Answer the following questions on a separate piece of paper.

1. What is public key infrastructure, and why is it receiving so much attention within the healthcare industry?

2. What are the benefits and drawbacks of using each of the following human features for authentication purposes: fingerprints, iris images, and facial images?

3. Firewalls protect network access by employing proxy and filtering services. What are proxy services and filtering services?

4. What are two practical ways to instill user trust in healthcare organizations when deploying information system audit trails?

Healthcare Informatics and Health Information Management

Health information management is the healthcare industry's professional field that ensures that high-quality data and information are available to every type of authorized user who depends on the data/information to deliver high-quality healthcare services and to make high-quality healthcare-related decisions. HIM professionals serve not only the healthcare industry, but also the public. By managing, compiling, analyzing, and utilizing data from many sources, HIM professionals identify ways to better utilize healthcare resources, more accurately provide patient billing and reimbursement services, reveal public health patterns, and establish new medical treatments vital for improved patient care and administrative purposes.

Trained HIM professionals manage the quality of the data/information content, including its timeliness, appropriateness, accuracy, relevance, and integrity. In addition, HIM professionals develop policies to meet information management standards as mandated by the government and other regulatory and accrediting organizations. Most important, HIM professionals work diligently to protect the privacy of the individual and the confidentiality of the data/information they make available to legitimate users.

Historically, healthcare and healthcare-related data and information have been collected, stored, and transmitted using paper technologies. Currently, paper technology is still used as the primary source for data/information management purposes. Consequently, having to maintain dual technologies and related systems—part manual, part electronic (often referred to as "hybrid" systems)—is providing the most angst for HIM professionals who are fighting hard to maintain their existing territories. However, as more and more healthcare and healthcare-related data/information are being collected, stored, and transmitted using computer technologies, the HIM discipline is increasingly becoming a professional field within the domain of healthcare informatics.

Because healthcare informatics is the healthcare industry's professional field that is concerned with the management of all aspects of health data and information, it includes and, in fact, cannot ignore HIM as one of its components. Because healthcare informatics is focused on the application of computers and computer technologies to support authorized users in their healthcare and related practices, processes, research, and education, HIM is the component of the healthcare informatics infrastructure by which authorized users' information needs are electronically created and managed.

As such, HIM professionals must continue to be viewed as intimate partners with HIT professionals, who, together, form strong alliances with each type of authorized user (physicians, nurses, clinicians, dentists, consumers, and administrators) to develop and implement the required hardware/software and to manage the data/information content. Also, HIM professionals must continue to be viewed as healthcare informatics professionals who support each type of authorized user's unique information needs and, concurrently, support the overall information needs of the healthcare organizations in which they work. Only in this context will HIM professionals continue to assume a leadership role in the development, implementation, and use of improved healthcare information systems, integrated patient information systems, accurate decision support tools, or any or all of the current and emerging information technologies and systems highlighted in this chapter.

Real-World Case

Six months after the merger of two of Chicago's large acute care organizations, Diane Samuels was appointed chief information officer (CIO) of the merged entity. The CIO from one of the merged acute care organizations had accepted an offer from an employer in the area of the country from which he had moved 2 years ago. The CIO from the other merged acute care organization resigned after 10 years of service when he was not chosen CIO of the merged entity.

In interviewing for the position, Diane learned that:

- One of her predecessors had recommended that the clinical information systems of the two acute care organizations be merged by 2005.
  - One of the CISs in one of the acute care organizations, City General (CG), was installed about 15 years ago. This system was not HIPAA security compliant and it lacked important CIS features, such as alerts and reminders.
  - It was estimated that $10 million would be saved following the merger of the two CIS systems.
- Her boss, the CEO of the merged entity, had committed to its board that expenses would be reduced during fiscal year 2004 by the $10 million that was expected to be saved following the merger.

When Diane began her new position, she knew she needed to make a number of critical decisions regarding the CISs. At first, she thought that in order to merge the two CISs, she could either implement into CG the existing CIS at the other acute care organization, University Medical Center (UMC), or implement an entirely new CIS in both facilities.

However, Diane quickly learned the following information:

- If the choice were made to implement the UMC CIS into CG, the existing UMC CIS would need to be significantly rewritten to "fit" into CG and its environment of existing systems. This appeared risky because there had been inadequate documentation of the many changes that had been made to CG's environment of existing systems that were interfaced to the old, current system. Further, UMC's existing CIS could create technical problems in CG's existing environment of "other" systems' operating systems.
- CISs are closely integrated with registration systems. Therefore, at UMC, extensive work had already been completed on a new registration system using IDX's Flowcast software, which had been specifically designed to integrate acute care facility inpatient and outpatient registration. UMC's objective was to eventually integrate this hospital registration system with the UMC physician offices' registration system. Therefore, implementing UMC's CIS into CG would require that CG's existing registration system also be converted to IDX's Flowcast. The usual time to undertake such a project is two years.
- Both UMC's and CG's CIS hardware leases and software licenses were due to terminate in about six months. Both lease contracts forced the hospitals to both purchase the existing (and out of date) hardware and software (which may not allow system integration) at a cost of approximately $10 million.
- If the choice were made to implement an entirely new CIS in both facilities, a new system would cost approximately $50 million. However, it would serve both hospitals and, according to vendors, have a better chance of achieving full integration.
- Aside from the dollars, the IT staff at CG had a poor track record of implementing new systems. In addition, the IT department had a vacancy rate of 50 percent.

Diane met with her staff and, after researching several companies that offered both products and/or services, she solicited request for proposals (RFPs) from the following three companies:

- Dak Systems Consulting, the leading company in healthcare systems integration services, refused to bid on the systems integration required for a new CIS at both facilities. This was because of the risks and time constraints involved in designing, implementing, and testing the system before the leases and year terminated.
- IDX proposed that its new, recently redeveloped CIS be implemented in both facilities. After all, this system was developed to integrate into IDX's registration system, which was already installed at UMC and most likely would need to be installed at CG anyway. In addition, the merged entity would get a much better price than $50 million for purchasing this new system. Unfortunately, IDX was unable to provide evidence of successful installation of its recently redeveloped CIS not only at a similar, large delivery network, but anywhere.
- Cerner Corporation was the leading provider of CISs for large acute care facilities and integrated delivery networks. Cerner proposed that its CIS be installed in both acute care organizations and strongly recommended that its registration system replace CG's existing and old registration system as well as UMC's existing and new registration system. Unfortunately, aside from the UMC CIS's high price tag, Cerner's registration system had not been chosen the year before when UMC was evaluating new registration systems. This was because UMC believed that Cerner did not have as extensive experience as IDX in integrating both hospital and physician office registration systems.

Finally, Diane could outsource management of any new CIS, but it was unlikely that an outsourcing firm would guarantee that a new CIS would be in place before the leases expired and the year ended.

The stakes surrounding Diane's recommendation to her CEO could not be higher in terms of dollars or her career.

Summary

Making clearer the benefits of the current and emerging information technologies and systems and their application in the healthcare industry requires significant changes. Such changes are technological, organizational, social, and attitudinal.

Demonstrating the return on investment in computer technologies requires methodical planning. This comes in light of their staggering capital and operating costs as well as the expense of human resources in installing, integrating, managing, and maintaining increasingly complex systems.

Accepting the trade-offs associated with computer technologies requires massive education and training.

For example, EHR systems will never exactly replicate the flexibility of paper technology. However, increased legibility, increased access to the information, and the ability to use the information simultaneously for other purposes will be provided in return. All the confidential information cannot be locked in drawers and file cabinets. However, the growing volume of information stored electronically and accessed remotely results in the need for ongoing attention to privacy and security concerns.

Accomplishing the organization's visions for providing the highest-quality care in the most effective way requires providing healthcare professionals the authority to establish the links between the promised benefits and the key enablers of the benefits, the information technologies.

Depicting the art of the possible requires patience.

These requirements are how well-trained and highly skilled individuals with knowledge about both healthcare and computerized information technologies will design, develop, select, implement, and maintain tomorrow's healthcare information management systems and apply technology to the management of healthcare information. This is how HIM professionals will contribute to the important field of informatics in healthcare.

References

American Health Information Management Association. 2005. AHIMA e-HIM Personal Health Record Work Group: Defining the personal health record. *Journal of American Health Information Management Association* 76(6):24–25.

American Health Information Management Association. 2004. Practice brief: Delving into computer-assisted coding. *Journal of American Health Information Management Association* 75(10).

American Health Information Management Association. 2000. AHIMA's basic operational tenets for protecting the privacy of personal health information on the Internet. Available online from ahima.org/infocenter/guidelines/tenets.asp.

American Medical Informatics Association. 2005. amia.com.

Barnett, G.O., J. Cimino, J. Hupp, and E. Hoffer. 1987. DXplain: An evolving diagnostic decision-support system. *Journal of the American Medical Association* 258(1):67–74.

Borowitz, S. 2001. Computer-based speech recognition as an alternative to medical transcription. *Journal of the American Medical Informatics Association* 8(1):101–2.

Brailer, D.J. 2005 (Jan. 19). Interoperability: The key to the future health care system. *Health Affairs* Web Exclusive. Available online from content.healthaffairs.org/cgi/content/full/hlthaff.w5.19/DC1.

Bufton, M. 1999. Electronic health records and implementation of clinical practice guidelines. In *Electronic Health Records: Changing the Vision,* edited by G.F. Murphy, M.A. Hanken, and K.A. Waters. Philadelphia: W.B. Saunders Company.

California HealthCare Foundation. 1999. National survey: Confidentiality of medical records. Available online from ehealth.chcf.org.

Center of Information Technology Leadership. 2004. *The Value of Healthcare Information Exchange and Interoperability*. Boston: Partners HealthCare.

Department of Health and Human Services. 1993 (Nov. 23). A push toward paperless processing in healthcare. *HHS News* press release.

Dick, R., and W. Andrews. 1995. Point of care: An essential technology for the CPR. *Healthcare Informatics* 12(5):64–66, 78.

Dick, R.S., and E.B. Steen, eds. 1991. *The Computer-based Patient Record: An Essential Technology for Health Care,* 1st ed. Washington, DC: National Academy Press.

Dick, R.S., E.B. Steen, and D.E. Detmer, eds. 1997. *The Computer-based Patient Record: An Essential Technology for Health Care,* revised ed. Washington, D.C.: National Academy Press.

Drazen, E. 2001. Is this the year of the computer-based patient record? *Healthcare Informatics* 18(2):94–98.

Goldman, J., and Z. Hudson. 2000. Virtually exposed: Privacy and e-health. *Health Affairs* 19(6):140–48.

Hagland, M. 2001. Getting more personal. *Journal of American Health Information Management Association* 72(8):35.

Health Insurance Portability and Accountability Act of 1996. Public Law 104-191. Available online from access.gpo.gov/nara/cfr/index.html.

Henchey, P. 1998. Maximizing ROI in data warehouses. *Advance for Health Information Executives* 2(1):60–70.

Hunt, D., R. Haynes, S. Hanna, and K. Smith. 1998. Effects of computer based clinical decision support systems on physician performance and patient outcomes: A systematic review. *Journal of the American Medical Association* 280(15):1339–46.

Institute of Medicine, Committee on Quality of Health Care in America. 2003. *Patient Safety: Achieving a New Standard of Care.* Washington, DC: National Academy Press.

Institute on Medicine, Committee on Quality of Health Care in America. 2002. *Leadership by Example: Coordinating Government Roles in Improving Health Care Quality.* Washington, DC: National Academy Press.

Institute of Medicine, Committee on Quality of Health Care in America. 2001. *Crossing the Quality Chasm: A New Health System for the 21st Century.* Washington, DC: National Academy Press.

Kelly, F. 2001. Implementing an executive information system (EIS). Available online from dssresources.com.

Kohn, L.T., J.M. Corrigan, and M.S. Donaldson, eds. 1999. *To Err Is Human: Building a Safer Health System.* Washington, DC: National Academy Press.

Krohn, R. 2004. Clinical decision support systems. *Journal of Healthcare Information Management* 18(4):10–11.

National Committee on Vital and Health Statistics. 2001. Information for health: A strategy for building the NHII. Available online from aspe.hhs. gov/sp/nhii/Documents/NHIIReport2001/default.htm.

Nussbaum, G. 2001. Bitten by the ASP: Application service providers. *Proceedings of the Healthcare Information and Management Systems Society,* Vol. 1 (Session 7), pp. 1–9. Chicago: HIMSS.

Power, D.J. 1997. What is a DSS? *DS*, The On-Line Executive Journal for Data-Intensive Decision Support* 1(3). Available online from taborcommunications.com/dsstar/971021/100015.html.

Schnitzer, G. 2000. Natural language processing: A coding professional's perspective. *Journal of American Health Information Management Association* 71(9):95–98.

Siwicki, B. 1996. Artificial intelligence: A new generation of health care applications. *Health Data Management* 4(4):47–52.

Stead, W., and M. Lorenzi. 1999. Health informatics: Linking invest-ment to value. *Journal of the American Medical Informatics Association* 6(5):341–48.

Tabar, P. 2003. Get the message? *Healthcare Informatics* 20(5):50.

Turley, J., C. Johnson, T. Johnson, and J. Zhang. 2001. A clean slate: Initiating a graduate program in health informatics. *MD Computing* 18(1):47–48.

Walker, J., E. Pan, D. Johnston, J. Adler-Milstein, D. W. Bates, and B. Middleton. 2005 (Jan. 19). The value of health care information exchange and interoperability. *Health Affairs* Web Exclusive. Available online from content.healthaffairs.org/cgi/content/full/hlthaff.w5.10/DC1.

Warner, H. 2000. Can natural language processing aid outpatient coders? *Journal of American Health Information Management Association* 71(8):78–81.

Chapter 4
The Health Information Management Profession

Sandra R. Fuller, MA, RHIA

Learning Objectives

- To understand the professional definition of health information management (HIM)
- To recognize the components of HIM
- To differentiate HIM from information technology and health library science
- To identify the types of data relevant to the HIM profession
- To identify the functions within the HIM professional domain
- To understand the media and forms in which health information is found
- To recognize the components of the HIM body of knowledge
- To identify the characteristics of a profession that apply to HIM
- To identify the key HIM professional associations
- To understand the importance of a professional code of ethics and what the HIM Code of Ethics means
- To recognize the importance of lifelong learning in the HIM profession
- To understand the process and benefits of certification and the requirements for maintaining certification
- To recognize the importance of continuing education and the options available to HIM professionals

Key Terms

Access control
American Association for Medical Transcription (AAMT)
American Health Information Management Association (AHIMA)
American Medical Informatics Association (AMIA)
Certification
Certified coding associate (CCA)
Certified coding specialist (CCS)
Certified coding specialist—physician based (CCS-P)
Certified in healthcare privacy (CHP)
Certified in healthcare privacy and security (CHPS)
Certified in healthcare security (CHS)
Certified professional in health information management systems (CPHIMS)
Clinical data
Coded data
College of Healthcare Information Management Executives (CHIME)
Commission on Accreditation for Health Informatics and Information Management Education (CAHIIM)
Continuing education
Data capture
Data dictionary
Data display
Data modeling
Data quality management
Demographic data
e-HIM
Epidemiological data
Financial data
Healthcare Information Management and Systems Society (HIMSS)
Health science librarians
Informatics
Information technology professionals
International Federation of Health Record Organizations (IFHRO)
International Medical Informatics Association (IMIA)
Medical informatics professionals
National Cancer Registrars Association (NCRA)
Nosology
Process and work-flow modeling
Reference data
Registered health information administrator (RHIA)
Registered health information technician (RHIT)
Research data

Introduction

In 1928, the Association of Record Librarians of North America was organized under the sponsorship of the American College of Surgeons. The objective of the new organization was "to elevate the standards of clinical records in hospitals, dispensaries, and other distinctly medical institutions" (Huffman 1941, p. 18). This precursor to the American Health Information Management Association (AHIMA) began to define the qualifications, duties, and training for individuals working in medical records. In 1941, Huffman (pp. 185–87) categorized the responsibilities of the medical record librarian as:

- Organization and management
- Numbering, filing, and cross-indexing
- Ethics and medicolegal
- Statistics, comparative studies, and research
- Secretarial duties
- Correlation of the medical records library and the medical reference library

Many of these elements are still included in today's professional definition of health information management (HIM). Other elements of the 1941 definition are irrelevant or of limited importance. The longevity of this professional definition documents the unique role of the health information manager and the resilience of the profession through time.

This chapter focuses on the professional definition and scope of HIM practice. It also discusses the characteristics of a profession, such as belonging to professional organizations, and provides specific examples that apply to HIM.

Theory into Practice

Joe was faced with a dilemma. For the past 15 years, he had been director of medical records in the largest community hospital in the small city where he lived. During that time, he had completed his master's degree in HIM and was now looking for a new challenge. However, Joe already had the most senior-level HIM job in his organization. Moreover, moving to another city was out of the question because his wife had a great job, and they did not want to relocate their family.

Then Joe learned that a new position was being created in the information systems (IS) department. The hospital was planning to acquire a new clinical IS and the chief information officer (CIO) was looking for someone to lead the project. Joe had worked with the IS department on a number of projects in the past and had always liked project management, application specification, and ensuring that new systems met the organization's needs. He felt that the IS position was just what he was looking for, but there were a few obstacles. First, the CIO was looking for a nurse to fill the position. Second, Joe did not want to leave HIM. And third, he was uncertain how the IS role would prepare him for the future.

Joe decided to gather some information. He spoke with someone from his master's program who had a made a similar move, talked with a friend at the annual convention about nontraditional roles, met with a recruiter to discuss career paths, and did some reading on evolving HIM careers.

Finally, Joe applied for the job. Despite his skepticism, the CIO agreed to interview Joe because of his strong performance with the organization. However, Joe explained how his education had prepared him for both the technical and project management elements of the job. Also, he pointed out that he already had established relationships with a number of the clinical staff with whom he would be working. Moreover, he had excelled at putting together a team with diverse skills and getting the job done. Joe was offered the job and began two months later.

Because of the job's critical nature, the system's high profile, and Joe's qualifications, he was able to make the move without a salary cut. Further, he could negotiate an increase in six months if the implementation was on schedule and within budget. His talks with friends and colleagues had persuaded him that he would not be leaving HIM but, rather, would be moving into a different phase of his career and the profession. A growing number of HIM professionals are working outside their departments within hospitals and outside hospitals altogether.

What's more, Joe now sees new possibilities for his future. Working with the IS department continues to develop his technical expertise. He is fine-tuning his project management skills, and the new position has already provided opportunities to practice his presentation skills. He is planning ahead and considering how he might leverage these new talents to apply for the CIO role at another healthcare organization in town or perhaps go into consulting to help other organizations with their system implementations.

Professional Definition

In the past 50 years, numerous changes have affected the responsibilities of the health information manager. The advent of computers, government sponsorship and regulation of healthcare, advances in medical practice, and socioeconomic changes and progress in higher education have all affected the HIM profession. In 2000, AHIMA's Committee on Professional Development completed the most recent update of the professional definition for HIM. (See figure 4.1.) Changes in the healthcare environment, information technology, and information management continue to have an impact on the practice of health information management. The new definition reads:

> Health information management improves the quality of healthcare by ensuring that the best information is available to make any healthcare decision. Health information management professionals manage healthcare data and information resources. The profession encompasses services in planning, collecting, aggregating, analyzing, and disseminating individual patient and aggregate clinical data. It serves the healthcare industry including: patient care organizations, payers, research and policy agencies, and other healthcare-related industries (Russell 2001, p. 48B).

Figure 4.1.   Update of the professional definition of health information management

Health Information Management: Professional Definition
Developed by the 1999 and 2000 Committees on Professional Development

Effective January 2001

Health information management improves the quality of healthcare by ensuring that the best information is available to make any healthcare decision. Health information management professionals manage healthcare data and information resources. The profession encompasses services in planning, collecting, aggregating, analyzing, and disseminating individual patient and aggregate clinical data. It serves the following healthcare stakeholders: patient care organizations, payers, research and policy agencies, and other healthcare-related industries.

HEALTH	Domain Description	Unique Impact
The field of health is broad, including everything from birth to death and wellness to illness. Health information management deals largely with patient data.	Health information includes: • **Clinical data** captured during the process of diagnosis and treatment. • **Epidemiological databases** that aggregate data about a population. • **Demographic data** used to identify and communicate with and about an individual. • **Financial data** derived from the care process or aggregated for an organization or population. • **Research data** gathered as a part of care and used for research or gathered for specific research purposes in clinical trials. • **Reference data** that interacts with the care of the individual or with the healthcare delivery systems, like a formulary, protocol, care plan, clinical alert or reminder, etc. • **Coded data** that is translated into a standard nomenclature or classification so that it may be aggregated, analyzed, and compared.	Health information professionals manage a variety of types of information across the healthcare industry. Their expertise uniquely impacts the value of this data as evidenced in the examples below: • **Clinical Data**—Organization of information supports direct patient care and serves a variety of industry needs like reimbursement, planning, and research. • **Epidemiological Databases**—Aggregate statistics reveal disease trends. • **Demographic Data**—Attention to data quality provides unique identification of patients in a healthcare enterprise and accurate information available to run the business of healthcare. • **Financial Data**—Understanding the clinical context of costs and the rules for reimbursement improves organizational decision making. • **Research Data**—Planning for future use of data improves the quality and reduces the cost of data capture and analysis. • **Reference Data**—Providing current literature and research outcomes enhances clinical knowledge at the point of care and in operational decision making. • **Coded Data**—Aggregate statistics enhance analysis for epidemiological patterning. Combining knowledge of the clinical content, documentation principles, coding systems, and data use provides accurate information for the industry.
INFORMATION	Domain Description	Unique Impact
Health information is captured and stored in a variety of media and forms.	The management of information relates to all of these forms: • **Data**—Individual and aggregate • **Reports** • **Medical records**—An aggregation of reports and data that describe an individual patient usually within one delivery site or system • **Data dictionaries** • **Vocabularies** Information may be stored using a variety of media: • **Paper** • **Databases** • **Microfilm/microfiche** • **Computer stored**	**FORMS** **Data** • Healthcare generates enormous amounts of data that are only useful if well managed. **Reports** • Summarization of data into relevant reports quickly communicates vital information. **Medical Records** • Developing uniform definitions of the most critical information gathered about a patient to create a legal document. **Data Dictionary** • Creating standards to define critical content. **Vocabularies** • Defining the language of healthcare. **MEDIA** **Paper** • Managing the historic and pervasive method of healthcare communication. **Databases** • Constructing relevant collections of data. **Microfilm/Microfiche** • Reduction of storage space required for maintaining legal documents. **Computer Stored** • Assuring preservation of a legal standard when applying new technologies.

(Continued on next page)

Figure 4.1.   (Continued)

MANAGEMENT	Domain Description	Unique Impact
Management of health information uniquely stems from a knowledge of clinical, management, and informatics principles and is performed by individuals focused at the strategic, management, and technical levels.	**PLANNING** **Administration** • Managing data collection and storage • Managing information retrieval and release **Policy Development** • Establishing security, confidentiality, retention, integrity, and access standards • Developing training programs that empower others to carry out the information policies • Advocating for privacy, confidentiality, and access **Strategic Planning** • Identifying the organization or projects that need information support for current and future strategic operations and initiatives • Planning capture, storage, and display of data to ensure operational effectiveness, including use of technology **INFORMATICS** **Data Modeling** • Determining data needs and identifying the relationships among these data **Process and Work-Flow Modeling** • Identifying the flow of work and information required to perform a function including: decomposition diagrams, dependency diagrams, and data flow **Data Capture and Display Design** • Focusing on system design, screen design, report design, and forms design **Data Dictionary Maintenance** • Maintaining dictionary design, standardization, update, and dissemination **Access Control** • Designing, implementing, and monitoring the map between information and user access **Data Quality Management** • Effecting the collection, application, warehousing, and analysis of data to improve information quality **Nosology** • Analyzing and interpreting disease and procedure classifications and terminologies for accuracy of translation of healthcare data **TECHNICAL** **Classification and Coding** • Assigning the appropriate code or nomenclature term for categorization **Abstracting** • Compiling the pertinent information from the medical record based on predetermined data sets **Registry Development** • Assembling a chronological set of data for an express purpose **Storage** • Implementing and providing oversight of electronic and paper-based filing systems **Retrieval** • Making accessible information that is stored in various media and sites **Release** • Appropriately responding to requests for information based on laws and policy **Analysis** • Performing qualitative and quantitative analysis of documentation against standards and policy	**PLANNING** **Administration** • Reducing the cost of health information • Successfully implementing an enterprisewide master person index **Policy Development** • Participating in national policy discussions on health information privacy • Drafting organizational policies that conform with state and federal regulations **Strategic Planning** • Initiating market position strategies influenced by sound outcomes data • Ensuring easy access to health information by care providers across an enterprise **INFORMATICS** **Data Modeling** • Improving access to healthcare data • Improving the quality of information **Process and Work-Flow Modeling** • Ensuring faster access to cash through improved revenue cycles • Providing for less time spent by clinicians in charting; more time for patient care **Data Capture and Display Design** • Improving patient safety through reduced documentation error • Reducing training time for clinicians in how to chart **Data Dictionary Maintenance** • Making accurate and timely data available for clinical and business decisions • Increasing access to data **Access Control** • Protecting patients' right to privacy • Complying with state and federal laws and regulations • Improving access when appropriate **Data Quality Management** • Consistently and methodically improving the quality of data • Improving decision making influenced by reliable information **Nosology** • Providing access to clinically relevant aggregate data **TECHNICAL** **Classification and Coding** • Reducing the threat of fraud and abuse litigation • Improving data accuracy • Establishing processes for accurate reimbursement **Abstracting** • Providing access to key data at the patient and aggregate levels **Registry Development** • Providing information to support long-term care of chronic disease • Providing research information for the value of treatment of chronic disease **Storage** • Reducing costs of storing records • Complying with state and federal laws **Retrieval** • Making information available for healthcare emergencies • Providing the most cost-effective access to information **Release** • Protecting patients' rights to privacy of health information • Reducing risk of litigation from inappropriate release **Analysis** • Allowing for meaningful interpretation of statistical data • Presenting both business and clinical information with appropriate content and context review **EXTENDED ROLES** *As with any robust profession, individuals evolve into divergent roles to develop, support, and nurture aspects of the profession. Although related to the profession, additional skills are developed to contribute to health information management without directly managing health information. For example, they support the core definition by:* • *Teaching others to manage health information* • *Developing and marketing products and services that help to manage health information* • *Developing software that manages health information* • *Consulting with others in the management of health information*

Source: AHIMA 2005a.

HIM deals primarily with information that is created during the diagnosis and treatment of individual patients. Closely related, but different, fields include information technology (IT), health science libraries, and medical **informatics.**

The IT field provides computing hardware, software, and data transmission technology for all industries, including healthcare. Although HIM professionals routinely work with **information technology professionals** and study some computer science topics, HIM does not require the same depth of computer knowledge and skill that IT does. However, HIM's unique healthcare focus requires knowledge about clinical information and the healthcare industry, in addition to the core HIM curriculum described later.

Health library science is a specialized area of library science that evolved from the enormous volume of reference materials published in medical and health literature. **Health science librarians** provide access to library resources and teach people how to use them (Chronicle Guidance Publications 1999, p. 8). The provision of reference material to aid in health decision making is an increasingly important function of computer-based patient records (IOM 1997, p. 88). As the demand for faster access to health literature increases, HIM professionals will continue to work closely with health science librarians to integrate these information resources with information on a specific patient or patient population.

Medical informatics is the "field that concerns itself with the cognitive, information processing and communication tools of medical practice, education and research including the information science and technology to support these tasks" (Greenes and Shortliffe 1990). **Medical informatics professionals** are physicians who specialize in medical information processing. Other disciplines also are developing postgraduate informatics specialties such as nursing informatics, dental informatics, and pharmacy informatics. Applied health informatics and graduate HIM education lead to new problem-solving techniques, analytic methods, and systems thinking combined with an understanding of technology that are focused on the information needs of healthcare.

Scope of Health Information

Health information includes information from birth to death. It also includes information from the individual patient record as well as aggregate data on a patient population that can span the globe. Within the professional definition of HIM, health information includes the following types of data:

- **Clinical data,** the most common type of health information, document the signs, symptoms, diagnoses, impressions, treatments, and outcomes of the care process. They are captured during diagnosis and treatment and are stored in the medical record. Clinical data serve a variety of industry needs beyond direct patient care, including reimbursement, planning, and research. They may be collected and stored in paper or computer formats. Although the health information manager rarely collects or uses clinical data directly in the delivery of care, one of his or her principal roles is that of developing systems that collect accurate and timely information and make it available to decision makers.

- **Epidemiological data** are used to describe health-related issues or events, such as disease trends, found in specific populations. The information then may be used to inform the public or to generate actions that could affect a trend. For example, data on the incidence of sexually transmitted diseases might be used to measure the impact of a teen education program. HIM professionals could establish systems to transmit such information accurately and appropriately while maintaining patient confidentiality. They also could be involved in data analysis and display.

- **Demographic data** provide statistical information about a population, such as age, place of residence, gender, and so on. Accurate and complete demographic data perform two important information functions in healthcare. First, data such as age and gender have their own value when combined with clinical information. For instance, a gender designation can make a diagnosis commonplace, rare, or impossible. Breast cancer, a common diagnosis in a certain age of female, is rare, albeit possible, in males. However, pregnancy is only possible in females. Second, demographic data may be used to uniquely identify individuals so that all the other health information attributed to them can be collected and accessed accurately.

- **Financial data** are either derived from the care process or aggregated for an organization or population. Healthcare is a business. It is, in fact, a business that consumed $1.7 trillion or almost 15 percent of the gross domestic product from 2000 to 2005 (Sager and Socolar 2005). Although accounting and financial management are not within the HIM domain, understanding the rules for reimbursement and the relationship between clinical services and costs is important to the health information manager role.

- **Research data** may be collected as a part of care and then used in research or collected for specific research purposes in clinical trials. HIM professionals play a role in the collection and use of research data from existing records. In addition, they consider research needs when planning for future types and uses of data as a research tool. In this way, HIM professionals improve access to data and reduce the costs of research at the same time.

- **Reference data** are commonly created and maintained by someone outside health information management. They interact with the care of the individual or with the healthcare delivery system in the form of a formulary, protocol, care plan, clinical alert, or reminder. The nursing staff or the medical staff generally create care plans; the pharmacy normally administers the formulary, although ensuring that reference data are available for the care provider is a critical HIM role. Health information managers also are responsible for incorporating elements of this static information into the patient's medical record to support clinical documentation and to create a complete record.

- **Coded data** are data that have been translated into a standard nomenclature of classification so that they can be aggregated, analyzed, and compared. To facilitate the analysis of large amounts of information, coded data frequently are grouped into meaningful categories. The categories may be as simple as M for male and F for female or as extensive as those used to code diagnoses and procedures. The grouping may be age range or the complex methodology used for prospective payment systems.

HIM professionals may have responsibilities that require that they specialize in working with one data type or engage with multiple data types. Whatever the type of health information or the type of data it is derived from, HIM professionals perform a variety of tasks associated with ensuring the availability of high-quality data and information to support the healthcare industry.

Check Your Understanding 4.1

Instructions: Answer the following questions on a separate piece of paper.

1. What factors have influenced the change in the professional definition of health information management?

2. What are the differences between HIM professionals and information technology professionals?

3. What role does the HIM professional play in working with clinical data? How does the HIM professional's role differ from roles assumed by other healthcare professionals?

4. How are reference data different from other types of healthcare data?

Domains of Health Information Management Practice

The management of health information is based on a knowledge of clinical practice, information management principles, and informatics concepts. HIM can be practiced at the planning level, addressing the administrative aspects of health information systems, including policy development. When focused on informatics, HIM includes several functions that are required to develop and administer computer-based information systems. When practiced at a technical level, HIM manipulates data to be used by others for a variety of decision-making purposes. (See figure 4.1.)

Planning

The practice of HIM at the planning level involves the administration of information systems and the development of policies to ensure that those systems are administered effectively and confidentially today and in the future.

Administration

HIM involves the administration of systems that collect and store data and the management of information retrieval and release. Effective administration of these systems makes information available and ensures appropriate access, security, and confidentiality. Effective administration of health information systems also makes healthcare delivery more efficient because of reduced waste in clinical time and business processes. Administrative responsibilities may involve staff, space, equipment, and procedures for a large integrated delivery system or may be focused on ensuring the effective utilization of a single information resource, such as managing a cancer registry.

Policy Development

Along with the administration of systems and people, the development of policies specific to health information is among the HIM professional's job functions. Policy development includes:

- Establishing data security, confidentiality, retention, integrity, and access standards
- Developing training programs that empower others to carry out the information policies
- Advocating for data privacy, confidentiality, and access

Strategic Planning

Finally, strategic planning for future information needs is a role for the HIM professional involved in the planning function. This role involves identifying information needs for an organization or a project to support current and future strategic operations or in support of compliance with regulations or laws. It also involves planning the capture, storage, and display of data to ensure operational effectiveness, including the use of technology.

Informatics

Informatics is the science of information management in a computer-based environment. It involves the use of computers to automate the collection, storage, utilization, and transmission of information.

Those information management tasks that actually involve handling data and information fall into the arena of informatics. These tasks include:

- *Data modeling:* The process of determining data needs and identifying the relationships among the data
- *Process and work-flow modeling:* A method for identifying the flow of work and information required to perform a function, including decomposition diagrams, dependency diagrams, and data flow
- *Data capture and display:* A function that includes system design, screen design, report design, and form design
- *Data dictionary maintenance:* A task that encompasses dictionary design, standardization, update, and dissemination

- *Access control:* The process for designing, implementing, and monitoring the map between information and user access
- *Data quality management:* A function that encompasses the collection, application, warehousing, and analysis of data to improve information quality
- *Nosology:* The function of analyzing and interpreting disease and procedure classifications and terminologies for accurate translation of healthcare data

These informatics functions can be illustrated using a simple IS example. A patient presents to the emergency department and needs to be registered. Data modeling would indicate what information is needed to identify the patient, to collect insurance information for payment, to provide demographic information needed for patient care, and to identify the person the patient would want contacted in the event his or her condition worsened. An example of the relationship among the data might be that the patient's address is the same for identification, billing, and contact purposes. Thus, this information would need to be collected only once.

Continuing with the example, process and work-flow modeling would involve identifying how this information is collected. In the emergency department, a critical patient may have a different process model than a patient with a less serious condition. Certain information, such as name and date of birth, might need to be collected before any clinical treatment could begin, whereas insurance information could be collected prior to disposition.

Data capture and data display for collecting the registration information might involve a form the patient fills in and returns to the registration clerk. It is easy to see how such a form should be designed to easily transform written patient information to the data fields on a computer screen. Also, information should be collected in the most convenient manner for the patient. For example, all the insurance information should be collected at one time, rather than making the patient repeatedly refer to his or her insurance card throughout the interview.

A data dictionary defines all the unique data elements in the data set. For instance, the data field for a Social Security number would indicate that it is nine characters long, numeric, and the unique identifier assigned by the Social Security Administration. Having a complete and specific data dictionary allows for data field design and editing. An edit for the Social Security number would be to ensure that all the characters are numbers. A data dictionary also may record other types of data attributes (for example, weight recorded in pounds rather than grams) or stipulate that an entry must be authenticated or signed by the person collecting the information.

Access control is a critical function within HIM relative to information security. This function maps the relationship between information and the individuals authorized to use it. It may be established at a variety of levels. For instance,

an attending physician may have access to a patient's entire medical record, but a lab technician may have access to lab data only. Understanding the information contained in the medical record and the roles of the different individuals authorized to use it allows the health information manager to design mechanisms that enable users to access the information they need and also safeguard patient confidentiality.

In the emergency department example, it is clear how data quality management plays a key role in high-quality care and the effective delivery of medicine. Data quality management considers each of the steps of the data cycle: collection, application, warehousing, and analysis. HIM professionals first look at how the data are used and then design the required data set, through data modeling, to ensure that they are collected at the most logical point. Application (use) of the data is considered to ensure that the information is available when and where it is needed. Warehousing (storage) of the data ensures that the information from this emergency visit is available for a follow-up visit to either the patient's primary care provider or the hospital inpatient unit should the patient require hospitalization. Making the data available for analysis may be required to determine staffing levels in the emergency department, to address quality of care concerns, or to improve patient satisfaction questionnaires.

Nosology, the final informatics function in the HIM professional definition, does not deal directly with the information collected in the emergency department encounter. As a nosologist, the HIM professional puts in place a standard terminology or description of the diagnoses and procedures used so that information can be stored and analyzed. Suppose the HIM professional wanted to find all the patients who came to the emergency department for a myocardial infarction. Care providers use a number of different terms to refer to a myocardial infarction, including an MI, a heart attack, a coronary, and so on. By developing and using a standard terminology to describe this condition, the nosologist can ensure that every case of myocardial infarction will be found.

Technical Functions

There are many technical functions that fall into the HIM scope of practice. Much of this technical work is the focus of the associate-level education in the HIM field. For example, HITs are commonly engaged in the following activities:

- *Classification and coding:* the process of assigning the appropriate code or nomenclature term for categorization
- *Abstracting:* The function of compiling the pertinent information from the medical record based on predetermined data sets
- *Registry development:* The process of assembling a chronological set of data for an express purpose

- *Storage:* Implementation and oversight of computer-based and paper-based filing systems
- *Retrieval:* The process of making information stored in various media and sites accessible
- *Release:* The function of appropriately responding to requests for information based on laws and policy
- *Analysis:* The process of conducting qualitative and quantitative analysis of documentation against standards and policy

Health Information Media and Forms

The final domain of HIM professional practice concerns the forms in which health data are captured and stored. The management of information relates to all the following forms:

- Data (individual and aggregate)
- Reports
- Health records
- Data dictionaries
- Clinical vocabularies

Information may be stored using a variety of media, including paper, database, microfilm/microfiche, and electronic (computer systems).

Check Your Understanding 4.2

Instructions: Answer the following questions on a separate piece of paper.

1. What benefits are gained from HIM planning?
2. How are data modeling and process or work-flow modeling related?
3. What are some of the elements of a data dictionary?
4. What are some examples of how understanding the content of health information relates to the informatics functions?

Health Information Management Body of Knowledge

To carry out the professional definition, HIM professionals study a defined curriculum or body of knowledge. There are distinct curriculum models for each educational level within the field: associate, baccalaureate, and master's degrees. The health information administration (HIA) model (baccalaureate level) is presented in figure 4.2 (p. 88) and can be categorized into 16 topics:

- Health data structure, content, and standards
- Healthcare information requirements and standards
- Clinical classification systems
- Biomedical sciences
- Reimbursement methodologies
- Healthcare statistics, biomedical research and quality management—healthcare statistics and research
- Quality management and performance improvement
- Health services organization and delivery
- Healthcare privacy, confidentiality, legal, and ethical issues
- Information technology and systems

- Applied health informatics
- Organization and management
- Human resources management
- Financial and resource management
- Strategic planning and organizational development
- Project and operations management

Like the professional definition of HIM, the HIM curriculum is examined and updated periodically to ensure its relevance to the demands of the field. **The Commission on Accreditation of Health Informatics and Information Management Education (CAHIIM)** accredits educational institutions that offer associate and baccalaureate degrees in health information administration and health information technology. This accreditation process ensures that the appropriate curriculum is being taught, along with other essential elements of a high-quality educational experience.

Two elements make this curriculum unique: (1) the specialization to healthcare throughout the curriculum, and (2) the combination of studies in the biomedical sciences, management, and information fields. In addition to this specific HIM curriculum, HIM students are required to have an understanding of additional general education topics to prepare them for the workplace, including:

- Oral and written communications
- Social sciences
- Arts and humanities
- Microcomputer literacy, including word processing, spreadsheets, database management, and graphics and presentation
- Natural sciences
- Mathematics

These content areas do not represent individual courses but, rather, define the scope of instruction required of all accredited HIA programs.

Check Your Understanding 4.3

Instructions: Answer the following questions on a separate piece of paper.

1. What is the purpose of health services organization and delivery in the HIA curriculum?
2. Accreditation standards are included in what topic of the curriculum?
3. What are the elements within health data structure, content, and standards?
4. List all the curriculum topics that are important to performing research.

Characteristics of a Profession

The term *profession* may be defined in a number of ways. *Merriam-Webster's Collegiate Dictionary* (1995) defines it as "a calling requiring specialized knowledge and often long and intensive academic preparation." In *The Qualifying Association,* Millerson describes a profession as "a type of higher grade, non-manual occupation, with both subjectively and objectively recognized occupational status, possessing a well-defined area of study or concern and providing a definite service, after advanced training and education" (1964, p. 10). There are certainly characteristics of a profession that apply to health information management:

- Professional associations
- A code of ethics
- A unique body of knowledge that must be learned through formal education
- A system of training with entry by examination or other formal prerequisites (certification)
- Professional cohesion
- Professional literature

Professional Associations

Accepting the rewards of a profession means accepting its responsibilities. One of the ways to ensure professional success is through membership in a professional association. The following professional associations are particularly important to individuals working in the field of health information management.

American Health Information Management Association

AHIMA represents more than 50,000 HIM professionals who work throughout the healthcare industry. HIM professionals serve the healthcare industry and the public by managing, analyzing, and utilizing data vital for patient care and making them accessible to healthcare providers when they are needed most.

AHIMA members play many diverse roles, yet share a common purpose: to provide reliable and valid information that drives the healthcare industry. They are specialists in administering information systems, managing medical records, and coding information for reimbursement and research. As leaders in the field of HIM, AHIMA members work to ensure that healthcare is based on accurate and timely information. AHIMA is the oldest and largest of the membership associations in health information. Since its creation in 1928, AHIMA has undergone numerous changes and significant development. (See figure 4.3, p. 94.) Building on the profession's strong tradition, AHIMA members also are prepared to be a driving force in a changing healthcare industry.

AHIMA works not only to strengthen the profession, but also to improve healthcare by:

- Supporting members with practice guidance and life-long learning opportunities
- Providing a professional network through Communities of Practice for members to reach out to their colleagues
- Guaranteeing excellence to the healthcare industry through certification and relevant resources
- Disseminating best practices and innovations
- Promoting education and research in the field

- Providing public policy leadership
- Advocating for the profession and for HIM issues

AHIMA supports a system of component organizations in every state plus Washington, DC, and Puerto Rico. Component state associations (CSAs) provide their members with local access to professional education, networking, and representation. They also serve as an important forum for communicating national issues and keeping members informed of regional affairs that affect HIM. For more information, visit the AHIMA Web site at ahima.org.

American Medical Informatics Association

The **American Medical Informatics Association** (AMIA) is a membership organization composed of individuals, institutions, and corporations that develop and use ITs to improve healthcare. Founded in 1990, AMIA was created when the American College of Medical Information and the Symposium on Computer Applications in Medical Care merged. Its members include physicians, nurses, computer and information scientists, biomedical engineers, medical librarians and academic researchers, and educators. AMIA represents the United States at the **International Medical Informatics Association** (IMIA). Further, AMIA sponsors educational sessions and publishes the *Journal of the American Medical Informatics Association (JAMIA)*. For more information, visit the AMIA Web site at amia.org.

American Association for Medical Transcription

The **American Association for Medical Transcription** (AAMT) is the largest association for medical transcription. Its mission is to lead the evolution of medical transcription and to represent and advance the profession and its practitioners. AAMT has chapters around the country that provide local educational opportunities as well as an annual national conference. AAMT also certifies medical transcriptionists. For more information visit the organization's Web site at aamt.org.

College of Healthcare Information Management Executives

The **College of Healthcare Information Management Executives** (CHIME) was formed in 1992 through a collaborative effort by the **Healthcare Information Management and Systems Society** (HIMSS) and the Center for Health Information Management (CHIM). CHIME serves two purposes: (1) to serve the professional development needs of healthcare chief information officers (CIOs), and (2) to advocate more effective use of information management within healthcare.

CHIME offers its members professional development opportunities through its biannual CIO Forums and through courses in IT strategies, architecture, and best practices. Other resources include member-to-member surveys, online reference documents, and various presentations made available online. For more information, contact cio-chime.org.

Figure 4.2.   HIM baccalaureate degree knowledge cluster content and competency levels (2005)

Health Data Structure, Content, and Standards
- Structure and use of health information (individual, comparative, aggregate) (5)
- Health information media (paper, electronic/computer-based; e-health-personal, Web based) (5)
- Type and content of health record (paper, electronic, computer-based, e-health, personal, Web based) (5)
- Data quality assessment and integrity (5)
- Secondary data sources (registries and indexes; databases such as MEDPAR, NPDB, HCUP) (4)
- Healthcare data sets (such as OASIS, HEDIS, DEEDS, UHDDS, UACDS, NEDSS, NMMFS) (4)
- Health information archival systems (5)
- National Healthcare Information Infrastructure (NHII) (5)
- Data collection tools (such as forms, computer input screens, other health record documentation tools) (5)

Healthcare Information Requirements and Standards
- Standards and regulations for documentation (such as JCAHO, CARF, COP, AAAHC, AOA) (5)
- Health information standards (such as HIPAA, ANSI, ASTM, LOINC, UMLS, MESH, Arden Syntax, HL-7) (5)

Clinical Classification Systems
- Healthcare taxonomies, clinical vocabularies, terminologies/ nomenclatures (such as ICD-9-CM, ICD-10, CPT, SNOMED-CT, DSM-IV) (4)
- Severity of illness systems (4)

Biomedical Sciences
- Anatomy (3)
- Physiology (3)
- Medical terminology (5)
- Pathophysiology (4)
- Pharmacotherapy (4)

Reimbursement Methodologies
- Clinical data and reimbursement management (5)
- Compliance strategies and reporting (e.g., National Correct Coding Initiative) (4)
- Chargemaster management (4)
- Case-mix management (4)
- Audit process such as compliance and reimbursement (5)
- Payment systems (such as PPS, DRGs, APCs, RBRVS, RUGs) (4)
- Commercial, managed care, and federal insurance plans (4)

Healthcare Statistics, Biomedical Research, and Quality Management—Healthcare Statistics and Research
- Statistical analysis on healthcare data (5)
- Descriptive statistics (such as means, standard deviations, frequencies, ranges, percentiles) (5)
- Inferential statistics (such as t-tests, ANOVAs, regression analysis, statistical process control, reliability, validity) (5)
- Vital statistics (5)
- Epidemiology (4)
- Data reporting and presentation techniques (5)
- Computerized statistical packages (5)
- Research design/methods (such as quantitative, qualitative, evaluative, outcomes) (5)
- Knowledge-based research techniques (such as Medline, CMS, libraries, Web sites) (5)
- National guidelines regarding human subjects' research (4)
- Institutional review board process (5)
- Research protocol data management (4)

Quality Management and Performance Improvement
- Quality assessment and management tools (such as benchmarking, ORYX, SQC) (5)
- Utilization and resource management (4)
- Risk management (4)
- Disease management process (such as case management, critical paths) (4)
- Outcomes measurement (such as patient, customer satisfaction, disease specific) (5)

Health Services Organization and Delivery
- Organization of healthcare systems (5)
- Components and operation of healthcare organizations including e-health delivery (5)
- Accreditation standards (such as JCAHO, AOA, NCQA, CARF, CHAP, URAC) (5)
- Regulatory and licensure requirements (such as COP, state health departments) (5)

Healthcare Privacy, Confidentiality, Legal and Ethical Issues
- Legislative and legal system (4)
- Privacy, confidentiality, security principles, policies and procedures (5)
- Health information laws, regulations, and standards (such as HIPAA, e-health, JCAHO, state laws) (5)
- Elements of compliance programs (5)
- Professional and practice-related ethical issues (5)

Information Technology & Systems
- Computer concepts (hardware components, systems architectures, operating systems and languages, and software packages and tools) (4)
- Communications technologies (networks—LANS, WANS, VPNs; data interchange standards—NIST, HL7) (4)
- Internet technologies (Intranet, Web-based systems, standards—SGML, XML) (4)
- Data, information, and file structures (data administration, data definitions, data dictionary, data modeling, data structures, data warehousing, database management systems) (5)
- Data storage and retrieval (storage media, query tools/applications, data mining, report design, search engines) (5)
- Data security (protection methods—physical, technical, managerial, risk assessment, audit and control program, contingency planning, data recovery, Internet, Web-based, and e-Health security) (5)

Applied Health Informatics
- Leading development of health information resources and systems (4)
- Brokering of information services (5)
- Clinical, business, and specialty systems applications (administrative, clinical decision support systems, electronic health record and computer-based health record systems, nursing, ancillary service systems, patient numbering systems at master and enterprise levels) (5)
- Systems development (planning, analysis and design, customization, selection/procurement, implementation, integration, support, testing and evaluation, auditing and monitoring) (5)
- Human factors and user interface design (4)
- Systems Life Cycle (systems analysis, design, implementation, evaluation, and maintenance)

Figure 4.2.   (Continued)

Organization and Management
- Principles of management (5)
- Negotiation techniques (4)
- Communication and interpersonal skills (5)
- Team/consensus building (5)
- Professional development for self and staff (4)
- Problem-solving and decision-making processes (5)

Human Resources Management
- Employment laws (4)
- Principles of human resources management (recruitment, supervision, retention, counseling, disciplinary action) (5)
- Workforce education and training (4)
- Performance standards (5)

Financial and Resource Management
- Healthcare finance (payer mix, bond rating, investment, capitalization) (3)
- Accounting principles (4)
- Budget process (capital and operating) (5)
- Cost-benefit analysis (5)

Strategic Planning and Organizational Development
- Strategic leadership, management, and planning (4)
- Organizational behavior (4)
- Business building (entrepreneurialism—building your own business; intrapreneurialism—championing best practices, processes, services within your organization) (3)
- Change management (4)
- Organizational assessment and benchmarking (4)

Project and Operations Management
- Process reengineering and work redesign (4)
- Project management (5)

Competency Levels

1 = Awareness	Introductory recall and recognition
2 = Literacy	Knowledge of framework and content
3 = Concept	Comprehension, translation, extrapolation, and interpretation of meaning
4 = Detailed Understanding	Appropriate application of knowledge in a structured or controlled context
5 = Skilled Use	Application using analysis, synthesis, and evaluation in new situations

Source: AHIMA 2005b.

Healthcare Information and Management Systems Society

HIMSS provides leadership in healthcare for the management of technology and management systems. Members include healthcare professionals in a variety of healthcare settings, including hospitals, corporate healthcare systems, clinical practice groups, vendor organizations, and consulting firms. HIMSS also represents some 220 member corporations. Although HIMSS offers a variety of benefits, it is best known for its annual conference and exhibition, which is the largest in the industry. HIMSS has 42 chapters organized in geographical areas. HIMSS also offers the following certification: **certified professional in health information management systems** (CPHIMS) and **certified in healthcare security** (CHS). For more information, visit the HIMSS Web site at himss.org.

International Federation of Health Record Organizations

The **International Federation of Health Record Organizations** (IFHRO) supports national associations and health records professionals to improve health records. Established in 1968 as a forum to bring together national organizations, IFHRO continues to focus on global issues affecting health information. IFHRO is organized into four regions: the Americas, Europe, Africa/Eastern Mediterranean/South-East Asia, and the Western Pacific. Although national membership is reserved for one association per country, individuals may be associate members of IFHRO. A world congress is sponsored every three years and attracts HIM professionals from all over the globe. For more information, visit ifhro.org.

International Medical Informatics Association

The mission of IMIA is to promote informatics in healthcare and biomedical research; advance international cooperation; stimulate research, development, and education; and disseminate and exchange information. Generally, membership to IMIA is limited to organizations, societies, and corporations. IMIA sponsors a conference, MEDINFO, every three years and engages multiple working groups to advance its mission. For more information, visit imia.org.

National Cancer Registrars Association

The **National Cancer Registrars Association** (NCRA) was chartered in 1974 and its almost 4,000 members represent the various types of institutions that have an interest in cancer management. NCRA sponsors an annual conference designed to improve registrars' professional expertise. NCRA also sponsors a certification, the certified tumor registrar (CTR®.), for individuals working in this field. For additional information, visit ncra-usa.org.

Code of Ethics

An important element of any profession is its commitment to a code of ethics. Today's HIM professionals can face a variety of ethical dilemmas regarding payment and reimbursement systems, confidentiality and privacy, facility accreditation and licensure, and fair employment practices. A formal code of ethics ensures that professionals understand and agree to uphold an ethical standard that puts the best interests of the profession before their personal best interests.

AHIMA has developed a code of ethics for certified HIM professionals. (See Appendix E.) A violation of the code of ethics is grounds for disciplinary action, including revocation of credentials. AHIMA's professional ethics committee evaluates and responds to reports of ethical violations through a formal hearing process.

Education

An educational requirement is part of the definition of a profession. Indeed, completing a profession's educational requirements is fundamental to gaining entry into the field. Additionally, ongoing education is a responsibility of any professional. This is especially true of HIM professionals challenged by new regulations, revolutionary technologies, and an industry in transition. In October 2004, the AHIMA House of Delegates passed a resolution calling for its members to embrace lifelong learning:

> That AHIMA members make the commitment to lifelong learning and professional development so that HIM professionals continue to be vital players in ensuring quality healthcare through quality information.

This learning may be formal education through the pursuit of a master's or doctoral degree. Ongoing professional development also can be demonstrated through **continuing education** (CE) gained from conferences, workshops, reading, or distance learning activities. Seeking challenging work assignments and making professional development a goal when making career choices all contribute to an individual's professional development.

Certification

Certification is a process by which a nongovernment agency or association recognizes the competence of individuals who have met certain qualifications as determined by the agency or association. In HIM, AHIMA certification provides both personal validation and validation to employers and consumers of professional competence. Specifically, certification:

- Demonstrates to colleagues and superiors a dedication to high-quality healthcare and to the highest standards of HIM.
- Presents solid evidence to employers that an employee has trained and been tested to implement best practices and apply current technology solutions, abilities that in turn advance the organization.
- Sets a person apart from noncredentialed job candidates. In recent AHIMA-sponsored research groups, healthcare executives and recruiters cited these reasons for preferring credentialed personnel: (1) assurance of current knowledge through continued education, (2) possession of field-tested experience, and (3) verification of base-level competency.
- Has value for employers because it supports a worker's ability to uphold industry standards and regulations, thereby potentially saving organizations from fines and penalties due to errors or noncompliance.

- Catalyzes career development by augmenting resumes and adding recognition to candidates' capability. Because credentials appear after a person's name, they announce expertise with every signature.

To achieve AHIMA certification, individuals must meet certain eligibility requirements and successfully complete an examination. AHIMA currently awards seven credentials, as described in the following subsections.

Registered Health Information Administrator

Registered health information administrators (RHIAs) are skilled in the collection, interpretation, and analysis of patient data. Additionally, they receive the training necessary to assume managerial positions related to these functions. RHIAs interact with all levels of an organization—clinical, financial, administrative—that use patient data in decision making and everyday operations.

In a recent membership survey, AHIMA found that more than half the RHIA respondents were directors, managers, or consultants, with nearly 31 percent serving as HIM directors. Historically, most RHIAs have held the title of director of the HIM department of an acute care facility, but today other career opportunities abound. As patient records evolve toward computerization and as more entities such as third-party payers require health data, RHIAs benefit from a wide selection of roles in the industry. Information security and storage, data quality assurance, and advanced assistance to consumers with their health information are among the new domains. AHIMA's Vision 2006 (discussed later in this chapter) identifies and describes emerging HIM roles that parallel changes in the healthcare industry.

RHIAs enjoy job placement in a broad range of settings that span the continuum of healthcare, including office-based physician practices, nursing homes, home health agencies, mental health facilities, and public health agencies. The growth of managed care has created additional job opportunities in health maintenance organizations (HMOs), preferred provider organizations (PPOs), and insurance companies. Prospects are especially strong in these settings for RHIAs who possess advanced degrees in business or health administration.

To become eligible to take the RHIA examination, applicants must meet one of the following educational requirements:

- Hold a baccalaureate degree from a health information administration (HIA) program accredited by CAHIIM
- Hold a baccalaureate degree from an accredited college or university and a certificate in HIA from an accredited program
- Hold a degree from a foreign HIA baccalaureate program with which the CAHIIM has a reciprocal agreement (the CAHIIM currently has an agreement with

the Health Information Management Association of Australia at the baccalaureate level)

The RHIA exam is offered continually at computer testing sites located throughout the country. An application must be filed with AHIMA, and then an identification number and password are assigned.

Registered Health Information Technician

Registered health information technicians (RHITs) are health information technicians who ensure the quality of medical records by verifying their completeness, accuracy, and proper entry into computer systems. RHITs also may use computer applications to assemble and analyze patient data for the purpose of improving patient care or controlling costs. These technicians often specialize in coding diagnoses and procedures in patient records for reimbursement and research. Moreover, they may serve as cancer registrars, compiling and maintaining data on cancer patients. In a recent AHIMA membership survey, the majority of RHIT respondents held job titles in one of the following categories: coding/technician or manager/supervisor. With experience, the RHIT credential holds solid potential for advancement to management positions, especially when combined with a bachelor's degree.

Although most RHITs work in hospitals, they also work in a variety of other healthcare settings, including office-based physician practices, nursing homes, home health agencies, mental health facilities, and public health agencies. In fact, employment opportunities exist for RHITs in any organization that uses patient data or health information, including pharmaceutical companies, law and insurance firms, and health product vendors.

RHITs can look forward to expanding career opportunities in health information technology. According to the Bureau of Labor Statistics, HITs occupy one of the top 10 health occupations, with the fastest potential growth between now and year 2010 (Wing and Salsberg 2002, p. 40).

Certified Coding Associate

Certified coding associates (CCAs) are entry-level coders certified in the knowledge required to code. They are tested in their understanding of anatomy and physiology, pathophysiology, medical terminology, medical documentation, and the principles of classification systems. This credential was developed to address the shortage of qualified coders. It creates the first step of a coding career ladder that could lead to a CCS or a CCS-P with more training and experience. Moreover, CCAs may choose to diversify their interests in HIM beyond coding and continue their education by applying for the RHIT or RHIA credential.

Certified Coding Specialist

Certified coding specialists (CCSs) are professionals skilled in classifying medical data from patient records, generally in the hospital setting. CCSs review patient records and assign numeric codes for each diagnosis and procedure. To perform this task, they must possess expertise in the ICD-9-CM coding system and the surgery section within the CPT coding system. In addition, the CCS must be knowledgeable in medical terminology, disease processes, and pharmacology.

Hospitals or medical providers report coded data to insurance companies or the government (in the case of Medicare and Medicaid recipients) for reimbursement of their expenses. Researchers and public health officials also use coded medical data to monitor patterns and explore new interventions. Thus, coding accuracy is highly important to healthcare organizations because of its impact on revenues and in the description of health outcomes. Accordingly, the CCS credential demonstrates tested data quality and integrity skills in a coding practitioner. The CCS certification exam assesses mastery or proficiency in coding rather than entry-level skills.

Certified Coding Specialist–Physician-Based

The **certified coding specialist–physician based** (CCS-P) has expertise in physician-based settings such as physician offices, group practices, multispecialty clinics, or specialty centers. The CCS-P reviews patient records and assigns numeric codes for each diagnosis and procedure. To perform this task, he or she must possess in-depth knowledge of the CPT coding system and familiarity with the ICD-9-CM and HCPCS Level II coding systems. The CCS-P is also expert in health information documentation, data integrity, and quality. Because patients' coded data are submitted to insurance companies or the government for expense reimbursement, the CCS-P plays a critical role in the health provider's business operation. Moreover, the employment outlook for this coding specialty looks highly favorable with the growth of managed care and the movement of health services delivery beyond the hospital.

AHIMA will continue to develop relevant certification programs in response to market demand. Future initiatives will likely lead to other advanced specialty certification in focused HIM topics.

Certified in Healthcare Privacy

The **certified in healthcare privacy** (CHP) credential is a specialty credential denoting advanced competency in designing, implementing, and administering comprehensive privacy protection programs in all types of healthcare organizations. Becoming certified in healthcare privacy demonstrates a focus and advancement by specializing in the privacy dimension of HIM. By being recognized for special expertise, it signifies a commitment to advancing privacy management practices and to lifelong learning and professional development.

Certified in Healthcare Privacy and Security

The **certified in healthcare privacy and security** (CHPS) credential denotes advanced competency in designing, implementing, and administering comprehensive privacy and security protection programs in all types of healthcare organizations. AHIMA and HIMSS jointly sponsor this credential. Those wishing to earn this credential will need to successfully pass both the CHP and the CHS exams.

Certification Maintenance

The purpose of a CE program is to offer the public a form of assurance that individuals practicing a profession maintain competence following certification in that profession. In the health professions, maintaining competence is especially critical because of the rapid growth in technology, changes in social policies, and the expanding roles of health professionals in all areas of healthcare.

Participants are responsible for self-assessment of their personal strengths and weaknesses and for developing individual CE programs designed to ensure their own professional competence. The number of CE hours that can be obtained in any particular activity is unlimited. It is recommended that participants attempt to increase their knowledge and skills through a balanced variety of educational methods.

Continuing Education Requirements

All RHIAs and RHITs, including active, inactive, and student members of AHIMA as well as nonmembers, maintain their credentials through:

1. *Completion of acceptable CE credits during a two-year period (cycle):* RHIAs must earn 30 CE clock hours/ credits, and RHITs must complete 20 CE clock hours. Eighty percent of all CE units must be earned within the educational core content areas. (A current definition of the core content areas is available on the AHIMA Web site.)

   To receive credit, activities must be completed within the assigned cycle period. All cycles begin on January 1 and end on December 31 the following year. Individuals holding multiple credentials must earn 10 CE credits for each additional certification above the number required for their initial certification, not to exceed 60.

2. *Payment of CE assessment fees:* AHIMA members are charged a CE assessment with annual membership dues. Nonmembers pay a CE fee set by the AHIMA Board of Directors at the end of each CE cycle.

3. *Validation of CE report:* Participants must submit their CE report forms to AHIMA by January 31, following the end of the CE cycle. The report may be completed online or using the paper form and returning it to AHIMA. (Participants should keep a photocopy or a printout of the form.) Participants who are not audited will receive a CE validation certificate to retain as evidence of meeting CE requirements. Participants selected for audit do not meet requirements until they have complied with the audit procedures. A CE validation certificate will be forwarded to audited participants after documentation has been received and approved.

Reporting Requirements and Cost

Four to six weeks prior to the end of the CE cycle, participants will receive a CE report form from AHIMA. Participants must record the number of clock-hour credits received in each of the core content areas, the number of hours received in other HIM areas, and the total hours earned during the reporting period.

Although only the number of hours earned needs to be reported, it is important that participants maintain complete personal files of CE activities in case they are audited. AHIMA provides a CE tracking form that members may use to track their hours throughout the reporting period.

Currently, non-AHIMA members pay a $100 CE assessment per cycle. AHIMA members currently pay an annual $10 assessment with their membership dues.

Revocation and Restoration of Certification

The RHIA or RHIT credential will be revoked for failure to comply with CE requirements. Revocation is effective the year following the end of the applicable CE cycle. Before revocation, a Notice of Intent to Revoke is sent to the participant. If there is no response to the notice of intent, credentials are revoked.

After four years, or two consecutive CE cycles, candidates must apply and retake the applicable examination. Candidates must complete the Intent to Restore Credential application and pay all appropriate examination and restoration fees to reinstate a credential. During restoration, an individual is listed as a restoration candidate for a maximum period of one year.

No one may use the RHIT or RHIA credential after it has been revoked.

Continuing Education Audits

As CE hours are entered into the membership files, approximately 2 percent of the candidates are randomly selected for audit. An individual selected for audit is required to submit verifiable documentation for each activity listed on the CE report form. Auditors will seek verification of attendance or participation, content description, and CE credits earned. Thus, CE participants are advised to retain all records in their files for at least one year following the cycle end date.

Prior Approval of Activities

Unless otherwise indicated, programs or activities do not need prior approval from AHIMA. If the program or activity has not received AHIMA prior approval, candidates can judge for themselves whether it meets AHIMA requirements.

Professional Cohesion

Another aspect of a profession is professional cohesion, which is characterized by the members of a profession acting in a unified way. The existence of a professional association is one expression of professional cohesion as it embodies the members of the profession who act as a profession rather than as individuals. Professional cohesion can be witnessed in AHIMA's position statements or in advocacy positions that are taken with regulators or legislators. The recognition and adoption of best practices is another example of professional cohesion.

Professional Literature

The final element of a profession is the existence of professional literature. This textbook is one example of professional literature. The *Journal of the American Health Information Management Association* is the best-known source of HIM knowledge. Published since the 1930s, it is distributed to all AHIMA members and is available by subscription to nonmembers. Despite the fact that several other companies publish books and periodicals dealing with HIM, research and publication of HIM topics is in short supply when compared to other professions. This is an area of concern and opportunity for HIM professionals.

Check Your Understanding 4.4

Instructions: Answer the following questions on a separate piece of paper.

1. Which professional HIM associations offer professional certification to their members?
2. Why might someone belong to more than one professional association?
3. What are some of the key services provided by professional associations?
4. What are examples of international health information associations?
5. Why is it important to understand the HIM Code of Ethics?
6. How is the importance of continuing education addressed in the AHIMA's Code of Ethics?
7. What elements of the Code of Ethics relate to the individual's participation in AHIMA?
8. What are the benefits of certification, and how does one maintain it?
9. Who is eligible for RHIA certification?
10. How frequently are certification records audited?
11. How does someone report CE activities?

Current and Evolving Professional Roles

Workforce research has confirmed that HIM professionals hold 200 different job titles in 40 types of organizations ranging from hospitals to veterinary clinics (Wing and Langelier 2004). This underscores how fundamentally HIM is changing. Just 20 years ago, almost all HIM professionals worked in acute care hospitals. Today that number is just over 50 percent. For decades, we differentiated "traditional" from "nontraditional" practice; today, this distinction is irrelevant. HIM skills and competencies are needed by all organizations that use person-specific or aggregate patient data. The national push to adopt health IT will accelerate demand for a qualified HIM workforce

In 1996, AHIMA's Board of Directors took on an ambitious project: looking into the future and envisioning HIM practice and roles in the next millennium. Logically, the board's first step was to ask, "Exactly what does a health information manager do?" To answer that question and to continue to build a definition of the profession, the association began an initiative called Vision 2006. Vision 2006 is built on the work of a prior initiative, Vision 2000, which in 1991 sought to describe how HIM practice would evolve in the 1990s. Then in 2003, AHIMA convened a task force to articulate a vision for an **e-HIM** future. Electronic health information management (e-HIM) looks ahead to and embraces the real benefits that will accrue when healthcare comes fully into the information age (AHIMA 2003).

Traditional HIM practice has been based on physical records, files filled with paper forms and documents. Although some information based on current health records may be electronically stored and manipulated, most HIM functions today are still built around the existence of a physical record. New practice will be based on data management. As HIM practice evolves from its traditional base and aligns itself with changes in the healthcare delivery system and information technology, exciting career opportunities will emerge. Vision 2006 defines seven roles for the future. (See figure 4.4, p. 94.) These roles were confirmed in the e-HIM report, but have been extended to include the following additional titles:

- A *health information manager* in an integrated delivery system is responsible for the organization-wide direction of HIM functions. The role may be a line or staff management position. It includes working with the CIO and IS users to advance systems, methods, and applications support and to improve data quality, access, confidentiality, security, and usability.
- A *clinical data specialist* concentrates on data management functions in a variety of applications, including clinical coding, outcomes management, specialty registries, and research databases.
- A *patient information coordinator* helps consumers manage their personal health information, including personal health histories and release of information. This individual also helps customers understand managed care services and access to health information resources.
- A *data quality manager* is responsible for data management functions that involve formalized continuous quality improvement activities for data integrity throughout the organization, beginning with the data dictionary and policy development, as well as data quality monitoring and audits.
- A *data resource administrator* represents the next generation of records and data management and uses technological tools such as the computer-based patient record, data repositories, and data warehouses to meet current and future care needs across the continuum, provide access to the needed information, and ensure long-term data integrity and access.
- A *research and decision support analyst* ensures the quality of data and information generated through clinical investigations and other research projects.

Figure 4.3.   AHIMA timeline (name changes, credentials awarded)

1928 (Oct. 11)	Association of Record Librarians of North America (**ARLNA**) founded.	**1980** (Aug)	*Journal of the American Medical Record Association* replaces *Medical Record News.*
1929	*Bulletin of the Association of Record Librarians of North America* published.	**1991**	Name of association changed to American Health Information Management Association (**AHIMA**).
1933	Registered Record Librarian (**RRL**) credential established.	**1991** (Nov)	*Journal of the American Health Information Management Association* (*Journal of AHIMA*) replaces *Journal of the American Medical Record Association.*
1938 (Dec)	*Bulletin, American Association of Medical Record Librarians,* replaces the *Bulletin of the Association of Record Librarians of North America.*	**1992**	Certified Coding Specialist (**CCS**) credential established.
1944	Name of association changed to American Association of Medical Record Librarians (**AAMRL**) when Canadian members formed their own organization.	**1997**	Certified Coding Specialist–Physician-based (**CCS-P**) credential established.
1944 (Dec.)	*Journal of the American Association of Medical Record Librarians* replaces *Bulletin, American Association of Medical Record Librarians.*	**1999**	Fellow of the American Health Information Management Association (**FAHIMA**) designation established to recognize members who have made significant and lasting contributions to the HIM profession.
1953	Accredited Record Technician (**ART**), credential established.		
1954	Certified Record Librarian (**CRL**) designation established to recognize RRLs who had been in the field for at least 15 years and had made significant contributions to the profession. It was discontinued in 1964 because the general membership thought its use detracted from that of the RRL.	**2000**	Registered Health Information Technician (**RHIT**) credential replaces the Accredited Record Technician (ART) credential; Registered Health Information Administrator (**RHIA**) credential replaces the Registered Record Administrator (RRA) credential.
1964 (Jan)	*Medical Record News, the Journal of the American Association of Medical Record Librarians* replaces *Journal of the American Association of Medical Record Librarians.*	**2001**	Certified Coding Associate (**CCA**) entry-level coding credential established.
1970	Name of association changed to American Medical Record Association (**AMRA**).	**2002**	Certified in Healthcare Privacy (**CHP**) credential created.
1970 (Feb)	*Medical Record News, the Journal of the American Medical Record Association* replaces *Medical Record News, the Journal of the American Association of Medical Record Librarians.*	**2002**	Certified in Healthcare Security (**CHS**) credential, sponsored by HIMSS and administered by AHIMA created.
1978	Registered Record Administrator (**RRA**) credential replaces the Registered Record Librarian (RRL) credential.	**2002**	Certified in Healthcare Privacy and Security (**CHPS**) credential, sponsored jointly by AHIMA and HIMSS, created.

Source: AHIMA 2004.

Figure 4.4.   e-HIM professional roles

Business process engineer
Clinical research protocol designer and manager
Clinical trials manager
Clinical vocabulary manager
Consumer advocate
Data analyst
Data facilitator
Data information broker
Data/information presenter
Data sets, nomenclature, and classification standards developer
Data miner
Data navigator
Data quality and integrity manager
Data resource manager
Data security, privacy, and confidentiality manager
Data translator
Information system designer
Work and data-flow analyst

Source: e-HIM Task Force 2003.

The decision support specialist provides clinicians and senior managers with information for decision making and strategy development. Both specialists use a variety of analytical tools.

- A *security officer* is responsible for managing the security of electronically maintained information, including promulgation of security requirements, policies and privilege systems, and performance auditing.

Since the launch of Vision 2006 in 1996, new roles have emerged: compliance officer and privacy officer. Roles for HIM professionals are developing in e-health companies and the pharmaceuticals industry. The key is that the profession continues to respond to the needs of the healthcare industry and to advance the quality of health information.

Real-World Case

Jane Rogers, age 31, is supervisor for clinical coding in the health information service at Memorial Medical Center in Chicago. She left her job as a clinical coder at Community

General Hospital six months ago to take this newly created position. Jane graduated from the Health Information Administration program at Chicago University 10 years ago and is credentialed as a registered health information administrator (RHIA) and clinical coding specialist (CCS) by AHIMA. She is an active member in good standing of the association and serves on the Coding Roundtable for the Chicago Area Health Information Management Association. The position at Memorial was a significant promotion, increasing her salary by $11,000 a year and offering her a chance to be a supervisor. The new level of earnings allowed Jane to live on her own and to purchase her own car, a four-year-old bright-red Saturn.

Jane reports to Steve Murray, manager of patient accounts and the health information service. Steve is the nephew of Memorial's chief financial officer, John Murray III, who was brought in to turn around the medical center, which was in significant financial trouble in the mid-1990s. Steve has an MBA from the University of Chicago but, unlike most managers at Memorial, including his uncle, no formal training in healthcare administration, health information, or financial management. However, he is young and ambitious and has shown himself to be an effective manager. He has streamlined operations in patient accounts and health information services, increasing revenues by 20 percent, increasing collections and cash flow, automating many functions, and reducing clerical staff.

Jane is responsible for the staff that review medical records of patients treated at Memorial to identify the diagnoses and procedures involved in inpatient, outpatient, and emergency treatment. Staff assign codes that are the basis for the bills submitted for reimbursement to the federal and state government and to private insurance companies.

Steve told Jane that her first priority was to make coding functions more current. Further, he wanted to cut in half the 20 or more days that it currently took to complete coding and billing functions. To that end, Jane reorganized processing procedures, taught staff new techniques for speeding up record review, and within three months had achieved her goal. In a meeting with Steve at the end of her three-month probationary period, Jane was awarded a $1,000 spot bonus for her achievement. Even John Murray stopped by to congratulate her. Jane was so proud of her achievement that she presented her approaches at the monthly meeting of the Coding Roundtable and received words of encouragement from many of her colleagues.

With processing now running smoothly, Jane turned to coding accuracy. She undertook a study in which she randomly sampled the coded records of all six of her coding staff and recoded them herself without looking at the original codes. She found that accuracy rates ranged from 78 to 92 percent. Although benchmark standards are difficult to come by, Jane knew that the coders at Community General met a standard of 90+ percent and that their evaluations and merit increases depended on maintaining it. Despite standard guidelines for correct code assignment, payer requirements do not always conform to them. Payers are constantly issuing instructions about what codes they will and will not accept, and coders sometimes do not have the latest instructions. Further, medical record documentation is not always clear or complete and accurate code assignment requires some individual judgment. Because the codes assigned to a case determine reimbursement, it is possible to increase the organization's revenue by using codes representing more complex diagnoses or procedures. These must be supported by documentation in the medical record. However, code assignment is seldom a black-and-white decision, and thus it is possible to assign unsupported codes, thereby increasing reimbursement, and to fail to assign an appropriate code, thereby decreasing reimbursement.

In her weekly meeting with Steve, Jane reviewed the findings and proposed a plan for retraining and ongoing data quality control, including an adjusted compensation plan that would reward accurate work by her staff members. Her plan also called for developing a set of written guidelines that would reinforce Memorial's official guidelines and be presented to administration and the medical staff for approval. In this way, the coders would know the ground rules and the basis on which their performance was to be measured. Steve indicated that he would support the plan provided it did not result in slower processing time or reduced levels of reimbursement. Jane agreed to make certain that training did not slow down processing. She also suggested that improving accuracy would likely have a neutral effect on reimbursement because coders were undoubtedly missing reimbursable diagnoses and procedures.

With her plan in hand, Jane thought it would be wise to focus on the clinical areas most vulnerable to inaccurate coding. She began by conducting another interrater reliability study of cardiac surgery cases because these cases always present a challenge to coders. Again, she found wide variability in coder performance, this time ranging from 68 to 89 percent. She developed guidelines and obtained approval for them from the cardiac surgery clinical staff and administration. Then, she conducted a training program for her staff, who were paid overtime to attend so they did not fall behind in their work.

With another success under her belt, Jane next tackled the area of respiratory disease, another area of coding complexity and a major clinical service at Memorial, representing nearly 10 percent of its discharges. Further, Jane knew from reading her *Journal of the American Health Information Management Association* that bacterial pneumonia was the focus of investigations of Medicare fraud and abuse being conducted by the Department of Justice (DOJ). In fact, a number of healthcare organizations had paid substantial fines for having coded pneumonia cases with codes not supported by documentation in the medical records. Jane pulled a sample of records coded as "bacterial pneumonia," "other bacterial pneumonia," and "viral pneumonia." She worked late into the night for a week coding, recoding, checking, and double-checking her findings, which showed that cases were being consistently coded with the "bacterial" and "other bacterial" codes even though very few of the records had culture reports verifying bacterial infection. She calculated that with 150 cases a year and $5,000 in additional billings per case, this pattern of inaccurate coding was resulting in $750,000 in unsubstantiated revenue. The sheer volume of such cases made it unlikely that Memorial could claim random error if the DOJ chose to investigate.

Jane spent the weekend rechecking her findings and preparing a report with guidelines for accurate coding. She decided she had better talk to the coding staff before her regular weekly meeting with Steve on Monday afternoon. So first thing Monday morning, she met with her staff and reviewed her findings. Jane was shocked when Sally, the most tenured coder nodded and said, "We're just doing what we're told." When pressed, Sally acknowledged that the chief of respiratory medicine, Dr. Barrows, and Steve Murray had met with the coding staff the year before to discuss the coding of pneumonia cases. Jane asked, "Do you have anything in writing from the meeting?" "No," Sally replied, "they just told us that there were other ways to determine bacterial pneumonia than by culture and that Memorial was the major referral center for treating bacterial pneumonia." Needing time to digest what she had learned, Jane rescheduled her meeting with Steve, claiming a headache and upset stomach. She went home early to consider what to do next.

Concluding that the best approach would be to let the facts speak for themselves, Jane presented her report to Steve the next day along with her pneumonia coding guidelines. Steve was quiet and did not interrupt her, taking notes as she went through her findings. She concluded by saying, "Steve, we must implement the new guidelines at once, and we must also submit corrected bills for the cases we inaccurately submitted over the past year. This is the only way we can be sure that a fraud and abuse investigation will not be brought against Memorial." Steve replied, "Thank you, Jane. I'd like a copy of the report, and I'll discuss it with Dr. Barrows and John Murray. We'll get back to you. In the meantime, don't say anything about this to anyone."

Three weeks have passed, and Steve has canceled three weekly meetings in a row and barely spoken to Jane when they meet informally in the hallway or cafeteria. He has asked no further questions and has given no indication of his intention to act on Jane's findings or proposals for action.

Summary

Health information managers work with clinical, epidemiologic, demographic, financial, research, reference, and coded healthcare data. Health information administrators plan information systems, develop policy, and identify current and future information needs. In addition, they apply the science of informatics to the collection, storage, use, and transmission of information.

HIM professionals prepare for their careers by mastering a well-defined body of knowledge expressed in a formal curriculum. This curriculum covers, though is not limited to, content that addresses biomedical sciences, informatics, management, and research principles. When they are finished with their formal education, most HIM professionals achieve certification by passing a certification examination offered by AHIMA. Maintenance of certification demonstrates a lifelong commitment to continuing education and adherence to the HIM Code of Ethics.

As the professional association that represents most health information managers, AHIMA provides numerous services to its members and to the healthcare industry. Through accreditation of academic programs and certification of individual members, AHIMA ensures a qualified workforce. AHIMA works to improve healthcare by disseminating best practices, promoting research, and providing public policy leadership.

The HIM profession continues to evolve and change in response to healthcare trends, information technology, and government regulation. In the 1980s, most HIM professionals worked in hospitals; today, almost half of AHIMA's members work outside hospitals in a growing variety of health information practice sites. Health information management is a dynamic profession facing many current and future challenges, transitions, and opportunities. The ongoing conversion from paper files to computer-based records has brought with it a shift in roles (from managers and supervisors to more high-level technical specialists) for HIM leaders.

References

AHIMA e-HIM Task Force. 2003. Vision of the e-HIM future: A report from the AHIMA e-HIM Task Force. Supplement to *Journal of American Health Information Management Association.*

American Association for Medical Transcription. 2005. aamt.org

American Health Information Management Association. 2005a. Health information management: Professional definition. ahima.org/infocenter/.

American Health Information Management Association. 2005b. HIM baccalaureate degree knowledge cluster content and competency levels. ahima.org/academics/.

American Health Information Management Association. 2004. AHIMA timeline. library.ahima.org.

American Medical Informatics Association. 2005. amia.org.

College of Healthcare Information Management Executives. 2005. cio.chime.org.

Chronicle Guidance Publications. 1999. *Health Sciences Librarians Brief 516,* pp. 8–11. Moravia, NY: Chronicle Guidance Publications.

Greenes, R.A., and E.H. Shortliffe. 1990. Medical informatics: An emerging academic discipline and institutional priority. *Journal of the American Medical Association* 263(8):1114–20.

Health Information Management and Systems Society. 2005. himss.org.

Huffman, E.K. 1941. *Manual for Medical Records Librarians.* Chicago: Physicians' Record Company.

Institute of Medicine, Committee on Improving the Patient Record in Response to Increasing Functional Requirements and Technological Advances. 1997. *The Computer-Based Patient Record: An Essential Technology for Health Care.* Washington, DC: U.S. National Academy of Sciences.

International Federation of Health Records Organizations. 2005. ifhro.org

International Medical Informatics Association. 2005. imia.org

Merriam-Webster's Collegiate Dictionary. 1995. Springfield, MA: Merriam-Webster.

Millerson, G. 1964. *The Qualifying Association: A Study in Professionalization.* London: Routledge & Paul.

National Cancer Registrar's Association. 2005. ncra-usa.org.

Russell, L.A. 2001. Not what we were in 1928: A new professional definition. *Journal of American Health Information Management Association* 72(4):48A–48D.

Sager, A., and D. Socolar. 2005. Health care costs absorb one-quarter of economic growth, 2000–2005. Boston University School of Public Health, Health Reform Program. healthreformprogram.org.

Wing, P., and M.H. Langelier. 2004. The future of HIM: Employer insights into the coming decade of rapid change. *Journal of American Health Information Management Association* 75(6):28–32.

Wing, P., and E. Salsberg. 2002. How trends shape the work force today and tomorrow. *Journal of American Health Information Management Association* 73(4):38.

Chapter 5
Data and Information Management

Frances Wickham Lee, DBA, RHIA

Learning Objectives

- To understand the differences among data, information, and knowledge
- To discuss the basic principles of information management
- To discuss the JCAHO-based information management model
- To list and give examples of seven characteristics of quality data as outlined by AHIMA
- To list and give examples of the Essential Principles of Healthcare Documentation as developed by the Medical Record Institute Consensus Workgroup on Health Information Capture and Report Generation
- To discuss how the design of a database can affect data quality
- To compare a relational database and its characteristics with other database models

- To discuss how data modeling, particularly using an entity relationship diagram (ERD), can help ensure high-quality data
- To discuss the role of a data dictionary in ensuring both the quality of enterprise-wide data and data within a specific database application
- To apply appropriate visual data display techniques
- To apply techniques for improving presentation of data
- To describe and compare the roles of database administrator, data administrator, and data resource manager
- To discuss how to ensure the integrity and security of data within a database
- To apply principles of effective data display
- To apply principles for making effective presentations

Key Terms

Aggregate data
Attributes
Authorization management
Comparative data
Conceptual data model
Data
Data administrator
Data definition language (DDL)
Data dictionary
Data integrity
Data manipulation language (DML)
Data modeling
Data models

Data quality model
Data resource manager
Database
Database administrator
Database life cycle (DBLC)
Database management system (DBMS)
Derived attribute
Entity
Entity relationship diagram (ERD)
Foreign key
Information
Information capture
Information management

Integrity constraints
Key attributes
Knowledge
Knowledge-based data
Logical data model
Many-to-many relationship
Normalization
Object
Object-oriented database (OODB)
Object-oriented database management system (OODBMS)
One-to-many relationship
One-to-one relationship

Patient-specific data
Physical data model
Primary key
Relational database
Relational database management system (RDBMS)
Report generation
Seven dimensions of data quality
Structured query language (SQL)
System catalog
Unified modeling language (UML)

Introduction

Health information managers have numerous roles within the healthcare industry. Most, if not all, of these roles involve managing **data** and information shared by a diverse and sometimes widely dispersed group of users. Meeting the challenge of managing the data and information needed to deliver or support high-quality healthcare is not a simple task. Users have different information needs and may even have different data definitions. These different needs and definitions must be dealt with in developing effective healthcare information systems.

This chapter introduces data and information as organizational assets that must be managed effectively to provide and sustain their value. It looks at the relationship between data and information, a JCAHO-based model for managing healthcare information, other principles of healthcare **information management,** issues related to measuring data quality in a healthcare setting, basic database design, a few key concepts related to database management (**data dictionaries,** data management roles, ensuring the security and integrity of databases), and some basic principles of effective data and information display and presentation.

Theory into Practice

The following true story appeared in "Tools for Defining Data," an article written by Abdul-Malik Shakir and published in the *Journal of American Health Information Management Association* in September 1999. It clearly illustrates the need for users to agree on data definitions and some of the problems that can be created when definitions are not in place.

A large national health maintenance organization (HMO) was planning to create a disease management program for pediatric care. As part of the planning effort, the HMO decided to conduct a survey of its regional sites to determine the utilization pattern for pediatric care. It sent a questionnaire to the 12 regional offices asking these two questions:

1. How many pediatric members were enrolled as of year-end?
2. How many pediatric visits took place in one year?

On the surface, the questions seemed simple and appropriate. The HMO would determine the number of pediatric members and the number of pediatric visits by region. It then could compute pediatric utilization by region and across the program as a whole. These data then would be used to determine a baseline for development of utilization management programs and would assist in comparative analysis of pediatric utilization across regions.

There was only one problem: the absence of common data definitions. Each of the regions operated somewhat autonomously and interpreted the request for information differently. As a result, the regional offices raised a number of questions and revealed numerous discrepancies in their interpretations of data definitions:

1. What is a pediatric member?
   —A dependent member under the age of 18
   —A dependent member under the age of 21
   —A dependent child member, regardless of age
   —A patient under the age of 18

2. What is a pediatric visit?
   —A visit by a pediatric member
   —A visit by a patient under the age of 18
   —Any visit to the pediatric department
   —A visit with a pediatrician

Attempts to answer these questions only raised more questions. What is a member? What does it mean to be enrolled? What is a dependent? How is patient/member age calculated? What is a visit? What is a patient, and how does a patient differ from a member? What is a department? What are the department types? What is a pediatrician?

This story shows how important it is that suppliers and consumers of data agree on data definitions before exchanging information. Had the regions not revealed their assumptions, the discrepancies in their interpretations of the data definitions might never have been recognized, and the organization would have unknowingly compared apples to oranges. In the long term, a business strategy with significant implications would have been based on invalid information.

From Data to Information

Where does **information** come from? The simple answer is that information is processed data. Data are the raw facts, generally stored as characters, words, symbols, measurements, or statistics. Unprocessed data are not very useful for decision making. Take, for example, the numerals 6, 5, and 0. What do they mean? If seen together as 650, the data might be processed into the number six hundred and fifty. When processing this number further by looking it up in the ICD-9-CM codebook or entering it into an encoder software program, it takes on even more meaning. It is now known that 650 is the code that represents a completely normal delivery. Is this information? That depends. When looking for a particular patient's diagnosis to process a claim, 650 may, in fact, be providing the information an insurance clerk needs. However, for the medical researcher looking for patient characteristics that contribute to completely normal deliveries, 650 on one patient's chart is not yet "processed" enough to provide useful information. (See figure 5.1.)

Some texts include a third, higher level in the data-to-information hierarchy: **knowledge.** Johns (1997, p. 53) defines knowledge as "a combination of rules, relationships, ideas, and experience." People use knowledge to make decisions. In the 650 example above, the medical researcher might use his or her experience, diagnostic rules (written or not), and statistical rules to determine the relationships between patient characteristics and the 650 diagnosis. Computer systems that combine an expert knowledge base and some type of rule-based decision analysis component are sometimes referred to as knowledge systems to differentiate them from more traditional transaction-based or analytical information systems. Although computerized decision support systems (DSSs) in healthcare are not always knowledge systems, knowledge systems are almost always used for decision support. (See chapter 19 for more information on decision support systems.)

Where does data end and information begin? How are the two concepts related? Do the data collected and stored affect the information available within the organization? To answer these questions, one must first know who needs the data/information to perform what job function or functions. What people and what decisions are involved?

Information is a valuable asset at all levels of the healthcare organization. Personnel, both clinical and support staff, who perform the day-to-day operations related to patient care or administrative functions rely on information to do their jobs. This is truly the information age, and nowhere is this more apparent than in healthcare. Healthcare managers at both the middle management level and the executive level make extensive use of information, both to carry out day-to-day operations and in strategic planning for the organization. An interesting point to think about is that the same data may actually provide different information to different users.

In other words, one person's data may be another person's information.

To illustrate this point, consider a small data set that represents some patient demographic data. It might be a subset of data from a hospital master patient index (MPI) system. (See table 5.1.)

This single set of data could be used at all levels of the hospital, beginning with the admissions process, a day-to-day operation of the facility. Admission personnel would use the data set to verify previous admissions or the spelling of a name. They also would be responsible for data entry and updating the MPI to ensure that it contains accurate, timely data. The MPI data set, as is, would provide useful information to the admissions personnel.

At the middle management level, the director of outpatient services might want information about where recent patients live and how far they travel to use this hospital. He or she might further process or query the data set to classify patients by zip code. After the query is completed, the director of outpatient services has useful information to help identify where patients live.

The CEO is interested in patient mix as well but wants to see trend data over time showing the percentage of Medicare patients versus the percentage of private-pay and nonpaying patients. Again, the same data set is used, but the query process is more complex and the data set must be linked to another data set that contains payment information. The data in the MPI data set must be processed more extensively before any truly useful information is available to meet the CEO's needs.

Moreover, the data from the MPI might be used in strategic planning for the hospital. Any number of complex queries about the patient population could contribute to strategic marketing or development decisions. The organization might even combine the MPI data set with external data sets using sophisticated DDSs that compare its performance with the performance of other facilities in the region or state.

Figure 5.1.   From data to knowledge

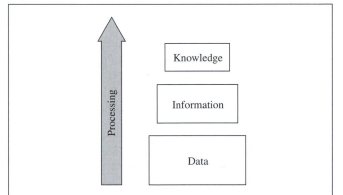

Check Your Understanding 5.1

Instructions: Answer the following questions on a separate piece of paper.

1. Give an example of data that are found in a patient medical record. How could these data become information?

2. Explain the statement that "one person's information can be another person's data."

Table 5.1.   Subset of a master patient index table

MRN	SSN	Last Name	First Name	Middle Name	DOB	Payment Type	Zip Code
096543	123-23-2345	Jones	Georgia	Louise	11/21/1957	Self	29425
065432	789-99-3456	Lexington	Milton	Robert	08/12/2000	Private	29425
467345	022-45-5378	Lovingood	Jill	Karen	10/14/1992	Medicaid	29401
678543	222-56-7777	Martin	Chloe	Mary	05/30/1978	Private	29465
234719	654-33-2222	Martin	John	Adams	06/22/1961	Private	29401
786543	435-89-0034	Nance	Natalie	JoAnn	11/27/1902	Medicare	29464

Joint Commission on Accreditation of Healthcare Organizations Model for Managing Information

In the 2005 *Comprehensive Accreditation Manual for Hospital: The Official Handbook,* the JCAHO introduces the Management of Information (IM) standards by emphasizing that information is a resource that must be managed carefully and deliberately, just as other categories of resources such as financial, material, and human resources are managed. The healthcare environment is complex and highly dependent on information. Therefore, the JCAHO states that "managing information is an active, planned activity" (p. IM-1). The JCAHO model for managing information displayed in figure 5.2 includes four types of healthcare data shown as inputs: **patient-specific, aggregate, comparative,** and **knowledge-based.**

Patient-specific data and information can be linked to a specific patient through a unique identifier, such as a medical record number or Social Security number. Patient-specific data and information are used to "facilitate patient care, treatment, and services, serve as a financial and legal record, aid in research, support decision analysis, and guide professional and organization performance improvement. This information may be maintained as a paper record or as electronic health information" (JCAHO 2005, pp. IM-15–16).

Aggregate data and information come from patient-specific information, but generally there are no patient identifiers and the data or information is presented in summary form. Results of a quality improvement study using summarized patient data is an example of aggregate information.

Comparative data and information are used for benchmarking or other comparisons within or across healthcare organizations. They do not include patient identifiers and are generally presented as summary data or statistics. The data and information falling into this category (unlike simply aggregate) are generally used to measure performance against an internal or external standard.

Knowledge-based information is a "collection of stored facts, models, and information that can be used for designing and redesigning processes and for problem solving." When the term is used by the JCAHO IM standards, it refers to the information found in the relevant clinical, scientific, and management literature (JCAHO 2005, p. GL-10).

All four types of healthcare data must be considered in the healthcare facility's overall plan for managing information.

The JCAHO model for managing information begins with a needs assessment and ends with information use. The ultimate goal of any healthcare information system is to produce high-quality information that can be used effectively to meet the organization's needs. There are many different, specific uses of healthcare information. The JCAHO identifies five categories of uses: clinical decision making, organizational decision making, research, performance improvement, and education (of patients, families, and healthcare providers).

The needs assessment is organization specific. Clearly, although they likely have some data and information needs in common, a 50-bed critical care hospital has different needs than a multifacility academic healthcare center. There is no "one size fits all" in planning how to manage a healthcare organization's information. After determining its information needs (based on the inputs identified in the model), the healthcare organization must plan and design its information systems (ISs). JCAHO does not dictate that the ISs must be computer based, but it does expect them to meet certain standards, whether they are paper based or fully electronic. In planning and designing ISs that will meet its identified needs, the healthcare organization must consider not only how to capture and report its information, but also how to process, analyze, store, retrieve, disseminate, display, and, finally, use it (JCAHO 2005).

Basic Principles of Information Management

With so many different uses of healthcare data and information, it is critical that healthcare organizations manage their information resources wisely. Before the design and development of any IS, it is important to understand and embrace some basic principles of information management beyond the JCAHO model.

In one well-known source, Austin and Boxerman (1998) cite three "overarching" principles for managing information resources:

1. Treat information as an essential organizational resource, on a par with human resources, financial resources, and capital facilities and equipment.
2. Obtain top executive support for IS planning and management.
3. Develop an IS strategic vision and plan.

These three principles may be considered steps in setting the stage for effective information management within the healthcare organization. However, planning for information systems involves other important considerations, including:

- The value of information lies in its application to decision making within the organization.
- High-quality data is the foundation of high-quality information.
- Integration of systems enhances IS quality and efficiency.
- Information users must be involved in defining needs and designing information systems.

All these principles are highly intertwined. Strategic IS planning is key to managing information resources wisely and ensuring that systems are compatible with one another

Figure 5.2. JCAHO IM model

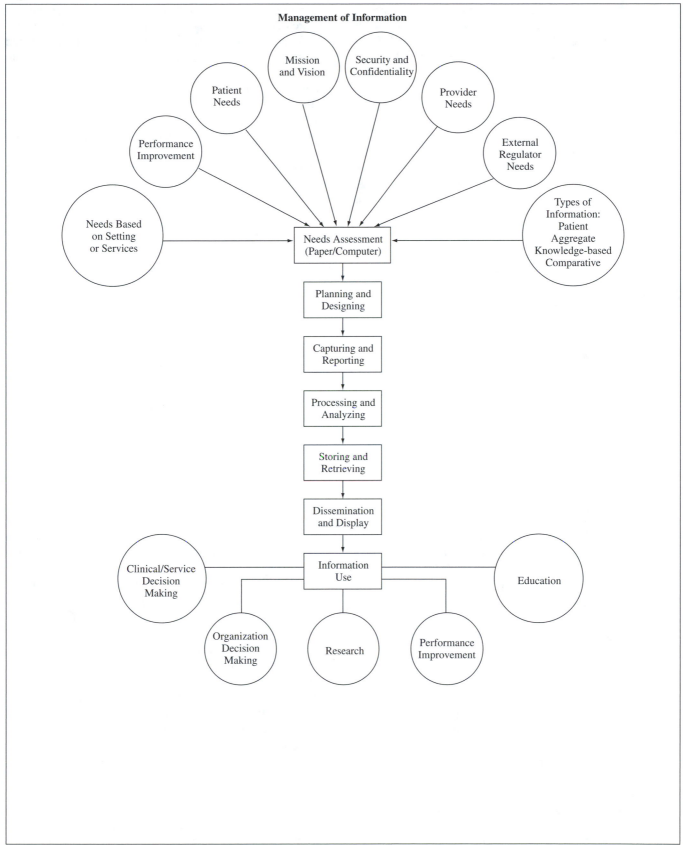

Source: JCAHO 2005.

and can be integrated. Moreover, planning ensures that the ISs the organization is developing are in line with its overall mission, goals, and strategic plan. The entire strategic IS planning process is only effective if the organization's top-level executives are supportive and actively involved.

It is the enterprise-wide nature of information that dictates the importance of systems integration and user involvement in defining and designing ISs. Too often, ISs are built for one particular unit within the organization, which can lead to inefficient management of information or even inaccurate information. If the users are not involved in every aspect of systems design and development, the resulting IS may function very well technically but be of no use to anyone. Which is worse, a technically weak and cumbersome computer system that provides the information needed or a technically savvy system that does not? Invariably, end users choose the cumbersome system that provides the "right" information. (See chapter 6 for a more complete discussion of strategic IS planning.)

Check Your Understanding 5.2

Instructions: Answer the following questions on a separate piece of paper.

1. Why does the JCAHO IM model begin with a needs assessment?

2. What basic types of information go into the JCAHO model? What are the basic categories of information used in the model?

3. What are the basic principles of information management?

4. Why is it particularly important for healthcare organizations to understand the basic principles of information management?

Data Quality

The concept of data quality is closely tied to the ability of a healthcare IS to support decision making at all levels of the organization. The adage "Garbage in, garbage out" is very true. This section discusses the importance of establishing data quality standards and introduces two sets of guidelines that can be used for this purpose.

How can one know when data quality has been achieved? The quality of data is tied to the use, or application, of the data. Again, high-quality data is the foundation of high-quality information and the value of information lies in its application to decision making within the organization.

Consider for a moment an organization with sophisticated healthcare ISs that affect every type of healthcare information, from patient-specific to knowledge-based. What if the quality of the documentation going into the systems is poor? What if there is no assurance that the reports generated from the systems are accurate or timely? How would the users of the systems react? Are those ISs beneficial or detrimental to the organization in achieving its goals (Wager, Lee, and Glaser 2005)?

A healthcare organization cannot have high-quality healthcare information without first establishing that it has high-quality healthcare data. We know that clinical providers and administrative staff gather healthcare information. Much

of this clinical information is recorded in patient records and subsequently coded for purposes of reimbursement and research. As noted in the discussion of the JCAHO model for managing information, patient record information is shared across many providers and payers, aggregated, and used to make comparisons relevant to healthcare and related issues (Wager, Lee, and Glaser 2005).

Poor-quality data collection and reporting can affect patient care, communication among providers and patients, documentation, revenue generation (due to problems with reimbursement), outcomes evaluation, or research activities.

The problems with poor-quality patient care data are not strictly limited to the patient medical record. In a recent well-circulated report, the Medical Records Institute (MRI) identified five major functions that are affected by poor-quality documentation (MRI 2004). These functions are found not only at the healthcare organizational level, but also throughout the healthcare environment.

Patient safety is affected by inadequate information, illegible entries, misinterpretations, and insufficient interoperability.

Public safety, a major component of public health, is diminished by the inability to collect information in a coordinated, timely manner at the provider level in response to epidemics and the threat of terrorism.

Continuity of patient care is adversely affected by the lack of shareable information among patient care providers.

Healthcare economics are adversely affected, with information capture and report generation costs currently estimated to be well over $50 billion annually.

Clinical research and outcomes analysis are adversely affected by a lack of uniform information capture that is needed to facilitate the derivation of data from routine patient care documentation.

The MRI report identifies healthcare documentation as having two basic parts: **information capture** and **report generation.** Information capture is "the process of recording representations of human thought, perceptions, or actions in documenting patient care, as well as device-generated information that is gathered and/or computed about a patient as part of health care" (MRI 2004, p. 2). Some means of information capture in healthcare organizations are handwriting, speaking, typing, touching a screen, pointing and clicking on words or phrases, videotaping, audio recording, and generating images through x-rays and scans.

Report generation "consists of the formatting and/or structuring of captured information. It is the process of analyzing, organizing, and presenting recorded patient information for authentication and inclusion in the patient's healthcare record" (MRI 2004, p. 2). In order to have high-quality documentation that results in high-quality data, both information capture and report generation must be considered.

Data Quality Standards

Before an organization can measure the quality of the information it produces and uses, it must establish data standards. That is, data can be identified as high quality only when they conform to a recognized standard. Ensuring this conformance is not as easy as it might seem because no universally recognized set of healthcare data quality standards exists today. One reason for this is that the quality of the data needed in any situation is driven by how the data or the information that comes from the data will be used. For example, in a patient care setting the margin of error for critical lab tests must be zero or patient safety is in jeopardy. However, a larger margin of error may be acceptable in census counts or discharge statistics. Healthcare organizations must establish data quality standards specific to the intended use of the data or resulting information.

Although no universally adopted healthcare data quality standards exist, two organizations have published guidance that can assist healthcare organizations in establishing their own data quality standards. In *Healthcare Documentation: A Report on Information Capture and Report Generation,* the MRI has published a set of "essential principles of healthcare documentation," and the American Health Information Management Association (AHIMA) has published data quality management guidelines (Wager, Lee, and Glaser 2005.)

MRI Principles of Healthcare Documentation

The MRI report states that many steps must be taken to ensure the quality of healthcare documentation (and, thus, the quality of healthcare data). It lists the essential principles that healthcare organizations should adhere to as they establish healthcare documentation and information systems (and their accompanying policies). (See figure 5.3, p, 106.) The MRI recommends that these principles be uniformly adopted by healthcare organizations.

It is noteworthy that the MRI takes the position that when practitioners interact with electronic resources, their ability to adhere to these principles is increased. All documentation records data and information, which needs to be retrieved in order to be used. The MRI argues that all healthcare information should be indexed "to facilitate both clinical and administrative retrieval" (MRI 2004, p. 16). This is difficult to do with unstructured, free text, such as handwriting, e-mails, and transcription. As electronic medical records are implemented and information capture methods become more interactive, the ability to retrieve information will improve. Table 5.2 (p. 107) shows documentation styles and major information capture methods.

AHIMA Data Quality Model

AHIMA has published a **data quality model** and an accompanying set of general data characteristics. There are some similarities between the AHIMA characteristics and the MRI key principles. However, one difference is that AHIMA strives to include all healthcare data and limits characteristics to clinical documentation. (See figures 5.4 and 5.5, pp. 107 and 108.)

The AHIMA model includes the following **seven dimensions of data quality:**

- *Relevancy:* Data must be relevant to the purpose for which they are collected. Very accurate, timely data

may be collected about a patient's color preferences or choice of hairdresser, but are they relevant to the patient's care?

- *Granularity:* Data granularity is sometimes referred to as data "atomicity," which means that the individual data elements cannot be further subdivided; they are "atomic." For example, a typical patient's name should generally be stored as three data elements—last name, first name, middle name ("Smith," "John." and "Allen")—and not as a single data element ("John Allen Smith"). Again, granularity can be related to the purpose for which the data are collected. Although it is possible to subdivide a person's birth date into separate fields for the month, date, and year, this is usually not desirable. Birth date is at the lowest level of granularity when used as a patient identifier.

- *Precision:* Precision often relates to numerical data. It denotes how close to an actual size, weight, or other standard a particular measurement is. Some healthcare data must be very precise. For example, in figuring drug dosage, it would be unacceptable to round up to the nearest gram if the drug were to be dosed in milligrams.

- *Timeliness:* Timeliness is a critical dimension in the quality of many types of healthcare data. Take, for example, a patient's discharge diagnoses recorded as ICD-9-CM codes. These codes must be recorded in a timely manner in order to facilitate reimbursement for the healthcare facility.

- *Currency:* Many types of healthcare data become obsolete after a period of time. A patient's admitting diagnosis is often changed by the time he or she is discharged. If a clinician needed a current diagnosis, which one would he or she choose?

- *Consistency:* Data quality needs to be consistent. A difference in the use of abbreviations provides a good example of how the lack of consistency can lead to problems. For example, a nurse may use CPR to mean cardiopulmonary resuscitation one time and computer-based patient record another time, leading to confusion if the chart were audited.

- *Accuracy:* Data that are free of errors are accurate. Typographical errors in discharge summaries or misspellings of names are examples of inaccurate data.

Data Quality Requirements for Information Systems

It already has been noted that users must be involved in defining their information needs and designing information systems. One of the first steps in systems analysis is to identify the users' specific data needs. As a part of this process, it is important to identify the level of quality the user requires for each data element. Another way to view this is to evaluate the use of the data along the seven dimensions of quality. This evaluation eventually will be translated into technical performance requirements for the IS.

Figure 5.3.   MRI consensus workgroup essential principles of healthcare documentation

For optimal information capture and report generation, it is important to establish a set of documentation principles to be implemented on a national/international basis. This report recommends that all healthcare documentation must meet the following "Essential Principles of Healthcare Documentation."

Unique identification of patient
Systems, policies, and practices should:
- Provide unique identification of the patient at the time of recording or accessing the information.
- Provide within and across organizations:
  –Simple and easy methods to identify individuals and correct duplicate identities of the same individual.
  –Methods to distinguish among individuals, including those with similar names, birth dates, and other demographic information.
  –Linkages between different identifications of the same individual.

Accuracy
Systems, policies, and practices should:
- Promote accuracy of information throughout the information capture and report generation processes as well as during its transfer among systems.
- Require review to assure accuracy prior to integration in the patient's record.
- Include a means to append a correction to an authenticated document, without altering the original.
- Require the use of standard terminology so as to diminish misinterpretations.

Completeness
Systems, policies, and practices should:
- Identify the minimum set of information required to completely describe an incident, observation, or intent.
- Provide means to ensure that the information recorded meets the legal, regulatory, institutional policy, or other requirements required for specific types of reports (for example, history and physical, operative note).
- Link amendments to the original document (that is, one should not be able to retrieve an original document without related amendments [or vice versa] or notification that such amendments exist and how to access them).
- Discourage duplication of information.
- Discourage nonrelevant and excessive documentation.

Timeliness
Systems, policies, and practices should:
- Require and facilitate that healthcare documentation be done during or immediately following the event so that:
  –Memory is not diminished or distorted.
  –The information is immediately available for subsequent care and decision making.
- Promote rapid system response time for entry as well as retrievability through:
  –Availability and accessibility of workstations.
  –User-friendly systems and policies that allow for rapid user access.
- Provide for automatic, unalterable time, date, and place stamp of each:
  –Documentation entry, such as dictation, uploading, scanning (original, edits, amendments).
  –Access to the documentation.
  –Transmittal of the documentation.

Interoperability
Systems, policies, and practices should:
- Provide the highest level of interoperability that is realistically achievable.
- Enable authorized practitioners to capture, share, and report healthcare information from any system, whether paper- or electronic-based.
- Support ways to document healthcare information so that it can be correctly read, integrated, and supplemented within any other system in the same or another organization.

Retrievability (the capability of allowing information to be found efficiently)
Systems, policies, and practices should:
- Support achievement of a worldwide consensus on the structure of information so that the practitioner can efficiently locate relevant information. This requires the use of standardized titles, formats, templates, and macros, as well as standardized terminology, abbreviations, and coding.
- Enable authorized data searches, indexing, and mining.
- Enable searches with incomplete information (for example, wild card searches, fuzzy logic searches).

Authentication and accountability
Systems, policies, and practices should:
- Uniquely identify persons, devices, or systems that create or generate the information and that take responsibility for its accuracy, timeliness, etc.
- Require that all information be attributable to its source (that is, a person or device).
- Require that unsigned documents be readily recognizable as such.
- Require review of documents prior to authentication. "Signed without review" and similar statements should be discouraged.

Auditability
Systems, policies, and practices should:
- Allow users to examine basic information elements, such as data fields.
- Audit access and disclosure of protected health information.
- Alert users of errors, inappropriate changes, and potential security breaches.
- Promote use of performance metrics as part of the audit capacity.

Confidentiality and Security
Systems, policies, and practices should:
- Demonstrate adherence to related legislation, regulations, guidelines, and policies throughout the healthcare documentation process.
- Alert the user to potential confidentially and security breaches.

RECOMMENDATION #1: Fund, create, and promote a practical implementation guide for the dissemination, teaching, and adoption of the "Essential Principles of Healthcare Documentation" by practitioners, providers, vendors, and healthcare organizations, as well as regulatory bodies and medical schools.

Source: MRI 2004.

Table 5.2.   Documentation styles and major information capture methods

	Free Text	Structured Text	Interactive Text
Handwriting	Mostly free text	Paper forms	N/A
Transcription	Mostly free text	Macros and normals	N/A
Speech Recognition	Free text	Templates	Interactive templates
Direct Input	Free text	Mostly structured text	More interactive

Source: MRI 2004.

Figure 5.4.   AHIMA data quality management model

Application—The purpose for which the data are collected.

Collection—The processes by which data elements are accumulated.

Warehousing—Processes and systems used to archive data and data journals.

Analysis—The process of translating data into information utilized for an application.

Source: AHIMA 1998.

Consider a billing IS. A patient's principal diagnosis is a critical piece of data that must be contained in the billing system. Which of the seven dimensions of quality must this principal diagnosis meet when it is recorded on the patient's bill? A principal diagnosis code is relevant to the bill and is, by nature, a granular, or atomic, data element. It is precise because it has only one meaning. However, the remaining dimensions of timeliness, currency, consistency, and accuracy also must be achieved. A billing system would be considered functioning well only if these quality dimensions for the principal diagnosis could be demonstrated.

Check Your Understanding 5.3

Instructions: Answer the following questions on a separate piece of paper.

1. Compare and summarize the similarities and differences between the AHIMA Data Quality Model and the MRI Essential Principles of Documentation.
   a. What data quality characteristics do they both list?
   b. What is the major difference between these two sets of guidelines? Are they compatible with one another?
2. List the seven dimensions of data quality.
3. Give one example of the importance of each dimension in ensuring the quality of patient information

Database Design and Management

Today's healthcare information systems are generally built on an underlying **database** structure. A database is a collection of data that is organized so that its contents can be easily accessed, managed, and updated (Whatis.com 2005). This type of IS structure can be found in computer applications ranging from an enterprise-wide clinical data repository to a small desktop application designed to track delinquent signatures on patient records. Regardless of the scope or size of the database used in an application, the theoretical constructs are the same and a good database design is equally important.

"A good database does not just happen" (Rob and Coronel 2002). The structure of the database must be designed carefully. A poorly designed database can lead to redundant data and information errors, which in turn can lead to poor management or patient care decisions. Redundant data within a database result from storing unnecessarily duplicated data.

Revisit the master patient index (MPI) subset described earlier. Think of it as representing a portion of a table within a database that provides the data for an integrated hospitalwide IS. Assume that this table stores all patient demographic information. This should be the only place where the patient's name, date of birth, and address are stored. If this information is needed in other applications, such as billing, the unique identifier (in this case, the medical record number [MRN]) should be used to link the table to other tables with the accounting and billing information. Storing a data element in one location within the database enables accurate data updates and deletions.

Suppose there was a separate storage table for patient demographic information for each department-level application. The patient's demographic information would be stored in a billing database and in the MPI database. What if a patient's name was misspelled or a birth date was incorrect? Someone would have to go to each table separately and update the information. Updating the MPI without also updating the billing database would lead to reports yielding inconsistent, if not inaccurate, results. How would anyone know which table had the correct information?

It is no exaggeration to say that a poorly designed database can lead to poor decision making. The database is the source from which information is created. To repeat, one of the basic principles of information management is that the value of information lies in its application to decision making within the organization.

Figure 5.5.   AHIMA characteristics of data quality

Characteristic	Application	Collection	Warehousing	Analysis
Data Accuracy Ensure data are the correct values and are valid.	To facilitate accuracy or to determine the application's purpose, the question to be answered, or the aim for collecting the data element.	Ensuring accuracy involves appropriate education and training and timely and appropriate communication of data definitions to those who collect data. For example, data accuracy will help ensure that if a patient's sex is female, it is accurately recorded as female and not male.	To warehouse data, appropriate edits should be in place to ensure accuracy. For example, error reports should be generated for inconsistent values such as an inappropriate diagnosis for age or gender. Exception or error reports should be generated and corrections should be made.	To accurately analyze data, ensure that the algorithms, formulas, and translation systems are correct. For example, ensure that the encoder assigns correct codes and that the appropriate DRG is assigned for the codes entered. Also, ensure that each record or entry within the database is correct.
Data Accessibility Data items should be easily obtainable and legal to collect.	The application and legal, financial, process, and other boundaries determine which data to collect. Ensure that collected data are legal to collect for the application. For example, recording the age and race in medical records may be appropriate. However, it may be illegal to collect this information in human resources departments.	When developing the data collection instrument, explore methods to access needed data and ensure that the best, least costly method is selected. The amount of accessible data may be increased through system interfaces and integration of systems. For example, the best and easiest method of obtaining demographic information may be to obtain it from an existing system. Another method may be to assign data collection by the expertise of each team member. For example, the admission staff collects demographic data, the nursing staff collects symptoms, and the HIM staff assigns codes. Team members should be assigned accordingly.	Technology and hardware impact accessibility. Establish data ownership and guidelines for who may access data and/or systems. Inventory data to facilitate access.	Access to complete, current data will better ensure accurate analysis. Otherwise results and conclusions may be inaccurate or inappropriate. For example, use of the Medicare case-mix index (CMI) alone does not accurately reflect total hospital CMI. Consequently, strategic planning based solely on Medicare CMI may not be appropriate.
Data Comprehensiveness All required data items are included. Ensure that the entire scope of the data is collected and document intentional limitations.	Clarify how the data will be used and identify end users to ensure complete data are collected for the application. Include a problem statement and cost-benefit or impact study when collected data are increased. For example, in addition to outcome, it may be important to gather data that impact outcomes.	Cost-effective comprehensive data collection may be achieved via interface to or download from other automated systems. Data definition and data precision impact comprehensive data collection (see these characteristics below).	Warehousing includes managing relationships of data owners, data collectors, and data end users to ensure that all are aware of the available data in the inventory and accessible systems. This also helps to reduce redundant data collection.	Ensure that all pertinent data impacting the application are analyzed in concert.
Data Consistency The value of the data should be reliable and the same across applications.	Data are consistent when the value of the data is the same across applications and systems, such as the patient's medical record number. In addition, related data items should agree. For example, data are inconsistent when it is documented that a male patient has had a hysterectomy.	The use of data definitions, extensive training, standardized data collection (procedures, rules, edits, and process), and integrated/interfaced systems facilitate consistency.	Warehousing employs edits or conversion tables to ensure consistency. Coordinate edits and tables with data definition changes or data definition differences across systems. Document edits and tables.	Analyze data under reproducible circumstances by using standard formulas, scientific equations, variance calculations, and other methods. Compare "apples to apples."

Figure 5.5.   (Continued)

Characteristic	Application	Collection	Warehousing	Analysis
Data Currency The data should be up-to-date. A datum value is up-to-date if it is current for a specific point in time. It is outdated if it was current at some preceding time, yet incorrect at a later time.	The appropriateness or value of an application changes over time. For example, traditional quality assurance applications are gradually being replaced by those with the more current application of performance improvement.	Data definitions change or are modified over time. These should be documented so that current and future users know what the data mean. These changes should be communicated in a timely manner to those collecting data and to the end users.	To ensure current data are available, warehousing involves continually updating systems, tables, and databases. The dates of warehousing events should be documented.	The availability of current data impacts the analysis of data. For example, to study the incidence of diseases or procedures, ICD-9-CM codes may be used. Coding practices or the actual code for a disease or procedures may change over time. This should be taken into consideration when analyzing trends.
Data Definition Clear definitions should be provided so that current and future data users will know what the data mean. Each data element should have clear meaning and acceptable values.	The application's purpose, the question to be answered, or the aim for collecting the data element must be clarified to ensure appropriate and complete data definitions.	Clear, concise data definitions facilitate accurate data collection. For example, the definition of patient disposition may be "the patient's anticipated location or status following release or discharge." Acceptable values for this data element should also be defined. The instrument of collection should include data definitions and ensure that data integrity characteristics are managed.	Warehousing includes archiving documentation and data. Consequently, data ownership documentation and definitions should be maintained over time. Inventory maintenance activities (purging, updates, and others), purpose for collecting data, collection policies, information management policies, and data sources should be maintained over time also.	For appropriate analysis, display data needs to reflect the purpose for which the data were collected. This is defined by the application. Appropriate comparisons, relationships, and linkages need to be shown.
Data Granularity The attributes and values of data should be defined at the correct level of detail.	A single application may require varying levels of detail or granularity. For example, census statistics may be utilized daily, weekly, or monthly depending upon the application. Census is needed daily to ensure adequate staffing and food service. However, the monthly trend is needed for long-range planning.	Collect data at the appropriate level of detail or granularity. For example, the temperature of 100° may be recorded. The granularity for recording outdoor temperatures is different from recording patient temperatures. If patient Jane Doe's temperature is 100°, does that mean 99.6° or 100.4°? Appropriate granularity for this application dictates that the data need to be recorded to the first decimal point while appropriate granularity for recording outdoor temperatures may not require it.	Warehouse data at the appropriate level of detail or granularity. For example, exception or error reports reflect granularity based on the application. A spike (exception) in the daily census may show little or no impact on the month-to-date or monthly reports.	Appropriate analysis reflects the level of detail or granularity of the data collected. For example, a spike (exception) in the daily census resulting in immediate action to ensure adequate food service and staffing may have had no impact on analysis of the census for long-range planning.
Data Precision Data values should be just large enough to support the application or process.	The application's purpose, the question to be answered, or the aim for collecting the data element must be clarified to ensure data precision.	To collect data precise enough for the application, define acceptable values or value ranges for each data item. For example, limit values for gender to male, female, and unknown; or collect information by age ranges.		

(Continued on next page)

Figure 5.5.   (Continued)

Characteristic	Application	Collection	Warehousing	Analysis
Data Relevancy The data are meaningful to the performance of the process or application for which they are collected.	The application's purpose, the question to be answered, or the aim for collecting the data element must be clarified to ensure relevant data.	To better ensure relevancy, complete a pilot of the data collection instrument to validate its use. A "parallel" test may also be appropriate, completing the new or revised instrument and the current process simultaneously. Communicate results to those collecting data and to the end users. Facilitate or negotiate changes as needed across disciplines or users.	Establish appropriate retention schedules to ensure availability of relevant data. Relevancy is defined by the application.	For appropriate analysis, display data to reflect the purpose for which the data were collected. This is defined by the application. Show appropriate comparisons, relationships, and linkages.
Data Timeliness Timeliness is determined by how the data are being used and their context.	Timeliness is defined by the application. For example, patient census is needed daily to provide sufficient day-to-day operations staffing, such as nursing and food service. However, annual or monthly patient census data are needed for the facility's strategic planning.	Timely data collection is a function of the process and collection instrument.	Warehousing ensures that data are available per information management policy and retention schedules.	Timely data analysis allows for the initiation of action to avoid adverse impacts. For some applications, timely may be seconds. For others it may be years.

Source: AHIMA 1998.

Database Life Cycle

Chapter 6 introduces the concept of a systems development life cycle (SDLC), which is used in systems analysis to illustrate the stages of development for an IS. The general SDLC provides a framework for developing any type of IS project. When dealing with a database project, the SDLC is often referred to as the **database life cycle** (DBLC) (Rob and Coronel 2002). The phases of the DBLC correspond to those of the general SDLC but include the specific tasks needed to develop an effective database.

Figure 5.6 illustrates a six-phase DBLC. The phases of this life cycle are as follows:

1. *Database initial study:* In the initial study phase, the database developer meets with key users and develops a list of user requirements. Technical requirements are discussed, and an analysis of how this database fits with existing systems is conducted.

2. *Database design:* In the design phase, the type of database is determined (relational or **object** oriented, for example). Conceptual-level and logical-level data models are developed during this phase. User interface also is designed. User–developer interaction is critical during this phase. Depending on the scope of the project, a prototype database may be developed and tested.

3. *Database implementation:* The database is actually loaded onto the network or workstation where it will reside. Test users are assigned user and access rights at the time of implementation.

4. *Testing and evaluation:* The importance of testing the database and evaluating the results of the testing cannot be overemphasized. Many times, even after careful design, problems are not discovered until the database is being used in a "live" environment.

5. *Database operation:* After the database is implemented, tested, and evaluated, it can be put into full operation.

6. *Database maintenance and evaluation:* In this last phase of the cycle, the database must be continually maintained, evaluated for its usefulness and efficiency, and updated as enhancements or changes are required.

It is important to recognize that this life cycle is an iterative, rather than a sequential, process. Each phase can lead to modifications in other phases. This chapter focuses on activities related primarily to the design phase, although the design phase is closely related to the other phases of the SDLC. For example, the importance of user involvement in defining the objectives and constraints of the database cannot be overemphasized. Moreover, users are critical to development of a complete and accurate data dictionary. (Data dictionaries

Figure 5.6.   Six-phase database life cycle

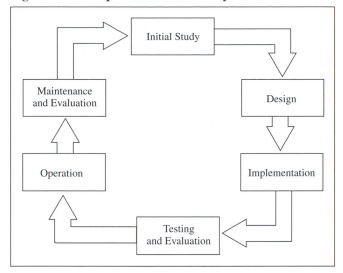

are defined and discussed later in this chapter.) Compare the database life cycle to the JCAHO IM model. The database life cycle or many life cycles would be contained within the iterative IM model. Each application selected by the organization that utilized a database would have included one or more database life cycles.

Data models, which are pictures or abstractions of real conditions, are used extensively during database design. A good analogy for a data model is a blueprint of a new building. No reputable builder would construct a building without a detailed blueprint. Of course, some changes may occur along the way, but the basic foundation and ways in which the building units will be put together are worked out in the blueprint. The use of data models facilitates communication between the technically oriented database designer and the end users. Data models also enable the individuals involved in database design to explore the features and characteristics of the database before actual implementation occurs.

Types of Databases

Before beginning a more detailed discussion of using and developing data models, the common types of databases and their associated **database management systems** (DBMSs) should be defined. This section defines and describes two database structures: **relational** and **object oriented.** Two other structures, hierarchical and network, are older types that no longer have a significant presence in the database market. They may be found as legacy systems within healthcare organizations but not in newer systems.

Relational Database Structure

The relational database model was developed in 1970 (Rob and Coronel 2002). It was not considered a practical design at the time because it required significant processing power. As computers became more powerful in the late 1980s and 1990s, the relational database became the predominant type used in

healthcare and in other industries. A relational database is implemented through a **relational database management system** (RDBMS). The major advantage of the RDBMS is that it allows a database designer to operate at a logical, rather than a physical, level. (See section on levels of data models.) Microsoft Access is an example of an RDBMS for developing desktop applications. Oracle, DB2, and Sybase are examples of more robust systems for developing larger applications.

The RDBMS consists of three distinct components: the interface, the data manipulation "engine," and the tables. (See figure 5.7.) The interface component is developed using a wide variety of software. In Microsoft Access, for example, Visual Basic for Applications (VBA) is built into the RDBMS and is used to create the forms and reports that comprise the majority of the user interface. The tables within a relational database are created using a special type of software, a **data definition language** (DDL). In between the user interface and the data tables is the database engine, the component that retrieves, edits, and updates the data from its underlying tables. The type of software used for these functions is called a **data manipulation language** (DML).

The most common language used for both DDL and DML for relational databases today is **structured query language** (SQL). All RDBMSs support SQL, and many RDBMS vendors have created extensions to the language that are specific to their product. The SQL used in Access looks slightly different from the SQL used in Oracle. SQL is a nonprocedural, or fourth-generation, language. The user specifies what must be done, but not how it is to be done. In other words, the SQL user does not have to know about the complex actions that actually are occurring when an SQL command is executed by the computer (Rob and Coronel 2002).

Tables (sometimes called relations) provide the foundation of a relational database. Each table consists of rows and columns. Rows represent each record within the table; columns represent the data fields or **attributes** of each table.

Tables in a relational database are related to one another by sharing a common field, or key attribute. In the earlier example involving the MPI and the billing system, these two tables could be linked by the key attribute, MRN.

Figure 5.7.   RDSMS components

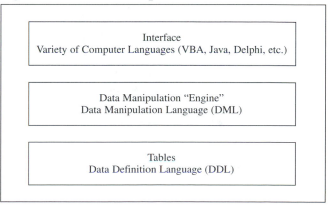

The relational database has several advantages over its predecessors, the network and hierarchical databases. The most important advantages include:

- *Structural independence:* It is possible to make changes to the database structure without affecting how the RDBMS accesses the data. In other words, data elements can be changed in the tables without affecting the data manipulation features or interface with the user.
- *Improved conceptual simplicity:* Through its use of logical tables, the relational database makes it easier for the developer and the user to understand the data.
- *Easier database design, implementation, management, and use:* Relational databases are much easier to design and manage than their predecessors were.
- *Ad hoc query capability:* The common data manipulation language, SQL, is simple to use and understand because it so closely resembles the English language.
- *A powerful database management system:* A good RDBMS makes it possible to hide a system's physical complexity from the developer and the user (Rob and Coronel 2002).

Object-Oriented Database Structure

The newest type of database structure is the object-oriented database (OODB). The basic component in the OODB is an object, not a table. An object includes both data and their relationships within a single structure; it is conceptually more difficult to understand than a table. **Object-oriented database management systems** (OODBMSs) utilize classes and subclasses that "inherit" characteristics from the parent class. The goal of using objects in programs and database management systems is to promote reuse of program codes and to store the data with the methods (procedures) that use the data. Object-oriented database concepts are beyond the scope of this chapter, but experts have predicted that they will have a definitive impact on healthcare applications in the near future (Duffy 1997). "Pure" object-oriented databases are not yet common in the healthcare market, but there are applications with object-oriented components built upon relational databases. This hybrid database type is referred to as an object-relational database.

Data Models

Data modeling serves as a link between "real" things about which the organization wants to collect and maintain data and the actual database structure. One of the problems with database design is that designers, programmers, and users do not necessarily see data the same way. Different users have different views of the organization's data, depending on their particular needs. Different views of data can lead to poorly constructed information systems that fail to meet the needs of many users. Ensuring that communication among designers, programmers, and users is as unambiguous as possible can prevent this. Data modeling is an excellent communication tool for reducing complex data structures to easy-to-understand pictures or abstractions.

Levels of Data Models

There are three levels of data models: conceptual, logical, and physical. These levels are based on the degree of abstraction represented by the data model. The **conceptual data model** is the one with the highest level of abstraction. In other words, it is neither hardware nor software dependent. In theory, the same conceptual model can be developed whether the organization develops its database as a relational database or an object-oriented database. The conceptual model also implies that it defines requirements for the entire enterprise or organizational unit under consideration. End users should be intimately involved in the development of conceptual data models. The level of abstraction should be high enough that end users with little or no computer programming experience can visualize the data requirements.

The next level of data model is the **logical data model.** The logical data model is still hardware independent but will be drawn to match the type of database management system (DBMS) that will be used. There are differences in the way logical models are depicted, depending on whether the DBMS is relational or object oriented. For example, the **entity relationship diagram** (ERD), described in detail in later sections of this chapter, was developed to depict relational database structures. It can be used to depict conceptual-level models for any type of database but would only be used to model a relational database at the logical level. A common notation used for modeling object-oriented databases is **unified modeling language** (UML). UML can be used to depict a conceptual data model and a logical OODB model.

Another characteristic of the logical data model is that it is drawn to represent a view of the data by a specific group within the enterprise, for example, a department or a unit within a department. Of course, the logical data model should be based on the conceptual model for the enterprise. Another way to think about logical data models is that they are components of the conceptual model with more DBMS-related detail.

The **physical data model** is concerned with the lowest level of abstraction, including how data are physically stored on storage media such as disks or tapes (Rob and Coronel 2002). This level of modeling is generally done by programmers or database developers with little interaction with users (Johns 1997). As relational and object-oriented databases have become more widely used, the physical data model has decreased in importance. One of the strengths of the relational and object-oriented databases is that they do not require the physical modeling details required by the older hierarchical and network database structures.

Data Modeling Process

The importance of data modeling cannot be overstated. Not only does the data model serve as a communication tool among IS developers and users, but it also provides the developer an opportunity to work out conceptual and design issues and problems prior to beginning the actual design process. This is an important step in ensuring the quality of the data and, subsequently, the quality of the information that can be gathered from the IS. The data themselves constitute the most basic units within an IS.

As stated earlier, one of most common data models, the ERD, is associated with relational database design. The ERD modeling technique is used to develop both conceptual and logical data models for relational databases. Several different sets of notations are used for drawing an ERD. Two of the most common methods are the Chen model and the Crow's foot model. Peter Chen developed his notation for ERDs in the 1970s (Rob and Coronel 2002). The Crow's foot model was developed by C. W. Bachman and is based on the same modeling concepts as the original Chen model. However, the Crow's foot model depicts the data relationships at a slightly higher level of abstraction than the Chen model does, making it a very effective communication tool for users and developers (Rob and Coronel 2002). The models used for illustration throughout this chapter are drawn using the Crow's foot symbols.

Figure 5.8 illustrates a simple ERD drawn using the conventions associated with the Chen model and the Crow's foot symbols. These models show that the relationship between the data table (or **entity**) HOSPITAL and the data table (or entity) DIVISION is one to many. This relationship means that for every instance of HOSPITAL stored in the database, many related instances of DIVISION may be stored. Reading the diagram in the other direction, each instance of DIVISION stored in the database is related to only one instance of HOSPITAL. Think about a multihospital system that has three hospitals—A, B, and C. Each hospital has multiple divisions within it, and each specific division (for example, the finance division in A) is related to only one hospital.

Although a detailed discussion of the conventions and steps associated with developing an ERD are beyond the scope of this chapter, the basic steps for developing an ERD for a simple end-user database is outlined. Readers desiring a more complete discussion should refer to a database development textbook, such as *Database Systems: Design, Implementation, and Management* (Rob and Coronel 2002).

An ERD is a graphical representation of the entities, attributes, and relationships that comprise a database. It is used as a planning and communication tool throughout the database development process. As stated earlier, an ERD can be used as a conceptual-level data model for any type of database and as a logical-level data model for a relational database. This discussion examines a simple ERD being developed for a patient-tracking system in a rural healthcare system that operates three clinics. The proposed tracking system will be developed as a relational database. Its purpose is to track patient visits within the three clinics.

Entities

Entities in the ERD are represented by a rectangle. An entity is a person, place, or thing about which data are to be collected in the database being designed. What would the entities for the patient-tracking database be?

Another way to think about entities is that they eventually will be transformed into the tables within the database. The entities for the visit-tracking database would be PATIENT, CLINIC, and VISIT. There could be more entities, depending on the data to be stored. For example, if one wanted to collect information about the provider of care for the visit, one would likely have an entity, PROVIDER, or even two entities, PHYSICIAN and NURSE. Selecting the entities for an ERD depends on the purpose of the proposed database. This example limits data collection to VISIT, PATIENT, and CLINIC.

Attributes

Attributes are the characteristics or data elements to be collected about each entity. They can be depicted in an ERD as oval shapes coming off an entity. This method is not practical when there are many attributes per table; therefore, many designers use a separate list to document attributes. In the Crow's foot notation, attributes are sometimes listed within the entity rectangle.

What would be some likely attributes in this example? For the PATIENT table, one would want to store a unique identifier for the patient, such as a Social Security number or a medical record number. This unique identifier is called a **primary key.** A primary key cannot be duplicated within the table and cannot contain a null value. Each table row or record within the database must have a unique primary key.

Figure 5.8.   ERD notations

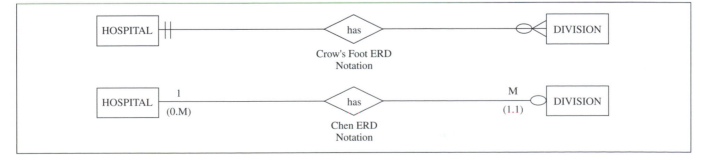

Continuing with the example, one also would want to store at least basic demographic information such as address, phone number, and date of birth. Figure 5.5 shows simplified, partial lists of attributes for the three tables. Attributes become the fields or column headings within the data tables of a relational database. Notice that the names of the attributes in figure 5.9 adhere to a common naming convention for database fields. The name of the table makes up the first part of the name followed by an underscore. This way, it is easy to identify where a particular data element is stored by looking at its names. Also note that these attributes are all "atomic," meaning they cannot be further subdivided.

Another type of attribute is a **derived attribute.** Derived attributes are not stored in the database table but, instead, are calculated when the database is accessed. An example of a derived attribute is age. A patient's age at the time of a visit could be calculated using the date of birth attribute, the admission date, and the visit date. A patient's current age could be calculated using date of birth and today's date.

In this example, the primary key (PK) for PATIENT, PATIENT_MRN, is repeated in VISIT, as is the PK for CLINIC, CLINIC_ID. These keys are called **foreign keys** (FK) in the VISIT table. By having the foreign keys in VISIT, the information in PATIENT and CLINIC is linked through the VISIT table. Figure 5.10 illustrates the ERD for this example.

Relationships

Relationships are represented in an ERD by a diamond shape or as text across the relationship line. The name of the relationship is usually a verb that describes the relationship between two or more of the entities in the diagram. A conceptual ERD contains three types of relationships:

- **One-to-one relationship**
- **One-to-many relationship**
- **Many-to-many relationship**

A one-to-one relationship exists when an instance of an entity (a row or record) is associated with one instance of another entity, and vice versa. This type of relationship is illustrated in figure 5.11. The relationships shown in figure 5.7 are taken from a current bed assignment database. There is only one bed per patient and one patient per bed. One-to-one relationships are rare in logical-level data models because they often indicate that a separate entity is unnecessary. Often a one-to-one relationship can be implemented as an attribute or field within a single table. In other words, a field, PATIENT_BED, could be added in the PATIENT table in this example to collect this information.

The one-to-many relationship exists when one instance of an entity is associated with many instances of another entity. In the example shown in figure 5.11, the relationship between PATIENT and VISIT is one to many. For each instance of PATIENT in the database, there could be many instances of VISIT. In other words, each patient may have many visits,

but each visit is associated with only one patient. The relationship between CLINIC and VISIT is also one to many. For each instance of CLINIC, there can be many VISITS, but each visit occurs in only one clinic. One-to-many relationships also can be optional. In this example, however, they are not because each patient must have a visit before he or she is entered into the database and each clinic must have visits before it is entered into the database.

Whether a relationship is optional is determined by the "business rules" of an organization. If one said that patients were entered into the database before they had any visits, this relationship would change to optional. This might occur in a family-oriented clinic where children or spouses of patients were registered but never seen.

Figure 5.9. Partial attribute lists for PATIENT, VISIT, and CLINIC

PATIENT Entity Attributes	VISIT Entity Attributes
PATIENT_MRN (PK) PATIENT_LNAME PATIENT_FNAME PATIENT_MNAME PATIENT_SSN PATIENT_STREET PATIENT_CITY PATIENT_STATE PATIENT_ZIPCODE PATIENT_PHONE PATIENT_DOB . . .	VISIT_ID (PK) VISIT_DATE VISIT_REASON PATIENT_MRN (FK) CLINIC_ID(FK) . . .

CLINIC Entity Attributes

CLINIC_ID (PK)
CLINIC_NAME
CLINIC_STREET
CLINIC_CITY
CLINIC_STATE
CLINIC_ZIPCODE
CLINIC_PHONE
CLINIC_FAX
. . .

Figure 5.10. Sample ERD

Figure 5.11. One-to-one relationship

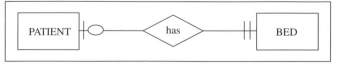

A many-to-many relationship occurs only in a data model developed at the conceptual level. In the example shown in figure 5.11, suppose the need for a separate VISIT entity was not recognized. The relationship between PATIENT and CLINIC is many to many. For each instance of PATIENT, there could be many instances of CLINIC because patients can be seen in more than one clinic. For each instance of CLINIC, there could be many PATIENTS because the clinic sees many patients. Figure 5.12 shows the many-to-many relationship between PATIENT and CLINIC.

Well-structured databases consist primarily of one-to-many relationships. Many-to-many relationships cannot be implemented in a relational database and, as discussed, one-to-one relationships are rare. The process of ensuring that the data model can be implemented as relational tables in a database is called **normalization.** By normalizing the data tables to ensure that data are stored in only one location, except for the planned redundancy inherent in **key attributes,** database developers decrease the possibility of data anomalies resulting from additions and deletions.

Check Your Understanding 5.4

Instructions: Answer the following questions on a separate piece of paper.

1. Which type of database is the most common today?

2. How does database design affect the quality of the data stored in the database?

3. What is a data model?

4. Discuss the differences among a conceptual-level, logical-level, and physical-level data model.

5. What are some common uses of an ERD? What is UML?

6. Define the basic components of an ERD.

7. How are the entities and relationships depicted in an ERD?

8. Using the Crow's foot notation, draw an ERD to depict the following relationship: Each patient has one physician, but each physician has many patients.

Data Dictionary Used as a Tool in Controlling Data Quality

An important tool in controlling the quality of data in healthcare is the data dictionary. Whenever a set of data is created, it should have an accompanying data dictionary. Revisit the brief scenario described at the beginning of this chapter. The problems encountered because of a lack of data definitions could have been avoided had the organization invested time and resources in developing a data dictionary.

Figure 5.12.   Many-to-many relationship

Types of Data Dictionaries

There are two general types of data dictionaries: the DBMS data dictionary and the organization-wide data dictionary.

DBMS Data Dictionary

The DBMS data dictionary is developed in conjunction with development of the database. Modern DBMSs have built-in data dictionaries that go beyond data definitions and store information about tables and data relationships. These integrated data dictionaries are sometimes referred to as **system catalogs,** reflecting their technical nature.

Figure 5.13 shows a portion of a designer-defined data dictionary developed in Microsoft Access for the simplified PATIENT table discussed earlier. The database developer would use this portion of the software to define the data to be stored in the database's system catalog.

A typical data dictionary associated with a DBMS allows for at least documentation of the following:

- Table names
- All attribute or field names
- A description of each attribute
- The data type of the attribute (text, number, date, and so on)
- The format of each attribute, such as DD_MM_YYYY for the date
- The size of each attribute, such as 11 characters in a Social Security number with dashes
- An appropriate range of values, such as integers 100000–999999 for the health record number
- Whether the attribute is required
- Relationships among attributes

Other descriptions that might be stored in the data dictionary associated with a database include:

- Who created the database
- When the database was created
- Where the database is located
- What programs can access the database
- Who the end users and administrators of the database are
- How access authorization is provided to all users

Organization-wide Data Dictionary

The second type of data dictionary is developed outside the framework of a specific database design process. This data dictionary serves to promote data quality through data consistency across the organization. Individual data element definitions are agreed upon and defined. It leads to better-quality data and facilitates the detailed, technical data dictionaries that are integrated with the databases themselves. Ideally, every healthcare organization will develop a data dictionary to define common data and their formats. This organization-wide document becomes a valuable resource for IS development.

Looking at the MPI example discussed earlier, what would need to be defined for each field? Although everyone

Figure 5.13.   Partial data dictionary for PATIENT table

may think they know the definition of a Last Name, can they all agree that it will be stored as no more than 25 characters? How should the Middle Name be handled? Will it be the maiden name for married women? Is the medical record number to be stored with leading zeros? Is the Social Security number required? If so, what will be used when it is not available? All these issues can be settled with the development of an organization-wide data dictionary.

Another challenge for healthcare managers results from interorganizational projects or the merger of healthcare organizations. Suppose a multifacility organization wanted to merge its MPI systems. Imagine the challenges involved in not only defining data elements, but also in uncovering existing definitions. What if the organizations in question had built other systems based on internal MPI definitions?

The true story of the HMO discussed at the beginning of this chapter could have been prevented if the HMO had developed an organization-wide data dictionary. Each regional office then would have been using the same definitions.

Development of Data Dictionaries

The health information manager would be a key member of any data dictionary project team. Developing a data diction-

ary can be an overwhelming task in light of the diversity of data users and the size and scope of some healthcare organizations. However, the following simple steps can be taken at the beginning of the data dictionary development project to get it under way:

1. *Define the scope of the project.* Is the project related to one application, one facility, or the entire organization?
2. *Determine the members of the project team.* The scope of the project will dictate who needs to be involved. If multiple facilities are involved, each one will need adequate representation on the team. The team should have representatives from all user groups, including clinicians and administrative personnel.
3. *Set priorities.* Which group of data elements is most critical to the project? Making this determination will clarify where to begin.
4. *Learn from the experience of others.* Investigate how other organizations have developed data dictionaries (Duffy 1997). The Internet and published journal articles, as well as personal contacts, can be helpful for this step.

Roles in Data Management

This chapter focuses on the importance of maintaining high-quality data that will lead to high-quality information and decisions. High-quality data do not just happen. Healthcare organizations must establish mechanisms and policies for managing their data resources. Such mechanisms and policies must encompass not only the technical aspects of implementing and maintaining the databases within the organization, but also ensure that the data conform to established standards of quality. Several roles within the healthcare IS team can be used to manage the quality of healthcare data. These include **database administrator, data administrator,** and an emerging role for HIM professionals, as defined by AHIMA (1999), **data resource manager.**

Database Administrator

The technical aspects of managing a database are usually assigned to a database administrator (DBA). Typical DBA functions include defining and developing the database, implementing the technical aspects of the DBMS, monitoring the performance of the database, creating and enforcing the security measures associated with the DBMS, and managing the system catalogs or data dictionaries that are internal to the DBMS (Johns 1997).

DBAs typically have information technology (IT) backgrounds and may not be equipped to deal with managing the less technical side of data quality, particularly healthcare data. This has led some healthcare organizations to create a new position—the data administrator (DA).

Data Administrator

According to Johns (1997), the functions of the data administrator include:

- Planning for the database, including identifying the major entities, attributes, and relationships among entities and developing the conceptual data models for the organization
- Evaluating and selecting an appropriate DBMS
- Managing an enterprise-wide data dictionary
- Training database users
- Developing and implementing database security policies and procedures

The DA must work closely with the DBA, but the focus of the DA role is on managing the data and the database rather than on the technical implementation and maintenance issues that are the DBA's responsibility.

Data Resource Manager

In 1998, AHIMA described an emerging data management role for HIM managers in its Vision 2006 document—the data resource manager (DRM). AHIMA (1999) defines a DRM as the person who "uses technical tools, such as computer-based health record systems, data repositories, and data warehouses . . . (to) ensure that the organization's information systems meet the needs of those who provide and manage patient services along the continuum of care and that the organization's data resources are secure, accessible, accurate, and reliable."

The role of the DRM is specifically defined as having two primary goals: (1) to provide leadership for the data resource management functions and (2) to ensure that the data are secure, accessible, accurate, and reliable.

The DRM role is very similar to the DA role described by Johns (1997), with a few differences in focus. As defined by AHIMA, the DRM is not only concerned with managing the quality and security of the healthcare data in an organization, but also very involved in retrieving data from the systems within the organization. The skill set required to perform the data resource management function in a healthcare organization includes a thorough understanding of health information administration and a working knowledge of the technical aspects of health information systems, particularly databases and DBMSs. The DRM should be comfortable as a participant in healthcare database management and design. Further, he or she should have a thorough understanding of HIM issues such as confidentiality, access, release of information, and security.

Safeguards for Ensuring Data Integrity and Security

Nowhere is ensuring the integrity and security of data more important than in healthcare. Healthcare organizations have an obligation to protect patient privacy and to maintain the confidential nature of the physician–patient relationship. Healthcare privacy and confidentiality are regulated by state and national laws and standards, as well as by standards of care. Other chapters in this text discuss confidentiality and privacy from a legislative and regulatory perspective. This section focuses on the safeguards that should be implemented in a healthcare database system.

Data Integrity

Data integrity is the assurance that data have been accessed or modified only by those authorized to do so (Whatis.com 2005). Databases contain conditions known as **integrity constraints** that must be satisfied by the data stored there. Database integrity constraints include:

- *Data type:* The data entered into a field should be consistent with the data type for that field. For example, if a field is a numeric field, it should only accept numbers. If it is a date field, it should only accept a legitimate date.
- *Legal values:* Many fields have a limited number of "legal" values. For example, a health record number may only be entered as 000001 through 999999.
- *Format:* Certain fields, such as Social Security numbers, must be entered in a certain format, such as 999-99-9999.
- *Key constraints:* Key constraints are the constraints placed on the primary and foreign keys within the database. A foreign key, for example, cannot be entered into the database unless a corresponding primary key already exists (Pratt and Adamski 2000).

These constraints help ensure that the originally entered data and changes to these data follow certain rules. DBMSs today include the functionality to enforce integrity constraints (Pratt and Adamski 2000). After the parameters for the types of integrity have been set within the database, users cannot violate them. For example, they cannot enter nonnumeric data into a number field. An error message will result. Likewise, a user cannot add a VISIT entry to the database described earlier unless a corresponding PATIENT has already been entered.

Data Security

Modern DBMSs also have built-in mechanisms to enforce security rules. Within healthcare organizations, most of the database systems are shared with multiple users. This makes implementing the security features of the DBMS critical.

Protecting the security and privacy of data in the database is called **authorization management.** Two of the important aspects of authorization management are user access control and usage monitoring (Rob and Coronel 2002).

User access control features within the database are designed to limit access to the database or some portion of it. They generally provide the DBA or DA responsible for security with the tools to:

- Define each user of the database. The DBA can create log-in information for each user.
- Assign passwords to users.
- Define user groups. By defining user groups, the DBA can limit access to certain groups. For example, some users may have read-only privileges. These users can see the data in the database but cannot enter or change them. Other users may be granted read-write privileges, so they can enter and change data.
- Assign access privileges. This can be done according to user groups as described above or on an individual basis. The highest level of privilege is the administrative level, which should be reserved for the DBA. Persons with administrative permissions can change the underlying structure of the database (Rob and Coronel 2002).

This list represents the security features that are part of the DBMS. The database also can be secured at the network operating system level. In many cases, a database user will first log in to the network system with one log-in and password and then log in to the database with a second log-in and password. The database also can be secured through physical security protections, such as locked rooms and password-protected workstations. The level of sensitivity of the data within the database should determine the level of security.

Usage monitoring is another aspect of authorization management. One of the most common ways that database administrators monitor database use is to use audit trails to determine whether there have been any actual or attempted access violations. The audit trails should be able to tell the DBA when and where the attempted breech occurred.

Check Your Understanding 5.7

Instructions: Answer the following questions on a separate piece of paper.

1. What is data integrity?
2. How is data integrity different from data security?
3. What do the authorization management features in a DBMS do?

Effective Data Display and Presentation

The MRI report on healthcare documentation reminds us that there are two major components to the documentation process: information capture and report generation. However, many methods are used for clinical and administration report generation and transmission in healthcare. For example, many reports are disseminated in a standard document format, such as Microsoft Word, rich text, or pdf. The reports also might be generated directly from the database system, a report-writing application such as Crystal Reports, or a spreadsheet such as Microsoft Excel. Moreover, different types of reports are suited for the different types of healthcare information. Patient-specific information to be filed in a paper-based medical record would commonly be printed in a document format with an individual focus; aggregate and comparative reports are more likely to include statistical and graphical information.

Health information managers also may be required to make presentations or provide information for others to make presentations based on aggregate and comparative data. These types of presentations often are supported by the use of presentation software such as Microsoft PowerPoint®. To fully explore the various technologies and best practices for preparing high-quality reports and presentations is beyond the scope of this chapter. However, the following section introduces some basic principles for displaying data, particularly graphical data, and for creating slides for presenting data.

Principles of Data Display

In his seminal work, The Visual Display of Quantitative Information, Edward Tufte (1983, p. 13) outlined the features of an "ideal" graph. Graphs should

1. Show the data
2. Induce the viewer to think about the substance rather than the methodology, graphic design, the technology or other things
3. Avoid distorting what the data have to say
4. Make large data sets coherent
5. Encourage the eye to compare different pieces of data
6. Reveal the data at several levels of detail
7. Serve a reasonably clear purpose
8. Be closely integrated with the statistical and verbal descriptions of the data set

---

Check Your Understanding 5.8

Instructions: Answer the following questions on a separate piece of paper.

1. What are the features of an "ideal" graph?
2. What are the basic guidelines for graphical excellence?
3. List and give examples of the guidelines for making effective presentations.

With the advent of easy-to-use software packages, such as Excel, any user can create a professional-looking graph with ease. However, this ease does not negate the need for the user to understand the data being displayed and to select the appropriate format. Examine the data set presented in table 5.3, which shows the average number of admissions per month to a healthcare facility for one year.

The graphs in figures 5.14 through 5.16 (pp. 120 and 121) were created using Microsoft Excel to represent these data. Which one is the most effective for showing a comparison of the average admissions for the year?

The bar graph is a clear, accurate representation of the data. No unnecessary information or misleading three-dimensional aspects are given. The scale begins at zero and is not distorted. What about the pie chart? This is a totally inappropriate use of a pie chart. A pie chart is only used to show part or percentages

Table 5.3. Average facility admissions by month

Month	Admissions
January	999
February	780
March	923
April	834
May	800
June	959
July	845
August	902
September	1,005
October	782
November	966
December	1,027

of a whole. What does this chart tell you? What is the "whole" you are comparing to? If you wanted to have a chart to show the breakdown for a month's admissions by race, a pie chart might be appropriate. (See figure 5.17, p. 121.)

What about the line chart? At first glance, you might have chosen this as the best graph. However, on closer look the scale for the chart is distorted, exaggerating the differences in average admissions. Consider the line graph in figure 5.18 (p. 122), which displays the same data. Which one adheres to Tufte's admonishment to avoid distorting what the data have to say?

Tufte (1983, p. 51) also provided a list of principles for graphical excellence. He stated that graphical excellence:

- Is the well-designed presentation of interesting data—a matter of substance, of statistics, and of design
- Consists of complex ideas communicated with clarity, precision, and efficiency
- Gives the viewer the greatest number of ideas in the shortest time with the least ink in the smallest space

Principles of Creating Effective PowerPoint Presentations

Any number of sources provide guidance in developing effective PowerPoint presentations. A search of the Internet or a trip to the library will yield a variety of resources. Victor Chen at the University of Iowa (2005) recently posted an excellent PowerPoint presentation, entitled "Designing Effective PowerPoint Presentations." (To view his full presentation, go to vetmed.iastate.edu/vetzone/pdfanddocs/ Effective_presentation.ppt).

Figure 5.14.   Bar chart created to show the average number of patient admissions in one year by month

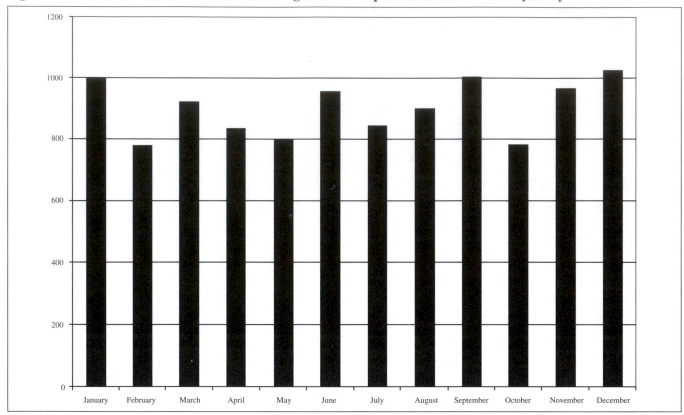

Figure 5.15.   Pie chart created to show the average number of patient admissions in one year by month

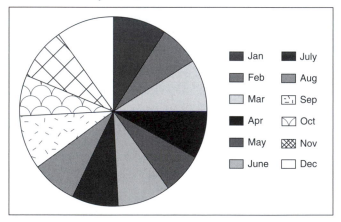

His approach is based on five criteria. The presentation should be:

1. *Big:* Make sure the font used is large enough to be seen from two meters away. Different fonts appear different, so it is best to test the font by moving away from the presentation. As a general rule, anything smaller than 24 points is too small. When in doubt, go larger!

2. *Progressive:* Start with the main point of the presentation and move to more detail for each point. Avoid giving the viewer all the information at one time.

3. *Consistent:* Differences should be planned. If the viewer sees a different size, color, or font, for example, he or she will interpret that as indicating importance. (See figure 5.19, p. 122.)

4. *Simple:* One of the most common mistakes with Power-Point presentations is that the creator feels he or she must include lots of detail, color, fonts, pictures, sounds, animations, or slide transitions. There is a general 6 × 7 rule to follow when creating the text for slides. There should be no more than six lines per slide and no more than seven words per line. (See figure 5.20, p. 123.) Avoid too many colors and unnecessary pictures on a slide. Fonts should be consistent. Animations and transitions should be used sparingly and only for important emphasis.

5. *Clear:* Generally, the creator of the presentation should avoid all capitals, use sans serif fonts, avoid italics, use color for emphasis rather than underlining, and use contrasting and complementary colors. (See figure 5.21, p. 123.)

Keep the purpose of the presentation in mind at all times. Added visuals should support and not distract from the presentation. Avoid adding extra features just because they are available. Just because you can do it does not mean you should!

Figure 5.16.   Line chart created to show the average number of patient admissions in one year by month

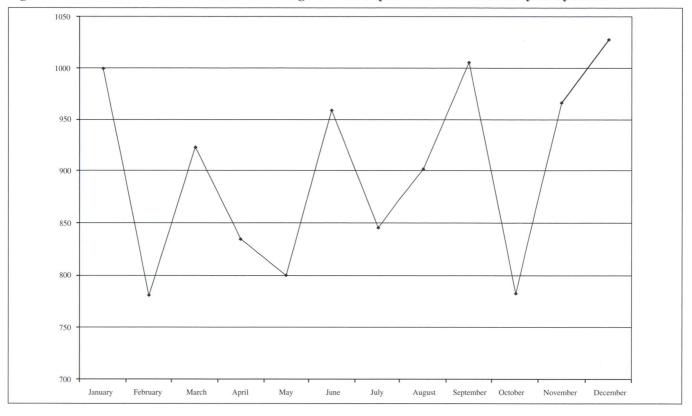

Figure 5.17.   Admissions by race

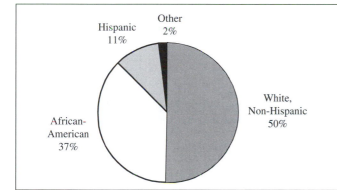

Real-World Case

Medical Associates (MA) is a physician group for a large academic medical center located in the southeastern United States. It provides services ranging from prevention and wellness to highly specialized care at outpatient clinics and facilities both on the medical center campus and in the surrounding community. Several years ago, after a major lawsuit involving the possibility of coding and billing inconsistencies, the MA executive committee voted to adopt a formal organizational compliance plan, with the goal of ensuring that the group's physicians, providers, and billing staff understood their legal responsibilities with regard to professional billing. One of the key features of the plan was to provide "coordinated training of clinical staff and billing personnel concerning applicable billing requirements and MA policies."

As outlined in the MA compliance plan, approximately 3,000 clinical and nonclinical employees need compliance education and training. Each of approximately 20 departments has a compliance coordinator responsible for tracking its employees' compliance education to ensure that all preestablished yearly requirements are met. Employees with patient care responsibilities must accrue four hours of training per year—one hour of general training and three hours of training related specifically to billing compliance. However, different categories of employees may have different training requirements. For example, some nonclinical employees need only one hour of general training. Any of this training can be obtained in a number of different settings: sessions offered by the employee's own department, departmental meetings with a compliance topic discussed, sessions offered by another department, sessions offered by the Compliance Office, videotape sessions, Internet sessions, or reading articles and other documents. Every employee must have documented evidence, including a signed attendance sheet, that he or she actually attended approved educational sessions to accrue the hours. Another complicating factor in maintaining quality-tracking records is that each training session may count for more than one type of training. Some sessions may last for only 15 minutes, others for three hours.

Figure 5.18.   Line chart without distortion

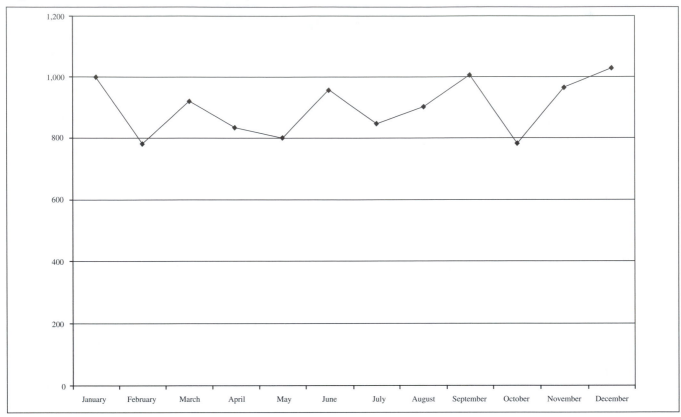

Figure 5.19.   PowerPoint text differences for emphasis

Figure 5.20. PowerPoint busy slide

Figure 5.21. PowerPoint clear slide

Originally, each department developed its own system for tracking employees. Recognizing that the education tracking and documentation would be an arduous task, several MA departments developed Excel applications for tracking and reporting; others developed small Access databases for this purpose.

Several significant issues emerged as compliance coordinators gained experience in tracking and reporting compliance education for their departments. They began to recognize a need to share their data across departments. As they began to share their spreadsheets and small databases, they soon realized that there were no standard definitions for the fields within the disparate tracking systems and no means for easily uploading one department's data into another's system. Multiple problems related to redundant data were identified. Any one employee might have education documented in more than one department's education-tracking system. The MA Compliance Office had to spend a great deal of time trying to clean and merge the data that came in from the various departments. The central Compli-

ance Office could not easily identify who actually needed what type of education. These issues and others led the MA Compliance Office to consider the development of a central, shared database for all coordinators to use.

After several months of planning, a centralized, shared compliance education database was developed. Figure 5.22 shows the underlying table structure of its final version. In addition, a user-friendly interface was developed for data entry and information retrieval. The database was designed as a relational database, and the relationships are included in the schema. The infinity symbol shows the "many" sides of each one-to-many relationship. Because of the relational nature of the database, redundancy was reduced and the chance for data-entry update and deletion errors was all but eliminated.

The centralized education database has worked well for the MA compliance coordinators since its implementation a year ago. Multiple standard reports have been developed. These can be customized to show data by department, by cost center, or by divisions within departments. The MA com-

Figure 5.22. Relational schema for compliance education database

pliance coordinators meet periodically to discuss multiple issues, including database issues. The database developer has continued to work under contract for MA compliance and has made various enhancements to the interface and standard reports. However, the underlying data structure has remained the same. The MA Compliance Office has expressed its confidence in the quality of the data and, consequently, in their reports since the database was implemented. The departmental coordinators also are happy in knowing that each employee for whom they are responsible is only in the database one time and that regardless of which department provided the education, they can track the total required hours accrued.

Summary

Health information managers must manage information that is shared by diverse and widely dispersed groups of end users. Information is derived from data, or raw facts, and then used by any number of individuals within a healthcare organization in making decisions about patient care. Thus, information is a valuable resource that must be managed carefully following certain basic principles. Essential to the management of information is the organization's ability to ensure the quality of the data it maintains. Data quality is evaluated by comparing its characteristics to recognized standards. Although no single set of nationally recognized standards for healthcare data quality exists, two organizations, the American Health Information Management Association and the Medical Records Institute, have published guidelines. Eventually, the evaluation of the data is translated into technical performance requirements for the information system.

Data quality can be controlled through multiple mechanisms. It can be controlled through effective database design found in computer applications. The design organizes the data in a way that facilitates their use. Two common types of database structures are the relational database and the object-oriented database. Each database structure is implemented through a specific management system. Key to database design is the process of data modeling, which links the "real" things about which the organization wants to collect and maintain data and the database structure.

An important tool in controlling data quality is the data dictionary. There are two general types: the DBMS (database management system) data dictionary, which is developed at the same time the database is developed, and the organization-wide data dictionary, which promotes data consistency throughout the organization.

To manage their data resources, healthcare organizations must set up mechanisms and policies that address not only database implementation and maintenance, but also standards of data quality. Three roles involved in data and information management are the database administrator, the data administrator, and the data resource manager. In 1998, AHIMA identified the latter as an emerging role for health information managers.

References

American Health Information Management Association. 1999. *Evolving HIM Careers.* Chicago: AHIMA.

American Health Information Management Association. 1998. Practice brief: Data quality management model. *Journal of American Health Information Management Association* 69(6).

Austin, C.J., and S.B. Boxerman. 1998. *Information Systems for Health Services Administration,* 5th ed. Chicago: Health Administration Press.

Chen, V. 2005. Designing effective PowerPoint presentations. Available online from vetmed.iastate.edu/vetzone/pdfanddocs/Effective_presentation.ppt.

Duffy, P.G. 1997. Data dictionaries: An overview. *Journal of American Health Information Management Association* 68(2):30–32, 34.

Johns, M.L. 1997. *Information Management for Health Professions.* Albany, NY: Delmar.

Joint Commission on Accreditation of Healthcare Organizations. 2005 *Comprehensive Accreditation Manual for Hospitals.* Oakbrook Terrace, IL: JCAHO.

Medical Records Institute. 2004. *Healthcare Documentation: A Report on Information Capture and Report Generation.* Boston: Medical Records Institute.

Pratt, P.J., and J. Adamski. 2000. *Concepts of Database Management,* 3rd ed. Cambridge, MA: Course Technology, Thomson Learning.

Rob, P., and C. Coronel. 2002. *Database Systems: Design, Implementation, and Management.* Cambridge, MA: Course Technology, Thomson Learning.

Shakir, A.M. 1999. Tools for defining data. *Journal of American Health Information Management Association* 70(8):48–53.

Tufte, E.R. 1983. *The Visual Display of Quantitative Information.* Cheshire, CT: Graphics Press.

Wager, K.A., F.W. Lee, J.P. Glaser. 2005. *Managing Health Care Information Systems: A Practical Approach for Health Care Executives.* San Francisco: Jossey-Bass.

Whatis.com. 2005. searchSQLServer.com definitions.

Chapter 6
Information Systems Development

Karen A. Wager, DBA

Learning Objectives

- To understand the importance of strategic information systems planning to healthcare organizations
- To describe the purpose and major activities within each phase of the systems development life cycle: analysis, design, implementation, and maintenance and evaluation
- To identify the resources needed to effectively manage information systems within healthcare organizations
- To discuss the roles and responsibilities of information system professionals
- To identify the health information manager's role in planning, selecting, and implementing healthcare information systems

Key Terms

Administrative information systems
Analysis phase
Application service provider (ASP)
Chief information officer (CIO)
Chief information security officer (CISO)
Chief information technology officer (CITO)
Chief medical informatics officer (CMIO)
Clinical information systems
Clinical systems analyst
Database administrators
Design phase
Electronic medical record (EMR)
Healthcare information systems steering committee
Implementation phase
Information system (IS)
Information technology (IT)
Maintenance and evaluation phase
Network administrators
Programmers
Request for information (RFI)
Request for proposal (RFP)
Strategic IS planning
Systems analyst
Systems development life cycle (SDLC)
Webmasters

Introduction

Healthcare organizations are under increased pressure to control costs and improve efficiency. At the same time, they are experiencing increased demands to ensure patient safety, reduce medical errors, improve the quality of care, promote access, and ensure compliance with privacy and security regulations. Many healthcare organizations are looking to **information system** (IS) technology to help them respond to these pressures and provide high-quality services in a more cost-effective manner.

Oftentimes, however, healthcare organizations have far more IS priorities than they have resources to allocate to them. How should decisions be made regarding which IS initiatives to support? How can healthcare administrators be reasonably assured that the information systems selected will meet their organization's current and future needs and be accepted by end users? What process will the organization use to select and implement a new system? After the decision is made to implement an IS, what resources are needed to adequately maintain and support it?

This chapter introduces a framework for addressing these important questions, including a description of the process that should be used to select a new IS, large or small. It also describes the people, policies, and organizational structure needed to maintain information systems and to manage information resources effectively. Finally, it discusses strategic information systems planning, the systems development life cycle, information resource management, and the role of the health information manager in planning, selecting, and implementing healthcare information systems.

Theory into Practice

This case is based on a comprehensive study of five primary care physician practices that implemented the same **electronic medical record** (EMR) product (Wager, Lee, and White 2001). Family Medicine Center (FMC) was the one practice out of the five studied that was dissatisfied with its choice of EMR. This brief synopsis provides a good illustration of how factors beyond the functionality of the healthcare IS may cause system failure or success.

FMC implemented its EMR system in the mid-1990s. The center purchased the system from a reputable vendor and expected that it would reduce personnel costs and enable FMC to realize numerous other efficiencies. Instead, FMC invested more than $400,000 in the system and spent several frustrating years trying to get it to work right. Now key personnel within the clinic want to pull the plug on the system and start over with a brand-new one (Wager, Lee, and White 2001).

What went wrong? As with most system failures, the authors of this case discovered that multiple factors, organizational and other, contributed to the frustration and dissatisfaction with the use of the EMR at FMC. One factor may have been the disastrous implementation phase. FMC's lead physician, Dr. Barron, selected the system based on the advice of a colleague in the field. The other physicians working in the practice knew very little about computers and trusted Dr. Barron's judgment. No planning group was identified and no real strategic decision process was used to make the EMR choice.

To complicate matters further, Dr. Barron agreed with the EMR distributor that it would be best to implement the scheduling and billing components of the system concurrently with the EMR components. It was the distributor's first sale, and he spent much of his time handling conversion problems from the old billing system to the new one, with little time left to train nurses, physicians, and support staff on proper use of the EMR.

Years later, common complaints among the nurses and physicians include:

- The initial training was grossly inadequate.
- The system is too cumbersome to use.
- Our patients do not like us typing in the exam room.
- Half the record is electronic and half is on paper.
- Rather than save time, the system has actually created more work.
- No one is available to help when we have problems with the system.

It would be easy to assume that FMC's EMR failed because the product was not appropriate for the facility. When examined within the context of the larger study in which the majority of practices were pleased or very pleased with the same EMR product that was installed at FMC, this conclusion seems too simplistic. What could FMC have done to improve its chances for a successful implementation of the EMR? Subsequent sections of this chapter outline some of the ways healthcare organizations can improve their chances of system success.

Definition of Terms

Two broad categories of healthcare information systems described in this chapter include administrative and clinical systems. **Administrative information systems** contain primarily administrative or financial data and are commonly used to support the management functions or general operations of a healthcare facility (Wager, Lee, and Glaser 2005). Examples include human resource management systems, materials management, patient billing, and staff scheduling. Administrative information systems were the first computerized systems implemented in most healthcare organizations. A recent survey by HIMSS Analytics shows that more than 90 percent of hospitals have in place administrative applications that support the patient revenue cycle (registration, billing, electronic claims, and credit collections) and nearly two-thirds have patient scheduling systems (HIMSS Analytics 2005). Additionally, nearly 100 percent of hospitals have accounts payable, general ledger, and materials management systems.

In contrast to these administrative systems, **clinical information systems** (or applications) contain primarily clinical or health-related data that are used to diagnose, treat, monitor, and manage patient care. Examples of clinical applications include ancillary departmental systems (such as pharmacy, radiology, and laboratory medicine) as well as EMR systems, computerized provider order entry, medication administration, and nursing documentation. Most U.S. hospitals have pharmacy, radiology, and laboratory information systems in place (HIMSS Analytics 2005). Far fewer, however, have EMR or computerized provider order-entry (CPOE) systems, only about half use emergency department software, and less than a third use more specialized software such as intensive care or cardiology. (See figure 6.1.)

Both administrative and clinical information systems may provide decision support capabilities to the end user. For example, one of the key attributes of an **electronic medical record** system (EMR) is its ability to alert the provider when two drugs should not be taken in combination or when a patient is due for a health maintenance examination. Decision support features such as these can serve as tools in enabling the provider to manage the patient's care more effectively. Furthermore, most health care organizations are grappling with how to effectively select and implement clinical decision support systems (such as EMR and CPOE systems) into the care process; thus, they are the focus of discussion in this chapter. The term EMR rather than the term EHR is used in this chapter because EMRs are unique to an organization. EHRs involve the sharing of information across organizations.

Today's Environment and the Growing Demand for Healthcare Information Systems

In 2003, healthcare spending reached $1.7 trillion, approximately 4.3 times the amount spent on national defense. Public funds account for just under half of healthcare expenditures (California HealthCare Foundation 2005). Coupled with rising healthcare costs is the fact that between 44,000 and 98,000 people die in hospitals each year as the result of medical errors (IOM 2000). Nearly 7,000 people die each year from medication errors alone, about 16 percent more deaths than the number attributable to work-related injuries. Even more staggering is the fact that more than 57,000 Americans die needlessly each year because they do not receive appropriate healthcare, and of this number, 90 percent die because of known conditions such as high blood pressure or elevated cholesterol that are not adequately monitored and controlled (NCQA 2003).

Containing healthcare costs and addressing patient safety issues have become national priorities. In response, President Bush has called for the widespread adoption of EHRs to become the standard within the next decade. To that end, he established the Office of the National Health Information Technology Coordinator (ONC) in 2004 and appointed Dr. David J. Brailer to coordinate and lead the effort. Numerous public and private agencies and organizations are currently working together to overcome the barriers that have impeded the widespread use and adoption of EHR (and related systems) in healthcare in the past. Examples of many initiatives under way can be found on the ONC Web site at http://www.hhs.gov/healthit/ and the e-Health Initiative Web site at http://ccbh.ehealthinitiative.org.

How achievable is the president's call? Although estimates vary, most studies show that only 5 to 20 percent of healthcare facilities have implemented EMR or other clinical decision support systems such as CPOE systems (Brailer and Terasawa 2003). It is not for their lack of benefit to patient care. Numerous studies have shown that the use of EMR-related systems can improve quality, decrease costs, and improve service and satisfaction (Bates and Gawande 2003;

Figure 6.1.   Current use of clinical information systems in hospitals

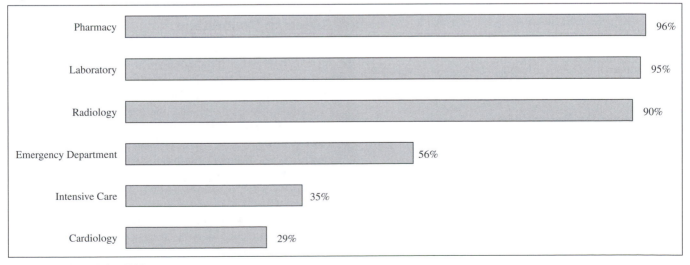

Pharmacy	96%
Laboratory	95%
Radiology	90%
Emergency Department	56%
Intensive Care	35%
Cardiology	29%

Source: HIMSS Analytics 2005.

Bates et al., 1999; Barlow, Johnson, and Steck 2004; Brailer and Terasawa 2003; Teich et al. 2000).

Despite the many benefits, major barriers to widespread adoption of EMR-type systems exist. The three primary barriers are the high cost of acquiring and supporting systems, a lack of sufficient standards and interoperability concerns, and organizational and behavioral resistance. Acquiring an EMR system (or other IS) is a significant investment of time, resources, and people. Besides the up-front capital needed to acquire the system, significant costs are associated with implementing and maintaining the system, not to mention the time, effort, and personnel resources devoted to redesigning processes and incorporating the system into the care process.

For the small physician practice (fewer than five physicians), it is very difficult to make a business case for EMR adoption. Coupled with the issue of cost is the fact that IS technology failures are common in healthcare. One-third to one half of all healthcare IS projects fail (Brailer and Terasawa 2003; Anderson 1997). Likewise, many healthcare organizations have diverse and competing IS priorities and many initiatives never get off the ground due to lack of sufficient buy-in from clinical staff.

Such barriers can—and will—be overcome. However, they require that healthcare managers and leaders assume an active role in ensuring that their organizations are well equipped and prepared for change. Healthcare managers need to ask themselves the following questions:

- What are the strategic goals of the organization? What type(s) of information systems are needed to enable the organization to achieve its goals? To what degree are the IS goals aligned with the organization's overall strategic goals?
- How should decisions be made regarding which IS initiatives to support? What criteria or methods will be used? How will the organization make capital budget decisions?
- How can the organization be reasonably assured that the IS selected will meet its current and future needs and be accepted by end users?
- After the decision is made to implement an IS, what resources are needed to adequately maintain and support it?

Strategic Information Systems Planning

No board of directors would ever recommend building a new healthcare facility without an architect's blueprint and a comprehensive assessment of community/market needs and resources. The architect's blueprint helps ensure that the new facility has a strong foundation, a well-planned organizational basis, and the potential for growth and expansion. The assessment helps ensure that there is a need for

the new facility and that adequate resources are available to support it.

Similarly, it is critical that the organization's IS plans be well aligned and integrated with its overall organizational strategic plans. To develop a blueprint for IS technology, the healthcare organization should engage in strategic IS planning. **Strategic IS planning** is the process of identifying and prioritizing IS needs based on the healthcare organization's mission and strategic goals.

Historically, few healthcare organizations have engaged in strategic planning for information systems. If an IS plan existed at all, it probably had been developed by the staff in the IS department, people who had not participated in the organization's overall strategic planning process. Having two separate plans often led to redundant systems, duplication of effort, and the acquisition of information systems that could not interact with each other.

Today, healthcare leaders recognize the importance of aligning business strategy with IT strategy (Wager, Lee, and Glaser 2005; Glaser 2002). Ross and Weill (2002) published an article in *Harvard Business Review* entitled "Six IT Decisions Your IT People Shouldn't Make." They studied IT management practices at hundreds of companies around the world and found that although a number of factors distinguish top-performing companies, the most important is that senior managers take a leadership role in a handful of IT decisions. Two of the key decisions include defining the strategic role that IT will play in the company and making clear decisions about which IT initiatives will and will not be funded. Glaser (2002) argues that these same principles apply to healthcare senior managers and organizations as well.

Different approaches or methods for developing a strategic IS planning process can be used. In the sections that follow, a generic approach is provided. Factors such as the type, size, and complexity of the organization as well as the decision-making philosophy of its leadership team are certainly important components in determining how IS priorities are established.

Role of the Healthcare IS Steering Committee

Strategic IS planning generally involves a range of senior-level managers and clinicians across the organization, including senior administrators, physicians, nurses, and key people from the ancillary services departments (for example, radiology, laboratory medicine, and pharmacy) as well as the **chief information officer** (CIO) and health information management (HIM) professional. Generally, these individuals are organized as a team or a committee known as the **healthcare information systems steering committee.** The committee's primary role is to identify and prioritize IS needs, ensure that all new IS initiatives support the organization's strategic goals, and monitor the progress of new system implementations and upgrades to existing systems.

Opinions vary as to who should lead the planning effort. Some people believe that the CIO or some other designated senior-level administrator should assume this role (Austin and Boxerman 2003). Others believe that it is better to have a clinician or medical staff leader who is "further removed" from the IS department. Whoever is chosen to organize or lead the planning effort should be someone who has strong communication and organizational skills, is well respected by clinicians and the administrative team, and is viewed as a leader within the organization. Ideally, the person chosen should have enough power or clout to make things happen.

Strategic Planning Process

The IS steering committee should begin strategic planning with a discussion of the organization's view of the role that IS technology will play in the organization's future. Historically, this has not been the approach to systems development within healthcare. Many information systems were developed or acquired by healthcare organizations in a rather piecemeal fashion. Early systems were primarily administrative or financial in nature and often developed in-house by what was then the data processing department. With the advent of microcomputers in the mid-1980s, healthcare organizations began to invest more extensively in clinical information systems. However, these systems were often purchased by outside vendors based on individual department needs and not on the needs of the organization as a whole or on its strategic plans. For example, the radiology department might have purchased the best radiology IS on the market and the laboratory department, the best laboratory IS, with little, if any, consideration of whether the organization had an appropriate **information technology** (IT) infrastructure to adequately support the two systems. The systems were thought of quite independently.

Today, it is vital that the leadership team adopt a system-wide perspective on information management and view each major IS acquisition within the context of the larger picture; that is, how the system supports the organization's overall mission and strategic goals. The goal is to build systems, not disparate applications. In fact, one of the major challenges facing IS staff is that of integrating data from disparate systems and getting the systems to "talk to each other." Clinicians are often frustrated at being unable to pull together clinical and financial data from among the various systems used within the healthcare enterprise.

To help ensure that information systems support the organization's strategic plan and not be acquired in isolation, healthcare managers examine both the external and internal environment and business plans before establishing IS priorities or making IS investments.

Generic Approach

The following steps represent a generic approach to developing a strategic IS plan. (See figure 6.2, p. 132.) This approach can be modified or adapted to meet the healthcare organization's individual needs. The steps include the following:

1. Review the organization's strategic plan and assess the organization's current external and internal environment.

2. Identify the organization's mission, strategic goals, and objectives and assess its IS needs.
3. Establish IS priorities.
4. Gain approval from the organization's leaders (executive management and board of directors) of the prioritized plan for completing IS projects.

Reviewing the Strategic Plan and Assessing the External and Internal Environment

To begin the planning process, the IS steering committee should review the organization's current strategic plans, goals, and objectives and evaluate its current external environment. The overall strategic plan should include an environmental assessment that analyzes the external forces that may affect the organization. External forces include changes in reimbursement methodologies, new government regulations, and changes in the demographics or healthcare needs of the community.

In addition, an environmental assessment should be performed to explore emerging ITs and their potential impact on the ways the healthcare organization delivers its services. In conducting this assessment, a subgroup of the committee may wish to review the literature, visit trade shows, network with colleagues in the field, or meet with leading vendors in the marketplace. A number of consultant groups also can provide vendor/product information to the organization.

In addition to the external environmental assessment, it is equally important that the IS steering committee conduct an internal environmental assessment of the organization's current IS environment. The committee should consider questions such as:

- Which information systems are currently used within the organization?
- To what extent do these systems meet the needs of end users?
- Which systems are likely to need replacement or upgrades? Which ones are likely to become obsolete within the next few years?
- To what extent is the organization able to support and maintain its current systems? Does it have the people, equipment, and network infrastructure needed to support its current systems?
- To what degree are the current systems cost-effective and efficient?
- How well do the existing information systems support the organization's strategic goals?

As part of the analysis of the current internal environment, the committee also may want to compare the organization's IT functionality and performance against external benchmarks. For example, the committee might compare the organization's ratio of end users to technical support personnel with industry averages. It also might compare the

Figure 6.2. Strategic information systems planning process

organization's performance in key areas with the performance of other, similar organizations. The committee might wish to consider the following questions:

- How secure are patient information systems?
- How much downtime does the facility experience?
- How much IT staff time is spent troubleshooting system problems?
- In what ways, if any, have the major systems adversely affected patient care?
- To what degree are existing systems in compliance with the Health Insurance Portability and Accountability Act (HIPAA) privacy and security regulations?

It is essential that the organization evaluate existing systems to accurately identify its needs, problems, and opportunities for improvement. Otherwise, it runs the risk of installing a new IS to fix a perceived problem only to discover that the new system never addressed the actual problem and, instead, created a host of new problems.

Identifying IS Needs and Prioritizing IS Projects

After the committee has developed a thorough understanding of the organization's strategic goals, environment, emerging information technologies, and existing information systems, it should begin to identify IS needs throughout the organization. This internal needs assessment can be formal or informal. For example, if the committee wants to conduct a formal assessment, it might conduct structured interviews with key users or administer surveys in key areas throughout the organization. A less formal approach would be to ask all IS steering committee members to list the information needs within their respective areas. The outcome of this assessment is a fairly comprehensive list of the organization's information management needs. Eventually, the list can be used to identify projects and establish IT priorities.

The next step in the planning process is to establish priorities. Again, the committee might take different approaches to accomplish this very important task. One approach is to identify all proposed IS projects and hold an intensive retreat where all interested stakeholders (IS steering committee members and other interested clinicians and staff) score and rank each project. Sufficient information concerning each project should be given to the stakeholders ahead of time to help them make informed choices. (See chapter 9 for a discussion specific to EMR planning considerations and migration strategies.)

Gaining Approval for the Plan

Whether the approach described above or another approach to priority setting is used, the strategic IS planning process should result in a list of identified project priorities. These priorities then should be developed further and forwarded to the senior administration and/or the board of directors for approval and funding. It is important to note that the priority list is not static. It should be reviewed periodically and modified accordingly based on changes in the environment and the growing needs of the organization.

Check Your Understanding 6.1

Instructions: Answer the following questions on a separate piece of paper.

1. Why is strategic planning for information systems important to organizations in today's healthcare environment? What risks are associated with not having an IS plan?

2. Who should be involved in the strategic planning process? Who should lead the effort?

3. Why is it important for the IS plan to be integrated with the healthcare organization's overall strategic plan?

4. Why is it important for healthcare organizations to examine their existing information systems? What aspects of the existing system(s) should be examined during the planning process?

5. How might a healthcare organization go about prioritizing its IS projects or needs?

Information Systems Development

After IS priorities have been established as part of the strategic plan, the healthcare organization should follow a structured project management process for selecting and implementing new systems. The structured approach enables the organization to identify viable alternatives, gain user buy-in, select a system that meets the needs of the users, and implement the system in a well-organized, systematic way.

Because several new system projects may be going on at the same time and people may be involved in more than one project, it is important that the projects be organized and managed consistently. Ideally, the IT staff or the project leader should maintain a project repository for every IS initiative. Included in the project repository would be all minutes, notes, survey results, and other relevant information used in managing the project. The project repository is particularly important in healthcare organizations that experience high turnover among IT staff. (See chapter 27 for a full discussion of project management principles, processes, and tools.)

Systems Development Life Cycle

One process for IS development is the **systems development life cycle** (SDLC). Although there are many different models of the SDLC, all generally include a variation of the following four phases: analysis, design, implementation, and maintenance and evaluation. As the activities that occur in each phase are discussed, it should become apparent that the process does not end when the new IS is implemented. Rather, the SDLC is an ongoing process that requires ongoing assessment and planning. Figure 6.3 illustrates the cyclical nature of the SDLC.

Like the strategic IS planning process, the SDLC involves the participation of numerous people with different backgrounds and areas of expertise. Depending on the nature and scope of the project, representatives from the key clinical and administrative areas should be involved. For example, if the organization plans to replace its pharmacy IS, in addition to key people from the pharmacy department, the process might include individuals from the medical staff, nursing, and other ancillary areas that depend on or use pharmacy information. Representatives from IT and HIM services also should be involved.

Analysis Phase

After senior administration or the board gives the go-ahead for the project, the **analysis phase** begins. During the analysis phase, the need for a new IS is explored further, problems with the existing system are solidified, and user needs are identified. The primary focus in this beginning phase of the SDLC is on the business problem, independent of any technology that can or will be used to implement a solution to that problem.

In this phase, it is important to examine the current system and to identify opportunities for improvement or enhancement. Even though an initial assessment was completed as part of the strategic information planning process, the analysis phase of the SDLC involves a more extensive evaluation. Typically, the existing system is evaluated by asking people who routinely use it to identify its strengths and limitations. Completion of this task can help to ensure that the organization does not make a significant investment in a new system only to later discover that what was needed

Figure 6.3. Systems development life cycle

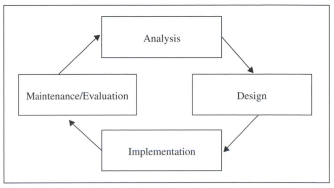

was better communication, additional training, and more extensive technical support, not a new information system.

When it is clear that a new IS is needed, the next step is to assess the information needs of users and to define functional requirements. It is best to have a structured method for accomplishing this task. For example, the project team might administer a questionnaire, conduct focus groups, or hold joint-requirements planning sessions. A joint-requirement planning session is a highly structured group meeting that is conducted to analyze problems and define functional requirements. Whatever method or combination of methods is used to solicit user input, the process should result in a detailed list of user specifications.

Design Phase

After the users' needs have been identified, the process generally moves into the **design phase.** During this phase, consideration is given to how the new system will be designed or selected. Questions to ask include:

- Will the new system be built in-house?
- Will the organization contract with an outside developer to build the system?
- Will the facility purchase an IS from a vendor, or lease it from a vendor or **application service provider** (ASP)? (An ASP is a company or firm that deploys, manages, and remotely hosts prepackaged software through centrally located servers, often on a fixed, per user basis or on a per transaction fee basis.)

Because of time, cost, and personnel restraints, most healthcare organizations first look at what IS products are available in the vendor community. For this reason, this discussion focuses on selecting an IS from a vendor rather than building one in-house. In the rare situation that a facility decides to build a system in-house, it is generally because the facility's needs are unique and it has the technical expertise to design and support the system.

A facility that wishes to explore the systems available in the vendor community might begin by obtaining information from exhibits at professional conferences, directories or publications, the Internet, vendor user groups, consulting firms, and contacts with colleagues in the health information systems (HIS) field. A **request for information** (RFI) is generally sent to a fairly extensive list of vendors that are known to offer products or systems that meet the organization's needs. The RFI is used to obtain general product information and to prescreen vendors. Responses to the RFI are used to narrow the list to a smaller number of vendors who will be invited to respond to the **request for proposal** (RFP).

The RFP generally includes much more detail on the system's requirements and provides guidelines for vendors to follow in bidding. For a major system acquisition, the RFP generally includes (Wager, Lee, and Glaser 2005):

- Instructions for vendors, including the proposal deadline and contract information, specific instructions for

completing the RFP, and any stipulations for which the vendor must comply
- Organizational objectives, including the type of system or application being sought, and how it will fit into the organization's strategic plans and goals
- Background of the organization, including a description of the facility (size, type of patient services, patient volume, and so forth) and an inventory of applications and the network infrastructure
- System goals and requirements, including a description of the system characteristics and the features that are desired or required
- Vendor qualifications, including background information, experience, number of installations, annual financial reports, and standard contract
- Proposed solution, including a description of how the vendor believes its product meets the organization's goals and needs
- Criteria to be used in evaluating the RFP
- General contractual requirements, including warranty information, payment, schedule, and penalties for failure to meet schedules specified in the contract
- Pricing and support

Moreover, it is a good idea to ask about the number of planned installations during the same time period and how staffing and other support issues will be managed if multiple implementations are under way at the same time.

After the RFP has been distributed to the vendors, the organization may wish to hold a bidders' conference to answer the vendors' questions about the RFP and to give all vendors the opportunity to receive the same information (Austin and Boxerman 2003).

Concurrent with development of the RFP, the project team should establish the criteria with which to evaluate the vendors' responses to the RFP. For example, the team may wish to evaluate the extent to which each vendor's product meets the functional requirements of the new system, the vendor's track record of performance, and the extent to which the vendor's philosophy of systems development is congruent with the organization's IT strategy. In addition, the team may wish to evaluate system reliability, costs, and projected benefits.

Evaluation of the vendor and its products should not depend solely on its response to the RFP. Other formal and informal mechanisms should be used to evaluate each vendor and its products. For example, the project team may hold vendor presentations, check references, attend user group meetings, and make site visits to other facilities that use the product. The purpose of these activities is to gather as much relevant information as possible to make an informed decision. Interested clinicians, administrators, and other end users, as well as members of the project team, should have the opportunity to participate in as many of these activities as possible.

As part of the system selection process, the project team should conduct a cost-benefit analysis for each viable alternative. Costs should include acquisition costs (for example, hardware, software, network, and training) in addition to operating or maintenance costs (for example, system upgrades, technical support, supplies, and equipment). Most costs can be identified and measured reasonably accurately. However, the benefits to implementing an IS can be much more difficult to identify. Some benefits, such as increased productivity or improved access to information, are tangible and can be measured (albeit not easily); others are intangible and very difficult to quantify. For example, a new EMR system might lead to improved employee morale or increased patient satisfaction, but these potential benefits might be more difficult to isolate and quantify. Consequently, when comparing different vendor systems or alternatives, it is important to evaluate and measure costs and benefits to the extent possible. A variety of standard cost-benefit analysis methods may be used to evaluate different IT options that are beyond the scope of this book. A fairly complete explanation of different cost-benefit analysis methods is provided in *Systems Analysis and Design* (Whitten, Bentley, and Dittman 2004).

When the top two or three vendors have been identified, leadership within the healthcare organization generally initiates the contract negotiation process. It is generally a good idea to begin contract negotiations with more than one vendor. This provides leverage during the negotiation process and affords the organization an alternative should it and the vendor not agree on the terms of the contract. A host of very detailed and technical issues are generally addressed in the contract, everything from when the system is to be delivered and installed, to warranties and guarantees, to who is responsible for ensuring that the product interfaces with other institutional systems. Internal legal counsel generally reviews the contract carefully before it is signed and commitments are made.

Implementation Phase

After contract negotiations have been finalized, the **implementation phase** begins. In this phase, a comprehensive plan for implementing the new system is developed. An interdisciplinary implementation team is generally established and led by a project manager. The implementation team will likely include some of the same individuals involved in selecting the new system, but other key people should be involved in the process as well.

Ideally, the project manager should be someone who is well respected and knowledgeable, has experience with implementing new systems, and has the political influence and power to make things happen. He or she also should have strong organizational and communication skills and be able to work effectively with the vendor. The importance of selecting the right person to lead the effort cannot be overemphasized. Even though a good implementation does not guarantee user acceptance of the new system, as illustrated in the FMC case study described earlier, a poor implementation can lead to frustration, dissatisfaction, and disillusionment. Some organizations never recover fully from a disastrous system implementation.

One of the implementation team's priorities is to identify all the tasks that must be completed before the go-live date. Depending on the type of system, the number of users, and the complexity of the conversion process, the tasks may vary in scope and complexity. However, many system implementation projects require at least the following tasks:

- Preparing the site (for example, work-flow patterns, noise, space, telephone lines, and electrical power)
- Installing the necessary hardware and software
- Preparing data tables
- Building interfaces
- Establishing an IT infrastructure (for example, stable network, secure database) to support the system
- Ensuring that adequate security and confidentiality practices are in place
- Training managers, technical staff, and other end users
- Testing the new system
- Identifying and correcting errors
- Preparing documentation to support system use (for example, procedure manuals)
- Implementing conversion plans
- Developing and testing backup and disaster recovery procedures

Although each of these major tasks is very important, a few should be highlighted to stress their relevance to the implementation phase. First, it is critical to thoroughly test any new system before the go-live date. This means testing, testing, and retesting the new system with real patient data, not sample data the vendor may have provided or your institution may have created. Even though it is nearly impossible to identify and correct all the errors before a system goes live, it is essential to identify and correct as many of them as possible. It is often much easier to correct a problem in the test mode than after the system is fully operational.

Second, adequate training is essential. As seen in the FMC case, a healthcare organization may be implementing a solid, highly reputable new system, but if the staff who will be using it are not thoroughly trained, the system's implementation can result in dissatisfaction and low morale. For any new system to be successful, it must be accepted and used by the staff. Different organizations and vendors might use different approaches to training, but one common approach is to train the trainer. This approach involves identifying key people in the various functional areas (for example, nursing units, laboratory, and billing), training them on the system, and then having them train others in their area (with guidance from the vendor or a "super user").

The train the trainer method can be effective because after the vendor is gone, staff must be available who are comfortable with the system and can assist others. It is equally important to allow adequate time for training. Staff should not have to squeeze in training on their lunch break, with little or no time to practice using the new system. Just as it is important to use real data in testing the system, it is critical to give staff practice using the new system with real patients or real data.

In addition to providing training, the organization must have the IT infrastructure and processes in place to support the system. The infrastructure should include a stable network, a sufficient number of workstations appropriately located throughout the organization, adequate security measures, up-to-date procedural manuals, and a process for reporting problems with the system.

Finally, it is important to develop plans for converting the old system to the new one. Conversion to a new system often requires major changes in the work flow and organizational structure and places increased demands on staff during this period. Therefore, it is essential to plan appropriately for the conversion and to ensure that adequate technical and support staff members are available to assist managers and end users, as needed.

Throughout the implementation process, many tasks or activities may occur simultaneously; others will need to be completed before other activities can begin. Because of the number of different tasks occurring, it is generally a good idea for the project manager to use a Gantt chart or project management tool that identifies the major tasks, their estimated start and completion dates, the individuals responsible for performing them, and the resources needed to complete them. Again, activities or tasks that depend on the completion of other tasks should be readily identified. Project management software such as Microsoft Project® is useful in creating Gantt charts, is easy to use, and enables the manager to track project resources (for example, staff, equipment) and expenditures.

Maintenance and Evaluation Phase

The final phase of the SDLC is the **maintenance and evaluation phase.** Regardless of how well designed and tested a new system may be, errors or bugs inevitably occur after it goes into operation. IT support staff must be available to find potential problems and take steps to correct them. Whether the technical staff are in-house or employed through a contract service, well-trained staff must be available to maintain or support the new system. For critical systems such as patient care or clinical information systems, technical support should be available 24 hours a day, seven days a week. Sufficient technical staff also should be available to oversee system backups and upgrades, replace outdated equipment, respond to new regulatory requirements, and provide ongoing training and assistance. Some experts estimate that at least 25 percent of the total technical staff time may be devoted to maintenance activities when several information systems are in place (Austin and Boxerman 2003).

As the organization hires new people, its technical or support staff must be available to train them on the system. Likewise, all staff will need additional training on a regular basis to ensure that they are current with system upgrades, enhancements, and new features or procedures. Ideally, the organization should have a plan in place outlining how staff will receive initial and ongoing training on any new or existing IS. Many healthcare organizations now appoint an individual within key clinical and administrative departments whose primary role is to ensure that the department staff have adequate training and technical support available to them. For example, the radiology department might have a radiological technician with strong computer skills who serves as the information technician and assists and trains other staff in the department. Such an approach can be effective in increasing response time to user requests and alleviating user frustration.

In addition to providing adequate training and support, the healthcare organization should monitor data quality and integrity and ensure that the system is secure and safe. Specifically, emergency backup procedures should be in place in the event the system fails or goes down for any reason. All staff should know what to do in such circumstances. The backup procedures should be well documented and readily available to staff. If forms are utilized during downtimes, clear instructions on what to do with them should be available when the system is restored.

However, maintaining and supporting the new systems is not enough. Information systems should be evaluated on an ongoing basis to determine whether they are contributing to the institution's overall goals and meeting user needs. Healthcare administrators today are demanding to know whether the return on investment (ROI) to the organization has been realized since system implementation. Being able to measure ROI is becoming increasingly important as healthcare institutions struggle to manage limited resources more effectively. Consequently, as a part of the system evaluation process, institutions are looking at the organizational, technological, and economic impact of information systems on the enterprise as a whole (Anderson, Aydin, and Jay 1994; Friedman and Wyatt 1997; Kaplan 1997).

HIM Contributions to IS Development

Health information managers can make unique contributions to the SDLC process. Because HIM professionals understand the origins and content of patient data contained in health records as well as the financial impact of coding, they are in an ideal position to speak to the need to integrate clinical and financial information. HIM professionals also have a broad understanding of healthcare organizations and their major components and frequently interact with clinicians and administrators who need access to relevant information for decision-making purposes.

Perhaps the best way to describe the different contributions HIM professionals could make to the SDLC is to walk through a simple example. Let's say that the healthcare organization has decided to select and implement an enterprise-wide EMR system within the next two years. During the analysis phase, the HIM professional could assist in identifying problems with the current health record system and in assessing the needs of various user groups. Because this individual understands the major components of an EMR system and many of the problems associated with paper-based health record systems, she or he could assist the project team in identifying user specifications for the RFP.

During the design phase, the HIM professional could share knowledge and insight into the EMR selection process. Most likely, he or she would attend several professional conferences each year to visit vendor exhibits, network with colleagues throughout the nation, and attend educational sessions on various aspects of EMR development and implementation. The HIM professional could bring back to the institution the insight and lessons learned from others in the field. Throughout the EMR selection process, the HIM professional could attend vendor demonstrations, conduct site visits, and evaluate vendor responses to the RFP. In addition, he or she could provide valuable input when security and confidentiality issues are addressed.

During the implementation phase of the EMR project, the HIM professional should become part of the implementation team or could participate in system-building activities such as:

- Developing a data dictionary
- Performing data mapping
- Designing electronic forms and reports
- Testing the system
- Training staff
- Identifying technical errors
- Developing backup and disaster recovery plans
- Ensuring that all staff members are aware of patient confidentiality and system security

Finally, in the maintenance and support phase, the HIM professional could evaluate the system's impact on the department's operations and on the quality of the data residing in the EMR, identify and communicate problems to the appropriate individuals, and develop an ongoing training program for staff. These are just a few of the many ways in which a HIM professional could make significant contributions to the SDLC of a new system.

Check Your Understanding 6.2

Instructions: Answer the following questions on a separate piece of paper.

1. What is the relationship between strategic information systems planning and the systems development life cycle?
2. Identify the four main phases of the SDLC and describe the purpose or intent of each.
3. What is the difference between an RFI and an RFP?
4. Briefly describe the HIM professional's contributions to the SDLC.

Management of Healthcare Information System Resources

Managing information resources is a vital function of any healthcare organization. Within hospitals or health systems, an in-house information services or information systems department often coordinates this function, although a growing number of healthcare organizations outsource IT functions to outside vendors. In fact, a recent survey of health information leaders revealed that two-thirds of healthcare organizations currently outsource at least some of their IT functions (HIMSS 2005). Web site development and management is the most frequently outsourced function, followed by applications development and workstation support. Advantages to outsourcing often include cost reductions and accessibility to highly competent IT staff.

Despite the trend to outsource some IT functions, however, many healthcare organizations have an IS department that provides a wide range of technical support functions to users throughout the organization. These functions include systems development and implementation, systems support/maintenance, user support, database administration, communications and network administration, and Web support. Figure 6.4 (p. 138) shows a typical organizational structure for an IS department, and the following sections describe some of the key positions within that structure.

IS Management Team Chief Information Officer

Generally, the IS department is managed by the CIO or director of IS, who in turn reports to the chief executive officer (CEO) or some other senior-level individual. The CIO is responsible for helping to lead the strategic IS planning process, managing the major functional units within the IS department, and overseeing the management of information resources throughout the enterprise.

Chief Medical Informatics Officer

An emerging position is that of **chief medical informatics officer** (CMIO). Individuals assuming CMIO positions are typically physicians who have medical informatics training. Generally, the role of the CMIO is to provide physician leadership and direction in the deployment of clinical applications in healthcare organizations.

Chief Information Technology Officer

Another relatively new position is that of **chief information technology officer** (CITO). The purpose of this role is to guide the organization's decisions related to technical architecture. For example, the CITO might be involved in determining which operating systems or network technologies the organization will support. This individual also typically keeps current on the latest technology developments and their applicability or potential use in the organization.

Chief Information Security Officer

Chief information security officer (CISO) is yet another emerging IT leadership role. The need for a CISO has grown as a direct result of the organization's need to be compliant with HIPAA security regulations. The CISO's primary responsibility is to ensure that the healthcare organization

Figure 6.4.   Typical organizational structure for IS department

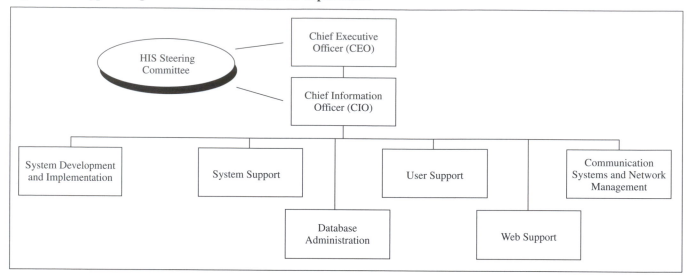

has an effective information security plan and that appropriate measures are in place to ensure that the organization's information systems are secure and safe from tampering or misuse (Wager, Lee, and Glaser 2005).

IS Technical Staff

In years past, most of the staff working in the IS department typically had backgrounds in programming and computer science. Today, the department is likely to include individuals with unique sets of skills and specialized areas of interest. These positions include:

- *Systems analysts:* Systems analysts investigate, analyze, design, develop, install, evaluate, and maintain the healthcare organization's information systems. These individuals typically are involved in all aspects of the SDLC and serve in a liaison role between end users and programmers, database administrators, and other technical personnel. Systems analysts with a clinical background in nursing, medicine, or other health professions, including HIM, are often called **clinical systems analysts.** They understand the language of clinicians and typically have an in-depth understanding of the patient care process.
- *Programmers:* Programmers are responsible primarily for writing program codes and developing applications. They typically perform the function of systems development and work closely with system analysts.
- *Network administrators:* Network administrators are involved in installing, configuring, managing, monitoring, and maintaining network applications. They are responsible for supporting the network infrastructure and controlling user access.
- *Database administrators:* Database administrators are involved in database design, management, security, backup, and user access. They are responsible for the technical aspects of managing a database.

- *Webmasters:* Webmasters are the most recent additions to the IS department. They provide support to Web applications and to the healthcare organization's intranet and Internet operations. Some of their responsibilities include designing and constructing Web pages, managing hardware and software, and linking Web-based applications to the organization's existing information systems.

All IS staff must have an opportunity to keep current in the IS field by attending conferences, gaining certification in specialized areas, and enrolling in formal academic or continuing education courses. IT applications serving the healthcare industry are emerging at a phenomenal rate, so the professional development of IS staff is critical.

HIM Professional Roles in Information Technology

As healthcare organizations move toward EMR system implementation, HIM professionals are finding career opportunities within the IT department. In June 2005, the American Health Information Management Association's (AHIMA's) HIM Practice Transformation e-HIM Work Group published an article titled "EHR Career Opportunities: Sample HIM Job Descriptions." This article identifies some of the types of positions closely aligned with the IT organizational structure that are held by experienced HIM professionals and by new graduates (for example, clinical applications coordinator, enterprise application specialists, and integration architect). (See figure 6.5.) Each of these positions reflects the valuable contribution the HIM body of knowledge brings to the healthcare organization's IT department as it implements EMR systems and is required to manage an increasing variety and volume of clinical data for numerous internal and external users.

Figure 6.5. EHR career opportunities: Sample HIM job descriptions

Clinical Analyst
- Format, design, and build relevant clinical content into appropriate workflows
- Lead discussions on clinical and functional design with multidisciplinary teams
- Provide key knowledge on implementation of standardized, streamlined clinical content
- Design clinical content for software applications across all care processes (including documentation, ordering, alerting and notification actions, reporting needs)
- Develop future state process and knowledge structures
- Test and troubleshoot problems within the applications
- Develop detailed content design documents
- Facilitate validation sessions with clinical researchers
- Develop and publish supporting documentation
- Exhibit excellent written and verbal communication skills

Clinical Applications Coordinator
- Implement and support multiservice software packages
- Manage the customization of site parameters
- Address integration issues with other software packages
- Review site parameters and local tables with each service for accuracy and completeness
- Coordinate implementation of new software products that cover these functions
- Analyze and evaluate processes related to information flow
- Provide training to all services on current software applications and new features
- Ensure training is scheduled for new users
- Coordinate efforts to correct deficiencies and errors that occur in the electronic record

Clinical Project Manager, Senior Project Manager
- Manage the scope of work, objectives, and other project management activities of assigned projects
- Finalize project budget and scope of work
- Act as primary project contact with sponsor to ensure appropriate communication channels are maintained and reporting schedules adhered to
- Manage project budget to meet financial and company goals (realization targets); identify and develop change orders
- Develop project plans, schedules, and other scope definition documents for assigned projects as outlined in the project operations database
- Maintain project management information and tracking systems
- Coordinate and evaluate the probability and impact of risks
- Develop plans for minimizing risk impact on project objectives
- Implement improvement processes for assigned projects

Clinical Research Associate
- Monitor activities at clinical study sites to ensure adherence to good clinical practices, standard operating procedures, and study protocols
- Review regulatory documents as required and prepare site visit reports
- Manage multiple projects
- Work both independently and in team environments
- Participate in the study development and start-up process, including reviewing protocols and designing or reviewing study follow-up
- Prepare informed consent forms
- Develop study documents
- Organize and present at investigator meetings
- Work with management on monitoring strategy
- Develop project-specific clinical research associate training
- Participate in clinical training programs and maintain awareness of developments in the field of clinical research

Clinical Vocabulary Manager
- Create, maintain, and implement terminologies, validation files, and maps for a variety of use cases in the EHR
- Perform ongoing review of the auto and manual encoder systems for terminology and classification systems, including methods and processes, and implement recommendations for improving and optimizing the encoding process
- Assist in the analysis of the enterprise's classification and grouping system assignment trends and use data from classification and grouping systems to assist in decision making
- Proactively monitor developments in the field of clinical terminologies and medical vocabularies
- Recommend the most appropriate classification or terminology systems to meet all required information reporting needs
- Possess expertise in clinical terminology, medical vocabulary, and classification systems and skill in mining, deriving, or engineering clinical ontologies

Enterprise Applications Specialist
- Possess knowledge of existing and emerging requirements related to privacy and confidentiality of health information
- Possess knowledge of existing EHR policies and procedures associated with the collection and distribution of clinical data via the repository
- Facilitate the identification, creation, implementation, and maintenance of organization policies and procedures related to the EHR
- Serve as a clinical information liaison to facilitate communication between clinical caregivers and technical implementation teams
- Maintain current knowledge of applicable federal and state EHR-related laws and accreditation standards; monitor and communicate changes to ensure organizational adaptation and compliance
- Serve as EHR consultant to the organization
- Manage multiple projects simultaneously
- Coordinate and assemble appropriate personnel for task force assignments related to EHR projects and issues
- Coordinate activities related to the integrity of the master patient index file
- Provide development guidance and coordination to ensure clinical data generated and stored in disparate clinical systems is made available in the EHR when appropriate
- Work cooperatively with the administrative director of HIM and other applicable organizational entities to ensure policies and procedures meet or exceed existing legal and regulatory requirements as related to the EHR and accepted medical record standards of practice
- Work cooperatively with privacy and security officer to ensure compliance with all existing and emerging requirements related to privacy and confidentiality of health information

Health Systems Specialist
- Possess knowledge of automated data processing
- Process file structures
- Implement applications
- Possess knowledge of data communication principles and techniques
- Develop and analyze data
- Prepare recommendations resulting from special studies

Health Information Services Department Technician
- Possess knowledge of hospital and departmental policies and procedures
- Exercise excellent communication skills
- Perform regulatory and accreditation review for the health information services department
- Summarize findings and report results
- Provide technical and administrative assistance for other health information services functions

(Continued on next page)

Figure 6.5.   (Continued)

Information Privacy Coordinator
- Monitor organizational information privacy compliance issues
- Work in collaboration with managers of technical information security to assess risks to health information security and privacy
- Establish policies and procedures to address privacy and security risks
- Draft information privacy policies and procedures and champion their approval and adoption by operational departments
- Develop training and monitoring programs to ensure employee awareness of and compliance with health information privacy policies and procedures

Integration Architect (Implementation)
- Manage the integration of all vendor applications at a single client site
- Work closely with client and installation teams to ensure the smooth and seamless flow of information and data across all client domains
- Manage the oversight and design of test scenarios, the installation process, and timely conversion of systems, which requires:
  −Clinical system integration experience
  −Installation experience with numerous clinical applications
  −Consulting experience
  −Clinical experience

Optical Imaging Coordinator
- Assist in the implementation of new systems
- Train users and provide follow-up training when required
- Monitor workflow
- Function as a liaison between health informatics and information services departments

Process Improvement Engineer
- Educate customers and transfer knowledge
- Diagnose and resolve problems
- Anticipate and address customer needs
- Function as an effective team leader
- Function as an effective team facilitator and methodology advisor
- Act as an effective team member
- Acquire and apply superior skills to achieve quality outcomes
- Respond to changing circumstances
- Manage highly complex projects

Records and Information Coordinator
- Provide reference services to all departments and levels of personnel and process incoming information
- Sort, classify, and verify coded material for integration into systems
- Create and maintain logs, computerized indexes, and databases to provide accurate status and retrieval information

Risk Management Specialist
- Assess and prevent risks that threaten the ongoing viability of the organization
- Analyze and improve patient safety and thorough managing functions
- Collect and disseminate patient safety lessons
- Lead the intervention of patient safety issues

Senior Document Coordinator
- Provide support for the processing of adverse event reports through tracking and data entry
- Generate reports
- Manage records
- Participate in continuous improvement of departmental processes and procedures
- Track timelines for completion of adverse event processing and enter data into safety database

Solution Analyst
- Provide support for clients and vendor associates working directly on client projects
- Possess expertise in field investigation and the successful resolution of service requests
- Develop education and knowledge transfer materials
- Provide documentation for requirements modeling and functional design, test products, which requires:
  −Background in healthcare, sciences, or information systems
  −Ability to work on multiple projects simultaneously
  −Effective written and verbal communication skills

Solution Consultant
- Provide in-depth solution and functionality knowledge support for the sales process
- Initiate contact with clients and make sales demonstrations of solution functionality, which are customized and specific to benefits sought by the client
- Provide input on the development of marketing materials
- Take part in knowledge transfer from the sales team to the project implementation team, requiring:
  −Strong understanding of a hospital organization
  −Background in clinical information systems
  −Formal presentation experience at the executive level as well as with physicians and nurses
  −Experience presenting IT solution demonstrations

Systems Analyst
- Determine client's business and technical requirements
- Identify appropriate stakeholders
- Consult with client on alternatives to target business needs and opportunities
- Evaluate, recommend, and redesign processes
- Collect and define requirements
- Translate functional design documents
- Participate in the technical design, test planning, and user documentation processes
- Participate in analysis of client-identified issues or problems, which may require changes to procedures, standards, or systems
- Analyze business and user needs, document requirements, and revise existing systems logic difficulties as necessary
- Work with users and peers in planning, developing, implementing, and supporting new or existing applications
- Analyze and re-engineer business processes

Source: AHIMA 2005.

That unique HIM body of knowledge includes knowledge of:

- Existing and emerging requirements related to privacy and confidentiality of health information
- Applicable federal and state EHR-related laws, accreditation standards, and data and vocabulary standards
- Critical activities related to the integrity of the master patient index file
- Clinical data requirements of both internal and external data users
- Interdepartmental and interdisciplinary clinical data and the information work flow

Figure 6.6 shows how HIM professionals' skills overlap to make them uniquely qualified for e-HIM roles.

Real-World Case

Brian Hutchinson, a graduate student at the Medical University of South Carolina, wrote the following original case study. It has been adapted for educational use and is used with permission.

Sunnybrook Medical Center (SMC) is an 850-bed acute and long-term care facility located in Inner City, California, that is composed of many departments, including surgery, rehabilitation, geriatric psychiatry, and long-term care. Its patient volume is approximately 100,000 visits per year, and the emergency department sees 20,000 visits a year. The medical staff is composed of 125 active attending physicians, 50 salaried (18 full-time, 32 part-time), and 100 residents. Most physicians admit solely to SMC and are single practitioners, located on-site or within 10 miles of SMC.

The hospital identified as one of its goals the desire to implement a computerized provider order-entry (CPOE) system. This goal emerged from that fact that the hospital had been experiencing high turnover of pharmacists who were unhappy with paper order system, long delays in medications reaching patients, patient safety concerns, and the fact that the clinic staff spent too much time dealing with the paper orders. Therefore, it was felt that implementation of a CPOE system would facilitate patient safety and enable providers to deliver higher-quality care. By defining a broad set of goals, SMC was able to define specific objectives of what it wanted the CPOE system to accomplish. Specifically, SMC wanted to reduce the turnaround time for patient medication, to eliminate transcription errors, to reduce the time clinical staff spent on paper orders, to improve the work flow among the different departments of the hospital, to provide decision support tools for physicians, and to increase pharmacists' job satisfaction and retention.

In 2000, SMC began implementation of a 100 percent CPOE system with an interface to the pharmacy computer system. SMC completed implementation in two phases.

Figure 6.6.   HIM skills overlap e-HIM roles

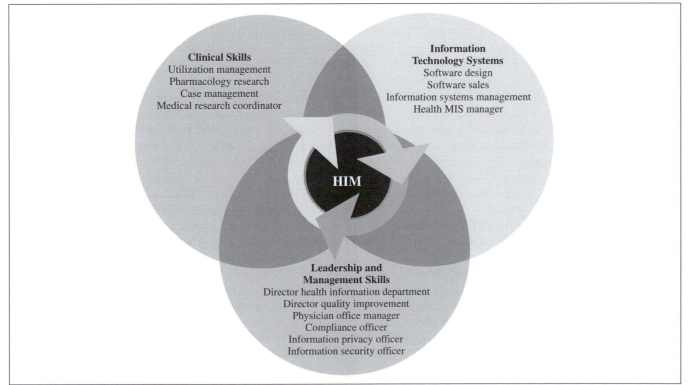

Source: AHIMA 2005.

The first took 18 months and was piloted in the Traumatic Brain Injury unit of rehabilitation medicine. This site was selected because it had a longer average length of stay, a small number of attending physicians and residents, and a dedicated core of nurses. All these factors allowed for a comprehensive evaluation of the CPOE system in this unit within a controlled environment. After successfully implementing the system in the pilot area, SMC implemented the CPOE in each area of the hospital. Then, in 2004, the last phase involved installation of an interface from the CPOE to the computerized pharmacy system.

Before implementation, SMC recognized the barriers that inhibit successful CPOE implementation. The barriers to quality transformation are: no ownership of the system, personnel shortages, fear of system failures, low expectations, poor senior leadership, little physician engagement, and lack of standardized work processes. SMC's solutions to these barriers started with a shared vision and support from upper management that the entire hospital could buy into; thus, the entire hospital could take ownership in implementation of the CPOE. Next, SMC built a bridge between the "suits and coats" (administrators/physicians) and developed a physician-led performance improvement structure that showed the medical staff that administration was concerned about their issues and that the staff could take ownership in improving the hospital. In SMC's case, its CEO and president happened to be a medical doctor, so the medical staff felt more connected to administration than they might otherwise feel in other organizations.

After the senior management and physicians were on board, SMC used model software with tools capable of adapting to the needs of SMC. However, in order to do this, SMC needed to select a vendor whose flexibility would allow the CPOE system to adapt to the people and processes of the organization. When this was established, the hospital could focus on creating an IT team, which would be careful to understand the importance of the clinical processes.

The IT team was composed of a system champion, who understood the CPOE system and had the capacity to support the clinical staff; representatives from management and line staff; and vendor support. Moreover, SMC involved the IT department in committees that helped manage change throughout their organization so that the IT staff would understand the needs of the hospital.

Lastly, SMC realized that for a CPOE system to meet its objectives, the work processes related to medication order entry had to be error free. Physicians at SMC had historically relied on nurses to administer orders in some cases. For example, an order written QAM for insulin should be administered before breakfast, not at 10 a.m. This might not seem like a hindrance, but computers are essentially dumb and correct information must be entered precisely. Moreover, the hospital wanted to have a more accurate audit trail to ensure that its practices were consistent with Leapfrog recommendations and Joint Commission on Accreditation of Healthcare Organizations (JCAHO) standards.

In 2004, the interface connecting the pharmacy system to the CPOE system was installed. Before this time, pharmacists had to reenter physician orders from a printout they received from the CPOE system into the existent pharmacy system. This was very labor and time intensive. The time it took to administer a medication to the patient could be as long as 48 hours, with it taking 8 to 24 hours for the pharmacist to review the medication. Needless to say, this was highly inefficient and costly in terms of patient satisfaction, quality of care, and financially. Yet, when the interface was implemented in 2004, the time it took for medication to be administered to patients decreased to approximately one hour for pharmacist review and another hour to reach the patient. This dramatic decrease in time was due to the reduction in the medical management work flow. Before the interface was implemented, the work flow consisted of 10 steps, of which ordering comprised 39 to 49 percent. After implementation, the ordering processes were simplified to include only the physicians and pharmacists, not the medication administration record (MAR) transcription, nurse review, and the time it took the chart copy to reach the pharmacy.

On top of this, the hospital experienced a $50 million loss during a two-year period. However, SMC remained committed to implementing the CPOE system. Eventually, its investment paid off with higher revenues and its objectives were satisfied.

Implementation decreased medical errors due to both improved legibility and clinicians being alerted to potential problems, such as allergic reactions and adverse drug interaction, from safeguards built in the CPOE system. In addition, the retention of pharmacists improved and job satisfaction increased. So SMC was left with a dedicated team of pharmacists, which eliminated its need for agency personnel. In addition, the pharmacists could now focus on patient care instead of dispensing activities, which resulted in a 50 percent increase in the number of medication-related interventions.

During the implementation process, SMC learned many lessons. First, the entire organization, including senior management, must be committed. Second, a phased-in approach offered SMC a chance to minimize the impact of glitches and technical problems. Third, having a strong partnership between the IS staff and the clinical staff was critical. SMC also found that it was important for the IS staff to understand the clinical and technical components of the clinicians' work. Fourth, it is important for an organization to plan for a high level of physical on-site support. Fifth, an organization should reengineer and streamline its work flow in order for a CPOE system to be successful. Sixth, having a system champion who is a clinician to aid in the transition process is critical. Last, the vendor must provide support and flexibility.

SMC's experiences provide valuable information for organizations seeking to implement a CPOE system. First, SMC shows how successful implementation must start with senior-level management arriving at a consensus on a vision and fully supporting it. Moreover, a relationship must exist between administration and the clinical staff that fosters understanding. In addition, SMC shows the importance of strategic planning when implementing any information system. If the CEO at SMC had not taken the bold step of acquiring the CPOE system, which put the hospital in financial crisis for two years, SMC would never have realized the gains in revenue and healthcare quality. In conclusion, it is necessary to have an IT vendor who is both flexible and knowledgeable throughout the entire implementation process.

Summary

In today's environment, healthcare organizations look to information systems (IS) technology as a way to help them provide high-quality care in a cost-effective manner. However, healthcare managers at all levels often find that they are competing with their colleagues for limited IS resources. Senior administrators are encouraging healthcare managers to work together to build integrated information systems that will support patient care and enable them to control costs across the enterprise. Clearly, in today's environment, information systems should not be developed or selected in isolation. Healthcare organizations should engage in strategic IS planning to ensure that systems are available to support their goals and plans and to prioritize IS needs. The IS plans should be well aligned and integrated with the organization's overall strategic plans. This process should involve key stakeholders throughout the organization, including clinicians/administrators and HIM and information technology leaders.

After the decision has been made to develop or select a new information system, a project manager should be appointed to oversee and manage the SDLC process. Again, key stakeholders throughout the organization should be involved in the analysis, design, implementation, and maintenance/support phases of the SDLC. Adequate technical and organizational resources should be in place to ensure that the new systems are sufficiently maintained and supported. Moreover, systems should be reviewed and evaluated on an ongoing basis to determine their technological, organizational, and economic impact on the enterprise.

References

AHIMA HIM Practice Transformation e-HIM Work Group. 2005. Practice brief: EHR career opportunities: Sample HIM job descriptions. *Journal of American Health Information Management Association* 76(6):56A–56D. Available online from www.ahima.org/infocenter/ehim/.

Anderson, J.G. 1997. Clearing the way for physicians' use of clinical information systems. *Communications of the Association for Computing Machinery* 40(8):83–90.

Anderson, J.G., C.E. Aydin, and S.J. Jay. 1994. *Evaluating Health Care Information Systems: Methods and Applications.* Thousand Oaks, CA: Sage Publications.

Austin, C.J., and S.B. Boxerman. 2003. *Information Systems for Health Services Administration,* 6th ed. Chicago: Health Administration Press.

Barlow, S., J. Johnson, and J. Steck. 2004. The economic effect of implementing an EMR in an outpatient clinical setting. *Journal of Healthcare Information Management* 18(1):46–51.

Bates, D., and A. Gawande. 2003. Improving safety with information technology. *New England Journal of Medicine* 348(25):2526–534.

Bates, D., G. Kuperman, J. Rittenberg, J. Teich, J. Fiskio, N. Ma'luf, et al. 1999. A randomized trial of computer-based intervention to reduce utilization of redundant laboratory tests. *American Journal of Medicine* 106(2):144–50.

Brailer, D.J., and E.L. Terasawa. 2003. *Use and Adoption of Computer-Based Patient Records.* Oakland, CA: California HealthCare Foundation.

California HealthCare Foundation. 2005. *Health Care Costs 101 Snapshot.* Oakland, CA: California HealthCare Foundation.

Friedman, C.P., and J.C. Wyatt. 1997. *Evaluation Methods in Medical Informatics.* New York: Springer.

Glaser, J.P. 2002. *The Strategic Application of Information Technology in Healthcare Organizations,* 2nd ed. San Francisco: Jossey-Bass.

Health Information Management Systems Society Analytics and HIMSS. 2005. *Annual Report of the US Hospital IT Market: An Industry Report.* Chicago: HIMSS.

Institute of Medicine, Committee on Quality of Healthcare in America. 2000. *To Err Is Human: Building a Safer Health System.* Washington, DC: National Academy Press.

Kaplan, B. 1997. Addressing organizational issues into the evaluation of medical systems. *Journal of American Medical Informatics Association* 4(2):94–101.

National Committee for Quality Assurance. 2003. *The State of Healthcare Quality: Industry Trends and Analysis.* Washington, DC: NCQA.

Ross, J.W., and P. Weill. 2002. Six IT decisions your IT people shouldn't make. *Harvard Business Review* 80(11):84–91, 133.

Teich, J., P. Merchia, J. Schimiz, G. Kuperman, C. Spurr, and D. Bates. 2000. Effects of computerized physician order entry on prescribing practices. *Archives of Internal Medicine* 160:2741–747.

Wager, K.A., F.W. Lee, and J.P. Glaser. 2005. *Managing Health Care Information Systems: A Practical Approach for Health Care Executives.* San Francisco: Jossey-Bass.

Wager, K.A., F.W. Lee, and A.W. White. 2001. Life after a disastrous electronic medical record implementation: One clinic's experience. *Annals of Cases on Information Technology* 3:153–68.

Whitten, J.L., L.D. Bentley, and K.C. Dittman. 2004. *Systems Analysis and Design Methods,* 6th ed. Chicago: McGraw-Hill.

Part II

Development of Healthcare Information

Chapter 7
Healthcare Information Standards

Kathleen M. LaTour, MA, RHIA, FAHIMA

Learning Objectives

- To explain healthcare data sets and to describe their purpose
- To recognize the basic data sets used in acute care, ambulatory care, long-term care, emergency care, and home care settings
- To describe the unique use of the Minimum Data Set for Long-Term Care and Resident Assessment Protocols in defining and addressing the care of residents in long-term care facilities
- To identify the purpose and use of the Health Plan Employer Data and Information Set (HEDIS)
- To explain the intent of the ORYX initiative and to give examples of the core measures identified through ORYX
- To recognize the key players in current efforts to develop standards for electronic health records
- To define the term healthcare information standards and to explain vocabulary standards, content and structure standards, technical standards (message format, electronic data interchange, transaction, communication), medication, and privacy and security standards
- To recognize the impact of the Health Insurance Portability and Accountability Act of 1996 (HIPAA) on the development of health informatics standards
- To explain the relationship of core data elements to healthcare informatics standards in electronic environments
- To describe current federal initiatives to support electronic health record development and to create a national health information network (NHIN)
- To explain the concepts of interoperability and connectivity as they relate to the federal initiatives to create a national health information data structure

Key Terms

Accreditation
Accreditation Standards Committee X12
Aggregate data
American College of Radiology–National Electrical Manufacturers Association (ACR-NEMA)
American National Standards Institute (ANSI)
American Society for Testing and Materials (ASTM)
ASTM Standard E1384-02a
Bills of Mortality
Center for Drug Evaluation and Research Data Standards (CDER) Manual
Centers for Medicare and Medicaid Services (CMS)
Certification Commission for Health Information Technology (CCHIT)
Consolidated Health Informatics initiative (CHI)
Continuity of care record (CCR)
Core data elements/core content
Core measure/core measure set
Data/datum
Data dictionary
Data elements
Data Elements for Emergency Department Systems (DEEDS)
Data set
Department of Health and Human Services (HHS)
Digital Imaging and Communication in Medicine (DICOM)
Electronic data interchange (EDI)
Essential Medical Data Set (EMDS)
Extensible markup language (XML)
FDA Unique Ingredient Identifier (UNII) Codes
Health Insurance Portability and Accountability Act of 1996 (HIPAA)
Health Level Seven (HL7)
Health Plan Employer Data and Information Set (HEDIS)

Healthcare information standards
Health care provider dimension (HCPD)
Health Information Exchange (HIE)
Hospital discharge abstract system
Identifier standards
Information
Inpatient
Institute of Electrical and Electronics Engineers (IEEE)
Joint Commission on Accreditation of Healthcare
     Organizations (JCAHO)
Long-term care
Medicare prospective payment system
Message format standards
Minimum Data Set for Long Term Care–Version 2.0
     (MDS 2.0)
National Alliance for Health Information Technology
National Center for Health Statistics (NCHS)
National Committee for Quality Assurance (NCQA)
National Committee on Vital and Health Statistics
     (NCVHS)
National Council on Prescription Drug Programs (NCPDP)
National Drug Code (NDC) Directory
National Health Information Network (NHIN)
National Information Infrastructure-Health Information
     Network Program (NII-HIN)
National provider identifier (NPI)
Office of the National Coordinator of Health Information
     Technology (ONC)
ORYX initiative
Outcomes and Assessment Information Set (OASIS)
Outpatient
Personal health dimension (PHD)
Population health dimension (PHD)
Privacy standards
Resident Assessment Protocols (RAPs)
Regional Health Information Network (RHIN)
Regional Health Information Organization (RHIO)
RxNorm
Security standards
Semantic Clinical Drug (SCD)
Social Security number (SSN)
Standards development organizations (SDOs)
Structure and content standards
Subnetwork organization
Transaction standards
Uniform Ambulatory Care Data Set (UACDS)
Uniform Hospital Discharge Data Set (UHDDS)
United Nations International Standards Organization (ISO)
Unique physician identification number (UPIN)
Unique identification number
Vocabulary standards
X12N

Introduction

Data and information pertaining to individuals who use healthcare services are collected in virtually every setting where healthcare is delivered. **Data** represent basic facts and measurements. In healthcare, these facts usually describe specific characteristics of individual patients. The term *data* is plural. Although the singular form is datum, the term that is frequently used to describe a single fact or measurement is *data element.* For example, age, gender, insurance company, and blood pressure are all data elements concerning a patient. The term ***information*** refers to data that have been collected, combined, analyzed, interpreted, and/or converted into a form that can be used for specific purposes. In other words, data represent facts; information represents meaning.

In healthcare settings, data are stored in the individual's health record whether that record is in paper or electronic format. The numerous data elements in the health record are then combined, analyzed, and interpreted by the patient's physician and other clinicians. For example, test results are combined with the physician's observations and the patient's description of his or her symptoms to form information about the disease or condition that is affecting the patient. Physicians use both data and information to diagnose diseases, develop treatment plans, assess the effectiveness of care, and determine the patient's prognosis.

Data about patients can be extracted from individual health records and combined as **aggregate data.** Aggregate data are used to develop information about groups of patients. For example, data about all of the patients who suffered an acute myocardial infarction during a specific time period could be collected in a database. From the aggregate data, it would be possible to identify common characteristics that might predict the course of the disease or provide information about the most effective way to treat it. Ultimately, research using the aggregated data might be used for disease prevention. For example, researchers identified the link between smoking and lung cancer by analyzing aggregate data about patients with a diagnosis of lung cancer; smoking cessation programs grew from the identification of the causal effect of smoking on lung cancer and a variety of other conditions.

The first known efforts to collect and use healthcare data to produce meaningful statistical profiles date back to the 17th century. In the early 1600s, Captain John Graunt gathered data on the common causes of death in London. He called his study the **Bills of Mortality.** However, few systematic efforts were undertaken to collect statistical data about the incidence and prevalence of disease until the mid-20th century, when technological developments made it possible to collect and analyze large amounts of healthcare data.

Modern efforts at standardizing healthcare data began in the 1960s. At that time, healthcare facilities began to use computers to process larger amounts of data than could be handled manually. The goal was to make comparisons among data from multiple providers. It soon became evident that healthcare organizations needed to use standardized, uniform data definitions in order to arrive at meaningful data comparisons.

The first data standardization efforts focused generally on hospitals and specifically on hospital discharge data. The intent of the efforts was to standardize definitions of key data elements commonly collected in hospitals. Discharge data were collected in **hospital discharge abstract systems.** These systems used databases compiled from aggregate data about all of the patients discharged from a particular facility. The need to compare uniform discharge data from one hospital to the next led to the development of **data sets,** or lists of recommended data elements with uniform definitions.

There is an old saying, "You can't compare apples and oranges." When we attempt to compare terms that do not have the same definition it is like comparing apples and oranges. Standardizing data elements and definitions makes it possible to compare the data collected at different facilities. For example, when data are standardized, the term "admission" means the same thing at City Hospital and at University Hospital. Because both hospitals define "admission" in the same way, then the hospitals can be compared with each other on such things as the number of admissions or the percentage of occupancy each has had.

Today, hospitals and other healthcare organizations collect more data and develop more information than ever before. Moreover, data and information from the health records of individual patients are used for more purposes than ever before. The demand for information is coming from users within the organizations as well as from external users such as third-party payers, government agencies, **accreditation** organizations, and others. The extensive use of information within and across organizational boundaries demands standards that promote interoperable electronic interchange of data and information. Information standards are critical in the migration to electronic health records (EHR), as described in Chapter 9.

The data sets originally developed to support uniform data collection are inadequate for an electronic environment and many public and private organizations have been actively engaged in the process of developing **healthcare information standards** to support EHR development and information interchange. Healthcare information standards development is a dynamic process that evolves on a continuous basis as key players in the standards development community negotiate, refine, and revise standards. The critical importance of healthcare information standards has been recognized in recent federal initiatives including the **Consolidated Health Informatics** (CHI) **initiatives** as well as efforts of the Office of the National Coordinator of Health Information Technology (ONC).

According to the **National Committee on Vital and Health Statistics** (NCVHS) in its initial 2000 report entitled Toward a National Health Information Infrastructure, "if information in multiple locations is to be searched, shared, and synthesized when needed, we will need agreed-upon information guardians that can exchange data with each other . . . we will need equitable rules of data exchange so that competitors (within or between healthcare provider systems, health information management companies, or health Web services) will be willing to connect and share data" (NCVHS 2000).

This chapter describes the initial efforts at developing standardized data sets for use in different types of healthcare settings, including acute care, ambulatory care, long-term care, and home care. It explores the recent national initiatives related to interoperability and connectivity of healthcare information systems that will support widespread implementation of electronic health records and the ultimate establishment of a national health information network that will improve patient care, increase safety, and optimize both clinical and administrative decision making. This chapter addresses the evolution of health information standards that are the foundation of this vision.

Theory into Practice

In a large Midwestern health system, the director of health information services leads the system's clinical data standards committee. The committee recently decided to develop a **data dictionary** as a first step toward implementing an electronic health record system (EHR).

Data dictionaries include the following components:

- A list of **data elements** collected in individual health records
- Definitions of the data elements
- Descriptions of the attributes of each data element
- Specifications for the size of the data field in the information system
- Descriptions of the data views to be accessed by various users

The committee began the process with what it considered to be a simple data element: patient gender. The committee members looked at the two standard references for patient data sets in acute care settings: the **Uniform Hospital Discharge Data Set** (UHDDS) and the **Uniform Ambulatory Care Data Set** (UACDS). Both data sets indicated that gender should be recorded as either "male" or "female." However, this either-or choice presented a problem.

The healthcare system included a number of hospitals and clinics. One of the hospitals offered a gender re-identification program that treated patients who were in the process of transitioning from one gender to the other. Another hospital provided neonatal intensive care services for a large geographical region. Some of the infants treated in the neonatal intensive care unit had been born with congenital defects that made it difficult to determine their gender.

During discussions of the problem, the clinical laboratory representative on the committee stressed the importance of documenting the gender of every patient. She explained that the normal range for most laboratory tests varies by gender. This information was a surprise to many committee members.

After the committee's initial discussion, the health information management director agreed to research other data sets and standards. He found that recent healthcare information standards for electronic and computer-based patient records recommended using four gender descriptors: male, female, undetermined, and unknown.

The committee decided to adopt the four descriptors for gender. In the data collection process, if the term undetermined or unknown was selected, the individual doing data entry would be referred to another screen that would explain the data choice in more detail and include another data element to describe the patient's genitalia.

The challenges the committee faced in defining this relatively simple data element raised its awareness of how difficult it is to adequately define every data element included in the new EHR system. The committee members gathered information on every available healthcare data set and healthcare information standard and carefully compared the data definitions recommended. They discovered that implementation of the EHR system would be a huge project. However, they were committed to the process because it would improve the quality of the data collected in the system. The collection of consistent, reliable, and valid data would improve administrative and clinical decision making and make it possible to perform meaningful performance improvement comparisons.

Standardized Healthcare Data Sets

The concept of data standardization became widely accepted during the 1960s, and, under the leadership of the **National Center for Health Statistics** (NCHS) and the NCVHS in collaboration with other organizations, data sets were developed for a variety of healthcare settings. Data sets for acute care, long-term care, and ambulatory care were the first to be created. In healthcare, data sets have two purposes: (1) to identify the data elements that should be collected for each patient and (2) to provide uniform definitions for common terms. The use of uniform definitions ensures that data collected from a variety of healthcare settings will share a standard definition.

The standardization of data elements and definitions makes it possible to compare the data collected at different facilities. Comparison data are used for a variety of purposes, including external accreditation, internal performance improvement, and statistical and research studies. However, data sets are not meant to limit the number of data elements that can be collected. Most healthcare organizations collect additional data elements that have meaning for their specific administrative and clinical operations.

Uniform Hospital Discharge Data Set

In 1969, a conference on hospital discharge abstract systems was sponsored jointly by the NCHS, the National Center for Health Services Research and Development, and Johns Hopkins University. Conference participants recommended that all short-term general hospitals in the United States collect a minimum set of patient-specific data elements. They also recommended that these data elements be reflected in all databases formulated from hospital discharge abstract systems. They called the list of patient-specific data items the Uniform Hospital Discharge Data Set (UHDDS).

In 1974, the federal government adopted the UHDDS as the standard for collecting data for the Medicare and Medicaid programs. When the Prospective Payment Act was enacted in 1983, UHDDS definitions were incorporated into the rules and regulations for implementing diagnosis-related groups (DRGs). A key component was the incorporation of the definitions of principal diagnosis, principal procedure, and other significant procedures, into the DRG algorithms. As a result, accurate assignment of a DRG is dependent on accurate selection and coding of the principal diagnosis and principal procedure and the appropriate sequencing of other significant diagnoses and procedures. The National Committee on Vital and Health Statistics revised the UHDDS in 1984. The new UHDDS was adopted for all federal health programs in 1986.

The intent of the UHDDS is to list and define a set of common, uniform data elements. The data elements are to be collected in the health records of every hospital inpatient. They are subsequently abstracted from the health record and included in databases that describe aggregate patient characteristics. Most short-term, general hospitals in the United States collect patient-specific data in the format recommended by the UHDDS.

The UHDDS has been revised several times since 1986. The current version includes the recommended data elements shown in figure 7.1.

Uniform Ambulatory Care Data Set

Ambulatory care includes medical and surgical care provided to patients who return to their homes on the same day they receive the care. It is provided in physicians' offices, medical clinics, same-day surgery centers, outpatient hospital clinics and diagnostic departments, emergency treatment centers, and hospital emergency departments. Patients who receive ambulatory care services in hospital-based clinics and departments are referred to as **outpatients.** (Note: Patients who are admitted to hospitals for overnight stays are referred to as **inpatients.**)

Figure 7.1.   UHDDS data elements

Data Element	Definition/Descriptor
01. Personal identifier	The unique number assigned to each patient within a hospital that distinguishes the patient and his or her hospital record from all others in that institution.
02. Date of birth	Month, day, and year of birth. Capture of the full four-digit year of birth is recommended.
03. Sex	Male or female
04. Race and ethnicity	04a. Race 　　American Indian/Eskimo/Aleut 　　Asian or Pacific Islander 　　Black 　　White 　　Other race 　　Unknown 04b. Ethnicity 　　Spanish origin/Hispanic 　　Non-Spanish origin/Non-Hispanic 　　Unknown
05. Residence	Full address of usual residence Zip code (nine digits, if available) Code for foreign residence
06. Hospital identification	A unique institutional number used across data collection systems. The Medicare provider number is the preferred hospital identifier.
07. Admission date	Month, day, and year of admission
08. Type of admission	Scheduled: Arranged with admissions office at least 24 hours prior to admission Unscheduled: All other admissions
09. Discharge date	Month, day, and year of discharge
10 & 11. Physician identification • Attending physician • Operating physician	The Medicare unique physician identification number (UPIN) is the preferred method of identifying the attending physician and operating physician(s) because it is uniform across all data systems.
12. Principal diagnosis	The condition established, after study, to be chiefly responsible for occasioning the admission of the patient to the hospital for care.
13. Other diagnoses	All conditions that coexist at the time of admission or that develop subsequently or that affect the treatment received and/or the length of stay. Diagnoses that relate to an earlier episode and have no bearing on the current hospital stay are to be excluded.
14. Qualifier for other diagnoses	A qualifier is given for each diagnosis coded under "other diagnoses" to indicate whether the onset of the diagnosis preceded or followed admission to the hospital. The option "uncertain" is permitted.
15. External cause-of-injury code	The ICD-9-CM code for the external cause of an injury, poisoning, or adverse effect (commonly referred to as an E code). Hospitals should complete this item whenever there is a diagnosis of an injury, poisoning, or adverse effect.
16. Birth weight of neonate	The specific birth weight of a newborn, preferably recorded in grams.
17. Procedures and dates	All significant procedures are to be reported. A significant procedure is one that is: • Surgical in nature, or　　　　• Carries an anesthetic risk, or • Carries a procedural risk, or　　• Requires specialized training. The date of each significant procedure must be reported. When more than one procedure is reported, the principal procedure must be designated. The principal procedure is one that is performed for definitive treatment rather than one performed for diagnostic or exploratory purposes or is necessary to take care of a complication. If two procedures appear to be principal, the one most closely related to the principal diagnosis should be selected as the principal procedure. The UPIN must be reported for the person performing the principal procedure.
18. Disposition of the patient	• Discharged to home (excludes those patients referred to home health service)　　• Discharged to other healthcare facility • Discharged to acute care hospital　　• Left against medical advice • Discharged to nursing facility　　• Alive, other; or alive, not stated • Discharged home to be under the care of a home health service (including a hospice)　　• Died All categories for primary and other sources are: • Blue Cross/Blue Shield　　• Health maintenance organization (HMO) • Other health insurance companies　　• CHAMPUS • Other liability insurance　　• CHAMPVA • Medicare　　• Other government payers • Medicaid　　• Self-pay • Worker's Compensation　　• No charge (free, charity, special research, teaching) • Self-insured employer plan　　• Other
19. Patient's expected source of payment	Primary source Other sources
20. Total charges	All charges billed by the hospital for this hospitalization. Professional charges for individual patient care by physicians are excluded.

Source: Adapted from Hanken and Water 1994.

Since the 1980s, the number and the length of inpatient hospitalizations have declined dramatically. At the same time, the number of healthcare procedures performed in ambulatory settings has increased. There are several reasons for this trend, including:

- Technological improvements in diagnostic and therapeutic procedures and the development of short-acting anesthetics have made it possible to perform many medical and surgical procedures in ambulatory facilities. Surgical procedures that once required inpatient hospitalization and long recovery periods are now being performed in same-day surgery centers.
- Third-party payers have extended coverage to include most procedures performed on an outpatient basis.
- The **Medicare prospective payment system** limits reimbursement for inpatient care and, in effect, encourages the use of ambulatory and/or outpatient care as an alternative to more costly inpatient services.

Like hospitals, ambulatory care organizations depend on the availability of accurate data and information. A standardized data set to guide the content and structure of ambulatory health records and data collection systems in ambulatory care was needed.

In 1989, the National Committee on Vital and Health Statistics approved the Uniform Ambulatory Care Data Set (UACDS). The committee recommended its use in every facility where ambulatory care is delivered. Several of the data elements that make up the UACDS are similar to those used in the UHDDS. For example, the UACDS data elements that describe the personal identifier, residence, date of birth, gender, and race/ethnicity of the patient are the same as the definitions in the UHDDS. The purpose of keeping the same demographic data elements is to make it easier to compare data for inpatients and ambulatory patients in the same facility.

However, the UACDS also includes data elements specific to ambulatory care, such as the reason for the encounter with the healthcare provider. The UACDS also includes optional data elements to describe the patient's living arrangements and marital status. These data elements (shown in figure 7.2) are unique to the UACDS. Ambulatory care practitioners need information about the living conditions of their patients because patients and their families often need to manage at-home nursing care, for example, activity restrictions after a surgical procedure. Hospital staff provides such nursing services in acute care settings.

The goal of the UACDS is to improve data comparison in ambulatory and outpatient care settings. It provides uniform definitions that help providers to analyze patterns of care. The data elements in the UACDS are those most likely to be needed by a variety of users. Unlike the UHDDS, the UACDS has not been incorporated into federal regulations. Therefore, it is a recommended, rather than a required, data set and, in practical terms, it has been subsumed by other data definition efforts, most notably the **core data elements**

Figure 7.2.   UACDS data elements

Data Element	Definition/Descriptor
Provider identification, address, type of practice	Provider identification: Include the full name of the provider as well as the unique physician identification number (UPIN).
	Address: The complete address of the provider's office. In cases where the provider has multiple offices, the location of the usual or principal place of practice should be given. Profession:
	• Physician, including specialty or field of practice • Other (specify)
Place of encounter	Specify the location of the encounter: • Private office • Clinic or health center • Hospital outpatient department • Hospital emergency department • Other (specify)
Reason for encounter	Includes, but is not limited to, the patient's complaints and symptoms reflecting his or her own perception of needs, provided verbally or in writing by the patient at the point of entry into the healthcare system or in the patient's own words recorded by an intermediary or provider at that time.
Diagnostic services	All diagnostic services of any type.
Problem, diagnosis, or assessment	Describes the provider's level of understanding and the interpretation of the patient's reasons for the encounter and all conditions requiring treatment or management at the time of the encounter.
Therapeutic services	List, by name, all services done or ordered: • Medical (including drug therapy) • Surgical • Patient education
Preventive services	List, by name, all preventive services and procedures performed at the time of encounter.

Disposition	The provider's statement of the next step(s) in the care of the patient. At a minimum, the following classification is suggested:
	1. No follow-up planned
	2. Follow-up planned
	  • Return when necessary
	  • Return to the current provider at a specified time
	  • Telephone follow-up
	  • Return to referring provider
	  • Refer to other provider
	  • Admit to hospital
	  • Other

Source: Adapted from Hanken and Water 1994.

recommended as part of the National Health Information Network (NHIN) which is described later in this chapter.

Minimum Data Set for Long-Term Care and Resident Assessment Protocols

Uniform data collection is also important in the **long-term care** setting. Long-term care incorporates the healthcare services provided in residential facilities for individuals who are unable to live independently owing to chronic illness or disability. Long-term care facilities also provide dietary and social services as well as housing and nursing care.

For a long-term care facility to participate in the Medicare and Medicaid programs, the **Centers for Medicare and Medicaid Services** (CMS) requires the development of a comprehensive functional assessment for every resident. From this assessment, a nursing home resident's plan of care is developed.

The **Minimum Data Set for Long-Term Care–Version 2.0** (MDS 2.0) is a federally mandated standard assessment form used to collect demographic and clinical data on nursing home residents. It consists of a core set of screening and assessment elements based on common definitions. To meet federal requirements, long-term care facilities must complete an MDS for every resident at the time of admission and at designated reassessment points throughout the resident's stay.

The MDS uses some of the same data elements and definitions used in other data sets. However, it is far more extensive and includes more clinical data than either the UHDDS or the UACDS. The data collected via the MDS are used to develop care plans for residents and to document placement at the appropriate level of care.

The MDS organizes data according to 20 main categories. Each category includes a structured list of choices and/or responses. The use of structured lists automatically standardizes the data that are collected. The major categories of data collected in the MDS include:

1. Demographic information
2. Identification and background information
3. Cognitive patterns
4. Communication/hearing patterns
5. Vision patterns
6. Mood and behavior patterns
7. Psychosocial well-being
8. Physical functioning and structural problems
9. Continence in past 14 days
10. Disease diagnoses
11. Health conditions
12. Oral/nutritional status
13. Oral/dental status
14. Skin condition
15. Activity pursuit patterns
16. Medications
17. Special treatments and procedures
18. Discharge potential and overall status
19. Assessment information
20. Therapy supplement for Medicare PPS

The data collected via the MDS are used to develop a **Resident Assessment Protocol** (RAP) summary for each resident. The MDS provides a structured way to organize resident information and develop a resident care plan. Problems identified through the assessment process are documented, and a RAP is triggered. For each triggered RAP, the facility must describe the following factors:

- Nature of the condition (may include presence or lack of objective data and subjective complaints)
- Complications and risk factors that affect the decision to proceed to care planning
- Factors that must be considered in developing individualized care plan interventions
- Need for referrals/further evaluation by appropriate healthcare professionals

Nursing home personnel use the data from the MDS and RAP to plan, carry out, and assess the care given to individual residents. Other practice settings, such as rehabilitation and postacute care, are considering versions of the MDS for use in patient assessment, but none has been implemented to date. The Department of Health and Human Services is currently in the process of developing MDS Version 3.0. The original target date for implementation of Version 3.0 was 2003 but, as of early 2006, Version 3.0 had not yet been implemented and no new implementation date had been published.

Outcomes Assessment Information Set (OASIS)

In 1999, the Health Care Financing Administration (HCFA) (renamed the Centers for Medicare and Medicaid Services [CMS]) implemented a standardized data set for use in the home health industry. The **Outcomes and Assessment Information Set** (OASIS) is designed to gather data about Medicare beneficiaries who are receiving services from a home health agency. OASIS includes a set of core data items that are collected on all adult home health patients. The data are used in measuring patient outcomes in order to assess the quality of home healthcare services. Under the prospective payment program for home health, which was implemented in 2000, data from OASIS also form the basis of reimbursement for provided services.

OASIS data are grouped into the following categories:

- Demographics and Patient History
- Living Arrangements
- Supportive Assistance
- Respiratory
- Neurological
- Psychological
- Integument
- Pain

- Activities of Daily Living (ADLs)/Instrumental Activities of Daily Living (IADLs)
- Medications
- Elimination Status
- General Information
- Emergent Care

Data collected through OASIS are used to assess the patient's ability to be discharged or transferred from home care services and to evaluate the quality and outcome of services given to the patient.

Data Elements for Emergency Department Systems

Emergency and trauma care in the United States have become very sophisticated over the past few decades. Emergency services represent a significant part of the healthcare delivery system. As emergency and trauma care services have been developed, it has become increasingly important to collect relevant aggregate data. Many states require the reporting of trauma cases to state agencies.

In 1997, the Centers for Disease Control and Prevention (CDC) through its National Center for Injury Prevention and Control (NCIPC) published a data set called **Data Elements for Emergency Department Systems** (DEEDS). This data set was developed with input from the American College of Emergency Physicians, the Emergency Nurses Association, and the American Health Information Management Association. Its stated purpose is to support the uniform collection of data in hospital-based emergency departments and to substantially reduce incompatibilities in emergency department records.

DEEDS recommends the collection of 156 data elements in hospitals that offer emergency care services. As with the UHDDS and UACDS, this data set contains recommendations on both the content and the structure of the data elements to be collected. The data are organized into the following eight sections:

- Patient identification data
- Facility and practitioner identification data
- Emergency department payment data
- Emergency department arrival and first-assessment data
- Emergency department history and physical examination data
- Emergency department procedure and result data
- Emergency department medication data
- Emergency department disposition and diagnosis data

DEEDS incorporates national standards for electronic data interchange so its implementation in an electronic health record system can facilitate communication and integration with other information systems (NCIPC 1997).

Essential Medical Data Set

The **Essential Medical Data Set** (EMDS) was created as a complement to DEEDS. It was developed as part of the **National Information Infrastructure-Health Information Network Program** (NII-HIN) in 1997. The EMDS gives healthcare providers a concise medical history data set for each individual patient. The goal is to enhance the effectiveness of emergency care. The EMDS is different from DEEDS in that DEEDS is designed to collect data about a specific emergency encounter while EMDS is designed to create a health history for an individual patient.

The EMDS is intended for use in electronic health record systems. During the course of an emergency, the emergency department's information system queries a data repository for the patient's past medical history. The documentation for the visit is recorded according to the DEEDS format, and the data are sent to a regional data repository when the emergency care episode is complete.

Emergency care often has a critical impact on patient survival. Therefore, it is important to collect standardized, comparable data. These data then can be used to assess the effectiveness of treatment modalities, response time, and patient survival rates.

Trauma registries and statewide trauma database systems have grown incrementally over the past several years. State departments of public health as well as the federal agencies involved in oversight of emergency care are interested in statistical data about the efficacy of emergency treatment. Collecting standardized data in the emergency care system is fundamental to meaningful analysis of information about emergency care.

Standardized Data Collection Efforts

The following three initiatives do not represent the development and promulgation of information standards; however, each is an initiative in which standardized data are collected and used in assessing utilization, quality, and cost of healthcare for selected populations. As such, they are worth addressing in this chapter. HEDIS and ORYX are addressed in detail in Chapter 17.

Health Plan Employer Data and Information Set

The **Health Plan Employer Data and Information Set** (HEDIS) is sponsored by the **National Committee for Quality Assurance** (NCQA). HEDIS is a set of standard performance measures designed to provide purchasers, and consumers of healthcare with the information they need for comparing the performance of managed healthcare plans.

HEDIS is designed to collect administrative and claims data as well as health record review data. The data are used to analyze and assess the outcomes of treatment. HEDIS collects standardized data about specific health-related conditions or issues so that the success of various treatment plans can be assessed and compared. HEDIS data form the basis of performance improvement efforts for health plans. HEDIS data also are used to develop physician profiles. The goal of physician profiling is to positively influence physician practice patterns.

HEDIS contains more than 50 measures related to conditions such as heart disease, cancer, diabetes, asthma, chlamydia infection, smoking cessation, and menopause counseling. It includes data related to patient outcomes in addition to data about the treatment process used by the clinician in treating the patient.

Standardized HEDIS data elements are abstracted from health records in clinics and hospitals. The health record data are combined with enrollment and claims data and analyzed according to HEDIS specifications.

The purpose of HEDIS is to collect standardized data about specific health-related conditions or issues so that the success of various treatment plans can be assessed and compared. HEDIS data form the basis of performance improvement efforts for health plans. HEDIS data also are used to develop physician profiles. The goal of physician profiling is to positively influence physician practice patterns.

An example of a focused HEDIS review is diabetes care and treatment. Other examples of HEDIS clinical measures include:

- Adolescent immunizations
- Smoking cessation programs
- Antidepressant medication management
- Breast cancer screening
- Cholesterol screening after a heart attack
- Prenatal care during the first trimester

Data from HEDIS studies are often released publicly by health plans to document substantial positive effects on the health of their clients. Results are compared over time and with data from other sources. From the data, health plans determine opportunities for performance improvement and develop potential interventions.

HEDIS is an example of a population-based data collection tool. It illustrates the need for developing standardized data definitions and uniform collection methods. It also emphasizes the importance of data quality management.

Core Measures for ORYX

The **Joint Commission on Accreditation of Healthcare Organizations** (JCAHO) is one of the largest users of healthcare data and information. Its primary function is the accreditation of hospitals and other healthcare organizations. In 1997, the JCAHO introduced the **ORYX initiative** to integrate outcomes data and other performance measurement data into its accreditation processes. (The initiative was named ORYX after an African animal that can be thought of as a different kind of zebra.) The goal of the initiative is to foster a comprehensive, continuous, data-driven accreditation process for healthcare facilities.

The ORYX initiative uses nationally standardized performance measures to improve the safety and quality of healthcare. The program's objectives include:

- Establishing a national comparative database to support benchmarking, health services research, and internal performance improvement activities

- Fostering standardization of performance measures
- Encouraging the use of evidence-based treatment protocols

The goal of the ORYX initiative is to develop data sets for each core measure so that data collection can be standardized among all healthcare facilities. The core measures are based on selected diagnoses/conditions such as diabetes mellitus, the outcomes of which can be improved by standardizing care. They include the minimum number of data elements needed to provide an accurate and reliable measure of performance. Core measures rely on data elements that are readily available or already collected. Chapter 17 explores current ORYX core measure studies.

National Health Information Network (NHIN)

As discussed above, the standardized collection of common data elements can provide valuable information about the effectiveness of interventions and treatments for specific diseases. Healthcare providers are able to compare their success rates with those of other providers to determine areas for performance improvement. This type of analysis can provide critical information that will eventually have a positive impact on clinical outcomes.

In 1998, NCVHS produced the concept paper "Assuring a Health Dimension for the National Information Infrastructure" that discussed a conceptual model of a nationwide network of health information. In 2001, NCVHS began to explore the feasibility of a national health information infrastructure (NHII) that would allow the electronic exchange of health information. The goal of this initiative was to offer a technology solution that would increase patient safety, reduce medical errors, increase efficiency and effectiveness of health care, and contain costs (Mon 2005). The NHII initiative launched an industrywide discussion on how to exchange information electronically in a secure and standard fashion (Mon 2005) and this discussion focused attention on the necessity of developing standards to facilitate the definition, collection, exchange, and use of data and information. There were diverging opinions on how to accomplish the objective and, to date, there is no consensus on a single method of developing this information network. However, many key public and private organizations are actively working on making the concept of a national health information network a reality.

According to the NCVHS report Information for Health: A Strategy for Building the National Health Information Infrastructure (2001), the NHII includes not just technologies but, more importantly, values, practices, relationships, laws, standards, systems, and applications that support all facets of individual health, health care, and public health. It emphasizes the criticality of implementing national health information standards as a foundation of a system that supports connectivity and interoperability. As this initiative has developed, the term **national health information network** (NHIN) has replaced the use of the term NHII. At the time of publication there were indications that the terminology would again change to **subnetwork organizations.**

Past efforts at standards development have been disparate with little industry leadership and little federal influence. There has been minimal coordination of efforts between standards organizations resulting in fragmented and, in some cases, competing standards from different organizations. Under the NHIN initiatives, efforts are focused on creating standards that define a universal language of health information and maintaining that universality as NHIN development and electronic health record implementation moves forward. A key tenet of the NHIN is that the ideal is to collect information only once at the point of care. The needs for data by multiple users for multiple purposes subsequently should emerge from the data that is initially captured at the original point of care.

Efforts in the development of NHIN led to President George W. Bush issuing Executive Order 13335 in April 2004. This order called for widespread interoperable electronic health records (EHRs) within 10 years and it established the **Office of the National Coordinator for Health Information Technology** (ONC). The directive to the National Coordinator was to develop and implement a strategic plan to guide the nationwide implementation of interoperable health information technology (HIT) in both the public and private sectors (Thompson and Brailer 2004). ONC was given the responsibility of moving forward the already existing National Health Information Infrastructure initiative and, in fact, it was ONC that replaced the term NHII with the more contemporary term, NHIN.

In 2004, ONC issued a request for information (RFI) to gather broad input from key stakeholders about how the U.S. national health information network (NHIN) should be designed. AHIMA responded as a member of a collaborative of major healthcare and information technology organizations. This collaborative recommended general adoption of a set of tools critical to achieving an interoperable environment that supports modern healthcare practice, including precisely defined and uniform technical standards and common policies and methods. This set of tool is called the Common Framework (Kloss 2005b).

As currently envisioned, the NHIN will be comprised of a "network of networks" that will be built incrementally using internet technology with particular emphasis on confidentiality and security of data. A key element is that the network is private, secure, and built on patient control and authorization. Personal information would remain with the healthcare provider and accessed and exchanged only as needed and with proper authorization and security. (Kloss 2005b).

The NHIN has supported and, in fact, given impetus to the development of local or **regional health information organizations** (RHIOs). RHIOs are also referred to as **regional health information networks** (RHINs), community health information networks and, most recently, as **health information exchanges** (HIE). An RHIO is a networked community (with the community defined at the local or regional level) that includes physician offices, hospitals, nursing homes, pharmacies, and, in some cases, payers, vendors, or other healthcare-related agencies. The purpose of an RHIO is to give regional healthcare providers access to clinical information for all patients in the defined region across a decentralized technology environment. There are several models for RHIOs with no accepted model. To date, each RHIO has developed in response to local and regional needs and each operates independently, both in the choice of network design and in its access model. The goal of RHIOs are consistent with the goal of NHIN: improved quality of care, increased patient safety, reduction of medical errors, and cost savings. RHIOs are also addressed in Chapter 9.

As a result of the health care industry input in response to the RFI, The Office of the National Coordinator for Health Information Technology (ONC) issued a series of three year government contracts focused on the four key areas identified by the healthcare industry as key to HIE development: EHR certification, data standards, NHIN architecture, and privacy and security (Carol 2005). In November 2005 contracts were awarded to public-private groups to address three of the key areas:

- A contract was awarded to the **Certification Commission for Health Information Technology** (CCHIT) to develop criteria and evaluation processes to certify electronic health records and the infrastructure or network components through which they interoperate.
- The American National Standards Institute (ANSI) was awarded a contract to convene the National Health Information Technology Panel to bring together U.S. standards organizations and others to develop, test, and evaluate a process for bringing together a set of health IT standards that will support interoperability among healthcare software applications, especially EHRs.
- The Health Information Security and Privacy Collaboration was charged with working collaboratively with the National Governors Association and industry experts to develop privacy and security solutions.

An additional contract to develop national health information network architecture will be awarded at a later time. (hhs.gov/news/press/2005pres/20051006a.html)

NHIN Dimensions and Core Data Elements
To support the development of networked health information systems, NHIN defines three dimensions of the infrastructure that provide a means for conceptualizing the capture, storage, communication, processing, and presentation of information for each group of information users:

- Personal health dimension
- Healthcare provider dimension
- Population health dimension

These dimensions are graphically represented in figure 7.3.

Figure 7.3.   Examples of content for three dimensions and their overlap

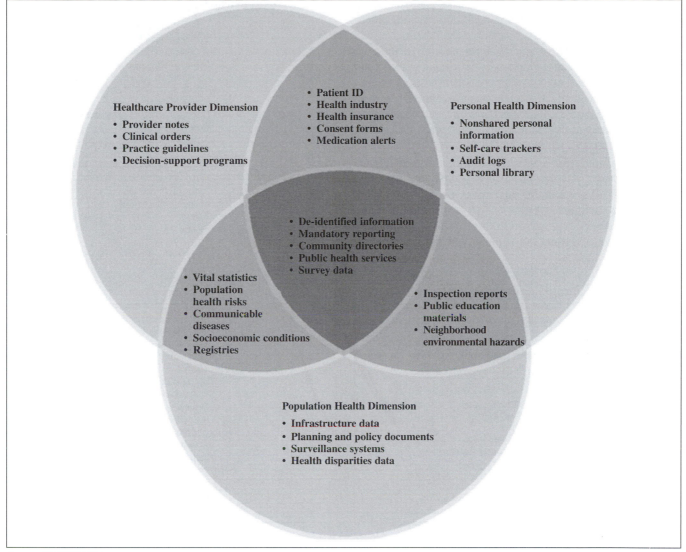

Healthcare Provider Dimension

- Provider notes
- Clinical orders
- Practice guidelines
- Decision-support programs

- Patient ID
- Health industry
- Health insurance
- Consent forms
- Medication alerts

Personal Health Dimension

- Nonshared personal information
- Self-care trackers
- Audit logs
- Personal library

- De-identified information
- Mandatory reporting
- Community directories
- Public health services
- Survey data

- Vital statistics
- Population health risks
- Communicable diseases
- Socioeconomic conditions
- Registries

- Inspection reports
- Public education materials
- Neighborhood environmental hazards

Population Health Dimension

- Infrastructure data
- Planning and policy documents
- Surveillance systems
- Health disparities data

Source: NCVHS 2001.

A set of core data elements has been developed for each of the dimensions of the NHII as part of the NCVHS report Toward a National Health Information Infrastructure (2000).

Personal Health Dimension: Core content of the **personal health dimension** (PHD) will be controlled by the individual both in the initial input of data and in the ability to edit personal data. The issues relating to patient input of data into the provider record and the ability to edit the provider record is still under discussion in the industry and no final recommendations have been agreed upon. Individuals will select data elements that are relevant to their specific age, gender, health history, health and wellness concerns, and other factors. The core content in table 7.1 (p. 158) represents a minimum data set; the intent of NHII is to develop standards for a personal health record and a data dictionary that supports a consistent format that will allow healthcare providers to access the data as needed and authorized by the individual.

Health Care Provider Dimension: The **health care provider dimension** (HCPD) includes information that is captured during the patient care process and concurrently integrates this information with clinical guidelines, protocols, and selected information that the provider is authorized to access from the personal health record, as well as information from the population health dimension that is relevant to the patient's care (NCVHS 2000). The HCPD would be useful to providers in any and all care settings.

Core content of the HCPD is delineated in table 7.2 (p. 158).

Population Health Dimension: The **population health dimension** (PHD) acknowledges the importance of population-based health data and resources that are necessary to improve public health. This data will help public health professionals to identify public health threats, assess population health, focus programs and policies on well-defined health problems, inform and educate individuals about health issues, evaluate programs and services, conduct research to address health issues, and perform other public health services (NCVHS 2000).

Core content of the population health dimension is identified in table 7.3.

According to the Nova Scotia Department of Health core data sets are "sharable electronic patient demographic and essential 'persistent' clinical information necessary to provide informed medical care." Data sets provide the means to record and communicate the most relevant and timely facts about a patient's health information and health care (AHIMA Workgroup 2004).

The transition from paper to electronic health records necessitates the transition from legacy data sets toward a comprehensive core data set that maps back to electronic health record functions. (AHIMA Workgroup 2004).

Table 7.1. Core content of the personal health dimension

Personal Health Record	• Personal identification information • Emergency contact information • Lifetime health history; summary of caregiver records from all sources of care, including immunizations, allergies, family history, occupational history, environmental exposures, social history, medical history, treatments procedures, medication history, outcomes • Lab results (e.g., EKGs) or links to results (MRI results at a radiology department data warehouse, digital images of biopsy slides, or digital video of coronary angiography) • Emergency care information (e.g., allergies, current medications, medical/surgical history summary) • Provider identification and contact information • Treatment plans and instructions • Health risk factor profile, recommended clinical preventative services, and results of those services • Health insurance coverage information
Other Elements	• Correspondence: records of patient–provider communication, edits made to PHR, or concerns about accuracy of information in health care provider medical records • Instructions about access by other persons and institutions • Audit log of individuals/institutions who access electronic records • Self-care trackers: nutrition, physical activity, medications, dosage schedules • Personal library of quality health information resources • Healthcare proxies, living wills, and durable power of attorney for health care
Elements from the Community Health Dimension	• Local public health contact information • Local healthcare services (e.g., walk-in clinics) • Environmental measures and alerts pertinent to an individual's home, neighborhood, school, and workplace

Source: NCVHS 2000.

Table 7.2. Core content of the health care provider dimension

Patient Record Elements	• Personal identification information • Sociodemographic identifiers (gender, birthday, age, race/ethnicity, marital status, living arrangements, education level, occupation) • Health insurance information (including covered benefits) • Legal consents or permissions • Referral information • Correspondence • Patient history information (may include longitudinal history from PHD, immunizations, allergies, current medications) • Stated reason for visit • External causes of injury/illness • Symptoms • Physical exams • Assessment of patient signs and symptoms • Diagnoses • Laboratory, radiology, and pharmacy orders • Laboratory results • Radiological images and interpretations • Record of alerts, warnings, and reminders • Operative reports • Vital signs from ICU • Vital signs from PHD • Treatment plans and instructions • Progress notes • Functional status • Discharge summaries • Instructions about access • Audit log of individuals who accessed patient record • Patient amendments to patient record • Provider notes, such as knowledge of patient, patient-provider interactions, patient's access to services
Other Elements That Support Clinical Practice	• Protocols, practice guidelines • Clinical decision-support programs • Referral history
Elements from the Community Health Dimension	Depending on the patient, the HCPD would include additional contextual information necessary for understanding, treating, and planning the care of the patient: • Aggregate data on the healthcare of community members • Community attributes affecting health (e.g., economic status and population age • Community health resources (e.g., home health services) • Community health (e.g., possible environmental hazards at home, work, school, or in the community at large)

Source: NCVHS 2000.

Table 7.3. Core content of the community health dimension

Public Health Data	• Infant mortality, immunization levels, and communicable disease rates • Environmental, social, and economic conditions • Measures related to public health infrastructure, individual healthcare providers, and healthcare institutions • Other summary measures of community health • Registries • Disease surveillance systems • Survey data • Data on Healthy People objectives and Leading Health indicators
Information from the HCPD (with personally identifiable information removed except under legally established public health protocols and strict security)	• Health status and outcomes, health events, health risks, health behaviors, and other individual characteristics • Healthcare utilization and access, health insurance status • Health care of community members
Other Elements	• Directories of community organizations and services • Planning, evaluation, and policy documents • Compendia of laws and regulations • Material to support public education campaigns • Practice guidelines and training materials for public health officials

Source: NCVHS 2000.

Check Your Understanding 7.1

Instructions: Answer the following questions on a separate piece of paper.

1. What is the difference between patient-specific data and aggregate data?

2. Why is it important for data from various sources to be defined in a standardized or uniform way?

3. How does a data set and/or core data elements make it possible to standardize data in healthcare organizations?

4. What organization initially took the lead in developing a minimum data set for hospitals and continues to play an active role in this area? NCHS

5. What role has the growth of technology played in the development of data sets and core content definitions?

6. How does the MDS indicate potential problems that must be addressed by the nursing home patient's caregivers? RAP

7. What is the primary difference between DEEDS and the EMDS?

8. What is the common purpose for the use of data generated through HEDIS and ORYX?

9. Why does each of these outcomes measurement systems focus on the collection of clinical data elements in their databases?

10. What is the purpose of the NHIN and how do the three core content areas support that role?

Standards to Support Interoperability and Connectivity

The original NCVHS uniform data sets (for example, UHDDS, UACDS) have been the industry standard for data collection, but they were created for use in paper-based (manual) health record systems. They were not designed to accommodate the data needs of the current healthcare delivery system or the demands of electronic health records and clinical information systems. The NHIN initiative has clearly identified the need to develop standards that support connectivity and interoperability. Thompson and Brailer (2004) state that "without an interoperable infrastructure to allow for the secure movement of health information, the adoption and use of EHRs will not realize their full benefits. . . . An interoperable infrastructure requires coordinated and secure health information exchange, including the business, governance, and technical delivery methods to support it; a set of intercommunication tools and services for common architecture development; the diffusion of product standards into deployed products; privacy and security assurances; and connectivity infrastructure.

To fulfill current demands for information and to implement the NHIN, information standards are critical, including **message format standards;** clinical data representation standards (including the vocabularies, clinical classification systems, and terminologies discussed in Chapter 13); technical standards such as electronic data interchange or e-commerce; medication standards; as well as data privacy and security standards, including those that were promulgated as part of The **Health Insurance Portability and Accountability Act of 1996** (HIPAA).

Data Needs in an Electronic Environment

Healthcare organizations often have several different computer systems operating at the same time. For example, a hospital's laboratory system might be entirely separate from its billing system. In fact, the various departments of large healthcare organizations often use different operating systems and are serviced by different vendors. In addition to operating multiple systems, it is an ongoing challenge to integrate information from legacy systems operating on old platforms with state-of-the art information systems.

Healthcare organizations must integrate data that originate in various databases within facilities as well as in databases outside the facility. They also must be able to respond to requests to transfer data to other facilities, payers, accrediting and regulating agencies, quality improvement organizations, and other information users. These goals can be accomplished only when every database system is either operating on the same platform or using common standards. It is impractical to require all systems to use a common operating platform; thus, the adoption of information/data standards is the method of choice for facilitating communication across information systems and supporting goals of interoperability and connectivity. Thompson and Brailer (2004) express the federal commitment to standards in their statement in the Framework for Strategic Action that "A key component of progress in interoperable health information is the development of technically sound and robustly specified interoperability standards and policies." They cite the development of the Consolidated Health Informatics (CHI): a joint initiative of the **Department of Health and Human Service** (HHS), the Department of Defense (DoD), and the Veterans Administration. CHI has endorsed 20 sets of standards to make it easier to share data among the collaborating agencies, and it serves as a model for the private healthcare sector.

Healthcare Information Standards

Healthcare information standards describe accepted methods for collecting, maintaining, and/or transferring healthcare data between computer systems. These standards provide a common language that facilitates and supports:

- Exchanging information
- Sharing information
- Communicating within and across disciplines and settings
- Integrating disparate data systems
- Comparing information at a regional, national, and international level
- Linking data in a secure environment

Standards are the key to exchanging data throughout the healthcare delivery system. They are the building blocks of effective health information systems and effective public health and healthcare delivery systems. They lay the foundation for disease surveillance, monitoring the health and healthcare of populations, performing outcomes research, providing for decision making, and policy development. The long-term vision is to enhance the comparability, quality, integrity and utility of health information from a wide variety of public sources through uniform data policies and standards. (NCVHS 2001).

As described earlier, health information standards fall into five categories: information standards, including content and structure of the electronic health record and message format standards; clinical data representation standards, including vocabularies, clinical classification systems, and terminologies as discussed in Chapter 13; technical standards such as electronic data interchange or e-commerce; medication standards; and data privacy and security standards, including those that were promulgated as part of HIPAA.

Content and Structure of Electronic Health Records

Structure and content standards establish and provide clear and uniform definitions of the data elements to be included in electronic health record systems. Moreover, they specify the type of data to be collected in each data field, the width of each data field, and the content of each data field.

Health Level Seven (HL7)

Health Level Seven (HL7) is a not-for-profit standards developing organization. It provides standards, guidelines and methodologies to enable healthcare information system interoperability and sharing of electronic health records. It focuses on the interface requirements of the entire health care organization. Technical Committees and Special Interest Groups made up of volunteers are responsible for defining the HL7 standard protocol. Its 2,000 members represent over 500 corporate members, including 90 percent of the largest information systems vendors serving healthcare. Both the organization and the standard itself are referred to as HL7. The HL7 standard consists of rules for transmitting demographic data, orders, patient observations, laboratory results, history and physical observations and findings. It also includes message rules for appointment scheduling, referrals, problem list maintenance, and care plans.

The original focus of HL7 was on messaging standards, but its scope has broadened to incorporate other types of health information standards, especially content and structure standards for electronic health records. According to its Web site, Health Level Seven, Inc. is a not-for-profit, ANSI-accredited, standards-developing organization dedicated to providing a comprehensive framework and related standards for the exchange, integration, sharing, and retrieval of electronic health information that supports clinical practice and the management, delivery, and evaluation of health services. As a result of their broadened mission, HL7 developed the HL7 Electronic Health Record System (EHR-S) Functional Model and Standards that address the content and structure of an EHR (HL7.org).

In April 2004, the EHR-S Functional Model and Standards passed an **American National Standards Institute** (ANSI) Draft Standards for Trial Use (see table 7.4). The purpose of the functional model is to provide a foundation for common understanding of possible functions of electronic health records systems. It does not include content of the EHR or a recommended technology platform (Shafarman and Van Hentenryck 2004).

The HL7 Clinical Document Architecture (CDA) provides an exchange model for clinical documents (such as discharge summaries and progress notes) and brings the healthcare industry closer to the realization of an electronic health record. The CDA utilizes XML, the HL7 Reference Information Model (RIM), and coded vocabularies to make documents machine readable, so they can be easily parsed and processed electronically. It also makes documents human readable so they can be easily retrieved and used by the people who need them. CDA documents can be displayed using XML-aware Web browsers or wireless applications such as cell phones. The CDA was adopted in May 2004 as the federal health information interoperability standard to identify standards and terminologies used to define the messaging architecture and syntax of clinical text documents. (NAHIT 2005).

Table 7.4.   A portion of the HL7 EHR functional descriptors

ID	Function Name	Function Statement
C.1	Care Management	
C.1.1.0	Health Information Capture, Management, and Review	
C.1.1.1	Enable the provider to identify and locate a patient record	Maintain and identify a single patient record for each patient.
C.1.1.2	Capture patient demographics	Capture demographic information that is reportable and trackable over time.
C.1.1.3	Manage problem list	Create and maintain patient-specific problem lists.
C.1.1.4	Manage medication list	Create and maintain patient-specific medication lists.
C.1.1.5	Manage allergy list	Create and maintain patient-specific allergies and reactions.
C.1.1.6	Manage other summary lists	Create and maintain patient-specific summary lists not otherwise specified.
C.1.1.7	Manage patient history	Capture, review, and manage medical, procedural, social, and family history, including the capture of pertinent negative histories.
C.1.1.8	Review chart summary	Make available a chronological, filterable, comprehensive review of the patient's entire clinical history, subject to confidentiality constraints.
C.1.1.9	Capture other key data	Capture, manage, and review other key data not otherwise specified and by a variety of caregivers.
C.1.1.10	Capture and create clinical documents and notes	Create, addend, and authenticate transcribed or directly entered clinical documentation and notes.
C.1.1.11	Capture external clinical documents	Capture clinical documents and notes originating from outside the EHR.
C.1.1.12	Capture patient-provided data	Capture patient-provided data.
C.1.1.13	Capture historical data	Capture and manage patient-reported or externally available patient clinical history.
C.1.2.0	Care Planning, Critical Paths, Protocols	
C.1.2.1	Present clinical guidelines	Present relevant information from knowledge resources to support data entry and clinical documentation
C.1.3.0	Medication Ordering and Management	
C.1.3.1	Enable medication ordering	Create prescriptions or other medication orders with detail adequate for correct filling and administration by pharmacy and clinical staff.
C.1.3.2	Support medication formularies	Provide information regarding compliance of medication orders with formularies.
C.1.3.3	Enable documentation of medication administration	Present to appropriate clinicians the medications that are to be administered to a patient and under what circumstances and permit documentation of administration details.
C.1.4.0	Orders, Referrals, and Results Management	
C.1.4.1	Enable ordering of diagnostic tests	Submit diagnostic test orders based on specific care provider input.
C.1.4.2	Enable placing of communication and other orders	Submit communicative or administrative orders based on specific care provider input.
C.1.4.3	Enable use of order sets	Provide order sets based on provider input or system prompt.
C.1.4.4	Enable ordering and tracking of referrals	Enable the origination, documentation and tracking of referrals between care provider or care settings, including clinical guidelines and administrative details of the referral.
C.1.4.5	Route and manage results	Route, manage, and present current and historical test results to appropriate clinical personnel for review, filtering, and comparison.
C.1.4.6	Enable the ordering of blood products	Communicate with regulatory-approved blood bank software to provide needed information on blood usage and orders for blood products.
C.1.5.0	Consents and Authorizations	
C.1.5.1	Manage consents and authorizations	Create, maintain, and verify patient data and treatment decisions in the form of consents and authorizations
C.1.5.2	Enable capture, maintenance, and access to patient advanced directives	Capture, maintain, and provide access to patient advanced directives
C.2	Clinical Decision Support	
C.2.1.0	Health information capture and review	
C.2.1.1	Support for standard assessments	Offer rule-based prompts to support the adherence to practice guideline standards at the point of information capture.
C.2.1.2	Support for Patient Context-enabled Assessments	Offer rule-based prompts based on patient-specific data at the point of information capture.
C.2.1.3	Support for identifying anomalies or potential problems	Identify anomalies and potential problems, or other patient "flags," and provide prompts for consideration at the point of information capture.
C.2.1.4	Patient and family preferences	Capture patient and family preferences at the time of information intake and integrate them into clinical-decision support at all appropriate opportunities.

American Society for Testing and Materials (ASTM) E31 Committee

The **American Society for Testing and Materials** (ASTM) develops standards for a variety of industries in the United States. The ASTM Technical Committee on Healthcare Informatics E31 is charged with the responsibility for developing standards related to the electronic health record. E31 works through subcommittees assigned to various aspects of this endeavor. An example is the Health Information Transcription and Documentation Committee (E31.22) that recently developed two new standards: E2344 Standard Guide for Data Capture through the Dictation Process and E2364 Standard Guide for Speech Recognition Products in Health Care. (Tessier 2004).

ASTM Standard E1384-02a identifies the content and structure for electronic health records. The scope of this standard is intended to cover all types of healthcare services, including acute care hospitals, ambulatory care, skilled nursing facilities, home healthcare, and specialty environments. The current version of the standard addresses all types of healthcare services, including acute care hospitals, nursing homes, skilled nursing facilities, home healthcare, and specialty care environments as well as ambulatory care. It applies to short term contacts such as emergency rooms and emergency medical care services) as well as long-term care such as primary care physicians with long-term contact (ASTM 2005) There are five purposes outlined for the ASTM Practice for Content and Structure of the Electronic Health Record:

- To identify the content and logical structure of the electronic health record
- To define the relationships of data coming from diverse source data systems and the data stored in the EHR
- To provide a common vocabulary, perspective, and references for those developing, purchasing, and implementing EHR systems
- To describe examples of a variety of views by which the logical data structure might be accessed or displayed
- To relate the logical structure of the EHR to the essential documentation currently used in the healthcare delivery system in order to support consistency and efficient data transfer (ASTM 2005).

ASTM Standard E1384-02a identifies basic information categories for health records and organizes the categories into segments. Specific data content is then identified for each segment.

Currently, ASTM Committee 31 is focused on the **continuity of care record** (CCR) initiative, which is categorized as Electronic Health Records standard E31.28. The CCR standard is a core data set of relevant current and past information about a patient's health status and healthcare treatment. The CCR was created to help communicate that information from one provider to another for referral, transfer, or discharge of the patient or when the patient wishes to create a personal health record (ASTM 2005). (See figure 7.4 for a list of the elements contained in the CCR.)

Data from the CCR may also be incorporated into a personal health record. Because it utilizes XML codes, it enhances interoperability and allows its preparation, transmission, and viewing in multiple ways. The CCR is described as organized and transportable. It is sponsored by a consortium of healthcare organizations, practitioners, and other stakeholders.

The CCR is intended to address the lack of appropriate, succinct, and up-to-date patient health information for practitioners as the patient seeks care in a new care setting. It improves continuity of care by providing a method to easily communicate the most relevant clinical information about a patient among practitioners, institutions, and other entities. Finally it enables a healthcare practitioner to readily access information about a patient's healthcare at any point in an encounter and to easily update the information at any point in time.

Because ASTM and HL7 are both involved in developing standards for electronic health records, the two organizations have negotiated a memorandum of understanding to bring into line ASTM's CCR initiative with HL7's EHR functionality and Clinical Document Architecture (CDA) standards. In October 2005 the HL7 Board of Directors issued a report on progress in this initiative, stating "The Continuity of Care Record . . . is rich in functionality and clinical utility. From a technical implementation perspective, however, it has not achieved the same degree of readiness for standardization. . . . We hope to continue to work with ASTM toward a common solution that leverages the strengths of both organizations" (HL7 2005).

Figure 7.4.   Continuity of care record core data set

- Patient administrative and clinical data
- Basic information about the patient's payer
- Advance directives
- Patient's sources of support
- Patient's current functional status
- Problems
- Family history
- Social history
- Alerts
- Medications
- Medical devices or equipment need by patient
- Immunization history
- Vital signs, as appropriate
- Results of laboratory, diagnostic, and therapeutic results
- Diagnostic and therapeutic procedures
- Encounters
- Plan of care
- Healthcare providers

Source: Adapted from HIMSS 2003.

Identifier Standards

Identifier standards recommend methods for assigning **unique identification numbers** to individuals, including patients, healthcare providers (for example, physicians and dentists), corporate providers (healthcare organizations), and healthcare vendors and suppliers. Identifiers usually use a combination of numeric or alphanumeric characters such as a hospital number or a billing number. At present, most identifiers are used only within one facility or within a single healthcare system. HIPAA regulations require the development of unique identification numbers that can be used across information systems.

It is generally agreed that unique identification numbers are needed for patients, but there is no consensus on the method of identification. Much of the controversy relates to the use of the **Social Security number** (SSN) as the identifier for patients. The Social Security Administration is adamant in its opposition to using the SSN for purposes other than those identified by law. AHIMA is in agreement on this issue due to privacy, confidentiality, and security issues related to the use of the SSN. As of this writing, AHIMA has formed a workgroup on patient identifiers that will explore this issue and will formulate recommendations related to a unique patient identifier.

As an alternative to the use of the SSN as a unique patient identifier, there have been proposals to develop a unique healthcare identifier number. For a variety of reasons, primarily related to confidentiality and security, these proposals have not been widely endorsed.

The most commonly used provider identifier is the **unique physician identification number** (UPIN). The UPIN was originally created by CMS for use by physicians who bill for services provided to Medicare patients.

In 1993, CMS initiated the National Provider Identification Initiative to develop a provider identification system to meet Medicare and Medicaid needs and, ultimately, the needs of all users. The workgroup investigated all existing identifiers and designed a new **national provider identifier** (NPI). The NPI uses an eight-character alphanumeric identifier. The CMS is working on implementing the NPI for the Medicare program. CMS announced a system whereby all health care providers, including Medicare providers, can apply for an NPI starting in May 2005. A CMS letter to providers indicates all providers must be using the NPI by May 23, 2007.

Clinical Representation Standards

Clinical representation standards include classification systems, vocabularies, terminologies, lab and clinical observation codes such as LOINC, drug codes, as well as standards for information modeling and metadata.

Vocabulary standards establish common definitions for medical terms to encourage consistent descriptions of an individual's condition in the health record. Medical terminology is extremely complex, and establishing medical

vocabulary standards is a challenging task. Various synonymous medical terms are often used in different areas of the country. In fact, medical terminology can vary among physicians working in the same organization, depending on where and when each physician was trained and which medical specialty he or she practices. For example, one physician might describe a patient's diagnosis as Parkinson's disease, another might describe it as Parkinsonism, and a third might use the term paralysis agitans. All three terms are correct, but using the terms interchangeably would adversely affect data quality. In addition, data comparison among the physicians' patients would be very difficult, if not impossible.

The use of clinical classification codes (for example, CPT and ICD-9-CM codes) to represent health-related conditions and procedures is common in healthcare. The use of standardized, uniform terminology is critical to accurate coding. Vocabulary standards not only provide guidance in code selection, but they also set the stage for future automated coding systems.

The development of vocabularies, terminologies, and classification systems as well as drug codes, laboratory and clinical observation codes, information modeling and metadata are thoroughly explored in Chapter 13.

Technical Standards

ANSI coordinates voluntary standards in the United States. Many standards developers and participants support ANSI as the central body responsible for the identification of a single consistent set of voluntary standards called American National Standards. ANSI provides an open forum for all concerned interests to identify specific business needs, plan to meet those needs, and agree on standards. Although ANSI itself does not develop standards, its approval of standards does indicate that the principles of openness and due process have been followed in the approval process and that a consensus of those participating in the approval process has been achieved.

Electronic data interchange (EDI) is the electronic transfer of information, such as health claims transmitted electronically, in a standard format between trading partners. EDI originated when a number of industries identified cost savings through the electronic transmission of business information. They were convinced that the standardization of formatted information was the most effective means of communicating with multiple trading partners. EDI allows entities within the healthcare system to exchange medical, billing, and other information and to process transactions in a manner that is fast and cost-effective. With EDI there is a substantial reduction in handling and processing time compared to paper, and the risk of lost paper documents is eliminated. EDI also can eliminate the inefficiencies of handling paper documents, which would significantly reduce administrative burden, lower operating costs, and improve overall data quality. In recent years the term EDI has often been replaced by the term e-commerce.

In 1979, ANSI chartered a new committee, known as the **Accredited Standards Committee** (ASC) **X12,** Electronic Data Interchange (referred to as ASC X12N or X12N). The charge of the committee is to develop uniform standards for the electronic interchange of business transactions.

X12N

One of the purposes of the HIPAA Administrative Simplification rules was to standardize information exchange, and in August 2000, the HHS published regulations for electronic transactions. These regulations apply to transactions that occur between healthcare providers and healthcare plans and payers (Rode 2001). The long-term goal of the **transaction standards** is to allow providers and plans or payers to seamlessly transfer data back and forth with little intervention. To do this, HHS has adopted the electronic transactions standards of ASC X12 Insurance Subcommittee (Accredited Standards Committee Health Care Task group **(X12N).**

The work of ASC X12 is conducted primarily by a series of subcommittees and task groups whose major function is the development of new, and the maintenance of existing, EDI standards. The standards adopted for EDI are called ANSI ASC X12N and include:

- Professional/institutional X12N 837 Healthcare Claim Transactions, version 4010
- X12N 835 Health Care Claim (HCC) Payment/Advice (or remittance advice, RA) transactions
- X12N 837 Coordination of Benefits (COB) transactions

To implement the HIPAA administrative simplification provisions, the above transaction standards are included under part 162 of title 45 of the Code of Federal Regulations (CFR) as the standard for processing electronic healthcare claims, coordination of benefits, and remittance advice (RA) transmissions.

Laboratory Logical Observation Identifier Name Codes (LOINC)

LOINC is a well-accepted set of standards that represents laboratory data for ordering lab tests and reporting results, including the electronic exchange of clinical laboratory results. It is managed by the Regenstrief Institute in Indianapolis, IN.

Institute of Electrical and Electronics Engineers (IEEE) 1073

IEEE 1073 provides for open systems communications in healthcare applications, primarily between bedside medical devices and patient care information systems, optimized for the acute care setting. The IEEE 1073 Series was adopted as a federal health information interoperability standard for electronic data exchange. (NAHIT 2005).

Digital Imaging and Communications in Medicine

Through a cooperative effort between the **American College of Radiology and the National Electrical Manufacturers Association** (ACR-NEMA), **Digital Imaging and Communications in Medicine** (DICOM) was originally created to permit the interchange of biomedical image waveforms and related information. These organizations define the health record to include not only textual, coded, and numeric information (linguistic), but also a detailed, structured record of image-related information (Bidgood 1997).

The information associated with each image is the standard administrative and billing information used today—patient name, procedure code, and so on. Combined with the open protocol, this only provides for data interchange, not data understanding. The people who developed the exchange standard now have taken another step and suggested a mapping/terminology resource to index the content of biomedical images in a clinically relevant manner (Bidgood 1997).

DICOM is used by most medical professions that utilize imaging within the healthcare industry including cardiology, dentistry, endoscopy, mammography, ophthalmology, and orthopedics. DICOM was adopted as the federal health information interoperability messaging standard for imaging in March 2003. (Alliance Standards Directory 2005).

Medication Standards

Medications are used extensively to prevent and treat medical conditions in the United States. Physicians, payers, and pharmacies communicate with one another to assure that correct medications are prescribed, administered, and reimbursed. Research studies are frequently conducted to determine the efficacy of various drugs; recent events relative to the removal of certain categories of drugs from the market due to unforeseen adverse effects has focused attention on medication issues and has underscored the need for accurate and accessible information about medications. A number of standards have been developed that address medication and drug issues.

Food and Drug Administration (FDA) Established Name for Active Ingredients and FDA Unique Ingredient Identifier (UNII) Codes

The FDA's UNII Codes were developed as a standard to enable the federal health care sector to share information regarding medication active ingredients. An active ingredient is a substance responsible for the effects of a medication. The UNII Codes were adopted in May 2004 as the federal healthcare information interoperability standard for active ingredients in medications. (Alliance Standards Directory 2005).

Semantic Clinical Drug (SCD) of RxNorm

RxNorm provides standardized names for clinical drugs (active ingredient + strength + dose form) and for dose forms as administered. It provides links from clinical drugs to their active ingredients, drug components (active ingredient + strength) and some related brand names. RxNorm is produced in consultation with the FDA, the Department of Veterans Affairs (VA), and the HL7 standards development organizations. RxNorm is only released in the UMLS Metathesaurus. (Alliance Standards Directory 2005).

The **Semantic Clinical Drug** is a subset of RxNorm for the ingredient plus strength and dose form. An example is: Fluoxetine 4MG/ML Oral Solution. The SCD of RxNorm was adopted as a federal healthcare information interoperability standard for clinical drug nomenclature. (Alliance Standards Directory 2005).

FDA Center for Drug Evaluation and Research Data Standards (CDER) Manual

The CDER Data Standards Manual is a compilation of standardized nomenclature monographs that have been reviewed and approved by the CDER Nomenclature Standards Committee (see table 7.5). The CDER standards are considered binding upon all existing automated databases when undergoing a major redesign. Use of the standards is strictly voluntary for static existing databases. In May 2004, the CDER Data Standards Manual was adopted as a federal healthcare information interoperability standard for sharing information regarding manufactured drug dosage forms. (Alliance Standards Directory 2005).

Some of the databases using the standards include the Center-wide Oracle Management Information System (COMIS), the Division Files System (DFS), and the Drug Product Reference File (DPRF), among others. (FDA 2002).

FDA National Drug Code (NDC) Directory

The FDA NDC Directory is a list of all drugs manufactured, prepared, propagated, compounded, or processed by a drug

Table 7.5.   Examples of FDA CDER drug nomenclature monographs

Drug Nomenclature Monographs	Monograph Number
Drug Classification	C-DRG-00101
Dosage Form	C-DRG-00201
Route of Administration	C-DRG-00301
Ingredient Name	C-DRG-00401
Proprietary Name	C-DRG-00402
Animal Common Names	C-DRG-00403
Animal Cell Tissue Fluid Biomolecule	C-DRG-00404
Biotechnology Origin	C-DRG-00405
Potency	C-DRG-00501
Indications	C-DRG-00601

Source: FDA 2005.

establishment registered under the Federal Food, Drug, and Cosmetic Act. The NDC serves as a universal product identifier for human drugs. It consists of prescription and selected over-the-counter, insulin, domestic, and foreign drug products that are in commercial distribution in the United States. It is updated quarterly within five working days after the end of March, June, September, and December. (Alliance Standards Directory 2005).

National Council for Prescription Drug Programs (NCPDP)

The **National Council for Prescription Drug Programs (NCPDP)** creates and promotes data interchange standards for the pharmacy services sector of healthcare. The NCPDP Provider Identification Number supplies 70,000 pharmacies with a unique identifying number for interactions with federal agencies and third-party processors. It was incorporated in 1977 and is a not-for-profit, ANSI-accredited standards development organization. Eleven working groups meet quarterly to develop and/or modify standards for the transmission of pharmacy data. NCPDP SCRIPT was developed for transmitting prescription information electronically between prescribers and providers. It covers the electronic transmission of new prescriptions, prescription refill requests, prescription fill status notifications, and prescription cancellations. NCPDP SCRIPT was adopted as the federal health information interoperability messaging standard for prescription data. (Alliance Standards Directory 2005).

LOINC Clinical Special Product Label (SPL)

The LOINC Clinical Special Product Label standard provides information found in the approved FDA drug label or package insert in a computer readable format for use in electronic prescribing and decision support. It is intended to make drug labeling more accessible, easier to read, and standardized. It was approved as an official ANSI-approved standard in September 2004 and as the federal health information interoperability standard for medication product labeling. Pharmaceutical companies must start submitting labeling in SPL to the FDA in 2005. It was adopted as a CHI standard upon gaining approval status by HL7 for the SPL specification and upon incorporation of the terminology into LOINC. (Alliance Standards Directory 2005).

Privacy and Security Standards

HIPAA mandated the adoption of privacy and security protection for identifiable health information. HIPAA **privacy standards** have been implemented throughout the healthcare industry. They are addressed thoroughly in Chapter 10.

Security standards ensure that patient-identifiable health information remains confidential and protected from unauthorized disclosure, alteration, or destruction. Effective security standards are especially important in computer-based environments because patient information is accessible to many users in many locations.

Security standards are addressed in detail in Chapter 9 as they relate to the electronic health record. Many standards organizations—most notably, the ASTM and Health Level Seven (HL7)—have developed security standards, but no single standard currently addresses all of the HIPAA provisions.

Standards Development

Many organizations are involved in the development of healthcare information standards. These organizations are referred to as **standards development organizations** (SDOs). Both private organizations and government agencies are involved in the process of developing standards. Many standards are created through a voluntary consensus process that involves identifying the need for a standard, negotiating the content of the standard, and drafting a proposed standard. The final standard is published after undergoing a comment and revision period.

A number of organizations play key roles in coordinating standards development. They do not develop standards but, rather, coordinate the efforts of other SDOs. ANSI coordinates the development of voluntary standards in a variety of industries, including healthcare. Most SDOs in the United States are members of the ANSI.

The United Nations International Standards Organization (ISO) coordinates international standards development. The ANSI represents the United States at the ISO.

Many organizations are involved in the process of setting standards within specific industries and areas of expertise. The U.S. healthcare industry is no exception. Table 7.6 (p. 167) provides a list of several of the organizations that are actively involved in developing standards for health-related information management. The ISO has several healthcare-related committees working on standards development for the healthcare industry.

Many private and government organizations influence the development of standards by taking positions on proposed standards and setting policies that lend credibility to standards. The government agencies that influence standards development include the Centers for Medicare and Medicaid Services, which is the overseer of the Medicare/Medicaid programs; the Food and Drug Administration (FDA); the Agency for Health Care Policy and Research (AHCPR); and the NCHS.

The **National Alliance for Health Information Technology** has developed a comprehensive list of health related standards, the Alliance Standards Directory (hitsdir.org). This extensive listing gives a flavor of the complexity of health information technology standards development. At present, one of the most challenge aspects of the standards movement is the area of standards harmonization. There are many initiatives occurring in the United States as well as in the international community, resulting in duplication and competition among organizations. Harmonization of these

efforts will be critical if the movement toward personal health records for individuals, electronic health records at all points of care, and networked health information systems at both the regional and national level are to move forward. The Office of the National Coordinator of Health Information Technology has been charged with the responsibility of leading efforts toward standards harmonization.

Check Your Understanding 7.2

Instructions: Answer the following questions on a separate piece of paper.

1. What is the difference between a data set and a healthcare information standard?

2. What changes in the healthcare industry have prompted the focus on developing healthcare information standards?

3. How would ASTM Standard E1384-02a and the HL7 EHR-S Functional Standard be helpful during the development of an electronic health record system?

4. What SDOs have been most active in developing structure and content standards for electronic health records?

Evolving Health Information Standards

The development of healthcare information standards is far from complete. The task is critically important to the development of an electronic health record systems and, ultimately, to implementation of a national health information infrastructure. Leading standards groups are continuously working to reach consensus on a variety of standards, but many issues are still to be resolved.

Development of Extensible Markup Language (XML)

Recent advances in standards development have occurred in the area of **extensible markup language** (XML). XML was developed as a universal language to facilitate the storage and transmission of data published on the Internet. Markup languages communicate electronic representations of paper documents to computers by inserting additional information into text (Sokolowski 1999). The best known markup language is hypertext markup language (HTML), which is used to convert text documents into Internet-compatible format.

Pothen and Parmanto (2000) describe XML as "an easy-to-learn, standardized mark-up language with customizable tags that describe data within documents." In other words, XML provides a context for data through the use of a tag. In the context of health data, XML tags each item of data with a descriptor that differentiates, for example, between a number that is a Social Security number from a number that represents the medical record number. XML allows data to be communicated from one computerized system to another without losing the integrity of the data. In addition, according to Sokolowski, XML provides structure and rules that are "important for healthcare informatics because they will

Table 7.6.   Standards development organizations

Organization	Types of Standards	Description
Accredited Standards Committee X12 Data Interchange Standards Association (DISA) 333 John Carlyle Street, Suite 600 Alexandria, VA 22314 Telephone: (703) 548-7005 www.disa.org	Electronic data interchange for billing transactions The committee's particular area of focus has been computer-to-computer communications between healthcare providers and third-party payers	Chartered in 1979 by ANSI, the X12N subcommittee develops and maintains X12 standards, interpretations, and guidelines. X12N is one of the standards for EDI that is specified in the regulations of the Health Insurance Portability and Accountability Act of 1996. Subgroups of X12N include: *WEDI: Workgroup on Electronic Data Exchange* WEDI has been the prime mover in the development of insurance industry standards. In 1995, WEDI became a private standards advocacy group. *HIBCC: Health Industry Business Communications Council*
American College of Radiology–National Electrical Manufacturers Association (ACR-NEMA) American College of Radiology 1891 Preston White Drive Reston, VA 20191 Telephone: (703) 648-8900 www.acr.org National Electrical Manufacturers Association 1300 N. Seventeenth Street, Suite 1847 Rosslyn, VA 22209 Telephone: (703) 841-3200 www.nema.org	Exchange of digitized images	ACR is a professional association, and NEMA is a trade association. They have worked collaboratively to develop the Digital Imaging and Communications in Medicine (DICOM) standard, which promotes a digital image communications format and facilitates development by the American College of Radiology of picture archive and communications systems. DICOM may be used for electronic exchange of x-rays, computed tomography (CT), magnetic resonance imaging (MRI), ultrasound, nuclear medicine, and other radiology images. Work is under way to support other diagnostic images.
American Society for Testing and Materials (ASTM) 100 Barr Harbor Drive West Conshohocken, PA 19428 Telephone: (610) 832-9585 www.astm.org	Multiple health informatics standards, including clinical content of patient records, exchange of messages about clinical observations, data security and integrity, healthcare identifiers, data modeling, clinical laboratory systems, Arden syntax (a coding system), and system functionality	Organized in 1898, the ASTM is one of the largest SDOs in the world. It provides a forum for vendors, users, consumers, and others to develop standards for a wide range of materials, products, systems, and services. It is composed of more than 140 subcommittees or working groups identified as E31 and E32. Since 1990, Committee E31 on Healthcare Informatics has developed standards for health information and health information systems. Standard E1384, discussed earlier, is a product of the E31 subcommittee of ASTM.
Health Level Seven (HL7) 3300 Washtenaw Avenue, Suite 227 Ann Arbor, MI 48104 Telephone: (734) 677-7777 www.hl7.org	Electronic interchange of clinical, financial, and administrative information among disparate health information systems	HL7 is an ANSI-accredited SDO. Level 7 refers to the highest level of the Open System Interconnection (OSI) model of the International Standards Organization. The HL7 standard addresses issues that occur within the seventh, or application, layer.
Institute of Electrical and Electronics Engineers (IEEE) 445 Hoes Lane P.O. Box 1331 Piscataway, NJ 08855-1331 Telephone: (732) 981-0060 www.ieee.org	Medical device information and general informatics format	The IEEE's Medical Data Interchange Standard (MEDIX) is a standard set of hospital system interface transactions based on the ISO standards for all seven layers of the OSI model. Another IEEE standard for a medical information bus (MIB) links bedside instruments in critical care with health information systems.
National Council on Prescription Drug Programs (NCPDP) 4201 N. Twenty-fourth Street, Suite 365 Phoenix, AZ 85016 Telephone: (602) 957-9105 www.ncpdp.org	Data interchange and processing standards for pharmacy transactions	The NCPDP has defined standards for transmitting prescription information from pharmacies to payers for prescription management services and for receiving approval and payment information back in near-real time. Other standards address adverse drug reactions and utilization review.

Adapted from Brandt 2000, p. 39.

provide context for narrative text, a document information model, agreement on high level structures, and a facility for standardizing formats" (Sokolowski 1999, p. 22).

As electronic health records continue to evolve in somewhat disjointed manner (as described by Amatayakul in chapter 9), XML has the potential to solve some of the difficulties posed by the lack of standardized vocabulary and the need to transmit data among disparate computer systems. Some of the characteristics that make XML relevant to the development of an EHR were described by Pothen and Parmanto (2000):

- XML combined with existing classification systems such as ICD-9-CM can improve the completeness of health records by providing a clear description of the content of data in the record
- XML allows data in the health record to be organized in a meaningful and searchable form

XML also can serve as a standard for exchange of health information over the Web because it is not impeded by disparate computer systems. A test project conducted in Canada utilized XML for data exchange among three remote health-related organizations that each used a different set of applications, databases, and technology. The organizations mapped each system to standard templates in XML and were able to seamlessly transfer data from one location to the other (Smith 2001). The implementation of XML within the healthcare industry has the potential to address many of the issues of both vocabulary and transmission.

Check Your Understanding 7.3

Instructions: Answer the following questions on a separate piece of paper.

1. What is the relationship between healthcare information standards and the coding of healthcare data?

2. What is the reason for creating a unique identification number for every healthcare consumer?

3. Why is use of the Social Security number as a unique identification number not appropriate?

4. What characteristics of XML make it a potential solution for many of the problems of storing and transmitting health information?

Real-World Case

In Winona, Minnesota, local healthcare providers and a healthcare information software vendor have developed a health information network that improves communication between patients and local physicians and other healthcare providers. The system relies on an already-existing high-speed network to provide interactive health records that can be used by local facilities, physicians, pharmacies, and patients. Patients are able to make appointments, check their health records for test results, and communicate with their physicians via the Internet. Physicians also will be able to communicate with one another and with local hos-

pitals, nursing homes, and clinics. The system was designed to ensure the security and confidentiality of data.

Because more than 60 percent of Winona residents use the Internet, the population is well prepared to use this health network to improve healthcare. Residents who do not own computers will have access to computer labs in schools, libraries, and other public locations.

Baseline data for the project will be gathered through health risk assessments, and patients will gain access to the health information network via a sign-in process. The results of the health risk assessments will provide a baseline of data about the community and also will allow the community to assess the impact of this project on its health status.

Summary

According to Brandt (2000), "The vision is clear: a longitudinal, or lifetime, health record for each person that is computer-based, secure, readily accessible when needed, and linked across the continuum of care [is needed]. In reality, we are a long way from that model." It is impossible to develop a longitudinal EHR that meets Brandt's specifications without standards that guide the development. The complexity of technology, the variations in computer platforms from one system to the next, and the differing (and sometimes conflicting) data needs of users demand flexible health data/information systems. The systems must be able to store volumes of data in a standardized format, communicate across vendor-specific systems, and keep data in a secure manner that protects individual privacy and information confidentiality.

The need for standardized data definitions was recognized in the 1960s, and the National Committee on Vital and Health Statistics took the lead in developing uniform minimum data sets for various sites of care. As technology has driven the development of the data/information systems, the early data sets have been supplemented with healthcare information standards that focus on electronic health record systems. A number of standards-setting organizations have been involved in developing uniform definitions, data fields, and views for health record content and structure. Standards for developing medical vocabularies, messaging/communications systems, and data/information security, privacy, and confidentiality are being created and implemented. These standards are dynamic and in constant development by various groups. Standards development generally takes place as a consensus-driven process among various interested parties. In most cases, implementation is voluntary. However, there are many groups involved in standards development and competition exists among those groups. One of the major efforts of the Office of the National Coordinator (ONC) is standards harmonization that consolidates a useful and accepted set of national IT standards. As discussed earlier, ANSI will convene the Health Information Technology Standards Panel to address standards harmonization

Some data sets and standards have been incorporated into federal law and are thus required for use by affected healthcare organizations. For example, in 1983, the standardized definitions of the Uniform Hospital Discharge Data Set were incorporated into the Prospective Payment Act (PL98-603) and are still required for reporting inpatient data for reimbursement under the Medicare program.

The Health Insurance Portability and Accountability Act of 1996 mandated the incorporation of healthcare information standards into all electronic or computer-based health information systems. Of particular importance under HIPAA are transaction/messaging standards for communication of data across systems, privacy standards that protect individual privacy and confidentiality, security standards that ensure that data is accessed only by those who have a specific right to access, and identifier standards that offer methods of identifying both individual patients as well as healthcare providers. The rules and regulations for HIPAA are still in development, and, to date, the transaction, privacy, and security standards have been implemented. Other standards are still under development.

The development of health information standards to support the development of electronic health record gained national support through recent federal initiatives aimed at developing a strategic plan to guide the nation's implementation of interoperable health information technology in both the public and private sectors. The Office of the National Coordinator of Health Information Technology (ONC) has been given a mandate to advance the development, adoption and implementation of healthcare information technology nationally through collaboration among public and private interests and to ensure that these standards are consistent with current efforts to set HIT standards for use by the federal government (Thompson & Brailer 2004).

Work will continue on the development of healthcare informatics standards well into the 21st century. It is a complex task and a dynamic one with constant activity in the development, modification, negotiation, and implementation process. The rapid growth of technology and the increasing need for healthcare data/information makes the task a daunting one. According to Kloss (2005) "The EHR is seen as essential for safe, effective care and a building block to wire the healthcare system. Now we need to better understand the prerequisites for interoperability so technology investments deliver on their promises. It is not sufficient to automate health records within organizations; there must be interconnectivity among providers and between providers and patients."

References

AHIMA. 2004. AHIMA Workgroup on Core Data Sets as Standards for the EHR. Practice brief: E-HIM strategic initiative: Core data sets. *Journal of American Health Information Management Association* 75(8):68A–D.

ASTM. 2005. astm.org.

Bidgood, W.D., Jr. 1997. Documenting the information content of images. Proceedings of the AMIA Annual Fall Symposium, pp. 424–28.

Brandt, M.D. 2000. Health informatics standards: A user's guide. *Journal of American Health Information Management Association* 71(4):39–43.

Carol, R. 2005. Short-term forecast: Experts speak up on ONC's RFI, RFPs and the year ahead. *Journal of American Health Information Management Association* 76(9):42–44, 46, 48, 50.

Food and Drug Administration Center for Drug Evaluation and Research (FDA CDER). 2005. National Drug Code Frequently Asked Questions. Available online from fda.gov/cder/ndc.

Food and Drug Administration Center for Drug Evaluation and Research. 2002. *CDER Data Standards Manual.* Available online from fda.gov/cder/dsm.

Hanken, M.A., and K. Water, eds. 1994. *Glossary of Healthcare Terms.* Chicago: AHIMA.

Health Information Management Systems Society. 2003 (December). Standards insight: An analysis of health information standards development initiatives: The continuity of care record standard initiative. Available online from himss.org/content/files/StandardsInsight/2003/12-2003.pdf.

Health level 7. 2005 (October). Board of directors report.

Kloss, L. 2005a. Standardized data: The difference for EHR solutions. *Journal of American Health Information Management Association* 76(2):23.

Kloss, L. 2005b. The NHIN comes into focus. *Journal of American Health Information Management Association* 76(3):23.

Mon, D.T. 2005. An update on the NHIN and RHIOs. *Journal of American Health Information Management Association* 76(6):56–57, 59.

National Association for Health Information Technology (NAHIT). Alliance Standards Directory. Available online from hitsdir.org.

National Center for Injury Prevention and Control. 1997. Data elements for emergency department systems, Release 1.0. Atlanta, GA: CDC and HHS. Available online from cdc.gov/ncipc/pub-res/pdf/deeds.pdf.

National Committee on Vital and Health Statistics. 2000. Toward a national health information infrastructure: Interim report. Washington, DC: HHS.

National Committee on Vital and Health Statistics. 2001. Information for health: A strategy for building the national health information infrastructure. Washington, DC: HHS. Available online from aspe.hhs.gov/sp/nhii.

Pothen, D.J., and B. Parmanto. 2000. XML furthers CPR goals. *Journal of American Health Information Management Association* 71(9):24–29.

Rode, D. 2001. Understanding HIPAA transactions and code sets. *Journal of American Health Information Management Association* 72(1):26–32.

Shafarman, M. and K. Van Hentenryck. 2004 (September). HL7 makes headway on version 3. *Healthcare Informatics* 50

Smith, D.A. 2001. Data transmission: a world of possibilities. *Journal of American Health Information Management Association* 72(5):26–27.

Sokolowski, R. 1999. XML makes its mark. *Journal of American Health Information Management Association* 70(10):21–24.

Tessier, C. 2004 (September). ASTM E31 committee. *Healthcare Informatics* 47.

Thompson, T.G. and D.J. Brailer. 2004. The decade of health information technology: Delivering consumer-centric and information-rich health care—Framework for strategic action. Washington, DC: HHS.

Chapter 8
Paper-Based Health Records

Mary Cole McCain, MPA, RHIA

Learning Objectives

- To describe the traditional (paper-based) health record and to identify its primary uses and users
- To describe the transition from the paper record to the hybrid record (combination of paper and electronic) to the fully electronic record and the impact of the transition on the flow of health record information
- To identify the organizations that publish standards on the content of the health record
- To describe the major content areas of the health record, including administrative and demographic data, clinical data, and specialized content
- To outline the flow of health record information from initial encounter to final format
- To contrast methods that providers use to contribute information to the health record
- To give examples of general requirements for the primary documentation required in most health records, including the history and physical, progress notes, orders, and discharge summary
- To define quantitative and qualitative record analysis
- To define the purposes of the following processes: concurrent analysis and discharge analysis, open-record review, records review, point-of-care review, and continuous record review
- To compare an incomplete health record and a delinquent health record
- To identify forms and documentation requirements specific to facilities other than acute care hospitals, including ambulatory care, home care, hospice care, rehabilitation care, and long-term care facilities
- To explain the role of the health information management professional in the forms control program
- To compare internal and contract word-processing services
- To summarize how new developments such as telecommuting and voice recognition technology will change the role of the **medical transcriptionist**
- To define the unit, serial, and serial-unit systems of record numbering and filing and the appropriate use of each, including methods of number assignment
- To explain the basic rules of terminal digit filing and the reasons why it is used
- To describe policies and procedures on health record storage, retention, and destruction
- To define the functions of the master patient index

Key Terms

Administrative information
Advance directive
American Association for Medical Transcription (AAMT)
American College of Surgeons (ACS)
Authentication
Authorization
Autoauthentication
Bar coding
Bylaws
Care path
Case manager
Certified medical transcriptionist (CMT)
Chart tracking
Closed-record review
Closed records
Compliance
Concurrent analysis
Conditions of Participation
Consent
Consultation
Continuous record review
Contract service
Delinquent health record
Demographic information
Digital dictation
Discharge analysis
Discharge summary
Disposition
Do not resuscitate (DNR) order
Electronic signature
Enterprise-wide master patient index (EMPI)
Family numbering
History
Hybrid record

Incentive pay
Informed consent
Integrated health record
Licensure
Longitudinal health record
Master patient index (MPI)
Master population index
Medical transcriptionist
Medicare
Microfilming
Notice of Privacy Practices
Ongoing records review
Open-record review
Optical imaging technology
Outsourcing
Point-of-care review
Principal diagnosis
Problem-oriented medical record (POMR)
Progress notes
Qualitative analysis
Quantitative analysis
Retention schedules
Scanning
Serial filing system
Serial numbering system
Serial-unit numbering system
Source-oriented health record
Telestaffing
Terminal-digit filing system
Transcription
Unique identifier
Unit filing system
Unit numbering system
Universal chart order
Voice recognition technology
Word-processing services

Introduction

The patient health record is in the process of transition from a paper-based to a computer-based format. Indeed, most healthcare facilities currently maintain their health records using a combination of the two formats (sometimes referred to as a hybrid health record system) in order to accommodate the many different ways in which patient information is provided. Today's health records include computer printouts as well as handwritten notes. Data now arrive via electronic transfer from computerized laboratory or radiological testing or examination, through direct voice entry into a word-processing system, and from provider wireless devices and/or handheld personal computers. But as this chapter describes, the paper-based health record is a long way from being obsolete. The momentum to move away from paper is increasing dramatically, but a fully operational electronic health record (EHR) for all types of healthcare providers and facilities remains a future goal for the health-care system.

This chapter traces the evolution of the health record and describes the different kinds of information it contains and the different formats in which it is kept. The chapter also focuses on the health information management professional's role in managing patient information, from the creation and storage of information to its long-term retention and eventual destruction, and in ensuring its accuracy, completeness, and security. Finally, the chapter describes the functions of the master or enterprise patient or person index.

Theory into Practice

The director of health information management (HIM) at one hospital was promoted to the newly created position of HIM director for the corporate system, which involved oversight responsibility for HIM services at five facilities located within a single metropolitan area. The purpose of the new position was to standardize patient health record procedures and formats and to create the foundation for the transition to a paperless record system.

The system's leadership recognized that computerization would not solve all its HIM problems. There first had to be an excellent manual system to computerize. At the largest facility, **optical imaging technology** had been purchased along with word-processing software to enable reports to upload directly into the imaging system. The laboratory and radiology results were entered into the system automatically.

The new director had to use her basic knowledge of HIM principles to assess the current systems in all five facilities. She found that although the facilities were a part of one system administratively, the individual HIM departments operated in different ways. The first phase of the process was to inventory forms and then standardize and index them so that records could be scanned into the imaging system immediately following patient discharge. This involved all the HIM professionals

at all five facilities working together as a team to review the forms. Imaging procedures then were implemented in all five facilities. The word-processing systems were standardized and upgraded, with experienced transcriptionists given the option of working from home. Further, all departmental policies and procedures were standardized for all five facilities. These myriad activities took three years to complete. When the Health Insurance Portability and Accountability Act (HIPAA) regulations were published, the focus of the job shifted from operational decisions for health information managers to the training of personnel in all five hospitals on the confidentiality and security of health information.

The HIM director's new job reflects the constant changes and opportunities for growth presented to many HIM professionals. Health information managers must be flexible and willing to grow professionally as technology changes the field and new challenges arise. The HIM professional's foundation of knowledge is important to ensure that excellent documentation and records management processes are instituted and continued in the transition steps to a computer-based patient record.

Evolution of the Health Record

The paper-based patient health record has evolved as medicine and medical technology have evolved. Once simply the notation of the patient's name and a brief description of his or her illness or injury, the health record today is a detailed collection of handwritten entries, typed reports, and computer printouts reflecting the contributions of numerous healthcare providers.

Historical Overview

Health records have existed as long as there has been a need to communicate information about patient treatment. Archeological evidence indicates that maintaining information on patient care and treatment techniques is an ancient art.

Health records are maintained by all organizations that deliver healthcare, including physician and provider offices, long-term care facilities, emergency clinics, rehabilitation facilities, home health, behavioral health, correctional institutions, and numerous types of delivery systems and organizations. Records vary depending on the type of facility. Healthcare records in acute care hospitals, for example, require rapid documentation by many providers. Patients are often in the hospital for life-threatening injuries or conditions, and many different providers access and record information in the patients' health records, on average, within a five-day time span. Records in nonacute care hospital settings have many of the same forms found in the acute care settings. The records also will contain many specialized forms to meet requirements related to those settings. Although format and content of the health record may differ among healthcare settings, all providers of care must maintain information to meet patient care needs and to comply with relevant laws, standards, and regulations.

Today's HIM professional is responsible for records that contain more paper than ever before and are maintained in a variety of formats other than paper. There is an increasing demand to share information among providers on a regional basis to improve continuity of care. The multiple formats of today's records are a challenge to plans for the uniform sharing of information. The skills of the HIM professionals are in great demand to ensure the quality of shared information.

Documentation and Maintenance Standards for the Health Record

Health records provide proof of what has been done for the patient. As the complexity of care has evolved, so has the need for improved documentation. Standards for record documentation and maintenance have been established and are refined and revised constantly.

The American College of Surgeons and the Joint Commission on Accreditation of Healthcare Organizations

The **American College of Surgeons** (ACS) provided the impetus for standardizing health records when it developed minimum standards for hospitals early in the 20th century. It was evident to the ACS that standards were needed because candidates for membership were unable to produce proof of their experience with various types of surgical cases. Records were either nonexistent or of poor quality. The ACS Minimum Standard of 1917 included specific requirements for maintaining patient health records. The Joint Commission on Accreditation of Healthcare Organizations (JCAHO) standards for documentation evolved from this original standard.

JCAHO (formerly called the Joint Commission on Accreditation of Hospitals) is the successor organization to the ACS in the area of standardization. It assumed responsibility for the accreditation process in 1952 as a joint effort of the ACS, the American College of Physicians, the American Medical Association, and the American Hospital Association. Initially responsible for the accreditation of hospitals, JCAHO has since expanded its accreditation process to home health, long-term care, and other types of healthcare facilities.

The major source of information on the work of the hospital or any healthcare facility is the health record. JCAHO surveyors routinely review the health records of current patients to obtain knowledge about the facility's performance and process of care.

Medicare Conditions of Participation

The federal government passed **Medicare** legislation in 1965 to provide healthcare insurance coverage to Americans over 65 years of age. Since then, the legislation has been expanded to cover persons disabled for two years as well as persons with chronic kidney disease. The Centers for Medicare and Medicaid Services (CMS), until 2001 known as the Health Care Financing Administration (HCFA), is the division of the federal Department of Health and Human Services responsible for developing and enforcing regulations regarding the participation of healthcare providers in the Medicare program.

The Medicare regulations for health record content and documentation were originally established in the **Conditions of Participation.** As health record documentation became increasingly important, CMS began to focus on reviewing it for medical necessity and compliance with the decision-making rules established by the federal government. In addition, CMS published guidelines for documenting **histories** and physical examinations and medical decision making that affect physician reimbursement.

State Licensure

Every state has certain **licensure** regulations that healthcare facilities must meet in order to remain in operation. Licensure regulations may include very specific requirements for the content, format, retention, and use of patient records. These regulations are established by state governments, usually under the direction of state departments of health.

Internal Standards

Bylaws, rules, and regulations are developed by the medical staff and approved by the board of trustees or governing body in every type of healthcare facility. In addition to describing the organization's manner of operation, bylaws delineate the content of patient health records, identify the exact personnel who can write or enter information in health records, and restate applicable JCAHO and Medicare requirements. In addition, bylaws describe the time limits for completing patient health records. Surveyors review the bylaws to ensure that healthcare facilities abide by their own established rules and regulations and that the bylaws are in agreement with current JCAHO standards.

The Modern Health Record

The modern health record includes the contributions of numerous healthcare providers. In addition, it includes information provided by the patient or a person acting on his or her behalf describing the reasons for the patient's visit to the healthcare provider and other pertinent background facts. The modern health record is patient centered, meaning that the patient is the focus of all documentation on the activities that revolve around him or her while under the provider's care.

Definition of the Health Record

The information in the health record must outline and justify the patient's treatment, support diagnosis of the patient's condition, describe the patient's progress and response to medications and services, and explain the outcomes of the care provided. As documentation of all the activities that revolve around the patient, the health record promotes continuity of care among all the providers who treat the patient.

The health record itself is the property of the healthcare facility. However, the patient has the right to be informed about the use of his or her personal health information (PHI). Federal HIPAA regulations require that the patient be notified of the uses of PHI through notices of privacy practices.

Functions of Health Records and Health Information

To providers, the health record is valuable as the principal source of information in determining care for the patient. To the healthcare facility, it is valuable as a key source of information in determining the reimbursement for care.

The primary functions of the health record are:

- To facilitate the ongoing care and treatment of individual patients
- To support clinical decision making and communication among clinicians
- To document the services provided to patients in support of reimbursement
- To provide information for the evaluation of the quality and efficacy of the care provided
- To provide information in support of medical research and education
- To help facilitate the operational management of the facility
- To provide information as required by local and national laws and regulations

Ongoing Care and Treatment of Individual Patients

The most important use of the health record is patient care and the person to whom the record is of most value is the patient. The care and treatment of individual patients reflected in the record is of paramount importance.

When physicians were the only caregivers, they knew the patient and family and decided how detailed the patient's records needed to be. Often a small card or a ledger listing the patient's problem at a particular time was all the record keeping physicians needed. As healthcare has come to depend on technology and the skilled personnel to use it, health records have become more complex. Providers cannot remember all the information provided by the available technology, and fast access to past information about the patient's care is vital to the continuity of care.

Clinical Decision Making and Communication

Health information serves the vital function of allowing all the patient's providers to enter and analyze information and to make decisions. Each member of the healthcare team has equal access to the information and can review what others are doing and communicate with them through the record. Thus, the health record is the healthcare team's primary reference and communication tool.

Reimbursement

Information in the health record is used to document the services provided to the patient so that payment for the care provided can be made by those responsible for the bill. Insurance companies, managed care organizations, and Medicare require that specific information be submitted to support the bill and to prove that the care provided was medically necessary.

Evaluation of the Quality and Efficacy of Care

The health record is used as a legal document to prove the quality of care rendered by the healthcare provider. The documentation in the record provides information for accrediting and licensing activities.

Medical Research and Education

Data from many health records can be aggregated and analyzed for research studies and to provide statistical information on medical conditions and treatment modalities. As an example, public health agencies need health information. Certain diseases and conditions must be reported to the department of health in order to develop prevention and control procedures and to monitor disease trends. Moreover, the information in health records serves to provide continuing education for students in a variety of health professions.

Operational Management

Information gathered from health records helps facilities plan for the future based on the types of patients and diagnoses treated. Aggregate statistical information provides data on the use of services, provider patterns, and other important issues. Management often uses the information to make comparisons with other facilities. Finally, the quality of information in the health record aids managerial decision making in terms of improving the quality of patient care.

Legal Purposes

The health record serves the legal interests of the patient, the provider, and the facility. It serves as evidence in legal cases addressing the treatment received by the patient. It serves to prove the patient's allegations in a malpractice case and also is used by the clinical provider and the facility to defend the care they provided the patient. The record is admissible as evidence because it is considered a business record in that documentation occurs routinely as part of the healthcare facility's daily operation.

The Longitudinal Health Record

The **longitudinal health record** is a record compiled about an individual from birth to death. It is valuable because all the information about a patient is maintained and accessible. It serves as a reference of past history and avoids repetition of details and duplication of testing for the same conditions. Moreover, the longitudinal health record helps to prevent medical errors because information on allergies, drug interactions, surgeries, and past medical problems can be made available before treatment decisions are made. The physician can review the details of a patient's care and retrieve information needed at a later date.

A longitudinal health record is difficult to achieve in a paper-based record system because the patient typically has records at a variety of provider locations, such as physician offices, clinics, and hospitals, each of which often has a totally separate paper system. The different records are not linked, making it difficult to access all needed patient information. A longitudinal electronic health record would be especially valuable because it would allow information to be accessed from different locations. Many efforts are under way at the present time to develop the capability to share patient information electronically to improve quality, safety, and continuity of care.

Responsibility for Quality Documentation

The provider of care is responsible for ensuring that entries made in the record are of high quality. Although the facility's medical staff bylaws establish the rules and regulations for record content, the individual care providers are ultimately responsible for the quality of entries they make and authenticate. Figure 8.1 presents general documentation guidelines that every provider who writes or enters information in the patient health record should follow.

The quality of provider entries includes legibility. If an entry cannot be read, it must be assumed that it cannot or was not used in the patient care process.

Figure 8.1.   Guidelines for documenting and maintaining the patient health record

These guidelines are considered standard or typical health information practices. Individual facilities develop their own policies based on institutional needs and laws and regulations.

1. All entries in the health record must be authenticated to identify the author (name and professional status) and dated.

2. No erasures or deletions should be made in the health record.

3. All entries in the paper health record should be in ink. Photocopying or scanning should be considered when colored ink or colored forms are used because some colors do not reproduce well.

4. Blank spaces should not be left in progress/nursing notes. If blanks are left, they should be marked out with an X so that additional information cannot be inserted on the paper out of proper date sequence.

5. If a correction must be made in a paper health record, one line should be neatly drawn through the error, leaving the incorrect material legible. The error then should be initialed and dated so that it is be obvious that it is a corrected mistake.

6. The original report should always be maintained in the health record. Cumulative laboratory reports or computerized nursing notes may be replaced with the latest cumulative report. Faxed copies of admission orders and histories and physicals may be used as originals in the record. The usual signature requirements should be followed.

7. All blanks on forms should be completed, especially on consent forms.

8. When health records are filed incomplete (as directed by medical staff/health record committee policy), a statement should be attached to indicate that this is the case. The statement should be signed by the chief of staff/chair of the health record committee as specified in the policy.

9. Chart folder labeling, dotting, or other methods of identifying at a glance a particular type of patient, such as one with a drug or alcohol diagnosis or HIV-positive status, should be discouraged to prevent inadvertent breaches of patient confidentiality.

The HIM professional is responsible for ensuring that providers understand the regulations and standards for proper documentation and for educating providers as changes occur. He or she should be involved in training residents and others who enter information so that standards are maintained and the record remains in its proper format.

The facility's administration is responsible for providing the equipment and support personnel to assist physicians in proper documentation. This includes computers and dictating and **transcription** equipment services, as well as HIM staff and other staff members who assist in creating a high-quality record and the proper coding and billing for reimbursement.

Except in facilities owned by individuals or the government, a board of trustees has ultimate legal responsibility for the quality of care rendered in the facility. However, responsibility for patient care decisions and documentation of these decisions is delegated to the physician responsible for the patient.

Check Your Understanding 8.1

Instructions: Answer the following questions on a separate sheet of paper.

1. What is the primary purpose of patient health information?

2. What are six other purposes or uses of patient health information?

3. What is the role of each of the following in the development of standards for health information: American College of Surgeons, Joint Commission on Accreditation of Healthcare Organizations, Centers for Medicare and Medicaid Services, state licensure, and medical staff bylaws?

4. Why is a longitudinal health record valuable, and why is a longitudinal health record in a paper-based system difficult to achieve?

5. Who is responsible for ensuring the quality of health record documentation?

Content of the Health Record

All health records contain information that can be classified into two broad categories: administrative/demographic data and clinical data. All health record entries must be legible, complete, dated, and authenticated according to the healthcare organization's policies. Health records may be paper based, electronic, or a combination of formats. As health records evolve from paper to electronic and imaging formats, the term *hybrid record* is used to describe the record information format.

Administrative and Demographic Information

Administrative and demographic information is generally found on the front page of the patient health record. The information entered provides facts that identify the patient and data related to payment and reimbursement and other operational needs of the healthcare facility.

Registration Data

Registration data represent one type of **administrative information.** Registration data are collected prior to, or at the time of, an inpatient admission treatment in an emergency department or outpatient facility or a physician or other provider office. This is the first information the facility collects. Payment information is part of the administrative information. Administrative information also includes the various **consents** for treatment and the use of patient information, notification of patient rights, and other nonclinical information.

Demographic information is a type of administrative information. Demographic information includes facts such as:

- The patient's name
- The patient's address
- The patient's telephone number
- The patient's date of birth
- The patient's next of kin
- Other identifying information specific to the patient

A **unique identifier** number is assigned to the health record that allows all information about the patient to be inserted in the correct record or to be accessed when a query is entered into the computer system. Demographic information helps to specifically identify the patient and provides statistical information that is vital for planning, research, statistics, and other needs.

Demographic information may be entered directly into the computer by admission or registration personnel. In cases where the patient is coming to the facility for elective, or voluntary, treatment and/or an operative procedure, he or she can provide this information prior to arrival at the facility. The patient usually provides the information directly, but in cases where the patient is a minor or is incapacitated or in an emergency situation, another individual may provide the information. In such cases, the record must state the name and relationship of the person providing the information in case the information has to be verified or amended.

The demographic information in a totally paper-based health record environment is usually on the first page, which is called the face sheet or front sheet. This term also is used to refer to the computer view containing the information in facilities that have a computer-based admissions and discharge system in which a printout of the computer screen becomes the face sheet of a paper record.

Consent to Treatment

Through the consent process, the patient agrees to undergo the treatments and procedures to be performed by clinical caregivers. This general consent is often part of the admission or entry process into the healthcare facility. However, the consent does not replace the individual consent forms the patient must complete and sign for each operation or special procedure to indicate that he or she is fully informed about the care to be provided. Written consents signed by the patient for experimental drugs and treatment and for participation in research must be included in the health record. Refusal of treatment or procedures likewise must be written

to ensure that the consequences of the decision have been explained and the patient is aware of them.

Consent to Use or Disclose Protected Health Record Information

With regulatory changes put into place under HIPAA, upon admission to the facility or prior to treatment by the provider, patients must be informed about the use of personally identifiable health information. This **Notice of Privacy Practices** must explain and give examples of the uses of the patient's health information for treatment, payment, and healthcare operations, as well as other disclosures for purposes established in the regulations. (See appendix C.) If a particular use of information is not covered in the Notice of Privacy Practices, the patient must sign an **authorization** form specific to the additional disclosure before his or her information can be released. (See figure A.21 in appendix A.)

Consent to Special Procedures

In cases where the patient is coming to the facility for a specific procedure, an **informed consent** spelling out the exact details of the treatment must be signed by the patient or his or her legally authorized representative. This consent must show that the patient or the person authorized to act for the patient understands exactly what the procedure, test, or operation is going to be, including any possible risks, alternative methods, and outcomes.

Advance Directives

An **advance directive** is a written document, such as a living will, that states the patient's preferences for care. It also can be in the form of a durable power of attorney for healthcare in which the patient names another person to make medical decisions on his or her behalf in the event he or she is incapacitated. When the patient has a written advance directive, its existence must be noted in the health record. Patients or family members may bring the document to the facility to show the patient's wishes in case of terminal disease, traumatic injury, or cardiac arrest. The advance directive can be included as a part of the health record, although its inclusion may not be required. There may be documentation by the physician of a discussion with the patient or the family about the patient's wishes, rather than a formal written document.

Patients must be informed that they have the right to have an advance directive. Further, they must be notified of the provider's policies regarding its refusal to comply with advance directives.

Acknowledgment of Receipt of Patient's Rights Statement

Medicare requires that patients be informed of their rights, including the right to know who is treating them, the right to confidentiality, and the right to be informed about treatment. The patient's rights statement also must explain the patient's right to refuse treatment, to participate in care planning, and to be safe from abuse. The patient must sign a statement that these rights have been explained, and the signed statement must be made part of the health record. States often have laws and regulations regarding the rights that must be explained to patients, such as the right to privacy in treatment, to refuse treatment, and to refuse experimental treatments and drugs.

Property and Valuables List

Although facilities encourage patients to leave jewelry and other valuables at home, patients will have with them needed property such as clothing, teeth, eyeglasses, hearing aids, and other personal articles. Patients may be asked to sign a release of responsibility form to absolve the facility of responsibility for loss or damage to their personal property. This form then becomes part of the patient health record.

Birth and Death Certificates

The collection of birth information is often the responsibility of admitting personnel, nursing, or HIM personnel who prepare the certificate for submission to the state department of health. Many states use birth certificate software that has the fields required for the collection of such information. Birth certificates do not necessarily require a physician's signature; some states allow each facility to select a designated person, such as an HIM professional, to certify births. In most states, official birth certificates are maintained permanently by the department of health.

The funeral home director or the coroner is responsible for completing the death certificate in many states. The funeral director must obtain the signature of the attending physician or the physician who declared the patient dead for the death certificate. Death certificates are usually maintained permanently by the department of health.

Clinical Data

Clinical data include information related to the patient's condition, course of treatment, and progress. The patient health record includes mainly clinical data.

Medical History

The history is a summary of the patient's illness from his or her point of view. Its purpose is to allow the patient or his or her authorized representative to give the physician as much background information about the patient's illness as possible. The physician usually tailors the physical examination to symptoms described in the patient's history and begins an assessment. Thus, the history provides a base on which the physician can develop a plan.

Documentation guidelines for histories and physical examinations and medical decision making published by CMS affect physician reimbursement and are discussed further in chapter 14.

Components of the Medical History

The medical history has several components, including:

- *Chief complaint:* Told in the patient's own words (or those of the patient's representative), the chief complaint is the principal reason the patient is seeking care.
- *Present illness:* This component addresses what the patient feels the problem is and includes a brief descrip-

tion of the duration, location, and circumstances of the complaint.
- *Past medical history:* This consists of questions designed to gather information about past surgeries and other illnesses that might have a bearing on the patient's current illness. The physician asks about childhood and adult illnesses, operations, injuries, drug sensitivities, allergies, and other health problems.
- *Social and personal history:* The social history uncovers information about habits and living conditions that might have a bearing on the patient's illness, such as marital status, occupation, environment, and so on. Consumption of alcohol or tobacco products also may affect a patient's health. This section also should address the patient's psychosocial needs.
- *Family medical history:* The questions in this component allow the physician to learn whether other family members have conditions that might be considered genetic. Common questions concern cardiovascular diseases or conditions, renal diseases, history of cancer or diabetes, allergies, health of immediate relatives, and ages of relatives at death and causes of their deaths.
- *Review of systems:* This component consists of questions designed to cue the patient to reveal symptoms he or she may have forgotten, did not think were important, or neglected to mention when providing the historical information.

It is important that the person recording the history document whether the information was given by the patient or by another person in cases where the patient is unable to communicate.

Physical Examination

The physical examination is the actual comprehensive assessment of the patient by the physician. Its purpose is to obtain initial signs and symptoms so that appropriate treatment can begin. The end of the physical examination should indicate the impression based on the information obtained and the initial plan for the patient's care while in the hospital.

Components of the Physical Examination

The physical examination is conducted by observing the patient, palpating or touching the patient, tapping the thoracic and abdominal cavities, listening to breath and heart sounds, and taking the blood pressure. The patient is examined thoroughly. If the patient is admitted for a particular procedure, a more focused physical examination will take place.

Time Frame of the History and Physical Examination

The facility must have a policy that establishes a time frame for completing the history and physical. Most facilities set the time frame as the first 24 to 48 hours following admission and require that the history and physical be completed by the provider who is admitting the patient. It is acceptable to JCAHO when the history and physical examination are completed within 30 days before the patient is admitted. Proposed Medicare rules specify that the history and physical examination be completed by the physician or other qualified individual who has medical staff privileges in accordance with state law. The history and physical examination must be completed no more than 30 days before or 24 hours after admission and the report must be placed in the record within 24 hours after admission. The proposed rules require that if the history and physical have been completed within the 30 days prior to admission, there must be an updated entry in the medical record that documents an examination for any changes in the patient's condition, and this entry must be included in the record within the first 24 hours of admission.

JCAHO requires the history and physical examination to be recorded and made part of the patient health record prior to any operative procedure. When the physician chooses to dictate the history and physical, the dictated report must be transcribed and attached to the chart before the procedure.

When the report is dictated but not transcribed, a written preoperative note covering the history and physical is acceptable only in an emergency. The physician must write an explanation of the emergency circumstances.

The HIM professional is responsible for ensuring that the most stringent time requirements are followed so that the facility is in **compliance** with state and federal laws and regulations, licensure standards, Medicare Conditions of Participation, and accreditation requirements for the specific type of facility. When the patient is readmitted within 30 days after discharge for the same condition, some hospitals allow the previous history and physical examination to be updated and signed and dated by the physician. This is called an interval history and is acceptable to JCAHO.

Table 8.1 lists the information usually included in a complete medical history, and table 8.2 (p. 179) shows the information usually documented in the report of a physical examination.

Table 8.1.   Information usually included in a complete medical history

Components of the History	Complaints and Symptoms
Chief complaint	Nature and duration of the symptoms that caused the patient to seek medical attention as stated in his or her own words
Present illness	Detailed chronological description of the development of the patient's illness, from the appearance of the first symptom to the present situation
Past medical history	Summary of childhood and adult illnesses and conditions, such as infectious diseases, pregnancies, allergies and drug sensitivities, accidents, operations, hospitalizations, and current medications
Social and personal history	Marital status; dietary, sleep, and exercise patterns; use of coffee, tobacco, alcohol, and other drugs; occupation; home environment; daily routine; and so on
Family medical history	Diseases among relatives in which heredity or contact might play a role, such as allergies, cancer, and infectious, psychiatric, metabolic, endocrine, cardiovascular, and renal diseases; health status or cause and age at death for immediate relatives
Review of systems	Systemic inventory designed to uncover current or past subjective symptoms that includes the following types of data: • *General:* Usual weight, recent weight changes, fever, weakness, fatigue • *Skin:* Rashes, eruptions, dryness, cyanosis, jaundice; changes in skin, hair, or nails • *Head:* Headache (duration, severity, character, location) • *Eyes:* Glasses or contact lenses, last eye examination, glaucoma, cataracts, eyestrain, pain, diplopia, redness, lacrimation, inflammation, blurring • *Ears:* Hearing, discharge, tinnitus, dizziness, pain • *Nose:* Head colds, epistaxis, discharges, obstruction, postnasal drip, sinus pain • *Mouth and throat:* Condition of teeth and gums, last dental examination, soreness, redness, hoarseness, difficulty in swallowing • *Respiratory system:* Chest pain, wheezing, cough, dyspnea, sputum (color and quantity), hemoptysis, asthma, bronchitis, emphysema, pneumonia, tuberculosis, pleurisy, last chest x-ray • *Neurological system:* Fainting, blackouts, seizures, paralysis, tingling, tremors, memory loss • *Musculoskeletal system:* Joint pain or stiffness, arthritis, gout, backache, muscle pain, cramps, swelling, redness, limitation in motor activity • *Cardiovascular system:* Chest pain, rheumatic fever, tachycardia, palpitation, high blood pressure, edema, vertigo, faintness, varicose veins, thrombophlebitis • *Gastrointestinal system:* Appetite, thirst, nausea, vomiting, hematemesis, rectal bleeding, change in bowel habits, diarrhea, constipation, indigestion, food intolerance, flatus, hemorrhoids, jaundice • *Urinary system:* Frequent or painful urination, nocturia, pyuria, hematuria, incontinence, urinary infections • *Genitoreproductive system:* Male—venereal disease, sores, discharge from penis, hernias, testicular pain, or masses; female—age at menarche, frequency and duration of menstruation, dysmenorrhea, menorrhagia, symptoms of menopause, contraception, pregnancies, deliveries, abortions, last Pap smear • *Endocrine system:* Thyroid disease; heat or cold intolerance; excessive sweating, thirst, hunger, or urination • *Hematologic system:* Anemia, easy bruising or bleeding, past transfusions • *Psychiatric disorders:* Insomnia, headache, nightmares, personality disorders, anxiety disorders, mood disorders

Table 8.2.   Information usually documented in the report of a physical examination

Report Components	Content
General condition	Apparent state of health, signs of distress, posture, weight, height, skin color, dress and personal hygiene, facial expression, manner, mood, state of awareness, speech
Vital signs	Pulse, respiration, blood pressure, temperature
Skin	Color, vascularity, lesions, edema, moisture, temperature, texture, thickness, mobility and turgor, nails
Head	Hair, scalp, skull, face
Eyes	Visual acuity and fields; position and alignment of the eyes, eyebrows, eyelids; lacrimal apparatus; conjunctivae; sclerae; corneas; irises; size, shape, equality, reaction to light, and accommodation of pupils; extraocular movements; ophthalmoscopic exam
Ears	Auricles, canals, tympanic membranes, hearing, discharge
Nose and sinuses	Airways, mucosa, septum, sinus tenderness, discharge, bleeding, smell
Mouth	Breath, lips, teeth, gums, tongue, salivary ducts
Throat	Tonsils, pharynx, palate, uvula, postnasal drip
Neck	Stiffness, thyroid, trachea, vessels, lymph nodes, salivary glands
Thorax, anterior and posterior	Shape, symmetry, respiration
Breasts	Masses, tenderness, discharge from nipples
Lungs	Fremitus, breath sounds, adventitious sounds, friction, spoken voice, whispered voice
Heart	Location and quality of apical impulse, trill, pulsation, rhythm, sounds, murmurs, friction rub, jugular venous pressure and pulse, carotid artery pulse
Abdomen	Contour, peristalsis, scars, rigidity, tenderness, spasm, masses, fluid, hernia, bowel sounds and bruits, palpable organs
Male genitourinary organs	Scars, lesions, discharge, penis, scrotum, epididymis, varicocele, hydrocele
Female reproductive organs	External genitalia, Skene's glands and Bartholin's glands, vagina, cervix, uterus, adnexa
Rectum	Fissure, fistula, hemorrhoids, sphincter tone, masses, prostate, seminal vesicles, feces
Musculoskeletal system	Spine and extremities, deformities, swelling, redness, tenderness, range of motion
Lymphatics	Palpable cervical, axillary, inguinal nodes; location; size; consistency; mobility and tenderness
Blood vessels	Pulses, color, temperature, vessel walls, veins
Neurological system	Cranial nerves, coordination, reflexes, biceps, triceps, patellar, Achilles, abdominal, cremasteric, Babinski, Romberg, gait, sensory, vibratory
Diagnosis(es)	

Diagnostic and Therapeutic Orders

Physicians' orders drive the healthcare team. Orders may be for treatments, ancillary medical services, laboratory tests, radiological procedures, drugs, devices, related materials, restraint, or seclusion. Orders change according to the patient's needs and responses to previous treatment. In the case of drugs, the physician orders a specific drug in a particular dosage stating how often the drug is to be given, by what means (orally, intravenously, or by other method), and for how long. Certain categories of drugs, such as narcotics and sedatives, have an automatic time limit or stop order. This means that these medications must be discontinued unless the physician gives a specific order. This prevents patients from receiving drugs for a longer period of time than is necessary.

Orders for tests and services must demonstrate the medical necessity and explain the reason for the order. The legibility of orders is important to ensure that they are clearly understood by the personnel who must carry them out. Some facilities use a computerized order-entry system. Verbal orders entered into the record or computer system by nonphysician personnel must be signed or authenticated by the provider authorized to give orders. If providers have not signed in a timely manner, the computer will not let them access the system until the orders are signed.

Clinicians Authorized to Give and Receive Orders

Orders must be written by the physician or verbally communicated to persons authorized to receive verbal orders either in person or by telephone. The person accepting the order should sign and give his or her title, such as RN, PT, LPN, as appropriate. In some states, certified registered nurse practitioners and physician assistants are allowed to write or give verbal orders.

Medical staff policies and procedures must specifically state the categories of personnel authorized to accept orders. Verbal orders for medication are usually required to be given to, and to be accepted only by, nursing or pharmacy personnel. Some categories of personnel that may accept verbal or oral orders for services within the specific area of practice include physical therapists, registered nurse anesthetists, dietitians, and medical technologists.

Moreover, orders for tests and treatments must justify the condition of medical necessity because payers may not reimburse the facility if the reason for the test or treatment is not properly documented.

The time the order was given should be in writing. Some facilities do not allow verbal orders for treatments or procedures that might put the patient at risk. Other facilities require verbal orders to be repeated by the person accepting them to verify that they are clearly understood.

Signatures on Orders

Generally, orders must be dated and signed, or authenticated by, the provider or providers responsible for the patient's care and who either wrote or gave the orders. In the case of verbal or telephone orders, the provider should sign them as soon as possible after giving them. Many facilities require the ordering provider to indicate that the telephone orders are accurate, complete, and final by signing them within 24 hours. The timing requirements for signatures on orders are governed by state law, facility policy, accreditation standards, and government regulations and may vary from facility to facility. Proposed Medicare rules state that in the absence of state law, the time limit for authentication will be within 48 hours.

For years, HIM department personnel carefully reviewed each order and marked those with missing signatures so that each could be individually signed by the responsible provider after discharge. However, signing orders after discharge does not affect the patient's care process, so many facilities no longer routinely review orders for signature following patient discharge. A review of orders is part of the concurrent or **open-record review** process; thus, orders can be signed in a timely manner and providers with patterns of unsigned orders can be detected. A comparison of orders to laboratory and other ancillary reports and to nursing documentation is another way to ensure that all orders are carried out.

Some facilities are developing standing, or standard, orders for certain procedures that all physicians can use when performing the particular procedure. Other facilities require an additional order to implement the standing orders, and still others allow a registered nurse to initiate the standing orders because the medical staff has previously approved them.

Proposed Medicare rules published in the *Federal Register* provide a five-year exception to the rules regarding signatures on verbal orders. This exception allows verbal (telephone or oral) orders to be signed by another provider responsible for the patient's care. The proposed Medicare rules retain the current requirements that the use of verbal orders should be infrequent and used only when the orders cannot be written or given electronically. The proposed rules further state that verbal orders must only be accepted by persons authorized by hospital polices and procedures and state and federal law.

Special Orders

Do not resuscitate (DNR) **orders** must contain documentation that the decision to withhold cardiopulmonary resuscitation (CPR) was discussed, when the decision was made, and who participated in the decision. This discussion is often documented in the **progress notes.** Generally, patients are presumed to have consented to CPR unless a DNR order is present in the record. This may be part of the advance directives in the record.

Orders for seclusion and restraint, including drugs used for restraint, must comply with facility policies and Medicare regulations, state laws, and JCAHO requirements. These should never be standing or as-needed orders but, instead, must be ordered only when necessary to protect the patient or others from injury or harm. Specific time limits for these orders must be followed, and there must be continuous oversight of the patient under restraint or seclusion.

Discharge Orders

Discharge orders for hospital patients must be in writing and can only be issued by a physician. When a patient leaves against medical advice, this fact should be noted in lieu of a discharge order because the patient was not actually discharged. In the case of death, some facilities require that a discharge to the morgue order be written.

Clinical Observations

Clinical observations of the patient are documented in the health record in several formats, including progress notes, **consultation** reports, and ancillary notes, as described below.

Medical Services

Progress notes are chronological statements about the patient's response to treatment during his or her stay in the facility. Facility procedures and policies must state exactly what categories of personnel are allowed to write or enter information into progress notes. Generally, these personnel include physicians, nurses, physical therapists, occupational therapists, respiratory therapists, social workers, **case managers,** dietitians, nurse anesthetists, pharmacists, radiologic technologists, speech therapists, and others providing direct treatment or consultation to the patient. Each person authorized to enter documentation into the progress notes must write or enter his or her own note, authenticate and date it, and indicate authorship by signing his or her full name and title.

Each progress note reviews changes in the patient's condition, findings based on the facts of the case, test results, and response to treatment, as well as an analysis of the findings. The final part of the note contains the decisions or actions planned for future care. When writing in a paper patient record, providers must avoid leaving blank spaces between progress notes to prevent information from being added out of sequence.

Flowcharts are an effective way to illustrate the patient's progress and can be computerized to demonstrate progress or to keep track of certain data. Many physicians and other providers use handheld personal computers to maintain ongoing flowchart information about patients, such as blood glucose levels over time.

How often progress notes are written depends on the patient's condition, and the frequency is generally established by the healthcare facility or payers of care. In a hospital, the physician primarily responsible for the patient's care is often required to write a progress note daily. Doing so shows the physician's involvement and that he or she is aware of changes in the patient's condition.

Consultations are additional opinions of specialists. The attending physician may request that the specialist see the patient and prepare a consultation report. Each consultant is responsible for writing, dictating, or entering his or her own report. The report should show evidence of the consultant's review of the record and the patient and any pertinent findings, opinions, and recommendations. Moreover, the documentation should show that the physician requesting the consultation reviewed the report.

Nursing Services

Nursing personnel have the most frequent contact with patients, and their notes provide the complete record of the patients' progress and condition and demonstrate the continuity of care. Licensed registered nurses, licensed practical nurses (sometimes called licensed vocational nurses), and nursing assistants record the facts of the physician's orders being carried out, observe the patient's response to treatment interventions, and describe the patient's condition and complaints as well as the outcome of care as reflected in the patient's status at discharge or termination of treatment. The method most commonly used by nurses to enter notes is narrative detailed documentation.

Nursing personnel begin recording information in the health record when the patient is admitted to the facility. They coordinate the patient's care to ensure that orders are carried out. The initial nursing assessment must summarize the date, time, and method of admission; the patient's condition, symptoms, and vital signs; and other information. Many nurses use a variation of the **problem-oriented medical record** format (discussed later in this chapter) when recording notes. All nursing notes must be signed by the individuals who provided the service or observed the patient's condition. Full names and titles are required.

Charting by exception, or focus charting, is a method of charting only abnormal or unusual findings or deviations from the prescribed plan of care. A complete assessment is performed every shift or every eight hours. When events differ from the assessment or the expected norm for a particular patient, the notes should focus on that particular event and include the data, intervention, and response. Flow sheets and care plans may be used to illustrate changes in the patient's condition. The purpose of charting by exception is to reduce repetitive record keeping and documentation of normal events. Bedside terminals and direct input of monitoring information and other computerization of nursing observations and medication distribution save nurses a great deal of time because information does not have to be rewritten numerous times.

Medication records are maintained for all patients and include medications given, time, form of administration, and dosage and strength. The records are updated when the patient is given his or her medication. The health record must reflect when a medication is given in error, indicating what was done about it and the patient's response. Adverse drug reactions must be fully documented and reported to the provider and to the performance improvement/risk management program according to guidelines established by the facility.

Flow sheets are often used in addition to narrative notes for intake and output records showing how much fluid the patient consumed and how much was eliminated. In addi-

tion, blood glucose records are often flowcharted for ease of comparison. Degree of pain is another aspect of the patient's condition that is commonly flowcharted.

Nurses are responsible for maintaining records of patient transfers (to surgery, to another room, or level of care) as well as visits to physician or treatment offices and other locations outside the facility.

Case managers are nurses, social workers, or other personnel who are responsible for assisting the patient through the care process. The case management process improves quality of care because care is scheduled in an orderly way and fragmentation is reduced. Hospitals, managed care organizations, and other facilities use case managers to improve coordination of care, scheduling, and discharge planning. Many facilities use predetermined **care paths** that are specific to diagnoses or conditions; case managers ensure that patients receive care according to the care path. Care paths are also called clinical pathways, critical paths, and clinical algorithms.

Ancillary Services

Laboratory and radiology reports and reports from other ancillary services, such as EKGs (electrocardiographs) and EEGs (electroencephalographs), must be signed by the physician responsible for the interpretations. A pathologist is responsible for the work of the clinical laboratory; a radiologist is responsible for the work of the radiology department. Many states have separate **retention schedules** for the actual x-rays that differ from the retention time frames for other health records. The typed interpretations of the radiology or other reports become part of the health record and are kept as long as the health records are kept. Images may be part of a computerized picture archiving communication system (PACS).

Laboratory results in a computerized environment are available to the provider as soon as they are entered into the computer. In most facilities, a laboratory summary is generated consistently throughout the patient's stay, with a final summary completed within 24 hours after discharge. These multipage summaries are printed and made part of the patient health record. Some facilities use manually completed laboratory forms divided into several sections. The original report is the one that should be included in the record. The laboratory conducts tests on blood, urine, sputum, and other body fluids. Many specialized tests are performed in the laboratory to provide information the physician can use to make a diagnosis, including analyses of specimens removed during surgery. Most facilities require the original laboratory report to be placed in the health record within 24 hours.

Healthcare facility policies and procedures must state that the practitioner approved by the medical staff to interpret diagnostic procedures, such as nuclear medicine procedures, MRIs, EEGs, and EKGs, should sign and date his or her interpretations. The interpretations then become part of the health record. Scans and videotapes, tracings, or other actual recordings are often fed directly into the computer system.

Providers may view such recordings, but the recordings do not become part of the permanent record. It is important that all tests or procedures ordered have corresponding reports in the health record.

Orders and records of services rendered to patients from rehabilitation, physical therapy, occupational therapy, audiology, or speech pathology should be included in the record as appropriate to the patient. These reports must contain evaluations, recommendations, goals, course of treatment, and response to treatment. Nutritional care plans need to be developed in compliance with a physician order, and information on nutrition and diet should be included in the discharge plan and transfer orders.

Surgical Services

The operative section of the health record includes the anesthesia record, the intraoperative record, and the recovery record. The history and physical examination, informed consents signed by the patient or his or her authorized representative, and the postoperative progress note also are part of the documentation about the operative procedure. Every patient's chart must include a complete history and physical examination prior to surgery or invasive procedure unless there is an emergency. When the history and physical report was dictated, it must be included in the record in a typed version.

Moreover, the anesthesiologist or the certified registered nurse anesthetist must write a preanesthesia evaluation or an updated evaluation prior to surgery. This evaluation must cover information on the anesthesia to be used, risk factors, allergy and drug history, potential problems, and a general assessment of the patient's condition. An intraoperative anesthesia record must be maintained of all events during surgery, including complete information on the anesthesia administration, blood pressure, pulse, respiration, and other monitors of the patient's condition. Finally, after surgery, the appropriate anesthesia personnel must write a postoperative anesthesia follow-up report. Outpatient surgical cases also must include postanesthesia evaluations. Records of postanesthesia visits should indicate any unusual events or complications. Proposed Medicare rules state that any individual qualified to administer anesthesia can complete the postanesthesia evaluation.

The operative report itself must be written or dictated by the surgeon immediately after surgery and must include the names of the surgeon and assistants, technical procedures performed, findings, specimens removed, estimated blood loss, and postoperative diagnosis. The surgeon must write a brief postoperative progress note in the record immediately after surgery before the patient leaves the operating suite. Most facilities have dictation areas set up near the operative suite or cardiac catheterization laboratories to allow surgeons to dictate the operative reports immediately. However, the written postoperative progress note must be completed to provide information for patient care until the typed report is placed in the patient record, usually 12 to 24 hours after surgery. Some facilities use a preprinted postoperative progress note form

with the required elements listed to remind the surgeon of the items that must be included. The postoperative progress notes and the dictation and transcription of operative reports must be carefully monitored to ensure that they are placed in the health record in a timely manner.

Pathology reports are required for every case in which a surgical specimen is removed or expelled during a procedure and must include a microscopic and gross evaluation of the tissue. These reports are part of the operative section of the health record and must be signed by the pathologist. The preoperative diagnosis and pathological diagnosis can then be compared.

Information on the patient's discharge from the postoperative or postanesthesia care unit must be documented and signed by the licensed independent practitioner responsible for the discharge or by the provider verifying that the patient is ready for discharge according to specific discharge criteria. The operative section also will contain data on implants, including product numbers, and additional information for follow-up.

Organ Transplantation

Medicare requires hospitals to inform families of the opportunity to donate organs, tissues, or eyes. Documentation showing that the organ procurement organization has been notified regarding a patient near death must be included in the health record so that anatomical gifts can be preserved and used. In the case of living donor transplants of kidneys or other organs, an operative report must be written for both donor and recipient following all the standards for operative records.

Conclusions at Termination of Care

The health record must summarize the patient's condition at the beginning of treatment and basic information about tests, examinations, procedures, and results occurring as a result of treatment. The conclusion at termination of care is called the **discharge summary.**

Discharge Summary

The discharge summary, also called the clinical resume, provides details about the patient's stay in the facility and is the foundation for future treatment. It is prepared when the patient is discharged or transferred to another facility or when the patient expires. The summary states the patient's reason for admission and gives a brief history explaining why he or she needed to be hospitalized. Pertinent laboratory, x-ray, consultation, and other significant findings, as well as the patient's response to treatment or procedures, are included. In addition to a description of the patient's condition at discharge, the discharge summary delineates specific instructions given to the family for future care, including information on medications, referrals to other providers, diet, activities, follow-up visits to the physician, and the patient's final diagnoses. The discharge summary must be signed and dated by the physician.

Some facilities require the final diagnoses to be recorded and the discharge summary to be dictated or written at discharge or they immediately consider the chart delinquent.

The information in the discharge summary is extremely important to meet the facility's coding, billing, and reimbursement needs. In some facilities, a paper discharge summary form with an outline of contents is used to ensure that all items are included. The form has three parts so that the part with follow-up instructions can be given to the patient.

When a patient dies in the hospital, hospitals often require the physician who pronounced death to write a note that gives the time and date of death. The death note is in addition to the discharge summary required in all death cases no matter how long the patient was in the facility. Most facilities do not require a discharge summary for normal newborns and obstetrical cases without complications, as long as there is a final progress note.

A discharge summary is not required for patients who are in the hospital for 48 hours or less. Such patients usually have a short-stay or short-service record or a final discharge progress note. This one-page form can be used to record the history and physical examination, the operative report, the discharge summary, and discharge instructions. When the patient is admitted to the facility, the reason for admission must be recorded. When the patient dies 48 hours or less after admission, the short-stay record is insufficient and a complete discharge summary must be prepared.

The discharge summary must be completed within 30 days after the date of discharge. When a patient is transferred, the physician should complete the discharge summary within 24 hours.

The **principal diagnosis** and other diagnoses should be recorded completely without symbols or abbreviations on the health record summary sheet (the face sheet) or discharge summary or on another form prescribed by the facility. The principal diagnosis is defined as the condition determined, after study, to be chiefly responsible for occasioning the patient's admission to the hospital.

Healthcare facilities must determine what information goes with the patient when he or she is transferred to another level of care. When the transfer is to an affiliated institution that is part of the same healthcare system, the original patient record is transferred with the patient and new orders are written at the receiving institution to initiate care. A discharge summary is generally required.

Discharge Plan

Discharge planning information regarding further treatment of the patient should be part of the acute care health record. The discharge planning process begins at admission and must include information on the patient's ability to perform self-care as well as other services needed by the patient. The case manager, the social worker, utilization review personnel, or nursing personnel may write this plan.

Records Filed with the Health Record

In the past, there was much debate about whether patient records received from other facilities should be made part of the receiving facility's health record. Some facilities released all the information because all of it was used in treatment decisions. Other facilities maintained that they were responsible only for the information originating in their own facilities and had requestors obtain original records from the originating facility. HIPAA regulations now require that all information, including information from other facilities, is part of the health record. It is important for healthcare facilities to develop polices to determine exactly what health information mailed, faxed, or personally brought to the facility by the patient or patient's family becomes part of the receiving facility's designated health record. A good practice is to have the attending physician review copies and note which documents should be made permanent parts of the record. Any extraneous copies, x-rays, or other information should be returned to the patient.

Facilities maintain information on the release of information from the patient record explaining what was released, to whom the information was released, and the date. This required information is often filed with the health record but should not be released when the patient record is released. Federal regulations now require that facilities provide an "accounting of disclosure" under the HIPAA regulations, but most facilities have traditionally maintained this type of information. (See figure A.22 in appendix A.)

Specialized Health Record Content

The format of the patient health record varies according to the type of care provided. Many facilities offer specialized services requiring special documentation that is not found in every patient's record. JCAHO standards and regulations often specify particular content to include in the record. The following sections describe various specialized services and their records.

Obstetrical Care

The prenatal record, which is kept in the physician's office, serves as the history and physical for an obstetrical patient. When the patient requires a Cesarean section, the record must include a full history and physical or a detailed admission progress note explaining the need for a C-section.

A labor and delivery record indicates the name of the patient, maiden name, date of delivery, sex of infant, name of physician, name of persons assisting, any complications, type of anesthesia used, name of person administering anesthesia, and names of others present at delivery. In the case of a stillborn infant, a separate patient record is not created; rather, information is recorded in the mother's delivery record. A fetal death certificate is completed on the appropriate form.

Neonatal Care

Newborns are considered separate patients with separate health records. The newborn patient record must include an admission examination and a discharge examination. Usually, special chart forms for progress notes, orders, and nursing notes are included. When the patient has been in the newborn intensive care unit, a complete discharge summary is required.

Emergency Care

Emergency health records may be filed separately or incorporated into the health record when the patient is admitted to the same facility. When the records are filed separately, the emergency record must be available when the patient is readmitted or seeks care in the future. Most of the emergency information is recorded on one sheet in a paper health record format. Additional sheets include laboratory, radiology, and other tests; consent forms; and follow-up instructions.

The content of the emergency health record should include:

- Identification data
- Time of arrival
- Means of arrival (by ambulance, private automobile, or police vehicle)
- Name of person or organization transporting patient to the emergency department
- Pertinent history, including chief complaint and onset of injury or illness
- Significant physical findings
- Laboratory, x-ray, and EKG findings
- Treatment rendered
- Conclusions at termination of treatment
- **Disposition** of patient, including whether sent home, transferred, or admitted
- Condition of the patient upon discharge or transfer
- Diagnosis upon discharge
- Instructions given to the patient or the family regarding further care and follow-up
- Signatures and titles of the patient's caregivers

When the patient leaves before being seen or against medical advice, this fact should be noted on the emergency department form. Consent forms for treatment must be included. In cases where there is an emergency or the patient is in critical condition or otherwise unable to sign the consent, an explanation should be documented. A copy of the emergency record should be made available to the provider of follow-up care.

Most states require facilities to maintain an additional chronological record or to register all patients visiting the emergency department with name, date, time of arrival, and record number. This registration also includes the names of patients who were dead on arrival.

Emergency patients must be made aware of their rights. Transfer and acceptance policies and procedures must be delineated to ensure that facilities comply with the Emergency Medical Treatment and Active Labor Act (EMTALA) and state regulations regarding transfers. Patients cannot be transferred or refused treatment for reasons related to ability to pay or source of payment nor can hospitals determine that space is unavailable based on ability to pay or source of payment. Anyone who requests or requires an examination must be provided an appropriate medical screening examination by hospital staff to determine whether a medical emergency exists. Further, the hospital must stabilize the medical emer-

gency by ensuring an airway and ventilation, by controlling hemorrhage, and by stabilizing and/or splinting fractures before a patient can be transferred. The hospital must maintain screening examinations for a period of five years.

Appropriate transfer means that the receiving hospital agrees to receive the patient and provide appropriate medical treatment. Records must be provided to the receiving hospital, and the patient or responsible person must understand the medical necessity of the transfer.

Ambulatory or Outpatient Care

Ambulatory or outpatient care means that patients move from location to location. Patients arrive for treatment and leave after treatment has been administered; they do not stay overnight. Ambulatory or outpatient care may be given in a free-standing clinic, a clinic that is part of a larger hospital system, or a physician or other provider office. When patients are in a clinic affiliated with a hospital, the entire health record should be available. JCAHO requires ambulatory patients to have a summary list by the third visit that includes known diagnoses, conditions, procedures, drug allergies, and medications. It also requires each ambulatory care record to contain a history and physical examination, operative reports, diagnostic and therapeutic procedures, consultations, follow-up notes, observations of patients, and discharge notes at the conclusion or termination of treatment. Contents vary depending on the treatment received.

Ambulatory facilities that only perform surgery are called ambulatory surgery clinics (ASCs). Patients having surgery at any type of ambulatory facility must have a history and physical examination prior to surgery, consents, an operative note, a postoperative progress note, and the same anesthesia information as an operative patient in the hospital. In addition, the record must document instructions for postoperative care and postoperative follow-up. Clinics often call patients after surgery, and these calls should be documented in the record. The Accreditation Association for Ambulatory Health Care requires that the history and physical examination, laboratory reports, radiology reports, operative reports, and consultations be signed in a timely manner. Laboratory and other reports must be included in the patient record as soon as possible.

Traditionally, physician office records have been less comprehensive than hospital medical records. Physicians must develop standardized formats and comprehensive documentation practices.

The focus of ambulatory care is to see or treat patients quickly and then move them efficiently out of the facility. Because of the brief nature of ambulatory care, rapid access to information is vital.

Behavioral Health Care

Behavioral health records, also known as mental health records or psychiatric records, must include diagnostic and assessment information. Medicare requires that the records contain a provisional or admitting diagnosis and the reason for admission, as well as the names of the persons involved in making the admission decision. In addition, a goal-oriented treatment plan must be in place.

Medicare further requires that social service records assess family and home information and community resources available to the patient. Special requirements for a psychiatric evaluation include history, mental status, information on the present illness, and intellectual and memory function. Progress notes must be recorded at least weekly for the first two months and at least once monthly thereafter. Finally, a discharge summary should be written. Special attention must be paid to orders for restraint and seclusion as noted in the discussion on orders.

Home Health Services

According to the National Association for Home Care, the term *home care* covers many types of services "delivered at home to recovering, disabled, chronically or terminally ill persons in need of medical, nursing, social, or therapeutic treatment and/or assistance with the essential activities of daily living" (NAHC 2005). Physicians order home care services that may include visits from many types of healthcare providers, including physicians and nurses. Patient health records must contain a legible record of each visit describing what was done to or for the patient during the visit.

The providers working with patients must develop and document periodic plans of care. Specific forms developed by CMS are used in home care to document and update the plan of care. Verbal orders must be signed before the home health agency submits a bill for payment.

Hospice Care Services

The National Hospice and Palliative Care Organization (NHPO) defines hospice care as a "team-oriented approach to expert medical care, pain management, and emotional and spiritual support expressly tailored to the patient's needs and wishes." Because hospice care is delivered to patients with all types of terminal illnesses, the family is involved in the care and support is given by the hospice organization. Hospice services are provided in numerous types of settings, including homes, hospitals, and long-term care facilities (NHPO 2005). Special documentation for the election of hospice care is required for Medicare to pay it.

Rehabilitation Services

Rehabilitation covers a wide range of services provided to build or rebuild the patient's abilities to perform the usual activities of daily life. Among these services are physical therapy, occupational therapy, and speech therapy.

Physical therapists work in numerous types of facilities, ranging from acute care to long-term care and patient homes, setting goals for patients and helping them reach their goals by building muscle strength and respiratory and circulatory efficiency. Their patients include those who have been disabled for a number of reasons, including birth defect, trauma, and illness. Treatments include exercise, manipulation, heat therapy, light therapy, the use of electricity, and therapeutic massage. In addition to setting treatment goals, physical therapists have to document patient progress.

Occupational therapists are part of the rehabilitation team and work with patients to restore their ability to perform the usual functions of daily life, such as eating, dressing, preparing food, working, and handling other activities specific to the patient. Speech therapists and other specialized therapists are important members of the rehabilitation team and work together to achieve a variety of patient goals.

Long-Term Care

Long-term care describes the care provided for extended periods of time to patients recovering from illness or injury. Long-term care facilities offer a combination of services, ranging from independent living to assisted living to skilled nursing care. Rehabilitation services are often part of the long-term care plan. The long-term care record must document a comprehensive assessment that includes items in the Minimum Data Set (MDS) to meet Medicare requirements stated in 42 CFR 483.20. (Chapter 7 addresses MDS standards for data collection.)

In addition, long-term facilities must meet state requirements. Individualized patient care plans must be developed and included in the health record. These plans must cover the potential for rehabilitation, the ability to perform activities of daily living, medications prescribed, and other aspects of care.

As with acute care facilities, the frequency of notes depends on the patient's condition. The focus in long-term care is on the achievement of goals. The HIM functions are similar to those in other types of facilities, but a great deal of concurrent review is required. Paper records of patients who have been in the facility for an extended period of time must be divided with the most current information maintained on the nursing unit, with the rest filed elsewhere to save space at the nursing station.

Check Your Understanding 8.2

Instructions: On a separate piece of paper, match the contents with the appropriate part of the record by placing the letter for the form in the blank preceding the description of the form's content.

a. Care path
b. History
c. Physical examination
d. Orders
e. Consultations
f. Nursing notes
g. Advance directives
h. Emergency record
i. Discharge summary
j. Ancillary notes

1. ___ Directions given for drugs, devices, and healthcare treatments

2. ___ Comprehensive assessment of patient to determine signs and symptoms

3. ___ Records maintained by physical therapists, speech therapists, respiratory therapists, and other providers of special services

4. ___ Protocol for the process of care

5. ___ Summary of background information about the patient's illness

6. ___ Statement of patient's wishes and/or instructions for care

7. ___ Conclusions at the termination of care

8. ___ Observations of the patient's response to treatment

9. ___ Record that must contain the time and means of arrival and the name of the person transporting the patient to the facility

10. ___ Opinions of specialists

Format of the Paper-Based Health Record

The term *format* refers to the organization of information in the health record. There are many possible formats, and most facilities use a combination of arrangements.

Source-Oriented Health Records

The **source-oriented health record** is the conventional or traditional method of maintaining paper-based health records. In this method, health records are organized according to the source, or originating, department that rendered the service (for example, all lab reports are filed together, all radiological reports are filed together, and so on).

When the patient is in active treatment in the hospital, for example, the record is often maintained in reverse chronological order, with the most recent information on top. Tabs allow easy reference to the grouped reports, enabling staff to quickly find the patient's response to treatment.

After the patient is discharged, many facilities rearrange the record in chronological order. However, the arrangement is still source oriented with all labs together, all progress notes together, and all other related reports filed together in date order. Figure 8.2 (p. 188) shows the arrangement of forms for records maintained in a large acute care hospital. Sometimes facilities leave the record in the same format as it was maintained while the patient was in the facility rather than spend the time rearranging the forms. This is called **universal chart order.**

Problem-Oriented Health Records

Lawrence Weed developed the problem-oriented medical record (POMR) in the 1970s. The POMR comprises the problem list, the database (the history and physical examination and initial lab findings), the initial plan (tests, procedures, and other treatments), and progress notes organized so that every member of the healthcare team can easily follow the course of patient treatment.

A distinctive feature of the POMR is the problem list, which serves as the record's table of contents. All relevant problems—medical, social, or other—that may have an impact on the patient are listed with a number. As problems are resolved, the resolution is noted; new problems are added as they occur. The problem list serves as a permanent index that providers can quickly check to review the status of past

and current problems. JCAHO requires ambulatory records to have a problem list.

The most recognizable component of the POMR is the SOAP format, which is a method for recording progress notes. SOAP is an easy acronym that helps providers remember the specific and systematic decision-making process. *S* stands for subjective findings and includes statements about the patient and symptoms. The subjective findings are followed by objective findings (the *O* in the acronym) such as laboratory and test results and observations and findings from the physical examination. *A* stands for analysis, which consists of appraisals and judgments based on the findings and observations. The *P* stands for plan, which states the need for continuing care or revision of care. Although the full POMR as championed by Weed has not been adopted universally, many physicians and providers routinely use the SOAP method or an adaptation of it to document progress notes and include a problem list in the record.

Integrated Health Records

The content of the **integrated health record** is arranged in strict chronological order. Different types of information and sources of information are mixed together according to the dates on the entries. The order of the record is determined by the date the information was entered, the date of the service, or the date the report was received, not by the source department; and the record gives the sequence of the patient's care as delivered. Although this system makes it difficult to find a particular document unless one knows the date, it does provide a better picture of the story of the patient's care. Physician offices often use this format.

Strengths and Weaknesses of Paper-Based Health Records

The main benefit of paper-based health records is that they are the usual way that records are maintained and, therefore, familiar to all users. Providers do not need technological training to begin documenting in the record. Written documentation is not affected by system outages.

However, paper-based records have numerous disadvantages. The main disadvantage is that only one person at a time can access information. In addition, there are problems with tracking and monitoring locations of the paper record when it is checked out of the HIM department. The filing of loose and/or late-arriving reports also presents a problem. Attaching loose reports is not always a priority in a busy patient care area, and this can result in numerous loose pieces of paper arriving in the HIM department. HIM personnel must route or deliver the forms to the patient care treatment area if the patient is still present in the facility or personnel must sort and file stacks of loose paper forms. Organizing loose reports and attaching them to many individual records can be a formidable job. An entire record or a volume of a paper record can be lost or misfiled, making important patient information unavailable to providers when they need it.

Figure 8.2.   Patient record content

This is not a complete list but does show the types of forms found in most acute care hospitals.

Admission record (face sheet)
Discharge diagnosis information
Identification data
General conditions of admission form
Medicare statements
History
    Chief complaint
    Present illness
    Review of systems
    Past history
    Family history
    Social history
Physical examination
Impression or working diagnosis (part of history and physical or
        admission note)
Plan of care (part of history and physical or admission notes)
Prenatal and labor record
    Labor and delivery summary
    Admission assessment
    Labor progress record
    Infant identification sheet
Physician office record
Copies of records from other facilities
Reports of tests and results
    Laboratory
        Transfusions
        Bone marrow
        Toxicology
        Other special reports
    Radiology includes scans, ultrasounds, arteriograms, MRI, and so on
        EEG
        EKG
        Echocardiograms
        Treadmills
        Holter monitor
        Doppler
Therapy reports
    Physical therapy
    Occupational therapy
    Cardiac rehabilitation
    Respiratory therapy
    GI lab
    Cardiac catheterization
    Other specialty areas
Progress notes, clinical observations, and patient's response to care
Consultation reports
Informed consent
Anesthesia record
Operative room clinical record
Intraoperative report
Postoperative or recovery record
Pathology report

Discharge summary
Final diagnosis
Death
    Consent for autopsy
    Autopsy report, if done
    Release of body
Discharge instructions
Discharge medication orders
Nursing notes and observations
    Medication administration records
    Graphic charts
    Intake-output, temperature, pulse, respirations (vital signs)
Nursing assessments
    Admission assessments
    Care plans
    Critical pathways
Records of donation or receipt of transplants or implants
Advance directives (if brought to the facility by the patient)
Living will (if brought to the facility by the patient)
Power of attorney
Special consents
    Anatomical gifts
    AMA release
    Leave of absence
    Consent to photograph
Emergency record
    Demographic information
    Treatment record
        Triage assessments
        Nurses' notes
        EKG
Newborn records
    Admission record
    Discharge summary
    Consultation
    Consents
    Physician orders/progress notes
    Lab
    Radiology
    Newborn record
    Estimated gestational age
    Medication record
    Initial assessment
    Labor and delivery record
    Infant identification—footprints and photographs
    Newborn ICU delivery room
    Flow sheet
Observation, neonatal, ICU
Nursery progress record
Pediatrician selection form

Source: Methodist Health Systems, Memphis, TN.

The creation of shadow or duplicate systems is also a problem with paper-based health record systems. Some providers are so concerned about the possibility that records can be lost or not located in a timely manner that they create additional records by copying the original records or keeping a separate set of notes. Providers may want to maintain duplicate information for billing purposes. These notes may never become part of the original record or the provider may rely on only the duplicate shadow record without referencing the entire original record, which may have additional information.

Figure 8.3 lists the steps in the usual flow of the paper-based health record in a traditional acute care facility.

Check Your Understanding 8.3

Instructions: On a separate piece of paper, fill in the blanks with the appropriate terms.

1. ____ This is the conventional or traditional method of maintaining paper-based health records.

2. ____ This record is maintained in the same format while the patient is hospitalized and after discharge.

3. ____ This record is maintained in strict chronological order.

4. ____ This record begins with a problem list that serves as the table of contents for the record.

5. ____ This organization provides care to patients who are terminally ill.

6. ____ These services include physical therapy, occupational therapy, and speech therapy.

7. ____ These services range from independent living to assisted living and skilled nursing care.

8. ____ These duplicate notes or copies often do not become a part of the original record.

Figure 8.3. Steps in the flow of the paper-based patient health record following discharge

1. Records of discharged patients arrive or are delivered to HIM department.

2. Receipt of records is verified by comparing discharge lists to actual charts received.

3. Folder corresponding to records is pulled.

4. Record is assembled according to prescribed format ensuring that all pages belong to the correct patient and that forms are in correct date order.

5. Deficiencies such as signatures, reports needing completion, and so on are assigned to the responsible provider.

6. Diagnoses and procedures are coded.

7. Record is held for final completion by providers either in incomplete chart area or some other filing area.

8. Charts are rechecked after the providers have done their work to ensure that all have been completed.

9. The complete record is filed in the permanent filing area.

Staffing of the Health Information Department

The HIM department's organization varies according to the type of organization. Long-term care facilities may have a very small HIM department with one person in charge or with responsibility for records that are assigned as part of an administrative position. Some long-term care facilities use outside consultants to handle the functions of record keeping.

In contrast, large acute care facilities often employ many HIM professionals, including a department director. Other HIM professionals manage specific areas or functions such as coding, analysis, assembly, transcription, release of information (ROI), imaging, storage, filing, and retrieval. In addition, large facilities sometimes use contract personnel to perform transcription, coding, ROI, and other activities.

In facilities with large ambulatory patient populations and paper-based record systems, health records frequently move in and out of the HIM department. Records must be pulled from the file for clinic appointments and for walk-in patients without appointments; the records need to be delivered and picked up, and then refiled. Any reports of tests or treatments that arrive separately from the record must be attached to the record quickly. Patients may have several appointments in several different clinics, resulting in many transfers of patient records to various providers. Tracking chart location is critical because so many providers, including resident physicians, use the record.

Management of Health Record Content

The HIM professional manages health record content through oversight responsibilities of transcription, in which dictated information is converted into usable output—for example, clinical reports—that become part of the record. The responsibilities for incomplete records include analyzing and monitoring incomplete records to ensure that they are properly completed to meet facility standards and patient healthcare needs and controlling the design and production of forms to ensure that all records are in a standardized format.

Transcription

Completion of the health record is greatly enhanced by the sophisticated dictation and transcription equipment in use today. Physicians and other providers first dictate the necessary reports, including, but not limited to, history and physical examinations, operative reports, discharge summaries, consultations, progress notes, clinic notes, pathology reports, and radiology reports. The dictation then is converted to final printed output to become a part of the legal health record. Personnel who type, that is, transcribe, the dictation are called medical transcriptionists. Facilities should encourage providers to dictate so that reports can be accessed electronically.

Components of a Transcription System

The system encompasses both the dictation and transcription process. The physician or provider dictates into a variety of devices, including a telephone by calling a special number connected to the facility's dictation system or by using a special phone dedicated only to dictation. The dictation also may be recorded using a separate handheld recorder onto a cassette tape that is delivered to the department. Input from personal computers (PCs) or handheld personal computer devices called Personal Digital Assistants (PDAs) is becoming more prevalent. Whatever the means of input by the dictator, a transcriptionist retrieves the dictated voice and transcribes the content. The transcription may be performed on-site at the facility or off-site from a remote location. The final product, the transcribed report, is sent for review to the physician or provider, who signs the report authenticating it as the final approved original for inclusion in the legal health record. **Authentication** may be done on the printed report or electronically in the computer system. The facility's policies must specify that the signature indicates that the physician or provider who dictated the report has reviewed and corrected it (if necessary) and approves the content of the report..

Digital dictation is the process by which voice sounds are recorded and coverted into a digital format. The physician or provider begins the dictation process using a telephone, a microphone attached to a PC, or a hands-free microphone. The dictator enters digits to indicate certain basic information, such as identification of the dictator, identification of the patient, and the type of report to be dictated (a history and physical examination, a discharge summary, an operative report, and so on).

The dictation then is transmitted to a computer that digitizes the voice. After the voice sounds have been digitized, the dictation is accessed by the transcriptionist who transcribes the report by listening to the voice and converting it to typed output. Special software features allow the transcriptionist to produce reports with as few keystrokes as possible, using techniques such as word expanders. Word expanders are shortened versions of phrases. For example, the keystrokes WDWN are changed to produce typed output as "well-developed, well-nourished." Some facilities use normal reports or macros that the dictator can direct the transcriptionist to edit and tailor to the individual patient.

Digital systems allow the dictated information to be managed in order so that emergency reports that have to be completed quickly are produced first. The dictation can be easily located by utilizing any pieces of information that are provided by the dictator. Digital systems automatically time-stamp the date and time the work was dictated and the time the transcription was started and completed. Random access by the transcriptionist allows the workload to be shared and distributed among several transcriptionists. Providers and other appropri-

ate staff can dial in and listen to the recorded information rather than wait until the final report is transcribed. Coders can listen to the dictated recorded information and code from the discharge summary and other dictated reports rather than wait for the actual transcribed reports. The typed output can be faxed automatically to the physician's office, printed out in the transcription area, printed out to clinics or patient floors, uploaded into the electronic medical record (EMR), and tied into the chart completion system.

Providers can review transcribed documents online and may have editing capabilities. In some systems, both the original and the final edited versions become part of the legal patient health record.

PCs may also be used as recording devices rather than using a dedicated dictation station. A radiologist can view an image on the PC monitor and dictate into either a headset or an attached handheld microphone. One advantage is that the computer equipment may be used for multiple purposes other than dictation.

Speech recognition, or **voice recognition technology,** is used increasingly as the accuracy of input improves. In voice recognition technology, the spoken word is transmitted immediately to a database and converted to typed output, which eliminates the need for the transcriptionist to listen to and type the information. The quality of the output is very dependent on the quality of the dictation. The speaker must speak clearly and distinctly. The role of the transcriptionist will change as this new technology increases in accuracy. In time, the transcriptionist will become primarily an editor and proofreader. Speech recognition technology may be utilized on the front end where the person dictates through a microphone or headset apparatus connected to a PC. As the person dictates, the words appear on the screen and are corrected if they are not displayed correctly. The document is correct when completed and the dictator controls the entire process. The facility may still require the document to be sent to a transcriptionist or other person who controls its distribution. This method also requires training of the individual who is dictating and the dictator may feel that this process is too slow and takes too much physician time. In back-end speech recognition, the physician dictates in the usual manner, the audio is sent as a draft text along with the speech file to the transcriptionist who serves as an editor to listen to the audio in comparison with the displayed text and to make changes to the text document. This document then goes back to the dictator for approval. The advantage is that the person dictating does not have to change dictation behavior. Back-end speech recognition (also called server-based speech recognition) does not improve productivity because editing is as time-consuming as transcribing. Radiology departments and other departments that have many repetitive reports can utilize speech recognition technology more effectively than the general facility as a whole.

Turnaround times for transcribing dictated reports for different types of work are developed by the HIM department, administration, and physicians in order to meet patient care needs. For example, history and physical examination reports have a strict turnaround time due to JCAHO requirements that required them to be attached to the record prior to surgery. Consultation reports also often have a very short turnaround time. Operative reports, on the other hand, may be assigned a turnaround time of two to three days. And discharge summaries may have a lower priority for transcription if the digital system allows coders and other personnel to access and listen to them. Turnaround times are utilized as key indicators in assessing the quality and productivity of the transcription area.

Planning for and Selecting Transcription Equipment

When purchasing or upgrading a dictation and/or transcription system, the HIM professional must be aware of the long-range consequences of this important decision. Equipment vendors can provide a wealth of information based on their experience and work in various facilities. They can help the HIM department determine the number of ports, or entry points, that need to be available based on the number of dictators and transcriptionists requiring simultaneous access. The system needs to have sufficient accessibility to avoid collision, which would prevent a dictator or transcriptionist from gaining access to the system. Immediate access for all users, whether dictating or transcribing, is critical to the system's success. When dictators call in, a digital channel selector automatically selects an available line without input from the dictator.

In addition, it is important to anticipate the amount of recording time necessary to meet current needs and to have sufficient space available to meet future needs. Recording time is often stored on two drives so that backup, or redundancy, is available in case one drive fails. Dictation/transcription systems need to interface with existing facility information systems (ISs) to ensure that a method exists to automatically download identification information from the **master patient index** (MPI). Physicians or providers and transcriptionists do not have to enter a great deal of information, and this promotes accuracy and consistency in patient identification. Password protection also needs to be in place to ensure that only authorized persons can access the system.

The facility must have vendor support to keep the system operational at all times. Transcription systems should be designed so that the transcriptionists can work independently if the general facility information system is not working. Although entering patient information without the connection will require greater effort, the work can continue to be generated.

Transcription systems may be designed to archive, or save, dictated information for any length of time. Some facilities archive for 90 days and others for six or more months. Long periods of storage may cause the system to work more slowly, but the advantage is continued access. Even if dictated reports are not attached to the paper health records, the people who need the information for coding and billing purposes, quality studies, indexes, registries, and other operational needs can still access and utilize the information.

Transcription can be centralized or decentralized. In a decentralized system, pathology, radiology, and other departments may have their own transcriptionists. Some HIM departments have centralized transcription areas that type reports for the whole facility or for all facilities in an integrated system. Moreover, some transcription departments perform work for physician offices in order to generate revenue. The transcription department must consider every possible customer and analyze every possible location for a dedicated dictation station, including nurses' stations, clinics, operative areas, and workrooms in the HIM department. Further, every acceptable format (for example, separate tapes of different sizes or downloads from PCs or PDAs) must be determined and policies established for the types of recordings that are allowed. Using a variety of input devices will cause productivity problems and prevent full utilization of the dictation and transcription system's capabilities. In physician offices and clinics, cassette tapes are used more often for dictation purposes than in larger facilities.

The HIM professional must fully understand the dictation and transcription system application. A **certified medical transcriptionist** (CMT) may supervise the transcription area, but the manager of the HIM department is ultimately responsible for the work. Before purchasing any large system, the HIM professional should interview references and visit similar facilities to see the system in action. Often the vendor will arrange these site visits. The HIM professional also might visit facilities that are using the equipment under consideration but have not been specifically recommended by the vendor. Further, he or she might attend trade shows and seminars and narrow the field to avoid confusion. In addition, he or she should include the people who will actually use the system in the decision-making process.

Finally, transcription equipment lasts five to seven years. Vendors play an important role in keeping the HIM professional aware of system upgrades and enhancements to ensure that the department gets as much use out of its system as possible.

Issues in the Management of Transcription

Although transcription, is just one function of the HIM department, it often requires a great deal of the department's attention. A backlog of dictated minutes waiting to be transcribed is an issue that needs constant monitoring to be sure turnaround times are met. History and physical examination reports and operative reports have accreditation and regulatory time limitations. Turnaround time from dictation to transcribed report is important because providers must be able to retrieve information when it is needed for patient care.

Recruitment and retention of qualified medical transcriptionists are major problems for HIM professionals.

Transcription equipment is expensive to acquire and to maintain, and the equipment and technology are changing rapidly. Skilled medical transcriptionists who can accurately transcribe dictation are in short supply, and the role of the medical transcriptionist is evolving. This evolution is discussed in the following sections.

Internal versus Outsourcing Transcription

The facility must decide whether to handle transcription services in-house, to contract with (or outsource to) transcription companies outside the facility, or to use a combination of internal and **contract services.**

Outsourcing to transcription service companies, or contract services, is on the rise. Some healthcare facilities routinely contract all or a portion of their workload; others use the contract service on an as-needed basis. The major advantage to a contract service is that it can save the facility money in terms of salaries, fringe benefits, equipment, depreciation, floor space, maintenance, workstations, supplies, and reference materials. Further, use of an outside service can eliminate problems associated with overloading the system with increased dictation prior to a JCAHO survey or at times when medical residents change clinical service rotations in a teaching facility. Although outsourcing transcription services is an attractive option, it must be analyzed carefully. The major disadvantages to outsourcing are the loss of control over the transcription service and the high cost of contract transcription services.

When selecting a contract service, the HIM professional should become as familiar with the company as possible. A growing number of offshore companies or U.S.-based companies send work via the Internet to transcription personnel in other countries. Such companies must provide assurance that their transcriptionists are bonded, trained in confidentiality, and well supervised.

The manner in which the company handles a sudden influx of work is important because this is one of the major reasons why healthcare facilities use outside transcription companies. The exact method and rationale for billing and counting the final product also is extremely important. The HIM professional should question the exact definitions of a line, word, page, keystroke, minutes, or bytes or whether style requirements such as capitalizing, boldface, or underlining are an additional charge.

The counting method should be fully explained in the contract. Most companies charge by the line, but the definition of a line may be 65 characters rather than a physical line. For example, if physical lines are counted and the facility is paying $0.13 to $0.18 per line, the costs can add up in situations where one word on a line is considered a line. Using a smaller font to increase the amount of typing per line may be more costly because a smaller type may scan into an imaging system and or microfilm poorly. Some companies base their charge on turnaround time, with an increased cost per line when transcription is completed within a shorter time frame.

For example, the charge for transcription within 48 hours would be $0.10 a line; within 24 hours, $0.12 a line; and within 8 hours, $0.18 a line. In addition, the company may include disk storage costs of $2.00 to $6.00 per five minutes of dictation.

Billing can be complicated, and the HIM professional must determine the true cost of the outside contract company's service so that he or she can compare alternatives accurately. The distribution and delivery method and the number of copies provided by the company must be evaluated because reprints might cost as much as the original transcribed document. Some companies transmit information back to the facility to be printed by the facility or send information via the Internet, fax, overnight delivery service, or courier. The contract needs to state whether the facility or the company will pay for the service. Also, there may be an additional charge for corrections. If the facility allows physicians or providers to dictate on other devices instead of directly into the dictation system, this may affect the cost.

The facility also must assess how the outside company's equipment will integrate with the facility's current system, for example, with regard to phone lines, software, and interface with the electronic record system, if one exists. If the printing is to be done in-house (in the facility), responsibility for printer maintenance and supply costs must be determined. The quality of the work performed by the contract company must be evaluated in terms of content, proper abbreviation use, typing and spelling errors, general appearance, correction of grammatical errors, and correct spelling of physician names. Some companies provide several levels of proofreading, including by a physician. However, proofreading also must be performed by the healthcare facility, and the facility must maintain the dictation sound so that quality checks can be performed on the outside service's work to ensure that what was dictated was what was actually typed. The HIM professional must make sure the work is closely monitored.

Even with a contract service, the health information manager still has oversight responsibility for the outside contract service and quality control. Facility personnel must file the printed reports in the health record and distribute them to residents, referring physicians, and consultants, as appropriate. Further, contracts must be carefully reviewed to ensure that contract services provide for the security of patient information.

The HIM professional also must ensure fast and easy access to the system. If physicians and coders have the ability to listen to dictation prior to transcribing, this should not change when transcription is outsourced.

Staffing of the Transcription Area

When the healthcare facility chooses to do transcription internally, the staff must be carefully selected to ensure that transcription is of high quality. Each applicant for a transcription position should be tested using the kind of work to be performed to confirm that he or she can type from the dictated word. In addition, the applicant must have excellent concentration skills, excellent hearing skills, and excellent proofreading and editing skills.

Applicants who are CMTs are in great demand. The Medical Transcription Certification Commission grants certification upon the successful completion of an examination. The requirements for this voluntary examination are experience or formal education or both. The CMT must maintain currency and certification by earning continuing education (CE) hours. Proprietary business schools and community colleges offer formal educational programs and are excellent sources for transcriptionists. A healthcare facility's offer to allow students to obtain clinical experience at the facility is an excellent way to attract applicants. Some healthcare facilities offer on-the-job training to persons with excellent typing skills.

The **American Association for Medical Transcription** (AAMT) has a model curriculum for formal educational programs. The curriculum includes the study of medical terminology, anatomy and physiology, medical science, operative procedures, instruments, supplies, laboratory values, reference use and research techniques, and English grammar. All applicants should have knowledge of the areas of the model curriculum.

In addition, the AAMT produces a bimonthly journal and has excellent reference materials. CE opportunities are available for transcription professionals. Transcriptionists must be given the opportunity to participate in CE activities and to be updated in new medical procedures, tests, and terminology.

The AAMT has a model job description with three defined levels for the professional transcriptionist. Some facilities may use these levels as a guide for levels of classification of personnel and promotions.

Telestaffing, or telecommuting, is a growing alternative to transcriptionists working in-house (in the facility). In telestaffing, personnel are allowed to work from home or some other remote location. This has been very successful for healthcare facilities, although remote transcriptionists require special supervisory attention. They need to feel that they are part of the HIM department. The supervisor must ensure ongoing communication with telestaffing employees via e-mail or by bringing them to the facility for CE meetings and interaction with other departmental personnel. Some healthcare facilities offer telecommuting only to employees who have been with them for a period of time, fully understand the system, and are known to be responsible and dependable. Transcriptionists working outside the healthcare facility use a telephone line or cable connection to access the system. The facility supplies the transcriptionist with the telephone line, the computer workstation, and reference materials. Transcriptionists working from home must be held to the same production and quality standards as in-house transcriptionists and must be fully trained in the security and confidentiality of healthcare information.

Determining the number of transcriptionists needed in relation to the number of providers dictating is challeng-

ing and depends on the types and amount of information typed, the specialties of the facility, whether the facility is a teaching hospital or a clinic, and the types of nontranscription duties assigned to the transcriptionists, among other factors. In a clinic or physician office, transcription may be done as part of a larger job. Vendors can be of assistance in determining the volume of work. The type and length of work also must be evaluated. A random sample of each type of work should be selected and counted. Some vendors suggest that lines be counted for 10 reports of each type to determine an average number. A line is defined as 65 characters. Generally, the average transcriptionist on an eight-hour shift can produce 1,200 lines per day. There are approximately 10 lines per one minute of dictation; 5 minutes equals 50 lines; 10 minutes equals 100 lines. These averages, which represent the standard used by many equipment vendors, will assist the HIM professional in determining staffing needs.

Fluctuations in work flow may occur for numerous reasons depending on the healthcare facility. Hospitals have peak times, for example, before an accreditation survey, after notices are sent to physicians to complete charts, and when residents and medical students change service rotations. Teaching hospitals often have much longer hours of dictation to transcribe as medical students learn the art of taking histories and performing physical examinations. Medical students dictate much more detailed information than more experienced physicians. Transcription backlogs and turnaround times are constant issues that must be examined.

Productivity Management

Pay for transcription varies depending on whether the transcriptionist works for a healthcare facility or a contract service. Entry-level transcriptionists may be paid by the hour. Some contract services pay transcriptionists more per hour for straight production typing, but the transcriptionists may not have the benefits that are available to the employees of a healthcare facility. The AAMT has excellent current information about productivity on its Web site at www.aamt.org.

Quality is vitally important in transcription. The supervisor must review the quality of work produced on a regular basis. Among the items to review are punctuation errors, omitted dictation, misspelled words or medical terms, and formatting errors. An analysis of each transcriptionist's errors will target those areas that need improvement.

The facility may use numerous possible standards. For example, 10 lines of typing produced for every one minute of dictation might be translated into three or four minutes of typing for every minute of dictation. There is a great deal of debate over what the standard production, or even the best unit of measurement, should be.

Incentive Programs

Because of the competition for CMTs, many healthcare facilities offer **incentive pay** plans to reward transcriptionists for high productivity. For example, a hospital may require a transcriptionist to type eight hours a day and produce 1,200 lines of typed output for a base monthly salary. Beyond 1,200 lines, the transcriptionist may earn a bonus of $0.06 per line, with the bonus cents per line increasing to the point where a transcriptionist typing 2,001 lines would receive a bonus of $0.12 per line. However, the quality of the work must remain at 98 percent accuracy based on regular quality review.

For fairness in the incentive system, work must be rotated so that each transcriptionist has the opportunity to perform different kinds of work from different providers. Providers for whom English is a second language may produce dictation that is more difficult to transcribe. Moreover, some providers are not careful in their dictation, which requires more listening and replaying.

The proponents of incentive pay plans believe that monetary incentives increase productivity, reduce turnover, provide fair and equitable pay, and motivate employees. Highly productive transcriptionists are paid for what they produce.

Evaluation of the Effectiveness and Efficiency of Transcription Services

The effectiveness and efficiency of transcription services are judged primarily by turnaround time and accuracy in typing the dictation. History and physical examinations and operative reports have time limitations set forth in JCAHO regulations. Discharge summaries are valuable sources of information for coding, billing, and reimbursement. With EMR systems, the dictated information and transcribed documents are accessible to all providers and healthcare personnel who need to refer to them. The success of the transcription service depends on both the cooperation of the providers who dictate and the skills of the medical transcriptionists.

Check Your Understanding 8.4

Instructions: Answer the following questions on a separate sheet of paper.

1. What are the advantages of using a contract transcription system? What are the advantages of having transcription performed in-house?

2. What are the formal educational requirements for a certified medical transcriptionist?

3. How will speech recognition technology change the job of the medical transcriptionist?

4. What are the four benefits of an incentive pay plan?

5. What factors must be considered when determining the number of transcriptionists a healthcare facility needs?

Incomplete Record Control

Health records must be completed in order to provide all the information that is needed for patient care, billing, and reimbursement. The HIM department must verify that all records are received from the nursing floor, including records of any previous admissions that were sent to the nursing unit. After the records arrive in the HIM department, their location must be carefully tracked until they reach final storage in the filing area.

The financial office notifies the HIM department of bills that are waiting for information from the physician so that the record can be coded and the bill prepared. The administration places a great deal of pressure on the HIM department to process bills in a timely manner so that revenue can be generated for the facility. In turn, the HIM professional must motivate physicians to provide the information the department needs to do its work. Incomplete records are a chronic problem in most healthcare facilities, and monitoring them is a constant challenge for the HIM professional.

Quantitative Analysis

Quantitative analysis, often called **discharge analysis,** is a review of the health record for completeness and accuracy. It is generally conducted retrospectively, that is, after the patient's discharge from the facility or at the conclusion of treatment. Quantitative analysis also may be done while the patient is in the facility, in which case it is referred to as concurrent review or **concurrent analysis.**

One component of the discharge analysis process is to rearrange the forms in the paper-based health record in a standard permanent sequence for filing. This order differs from the sequencing of forms while patients are under active treatment when convenient reference to certain information is needed. While in active use, the health record is arranged with the most current information on top as follows: orders, progress or clinic notes, operative notes, medications, graphic sheets, nursing notes, consultations, ancillary forms, consents, history and physical, demographic information, and face sheet. The order differs according to the facility, but the record forms the provider prepares and writes on most frequently are on top to allow for quick entry of orders and progress notes. Labeled tabs divide the chart into sections to assist in finding needed documents.

When the patient is discharged or treatment is terminated, the record arrives in the HIM department, where it is immediately rearranged in reverse order. The face sheet and demographic information are on top, followed by the history and physical examination, the discharge summary, ancillary reports, consents, operative reports, progress notes in date order with the earliest orders first, orders in date order, nursing notes in date order, and so forth. Many facilities leave the record in the order in which it arrives in the HIM department rather than spend the time to rearrange it. This system is called universal chart order or uniform chart order. The benefits of the system are that time is saved in the HIM department and providers can more easily find the parts of the record they need because the arrangement remains the same.

A facility moving to universal chart order must involve nursing and physicians in the decisions about chart arrangement because they use the record as a reference for patient care every day. Labeled dividers and a standard table of contents help ensure that everyone who works with the chart knows the proper arrangement.

Quantitative analysis involves several additional steps. The record forms must be reviewed individually to make sure they belong in the record and belong to that particular patient. Organizing the paper forms is an important step. Forms are often intermingled and usually separated into a source-oriented format. Preliminary laboratory reports may be discarded when there is a final cumulative summary report.

Each facility must develop its own procedures for quantitative analysis. Responsibility for completion of the record must be assigned to each responsible provider. This is called deficiency assignment. The deficiencies, or parts of the record needing completion or signature, are entered into a computer software program or on paper worksheets attached to the incomplete, or deficient, health record.

Moreover, the record must be reviewed to ensure that certain basic reports that are common to all patient records are present, including the history and physical, progress notes, orders, nursing notes, and discharge summary. Other reports (for example, operative reports, diagnostic tests, consultations, and so on) may be included depending on the patient's course of treatment. Quantitative analysis also includes a review for authentication that may be done by written signature, rubber stamp facsimile, computer password, or initials, and must include the professional title of the responsible individual.

Any corrections to the record must be entered properly. The provider should draw a single line through the error, add a note explaining the error, initial and date the error with the date it was discovered, and make the correct entry in chronological order. The entry being replaced also must be indicated. For computer entries, a procedure should be followed that explains how to correct errors and make addenda to the health record.

Criteria for Adequacy of Documentation

Documentation must reflect the care rendered to the patient and the patient's response. It must be timely and legible and signed by the person who wrote it. The health record is considered a legal document and a business record because it records events at or about the time they happen. Timeliness and legibility are two of the main areas of focus for accreditation and licensure bodies.

Moreover, the record must be analyzed to ensure that symbols and abbreviations used in documentation have been approved by the medical staff and have only one clear meaning.

Concurrent analysis means that the record is analyzed during the patient's stay in the healthcare facility. It has the advantage of HIM or other personnel being present on the floors where the physicians see patients. HIM personnel can remind providers to complete items in the record and to sign orders and progress notes. Some facilities have HIM personnel physically located on the nursing floors to monitor record completion closely. Other facilities have HIM personnel visit patient care areas to obtain signatures and ensure that loose reports are placed in the health record.

After the patient is discharged, the record is brought to the HIM department by delivery or by HIM personnel who pick up records. Discharge analysis serves as an additional check to ensure that the record is complete and that all information belongs to the patient. Concurrent review and discharge analysis review the records for the same documentation.

Record Completion Policies and Procedures

The health record is not complete until all its parts are assembled, organized, and authenticated. The HIM professional, the administration, and the medical staff must develop record completion policies and procedures and include them in the medical staff bylaws. Although the facility's governing body has overall responsibility for patient care, responsibility for the delivery and documentation of patient care is delegated to the medical staff. The medical staff and the individual physician have primary responsibility for completing the health record to document the process of care that was rendered.

Most facilities have a committee in place composed of members of the medical staff, the administration, nursing, and other provider disciplines with responsibility for ensuring that medical staff members follow the established rules and regulations for health records. This committee may be the health record committee, the quality committee, or some other committee responsible for ensuring compliance with rules and regulations. The HIM professional should serve on the committee and generally assist the physician or provider committee chair by preparing the agenda and minutes for meetings.

The HIM professional also assists the committee by preparing reports on the status of record completion and problems with the flow of the record through the facility. Reports regarding the percentage of records are important to ensure that accreditation standards are met on an ongoing basis. The findings from various types of record review, including concurrent reviews and retrospective reviews, are presented to the committee and discussed. The committee often plays a key role in the approval of forms so that the standard form and format of the record can be maintained.

The committee chair may communicate directly with physicians or other medical staff members to solve problems related to record completion. The committee can be a valuable resource to the HIM professional because it has representation from every area that enters documents into the patient record. Committee members can often assist the HIM department in acquiring equipment and personnel needed to properly perform its responsibilities. The committee generally reports to the executive committee of the medical staff and makes recommendations for executive staff action to improve patient record services.

Qualitative Analysis

In **qualitative analysis,** HIM personnel carefully review the quality and adequacy of record documentation and ensure that it is in accordance with the policies, rules, and regulations established by the facility, the standards of licensing and accrediting bodies, and government requirements. Like quantitative analysis, qualitative analysis may be done concurrently or retrospectively.

Qualitative analysis is a more in-depth review of health records than quantitative analysis is, although the processes may overlap somewhat, depending on the facility. When qualitative analysis is done while the patient is in the facility or under active treatment, it is called open-record review, **ongoing records review, point-of-care review,** or **continuous record review.** JCAHO requires an open-record review to ensure that its documentation standards are met at the point of care delivery. A specific format for open-record review covers all types of records. HIM personnel or case management personnel, nurses, physicians, and other providers should participate in the open-record review process. This review process looks at requirements such as presence of the history and physical examination prior to surgery, completion of the postoperative note, and many other aspects of the care process as documented in the health record. Open-record review should be done on an ongoing basis.

Qualitative review also is performed on **closed records. Closed-record review** means that the qualitative review is done retrospectively following discharge or termination of treatment. The benefit of open-record review is that problems in the care process that are revealed through the review can be corrected immediately. Closed-record review is an important way to obtain information about trends and patterns of documentation.

Role of Health Information Management Professionals
Medicare and state licensure standards require healthcare facilities to have an HIM department with administrative responsibility for health records. This includes having the staff, equipment, and policies and procedures to ensure that records are current and accurate and that information is accessible.

The HIM department works closely with the finance department regarding chart completion. The finance department and the entire organization depend on the HIM staff to work with physicians and other healthcare professionals to provide the necessary information so that bills can be finalized. Bills are usually sent within two to three days after discharge. The health information manager receives daily notification of accounts that need information, and procedures must be established to expedite the flow of information for payment purposes.

Role of the Medical Staff
Medical staff members are responsible for developing bylaws governing their operation. The requirements for documentation and completion of health records as well as penalties for not adhering to them are included in the medical staff bylaws. Each member of the medical staff signs a statement that he or she will abide by the bylaws, and each is responsible for documentation.

Management of Incomplete Records

The HIM professional is responsible for ensuring that health records, whether manual or electronic, are readily accessible and that adequate equipment and personnel are available to facilitate record completion. No matter how well staffed and well organized the HIM department is, it can only facilitate the process. The providers are responsible for the documentation and must dictate, sign, and otherwise complete the patient health record.

Storage, Retrieval, and Tracking of Incomplete Records
Facilities provide access to incomplete records in various ways. Paper-based records needing completion are maintained in an area that is easily accessible to physicians. They may be arranged alphabetically by the last name of the responsible physician or filed in numerical order. Filing by physician name enables physicians to go directly to their own boxes to access and complete their own records.

One disadvantage is that completion is often delayed because the record may remain in one physician's box until it is completed and moved to the next box. In a facility with many specialists or many residents, maintaining incomplete records in numerical order by the patient's record number works well because the records are accessible to all providers who need to complete them. Other facilities file incomplete records alphabetically by the patient's last name. Still other facilities immediately file the records into the general file area, using a combination of filing methods. When only one provider needs to work on a record, it is filed under that provider's name; when several physicians need to work on the records, a numerical system is used. The advantage is that records are all filed in one area for ease of location by the clerical staff.

In any of these arrangements, clerical staff must be available to assist providers and to ensure that the portions of the record that need to be completed are actually done. When incomplete records are filed numerically, the facility might require physicians to call before arriving at the department so that the needed records can be pulled. Some HIM personnel speed up record completion by taking records to physicians' offices located on the hospital campus.

The completion time clock begins running when the patient is discharged or expires or when treatment is terminated. Records are considered deficient or incomplete immediately at discharge. Some facilities choose to begin the time clock after the records are reviewed quantitatively by the HIM staff and made available to the providers; however, regulations and standards do not provide for "extra" time for analysis or transcription delays, computer system downtime, or physician unavailability. Healthcare facility policies and medical staff bylaws must define when incomplete or deficient records become delinquent.

Delinquent health records are those records that are not completed within the specified time frame, for example, within 14 days of discharge. The definition of a delinquent chart varies according to the facility, but most facilities require that records be completed within 30 days of discharge as mandated by Medicare regulations and JCAHO standards. Some facilities require a shorter time frame for completing records because of concerns about timely billing. **Chart tracking** of the location of incomplete and delinquent records as they move through the completion process is vital because many people need access to the records of recently treated patients.

Policies and Procedures on Record Completion
When analyzing the record, HIM personnel list what needs to be done to complete it. This may be done by filling in a form listing the providers and items needing completion or signatures or by entering information into a computerized deficiency system. Physicians can then access the system to determine what they need to do.

Numerous other methods may be used to encourage the timely completion of records. JCAHO specifies that the number of delinquent records cannot exceed 50 percent of the average number of discharges, so keeping the number of delinquent charts as low as possible is a constant challenge for HIM staff. Concurrent analysis by HIM personnel can help speed up completion time. Using case managers to work with physicians on chart completion issues while the patient is in the facility also helps reduce the burden on the HIM department. HIM professionals rely on medical staff committees, such as the health record committee, chiefs of medical services, and medical staff leaders to motivate providers to complete records. They and healthcare administrators are willing to try any creative ideas that will motivate physicians to complete patient health records.

Many facilities limit the retrospective checking and flagging of incomplete items in the HIM department to the discharge summary, history and physical examination, operative reports, consultations, and clinical reports. Nursing information is not reviewed nor are signatures on progress notes and orders checked. Less detailed analysis is done after discharge due to the increased emphasis on open-record review when patients are in the facility under active treatment. Requiring physicians to sign notes and orders retrospectively does not affect the process of patient care and treatment. The HIM department should continue to monitor a sample of notes and orders to ensure that signatures are present to comply with established facility policies, accreditation standards, and regulations. Corrective measures should be developed when there is a pattern of missing signatures.

As mentioned above, penalties for noncompletion of health records must be included in medical staff bylaws. Penalties such as suspension of admission privileges or surgical privileges for the individual physician and/or group and the levying of fines per incomplete chart or per day must be explained in the bylaws. Some hospitals make health record completion a condition of continued membership on the medical staff and suspend physicians who do not comply with the rules regarding completion. Suspended physicians must reapply for staff membership. Some states require that physicians suspended three times in a year be reported to the state medical board. However, in some small facilities or in facilities where the physician is responsible for many admissions, it is difficult to enforce the rules regarding suspension of admitting privileges.

Each facility must have a policy in place for dealing with situations where records remain incomplete for an extended period. The HIM director can be given authority to declare that a record is complete for purposes of filing when a provider dies or has an extended illness that would prevent the record from ever being completed. Every effort should be made to have a partner or physician in the same specialty area complete the chart so that coding, billing, and statistical information is available. In teaching hospitals, residents sometimes leave before charts are completed and become difficult to locate. Thus, many facilities require departing residents to obtain clearance from the HIM department before the end of the residency period. The medical staff committee responsible for health record functions may review long-standing incomplete charts and direct that they be filed even though incomplete.

Physician Notification Processes
Most healthcare facilities notify physicians of charts that need completion on an escalating basis. For example, the first notice reminds the physician that records need completion, the second describes the penalties for noncompletion, the third limits the admission or operative privileges of the physician and his or her partners and might include suspension of even emergency admission privileges, and the fourth gives a warning regarding suspension or removal from the medical staff. Finally, the physician may be considered to have forfeited staff membership and would have to reapply for membership. Some teaching facilities withhold paychecks for residents or refuse to approve vacations until all the physician's charts are complete.

The HIM department is responsible for counting incomplete charts and preparing lists of those providers who have delinquent records and those whose privileges have been suspended. Extensions are often granted when physicians are out of town, sick, have a death in the family, and so on. The handling of physician suspensions requires a great deal of cooperation among the HIM professional, the medical staff leadership, and the administration.

Authentication of Health Record Entries
Authentication means to prove authorship by signing a document and can be done in several ways. Signatures handwritten in ink are the most common method for signing paper-based health records. JCAHO allows rubber-stamp facsimile signatures when there is a statement verifying that the physician is the only one who will use the stamp and will maintain control of it.

Autoauthentication is a policy that allows the physician or provider to state in advance that dictated and transcribed reports should automatically be considered approved and signed when the physician does not make corrections within a certain period of time. Another variation of autoauthentication is that physicians authorize the HIM department to send a weekly list of documents needing signatures. The list is then signed and returned to the HIM department. Some facilities use autoauthentication even though JCAHO does not approve it. The objection is that evidence cannot be provided that the physician actually reviewed and approved each report. Facilities that use these methods of authentication state that the physician offices automatically receive copies of transcribed reports and thus providers have the ability to review the reports before the deadline or before signing the list of reports.

An **electronic signature** or e-signature is defined by AHIMA as, "The system for assigning electronic documents by entering a unique code or password that verifies the identity of the healthcare practitioner and creates an individual signature on the record" (AHIMA 2003). A statement ensuring that the password is controlled and used only by the responsible provider should be required to protect patient confidentiality and to ensure that others do not use it. Password security is critical. Electronic signatures will be used more frequently as more documents in the record are produced by, and remain in, the computer and do not become part of the paper record. Facilities that scan paper records of discharged patients into imaging systems must make it clear to physicians that these are images of papers that can be viewed but not edited or signed.

Signatures in teaching hospitals are especially important to show that the attending physician responsible for the patient is actively involved in the patient's care. Signatures are generally required on all reports completed by residents and medical students. In electronic signature programs, the attending physician's cosignature should be entered after the resident has reviewed and signed the report to confirm the attending physician's participation.

Forms Design and Management

The management and design of forms used in the healthcare environment is a concern of all providers. Forms must be developed and approved in a careful, systematic process to ensure that they meet facility standards, are compatible with imaging and **microfilming** systems, and do not duplicate information on existing forms. (Examples of commonly used health record forms are provided in appendix A of this book.) HIM department personnel must be constantly vigilant to ensure that only approved forms become part of the permanent health record. Unapproved forms do not have the necessary form numbers or bar codes needed for imaging and indexing systems. Small forms and folded flowcharts create problems when records are handled and utilized. Oversize forms create problems in microfilming or optical imaging because special preparation is required to ensure that all information is filmed or scanned. As health records move toward a computer-based format, the forms design process becomes the process of designing computer views for entry of data, but the principles of control still apply.

Principles of Forms Design

A well-designed form improves the reliability of the data entered on it. A form should be designed to collect information in a consistent way and to remind providers of information that needs to be included. Many paper record forms consist of a single sheet. Other specialty forms, such as a unit-set form or a multipart form, have multiple-sheet forms preassembled in either carbon or carbonless sets. With spot carbons in unit-set forms, only part of the information on the original is visible on the copy. When the face sheet is the first page of a unit set and is printed on the computer, the carbon can be positioned so that the copy for a clinical department would have only the patient identification information and not the financial information.

Continuous-feed forms use a series of forms separated with perforations that can be printed by a printer without having to load the paper for each form printed. The forms then can be separated and distributed. Continuous-feed forms can be used for both single sheets and multiset forms.

Most forms include similar basic components and at least a heading to describe the contents and purpose, instructions on how to fill out the form, and spaces to enter required and/or optional information. General guidelines to follow when designing forms include:

- The form should be easy to complete.
- Instructions on completion and use of the form should be included.
- The form should have a heading with a title that clearly identifies its purpose.
- The facility's name and address should appear on each page of the form.
- The name, patient identification number, and other identifying information should be present on each form. Most facilities now use **bar coding** as identifying information.
- Bar coding also should be included in indexing the form for random access in an optical scanner or microfilming system. Bar codes are generally printed directly on the document or on a label affixed to the document.
- The form number and date of revision should be included to ensure that the form being used is the correct and most current version.
- Outdated forms should be recalled and eliminated.
- The physical layout of the form should be logical. When a clerk is entering information as the patient gives it, the form should be organized to match the way the information is requested (for example, the patient's city, state, and zip code).
- Personal and address data and other items of information that relate to one another should be put together.

- Font selection should be standardized. Some experts recommend all capital letters.
- Margins should be left for hole punches to allow the documents to be placed in folders or chart holders. The holes may be on the left-hand side of the form, at the top, or both, depending on the types of folders or binders used.
- Ruled lines may be used to outline sections of forms to allow for easy entry of data or to separate areas of the form.
- Shading can be used to separate and emphasize areas of the form.
- Check boxes and fields can be used to provide space for the collection of data.

Careful consideration also should be given to including information on the backs of forms. There is the possibility that another patient's information might be recorded on the back of the form. Facilities that are **scanning** and imaging paper records must have the bar-coded patient identification information on the back of the form to ensure proper indexing into the imaging system. Even though scanners can scan both sides of a document, the ability to index and thus access the information must be ensured.

Forms Control Systems

Facilities must develop strict guidelines and processes for forms control. Word-processing programs and programs specifically designed for forms design have made the process easier than in the past. Providers often design their own non-approved forms, which may appear in the paper record when it arrives in the HIM department. This affects procedures and the patient care process as well as procedures in the department. The person who designed the form may be unaware of the interrelated processes that are affected by changing it.

Forms control systems must:

- Provide for the development of forms according to established guidelines
- Control the printing and use of forms
- Guide providers in designing forms according to established guidelines
- Prevent staff from changing or designing forms that duplicate existing forms or could be combined into other forms

Forms control is critical as the transition toward image- and computer-based record systems continues. The transition usually begins with using an imaging system to gather information about existing forms and to ensure that all forms can be properly scanned and indexed. Without indexing, the information cannot be retrieved. The forms control process also should establish processes for forms inventory, forms identification, forms analysis, and forms purchasing.

Forms Inventory

The first step in the forms control process is the forms inventory. This process involves gathering each form and all of its

editions to ensure that the most current version is used. A subject file is a good idea for bringing together all the forms used by each of the areas, such as all admissions or registration forms, all operative forms, and all nursing forms. Organizing in this manner would prevent new forms from being developed when current forms have the needed information, assist in finding ways to combine forms with related information, and serve as a reminder that information changed on one form must be changed on related forms.

Forms Identification

The second part of the forms control process is forms identification. This involves assigning each form a distinct title that reflects its use. In paper systems, a forms number indicates that the form has been approved. The date and the source department are usually included with the number. Bar coding and labels with complete bar-coded information about the form are becoming more prevalent as facilities prepare for the eventual computerization of forms. A numerical listing of forms should be maintained.

Forms Analysis

Forms analysis involves the continuous review and revision of forms. The forms analysis process is often initiated because of procedural problems, for example, when providers are not receiving the information they need to do their work. Forms assist in guiding processes and ensuring that information is obtained and recorded. Flowcharting the development and distribution of the forms is helpful in determining whether a form is still useful, whether the information it contains is current, and whether it meets the current requirements of the facility.

Forms Purchasing

Purchasing and printing comprise the fourth part of the forms control process. A policy should be in place stating that forms cannot be ordered or reordered without approval of the forms committee or some other group or individual responsible for purchasing and printing approval.

Check Your Understanding 8.5

Instructions: Answer the following questions on a separate sheet of paper.

1. What are quantitative analysis and qualitative analysis? What purpose do they serve?
2. How does concurrent review facilitate record completion?
3. What is universal chart order, and why is it being adopted by healthcare facilities?
4. What is the difference between open- and closed-record review?
5. Why is the finance department concerned about the timely completion of records?
6. In what two ways do HIM departments store incomplete health records? How do the two storage systems work?
7. What is the difference between an incomplete record and a delinquent record?
8. How does the HIM professional help providers to complete health records?

9. What three methods do facilities use to authenticate health records? How does each method work?

10. Why have some facilities stopped notifying providers about orders and progress notes needing signatures?

11. Why is forms control a critical responsibility of the HIM professional?

12. What are the four parts of the forms control process?

13. Why is it important for those providers wanting a new form to go through the approval process?

14. How are bar codes and labels used in forms?

Creation, Storage, and Retention of Paper-Based Health Records

Healthcare organizations need policies covering the circulation and storage of health records to ensure that the records can be located quickly when they are needed for patient care and other uses. Controlling the storage of paper-based health records is critical to patient care. The quality of patient care as well as the image and reputation of the HIM department may depend on the speed with which patient health information can be retrieved.

Management of paper-based health records includes three processes: creation and identification, storage and retrieval, and retention and disposition.

Health Record Creation and Identification

As discussed earlier, the health record is created when the patient is first admitted to or treated in a healthcare facility. Every patient is assigned a specific identification number, and the health record is initiated with the collection of admission or registration information. As data and information about the patient's care and condition are documented, the record grows. The record remains in active use for the purposes of patient care, clinical coding, billing, statistical analysis, and other operational processes until the episode of care ends.

Health Record Identification Systems

For the correct health record to be quickly retrieved when it is needed, each record must be assigned a unique identifier. The choice of record identification system is tied to the organization's filing system.

Alphabetic versus Numeric Patient Identifiers

Small healthcare facilities, such as physician offices, often use a simple alphabetical identifier: the patient's last and first names. This identifier is also used for filing of medical records in strict alphabetical order by the patient's last name. Some experts suggest that alphabetical systems are most appropriate for facilities with fewer than 10,000 individual records

Most healthcare organizations use a record identification system that assigns a numerical identifier to each patient.

Serial Numbering System

In a **serial numbering system,** each patient receives a new number at each visit, and numbers are assigned in straight numerical sequence to consecutive patients in the order in which they arrive for treatment. Each time a patient is treated by the facility, a new number is issued to link the patient to that particular visit or admission. This system is often used by clinics and physician offices. Experts suggest that straight numerical systems can efficiently accommodate no more than 25,000 records.

Unit Numbering System

In a **unit numbering system,** the patient is assigned a number during the first encounter for care and keeps it for all subsequent encounters. The number may be assigned automatically by the computer system. Some facilities, such as Veterans Affairs facilities, use the patient's Social Security number as the unit number because it is a unique permanent number already assigned to the patient. Most large facilities use a unit numbering system.

Serial-Unit Numbering System

In a **serial-unit numbering system,** the patient is issued a different number for each admission or encounter for care and the records of past episodes of care are brought forward to be filed under the last number issued. This creates a unit record that contains information from all the patient's encounters. Because this system requires a great deal of shifting of records and changing of numbers, it is not as commonly used as the unit numbering system.

When facilities change from a serial to a unit numbering system, it is important to pick a start date and move forward from that point. As patients are readmitted, they are assigned a new number that then becomes the permanent unit number and all records are brought forward and linked under the new number.

Family Numbering System

Family numbering is a type of unit numbering system. In this system, the entire family is assigned one number and all information on visits by any family member is filed in one location. This system may be appropriate for use in family practice settings, but care must be taken to preserve patient privacy.

Health Record Filing Systems

Most healthcare facilities use numerical filing systems for paper-based health records. Small facilities, such as physician offices and clinics, often use alphabetic filing; larger facilities generally use numerical filing systems.

Serial Filing System (Straight Numeric)

In a **serial filing system,** records are filed according to the number assigned to a particular encounter or visit. The major shortcoming of serial filing is that the records for patients who received services multiple times at the facility would have different numbers, and the different records would be filed in multiple places in the filing system. Therefore, a serial filing system requires more searching and more retrieval time than a unit filing system does.

Unit Filing System

A true **unit filing system** arranges the records for all inpatient and outpatient visits and procedures for a single patient together under a permanent unit number. The individual patient's unit record grows in size as new information is added. There is only one record for the patient, and it is kept in one specific location in the file room.

Terminal-Digit Filing System

In a **terminal-digit filing system,** records are filed according to a three-part number made up of two-digit pairs. The basic terminal-digit filing system contains 10,000 divisions, with 100 sections ranging from 00–99 and 100 divisions within each section ranging from 00–99.

Terminal-digit filing is not difficult to learn, but it is different from straight numerical filing. In straight numerical filing, the first numbers (those farthest to the left) are considered first. The number itself can be a permanent unit number or a serial number.

In terminal-digit filing, the record number is placed into terminal-digit order when the health record is ready for filing. The number is broken down into two-digit pairs and is read from right to left. For example, the number 670187 would be written as 67-01-87. The first pair of digits on the right (87) is called the primary number or the terminal-digit number, the second pair of digits (01) is called the secondary number, and the third pair of digits (67) is called the tertiary or final number.

The primary number is considered first for filing. The primary numbers range from 00 to 99 and represent the 100 sections of the filing area. Because many records will be filed in each section, each section needs to be further subdivided, first according to the secondary number and then according to the tertiary number. As shown in figure 8.4, a

record numbered 67-01-87 would be filed in section 87, in subsection 01, and then in numerical sequence for 67 (after 66-01-87 and before 68-01-87). All records with the tertiary and secondary numbers of 01-87 would be filed within this part of the file.

Consider three patients who were admitted to a facility and were issued the following numbers in sequence: 67-01-87, 67-01-88, and 67-01-89. In a terminal digit system, these records would be added to three different filing sections of the 100 sections of the file rather than all being filed at the end as in a straight numerical system. (See figure 8.5).

The advantage of terminal-digit filing is that filing shelves fill equally rather than at the end, as is the case with conventional straight numerical filing. There will be one record with the primary number 00, one with 01, and so on through 99 for every 100 consecutive numbers issued to patients. For every 100 records added to the file, each section of the file will be increased by only one record. The task of moving charts to alleviate overcrowding at the end of the file is reduced because consecutively numbered charts can be moved from each section periodically. One hundred consecutively numbered folders would be removed from 100 separate locations. Thus, the even distribution of records throughout the filing space can be maintained, and misfiles can be reduced because clerks need to remember only two numbers at a time.

Another advantage of terminal-digit filing is that the department's workload can be evenly distributed among filing personnel. Certain sections can be designated for each employee. For example, if a department has five file clerks, each could be given responsibility for a specific section, with clerk one responsible for section 00–19, clerk two responsible for section 20–39, and so on. In addition to maintaining each section, each clerk would file loose reports and keep the records in order, handle requests for information from patient records, and perform other duties.

Terminal-digit filing can be adapted to various types of numbering systems. A six-digit number is most common, but some facilities, such as VA facilities, use a longer number. The VA uses the Social Security number as the basis

**Figure 8.4.   Filing of patient record 67-01-87
in a terminal digit system**

6	6	6	6	6	6	7	7	7
7	5	6	7	8	9	0	1	2
0	0	0	0	0	0	0	0	0
1	1	1	1	1	1	1	1	1
8	8	8	8	8	8	8	8	8
7	7	7	7	7	7	7	7	7

**Figure 8.5.   Filing of three consecutive patient records
under the terminal digit system**

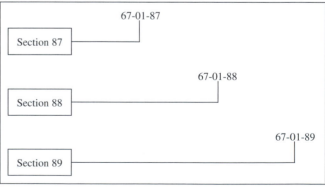

for terminal-digit filing. For example, number 401-80-1530 could be adapted to serve as a terminal digit by dividing it so that 30 is the primary number, 15 is the secondary number, and 40180 is the tertiary number. The files do not expand evenly because there is no facility control over the assignment of numbers to patients.

Generally, open-shelf filing is used for terminal-digit filing. The shelves are set up with guide tabs and folder tabs on the ends of the folders or guides so that they can easily be seen. In a standard terminal-digit filing area, there will be 10,000 guides to index the primary number sections and secondary number subdivisions so that behind each guide, all records will have the same final four digits. The guides are set up vertically with the digits above the line on the guide representing the division (secondary number) and the digits below the line representing the section (primary number). An index guide tab marked with 67 above the line and 80 below would indicate the 67 division of the 80 section.

Many facilities use color coding in their filing system—different colors to represent each of the 10 primary numbers 0 to 9—and the colors appear on the folders and guides. The records in a particular section are in blocks of color. This allows misfiles to be identified quickly. Vendors of file folders have endless possibilities of color-coding different pairs of numbers. The colors selected to represent particular digits must be permanent and continued when new folders are ordered or else the advantage of color-coding will be lost.

Even distribution of paper-based health records is difficult in today's environment. Patient records contain myriad information, including graphic tracings, photographs, and cumulative laboratory report printouts. Records are bulkier than in the past because of the large quantity of paper produced as documentation of care delivery.

Health Record Storage and Retrieval

The HIM department is responsible for ensuring that the paper record is available when needed by the provider for patient care. No matter how well organized and well managed the HIM department is, the timeliness of record delivery to providers is the measure of the quality of the department's services.

Health Record Storage

Storage is the application of efficient procedures for the use of filing equipment and storage media to keep records secure and available to those providers and other healthcare personnel authorized to access them. Record storage equipment can range from numerous types of file cabinets to open shelves of various heights and types.

Planning for record storage is a major responsibility for the HIM professional. He or she must maintain a leadership role in ensuring that sufficient, conveniently accessible space is available for the storage of paper records. Ways must be provided to consistently maintain sufficient filing room by moving inactive records or by microfilming or imaging records.

Because space is expensive, administrators and facilities management personnel are always looking for ways to better use it. The HIM professional must make sure that records are not located in poor environmental conditions where they can be either damaged or difficult to locate. For example, health records should not be stored in areas where pipes and flammable substances are located. Subbasements without proper flooring and temperature control, parking garages, and non-temperature-controlled commercial storage units are not appropriate storage locations for patient records.

Many companies specialize in the storage of vital records and provide the proper conditions for the protection of records as well as access to records. Water, pests, and mold are all potential problems. HIM professionals have had to deal with the restoration of paper records damaged by water resulting from hurricanes, earthquakes, and tornadoes. There are companies that specialize in the restoration of records and can handle disaster recovery. Moreover, some companies negotiate contracts ensuring that the healthcare provider is first in line for recovery efforts should a disaster occur. Paper is extremely fragile when wet and indirect circulation of air is critical; dehumidification and perhaps vacuum freezing are considerations in the restoration process. Storage space for patient records is often not a priority, and records sometimes are in the cheapest possible storage space. Temperature and humidity control are important to prevent mold. The storage area must be clean and dust free and located away from food and trash in order to prevent bugs such as paper mites. Chemical treatments for mold and pests can cause problems for workers who must sort through and locate records for patient treatment. The HIM professional must be firm in the need to protect the original records for the duration of the legally required period.

Health Record Retrieval

Retrieval is concerned with locating requested records and information. It involves signing out or checking out records from the filing area and tracking those that are not returned within the specified time period. A number of excellent software systems are available for tracking patient records.

HIM personnel must be able to quickly determine the exact location of a specific health record at any time. Facilities should have strict policies and procedures in place that specify who is permitted to check out records from the filing area. Past records are generally requested when patients are readmitted or appear for appointments. Large clinics create a lot of activity in the filing area because records must be pulled in advance for patient appointments. Acute care facilities must provide past records for readmitted patients.

The filing area should be audited periodically to ensure that files are in correct order, regardless of the filing system used. Loose reports should be attached, and those awaiting attachment should be sorted and organized to facilitate retrieval. It should be possible to locate charts in emergency situations within 15 minutes. The charge-out system should be reviewed to make sure the charged-out record is still under the responsibility of the person named in the system or on the charge-out form.

Statistics on the ratio of number of requests to number of records in the file should be maintained to demonstrate the activity in the filing area. Statistics on the ratio of the number of records located to the number of records requested provide evidence of the filing function's accuracy and quality.

Health Record Filing and Storage Equipment

Filing equipment vendors are the HIM professional's best resource in planning a filing area that makes the best use of the available space. Open-shelf filing is the least expensive option for health record storage. Shelves are usually arranged back to back just as is shelving in a library. Shelving uses space more efficiently because only 30 to 36 inches are needed for each aisle. When standard file cabinets are used, aisles should be at least five feet wide to allow two facing file cabinets to be opened at the same time and to allow personnel who need to work in the same area to pass. Lateral files with drawers and doors also require sufficient aisle space for opening the individual drawers and allowing personnel to pass.

Many facilities use open-shelf files mounted on tracks to conserve valuable space. These are referred to as movable files, and many different styles are available. The main consideration is whether the files open electronically or manually. With movable files mounted on tracks, more sections of files can be installed because the floor space for many fixed aisles is not needed. The files in a mobile unit can be opened one aisle at a time. With permanently installed open shelves, there are fixed aisles between each shelf. Whatever type of shelving is selected, the shelves must be able to handle the heavy weight of paper-based health records.

Vendors estimate the amount of file shelves needed based on several factors. One consideration is the average size of individual records. The volume of patients and the number of repeat visits or readmissions affect the potential expansion of each individual patient record. The type of facility also affects the size of individual records. Acute care facilities with extensive ancillary services and more acutely ill patients have larger individual patient records, as do facilities specializing in transplants, cancer, and other chronic diseases. When unit records are organized in a terminal-digit filing system, there must be adequate expansion space in each division of the filing area to allow for expansion of individual records.

It is the responsibility of the HIM professional to ensure that the vendors' estimates are adequate. The number of linear filing inches is the key factor. When there are existing records, the average size of the individual records can be easily calculated by measuring the number of files on a random sampling of shelves. The vendor should subtract for the side panels of the open-shelf filing units. The usable space must be measured from the inside of the panels, not from the outside

of the shelves, so that the true number of linear filing inches is reflected. For example, one standard three-foot-wide shelf would have approximately 33 linear inches available for filing. Allowance also should be made for file guides, which also reduce the number of linear filing inches.

An example might be that of a department expanding into another filing area. The department has selected eight-shelf open shelves that are 36 inches wide with 33 inches of actual filing space on each shelf. The department's present health records have been measured in random areas of the existing files and average two inches in thickness. With 5,000 discharges anticipated each year and a projection of five years, 25,000 records will need to be stored. Because records average a two-inch thickness, 50,000 filing inches are needed. Because each eight-shelf unit will have 264 linear filing inches available, the number of inches needed, 50,000, must be divided by 264 to determine the number of filing units that must be purchased, which will be 190.

Storage space is at a premium, and many facilities have several locations for storage of medical records. This can create retrieval problems when records are in distant locations or off-site. Much personnel time can be spent walking or driving to off-site locations. Some facilities contract with commercial storage companies to store inactive records; commercial storage companies can provide transportation of records to the facility.

Health Record Retention and Disposition

Disposition involves determining the retention schedule to be followed to protect and preserve active and inactive records. Establishing policies that incorporate state and federal laws and maintaining a disaster plan are part of the disposition process. The transfer and destruction of records, optical scanning, and microfilming are all part of this stage. Facilities must be careful to monitor record maintenance so that records are moved continuously out of active storage as they become inactive or reach maximum retention periods. Records cannot be stored indefinitely because storage areas fill up. Older records may not be as useful in the patient care treatment process.

Accreditation and Legal Record Retention Requirements

JCAHO asserts that the length of record retention depends on laws, regulations, and the use of health records for care and for other purposes such as research and education.

State laws, Medicare regulations, and other federal regulations, accreditation standards, and facility policies and procedures all must be reviewed when establishing a retention schedule. The HIM professional must adhere to the strictest time limit. In addition to the length of time for maintaining health records, the HIM professional must consider the required length of retention for immunization records, mammography records, x-rays and radiographs, and the records of minors and incompetent patients.

Medicare requires records to be maintained for at least five years, according to 42 CFR 282.26(d). This includes committee reports, physician certification and recertification reports, radiologist records (printouts, films, scans, and other images), home health agency records, long-term care records, laboratory records, and any other records that document information about claims. When state laws or licensing standards require a longer retention period, the longer requirement must be followed. State law should be reviewed to determine the handling of other images. In many states, these are handled the same way that radiologist records are handled.

State agencies also may have retention requirements. The Occupational Safety and Health Administration (OSHA) requires records of employees with occupational exposure to be maintained for the duration of employment plus 30 years. The statutes of limitation (deadline for filing a lawsuit) in various types of legal actions are important considerations in developing a retention schedule.

The facility or provider is responsible for maintaining the record. When the facility or provider cannot produce a record, it must be able to prove that the loss was unintentional and that there was no negligent treatment. AHIMA recommends that retention of health information be based on the needs and requirements of the facility, such as legal requirements, continued patient care, research, education, and other legitimate uses. Primary records are the original records in whatever form they are kept; secondary records are by-products of the original information, such as indexes, physician profiles, databases, billing information, and other reports or queries. Other departments rely on the expertise of the HIM professional to assist them in developing record retention procedures.

Retention Requirements for Ancillary Materials

E-mail messages and faxes are used for instructions, information about appointments, and the reporting of information. These must be printed and attached to the health record folder.

Images, such as complete readouts or "strips" from EEGs, EKGs, fetal monitors, Holter monitors, treadmill tests, EMGs, echocardiograms, videotapes, and other imaging records, do not have to be kept within the physical health record but must be retrievable for as long as legally required. The original interpretations of the results must actually be part of the physical patient health record. Facilities may have computerized systems that directly feed the results of some systems into the imaging system so that the actual images are available to physicians and other providers. These scanned images are not always of diagnostic quality in some scanning systems, so ancillary departments should maintain the information for the appropriate retention period.

Fetal monitoring strips create storage problems for many HIM departments. They are part of the mother's record, but because the strips relate to the newborn, they should be maintained according to the length of time stipulated for a minor's records. Because these strips are not compatible with scanning systems, some facilities have specific computer software to maintain and store fetal monitoring strips within the labor and delivery area.

Magnetic tapes containing the digital versions of MRI and CT studies are not considered permanent health records as long as a hard copy of the final images (radiographic film) is placed in the patient's health record. The signed interpretation of the studies must be maintained in the record for the full retention period required by law. According to 21 CFR 900.12 (c)(4), mammograms must be maintained for 5 to 10 years, depending on whether additional mammograms are performed. State laws may require a retention period for mammograms of 20 to 30 years. This is another example of the HIM professional having to ensure that the longer time period is followed when retention schedules are determined.

Microfilming or optical and electronic imaging technology is allowed by most state laws and is an acceptable method of maintaining patient health records. Because the images are of some documents, computerized results, and other test results, each type of work to be imaged must be carefully considered.

Destruction and Transfer of Health Records

The destruction of records after time limits for retention have been reached must ensure that records are burned, shredded, or destroyed in such a way that personal health information is not revealed. A retention plan must be carefully written and included in the departmental policy and procedure manual to ensure that record destruction is part of the normal course of business and that no one particular record or group of records is singled out for destruction.

When the facility is closed or sold, its health records are transferred to the successor provider, meaning the entity or individual that purchases the facility. In ambulatory care settings or physician offices, patients are informed of their options to transfer their records to another provider of choice before their records are transferred to the successor provider. When a physician leaves a group practice, patients should be given the choice to transfer their records and move with the physician or to have the records and the responsibility for care transferred to another provider in the group.

Development of a Record Retention Program

Figure 8.6 lists the objectives of a record retention program. The program must ensure that health records are retained;

Figure 8.6.   Objectives of a record retention program

To ensure retention and preservation of all valued health records

To maintain noncurrent records of continuing value for uniform time periods and in designated locations

To ensure cost-effectiveness in record storage space, equipment, and personnel

To dispose of unnecessary records by developing an orderly, controlled, and confidential system of record destruction

To establish record retention periods consistent with patient care, regulatory requirements, and other legal considerations that inactive records are maintained; that retention is cost-effective in terms of storage space, equipment, and personnel; that a formal record destruction process is in place; and that retention periods are established. A task force or committee might be established with representation from administration, medical staff, health information services, risk management, and legal counsel to give consideration to the needs of all groups who use patient health information. Figure 8.7 lists some of the elements to consider. These include looking carefully at all of the record's uses and the cost of space.

The HIM director is generally responsible for implementing the retention program. However, other individuals may be charged with the shared responsibility of implementing the program in some facilities. Some facilities establish a task force to oversee the record retention program, sometimes chaired by an HIM professional.

The steps in developing a record retention program include:

1. Conducting an inventory of the facility's records
2. Determining the format and location of storage
3. Assigning each record a retention period
4. Destroying records that are no longer needed

Conducting an Inventory of Records
The first step in establishing a record retention program is to carefully and completely inventory the records or categories of records that are maintained. In this phase, it is important to determine all the locations and formats of patient information, including images, videotapes, e-mails, tracings, computerized records, and other formats. The inventory also must include the records and registries maintained by all departments. A comprehensive list of all software and versions used also should be maintained so that records, documents, and images can be retrieved in the future. Specialized computer systems used by individual departments should be included.

Determining Storage Format and Location
Determining the format and location of storage is the second step in retention program development. Facilities may choose to retain records in paper format or on hard copy and store

Figure 8.7.   Elements to consider in the preservation of records

Patient value for continued care
Record usage in the facility as guided by the patient population and activity of its medical staff
Legal value as determined by the statute of limitations
Research value
Historical value
Volume and cost to maintain hard-copy storage versus microfilm, optical disk, or remote storage
Storage and safety standards
Contractual arrangements with payers

them either on-site or in off-site contract storage. Off-site contract storage should be located at a distance far enough away from the facility to ensure that a disaster affecting the facility will not also affect the storage location.

One storage mechanism for inactive records is microfilming. Microfilming is the process of recording miniaturized images of a patient health record on film. The images are usually filmed by a special camera onto rolls of 16-millimeter film. The microfilmed images may be stored permanently on the rolls, which may be stored either in boxes labeling the first and last patient numbers on a roll or inserted into special cartridges. Roll film contains information on many patients and cannot be changed. The images are often indexed at the time of filming to allow for quicker retrieval of information.

An alternative to storing microfilm rolls in cartridges is to store images in microfilm jackets. The roll film would be cut into strips and inserted into the channels of the jackets. The microfilm jacket has the advantage of serving as an individual folder for storing the records of one patient. Additional filmed images can be added to the jacket or changed. The jackets are usually four by six inches and have a strip at the top on which to record the patient's name and number. Because the strips can be color-coded, the jackets can be filed in filing cabinets or electric files using the same filing and numbering system the facility uses for paper records.

Microfilm cameras also can film directly onto a microfiche film format. Like the microfilm jacket, the microfiche has the advantage of having only one patient's information available on the fiche. However, its disadvantage is that patient information cannot be updated because the images are filmed directly onto the microfiche itself. The most common size of fiche is a four-by-six-inch sheet, with space for the patient's name and number.

The microfilming of records has many advantages, including:

- Microfilming saves space, which is the primary reason why facilities use it.
- Health records can be retrieved and retained for a long period of time.
- It is simple to duplicate microfilm records in order to provide security or backup copies, and paper copies can be printed from reader printer equipment.
- Microfilm is legally admissible as the original document.

Many facilities use a combination of microfilm formats to accommodate technology and equipment changes.

The facility must consider many issues when deciding whether to microfilm records. These issues include:

- Although microfilming saves a great deal of storage space, it is expensive. For example, preparing the records for filming is a major cost that involves removing staples, checking identification, adjusting oversized or overlapping forms for filming, repairing sheets, and other tasks.

- Special equipment is needed to read and copy microfilm.
- Personnel must be available in patient care areas or in the HIM department to find the microfilm jackets, microfiche, or roll microfilm and to locate the exact information needed.

Microfilming can be done on-site by facility personnel or under contract with a microfilming company. When the facility decides to have the microfilming done in-house, it must take into account the costs of labor and training, supplies, and maintenance.

On the other hand, when the facility decides to use an outside contract microfilming company, the contract should specify who performs the preparation and packs the boxes of records. After records have been transported to the outside contract company, the facility must be able to retrieve the patient's information at any time in case he or she is readmitted or appears for treatment. When records are to be indexed, the contract should fully explain the indexing procedure to ensure that needed documents are accessible. The contract also should specify the turnaround time for filming. Moreover, film returned to the facility must be carefully analyzed to ensure its quality and legibility before the original record is destroyed. The company microfilming the records usually handles their destruction after the facility has audited the returned film. The cost of microfilming is generally based on the number of images filmed.

A second storage mechanism is optical scanning. Records can be scanned into optical scanning equipment or digitally transferred. The imaging process converts paper or microfilm documents into a computer-readable digital format. The facility must determine what information can be fed directly into the imaging system, for example, registration and face sheet, discharge summary, and all other dictated and transcribed reports. Digitized information, including that produced by laboratory and radiology can be "COLD-fed" into the imaging system. COLD is the acronym for "computer output to laser disk" and now refers to a variety of technologies related to digitized input and output. Optical scanning produces an image of the record that can be indexed and quickly retrieved and simultaneously viewed by many providers. This is not a true electronic record because the image cannot be changed after it has been permanently archived.

Imaging involves preparing, or prepping, the documents, which must be done before the records are scanned. Staples must be removed, papers repaired, and each page checked to ensure the presence of a bar code on both the front and back of every form in the record. The scanning process involves inserting the paper into the optical scanner so that both the front and back pages are scanned at the same time. Two types of scanners are usually used for health records: flatbed scanners and automatic document-feed scanners. The type of scanner used depends on the volume to be scanned. Flatbed scanners are usually slower than automatic document-feed scanners but require less preparation of individual documents.

Indexing involves identifying each individual page. Indexing is critical. If the image is not indexed to the proper patient and the proper form for that admission, the information cannot be retrieved. Image and indexing inspection is important to make sure the image is legible.

The scanner is the device that actually scans a human-readable document and uses optical character recognition software to convert the document into a machine-readable format. After being scanned, records must be verified and generally are not submitted to the final stored archive until the physician completes them. After records are archived in the imaging system, they cannot be changed. While waiting to be archived, images can be added or indexing changed.

Facilities assign personnel to handle the tasks of preparation and scanning. Emergency department reports, outpatient reports, and reports submitted from physicians often do not have the proper patient numbers or encounter numbers, and all of this identifying information must be entered so that each form in the record can be properly indexed and retrieved. A concern for HIM professionals is that scanning equipment from one vendor may not work with equipment from another vendor. The long-term storage capability of optical disk has not been evaluated for long-term quality because the technology is still evolving.

Beginning an imaging system requires detailed planning. Decisions must be made about converting existing records or whether only information from a certain date forward will be imaged. In addition, security backups of images should be available. Health records should be on the type of optical disk storage using WORM, "write once, read many," technology. This means that the data cannot be erased or altered. Rewritable or erasable optical disk technology is not appropriate for health records.

Although imaging has the advantages of rapid retrieval and simultaneous access, it is not an easy process to implement. Loose materials and late-arriving information still must be scanned and indexed. Moreover, problems still exist with recovering charts from the nursing areas after discharge and with unapproved forms being developed and included in the record that cannot be indexed because they do not have bar coding. The HIM department still must perform open-record review and check forms for signatures. In other words, the traditional functions of the HIM department do not change. While the patient is in the facility or in active treatment, the record is paper. The imaging system does not convert the paper into images until after patient discharge or termination of treatment. Imaging is a key part of the progression to an electronic document management system and ultimately to the computerized health record because it provides providers with quick access to pictures such as x-rays, MRIs, and other documents rather than having to wait for the paper copy. This type of quick access to images improves safety and quality of care.

Assigning a Retention Period

After all departments have been inventoried, the third step is to assign a retention period for each type of record. The retention period should be defined as time in active files, time in inactive storage, and total time before destruction.

As discussed previously, state and federal laws and regulations must be reviewed to ensure that records are maintained for the longest length of time required. Many states recommend that patient health records be retained for 10 years following patient discharge or death. There are usually special requirements for minor patients. For example, the state of Tennessee requires that the records of minors or mentally disabled patients be maintained until the age of majority plus one year, or a total of 10 years, whichever is longer. Therefore, the record of a newborn in Tennessee would be maintained until the patient reaches the age of majority, which is 18 years plus one year or a total of 19 years.

Analysis of the retention period should reflect the scope and needs of the facility, along with the preliminary costs associated with microfilming, imaging, and other methods of maintaining and storing records. Storage mechanisms should be selected that protect records and provide ease of access and employee safety.

Protection of paper and microfilmed records during the legally required retention period is extremely important and needs to be considered before a disaster occurs or a situation occurs where a record in storage cannot be found. In addition, as discussed earlier, records can be destroyed or may be unusable due to water damage, extremes of heat and humidity, and damage caused by airborne chemicals and insects. Natural disasters such as floods, hurricanes, and earthquakes should also be considered when determining how and where to store paper medical records. Records should be stored in areas that have clear aisles and doorways and boxes or shelves should be well marked so that needed records can be found. Fire extinguishers should be easily accessible. Transportation and availability of records also must be considered.

Commercial storage vendors should be selected carefully to ensure that records are protected from unauthorized access. Policies for security of all satellite record storage areas must be developed and agreements signed regarding timely access to, and retrieval of, records.

Destroying Unnecessary Records

Destroying records that are not needed is the fourth step in developing a record retention program. There must be a rule that no patient health information can be destroyed or thrown away without approval of the HIM director or other authorized committee or person according to facility policy. The HIM professional must be alert to changes in departmental administration or departmental relocation or remodeling because departments often use these events to clean out files, which could result in the destruction of needed patient information.

The destruction of patient records must be done as part of the facility's usual business. When the required retention schedule has been satisfied, a complete list of records to be destroyed should be compiled and submitted to the individual designated to authorize the destruction. Outsourcing of destruction to shredding companies should be carefully monitored to protect patient confidentiality. The destruction of computerized records should follow security guidelines to ensure that the information is destroyed permanently. Facilities must maintain basic information about the patient in the MPI, which is maintained permanently even though the corresponding health record is destroyed.

AHIMA recommends that records be destroyed in such a way that the information cannot possibly be reconstructed. The destruction should be documented, and the documentation should include:

- Date of destruction
- Method of destruction (shredding, burning, or other means)
- Description of the disposed record series of numbers or items
- Inclusive dates covered
- A statement that the records were destroyed in the normal course of business
- The signatures of the individuals supervising and witnessing the destruction

AHIMA further recommends that facilities maintain destruction certification documents permanently. Such certificates may be required as evidence that records were destroyed in the regular course of business. When facilities fail to apply destruction policies uniformly or when destruction is contrary to policy, courts may allow a jury to infer that the facility destroyed its records to hide evidence of negligent care.

Check Your Understanding 8.6

Instructions: Answer the following questions on a separate piece of paper.

1. What is the difference between a serial numbering system and a unit numbering system?

2. What are two advantages of terminal-digit filing over straight numerical filing?

3. What are the main factors in determining how long to maintain a health record?

4. What is the major advantage of microfilming health records?

5. What is the major advantage of optical imaging in the chart completion process?

6. What are the four primary steps in a record retention program?

Master Patient Index

The MPI is a permanent database including every patient ever admitted to or treated by the facility. Even though patient health records may be destroyed after legal retention periods have been met, the information contained in the MPI must be kept permanently. The MPI is also referred to as the master person index, the **master population index,** the master name file, the **enterprise-wide master person or patient index** (EMPI), regional master patient index (RMPI) and the master patient database. Whatever it is called, the MPI is an important key to the health record because it contains the patient's name and health record number.

As electronic information exchange becomes more prevalent, it is critical that the master patient indexing system correctly identifies the patient. Each facility has an MPI, which is used as the key to locating patient information, for all patients who have been registered and/or treated at any location in the facility. One possible way to exchange healthcare information among facilities would be to utilize an MPI as an additional technical layer infrastructure serving as an umbrella to connect and provide access to computerized patient information at different facilities. Although the MPI consists of demographic information, it is the first step in ensuring that correct clinical information about the correct patient is shared. The MPI becomes the link among multiple computer systems that must be able to share information with each other. This is complicated within one facility with many computer systems, but when multiple facilities try to share information, the EMPI or RMPI is a prerequisite to linking together the data within their various computer systems.

In a totally manual system, the MPI can be a simple file containing cards with basic identification information about the patient or it can be a sophisticated computerized system. In a computer-based MPI, the database associates the patient with the particular number under which patient treatment information can be located. The index also helps to control number assignments to ensure that former patients are not inadvertently assigned an additional number.

The challenges are many. For example, patients may not remember previous admissions or may have been admitted under a different name. A person other than the patient may have provided incorrect information, resulting in a new number being assigned when the patient returns for an appointment or is readmitted to the hospital. Sometimes patients use different middle initials or a nickname rather than a given name, or their names may have many possible spellings or may be hyphenated. Babies may have names changed, first and last names can be reversed, and outside laboratories may use different data. Basic demographic information such as addresses can be abbreviated incorrectly. In some cases, patients do not speak the same language as the clerk entering the information, resulting in miscommunication and incorrect data. Facilities that have either merged or separated must keep information on patients treated and often have problems combining information from two computer systems. Facilities may have manual card files that have been microfilmed in the past or may use a variety of formats, from index cards, to microfilmed cards on rolls or microfiche, to a computerized database.

The challenge for facilities is to maintain a correct and current MPI so that each patient has a unique identifier number. Duplication and overlaps are a major problem. The goal is to have a true longitudinal record from birth to death, and the MPI serves as the link to information and certainty of identification that are critical to the quality and safety of patient care. Healthcare facilities have hired HIM professionals as EMPI coordinators or have hired consultants to clean and maintain EMPI systems to ensure that the correct information on the correct patient is available to the provider and others who need it. The sharing of data is a worthy goal, but incorrect information can adversely affect the quality and safety of care; thus, accuracy of the MPI is a critical issue. There is a movement toward a patient identifier that would be used nationwide, although the notion of a universal patient identifier raises concerns about compromising patient confidentiality.

Information contained in the MPI includes:

- The patient's full name and any other names the patient uses
- The patient's date of birth
- The patient's complete address
- The patient's health record number
- The patient's billing or account number
- The name of the attending physician
- The dates of the patient's admission and discharge or the date of the visit or encounter
- The patient's disposition at discharge or the conclusion of treatment
- The patient's date of death, if applicable
- The patient's marital status
- The patient's gender
- The patient's race
- The name of the patient's emergency contact

Other information may be included to further identify the patient and ensure that his or her name is linked to the proper record number. Some facilities include the mother's maiden name as another way to link the patient health record number and information to the proper patient.

Controls for accuracy include limiting access to the index and limiting the ability to make changes to the index to a few key personnel. The first key to maintaining an accurate index is to obtain the correct information in the beginning, but there are numerous problems, such as situations when the patient is unable to provide the correct information or when items are entered improperly. In the past, when only HIM personnel assigned numbers, there was more control; today, numbers are entered by many different personnel. The more people involved in entering data, the greater the potential for error.

When a patient's record or healthcare information cannot be located, his or her care may be compromised. Without prior information, the physician and other providers might duplicate tests or treatments. A second record for the same patient is then created under a new number, which adds to the problem of bringing the parts of the patient record together. Research to "clean up" duplicate numbers and other errors is among the HIM professional's responsibilities.

Check Your Understanding 8.7

Instructions: Answer the following questions on a separate piece of paper.

1. Why is the MPI considered the key index in the HIM department?
2. Why is accurate information critical for the MPI?
3. What are some of the reasons why incorrect information is obtained?
4. What is the consequence of a patient having duplicate health record numbers?

Real-World Case

A recently hired director of health information management is facing a difficult challenge. The hospital's inefficient record-tracking system has produced a tremendous backlog of incomplete records.

Three eight-shelf-high, open-filing shelves currently house the incomplete records of residents and attending physicians. The records are filed in straight numerical order because so many physicians are responsible for each record. The shelving cannot hold the vast number of delinquent records; thus, stacks of records are piled on the floor and in the dictation area booths. These piles of charts were not there when the new HIM director interviewed for the job.

Deficiencies are listed on index cards filed alphabetically by physician name and kept in a box on a table next to the shelving units. Physicians must ask someone in the department to pull their cards and then wait while the charts are pulled. Medicare charts or charts with high charges are filed in red folders to remind the physicians to do them first. The physicians complain about being unable to complete their charts unless a clerk is available to help them. The department is open from 8 a.m. until 4:30 p.m., Monday through Friday, and is closed on weekends.

Mary Jones is responsible for the incomplete files. She counts charts that are two weeks old every two weeks and sends out cartoon notices she designs herself. For example, one card has a picture of a dog in a doghouse with the message, "Get out of the doghouse. Do your records." She also sends out seasonal messages. For example, at Thanksgiving, she sends out cards that say, "Don't be a turkey. You have 14 records to complete." There are more than 4,500 delinquent records, which is well over the JCAHO rule for the number of discharges. The hospital definition of a delinquent record is one that is incomplete over 14 days following discharge.

Mary suggests hiring two or three people to serve as runners to deliver health records directly to the physicians' offices for signature. This, she claims, would reduce the number of charts dramatically.

Several physicians on the Medical Record Committee commented that they find the notes irritating and offensive, especially when the service in the HIM department is so bad when they come in to do the charts. The chief of the medical staff claims that some hospitals in town do not make physicians come in to sign charts that just need signatures on dictated reports. He wants to know why this facility cannot come up with an "automatic signature" policy like the one used at these facilities.

Summary

The patient health record is the foundation for most of the decisions made in any healthcare facility. Decisions relative to patient care and financial reimbursement depend on the quality of documentation in the health record. The record is the communication tool among the members of the patient's healthcare team. It is evidence of what was done for the patient, and the information it contains is used to evaluate the quality of care and to provide important information for research and public health needs. The information in the health care record protects the legal interests of both the patient and the facility. The traditional saying, "if it wasn't documented, it wasn't done," is a reminder of how important the record is for the patient, the facility, and the numerous other users of the record and the information it contains.

Ensuring that the health record meets current regulatory, legal, accrediting, and licensing standards as well as the facility's bylaws and polices is an ongoing challenge for the HIM professional. He or she must continuously educate and update providers on changes affecting documentation. Records must be reviewed both while the patient is in active treatment and after treatment to ensure that they meet the current requirements. Analyzing and processing paper records efficiently is important to ensure that complete information is available for billing and reimbursement purposes. Facilitating the completion of records by providers is a key factor in ensuring that needed information can be provided to all authorized users.

Facilities use a variety of formats for storing patient records to ensure that they are available for future use. As technology has changed, so have the methods of maintaining and storing patient records. Records may be copied onto different types of microfilm stored in cabinets on rolls or on microfiche.

The master patient index may be maintained partially on cards that have been microfilmed and on different types of microfilm. The facility may have a recently installed imaging system. Healthcare information includes videotapes, graphic results, videotapes, and images from specific computerized test results.

The HIM professional has been incrementally transitioning from managing paper health records to managing information in a variety of media and formats. The transition is ongoing, and HIM professionals must take a leadership role in ensuring that needed health information from the patient's past continues to be available for use in the future.

References

Abraham, P.R. 2001. *Documentation and Reimbursement for Home Care and Hospice Programs.* Chicago: AHIMA.

AHIMA Ambulatory Care Section. 2001. *Documentation for Ambulatory Care,* rev. ed. Chicago: American Health Information Management Association.

AHIMA e-HIM Work Group on Implementing Electronic Signatures. 2003 (Oct. 20). Practice brief: Implementing electronic signatures. *Journal of American Health Information Management Association* Web exclusive.

AHIMA e-HIM Work Group on Speech Recognition in the EHR. 2003 (Oct. 20). Practice brief: Speech recognition in the electronic health record. *Journal of American Health Information Management Association* Web exclusive.

AHIMA MPI Task Force. 2004. Practice brief: Building an enterprise master person index. *Journal of American Health Information Management Association* 75(1):56A–56D.

American Association for Medical Transcription. 2005. aamt.org

American Health Information Management Association. 2005. *Documentation and Reimbursement for Behavioral Healthcare Services.* Chicago: AHIMA.

Burrington-Brown, J., and G. Hughes. 2003 (June). Practice brief: Disaster planning for health information. *Journal of American Health Information Management Association* Web exclusive.

Clark, J.S., ed. 2004. *Documentation for Acute Care.* rev. ed. Chicago: AHIMA.

Code of Federal Regulations. 2004. 42 CFR 482.54: Centers for Medicare and Medicaid Services, conditions of participation for hospitals. Available on-line from gpoaccess.gov/cfr/index.html.

Federal Register 70(57). 2005 (March 25). Proposed rules: Centers for Medicare and Medicaid Services, conditions of participation for hospitals: Requirements for history and physical examinations; authentication of verbal orders; securing medications; and postanesthesia evaluations.

Horton, L. 2004. *Calculating and Reporting Healthcare Services.* Chicago: AHIMA.

Hughes, G. 2002 (Nov.). Practice brief: Destruction of patient health information. *Journal of American Health Information Management Association* Web exclusive.

James, E. 2004. *Documentation and Reimbursement for Long-Term Care.* Chicago: AHIMA.

Joint Commission on Accreditation of Healthcare Organizations. 2005. *Comprehensive Accreditation Manual for Hospitals.* Oak Brook Terrace, IL: JCAHO.

Marrelli, T.M. 2000. *Nursing Documentation Handbook,* 3rd ed. St. Louis: Mosby/YearBook.

National Association for Home Care. 2005. nahc.org.

National Hospice and Palliative Care Organization. 2005. nhpco.org.

Peden, A. 2005. *Comparative Records for Health Information Management,* 2nd ed. Clifton Park, NY: Thompson Delmar Learning.

Rhodes, H. 2002 (June 24). Practice brief: Retention of health information. *Journal of American Health Information Management Association* Web exclusive.

Tegan, A., et al. 2005. Practice brief: The EHR's impact on HIM functions. *Journal of American Health Information Management Association* 76(5):56C–H.

Chapter 9
Electronic Health Records

Margret Amatayakul, MBA, RHIA, CHPS, FHIMSS

Learning Objectives

- To describe the evolution of the electronic health record (EHR) and its supporting technologies
- To identify terms and concepts associated with EHRs
- To describe technologies that support and supplement EHRs
- To discuss EHR system challenges and the supporting roles of health information management professionals in addressing them
- To develop an appreciation for the planning and implementation aspects of EHRs
- To provide examples of EHR systems as they may be implemented in various types of care settings

Key Terms

Ancillary system
Application service provider (ASP)
Architecture
Bridge technology
Client/server architecture
Clinical data repository (CDR)
Clinical data warehouse (CDW)
Clinical decision support (CDS)
Clinical messaging
Computerized provider order entry (CPOE)
Computer output to laser disk (COLD)
Confidentiality
Connectivity
Continuity of care record (CCR)
Data exchange standards
Discrete data
Document imaging
Electronic health record (EHR)
Electronic medication administration record (EMAR)
Heuristic thought
Hospital information system (HIS)
Human–computer interface

Hybrid record
Integration
Integrity
Interface
Interoperability
Knowledge base
Legacy system
Message format standards
Migration path
Patient care charting system
Personal health record (PHR)
Practice management system (PMS)
Protocol
Redundant arrays of independent (or inexpensive) disks (RAID)
Risk analysis
Semantics
Server redundancy
Source systems
Syntax
Vocabulary
Web portal

Introduction

Although the concept of the **electronic health record** (EHR) has been around since the late 1960s, it has only been since the late 1990s that it has become a serious goal for many provider organizations. This goal was further solidified by reference to the importance of EHRs in the 2004 State of the Union address by President Bush and subsequent federal government initiatives. The concept of capturing clinical data from multiple sources for use at the point of care and in clinical decision making has been difficult to achieve because there are many unique challenges in health information computing.

Health information computing is not just about quickly "crunching" a lot of numbers to produce a bank balance or to calculate an airplane weight for takeoff. Health information is largely textual. Narrative text is not as easy to manipulate by computer as numbers are. Moreover, health information is contextual. A given word may have different meanings when associated with other words (for example, red may indicate embarrassment when describing a face or infection when describing a lesion).

Further, healthcare professionals who need to use computers are very mobile. They move to examining rooms, to the surgery suite with a patient on a gurney, or even to patients in their homes. Other workers are mobile, but their data requirements are generally more limited (such as in the package delivery industry). It has only been very recently that handheld, wireless devices have begun to be deployed successfully in healthcare computing.

Finally, most computerization has been built on the assumption that there are standard ways of doing things. Computers can process an enormous amount of data very rapidly when standard terms and standard processes are being used. However, the human body is anything but standard. Healthcare is as much an art as a science. It has taken time for sophisticated computational processes to be developed that essentially allow the computer to "learn" processes through pattern analysis thus supporting humans when they engage in **heuristic thought** processes when diagnosing and treating patients.

This chapter focuses on the emergence of the EHR and its supporting technologies. It also discusses how EHRs are created and how patient information is managed in an electronic environment. Finally, the chapter looks at future directions of health information technologies.

Theory into Practice

Dr. Smith is at home having breakfast with her family. Before heading off to the hospital to check on patients and then to the office, a quick check via the home computer starts her day in real time.

The EHR that Dr. Smith accesses provides an integrated inbox. The inbox reveals that one of her hospitalized patients is deteriorating rapidly. She also receives a message from a colleague, Dr. Jones, who is requesting a consult for a patient with an especially severe condition. He has forwarded the patient's continuity of1 care record to Dr. Smith for her review. In addition, Dr. Smith's office is requesting approval for renewal of a medication for a patient who is out of town. In responding to the renewal request, an alert informs Dr. Smith that the patient is also due for a checkup, so this information is sent back to the office scheduling system for contacting the patient within the next 10 days. Further checking today's schedule, Dr. Smith notes that a meeting with the local medical society is taking place this evening and there is an e-mail from another colleague wanting to chat before the meeting about a new treatment regime that appears promising. Not having seen literature on the new treatment regime, Dr. Smith checks the National Library of Medicine archives for any possible articles. Finding a few, she tags them for printing in the office.

Before logging off, Dr. Smith receives an instant message concerning the critical patient. Not wanting to wait until she arrives at the hospital, Dr. Smith engages the charge nurse in an exchange of information, including a streaming video of the patient's latest vital signs. Dr. Smith decides to move the patient to critical care and places a series of orders for the patient. She is aided by access to a comprehensive list of medications the patient is known to have taken in the past and with information about indications and contraindications from a drug knowledge base. In placing an order for a specific medication, Dr. Smith is alerted that the medication she entered is contraindicated with another drug the patient is taking, so she makes an adjustment.

This scenario reflects the growing trends of remote **connectivity;** clinical messaging; integrating voice, data, and video; use of knowledge sources; and clinical decision support that are all components of an EHR.

Evolution of the Electronic Health Record

The EHR is as much a concept as a product to buy or a system to build. In its landmark work, the Institute of Medicine (IOM) defined the EHR, what it then called the computer-based patient record (CPR), as a record "that resides in a system specifically designed to support users by providing accessibility to complete and accurate data, alerts, reminders, clinical decision support systems, links to medical knowledge, and other aids. This definition encompasses a broader view of the patient record than is current today, moving from the notion of a location or device for keeping track of patient care events to a resource with much enhanced utility in patient care (including the ability to provide an accurate longitudinal account of care), in management of the health care system, and in extension of knowledge" (IOM 1991, pp. 2–3). In addition, the IOM provided the caveat that "merely automating the form, content, and procedures of current patient records will perpetuate their deficiencies and will be insufficient to meet emerging user needs" (IOM 1991, p. 2).

As with any revolutionary system, the EHR has suffered somewhat from multiple different interpretations and rapid development of products that did not fully meet the vision. When the IOM first released its report, vendors rushed to market such products. They were often more vaporware than reality or were limited in true EHR functionality. In fact, some of them were so disappointing or cumbersome to use that they may have discouraged potential users to such an extent that they may be unwilling to try again.

Today, there is a much better understanding of the complexity of what an EHR is and how it may:

- Improve the quality of healthcare through data availability and links to knowledge sources
- Enhance patient safety with context-sensitive reminders and alerts, clinical decision support, automated surveillance, chronic disease management, and drug/device recall capability
- Support health maintenance, preventive care, and wellness through patient reminders, health summaries, tailored instructions, educational materials, and home monitoring/tracking capability
- Increase productivity through data capture and reporting formats tailored to the user; streamlined work flow support; and patient-specific care plans, guidelines, and protocols
- Reduce hassle factors/improve satisfaction for clinicians, consumers, and caregivers by managing scheduling, registration, referrals, medication refills, and work queues and by automatically generating administrative data
- Support revenue enhancement through accurate and timely eligibility and benefit information, cost-efficacy analysis, clinical trial recruitment, rules-driven coding assistance, external accountability reporting/outcomes measures, and contract management
- Support predictive modeling and contribute to development of evidence-based healthcare guidance
- Maintain patient confidentiality and exchange data securely among all key stakeholders

EHR Functionality

Two important work products have contributed significantly to today's better understanding of how an EHR should function. In 2003, the IOM again contributed to the body of knowledge surrounding EHRs when it responded to a federal government request to describe EHR key capabilities. It identified eight core functionalities and developed a spreadsheet of how they could be rolled out across four types of healthcare organizations (hospitals, ambulatory care, nursing homes, and care in the community [personal health record]) over an eight-year time frame. The core functionalities are (IOM 2003):

- Health information and data
- Results management
- Order entry/management
- Decision support
- Electronic communication and connectivity
- Patient support
- Administrative processes
- Reporting and population health management

The 2003 IOM work was then contributed to the Health Level Seven (HL7) standards development organization for them to enhance and ballot as a standard. This was done in 2004, as the EHR System Functional Model Draft Standard for Trial Use (DSTU). The model is depicted in figure 9.1, (p. 214).

The standard includes approximately 60 pages of functions, their descriptions, rationale for inclusion in the DSTU, and citations, where applicable. The DSTU is subject to a two-year trial period during which industry experience will offer modification for a final standard. The preface to the DSTU notes that the functions described are visionary and that not every vendor will, or would necessarily ever be expected to, incorporate all functions. This clearly recognizes that the EHR is still very much in development and that organizations must take a **migration path** through various applications and technologies to achieve the benefits cited for an EHR.

In order to assist organizations, a Commission on Certification Technology (CCHIT) has formed to establish baseline standards and provide certification of EHR products. The work is spearheaded by the Healthcare Information Management and Systems Society (HIMSS) and AHIMA and has now received federal government funding.

Migration Path

As the healthcare industry works through the steps to achieve recognition of what an EHR is and how it can best be implemented, each organization also should recognize that a migration path may be necessary to ultimately reach the goal of an EHR. This migration path should be carefully planned and well thought out. It should be a strategic plan that identifies the various goals the organization has for EHR along a time line that is realistic given its current culture, information technology (IT), financial capability, and other strategic imperatives. (See figure 9.2, p. 215.)

Many hospitals are rushing to adopt **bridge technology** such as **document imaging** and/or **clinical messaging** that provides some, but not all, the benefits of EHR, and many physician offices are rushing to market to buy an EHR that they really do not understand. Little study has been done on the impact that adoption of any of the technology has on the organization, whether it be the ability to move forward with other EHR components in a hospital or to actually use the EHR in the office. Indeed, many organizations are making

Figure 9.1.   HL7 EHR system functional model

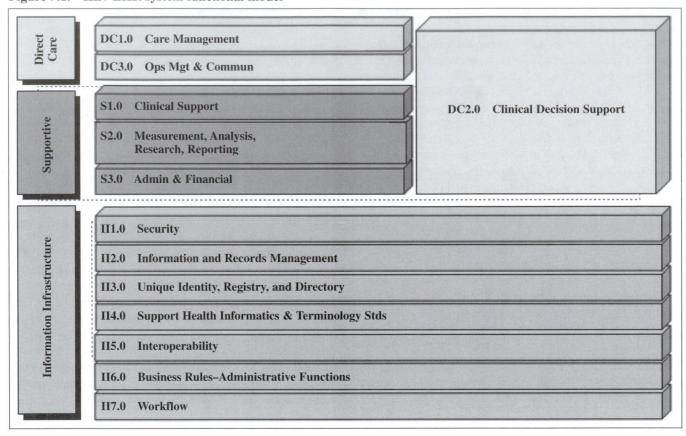

©2004 Health Level Seven (HL7), Inc.

investment decisions that will be difficult for them to change any time soon.

This is not to imply that bridge technology is inappropriate or that physician offices are not at all prepared for an EHR. Bridge technology serves a very useful purpose and may be the most appropriate strategy for a given organization. However, a formal review should be made of the EHR goals, current and planned applications, current and planned technology, and organizational culture and readiness. It should be understood that document imaging, for example, perpetuates the paper record, only making information more available. Some organizations actually believe that instituting document imaging sets an organization back in its quest for an EHR because it does not encourage use of data capture and retrieval technology.

Clearly, if the definition of EHR includes the ability to capture data from multiple sources, all source data must be in electronic form. (See figure 9.3.) Most hospitals and some physician offices have financial/administrative systems (such as patient accounting, registration-admission-discharge-transfer [R-ADT], chart tracking, and so on), and many have **ancillary systems** that are largely operational but also generate clinical information (such as laboratory information systems [LISs], radiology information systems

[RISs], pharmacy information systems [PISs], and so on). Still, many hospitals and physician offices do not have all source data automated or the ability for all source systems to communicate with one another or integrate all source data together. It may be prudent for an organization to address these issues prior to adopting additional applications or appropriate to consider strategic replacement of systems where current systems are old and there is little vendor support for a comprehensive EHR.

The next part of the EHR definition is for it to be used as the primary source of information at the point of care. Certainly, some of the bridge technology supports this part of the EHR definition, although in many cases the technology's intent is not always carried out. For example, documents may be scanned and other data fed into a repository for access at the nursing station, but clinicians may continue to use only printouts to review data and rely fully on paper for documentation.

The **clinical decision support** (CDS) element of the EHR definition is the one that is recognized as the greatest benefit, but it requires real-time entry of data and retrieval of information by clinicians for use. This is the greatest hurdle, which is not addressed by document imaging systems or most other bridge technology.

Figure 9.2.   An example migration path for an EHR

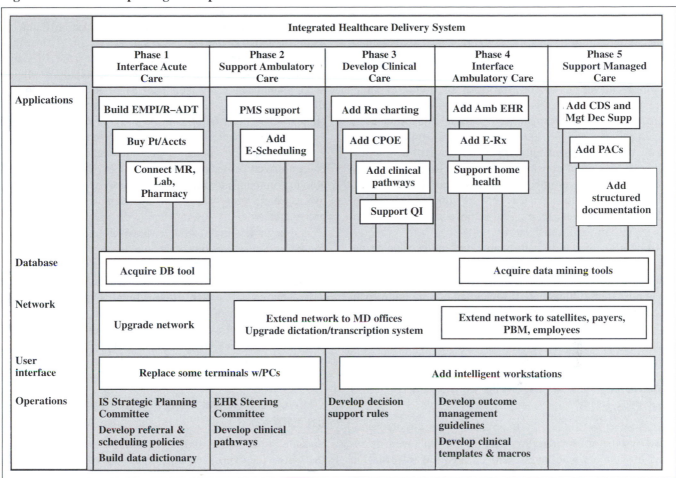

Integrated Healthcare Delivery System				
Phase 1 Interface Acute Care	**Phase 2** Support Ambulatory Care	**Phase 3** Develop Clinical Care	**Phase 4** Interface Ambulatory Care	**Phase 5** Support Managed Care

Applications, Database, Network, User interface, Operations rows as shown in figure.

Figure 9.3.   Source systems feeding data to the EHR

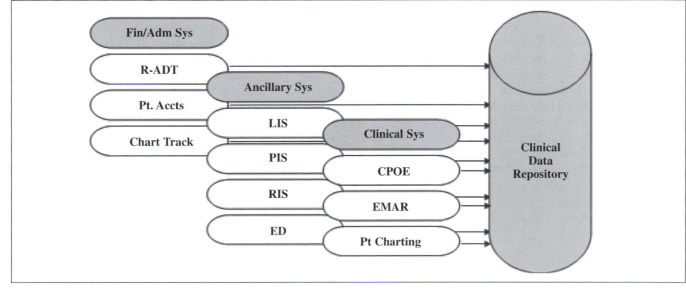

Every organization has its own migration path. There is no one right or wrong path, only one that is most appropriate for a given organization given its current situation and future goals. What is unfortunate, however, is that many organizations are not taking the approach of strategically planning for an EHR but, rather, are responding to external pressures to acquire whatever the vendor offers as a solution or to implement a system that is temporary, even though they have never retired any of their information systems. The investment not only in acquiring any IS, but also in taking the time and making the effort to implement and gain adoption of a system is immense and often considered too great to ever abandon. Even when a vendor retires a product, a healthcare organization is more likely to find a way to work with the system than to buy a replacement, fearing the effort it will take to get a new system to work satisfactorily.

Building a migration path begins with understanding the state of applications, technology, and processes that are used today and then building on those to identify the most appropriate next steps. Often there is something of a migration path in adoption of current applications, as they have typically included financial/administrative systems, ancillary support systems, systems to support access to clinical information, and finally systems to support provider–patient connectivity.

Financial/Administrative Systems and the EHR

Early efforts to develop EHR products were largely segregated by type of provider. Products for hospitals were developed by vendors who had developed **hospital information systems** (HISs) for financial and administrative purposes. Products for outpatient departments or physician offices were developed by vendors who had developed billing and practice management systems (PMSs).

Such development involved two primary issues. First, although there are distinct differences in work flow and computing needs for acute care versus ambulatory care, the fact that these products were being developed independently also meant that they were generally unable to exchange data seamlessly across the settings. Although Web-based technology can help exchange health information between hospitals and clinics or physician practices, systems have to be upgraded to accommodate this function. Second, the fact that vendors with financial/administrative expertise were developing clinical computing products often left much to be desired with respect to the products' ability to be used at the point of care and in CDS. Some of these vendors have subsequently addressed their clinical deficiencies by adding clinical staff and/or acquiring more clinically based products. Other vendors with specific clinical focus have emerged.

Ancillary Support Systems as Source Systems for the EHR

A critical step toward achieving the EHR is to automate all the systems in the hospital or clinic that provide source data to the EHR or must receive data from an EHR. These systems are often referred to as **source systems** or feeder systems. For example, patient demographic data are needed in financial/administrative, operational, and clinical systems. Lab results from the LIS, medication information from the PIS, and radiology reports and images from RISs and picture archiving and communications systems (PACS) all are required for the EHR. Furthermore, the data must not only be accessible to clinicians, but also be able to be integrated for processing. For example, a medication order should be compared with lab results to determine potential contraindications. Likewise, a **computerized provider order-entry** (CPOE) system must be able to communicate orders to each of these systems respectively. Charges also should be captured as source systems process the orders.

Although hospitals tend to have a greater number of source systems than physician practices or clinics, source systems are still an issue in these settings as well. Some physician practices started out with only a billing system. When they acquired a **practice management system** (PMS), the two systems needed to communicate demographic data. (In most cases now, the PMS incorporates billing.) Frequently, practices rely on external labs. Even though the results are generated electronically, they typically have been faxed to the provider.

Legacy Systems and Their Impact on EHRs

Virtually all hospitals and many clinics have some existing ISs before they approach adoption of an EHR. When these systems have existed solely for the purpose of financial and administrative functions and then are called on to support clinical computing, they are often referred to as **legacy systems.** In addition to the lack of **integration** between hospital and clinic systems and the focus on financial/administrative processes, legacy systems often pose additional issues for providers wanting to acquire an EHR.

One legacy system issue relates to the fact that all or most of the systems may be from a single vendor. They are likely to be well integrated among themselves, but highly proprietary. This scenario is often described as "best-of-fit." In a best-of-fit environment, it is very difficult to introduce an EHR from a different vendor into the mix of legacy source systems. Other organizations have approached automation from a "best-of-breed" situation, where many, if not all, source systems are from different vendors. Where necessary, the organization has interfaced these systems so that some data are passed from one to another (typically demographic data from the financial system to [some of] the administrative systems and charges from administrative systems to the financial system). In some cases, the different systems do not exchange data electronically, so data in one system that are needed by another system may have to be rekeyed. One solution to this situation is called "dual core," where the financial/administrative systems are retained in their legacy architecture and new technology, including a data repository, is acquired for the clinical components of the EHR. The two cores are then interfaced (Cohen and Amatayakul 2004). (See figure 9.4.)

Another legacy system issue is that many of these systems are truly "old" systems. They may be based on mainframe computer technology with terminals that use older (DOS-based, "green screens") operating system software. This frequently requires organizations to revamp their technology to newer, **client/server architecture** or to use other, third-party software to create a Windows™ environment.

Systems to Support Access to Clinical Information

The challenges posed by legacy systems are very significant. The cost of replacement and data conversion can be very great. As a result, a number of organizations have opted to approach their EHR through the use of bridge technology to improve access to data. They have adopted document-imaging and **computer-output-to-laser-disk** (COLD) systems. These systems make paper and transcribed documents as well as data in legacy systems available for review. Although data in image form are not processable in all CDS systems, they do have the benefit of making information available to multiple users simultaneously. Clinical messaging is another bridge technology, where Web-based systems are used to exchange scanned or COLD-fed documents or results from source systems as well as electronic mail messages among users, often remotely (such as from the hospital to a physician office).

Systems to Provide Provider–Patient Connectivity

Some of the clinical messaging systems utilize **Web portals** (secure gateways to a local area network [Internet] based on Internet technology) to provide secure connectivity. In addi-

tion to linking hospitals and clinics through provider portals, some are set up as patient portals. Patients may request appointments, manage preadmission processing, retrieve results, and submit health history information via such a portal. If the patient does not have access to the Internet at home or does not wish to use an employer's system, he or she may use a kiosk at the provider organization. **Personal health records** (PHRs) are becoming popular with some patients. They come in many forms, from paper copies of discharge summaries or printouts of instructions to systems coordinated with the EHR and accessible electronically (Connecting for Health 2003).

Health Information Systems for Other Types of Healthcare Institutions

Although hospitals and clinics have generally been the early adopters of EHRs, other types of healthcare providers, as well as payers, are adopting various forms of EHRs as well. Behavioral health facilities find the integration of data from multiple sources especially helpful in coordination of care. Home health agencies are adopting handheld devices to capture data in compliance with regulatory requirements. Long-term care facilities have a more difficult time affording systems, but their highly structured data-reporting requirements also make them good candidates for simple EHR systems. Finally, health plans collect a tremendous amount of data about individuals from claims as well as attachments. These health plans are creating EHRs for disease management and predictive modeling.

Still, it is important to note that the many forms of EHR that exist in the different health environments are generally stand-alone with respect to the organization in which they reside, with little exchange among different organizations. Even among components of an integrated delivery network (IDN), not all systems communicate with one another. This

Figure 9.4.   IS strategic options

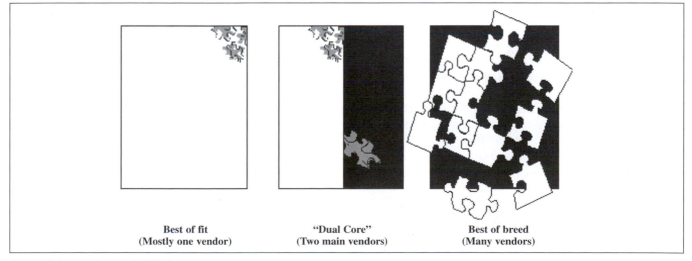

Best of fit **(Mostly one vendor)**	**"Dual Core"** **(Two main vendors)**	**Best of breed** **(Many vendors)**

Source: Cohen and Amatayakul 2004.

is changing as regional health information organizations (RHIOs) form. RHIOs are a fairly new concept intended to support care across the continuum within a geographical community, state, or region. Health information exchange within the RHIO is accomplished in a variety of ways, but frequently through portal technology. The federal government envisions a national health information network (NHIN) whereby health information may be exchanged securely and seamlessly to authorized parties across the country. In the absence of a national patient identifier, this will require a sophisticated record locator service. As the the national network develops, RHIOs are beginning to be referred to as health information exchanges (HIEs). (See chapter 7.)

Check Your Understanding 9.1

Instructions: On a separate piece of paper, match the EHR benefits with the functions that support them.

Benefits:
A. Enhance patient safety
B. Improve quality of care
C. Increase productivity
D. Maintain patient confidentiality
E. Reduce hassle factors
F. Support health maintenance
G. Support predictive modeling
H. Support revenue enhancement

Functions:
1. ____ Context-specific reminders
2. ____ Data availability
3. ____ Evidence-based health care
4. ____ External accountability reporting
5. ____ Medication refills
6. ____ Security
7. ____ Tailored instructions to patients
8. ____ Work flow support

EHR Terms and Concepts

Electronic health record (EHR) is the term used in this textbook to describe a comprehensive system of applications that afford access to longitudinal health information about an individual across the continuum of care, assist in documentation, support clinical decision making, and provide for knowledge building. Other terms have been used in the past, some specific to a vendor and others generic. As previously noted, the IOM coined the term *computer-based patient record* in 1991 but has subsequently migrated to using *EHR*. *Electronic medical record* has been a very popular term, in some contexts referring to physician office systems and in other contexts referring to document-imaging systems. In 2004, however, HL7 adopted *electronic health record,* which is the term most frequently used by the federal government in its efforts to promote adoption of health information technology. Although the term *record* still conveys a specific location, the

term *health* broadens the concept of the record containing only information about medical care to all information about the healthcare, wellness, and prevention of illness and injury important to an individual.

The EHR may be built on or complemented by technologies and systems that also have distinguishing names and features. Many EHRs, especially in hospitals, start out as component applications. For example, when most financial/administrative and ancillary systems are in place, results can be made accessible via workstations on the nursing units of a hospital. Consideration then may be given to adopting CPOE systems, **electronic medication administration record** (E-MAR) systems, and **patient care charting systems.** In the ambulatory environment, there may be electronic prescribing (e-prescribing) systems, CPOE (in larger clinics), and various work flow tools providing information about patient wait times, scheduling, referral management, and disease management.

When most of the components are in place, healthcare organizations typically look for tighter integration of data and adoption of CDS systems. CDS systems include context-specific templates that drive data collection; alerts about clinical conditions, such as indications and contraindications concerning medications or changes in patient vital signs; reminders, potentially about health maintenance and wellness protocols; and many other forms of clinical help. In general, CDS systems require two key things: a **clinical data repository** (CDR) and **discrete data.**

Many EHR systems are built on a CDR. The CDR is a type of database that organizes data from many different sources and makes it readily available to users. Data that go into a repository may come from various source systems or may be entered by a user directly. Data in a CDR may be structured, or "discrete," data, or it may be unstructured data. Discrete data are individual data elements entered into the computer, generally at the point of care by the clinician. The data are often encoded by the computer, with either a proprietary code system or a standard vocabulary.

For example, in the sentence, "This is a three-month-old female with a cough," the age, sex, and chief complaint are variables. If "three-month," "female," and "cough" are entered into fields for "age," "sex," and "chief complaint," they may be encoded by the computer for easy processing. The numeric age may be captured as is, with a code for a period of time. The sex may be designated as F or M, 1 or 2, or some other coding system as designated by the designer of the system. The chief complaint may be coded by ICD, SNOMED, or other **vocabulary.** When these three elements are entered, they may be processed in many ways in the CDR. For example, age may be used to calculate the appropriate dose of a medication. Calculating medication doses for pediatric patients is just one example of a use of CDS.

Unstructured data include narrative notes as well as images (of scanned documents or medical images). These data also may be captured in a repository, but highly robust CDS rules generally cannot be processed with such unstructured data.

However, a clinician may enter data, view them being processed (for example, in a graph or table), and also call up an image of an x-ray or report of a consultant simultaneously using a repository. When documents are scanned, certain data on them (for example, allergy information) may be individually indexed and then be available for the system to provide as a reminder.

The PHR has been mentioned as a means for individuals to compile information about their health, the care they have received, and other factors important to them. Personalizing healthcare is an important goal of federal government initiatives (Thompson and Brailer 2004). PHRs can be an important adjunct to EHRs. Many providers are looking at ways to provide patients with more information about their care and to receive information from individuals that may be useful for their care. Some providers are concerned that PHRs are not standardized and often not structured in a manner amenable to electronic processing in EHRs; others have expressed liability concerns. PHRs may contain more information than a provider has the ability to consume at any given care encounter or may be lacking information vital to the care of the patient. However, PHRs can be extremely valuable for patients with chronic illness, individuals who may be unable to relate health history except via a PHR carried by a caregiver, or individuals who are highly mobile. It is very likely that PHRs will see standardization and greater adoption in the near future.

Another relatively new concept is that of the **continuity of care record** (CCR), the content for which has been adopted as a standard by the ASTM International standards organization. The CCR is not intended to replace the EHR but, rather, to serve as an extraction of data for the purpose of providing health information about a patient when care is transferred from one provider to another.

Check Your Understanding 9.2

Instructions: On a separate piece of paper, indicate whether each answer below is true or false.

1. The CCR is the same as a CDR. True or false.

2. *EHR* is the term coined by the IOM to describe the function of capturing data from multiple sources for use in clinical decision support at the point of care. True or false.

3. Some providers are concerned about the liability that PHRs may introduce into their practice of medicine. True or false.

4. An example of discrete data would be the value of the diastolic blood pressure. True or false.

5. CDS depends on the integration of discrete data. True or false.

6. Hospital EHR systems tend to be built from many clinical computing components. True or false.

7. The federal government most commonly uses the term *electronic medical record* to distinguish physician office from hospital-based health information technology. True or false.

8. Discrete data are generally encoded by the computer for processing. True or false.

9. A repository does not contain unstructured data. True or false.

10. The purpose of the CCR is to transfer data among providers. True or false.

Technologies That Support the EHR

From the description of terms and concepts, it should be clear that an EHR is not simply a computer software package or program. Unlike laboratory information systems or admitting systems that basically perform one major function for one department, an EHR system may be viewed as the "engine" that integrates all other systems.

To serve its function of capturing data from multiple sources and converting them into timely, usable information, the EHR embodies many different technologies. These technologies include databases, data exchange standards, vocabulary standards, image processing, data retrieval technology, data capture technology, clinical decision support, communications and networking, storage, and security.

Databases

There are essentially two ways to integrate data for an EHR. One is to collect all the data needed in a central database, process them there, and disperse results from there; the second is to keep data in independent systems and use **data exchange standards** to access the data.

Integration of data from multiple independent systems into a central database is generally considered more appropriate for a comprehensive EHR. This not only provides access to data but integrates them in a manner that makes them more readily processable in real time and for CDS. In order to collect and process data in this integrated manner, a database is used that incorporates special indexing and management functions to capture, sort, process, and present information back to users—often in a split second! Such a database is called a data repository. To distinguish repositories that focus on clinical information (instead of financial and/or administrative data), the term *clinical data repository* is used.

Some EHR systems also include another form of database, called a **clinical data warehouse** (CDW). A data repository is typically used for processing transactions, which are the actions of entering, retrieving, and processing data for one specific patient and purpose at a time (such as entering an order or retrieving a lab result). Although many of these transactions are very complex, each transaction does not require processing an immense amount of data at one time. When complex analyses are to be performed on data, a data warehouse may be the more appropriate database structure to use. Data warehouses are designed to receive data (often as an extraction of data from a repository) and process them in aggregate form. Data can be mined and processed in many ways. For example, a data warehouse may be used for clinical quality improvement, best practice guideline development, or pay-for-performance (P4P) data reporting. Databases and their structures are more fully described in chapter 5.

Data Exchange Standards and Vocabulary Standards

The second way an EHR can be achieved is by retaining all the data in the various independent, departmental system databases and using data exchange standards to view data from each system. This approach to EHR is generally considered an interim approach because it primarily facilitates only viewing of information. As a result, processing the data is limited to the processing capability of only one application at a time. Thus different medications could be compared in a PIS, but lab results from an LIS could not be integrated into the PIS for processing.

However, data exchange standards may still be required to smoothly move data from an application system to a repository and back. For example, a hospital may have an LIS and a PIS. As it acquires a CPOE system, the data from the LIS and PIS flow into the repository. When an order is written, it also enters the repository. There, the order may be compared with data from the LIS and PIS. CDS rules may process the data to determine that a medication being ordered is contraindicated for the patient because of abnormal liver function studies. An alert will "fire" from the repository to the provider entering the order about this situation. The provider then can make whatever adjustments in the order that may be necessary. The repository then directs the medication order to the PIS where pharmacy operations can be performed, including generating a charge, updating the inventory, and so on. (See figure 9.5.)

Data exchange standards have typically been called message format standards because their primary intent was to move a "message" from one system to another. This is also called functional **interoperability.** For example, when the PIS sends a message that a drug has been removed from stock for a particular patient, it sends a charge message to the patient accounting system. (Note: As medication administration is becoming automated as well, some hospitals are shifting medication charge capture from the pharmacy to the bedside. In this way, the charge is not created until the drug is actually administered. However, wherever the charge is captured, a message must be sent to the patient accounting system.)

Message format standards make sure that the structure and format of data, as they are being transmitted from one system to another, are the same. This data structure and format is called **syntax.** Each proprietary system has its own syntax. For systems to exchange data or "talk" to one another, the syntax must be made the same. As an example, in figure 9.6, two different systems are attempting to convey the same information, but to use different field names (patient name versus individual name) and different element names (middle initial versus middle name) and to sequence the elements differently.

System developers use message format standards to create **interfaces** between systems. An interface is a **protocol** that maps data from one system to another so that the data can be sent either from one system to another (unidirectional interface) or between two systems (bidirectional interface). However, some of these standards, HL7 in particular, have a lot of optionality. As a result, even two systems that are HL7 compliant may not be fully interoperable (that is, able to exchange data). Writing an interface between two systems can be very challenging because it requires not only someone who knows how to do the computer programming involved, but also someone to negotiate between the two different vendors whose systems are being interfaced. It is for these reasons that interfaces have been very expensive, sometime costing tens of thousands of dollars (with some of that money to going to each of the two vendors). Additionally, interfaces must be kept up to date. Each time one of the two systems that have been interfaced is upgraded by its vendor, the interface must be modified to ensure that the change in one system is reflected in the capability to communicate the message to the other system. Of course, the problem is further compounded—and sometimes impossible to solve—when the vendors do not use HL7 at all. Although the syntaxes illustrated in figure 9.6 may seem subtle, they are sufficiently different as to render the two systems unable to communicate with one another without an interface.

Because of the cost and complexity of building interfaces between systems, some hospitals are reluctant to buy systems that have not been created by their primary vendor. However, it should be noted that buying systems from a single vendor may not necessarily mean they are fully integrated. (The term integration refers to the ability to exchange data without an interface.) A company may have bought another company in order to add a particular product to its product line. Although it will write an interface from the purchased product to its own product line in advance of selling the system, these interfaces may be limited in scope and/or may not work with other vendor systems a given hospital may have.

Figure 9.5.   Example of a data repository

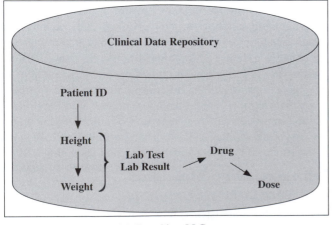

Figure 9.6.   Different systems attempting to convey the same information

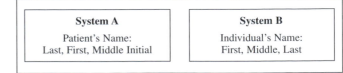

To date, message format standards have been limited to exchanging whatever data were sent from one system to another. There was no reconciliation that the terminology used in one system was the same in the other system. The data were not standardized. A common vocabulary was not used. Most recently, the industry has come to realize that for one clinical system to use another clinical system's data, terms must have the same meaning. **Semantics** is the term used to describe the fact that the content of a message has a common meaning. When a message format standard specifies the vocabulary with which the data are encoded, the functionality is called semantic interoperability. HL7 Version 3 has begun to embed vocabulary references into its message format standard.

Continuing the above example, the LIS may encode lab result data using the Logical Observations Identifiers Names and Codes (LOINC) vocabulary. The CPOE system may present clinical drug choices to the ordering provider via RxNorm vocabulary. The PIS may use National Drug Codes (NDCs) to maintain its drug inventory. However, knowing which vocabulary is used to express each data element in the process can ensure proper understanding by the respective user and system, and mapping can occur among the standard vocabularies. For example, a map from RxNorm codes to NDC codes ensures that both clinical treatment and pharmacy inventory needs are met. Data exchange standards are described more fully in chapter 7.

Electronic Document/ Content Management

Another set of technology that supports an EHR is electronic document/content management (ED/CM) and computer-output-to-laser disk/enterprise report management (COLD/ERM). Although the ultimate goal may be for clinicians to enter data directly into a system and to respond to CDS systems at the point of care, these are complex systems to build and require an enormous change in how clinicians work. As a result, many healthcare organizations are using various forms of document imaging and digital document management to automate the current paper charts to make them more readily accessible to clinicians. Document-imaging systems scan existing documents and store them for viewing through a computer workstation. As documents are scanned, they are indexed, assigning a description of the document and key contents for later retrieval. Documents that have been entered into an electronic transcription system or outputted in report-formatted digital documents (such as laboratory results from an LIS) can also be COLD-fed into a repository for viewing. The benefit of document imaging is greatly enhanced access to such documents. However, when content management and work flow tools are added to the document imaging, flow of work can be managed and many forms of documents can be accessible together, including the scanned and COLD-fed documents as well as e-mail, instant messages, Web pages, and so on. Work flow tools, for example, can not only pro-

vide access to scanned charts to coders at home, but also can direct different categories of charts to different coders and volumes managed. However, not all work flow systems have the capability of supporting both administrative (for example, coding and release of information) and clinical functions (for example, viewing the scanned documents in the emergency department).

Clinical images are pictures generated by medical devices such as x-rays, EKG monitors, and so on. Storage of these pictures is called PACS (picture archiving and communications systems). Clinical images from PACS can be viewed through standard monitors if great detail is not required. Diagnostic-quality viewing of such images requires special monitors with very high-resolution and/or full-motion video capability. Because of their ability to be enlarged, rotated, and several images viewed simultaneously, many radiologists find PACS superior to standard radiology film.

Data Retrieval Technology

Because most ISs used today in hospitals are primarily data retrieval systems, technology to support this functionality is quite mature. Retrieval technology may be as basic as a lookup, where a query is made to access certain data from a specific system (for example, a lab result on a certain patient from the LIS). The desired patient may be selected from a list or by entering his or her name and/or medical record number. Navigational tools permit the user to select a specific data element, to make a customized table, or even to graph results.

More sophisticated retrieval technologies enable a user to access several different types of data from different source systems through a single application screen. Hence, a medication list may be viewed from the same application screen as the lab results. There may be windows for different types of data from different sources, or there may be predesigned or customizable screens that permit viewing a specific user's preferred set of data. The most sophisticated retrieval technology, coupled with a CDR, permits not only viewing of data by type, but also manipulation of several different types of data, such as plotting lab results on a graph against medication administration, vital signs, and so on.

One disadvantage to using a computer to view information is the inability to "flip" quickly through multiple "pages" of data. Clinicians have learned to rapidly scan a patient's record to both get an overall picture of the patient and to find specific data. Although this capability is available in a computer through specific search features, color, and other navigational tools, they are not yet everyday tools used by clinicians. Eventually, everyone will use such tools, much as a nurse's progress note can be distinguished from a physician's progress note today. Now, however, they are still somewhat foreign to many users. Most users find it easier to use a printout of the electronically stored data to look at results. Unfortunately, such printouts create a number of problems. Multiple copies of the same information may be printed and filed in the record, making it more voluminous. Worse is the situation where some of the printouts have been annotated so that two copies of the same printout may have different data on them. If one of the "duplicates" gets destroyed, vital information may be lost. Destruction of copies even with no documentation on them is an added burden. The situation where some data are on paper and some data are in electronic form is called a **hybrid record.**

As more clinicians become accustomed to the computer, however, the key to achieving true usability of an EHR is to pack as much information on a single screen as possible. Although it may seem "cleaner" or more user friendly to have fewer data on any given screen, the reverse has actually proved to be true, although the layout of such a dense screen must be very carefully designed.

Thus, an important characteristic of retrieval technologies is that of screen layout and the ability to customize or tailor the layout to the preference of the user. Many EHR systems display a tailored screen based on the user's log-on. Thus, when Dr. Jones logs on, his personally preferred screen layout is displayed. The ability to drill down to greater detail is also important; but, again, caution must be applied to avoid having so many pathways through data that the user gets lost and cannot effectively go back to an original screen. Research also has shown that three levels of screen layers are about the most anyone can use effectively.

A word about color, animation, icons, and sound is also appropriate in a discussion of retrieval technologies. Color can be very helpful in navigating a screen to find desired data, but the number of people (especially men) who are color-blind must be considered. Color should never be relied on solely to convey any critical alerts; instead, color should be accompanied by a special icon, animation, or sound. Icons can be very effective in guiding users, but they must be large enough to be seen clearly and should be very intuitive. Unfortunately, few standard symbols can be used in creating icons for health information systems. Of all the navigational elements available, sound may be the least used in healthcare because of the many medical devices that routinely emit sounds and have special sound alarms.

Data Capture Technology

If it is difficult to get clinicians to retrieve data from EHR systems, it is even more difficult to get them to enter data. With the exception of possibly the most current generation of users, most clinicians have never learned to type and consider typing or any other form of keyboard use to be a clerical function. Even clinicians who are willing and able to type still often find data entry on a computer more challenging and time-consuming than handwriting or dictating.

Unfortunately, no ideal solution has yet been found to support data capture effectively for all users in all environments. However, there are a few key considerations. Most important, data entry must return value to the user. If the user can obtain decision support at the time of data entry

that is valuable to him or her, data entry will be more palatable. However, the decision support must facilitate and not interfere with the flow of information processing. Clinicians are more inclined to do data entry when they can see that the direct result of their data entry is a benefit to their subsequent work (for example, it prompts for billing support data or automatically generates tailored instructions to the patient). However, if data entry is perceived to take longer than traditional recording, even if its purpose is laudable (such as to have more legible data to improve patient safety), it will be a hard sell.

However, several technologies can help make data capture easier. Collectively, these are often called **human–computer interfaces** because of their importance in getting clinicians to perform data entry. They include:

- *Discrete data entry through point-and-click fields, drop-down menus, structured templates, or macros:* In addition to making data entry easier, structured data entry makes processing of the data easier. Devices supporting such data entry include the mouse, light pens, and touch screens. If the data are further codified to a standard vocabulary, that makes them much more valuable. However, many clinicians want to be able to convey more information than just that accommodated through such menus.
- *Speech and handwriting recognition:* Speech recognition can be very effective for certain clinicians. It is not the panacea every clinician dreams of, but where data entry is fairly repetitive and the vocabulary used fairly limited, speech recognition devices can be effectively trained. As speech recognition improves, it is becoming a replacement for dictation. In some cases, the user reviews the speech as it is being converted to type and makes any needed corrections; in other cases, the speech is sent to a special device where it generates type for a "correctionist" to review and edit. Handwriting recognition is similar to speech recognition, where the system is "taught" to recognize a user's handwriting. Some tablet computers have been able to convert handwriting to type fairly successfully, but because of the need for somewhat greater precision than normal handwriting, most tablet computers are used today to capture and retain the handwriting.
- *Handheld and wireless devices:* Handheld devices, such as tablet computers and personal digital assistants (PDAs), may utilize any of the other forms of data entry, from keying and selecting from a list to speech and handwriting recognition. Their use is growing in popularity, but still not necessarily the total answer for everyone. Tablets are generally easy for mobile professionals to have readily available, though they are still fairly heavy. PDAs may be limited in terms of the volume of data they can store and their processing capabilities. The size of both the screen and the keypad

also may be smaller than desirable. Unless tablets or PDAs are wireless, their ability to communicate or link to primary information systems is limited to when they are docked to a workstation. Handheld devices also can run out of battery power. Extra batteries and charging are required. However, handheld devices are ideal for certain limited functions, such as writing prescriptions or for use in capturing a home health data set, and as they are becoming more sophisticated and wireless, they are becoming very popular. Still, many healthcare organizations find it just as effective to mount a notebook computer to a cart and move it with the user. These sometimes are affectionately called COWs (computers on wheels). For the less mobile healthcare professional, desktop computer workstations are still the mainstay.

- *Direct data capture from a medical device attached to a patient:* This is yet another important means of capturing certain kinds of data, such as vital signs. Special medical devices (such as a pacemaker) are even able to be connected to a standard telephone for capturing data or checking on the device's status from a remote location.

- *Patient data entry:* Incorporating patient-generated data into the EHR is just now starting to be used. In some systems, patients can log on to a Web site from home, enter data in accordance with a context-specific template, and submit the data to their provider. At the provider site, the provider reviews and validates the information, and it becomes part of the patient record. In the past, providers have been somewhat reluctant to incorporate patient-generated information. There were misunderstandings that the patients could access and change the entire content of the provider's records. Moreover, there were misperceptions that the information may be too voluminous or erroneous. As patients continue to be seen by an ever-increasing number of providers, however, it is coming to be recognized that they are the only source of at least where all their information is located, if not what the information is.

- *Natural language processing (NLP):* NLP may be considered a special form of data entry. It is the capability of a computer to apply very sophisticated mathematical and probabilistic formulas to narrative text and convert the text to structured data. Although text processing is becoming more feasible, the technology has a long way to go before it can be used routinely.

Clinical Decision Support

Much importance has been placed on the role of CDS in EHRs. CDS systems directly address patient safety and healthcare quality improvement issues. They also aid in bringing value to the user. CDS systems depend on analytical tools that process discrete data in many sophisticated ways. Special analytical tools include reminders and alerts, clinical guideline advice, benchmarking, expert system resources, and diagnostic or procedural investigative tools. CDS systems often depend on an elaborate set of rules, or logical pathways, to trigger reminders or to direct data through a pathway. These rules may be defined by the healthcare organization using them, or they may be acquired from the EHR vendor, via subscription to a **knowledge base** (such as a drug knowledge base [DKB]), or through associations, government agencies, and/or health plans that compile evidence-based health research into best practice guidance. A full discussion of decision support technology is provided in chapter 19.

A critical element of maintaining an EHR is to keep CDS up to date. There are many ways such systems can become obsolete or not functioning properly. Obviously, if a rule directs a clinician to perform certain diagnostic examinations or studies that have been based on best practices and the best practices change, the rule needs to change as well. The medical literature is replete with examples of where new evidence has suggested that an old treatment modality is not as effective as a newer one or where a correlation once believed to have existed between certain factors no longer appears to be true. In addition to keeping rules current, it is important to ensure that each rule has the correct information to process. For example, in an emergency situation where a patient presents with chest pain, there are several possible diagnoses, each based in a different bodily system, including cardiac, respiratory, digestive, and so forth. If a CDS system requires a specific set of data to be collected for every patient presenting with chest pain and all data requirements are met, the CDS will operate properly. However, if one data element is not entered, part of the rule may not permit the clinician to advance to the next screen. If clinicians routinely override the rule, the purpose of the CDS is lost; thus, when the rule fires, it may be erroneous. In some cases, clinicians find certain rules annoying and may demand that a rule be changed to allow only optional entry of a specific data element without an override requirement. In evaluating whether rules should be changed, a designated clinical committee should review the rules to determine whether their impact on the ultimate result warrants the change. It is also possible, however, to fire rules in accordance with classes of users. For example, when a house staff member logs on, he or she could have more CDS than when an attending physician logs on.

Health information management (HIM) professionals can help audit the use of rules and trace the impact of a change in any data element to the ultimate use of the data in CDS. This should be a part of the organization's health information audit program and part of its information systems change control, or configuration management, processes.

System Communication and Networks

The backbone of an EHR obviously is the hardware and software on which the system runs. The term *architecture* refers to the configuration, structure, and relationships of all components of a computer system. Three main types of architecture are used in creating an EHR:

- *Mainframe architecture* utilizes a single large computer to process data received from terminals into which data are entered. Mainframe systems tend to be considered legacy systems because they are the configuration of older applications. In general, mainframe architecture is limited in its ability to support the extensive transaction processing required of an EHR.
- *Client/server architecture* uses a combination of computers to capture and process data. Server computers are powerful processors. They typically will house all the application software and store all active data captured by all the clients throug hout the network. They then "serve" multiple client computers, which have less powerful processors (and in some cases have minimal processing capability of their own, in which case they are called thin clients). (See chapter 3 for further discussion of architecture and networks.)
- *Web services architecture* (WSA) is the next generation of computing structures. It is a way of integrating Web-based applications using open standards over an Internet protocol backbone. WSA allows organizations to share data across different system platforms behind a firewall without being tied to one operating system or programming language.

Storage Technology

The volume of data captured by information systems in general, and in particular by EHRs, is becoming very great. In addition, there is a growing expectation that data should be accessible in real time for very long periods of time. Finally, as clinicians become dependent upon the computer for all their data needs, they will not tolerate downtime or delays for retrieving archived data.

As a result, managing data storage has become an increasingly important issue. Where in the past data were retained online for at most a matter of days after discharge or a visit and a backup was made daily and stored on tape, an EHR virtually demands that data be retained online forever, be instantaneously retrievable, and be backed up continuously.

A storage device is a machine that contains nothing but storage media. Tape drives are the oldest form of storage device and are rapidly becoming obsolete because data are stored sequentially, making retrieval slow. Generally, tapes must be mounted by a person to a tape drive and connected to the central processor for use. Disk drives are the most common storage device today. However, disk technology has moved rapidly from magnetic disks to optical disks of many different forms. Many servers contain optical disk drives that can store very large volumes of data. Still, the result of storing data on the same server that is used to process data in the various applications slows down the server. As a result, disks are being organized in **redundant arrays of independent (or inexpensive) disks,** called RAID, so that a great volume of data can be stored. Storage devices also are being organized into their own storage area networks (SANs) so that they can be accessible from any server in the network. When

such technology is deployed, however, there also must be software that manages the SAN, to keep track of where data are stored, and moves older data to less expensive but still accessible storage locations. Storage management is becoming an entire domain within IS management.

In addition to being accessible, data must be continuously available. As noted, when paper backup no longer exists in a paperless EHR environment, there must be assurance that the computer system is available to users at all times. To achieve such availability, an EHR should have full **server redundancy,** accomplished through "mirrored processing." This means that as data are entered and processed by one server, they are simultaneously being entered and processed by a second server. Should the primary server crash, the system "fails over" to the second server and can continue processing as if (at least from the user's point of view) nothing had happened. Obviously, the servers must be monitored and when the primary server goes down, someone must be ready to perform repairs or replace it as rapidly as possible. Most organizations do not invest in yet a third redundant server.

So, although storage media are cheap, healthcare has had a tendency to store all electronic data, making storage management an increasingly expensive proposition. The introduction of an EHR should trigger a review of the organization's retention schedule, with an eye toward potentially enabling a realistic retention schedule for electronic data. Another element of the retention schedule should be the retention of metadata, including both audit trails and the "data about data" that support the data dictionary. As noted in the discussion of CDS systems, it is important to manage how discrete data are captured and used. For example, it was noted that a discrete data element could originally be established as mandatory for documentation but changed to optional. A smart attorney could require evidence of when the change took place to substantiate that the organization either did not make the change or made it at a point in time relative to an event under investigation.

Check Your Understanding 9.3

Instructions: On a separate piece of paper, spell out each of the following abbreviations for technology used in the EHR:

1. CDR
2. CDS
3. CDW
4. COW
5. COLD
6. RAID
7. SAN

Define the following EHR technology concepts:

8. Client/server architecture
9. Full server redundancy
10. Integration
11. Interface
12. Semantic interoperability
13. Source systems
14. Storage management

Security Controls

Every individual has private information he or she does not share with anyone, including innermost thoughts, dreams, and feelings. When some of this information is shared with someone else in confidence, a condition called **confidentiality** is established. Sometimes this confidential information is written down or placed into a computer system. To ensure that confidential information can be accessed only by those to whom the individual has given permission, security measures are put into place. In healthcare, in addition to affording confidentiality to private information that has been shared with providers, security measures protect the **integrity** of the information (so that it is not altered in any way) and ensure its availability (so that it is accessible when needed for subsequent care and other legitimate purposes).

An EHR system can afford better security for confidential information because access controls, audit trails, authentication systems, and other measures exist where they do not in a paper environment. Attention to security and privacy is not new. The Hippocratic Oath has directed physician protection of private information for centuries. Moreover, every provider has instituted security measures as part of his or her standard business practices. The Health Insurance Portability and Accountability Act (HIPAA) of 1996 requires specific attention to security and privacy. HIPAA uses the term protected health information (PHI) to describe individually identifiable health information held by a covered entity or business associate on behalf of the covered entity and which is protected through confidentiality, integrity, and availability measures required under the HIPAA regulations.

HIPAA Privacy Requirements

HIPAA privacy requirements include specific policies and procedures on uses and disclosures of PHI, individuals' rights with respect to their information (including the right to access, restriction requests, amendment requests, and others) and privacy management. Although most of HIPAA's privacy requirements are accomplished through administrative and operational activities, EHR technology can assist in carrying out a number of the privacy standards. For example, because patients have the right to request restrictions on who may use and disclose PHI, a means to put special access provisions must be in place to allow access perhaps only to the creator of the data or to a given few users with special authorization. In the paper environment, restrictions may have been accomplished by putting a special note on the chart cover, which may not be very effective when many individuals involved in treating a patient have access to all parts of the medical record. An EHR provides highly effective controls on specific categories of information for specific categories of people who may access the information. In another example, when a patient requests confidential communication, there needs to be a way to notify providers that an alternate address

or phone number must be used to contact the patient concerning certain information. Again, a note on the chart cover may be the only available solution in the paper environment, but a flag that pops up on a computer screen or that automatically routes calls or correspondence would provide much greater assurance that the patient's request is being carried out. Many technical measures are available to help protect patient privacy. HIPAA privacy measures are also discussed in chapter 10.

HIPAA's security requirements are generally more technical than the privacy requirements, but they also require establishment of policy to direct how the technical tools will be applied. Again using the example of access controls, a policy will need to be established on how access is authorized, who establishes the access controls, and what each user is authorized to access. Access profiles are established as a matter of policy. For example, some hospitals decide to control nurse access to patient information by the floor on which the nurse is working. Within nursing, there may be controls on who may view information and who may view and enter information. Laboratory technicians may be given access only to those patients for whom a laboratory test order has been placed. Their access might be limited to viewing only certain information about the patient, such as diagnosis and current medications, and entering information only into the laboratory component of the information system.

HIPAA Security Requirements

HIPAA requires that every provider conduct a security **risk analysis** to determine the appropriate level of security controls to put into place. A risk analysis is a systematic process of identifying security measures to afford protections given an organization's specific environment, including where the measures are located, what level of automation they have, how sensitive the information is that needs protection, what remediation will cost, and many other factors.

Risk is the potential for harm. It is composed of vulnerabilities and threats. Vulnerabilities are potential avenues of attack. For example, in the paper environment, an unlocked back door to the file room is an avenue of attack. In a computer system, a vulnerability is not having a firewall on the network or not backing up a computer system.

Threats include targets, agents, and events. A target is what might be attacked. HIPAA identifies three targets: confidentiality, integrity, and availability (C-I-A). Many security experts include a fourth target—accountability. Accountability refers to the fact that a person who has accessed a system, entered data, or otherwise used a system is associated with that action and held responsible for it. HIPAA includes this as part of the other three forms of targets.

An agent is a means of attack. Frequently, agents are individuals who have access to PHI, knowledge of security weaknesses, and motivation to cause harm. However, it should be noted that there are other forms of agents that do not necessarily intend to do harm, do not result in harm, or are physical agents. For example, a person who has access to an IS may inadvertently do something that results in a breach of confidentiality, an integrity problem, or a lack of availability. Moreover, access, alteration, or unavailability could have resulted in harm but did not. Finally, there are acts of nature, such as fire or flood, that cause harm.

An event is the form of harm. Inappropriate access that causes a breach of confidentiality, modification of data that causes an integrity problem, denial of service that renders information unavailable, and repudiation that allows an individual to disavow responsibility for an action are forms of harm.

A risk analysis studies each vulnerability and determines its associated threats. Generally, when doing a risk analysis, the combination of threat and vulnerability is assigned a risk level to help determine what mitigation steps should be taken and in what priority order. The risk level may be a numeric score or a relative value statement, such as high, medium, and low. Obviously, those with the highest score or relative importance would receive the greatest resources and first attention (Amatayakul 2004). (See figure 9.7.)

HIPAA security requirements are categorized into standards and implementation specifications. Standards describe what must be addressed. The implementation specifications describe how the standards can be implemented. Some implementation specifications are marked "required," meaning they must be implemented as described in the regulation. Other implementation specifications are marked "addressable," meaning the organization may determine how it can best implement the standard. It is important to note that addressable implementation specifications are not optional; they must be addressed but can be addressed in accordance with organizational risk needs. The security requirements also fall into three sections: administrative safeguards, physical safeguards, and technical safeguards.

Administrative Safeguards

Administrative safeguards cover policies, procedures, contracts, and plans for security. In addition to the security risk analysis already mentioned, HIPAA requires ongoing risk management, application of appropriate sanctions against workforce members who fail to comply with the security policies and procedures of the covered entity (CE), and IS activity review, wherein audit logs, access reports, and security incident reports are regularly reviewed for problems. In addition to this ongoing activity, HIPAA's evaluation standard requires a periodic technical and nontechnical evaluation of security measures in response to environmental or operational changes affecting the security of PHI in electronic form (ePHI). The CE must assign responsibility for the development and implementation of security policies and procedures to a security official and must have a security awareness and training program in place.

Policies associated with information access management include appropriate clearance procedures and supervision of, and termination procedures for, members of the workforce. Policies and procedures must be in place to authorize, establish, and modify access when there is a change in the workforce member's duties. These access management standards are very important and often troublesome for healthcare organizations because of the many different types of workforce members (including full- and part-time employees, temporary staff, volunteers, students, and members of the medical staff).

Contingency planning is another administrative security requirement. Applications should be categorized by criticality and backup plans, disaster recovery plans, and emergency mode operations plans developed in accordance with the criticality of the application and its information. These plans should be tested and revised routinely in accordance with the results of the tests.

Figure 9.7.   A security risk analysis

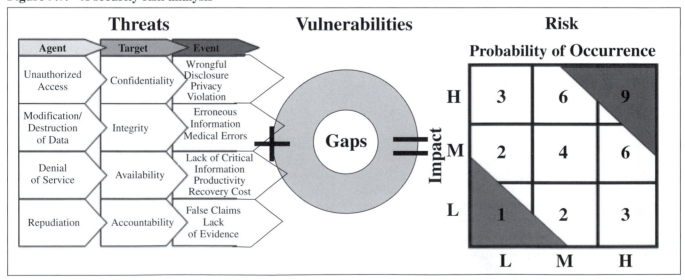

Just as in the Privacy Rule, the Security Rule requires business associate (BA) agreements with persons or entities that would have access to ePHI as part of their contractual responsibilities to the CE. The BA agreement relative to security requires the BA to appropriately safeguard the ePHI and to report to the CE any security incident of which it becomes aware.

Physical Safeguards

Physical safeguards obviously have to do with protecting the environment, including ensuring that applicable doors have locks that are changed when needed and that fire, flood, and other natural disaster preparedness is in place (for example, fire alarms, sprinklers, smoke detectors, raised cabinets). Other physical controls include badging and escorting visitors and other typical "security" functions such as patrolling the premises, logging equipment in and out, and camera-monitoring key areas. HIPAA does not provide specifics but does require a facility security plan with the expectation that these matters will be addressed.

Workstation use and security are important physical safeguards. CEs are expected to implement policies and procedures that specify the proper functions to be performed, the manner in which they are to be performed, and the physical attributes of the surroundings of a specific workstation or class of workstation that can access ePHI. Although HIPAA does not define *workstation,* healthcare organizations should consider a workstation to contain not only desktop computers, but also any human–computer interface that provides the ability to access, enter, or process ePHI. Members of the workforce who use workstations should know how to safeguard them, including ensuring that virus protection software is upgraded; that log-in failure is noticed; and how to create, change, and safeguard passwords.

Media and device controls also are very important parts of physical safety. Many providers are evaluating whether they really need all the printers they have, how to dispose of confidential trash (including nonrecyclable containers with labels, paper awaiting shredding, and so on), and whether all workstations need the capability of saving to disk drives. Tiny USB (universal serial bus) drives that can be carried on key chains or that are as small as the head of a pen have become a concern, and some organizations are disabling USB ports as a result. Certainly, whenever a device must be discarded, or even transferred to another user within the organization, it should have its disk drive thoroughly erased.

Technical Safeguards

There are five technical security standards. These include access controls, audit controls, integrity, person or entity authentication, and transmission security. The first four typically refer to data "at rest," that is, when data are stored in a database or even in a temporary location in a computer, such as cache memory. Transmission security obviously addresses the special needs to protect ePHI as it is being transmitted over an electronic communications network.

Access controls require unique user identification, emergency access procedures, automatic log-off, and encryption and decryption of data.

Although most organizations assign unique user identification to every user, often these unique "user IDs" are not always used. This requirement has met with concern in some hospital departments where it was common practice to share a single log-on for convenience sake and in some physician office settings where there may not even be a staff member who knows how to establish a unique user ID.

The user ID provides the access privileges for which a user has been authorized. HIPAA permits organizations to select the strength of the access controls they adopt. Some common examples include:

- *User-based access control* basically gives a person access by his or her name so that every user is assigned a specific set of privileges. This can be difficult to manage and frequently results in everyone being assigned the same access privileges.
- *Role-based access control* establishes parameters by what role an individual plays (nurse, physician, pharmacist).
- *Context-based access control* is the strongest form of access control. It not only establishes a profile based on who the person is and what role he or she is playing, but also on what specific information may or may not be accessed. In some cases, this can be linked to location and time of day as well. For example, "Nurse Jones may access patients on 3W during first shift, and in the emergency department on second shift if signed in for ED duty."

Emergency access procedures refer to procedures for obtaining necessary ePHI during an emergency. Many organizations have difficulty understanding or carrying out this requirement. However, if it is understood that the security access controls reflect the Privacy Rule minimum necessary requirements such that a treatment, payment, or operations (TPO) relationship must exist for access to ePHI, the emergency access procedure provides for access when such a TPO relationship has not existed but suddenly does exist. Sometimes emergency access procedures are carried out in a procedural manner, where the IT department or help desk must be called to provide access. This is clearly not very responsive if, in fact, there is a true medical emergency. More technical mechanisms to provide this access are called "break the glass." Much as when it becomes necessary to break the glass surrounding a fire alarm, the break-the-glass mechanism affords quick and easy access, often by perhaps only one additional keystroke that would provide the reason access is needed. Access is then provided, and a special audit trail is created that often is reviewed more frequently, perhaps by the information security official or even by a manager or attending physician. This can be a powerful disincentive for anyone trying to access information they do not have authority to access.

Unfortunately, many of today's ISs do not have break-the-glass capability, or if they do, the physicians are still resistant. Break the glass really only works effectively when access controls are very specific and when mechanisms are in place to clearly and always identify treatment relationships.

Person or entity authentication is closely related to access controls. Entity authentication refers to the password or other means to prove the identity of a person or other computer system (entity) needing access to ePHI. In most cases, a password has been used, although tokens, biometrics, call-back procedures, and PINs also are permitted. Although not the strongest method of authentication, passwords can be strengthened through several means. First, they should never be shared and strong sanctions should be in place to enforce this. A strong password is one that is extremely difficult to guess. If the password is strong, it does not need to be changed frequently. In fact, that will only encourage people to write a password down, making it accessible to others. Ideally, there should be a system of single sign-on, where one password will get a user into every application to which he or she is authorized access. Because of the great mix of old and new applications in healthcare, this is rarely achievable. However, users may be encouraged to synchronize their passwords to the extent possible. Systems also should log off automatically after a period of inactivity to prevent anyone from seeing what is currently on a screen and to prevent others from using someone's log-on.

Audit controls are the mechanisms that record and examine activity in information systems. HIPAA does not specify what form of audit controls must be used, how or how often they must be examined, or how long they must be retained (although HIPAA does require that all documentation associated with the standards be retained for six years). Ideally for an EHR, there should be the ability to audit both viewing of data as well as any entry of data, although most systems today can only audit data entry. (Note: Entry includes not only the entry of new data, but also the entry of any correction. Erroneous data can be hidden from normal viewing with only an annotation that there was an error, but the data must never be deleted.)

Integrity refers to the fact that data have not been altered or destroyed as they are captured, retained, processed, or transmitted in electronic form. Integrity is accomplished through technical measures, such as check-digits, hash totals, and other forms of edits on the underlying digital representation of the data to ensure that data are accurate and complete.

The transmission security standard requires the CE to guard against unauthorized access to ePHI being transmitted over an electronic communications network. It includes two addressable implementation specifications: integrity controls and encryption. As a matter of good business practices, most healthcare organizations have addressed security for their LAN through private cabling, their WAN through leasing private telephone lines, and for any network that utilizes the Internet through virtual private network (VPN) technology. A VPN is a security service that creates an encrypted tunnel in the Internet through which data can pass securely. The VPN requires special access controls and authentication procedures. When a healthcare organization permits access to the open Internet, it will utilize a firewall that examines each message and blocks those messages that do not meet specified security criteria.

HIPAA does not require use of a digital signature, although some healthcare organizations are beginning to experiment with this, especially for e-mail. It is important to note that three types of signatures may be used in computer systems:

- *Digitized signature* is generally considered the weakest type of signature. It is an image of a handwritten signature. Digitized signatures are commonly used in retail stores where they are captured on a signature pad and the clerk is supposed to compare the signature to the signature on the back of the credit card.
- *Electronic signature* is generally considered to be a userID and password or other form of authentication (such as token, biometric, callback procedure, and so on). In addition to the fact that HIPAA does not require more than this, the Electronic Signatures in Global and National Commerce Act (ESIGN) permits an electronic signature to be any "electronic sound, symbol, or process, attached to or logically associated with a contract or other record and executed or adopted by the person with the intent to sign the record." This definition encompasses digitized signature, even though it is considered very weak.
- *Digital signature* is a process that uses encryption to ensure that the elements that comprise the electronic signature are not altered. There are various forms of digital signature. The most common is an asymmetric key operation in which a pair of keys (passwords or other forms of authentication) is used, one on the sender side and one on the receiver side, to ensure that the signature is legitimate. When digital signature utilizes a digital certificate authorized by a certificate authority and other formal protocols to manage the keys, the process is called public key infrastructure (PKI). PKI is generally considered the strongest form of digital signature because the certificate authority acts as a notary to the keys and can revoke them at any time. PKI also may encrypt not only the passwords, but also the content of the message itself, thus affording both strong authentication and data integrity. Digital signatures and PKI are not yet widely adopted, primarily because there is no single standard for everyone to use. As a result, a hospital might not be able to transmit messages to a physician office if both used different digital signature technology.

EHR System Challenges

The greatest advantage of an EHR is its contribution to the quality of patient care. Greatly enhanced access to data is its current most important feature. Beyond the ability to retrieve data is the capability to use data. In the past, most clinicians did not truly value information as a tool to help them care for patients, except for limited, short-term results data. For the most part, recording information about patient care was viewed as a necessary evil. However, if such information could guide clinicians' work, communicate to others better, and help avoid errors, the EHR should truly become the much-enhanced utility that the IOM envisioned.

The greatest disadvantages of an EHR are directly related to its greatest advantages: Enhanced use and usability make the EHR a significant investment not only in direct cost, but also in gaining executive support, clinician adoption, system building, training, and maintenance. In addition, there are still some lingering concerns about legal and regulatory aspects.

Cost-Benefit, ROI, and Financing

EHR systems are undoubtedly expensive, even as costs are dropping. The cost of an EHR system for a hospital is very difficult to generalize because a single system is not purchased. Rather, source systems are integrated into a repository and other applications are acquired that collectively comprise the EHR. Costs also vary over time. However, estimates range from $3 to $4 million for a small community hospital with generally a single vendor, $10 to $15 million or more for a small to medium-sized community hospital with a best-of-breed situation, to upwards of $100 million for a large IDN to acquire the hardware, software, and human resources to fully implement an EHR. For physician offices, the cost is somewhat easier to estimate because the system being purchased is generally more self-contained. For very small practices (one to three physicians), an EHR may cost around $10,000 per physician (Monegain 2005). Costs go up as the practice increases in size because of the increase in complexity. There are generally more source systems to interface, and often the practices want greater customizability and more comprehensive functionality. Costs for such systems range from $25,000 to $50,000 or more per physician (also depending on whether a practice management system is acquired or replaced as part of the EHR acquisition).

As previously noted, the benefits of these systems are often difficult to quantify. Their primary benefits are quality and patient safety. However, there are other benefits that do accrue specific financial rewards. For hospitals, there can be an impact on the clerical workforce, admissions personnel, billers, transcriptionists, couriers, and other support staff. Storage of paper charts should be reduced. Although nurses are rarely, if ever, eliminated, overtime and temporary staff costs may be reduced or eliminated. The impact on nursing is much more that their time is freed up to perform more professional functions. This has a downstream benefit to patient safety and quality of care. Hospitals also generally find improvements in charge capture, reduced repetitive tests, use of lower-cost drugs, and other savings from clinical decision support. Bed turnover time may be reduced, discharge planning may be improved, and the ability to handle surges in patient load may be easier. Still, the greatest impact is the reduction in errors of all types, which ultimately impacts the bottom line through better positioning for contracting, improved likelihood of better accreditation and licensure outcomes, and so on. For physician offices, many of these same benefits apply. In addition, some offices find that they can see more patients because of productivity improvements. Others are able to add professional staff using paper storage space to enhance revenues to the group. Level of service (E&M) coding support generally improves revenues from 2 to 3 percent to as much as 20 to 30 percent, depending on the quality of coding performed prior to EHR adoption and sometimes the specialty of the practice.

However, the benefits must be weighed against not only the cost of the EHR, but also other factors that go into the total cost of ownership (TCO). For example, more staff trained in health informatics may be necessary. Other IT support staff needs may increase or be outsourced. Even the most rudimentary of EHR systems require some effort to implement. Data dictionaries must be created, rules must be reviewed, templates must be reviewed or developed, screen layouts potentially may have to be customized, reports have to be structured, and there is extensive testing. To gain adoption, there must be considerable process mapping and work flow analysis and redesign. Training is required for everyone, even for those who may have used another EHR system, because not only is each one different, but also every implementation is different due to the difference in source systems, customizations, and organizational preferences. Finally, because an EHR is a clinical system, it must be kept up to date with the latest evidence-based medicine, new and recalled drugs, new terms for new diseases, and new processes and work flows brought about by external factors, such as reimbursement or patient needs.

The result of a cost-benefit analysis should be the ability to perform return on investment (ROI) analysis. The easiest measure to calculate is the payback period. This is the cash flow (additional cash inflows less cash outflows due to the EHR) compared to the cost of the investment for the period of time it takes to achieve a positive difference. Generally, payback periods of from two to five years are tolerable. Longer payback periods are difficult to justify. Internal rate of return (IRR) and net present value (NPV) also may be calculated. These ROI measures require a financial calculator or a spreadsheet to factor into the cost-benefit equation the time value of money. If the IRR for an EHR investment is greater than the IRR on other investments, the EHR is considered a good investment.

Most vendors will attempt to provide ROI analysis for their clients. However, caution should be applied in interpreting these results because they typically assign a monetary value to every benefit, whether actual savings will result or the benefit will only yield greater value. For example, many vendors will calculate nurse full-time equivalent (FTE) savings, even though no nurses will be eliminated. Although this can provide a good comparison between systems, the expected savings cannot be "taken to the bank." And, in some cases, these savings do need to factor into bank loans or lines of credit for financing the investment.

Other financing options in addition to using cash reserves from operations or loans include acquiring the EHR through an **application service provider** (ASP) model, funding part of it through grants or even looking to philanthropy. The ASP model, sometimes called remote hosting, is both a financing and an acquisition strategy. With an ASP, the vendor hosts the hardware and software so that upfront and ongoing maintenance costs for the organization are minimized in return for usually a monthly fee. A good way to compare the ASP financing and acquisition model to the typical license agreement is to consider the ASP as renting an apartment and the license agreement the purchase of a house. In the ASP, rent accumulates over time to frequently be more than the actual cost of the license. The ASP generally offers less flexibility (you cannot paint the balcony on your apartment with pink and purple stripes when the rest of the building is green), but considerably less need for in-house IT expertise (you can call maintenance when there is a leaky faucet). However, the biggest concern providers have had about ASPs is that the data reside with the ASP. Again, this may actually be a more secure environment than a given provider could hope to provide. Unfortunately, however, many ASPs have been

known to go out of business, leaving providers in the worst case without access to their data or in the best case with their data and no application software to support them. Contractual agreements need to be very carefully worked out so that the provider is assured of getting access to the data and the software needed to at least continue processing until the data can be migrated to another application. Unfortunately, when an ASP goes out of business, it is often due to bankruptcy, so there is little hope of compensation for disruption of service or conversion.

Executive Commitment

Executives, obviously, are acutely aware and concerned about ROI and financing issues. They sometimes feel powerless to ensure that the EHR is adopted in a manner that will, in fact, achieve the expected benefits. However, executives can be the crucial factor in adoption and benefits realization if they demonstrate their commitment and support, establish appropriate expectations, and generally foster a culture of quality and productivity improvement. Implementing an EHR system into an adversarial environment is risky. In fact, many believe that implementing only a mediocre EHR product in a good environment can have better results than implementing the best EHR in a poor environment. People, policy, and process are the key to success. People, policy, and process are driven by executive leadership.

Therefore, many ask how executive support can be gained if it is not already present. (If it is present, it is highly likely that the organization is well on its way to achieving a successful EHR already.) Often, without executive leadership recognizing its own issues, little can be done from only a small segment of the organization desiring an EHR. There really needs to be a groundswell of support for the EHR before the executive posture is likely to change. This groundswell must include the medical staff and potentially even the community of patients, health plans, and businesses at large. One of the most successful implementations of an EHR engaged community leaders in helping to fund and motivate adoption.

Clinician Adoption

Although cost and executive commitment are essential ingredients in moving forward with an EHR, clinician adoption is the keystone to achieving results. Clinicians include physicians, nurses, pharmacists, technicians, therapists, and all others who use clinical information. Although each may be challenged in special ways, it is probably the physician community that is most challenged, followed by the nursing community that needs the most training.

Physician Concerns with EHR Adoption

For physicians, the EHR represents a monumental change to old habits. Virtually everything physicians do today concerning documentation is changed by an EHR. Consider only the need to select the patient for whom to write a medication order. In the paper environment, the correct patient's chart may have been presented to the physician by a member of the nursing staff or a blank sheet of paper could be used to write orders when the chart could not be immediately located. The physician did not have to select Mary Gonzalez from a list of patients that might also include Marie Gomez. The mere fact that care must be taken to distinguish between two relatively similar names is not the norm for the physician and requires a thought process that could be considered distracting from the processing of medication selection and dosage calculation, which is more likely uppermost in the physician's mind. This may seem a minor inconvenience in light of the fact that the system could return contraindication information that normally would have resulted in a phone call from the pharmacist, which simply delays the distraction to another point in time. Yet old habits die hard! The system, then, must be carefully programmed to be intuitive and include as many failsafe measures as possible, but not so many that they are distracting or delay the intended action on the system.

In many cases, physicians must be convinced of the value of the EHR through either using an EHR in their own practice or peer pressure. Typically, physician champions are identified and expected to lead the charge. Sometimes, however, physician champions can be looked upon as mavericks by their peers, or they may be brought into the picture too late in the process, which can cause resentment to build in the medical staff. In either case, physician leadership may be required to build trust in the system. Many organizations are beginning to identify the need for a medical director of information systems (MDIS) who would spend a good portion of time on EHR system selection and implementation and then maintenance, including training peers, ensuring the CDS system is appropriate and kept current, and troubleshooting system issues. Many MDISs recognize the importance of process improvement and support process mapping and other strategies to support change. However, hospitals must recognize that engaging the medical staff early is critical to success. Many hospitals still believe there are two strategic options to IT implementation: top down or bottom up. Many dictate that a CPOE system will be acquired and used. Unfortunately, this strategy is rarely successful with clinical information systems. (This strategy is not even successful when the system affects employees, such as an electronic medication administration record system expected to be used by nurses.)

It is interesting to note that physicians tend to be more willing to adopt EHR systems in their own office practice than they are in the hospital or hospitals with which they are affiliated. There are several reasons for this. Perhaps foremost is the fact that the hospital system is just that, a system designed to support an institution, not necessarily an individual. There are significant differences between systems designed for physician offices and hospitals. These differences reflect the many differences in workflow between these two kinds of care. (See table 9.1.)

A physician views the office EHR from an ownership perspective and the hospital EHR from an indentured servant perspective. Couple that with the fact that the hospital system is different from the office system, representing a second system to learn, and one can appreciate the challenge a physician has in using a hospital system. The most successful situation is one in which the office and hospital systems "look" and function very similarly. This, of course, can be aided by using a standard user interface (for example, Windows based) and providing remote connectivity to accustom the physician to the look and feel of the hospital system.

Physicians also are concerned about security and privacy issues, as well as patient perception issues. Today's ISs have typically been secured by virtue of the fact that they contain minimal patient data, few people know how to use them, and they are closed systems. They do not connect to the outside world. As use and users expand, security must be enhanced to better protect privacy. On the other hand, however, security measures must not be so onerous as to make EHRs even more formidable to learn and use.

Some physicians, and other clinicians, also have expressed concern about patient acceptance of computers. Will the patient perceive the computer to be a barrier between patient and clinician? Many clinicians are finding that patients actually expect them to use a computer, or at least are not surprised when they do. Many providers find that computers add value to the patient encounter. Clinicians who make the computer a barrier because they do not use it well will surely create a barrier for their patients. However, the computer can be used to engage and provide the patient with instantaneous information and instructions. Showing the patient a graph of personal data can be a powerful motivator. Instructions tailored specifically to the patient can improve his or her compliance with a treatment regime. Although its use is controversial and it must be specially secured, e-mail, or at least a patient portal to a secure Web site messaging system, can greatly contribute to patient–provider communications.

Table 9.1.   Differences in hospital and physician's office workflow

	Hospital	Physician's Office
Workflow	Tightly coordinated	Loosely coordinated
Communication	Formal	Informal
Primary user	Nurse	Physician
Data content	Comprehensive	Fragmented
Data volume	High density	Low density
Data source	Multiple, disparate	Patient/provider generated
Information flow	Location centric	Geographically dispersed
Data input	Mobile	Stationary
IS decision making	Administration	Physicians

Copyright ©2001. Margret/A Consulting, LLC.

Nursing Staff Concerns with EHR Adoption

Physicians are not the only users of EHRs. Certainly, their concerns are critical, but attention also must be paid to nurse issues, in both hospitals and physician offices.

In hospitals, nursing staff are the primary users of the EHR, yet very few nurses have the opportunity to learn about and evaluate various EHR systems from a nursing perspective. Although many physicians go to conferences and begin to see these systems and hear presentations from peers, nurses have less opportunity for such exposure. Moreover, physicians are starting to acquire EHRs for use in their own offices; hospital-based nurses have no such opportunity. Physician adoption is critical, but it should not be assumed that nurses will necessarily adopt the EHR without issues of their own. A good way to gain nurse support for the EHR is to engage them early in the process. They need to be prominent members of the EHR selection committee. They need the opportunity to see and hear from their peers what the issues are and how they can be overcome. Amazingly, many systems are not nurse-friendly. Care has not been taken to address special charting issues. For example, nurses depend on trended data to discern changes in their patients' status. If corrections made to data cannot be incorporated into the trend lines appropriately, their ability to monitor such trends is at risk. As an example, one system correctly identified where an error had occurred but placed the newly corrected information at the end of the trend line, not at the point of error. This was very difficult for nurses to use because they wanted to see the trend over time, not have to make mental adjustments for the fact that a certain data point should be somewhere else.

It is not uncommon to find nurses left out of the EHR decision-making process in physician offices (much as physicians are left out of the EHR decision-making process in the hospital). Again, this is a mistake because nurses are the ones who will likely use the EHR for a considerable portion of their work and will be expected to support the physician in learning to use the EHR.

Legal and Regulatory Issues

Although many states have not adopted specific statutes relating to EHRs, many have updated their statutes to address electronic health information in general. Other states are generally silent on whether health information is in paper or electronic form because the statutes are old and generally assumed a paper form. Every organization needs to review its own statutes, but EHRs are generally believed to be legally acceptable.

However, certain portions of EHRs may have to be converted to paper or signed on paper in certain circumstances and in certain states. For example, state boards of pharmacy generally control the form and format of a prescription. Standards for electronic prescribing are regulated by the federal government through the introduction of payment for outpatient drugs for Medicare beneficiaries under Part D, created by the Medicare Modernization Act (2003). However, a few states do not permit electronic prescriptions. Until these states change their statutes, they will not adopt electronic prescribing systems or will need to produce a paper prescription to be signed.

Hybrid Records and E-HIM

Some states specify that health information may be in electronic form but require special safeguards on their accuracy and integrity. HIM professionals are in the best position to advise their organizations on appropriate ways to carry out these safeguard procedures. As previously mentioned, they may include audits of how templates are completed and how CDS systems are used.

Safeguard procedures also may need to include how hybrid record situations are managed. If part of the official, legal record is deemed electronic and part paper, indications may need to be included in the paper record when content is in electronic form. HIM professionals must be vigilant about managing the use of printouts. Further, audits may need to be performed to verify that electronic portions of the record were reviewed prior to making clinical decisions.

Check Your Understanding 9.5

Instructions: Answer the following questions on a separate piece of paper.

1. List five areas of physician resistance that need to be overcome when adopting an EHR.

2. Differentiate between the payback period and internal rate of return for calculating return on investment for an EHR.

3. Compare the ASP and acquisition models of financing an EHR.

4. Discuss the importance of executive commitment in the adoption of an EHR.

5. What are the two key regulatory issues for EHR?

EHR System Planning and Acquisition

Dwight D. Eisenhower is quoted as having said: "In preparing for battle I have always found that plans are useless, but planning is indispensable." A recent study of chief technology officers indicated that 10 percent do not do strategic technology planning. They contend that strategic planning is a frustrating, time-consuming endeavor that distracts from, rather than contributes to, the real work of building and maintaining an adequate technology infrastructure. Still, the majority of those surveyed indicated that good planning helped achieve impressive outcomes with a minimum of frustration.

Many believe that an EHR is not a technology or an event but, rather, a journey toward goals aided by technology. Some call this a migration path; others view it as a strategic plan or an evolution along a set of generations (although some would prefer a revolution) (Gillespie 2003).

EHR Readiness

As an organization approaches the acquisition of an EHR, it is very important to assess its readiness, plot its migration path, and develop a plan of action. Organizations would be well advised to inventory their applications, technical capabilities, staffing resources, and reports. However, there is potentially nothing more important than taking a soul-searching look at the organization's culture of change management and process improvement. It cannot be emphasized enough that the organization's culture of responsiveness is a critical factor in EHR adoption.

Organizational Goals for EHR Systems

A large measure of an organization's readiness for the EHR is its understanding and articulation of goals for the EHR. Every member of the organization must understand what an EHR is. There should be a common understanding and clearly stated definition. The EHR is not an administrative or financial system; rather, it is a clinical system designed to support direct patient care. Clinicians who bypass the system for printouts or use clerical support for data entry are not achieving the benefit of the system and are undermining achievement of the system's goals. An organization that does not monitor achievement of goals to take corrective action is setting itself up for failure. EHRs can be powerful in helping an organization achieve its strategic initiatives, but they must be managed carefully.

After the organization establishes its EHR goals, it can better determine its overall approach to acquiring an EHR. An EHR migration path should be constructed, and all system selections should be made in relationship to the path. Organizations that develop a migration path are generally able to make support system selections that are more in line with their ultimate EHR requirements. An EHR migration path should address the following:

- What is the organization's current readiness? What applications does it currently have, what technology supports these applications, and what operational elements (EHR steering committee, physician champions, medical director of IS, nurse informaticists, e-HIM professionals, practice guidelines, evidence-based knowledge resource utilization, process mapping, and so on) are in place?
- What additional applications are needed, and in what sequence?
- What changes to existing applications must be made?
- Are interfaces required? Is there a repository? Is there a warehouse?
- Will the technical architecture support an EHR, or will a major investment in hardware need to be made first?
- Is the network sufficient to support all EHR users, or will this need to be enhanced?
- What operational changes need to be adopted? Will changes need to be made in policies and procedures

in support of an EHR? Are staff resources available to support both implementation and ongoing maintenance requirements?

It is not uncommon to find organizations without a migration path floundering in their EHR acquisition. They typically are reactive rather than proactive. Information systems have typically been requested and used by individual departments, and often this is expected to continue in an EHR environment. This stovepipe mentality must be changed in an EHR environment that requires all systems to work together, not be duplicative, and be acquired in the sequence that most appropriately addresses the organization's EHR goals. For example, a hospital with a document-imaging system should not approve a radiology department's request for a separate document-imaging system just because its PACS vendor is attempting to make a sale. Likewise, an HIM department would not need a chart-tracking system if a document-imaging system was going to be implemented within the next year. Yet, an organization without an EHR migration path might not be able to see the overall picture and focus the organization on working together.

EHR Planning and Project Management

An EHR migration path can be developed by an EHR steering committee or can be a precursor to the appointment of an EHR steering committee. If much infrastructure needs to be put into place prior to EHR acquisition, it may be appropriate to do that prior to forming an EHR steering committee. However, an EHR steering committee can begin to address the operational issues simultaneously with the technical infrastructure issues. Process mapping, gaining acceptance of practice guidelines, and adopting other standards can take considerable time.

An EHR steering committee should be composed of representatives of all direct users as well as those who support such users. The committee is often chaired by a clinician. Other clinical representatives must be present and representatives of IT and HIM are essential for representing the information management issues. Responsibility for information management does not shift from IT and HIM to others just because the EHR is a clinical system.

At some point, the organization will need an EHR project manager. When direct planning begins, someone needs to provide oversight that all elements are working together. Although an EHR project manager is critical during implementation, an organization is often best served when such an individual starts early in the planning stages and potentially remains in place at least through benefits realization. A project manager can be appointed from within the organization, hired from outside, or contracted with for a period of time. An internal candidate knows the organization but also may carry some "baggage." However, the position can be an excellent opportunity for someone interested in new challenges. An EHR is really a series of ongoing projects, so the project manager rarely needs to be concerned about finishing the project and not having a job. An external candidate has to get up to speed rapidly on the organization's culture but often is viewed as a more neutral party in negotiating among the different stovepipes that reflect current IS use today. The third option, contracting for a project manager, is often used in a small organization where the position of project manager is likely to be short term. The risks in using a contract project manager include that the project manager may not be devoted exclusively to one organization's project and may not impart the learning to existing staff necessary for them to continue to maintain the system. This can be guarded against by requiring staff to be trained but is often a secondary part of the project and frequently is not as successful as desired.

A project manager must have skills that may be different from those required of an operational manager. The project manager must have excellent communication, facilitation, negotiation, and leadership skills, while often not being the project leader (who is more likely the chair of the EHR steering committee). He or she must be skilled at delegating, diligent about following up, comfortable with escalating issues, and able to see the big picture yet be comfortable attending to highly detailed task monitoring. A project manager does not have to be highly skilled in information technology but should have a working knowledge of what can and cannot be accomplished. He or she will work with the vendor's implementation team, which will provide the IT expertise needed for the specific product. The project manager does not have to be a clinician but should have a thorough understanding of healthcare and the nature of clinical information and associated processes. Finally, the project manager should be well grounded in project management and process-mapping tools.

Vendor Selection

Healthcare organizations acquire EHR systems in a variety of ways. Some organizations build their own systems. This is especially true of more academic, research-based environments. Many of these have multiple source systems, some of which are homegrown and others of which are licensed from one or more vendors. If the organization does not believe a product exists on the market that addresses its needs, it may consider acquiring a repository and then creating the applications that will integrate data into the repository, run queries, provide CDS, and so on. Developing a system from scratch is becoming much less common as more sophisticated commercial products are introduced into the marketplace. Because it is difficult to hire and retain highly qualified IT staff, building a system from scratch is also costly and time-consuming. Vendors can provide economies of scale that simply are not available to individual organizations.

Other organizations buy a fully integrated HIS and upgrade as the vendor supplies more functionality toward the ultimate goal of the EHR. Many smaller hospitals and physician office practices find this to be a suitable solution.

The advantage is that the vendor provides a tried-and-true solution. The disadvantage is that these systems generally are fairly basic, meeting minimum requirements of everyone rather than trying to address any special needs or developing very advanced applications that are beyond the organizations' capabilities to implement and get adopted.

In general, most organization go to market to find an EHR vendor. An organization approaching EHR vendor selection typically goes through a lengthy process of analyzing EHR functionality. Although EHRs are not yet commodity products, organizations should be aware that most EHR vendors have a core set of functionality that does not vary considerably among vendors. What the organization should look for is the vendor's ability to be a good partner in EHR implementation. The vendor must have the core functionality desired and also should be ready to help the organization overcome adoption issues, address process changes, and support ongoing maintenance and upgrades well into the future. Organizations may review the IOM core functionality and HL7 EHR System Functional Model to help them determine their functional requirements. Beyond that, however, significant due diligence will be necessary to determine other key factors in deciding on a vendor.

Key selection criteria might include:

- Functionality
- Vendor viability
- Vendor support
- Training availability
- Implementation support
- Technology/architecture
- Vision (research and development momentum)
- Integration
- Vendor's clinical culture
- ROI potential

Except for the ROI potential, cost is not identified as a criterion for EHR selection. Cost is undoubtedly important, but it should not be used in the basic selection. Vendors have many ways to price products, and there are many financing options. The lowest bidder is likely to have the lowest ranking in most of the functionality. When the functionality does not support the user community, ROI will not be achieved.

Most organizations use a formal request for proposal (RFP) process to solicit information from vendors on how they can meet the criteria. This may then be accompanied by product demonstrations. From there, most organizations are able to narrow their choice down to a finalist and backup. Due diligence in the form of site visits, corporate visits, reference checks, credit checks on owners, and other steps need to be performed before a final contract is negotiated to ensure that the organization is getting the product it wants.

EHR System Implementation

After a system has been selected, system implementation includes system build, installation, testing, and user training.

Because the EHR directly affects clinical processes, process improvement, work flow redesign, and potentially even space layout are affected.

System Build

System implementation actually should begin with process mapping and work flow analysis. These will identify the data input and output requirements for system build. System build is the process whereby the organization's unique data and clinical standards are designed into the system.

System Installation

There are numerous ways in which installations can be phased in—by special users, by department, by nursing unit, by site, or by function. Often the vendor has the best recommendation and should be considered an important guide. This issue also should be evaluated during site visits and reference checks.

Paper chart conversion is a key issue for EHR implementation. There are several approaches. Some organizations use document imaging as both an interim solution to achieving improved access to information and a means to make old paper charts accessible in an EHR environment. This is the most common way to address the need to bring paper records into the EHR environment. The issue then becomes what parts of the paper record to scan and how far back to scan them. There are no right answers across the board; the organization needs to consider its readmission/revisit rate and use of records (for example, for patient care only or research and education as well). In some cases, the organization may decide to scan the entire records of active patients, but only parts of older records. In other cases, the organization may decide to scan only parts of active patients' paper records and pull the paper records if other information is needed.

If an organization is adopting an EHR where there are considerable discrete data and a repository supporting CDS, it may want to abstract some or all of certain records so that the data are not only accessible for viewing, but also are available for processing. In this case, the organization may hire abstractors or expect clinicians to perform their own abstracting. Again, issues arise concerning what data need to be abstracted and how far back the abstracting must be performed. Abstracting is generally more expensive than scanning, so it should be performed judiciously. Of course, a combination of scanning and abstracting can be used. For example, it may be desirable in an ambulatory environment to abstract the problem list, medication list, and immunizations and then scan other key documents.

Continuing to pull the paper charts is yet another possible way to address how old information is made available to clinicians. Some consider this the least expensive way to make information available, but it may not be if one considers the issues of the hybrid record raised in several locations throughout this chapter. Continuing to pull paper charts not only does not reduce this cost and creates patient safety risk if documentation continues to be performed in the paper chart, but also it continues a dependency on paper for those who are more resistant to using the computer.

It also is important to be aware that data conversion is required for all electronic data. Data housed in the various source systems need to be brought into the repository, and this process must occur not only in advance, but also at the point of go-live, when the switch is made from one system to another.

System Testing

It should be clear that a system as complex as an EHR system must be tested thoroughly. There may be several levels of testing, from evaluating that a screen has been built correctly to the fact that data can be passed from one component to another. Testing should follow the flow of data through all systems and through all decision points. Stress testing also may be performed to ensure that the system not only works in the test environment where there are minimal data and few users, but also will work when the system is live and many users are using it simultaneously. Generally, there is an "acceptance testing" process that addresses all aspects of the system, including adoption rates. This acceptance testing procedure usually triggers a final payment or sign-off on acceptance.

System User Training

The organization should provide user training throughout the implementation process. System builders are trained first. Then, super users are identified and trained so that they can perform train-the-trainer duties. However, every end user requires some form of training, which may involve considerable hand-holding and support, even when it is formal classroom instruction on use of the computer. It is important to recognize that users learn in different ways. For example, nurses may do well in a classroom session where the experience can be shared. On the other hand, physicians often require one-on-one, private instruction. In fact, physicians often learn best when a system is intuitive and they can learn on their own. Sufficient online help is critical. However implementation is managed, training is key to using the system and does not end at installation. Ongoing training of regular users hones their skills and helps them to learn new things on an ongoing basis. Finally, ongoing training also supports maintenance of the system.

The importance of system maintenance cannot be overlooked. As previously mentioned, a clinical system demands constant updating. New drugs, new procedures, new codes, new processes, and many other factors mean continual maintenance. Even things that may seem minor can be major factors in maintenance. For example, if a particular CDS system alert is set to page a physician and a given physician gets a new pager, the system will need to be reset to send the page to the correct pager. This example may seem minor, but it is major when the alert is a serious situation that is overlooked because the page was not received.

Future Directions of Information Technologies

This chapter represents both currently available technology and future directions. This is because all the technology described here is in use somewhere, but not necessarily adopted all in one place or very widely.

Today, it appears that information technology is beginning to be more broadly adopted for clinical information computing. Factors that are contributing to heightened interest and EHR use include a critical mass of support systems, more manageable human–computer interfaces, pervasive use of the Internet, the IOM patient safety reports, HIPAA standards, and, perhaps most important, federal government initiatives that have created new opportunities for EHR system use. The federal government is certainly promoting personalized care where the consumer is becoming much more knowledgeable and involved. Indeed, the government is more concerned than ever about public health and the need for surveillance systems to monitor for potential bioterrorism. If nothing else, the cost of healthcare is still a significant driver of the government's interest in productivity improvement. Its initiatives may drive pay for performance where the level of reporting data requires an EHR.

An EHR depends on having a critical mass of support systems. All patient care areas, ancillary departments, and support services must be automated and supply data to a CDR (or be fully integrated). More and more hospitals and physician offices are beginning to have all the necessary ISs in place to support a repository and eventually an EHR.

One of the most critical precursors to an EHR is the need for a user-friendly interface and other more manageable (and affordable) technologies. The healthcare industry has always been reactive rather than proactive when it comes to new technology. Even new medical technology undergoes years of testing before it is considered safe enough to use on patients. This reluctance to use new technology, coupled with the real lack of graphical user interfaces, mobile devices, data capture tools, and online application processing capabilities, truly has held back EHR adoption. Thanks to the Internet and e-commerce, many of new technologies are becoming more realistic for healthcare.

The explosion of Internet use and e-commerce has resulted in much more widespread use of computers in general and in particular by providers (who are realizing the value of enhanced communications through the Internet) and patients (who are demanding connectivity with their providers).

The biggest spurt of interest in EHR, and perhaps the most compelling for providers, grew out of the IOM reports on patient safety. As a result of these reports describing the extent of medical errors and their cause and potential cure, external pressure has been brought to bear on providers by employers and payer contracting groups. Caution must be applied, however, to recognize that many levels of automation can help reduce medical errors. CPOE can achieve greater legibility without a full EHR. However, a robust decision support system that is a component of an EHR identifies contraindications, provides information on more efficacious medications, and offers best practice guidelines (FCG 2003).

Interestingly, HIPAA has had minimal impact on achieving the EHR. The goal of HIPAA actually is to "encourage the development of a health information system." The transaction and code sets regulation has required a change in claims but has done little else in the way of promoting IS use. Privacy and security regulations are written to be more supportive of health information exchange in a secure manner, yet many organizations are either confused or concerned about potential breeches and, in some cases, have used the regulations as an excuse not to proceed with more clinical computing.

Patient medical record information (PMRI) standards, which were a part of HIPAA, have been recommended by the National Committee on Vital and Health Statistics (NCVHS) but have not as yet been made into regulations (NCVHS 2002). NCVHS has made specific recommendations for message format standards for achieving interoperability, standard vocabularies for data comparability, and data quality standards. Interoperability is critical to integrating data from disparate systems to support EHRs. Standard vocabularies ensure that content in disparate systems carries the same meaning. Data quality standards ensure internal consistency, accuracy, completeness, reliability, and timeliness.

There is every indication that the EHR's time has finally come. The future will include complete automation of support systems and use of Internet-based technology to make EHR adoption more affordable and easier to use. More than anything else, ROI is finally beginning to be recognized.

Real-World Case

A hospital already has a homegrown IS that includes basic patient registration and billing functions. It also supports nursing personnel in order entry and ancillary departments in managing order communications. An LIS is interfaced with the HIS so that laboratory results can be viewed from it. A special program was developed recently to supply clinical guidelines for the treatment of diabetes and heart disease that are printed out by nursing personnel for each applicable patient and placed in his or her paper health record. Physicians in their offices have access to the HIS and are able to maintain a patient problem list. The HIM department is scanning the contents of the medical record for coding and archival purposes. However, the scanned documents cannot be viewed through the HIS because the two systems do not communicate with one another. Access to archived documents is made available through dedicated workstations on the nursing units and selected other areas of the hospital. The hospital also has several other, smaller and independent ISs for its emergency department, nutrition services, surgery scheduling, and rehab. In response to several health plans that are offering pay-for-performance (P4P) incentives, the hospital is investigating the development or purchase of an EHR. It is important that whatever the hospital plans for helps reduce errors, is as easy to use as the current system, can be tailored to meet the network's specific needs, and interfaces with other major systems.

Summary

An EHR is both a reality today and a goal for tomorrow. For some organizations, the reality of an EHR is an interim solution or bridge technology, intended to support valid benefits of automation, yet falling short of the goals many have espoused for patient safety, quality of care improvements, productivity enhancements, rising healthcare costs, and homeland security issues. For others, the EHR reality is a continual migration path sometimes dictated by internal organizational issues and sometimes limited by vendor offerings. These migration paths often begin with the challenge of interfacing source systems, building a repository, getting clinicians to perform data entry, and building and achieving adoption of clinical decision support systems. Still, the EHR as envisioned by its early pioneers and carried forward by the Institute of Medicine and now federal government initiatives is very much a goal of all healthcare organizations.

References

Amatayakul, M.K. 2004. *Electronic Health Records: A Practical Guide for Professionals and Organizations,* 2nd ed. Chicago: AHIMA.

Amatayakul, M.K., S.S. Lazarus, T. Walsh, and C.P. Harley. 2004. *Handbook for HIPAA Security Implementation.* Chicago: AMA Press.

Cohen, M.R., and M. Amatayakul. 2004. EHR corner: Segmenting the EHR market. *ADVANCE for Health Information Executives* 8(6):22. Available online from health-care-it.advanceweb.com/common/EditorialSearch/AViewer.aspx?AN=HX_04jun1_hxp22.html&AD=06-01-2004.

Connecting for Health, Markle Foundation. 2003. The personal health working group final report. Available online from connectingforhealth.org/resources/final_phwg_report1.pdf.

First Consulting Group. 2003. Computerized physician order entry: Costs, benefits and challenges. Available online from fcg.com/healthcare/ps-cpoe-research-and-publications.asp.

Gillespie, G. 2003 (July). Helpful tips for CIOs who take on the universe. *Health Data Management* pp. 29–38.

Health Level Seven. 2004. *EHR System Functional Model.* Ann Arbor, MI: Health Level Seven.

Institute of Medicine. 1991. *The Computer-based Patient Record: An Essential Technology for Health Care.* Washington, DC: National Academy Press.

Institute of Medicine. 2003. Key capabilities of an electronic health record system, Letter Report. Washington, DC: IOM. Available online from nap.edu/books/NI000427/html/.

Medicare Prescription Drug, Improvement, and Modernization Act of 2003. Title I: Medicare Prescription Drug Benefit. Baltimore: CMS. Available online from cms.hhs.gov/medicarereform/MMAactFullText.pdf.

Monegain, B. 2005 (April). EHRs seen coming down in price. *Healthcare IT News.* Available online from healthcareitnews.com/NewsArticleView.aspx?ContentID=2705&ContentTypeID=3&IssueID=17.

National Committee on Vital and Health Statistics. 2002 (Feb. 27). Letter report to the secretary of HHS reporting on issues related to the adoption of uniform data standards for patient medical record information (PMRI). Available online from ncvhs.hhs.gov/020227lt.htm.

Thompson, T.G., and D.J. Brailer. 2004 (July 21). The decade of health information technology: Delivering consumer-centric and information-rich health care: Framework for strategic action. Available online from hhs.gov/healthit/frameworkchapters.html.

Chapter 10
Legal Issues in Health Information Management

Lynda A. Russell, EdD, JD, RHIA, CHP,
and Rita Bowen, MA, RHIA, CHPS

Learning Objectives

- To define terms specific to civil litigation
- To diagram the state and federal court systems
- To describe the sources of law
- To explain the difference between civil law and criminal law
- To describe the process for a civil case and the process for a criminal case
- To discuss liability for a tort as it relates to healthcare
- To discuss liability for breach of contract as it relates to healthcare
- To discuss the legal aspects of a health record
- To discuss the purposes for retaining health records
- To outline the basic principles for releasing confidential health information with or without patient authorization

- To identify the required elements of an authorization for the disclosure of confidential health information
- To analyze various requests for confidential health information and to determine whether patient authorization is required
- To elaborate on the role of the health record in medical staff appointments and privileges
- To discuss management of the use and disclosure of information process and function
- To explain the health information administrator's relationship with the risk manager in reducing facility liability

Key Terms

Administrative law
Case law
Circuit
Civil law
Common law
Contract law
Controlled Substances Act
Court of Appeals
Credentialing process
Criminal law
Default judgment
Defendant
Designated record set
Evidence
Federal Register
Felony
Freedom of Information Act (FOIA)
Health Insurance Portability and Accountability Act of 1966 (HIPAA)
Incident
Individually identifiable health information
Interrogatories
Judge-made law

Jurisdiction
Licensure
Litigation
Misdemeanor
Motion for summary judgment
National Practitioner Data Bank
Negligence
Plaintiff
Preemption
Privacy Act of 1974
Privacy Rule
Privilege
Privileging process
Prosecutor
Protected health information (PHI)
Request for production
Restitution
Standard of care
Statute of limitations
Statutory law
Tort
Trier of fact

Introduction

The U.S. legal system consists of three related subsystems: a judicial system, a regulatory system, and an administrative system.

The *judicial system* affords a person or entity the opportunity to bring a civil action against another person or entity believed to have caused harm to the original party. An individual can bring a wide variety of actions against an alleged wrongdoer. The judicial system also affords a person or entity charged with criminal wrongdoing the opportunity to defend himself or herself against those charges. In this way, the judicial system provides an avenue for a wronged party to seek retribution or to clear his or her name.

The *regulatory system* controls many activities related to industry, in particular, the healthcare industry. These controls exist as statutes or as regulations derived from, or promulgated pursuant to, statutes. Often the statutes set forth what action is required, and the regulations set forth how that action is to be met.

The *administrative system* controls governmental administrative operations. Federal and state administrative agencies enact regulations that have the same force of law that statutory laws do.

Understanding the American judicial, regulatory, and administrative subsystems within the legal system gives a health information management (HIM) professional an appreciation for the health record as a sublegal document and its role in each of these subsystems.

This chapter explains the basic workings of the U.S. legal system. It then identifies the legal principles that apply to healthcare in general and to health information administration in particular. Further, the chapter describes how health records are used in legal proceedings. Finally, it discusses medical staff appointments and privileging.

Because it is impossible to summarize the infinite variety of state laws, the text is based on applying the **Privacy Rule** under the **Health Insurance Portability and Accountability Act of 1996** (HIPAA). HIM professionals must consult their individual state statutes, codes, and regulations for specific applications that may have been declared more stringent than HIPAA and thus not preempted by HIPAA.

Theory into Practice

The Mid-America Medical Center (MAMC) is a 1,000-bed acute care hospital located somewhere in America. A Level III trauma center, it has several critical care units for adults, children, and newborns, and it offers a full range of services including heart, kidney, lung, and liver transplantation. In addition, it is a teaching hospital with residency programs in hand surgery, thoracic surgery, cardiac surgery, nephrology, internal medicine, orthopedics, general surgery, obstetrics, and pediatrics. MAMC has 7,500 staff members and 3,500 medical staff members, of which 2,500 are considered active.

The center's medical staff office (MSO) maintains all demographic, credentialing, and privileging information for every medical staff member in a physician database. The demographic information includes items such as the physician's name, educational degrees, professional license number, liability insurance information, office address, and office phone numbers, including any office facsimile (fax) numbers. The MSO has a policy and procedure for immediately updating the physician database upon receiving notice of any changed demographic information.

MAMC maintains all dictated medical reports, radiologic reports, lab/pathology reports, emergency department notes, and workers' compensation reports in a clinical data repository (CDR). It also maintains radiologic, EEG, and EKG images in digital format in the CDR. As the documents become available from medical transcription, they are uploaded immediately to the CDR and made available to caregivers. Further, as the digital images become available through the testing equipment, they likewise are uploaded immediately to the CDR and made available to caregivers. Upon loading into the CDR, the documents are autofaxed to the dictating physician and the attending physician (if different). The fax numbers in the CDR are updated on a real-time basis from the MSO physician database. This means that as soon as an MSO staff member updates the physician database with a new fax number, the number is automatically and immediately uploaded to the CDR for autofaxing purposes. The autofax cover sheet contains a confidentiality statement instructing anyone receiving material erroneously to call the director of the HIM department.

On December 28, a situation arose regarding the physician database. The HIM director/privacy officer received a call from an individual who had never been a patient at MAMC, but who indicated that he had just received a faxed history and physical, operative report, and discharge summary on a patient with AIDS and related conditions. It turned out that the patient was the mayor of the city where MAMC was located. He had acquired AIDS from a blood transfusion three years earlier during open-heart surgery. The HIM director/privacy officer instructed the caller to mail the documents to her attention by certified mail, and the caller complied.

However, before mailing the documents, the caller copied them and sold the copies to a local tabloid press. The information in the reports was "revised," and a printed story gave sordid details about how the mayor had acquired AIDS. The mayor called the HIM director/privacy officer in a rage. Further, the Department of Health and Human Services (HHS) Office of Civil Rights (OCR) notified the HIM director/privacy officer that the mayor had filed a HIPAA compliant alleging intentional breach of confidentiality.

The HIM director/privacy officer immediately contacted the risk manager and the chief executive officer (CEO). The HIM director/privacy officer and the risk manager investigated the matter together and ascertained that the dictating physician had notified the MSO of a fax number change on December 21. The MSO staff had not followed policy and procedure for updating this information in the physician database because the fax number was not changed until December 30. Thus, the CDR was not updated and reports continued to be autofaxed to the old fax number. The fax number had actually been valid for the physician until December 27 at midnight. On December 28, the phone company assigned the number to the anonymous caller at his request. The physician database had a feature that allowed entering information such as a fax number and inputting an effective date. On that date, the updated information would automatically be in effect and uploaded to the CDR.

The mayor suffered significant harm from the misleading publication. He filed a lawsuit in the state trial court, suing the hospital, the MSO director, and the MSO data-entry clerk personally for breach of confidentiality. After considerable pretrial discovery was conducted, the case went to trial. The jury found in favor of the mayor against the hospital and the MSO director, stating that MAMC had breached the mayor's confidentiality by failing to follow its own policies and procedures for protecting his confidential health information. The jury based its decision on the **tort** of **negligence.**

The jury also found the data-entry clerk personally liable because pretrial discovery showed that she was angry with the mayor and intentionally had not entered the physician's updated fax number into the physician database. She knew that any reports regarding the mayor would continue to be automatically faxed to the old fax number, which her boyfriend had taken as of December 28. She shared in the money received from the tabloid for the information. The jury's decision was based on the intentional tort of invasion of privacy.

The hospital's liability insurance paid the $4 million judgment on behalf of the hospital and the MSO director. However, its insurance company refused to pay the $8 million judgment against the data-entry clerk, reasoning that her actions were intentional and not within her scope of work.

The HIM director/privacy officer communicated the internal investigation findings to the OCR and an action plan detailing the process to ensure the MSO enters new fax numbers and effective dates on a timely basis. As of the printing of this text, it is unclear whether the OCR would have access to information gathered through the **litigation** pretrial and trial processes. If the OCR is permitted access to such information, the maximum penalty that could be assessed against the data-entry clerk would be a $250,000 fine and up to 10 years in jail for breaching confidentiality for personal gain.

Introduction to the Legal System

To understand the role of the HIM professional in protecting confidential health information, one must first understand the principles for disclosing such information. Because many disclosures are made as part of litigation, the HIM professional should be very comfortable with the legal process.

The following sections present the basics about the sources of American law, the court system, the legal process, and the types of actions encountered in healthcare.

Sources of Law

The laws that rule all Americans' lives come from many sources, which results in a rather complex legal system. Overall, there is a federal legal system and 50 individual state legal systems. Regardless of the source, the legal system is a process through which members of society settle disputes. These disputes may be between private individuals and organizations or between either of these entities and the government, whether state, federal, or both.

Constitutional Law

Much of the law governing society is set out in the state and federal constitutions. The Constitution of the United States is the highest law in the land. It takes precedence over constitutions and laws in the individual states and local jurisdictions (Pozgar 2004). The Constitution defines the federal government's general organization and grants powers to it. It also places limits on what federal and state governments may do. State constitutions have the same effect within the borders of each state. Some state constitutions are very elaborate and govern everything from state lotteries to retirement plans for state workers.

Common Law

English common law is the primary source of many legal rules and principles and was based initially on tradition and custom. **Common law,** also known as **judge-made** or **case law,** is regularly referred to as unwritten law originating from court decisions where no applicable statute exists. Before the Norman Conquest in 1066, English laws primarily addressed violent crimes. After the Norman Conquest, a legal system began to develop that included a jury hearing complaints from the king's subjects (Pozgar 2004).

After the American Revolution, most of the 13 original states adopted all or part of the existing English common-law principles in existence as of July 4, 1776 (Pozgar 2004). States created after the Revolution vary in their treatment of English common law, but most have adopted the common law in effect as of a certain date. As a matter of technical legal practice, this date of adoption can make a difference in how a lawsuit is resolved if the only source of law on the subject in the state is the English common law. These cases of "first impression" are rare. Louisiana is the exception because it bases much of its common law on the French (Code Civil des Français) and Spanish civil law systems (Pozgar 2004). States continue to add to the body of common law through court decisions when existing statutes do not apply to the issue before the court. Because each state adds to the common law within its boundaries, there is no body of national common law. Thus, a common-law principle established in one state has no effect in another state unless the second state also adopts the principle. Even then, it may be applied differently.

After a court establishes a new common-law principle, that principle becomes a precedent for future cases addressing the same issues. The body of common law in a given state is continually evolving through being modified, overturned, abrogated, or created by court decisions.

Statutory Law

By contrast, **statutory** (legislative) **law** is written law established by federal and state legislatures. It may be amended, repealed, or expanded by the legislature. Statutory law also may be upheld or found by a court to violate or conflict with the state or federal constitution. Further, it may be found to conflict with a different state law or a federal law.

Courts also interpret laws in terms of how they apply to a given situation. Thus, statutory law may be "revised" by a court ruling in terms of its constitutionality and applicability. However, if the legislature disagrees with the court's interpretation, it can revise the statute. The legislative revision then becomes the law versus the court's revision based on its interpretation.

Administrative Law

Federal and state legislatures often delegate their legislative authority to regulate in technical or complex areas to appropriate federal and state administrative agencies. These agencies are empowered to enact regulations that have the same force of law that statutory law has and can impose criminal penalties for noncompliance. Accordingly, **administrative law** is the branch of law that controls governmental administrative operations (Pozgar 2004). Such administrative agencies include licensing and accrediting bodies, Medicare, Medicaid, and other federal and state government programs.

Federal administrative agencies function under the Administrative Procedures Act, which sets forth the following (Pozgar 2004):

- The procedures under which administrative agencies must operate
- The procedural responsibilities and authority of administrative agencies
- The legal remedies for individuals or entities harmed by agency actions

The act also requires administrative agencies to make agency rules, opinions, orders, records, and proceedings available to the public (Administrative Procedures Act, §552). The publication used to accomplish this is the **Federal Register,** which is issued by the U.S. Government Printing Office every business day. The information that agencies must publish includes the following:

- Their organizational structure and the location where the public can obtain information
- Formal and informal procedures and forms and instructions for using them
- General statement of applicability
- Amendments, revisions, or repeals of any of this information

Furthermore, agencies must publish proposed administrative rules and revisions to existing rules for which they are delegated the responsibility and authority to enact. These rules and/or revisions are published in the *Federal Register* for a comment period during which the public is invited to make comments on the applicability and impact of the proposed rules on a given person, group of persons, or entity. After the comment period ends, the applicable administrative agency may or may not finalize the rules. If the rules are finalized, the notice and the final rule are published in the *Federal Register*. The final rule is also codified and published in the appropriate code section. The Medicare Conditions of Participation regulations and HIPAA's Administrative Simplification rules are examples of healthcare-related information published in the *Federal Register*. Most states have similar administrative procedure acts, but few have as elaborate a system for the adoption of new regulations as the federal government.

The Court System

The American court system is composed of the state court system and the federal court system. The nature of the issue determines which court has **jurisdiction** over the issue. Matters in the following three categories belong only to federal courts: federal crimes, such as racketeering and bank robbery; constitutional issues; and civil actions where the parties do not live in the same state. Other civil and criminal cases are heard in the state court system.

State Court System

Typically, the state court system has several levels. In most states, the lowest level consists of specialty courts or local courts that hear cases involving traffic, small claims, and justice of the peace issues. State civil and criminal cases are initiated in the lower-level trial courts. These are referred to differently in different states, for example, as district trial courts or superior courts. New York's trial courts are called the "Supreme Court." Some trial courts at this level have limited jurisdiction and include courts such as probate, family, juvenile, surrogate, and criminal. Other trial courts at this same level have general jurisdiction. Decisions made in a court at this level may be appealed to the intermediate courts, usually known as the state appeals courts. State appellate courts have general jurisdiction; however, some states (such as Texas) divide their appellate courts into civil and criminal appellate jurisdiction, and others divide appellate courts by legal and equitable jurisdiction.

State legal systems also include a court at the highest level. These courts of last resort also are known by different terms in different states. Many are simply the Supreme Court of the state; others are the Supreme Judicial Court as in Massachusetts, and New York has the **Court of Appeals** as its highest court. These higher courts also have general jurisdiction over all cases heard in the state's trial and appellate courts. Decisions coming from the highest state court hearing a case become the law of that state unless a state legislative process enacts a statute to override the court's decision, or unless it is overturned by another case.

Federal Court System

The trial-level federal courts are the U.S. district courts (trial courts). Included in the district courts are the bankruptcy courts. Special federal courts have jurisdiction over specific matters. These courts include the U.S. Tax Court (hears cases involving federal tax matters only), the U.S. Customs Court (reviews administrative decisions made by customs officials), the U.S. Court of Appeals for the Armed Forces (the jurisdiction of which is limited to hearing appeals from court martials under the Uniform Code of Military Justice), and the U.S. Court of Claims (hears certain claims against the government) (Pozgar 2004). The federal appellate level is composed of the U.S. Courts of Appeals, each covering a geographic area known as a **circuit.** The U.S. Supreme Court is the highest court in the U.S. legal system and hears appeals from the federal appellate courts and the various state courts of last resort.

The Legal Process

The HIM professional can better serve patient privacy interests if he or she has an understanding of the legal process. This understanding should cover both civil and criminal processes, as healthcare facilities sometimes are affected by criminal cases.

Civil Cases

Civil law involves relations between individuals, corporations, government entities, and other organizations. Most actions encountered in the healthcare industry are based in civil law. Typically, the remedy for a civil wrong is monetary in nature but also may include carrying out some action.

The party bringing the action or complaint in a civil case is the **plaintiff.** (In the Theory into Practice section of this chapter, the mayor was the plaintiff.) The plaintiff has the burden of proving the wrong, that the defendant did the wrong act, that the wrong did the plaintiff harm, the harm from the wrong, and the expected **restitution.** The plaintiff presents **evidence** before a judge or a jury that must be more compelling than that of the opposing side, the **defendant.** The plaintiff or an attorney on the plaintiff's behalf begins the process by filing a complaint in the appropriate court. Hereafter in this discussion, the term *plaintiff* will refer collectively to the individual or entity bringing the action and that individual or entity's attorney. The plaintiff has a summons, including a copy of the filed complaint, served on the defendant. The defendant or an attorney on the defendant's behalf prepares an answer and files it in the same court where the original complaint was filed. Hereafter in this discussion, the term *defendant* will refer collectively to the person or entity against whom an action has been brought and that person or entity's attorney.

A case may be resolved in five ways:

- A judge can dismiss the plaintiff's case for procedural reasons. The plaintiff's complaint may not set forth a claim recognized by law, the summons and complaint may not have been properly served on the defendant, or the defendant may not be subject to the court's jurisdiction (meaning that the court has no power to compel the defendant to do what it commands). The judge may permit the plaintiff to correct the error and refile the case.

- If the defendant fails to file a timely answer, the court will find in favor of the plaintiff and enter a **default judgment** against the defendant.

- A case may be settled out of court before it goes to trial or at any time during trial before the **trier of fact** (judge or jury) announces the decision.

- Presuming the case does not settle or is not dismissed or no default judgment is entered, the case will proceed with pretrial activities by both plaintiff and defendant. Such activities, known as pretrial discovery, include, but are not limited to, the taking of witnesses' depositions, the serving of **interrogatories** and **requests for production** on the opposing party, and the issuing of subpoenas, as necessary. The court (the judge assigned to the case) will set dates according to the law by which pretrial discovery must be completed. At the conclusion of this stage, in most cases one or both parties present **motions for summary judgment,** in which they argue that there are (or are not) any facts remaining in dispute and that one or the other is (or is not) entitled to a judgment being entered without the intervention of the trier of fact. If the judge grants such a motion, the case is over and has the same effect as if the case had proceeded to trial.

- If a motion for summary judgment is not successful or is not made, the case will proceed to trial before the trier of fact. In most civil cases, the plaintiff must prove his or her case by what is known as a "preponderance of the evidence." In simple terms, this means that there is enough evidence to tip the scales, even slightly, in favor of the plaintiff's case. This is a substantially lower standard of proof than a criminal case, in which the government must prevail "beyond a reasonable doubt." Upon conclusion of the trial, a verdict is given and a judgment rendered against the party determined to be wholly or partially liable for the harm. In civil cases, a verdict is more commonly referred to as being "liable" or "not liable." Either party may appeal the judgment to an appellate court and possibly even to the highest court in that state.

Criminal Cases

Criminal law addresses crimes that are wrongful acts against public health, safety, and welfare. Criminal laws also include punishment for those persons violating the law. Criminal cases involve matters between individuals or groups of people and the government. Crimes are either a felony or a misdemeanor as defined by state or federal law. **Felonies** are the more serious crimes and include, among others, murder, thefts of items or cash in excess of a certain set value (ordinarily $1,000), assault, and rape. **Misdemeanors** are lesser offenses and include disorderly conduct, thefts of small amounts of property, and breaking into an automobile. Information theft crimes (such as hacking, computer destruction, spamming, and the like) can be either misdemeanors or felonies. The criminal provisions of the HIPAA Privacy Rule have only felony crimes.

When law enforcement learns that a crime has or may have been committed, an investigation is begun. The government initiates a criminal action against those individuals or groups of people it believes have committed the crime based on the law enforcement investigation. When the **prosecutor** (prosecuting attorney), also known as the district or state attorney (depending on the state) or the U.S. attorney (in the federal system), determines sufficient evidence is present, he or she files charges against the defendant on behalf of the government. In some states, a grand jury must return an indictment for a felony crime to be prosecuted. The grand jury has the authority to issue subpoenas for its investigative process, and all evidence considered by the grand jury remains confidential unless an indictment is returned. The court arraigns the charged person on the prosecutor's charge, and the prosecutor prosecutes those charges against the defendant. The prosecutor has the burden of proving the charges against the defendant. In virtually all criminal cases, the government must prove the defendant's guilt beyond a reasonable doubt.

The accused defendant may plead guilty and be sentenced to probation or imprisonment and/or pay a fine. He or she also may plead not guilty, which results in a trial. Upon conclusion of the trial, a verdict of either guilty or not guilty is rendered. When a defendant is found not guilty, the charges are dismissed. A defendant found to be guilty is sentenced to probation or imprisonment and/or to pay a fine. In most jurisdictions, only a defendant who is found guilty at trial can proceed through the appellate process.

Actions Encountered in Healthcare

The healthcare industry is involved most often in civil cases and less often in criminal cases. Because government is increasing its investigations into and prosecutions for healthcare fraud and refusing to treat patients based on financial status, the healthcare industry will be faced with more criminal cases. However, this chapter focuses on civil actions. The types of civil legal actions that most typically affect the healthcare industry are torts and contracts. The vast majority of claims founded in tort and **contract law** are resolved without appearing in court, many before a lawsuit is filed.

Torts

A tort is an action brought when one party believes that another party caused harm through wrongful conduct and the party bringing the action seeks compensation for that harm. In addition to compensation, a second reason for bringing a tort action is to discourage the wrongdoer from committing further wrongful acts. Three categories of tort liability exist: negligent torts, intentional torts, and products liability (Pozgar 2004). Most healthcare **incidents** arise in the negligent tort category. (In the Theory into Practice section, the hospital and the MSO director were held liable for a negligent tort whereas the data-entry clerk was held liable for an intentional tort.)

Negligent Torts

Negligence results when a person does not act the way a reasonably prudent person would act under the same circumstances. A negligent tort may result from a person committing an act or failing to act as a reasonably prudent person would or would not in the given circumstances (Pozgar 2004). Typically, negligence is careless conduct that is outside the generally accepted standard of care. **Standard of care** is defined as what an individual is expected to do or not do in a given situation. Standards of care are established in a variety of ways: by professional associations, by statute or regulation, or by practice. Such standards are considered to represent expected behavior unless a court finds differently. Therefore, standards also are established by case law. Standards not established by a governmental body do not by themselves have the force of law.

In healthcare, the standard of care is the exercise of reasonable care by healthcare professionals having similar training and experience in the same or similar communities. However, some courts may define standards of care on a national level versus a community level.

Negligence also may occur in cases where an individual has evaluated the alternatives and the consequences of those alternatives and has exercised his or her best possible judgment. Thus, a person can be found negligent when he or she has failed to guard against a risk that he or she knew could happen. Furthermore, negligence can occur in circumstances where it is known, or should have been known, that a particular behavior would place others in unreasonable danger. Negligence may occur in the form of (Pozgar 2004, p. 33):

- *Malpractice:* Negligence or carelessness of a professional person, such as a nurse, pharmacist, physician, or accountant
- *Criminal negligence:* Reckless disregard for the safety of another; the willful indifference to an injury that could follow an act (in this respect, it is possible that conduct could at once create civil and criminal liability)

Negligence can further be categorized in other ways. For example, negligent torts can be categorized as (Pozgar 2004, p. 33):

- *Malfeasance:* The execution of an unlawful or improper act

- *Misfeasance:* The improper performance of an act resulting in injury to another
- *Nonfeasance:* The failure to act when there is a duty to act as a reasonably prudent person would act in similar circumstances

Applying this categorization to the Theory into Practice section, the hospital and MSO director would have committed nonfeasance, and the data-entry clerk would have committed either malfeasance or misfeasance.

Further, negligence can be categorized by the degree of wrongdoing. *Ordinary negligence* is failure to do what a reasonably prudent person would do, or doing something that a reasonably prudent person would not do, in the same circumstances (Pozgar 2004). *Gross negligence* is intentionally omitting care that would be proper or providing care that would be substandard or improper (Pozgar 2004).

To recover damages caused by negligence, the plaintiff must show that all four elements of negligence are present:

- There must be a *duty of care.* For this element to be present in a medical malpractice case, a physician–patient, nurse–patient, therapist–patient, or other caregiver–patient relationship must exist at the time of the alleged wrongful act.
- There must have been a *breach of the duty of care.* The plaintiff must present evidence that the defendant acted unreasonably under the circumstances.
- The plaintiff must have *suffered an injury* as a result of the defendant's negligent act or failure to act. Injury includes not only physical harm, but also mental suffering and the invasion of a patient's rights and privacy.
- The plaintiff must show that the defendant's conduct *caused* the plaintiff's harm. As an example, varying from a recognized procedure is insufficient to justify the plaintiff's recovery of damages. The plaintiff must show that the variance was unreasonable and that it caused the harm (Pozgar 2004).

Applying these elements to the Theory into Practice section, the MSO director had a *duty* to ensure that MSO staff followed policy. The director *breached that duty* by not ensuring that the data-entry clerk entered new physician information into the physician database immediately upon receipt. The mayor suffered *actual harm* from an inappropriate disclosure of confidential health information. The failure to change the fax number in the physician database *caused* the harm that the mayor suffered.

When no statute exists to define what is reasonable, the trier of fact determines what a reasonably prudent person would have done. The reasonably prudent person is generally defined in terms of the hypothetical person that a community believes exhibits ideal behavior in a given situation (Pozgar 2004). The trier of fact considers characteristics such as age, sex, training, education, mental capacity, physical condition, and knowledge in defining the reasonably prudent person. After the behavior of a reasonably prudent person is defined for the given circumstances, the trier of fact compares the defendant's behavior against that definition. If the defendant's behavior meets or exceeds the definition, no negligence has occurred. On the other hand, if the defendant's behavior does not meet the reasonably prudent person standard, negligence has occurred. In such a case, the trier of fact must determine whether:

- The harm that would result from the failure to meet the reasonably prudent person standard could have been foreseen.
- The negligent act caused harm to the plaintiff.

Intentional Torts

Although most torts experienced in healthcare are based on negligence, an occasional intentional tort is committed that includes actions such as assault, battery, libel, slander, invasion of privacy, and false imprisonment. The element of intent is the difference between the intentional tort and the negligent tort. *Intent* means the person committed an act knowing that harm would likely occur. (In the Theory into Practice section, the data-entry clerk's conscious and intentional decision not to enter the new fax number into the physician database in a timely manner is an example of an intentional tort.)

A quick review of several intentional torts gives the reader an idea of how they may occur in a healthcare setting. The intentional torts discussed below include assault and battery, false imprisonment, defamation of character, fraud, invasion of privacy, and reckless infliction of mental distress.

Assault is a deliberate threat that is combined with the apparent present ability to cause physical harm to another person (Pozgar 2004, p. 43). For example, a large male nurse in the emergency department tells a frail elderly woman that he will break her arm if she does not do what he tells her to do. His comment is a deliberate threat, and his size gives him the apparent ability to harm the woman. *Battery* is intentionally touching another person's body in a socially impermissible manner without that person's consent (Pozgar 2004, p. 44). In healthcare, laws regarding battery are especially important because of the requirement for consent for medical and surgical procedures. The hospital and the treating healthcare professionals may be held liable for harm caused by the lack of a proper patient consent. Even if the outcome of the procedure benefits the patient, touching the patient without proper consent may make the healthcare professional liable for battery.

False imprisonment is another intentional tort. A healthcare provider's efforts to prevent a patient from leaving a hospital may result in false imprisonment. This is not the case when a patient with a contagious disease or a mentally ill patient who is likely to cause harm to others is compelled to remain in the hospital (Pozgar 2004). There are limits to the actions staff can take to compel a patient not to leave a hospital. For example, staff may confine a person to protect them from harming themselves or others (Pozgar 2004). The patient's insistence on leaving the facility should be documented in his or her health record, and the patient should be asked to sign a discharge against medical advice form that releases the facility from responsibility. When excessive force is used to restrain a patient, the healthcare provider may be held liable for both false imprisonment and battery (Pozgar 2004).

Defamation of character is a false communication about someone to a person other than the person defamed that tends to injure that person's reputation (Pozgar 2004). The communication may be either oral or written. *Libel* is the written form of defamation, and *slander* is the spoken form. To recover in an action for defamation, the plaintiff must prove that:

- The defendant made a false and defamatory statement about the plaintiff.
- The statement was not a "privileged" publication and was made to a third person.
- At least negligence occurred.
- Actual or presumed damages occurred.

Proof of special damages, including economic losses, is not required to recover in a defamation case. Special damages include economic losses. Courts also may find that the defamation caused injury to a person's reputation. However, there are four exceptions regarding harm to reputation. In these exceptions, the plaintiff is not required to show proof of actual harm to his or her reputation when the defendant allegedly performs one of the following acts (Pozgar 2004, p. 47):

- Accuses the plaintiff of a crime
- Accuses the plaintiff of having a loathsome disease
- Uses words that affect the plaintiff's profession or business
- Calls a woman unchaste

When slander is alleged, the plaintiff usually must prove special damages. However, if the slander refers to the plaintiff in a professional capacity, the plaintiff is not required to show actual harm because slanderous references to a person's professional capacity are presumed to be damaging to that person's professional reputation (Pozgar 2004, p. 49). As to the second exception, healthcare professionals are protected against claims of libel when complying with laws requiring the reporting of communicable diseases that the patient may consider loathsome (Pozgar 2004).

The defendant (the one being accused of defaming another) has two defenses available to a defamation action. The person making an alleged defamatory statement that harms another's reputation will not be liable for that statement if he or she shows the statement was true (Pozgar 2004). Secondly, the person making the allegedly defamatory communication can claim privilege if he or she is making the communication:

- In good faith
- On the proper occasion
- In the proper manner
- To persons who have a legitimate reason to receive the information

The defense of privilege is based on the person making the communication being charged with a higher duty. For example, in one case, a director of nurses wrote a letter to a nurse's professional registry stating that the hospital wanted to discontinue a particular nurse's services because narcotics were disappearing whenever the nurse was on duty (*Judge v. Rockford Memorial Hospital* 1958). The court found the communication to be privileged because the director of nurses had a legal duty to make the communication in the interests of society. Thus, the court denied the nurse's claim for damages.

Fraud is a prevalent concern in today's healthcare environment. It is defined as "a willful and intentional misrepresentation that could cause harm or loss to a person or property" (Pozgar 2004, p. 51). For example, physicians can be held liable for fraud if they claim that a particular procedure will cure a patient's ailment when they know it will not, or if they charge a third-party payer for a medical procedure they did not actually perform.

Invasion of privacy is another major concern in healthcare. A person's right to privacy is "the right to be left alone—the right to be free from unwarranted publicity and exposure to public view, as well as the right to live one's life without having one's name, picture, or private affairs made public against one's will" (Pozgar 2004, p. 52). The right to privacy is also the right to control personal information (McWay 2003, p. 118). The courts recognize that absolute privacy is not a reality in the medical or nursing care of a patient (Pozgar 2004). However, they hold healthcare providers liable for negligent disregard for a patient's right of privacy, especially when patients cannot adequately protect themselves because of unconsciousness or immobility (Pozgar 2004). One major actionable offense of concern in healthcare involving invasion of privacy is the release or disclosure of health information without patient authorization in circumstances when it is required. (See figure A.22 in appendix A.)

The *intentional or reckless infliction of mental distress* for which a person can be held liable includes mental suffering resulting from such things as despair, shame, grief, and public humiliation (Pozgar 2004). If the plaintiff shows that the defendant (the one inflicting the distress) intended to cause mental distress and knew that his or her actions would do so, the plaintiff can recover damages even in the absence of physical harm (Pozgar 2004). Courts currently are struggling with the fine line between negligent and intentional infliction of mental distress, with most courts using the presence or absence of physical harm accompanying the distress (called the "impact rule" in most states) to determine whether damages can be awarded.

The distinction between negligence torts and intentional torts is far from academic. In most state legal systems, punitive damages (those damages awarded to punish or deter wrongful conduct over and above compensation for injury) are limited in negligence cases and may, in fact, be capped in medical malpractice cases. However, most states permit punitive damages as a matter of right in cases of intentional torts, and these damages usually fall outside the scope of state laws capping jury awards or damages. Consequently, it is possible for a battery case involving a failure to obtain surgical consent (an intentional tort) to have more economic value than a medical malpractice case (a negligence tort) due to the presence or absence of punitive damages.

Products Liability

A manufacturer, seller, or supplier may be liable to a buyer or other third party for injuries caused by a defective product (Pozgar 2004). The injured person may bring an action based in negligence, breach of warranty, or strict liability. To prevail in *negligence,* the plaintiff must show that there was a duty that was breached causing the injury. The manufacturer will not be held liable for injuries if they resulted from the user's negligent use of the product. Manufacturers will be held liable for injuries resulting from a bad product design (Pozgar 2004). Manufacturers often provide instructions on the proper use of their product. Should a manufacturer not provide these instructions, the manufacturer may be liable for negligence (Pozgar 2004). A manufacturer has a duty to warn of dangers associated with normal, proper use of the product.

To recover under the theory of *breach of warranty,* the plaintiff must show there was an express or implied warranty (Pozgar 2004). Through an *express warranty,* the seller makes specific promises to the buyer. Whereas an *implied warranty* exists when the law implies such a warranty exists "as a matter of public policy" to protect the public from harm (Pozgar 2004, p. 55).

The third basis on which a plaintiff may base a product's liability claim is *strict liability,* which is liability without fault. To prevail, the plaintiff only must show an injury resulted while using the product in the proper manner. The plaintiff does not need to show negligence by the manufacturer. The elements for a strict liability case are:

- Product must have been manufactured by the defendant;
- Product must have been defective at the time it left the hands of the manufacturer or seller;
- Plaintiff must have been injured by the specific product; and
- Defective product must have been the proximate cause of the injury (Pozgar 2004, p. 55).

However, a device manufacturer may be held strictly liable for injuries to a plaintiff, even though the plaintiff did not purchase the product. For strict liability to be imposed in this circumstance, the product must have been defective and the defect must have been the actual and proximate cause of the injuries (Pozgar 2004, p. 56). Under strict liability, the manufacturer also may be held liable pursuant to the concept of *res ipsa loquitur* (the thing speaks for itself). To recover, the plaintiff must show:

- The product did not perform in the way intended;
- Neither the buyer nor a third person had tampered with the product; and
- The defect in the product existed when it left the manufacturer (Pozgar 2004, p. 56)

Defenses

A healthcare provider may raise a number of defenses in response to a lawsuit (McWay 2003, pp. 55–60). These include the following:

- ***Statute of limitations:*** A statutorily set time frame within which a lawsuit must be brought or the court must dismiss the case.
- *Good Samaritan:* Statutes that protect physicians and other rescuers from liability for their acts or omissions in providing emergency care in a nontraditional setting such as at an automobile accident when no charge for services is made.
- *Contributory negligence:* The plaintiff's conduct contributed in part to the injury the plaintiff suffered and, if found to be sufficient, can preclude the plaintiff's recovery for the injury.
- *Comparative negligence:* The plaintiff's conduct contributed in part to the injury the plaintiff suffered, but the plaintiff's recovery is reduced by some amount based on his or her percentage of negligence.

The charitable immunity and governmental immunity defenses have been either significantly limited or abolished as defenses by state and federal laws.

Contract

Suits under contracts are the other type of civil claim arising in the healthcare industry. A contract is an agreement, written or oral, that, in most cases, is legally enforceable through the legal system. Contracts must not violate state or federal policy or state or federal statute, rule or regulation. Contract law is based on common law. However, some states have replaced common law with statutory law or administrative agency regulations. In those states, the statutes or administrative regulations control. One example of how contractual issues affect healthcare is a contract for services between the hospital and a contracting physician or a physician group, such as pathologists, radiologists, anesthesiologists, and emergency medicine physicians.

The elements of a contract must be stated clearly and specifically. A contract cannot exist unless all the following elements exist. There must be an *agreement* between two or more persons or entities. The agreement must include a valid offer, acceptance, and an exchange of consideration. In an *offer,* one party promises to either do something or not do something if the other party agrees to either do something or not do something (Pozgar 2004). The party making the offer must communicate it to the other party so that it can be accepted or rejected. There also must be *acceptance*. Communication of an acceptance is not necessary unless the offeror specifically requires that the acceptance be received for a contract to be formed (Pozgar 2004, p. 87); more often, commencing performance under the contract is sufficient to indicate acceptance. Finally, a contract must be supported by legal and bargained-for consideration. There is no common definition of consideration, but its essence is reflected by the term *price* (Pozgar 2004, p. 87).

The parties to a contract must have the capacity to enter into the agreement, such as being a competent adult, being of age of majority, not being incapacitated by medication or alcohol, and not being mentally incapacitated. The contract must be for a legal purpose. Finally, the contract must not violate public policy (Pozgar 2004, p. 90). A hospital contract with patients that attempts to limit their right to sue could be a contract to which a court would apply the unconscionable concept and hold the hospital liable.

A contract action arises when one party claims that the other party has failed to meet an obligation set forth in the contract. Another way to state this is that the other party has breached the contract. The resolution available is either compensation (money damages) or performance of the obligation. The defendant can raise a variety of defenses to a breach of contract action including waiver and default, conduct of the parties, and waiving rights under the agreement.

Check Your Understanding 10.1

Instructions: Answer the following questions on a separate piece of paper.

1. What are the four sources of laws governing Americans?
2. What types of cases are typically heard in the federal court system?
3. Which court is the court of last resort in the U.S. legal system?
4. What are the two most common types of civil cases experienced in healthcare?
5. In a court, who is the trier of fact?
6. What is the result of a trial called?
7. What types of cases are covered by criminal laws?
8. What are the roles of prosecutor and defendant in a criminal case? Who has the burden of proof?
9. What are the possible outcomes of a criminal case?
10. What are the three categories of tort liability? From which category do most healthcare cases arise?
11. What is the definition of a negligent tort?
12. What are the four elements of negligence?
13. How might false imprisonment occur in a hospital?
14. What defenses are available to a defendant accused of defamation of character?
15. Privacy is difficult to achieve in a healthcare setting. However, courts will hold healthcare providers liable for what type of invasion of privacy?
16. What is a contract?
17. What action must occur for a contract case to arise?

Legal Aspects of Health Information Management

The field of health information management must recognize and treat the patient's health record as a legal document. Thus, the HIM professional must have an understanding of all the regulations and statutes that affect the creation and maintenance of the health record.

Form and Content of the Health Record

The health record is a complete, accurate, and current report of the medical history, condition, and treatment that a particular patient receives during an encounter with a healthcare provider. (See chapter 9 for the definition of a legal health record.) In a hospital, the encounter may be on either an inpatient or outpatient basis. Moreover, it may be defined as one episode of treatment or an accumulation of all episodes of treatment in any setting that is part of the organization.

The health record is composed of two sections: the demographic section and the clinical section. Most of the information in the *demographic section* is collected at the time of admission or registration for treatment. It includes, among other items, the patient's name, sex, age, insurance information, and the person to contact in case of emergency. This information may be added to and changed throughout the patient's medical encounters. The *clinical section* comprises the patient's complaint, history of present illness, medical history, family history, social history, continuing documentation of ongoing medical care, report of diagnostic tests, x-ray reports, surgery and other procedure reports, consultant reports, nursing documentation, various graphs, and the final diagnoses. In some states, licensure regulations may specify the contents. In other states, the health record content is defined in broader terms.

Accrediting agency regulations or standards are one source for identifying health record content. (See appendix C.) The Joint Commission on Accreditation of Healthcare Organizations (JCAHO), the American Osteopathic Association (AOA), and other accrediting organizations include some level of requirements for health record content. The Medicare program's Conditions of Participation also include minimum requirements for health record content. However, some sources of regulations for health record content are more prescriptive than others are. For example, some regulations give details on the information to be retained, others specify the broad categories of information required, and still others state simply that the health record must be accurate, adequate, or complete. Most states have statutory or regulatory definitions of what a proper health record must contain, and many third-party payers also dictate how health records for their insured must be maintained and kept. The HIM professional must be aware of the most stringent definition of the health record content to which his or her particular organization is subject.

It also is important to heed requirements of agencies and laws that regulate hospitals and have an impact on the process of creating and maintaining health records. The healthcare industry in general and hospitals in particular are extensively regulated by all levels of the government and by numerous agencies within each level of government. Additionally, they are regulated for accreditation purposes by non-government agencies. Quite often, hospitals are faced with conflicting requirements because of this multiple-regulation environment.

Regulatory (Licensure) Agencies

Typically, state legislatures have granted authority to a state administrative agency to:

- Develop standards hospitals must meet
- Issue licenses to those hospitals that meet the standards
- Monitor continuing compliance with the standards
- Penalize hospitals that violate the standards

Licensure is issued for the organization as a whole. It addresses policies and procedures, staffing, and hospital building integrity among many other facets of the organization. Some states require additional licenses for specific services in the hospital. For example, laboratory, radiology, renal dialysis, and substance abuse services may require separate licenses in addition to the facility license. Additional state and federal laws apply to the use of drugs and medical devices.

Some states require separate licensure for hospital pharmacies whereas other states regulate hospital pharmacies through the general state hospital licensing system. Typically, the laws address dispensing and administering drugs to patients in the hospital and dispensing take-home drugs through an inpatient or outpatient hospital visit. Additionally, some regulations require sufficient staff members for the hospital pharmacy based on the hospital's size and scope of services.

Finally, some states require certain types of medical equipment to be separately licensed, such as x-ray equipment or medical waste disposal systems.

Hospitals cannot operate without a license. Those that violate the standards may lose their licenses or be penalized in other ways, such as with fines. Thus, licensure is government regulation that is mandatory for hospitals.

Accreditation Agencies

Accreditation is offered through nongovernment agencies. One of the most important accrediting agencies for hospitals is JCAHO. JCAHO develops standards that hospitals must meet to be accredited. The healthcare organization applies to JCAHO to be accredited, pays an accreditation fee, and submits to an extensive survey to ensure compliance with JCAHO's published standards. JCAHO addresses privacy, security, and confidentiality in a number of standards. Ethical behavior and patient rights are addressed in RI 1.10, 2.10,

2.20, 2.100, 2.120, and 2.180. Patient privacy, confidentiality, and information security are addressed in RI 2.50, 2.130, IM 2.10, 2.20, 2.30, MM 1.10, and EC 2.10. In LD 1.30, JCAHO addresses whether the hospital complies with applicable laws and regulations, and in HR 2.10 it addresses training.

Effective January 2004, JCAHO introduced a self-assessment approach to showing compliance with privacy and confidentiality standards and elements of performance. The organization uses 12 months of concrete data to score itself on the elements of performance. JCAHO verifies those scores during a regular accreditation visit.

Similarly, the AOA accredits osteopathic hospitals and functions in much the same way that JCAHO does.

Accreditation is considered voluntary and is not legally mandated, but it is very important to healthcare organizations. Some states accept JCAHO or AOA accreditation as a basis for partial or full licensure with limited or no additional survey by the state agency. This "deeming" authority gives JCAHO a significant amount of power it would not otherwise have.

Whereas JCAHO and the AOA focus on the entire hospital, other accrediting agencies focus on specific services of the hospital. For example, there is a separate accreditation process for laboratory and radiology services in addition to that of JCAHO and the AOA.

The federal Medicare program also sets standards for hospitals in its Conditions of Participation. Although these are government regulations, participation in the Medicare program is considered voluntary. However, few, if any, hospitals elect not to participate in this program. Thus, a hospital must comply with these standards to receive payment from the Medicare program for covered services provided to Medicare beneficiaries. The Medicare program also recognizes organizations that have JCAHO or AOA accreditation as meeting most of the Conditions of Participation, and it grants them deemed status. A hospital would typically undergo an additional survey only if a special Medicare inspection finds noncompliance.

Statutory and Regulatory Law

There are many sources of law mandating the privacy of confidential health information. Some of these sources are discussed below.

Privacy

There is no right to privacy specifically stated in the U.S. Constitution. However, in 1965, the Supreme Court recognized an implicit constitutional right of privacy in *Griswold v. Connecticut*. In this case, the court ruled that "the right to privacy limits governmental authority to regulate contraception, abortion, and other decisions affecting reproduction" (Miller 1986, pp. 6–7). Some states also have recognized the right to privacy in their state constitutions (California Constitution, Article 1, Declaration of Rights, Section 1; Arizona Constitution, 8 Right to privacy; Florida Constitution, Article I, Section 23, Right of privacy).

On August 21, 1996, Congress enacted HIPAA. This legislation initially focused on making it easier for employees to retain health coverage when they changed jobs or their family status changed. The HIPAA legislation addressed waste, fraud, and abuse in the healthcare system. It also focused on simplifying the administration of health insurance (HIPAA-b).

To address simplification, Congress added the Administrative Simplification provisions, which created a single federal standard electronic claims format for electronic data interchange (HIPAA-e). With these provisions, the legislature intended to improve the efficiency and effectiveness of the healthcare system (HIPAA-c). However, Congress continued to express concerns about privacy and security of patient information in an electronic environment (HIPAA-e). Consequently, HIPAA required HHS to develop and implement electronic transaction standards and to develop regulations to protect the privacy and security of **individually identifiable health information** (HIPAA-d). As a result, HHS issued three sets of standards: Transactions and Code Sets (45 CFR §§160, 162), Privacy, and Security (45 CFR §§160, 164). All rules for these three sets of standards have been promulgated and issued. Covered entities as defined in HIPAA were required to be in compliance with the Privacy Rule by April 14, 2003, and with the Transactions and Code Sets Rule by October 16, 2003. Covered entities were required to be compliant with the Security Rule by April 20, 2005. The compliance dates for small health plans were extended by one year for each set of rules. (HIPAA is covered in more detail later in this chapter.)

Another piece of federal legislation addressing a patient's right to privacy is the **Privacy Act of 1974.** This act gives individuals some control over the information collected about them by the federal government (Hughes 2002). It does not apply to records maintained by institutions in the private sector (McWay 2003). Under the Privacy Act of 1974, people have the right to:

- Learn what information has been collected about them
- View and have a copy of that information
- Maintain limited control over the disclosure of that information to other persons or entities (Hughes 2002)

This act also applies to federal government healthcare organizations such as the Veterans Health Administration (VHA) and Indian Health Services and to record systems operated pursuant to a contract with a federal government agency (Hughes 2002).

Further, the **Freedom of Information Act** (FOIA) is a federal law through which individuals can seek access to information without authorization of the person to whom the information applies. This act applies only to federal agencies and not the private sector. The Veterans Administration and Defense Department hospital systems are subject to this act, but few other hospitals are. The only protection of health information held by federal agencies exists when disclosure would "constitute a clearly unwarranted invasion of personal privacy" (Miller 1986).

Despite the need for patient privacy, healthcare providers disclose health information to subsequent healthcare providers to the extent necessary to ensure continuity of patient care (Hughes 2003). Federal legislation that specifically provides for such disclosures includes, but is not limited to:

- The Medicare Conditions of Participation for Hospitals
- Conditions of Participation for Clinics, Rehabilitation Agencies, and Public Health Agencies as Providers of Outpatient Physical Therapy and Speech-Language Pathology
- Conditions of Participation for Home Health Agencies
- Confidentiality of Alcohol and Drug Abuse Patient Records

As to privacy rights, the Conditions of Participation for Hospitals rule states that hospitals must have procedures to protect the confidentiality of patient records (Hughes 2002). Under this rule, hospitals must protect records against unauthorized access and alteration. Further, original records may be removed from the facility only in accordance with federal and state laws (Hughes 2002).

The Conditions of Participation for Clinics, Rehabilitation Agencies, and Public Health Agencies as Providers of Outpatient Physical Therapy and Speech-Language Pathology regulations permit the physician to provide medical information to the receiving facility (Hughes 2003).

The Conditions of Participation for Home Health Agencies also requires facilities to have written policies and procedures to safeguard health information against loss or unauthorized use (Hughes 2002). Furthermore, the Requirements for States and Long-Term Care Facilities give the resident or his or her legal representative the right to access information about the resident. Additionally, these regulations give the resident the right to personal privacy and confidentiality of personal and clinical records (Hughes 2002).

The Confidentiality of Alcohol and Drug Abuse Patient Records rule is a federal rule that applies to information created for patients treated in a federally assisted drug or alcohol abuse program (Hughes 2002). This rule specifically protects the identity, diagnosis, prognosis, or treatment of these patients (Hughes 2002). These rules generally prohibit redisclosure of health information related to this treatment except as needed in a medical emergency or when authorized by an appropriate court order or the patient's authorization (Rhodes and Hughes 2003). (See figure A.22 in appendix A.). The rule also specifies the circumstances under which information can be released without patient authorization and requires that language prohibiting redisclosure be attached to all released information concerning drug or alcohol treatment (Hughes 2002).

Other Federal Legislation

The Comprehensive Drug Abuse Prevention and Control Act of 1970, the **Controlled Substances Act,** controls the use of narcotics, depressants, stimulants, and hallucinogens (Pozgar 2004). Because this act affects the dispensing and administering of these specific drug categories, pharmacy staff must be well versed in this law and how it interacts with state licensing and regulatory laws and accrediting standards. The controlled substances are classified into schedules according to the extent to which they are controlled. Schedule I drugs are subject to the tightest controls; Schedule I–IV drugs may be dispensed only upon a practitioner's lawful order.

In the outpatient environment, a prescription that meets the requirements of the law is required. In the inpatient setting, an order in the health record satisfies this requirement for a lawful order. The practitioner signing the prescription or the order in the health record must be registered with the Drug Enforcement Administration (DEA) of the Department of Justice. State law determines which professionals may be classified as practitioners for this purpose.

The Food, Drug, and Cosmetic Act, which includes the Medical Device Amendments of 1976, covers products that are distributed in federal territory or transported in interstate commerce (Pozgar 2004, p. 275). Most equipment and supplies used in a hospital for patient care are regulated as devices under these regulations.

Retention of the Health Record

The health record serves several purposes and must be retained to meet those purposes. These purposes include:

- Most important, the health record is a tool used in the patient's continuing medical care because it provides complete and accurate information about the patient's previous care and treatment.
- It serves as a means of communication among the patient's healthcare providers—physicians, nurses, therapists, pharmacists, and technologists.
- It is used by the patient's healthcare providers as a basis for developing the plan of care. Further, the health record may be reviewed after care is rendered to evaluate the quality of the care.
- It is a source of information for statistical, research, and educational purposes.
- It serves as a source of billing and financial reports and information because billing records must be supported by the documentation in the health record.
- It is valuable in legal proceedings because it reflects the care given (the treatments, procedures, and medications the patient received), includes statements made by the patient about the cause of his or her illness or injury, and shows any errors in judgment or treatment made by healthcare facilities or professionals.

These varied purposes influence how long health records must be kept, or their retention period. Federal and state laws and regulations often determine retention periods. In the absence of such laws, professional organizations offer guidance (Davis, McConnell, and Shaw 2004; McWay 2003).

Further, the advent of technology, in particular the move toward an electronic health record, will influence retention periods (McWay 2003). For those periods determined by state law, the state defines what the minimum retention period will be. Some states are more specific than others. For example, some states base the retention period, at least partially, on the statute of limitations for bringing a legal action. Some state and federal statutes and regulations set specific retention requirements for particular parts of the health record (for example, x-rays or mammography studies) or for particular patient types (for example, minors, mentally ill, deceased) (Davis, McConnell and Shaw 2004).

The HIM professional must be aware of the retention statutes and retention periods in his or her state of employment. In some cases, the organization may define a retention period that is longer than the period required by the state. The organization should base its retention policy on hospital and medical needs and any applicable statutes and regulations.

Retention also includes the safeguarding of confidential information maintained in health records. All hospital staff members with the right to access a patient's health record have an obligation to protect the confidentiality of patient information.

Check Your Understanding 10.2

Instructions: Answer the following questions on a separate piece of paper.

1. What are the two sections of a health record? What type of information is contained in each section?
2. What is the primary difference between licensure and accreditation of healthcare organizations?
3. What national patient information confidentiality standards were promulgated in December 2000?
4. On what basis can a plaintiff claim unauthorized disclosure of health information against a hospital?
5. What was the holding regarding privacy issued by the court in *Griswold v. Connecticut?*
6. What information can the HIM professional use to determine how long to retain health records?
7. What are the three sets of standards included in the HIPAA Administrative Simplification provisions that are addressed in the text?
8. In addition to HIPAA, what other pieces of legislation are discussed that address privacy?

Ownership and Control of the Health Record

Patients often believe they own their health record. The HIM professional must be able to advise the patient regarding the actual ownership and control of the physical health record and the patient's rights to the information contained in it.

Ownership of the Physical Record

The physical health record is considered the property of the healthcare provider, the physician, or the hospital that maintains it because it is the healthcare provider's business record. Yet, the patient and others have an interest in the information contained within the health record. The patient and others, as authorized under state and federal laws, rules, and regulations, have the right to access the information as discussed below and to control the use and disclosure of that information.

Redisclosure of health information is of significant concern to the healthcare industry. As such, the HIM professional must be alerted to state and federal statutes addressing this issue (Rhodes and Hughes 2003). A consent obtained by a hospital pursuant to the Privacy Rule in Section 164.506(a)(5) does not permit another hospital, healthcare provider, or clearinghouse to use or disclose information. However, the authorization content required in the Privacy Rule in Section 164.508(c)(i) must include a statement that the information disclosed pursuant to the authorization may be disclosed by the recipient and thus is no longer protected.

Use and Disclosure of Patient Information

The HIPAA Privacy Rule addresses how and for what purposes **protected health information** (PHI) can be used. PHI is individually identifiable health information that covered entities or their business associates transmit or maintain in any form or format. The Privacy Rule covers information in oral, electronic, and paper formats (45 CFR §§164.500, 164.501, 165.514). The covered entities include:

- Health plans that pay for medical care
- Healthcare clearinghouses that receive health information in a nonstandard format and convert the information into a standard format; or healthcare clearinghouses that receive health information in a standard format and convert the information into a nonstandard format
- Healthcare providers that electronically transmit any health information (45 CFR §§160.102, 160.103)

The Privacy Rule is the first attempt at a national set of privacy protections. Although the HIPAA rules provide for preempting state law, it is not a true national standard for patient information privacy. In other words, it is not a ceiling. It is considered a floor because it permits exceptions to the state law **preemption** provisions (45 CFR §160.201–205).

Prior to HIPAA, many states recognized patients' rights to access their own health records. Many states also recognized that various third parties have a legitimate need to access the confidential health information contained in a health record. These third parties include insurance companies for payment purposes, insurance companies when coverage has been applied for, government agencies to determine eligibility for healthcare programs, and so on. Further, prior to HIPAA, many states also permitted patients to control access by all third parties except those to which the hospital is required to report information of a medical nature or as otherwise required by law.

The standard HIPAA rule is that it preempts state law if it is contrary to that state law except if one or more of the following conditions is met (45 CFR §§160.201–205):

- The secretary of HHS determines that the provision of state law is necessary to prevent fraud and abuse related to providing or paying for healthcare; to ensure appropriate state regulation of insurance and health plans; for state reporting on healthcare delivery or costs; or for public health, safety, or welfare if the intrusion into privacy is warranted when balanced against this need.
- The secretary of HHS determines that the provision of state law is for the purpose of regulating the manufacture, registration, distribution, dispensing, or other control of controlled substances.
- The provision of state law relates to the privacy of individually identifiable health information and is more stringent than a provision in the HIPAA Privacy Rule.
- The provision of state law provides for reporting disease or injury, child abuse, birth, or death, or for the conduct of public health surveillance, investigation, or intervention.
- The provision of state law requires a health plan to report, or to provide access to, information for management audits, financial audits, program monitoring and evaluation, or licensure or certification of facilities or individuals.

For purposes of the HIPAA preemption analysis, a state law is more stringent when, in general terms, it affords a patient more access to his or her medical information or more control over the disclosure of his or her medical information to third parties. As an example, a state statute that requires a patient to consent to any disclosure of his or her medical information to an insurance company for purposes of payment would survive HIPAA's implementation, but a statute that prohibited a mental health patient from receiving a copy of his or her health record (other than psychotherapy notes) would not.

Even though HIPAA is the first attempt at national privacy legislation, the HIM professional also must be aware of state laws affecting the use and disclosure of PHI. The Privacy Rule is discussed below in terms of patient rights, the types of disclosures that require the patient be given an opportunity to agree or object, uses and disclosures that require patient authorization, and uses and disclosures that do not require patient authorization.

Patient Rights

HIPAA provides patients with certain rights related to protecting their privacy and their PHI. It requires that every patient be provided a Notice of Privacy Practices (Notice) setting forth the following (45 CFR §164.520):

- How covered entities may use and disclose PHI
- The patient's rights regarding the covered entities' uses and disclosures
- The covered entities' obligations for protecting the patient's PHI

The Privacy Rule is very specific about the required contents of the Notice. The Notice must be provided upon request.

Covered entities having a direct patient relationship with the patient must provide the patient a copy of the Notice at the time of the first service delivery, including service delivered electronically. In emergency situations, covered entities providing care must provide the Notice as soon as practicable after the emergency treatment situation is resolved. The covered entity (CE) is to make a good faith effort to obtain the patient's written acknowledgment of receipt of the Notice. This requirement also is delayed until practicable in emergency treatment situations. If receipt is not obtained for any reason, including patient refusal to provide the acknowledgment, the CE is required to document its good faith efforts and the reason why the acknowledgment was not obtained.

With reference to the previous discussion of more stringent state privacy laws, the Notice must be tailored specifically to disclose the effect of these more stringent standards. A generic disclosure that "state laws may affect your rights" is not sufficient.

A second right that the Privacy Rule provides patients is the right to *access their own patient information* (45 CFR §164.524). Although, as stated earlier, some states had given patients this right, under HIPAA all patients now have it. The information that patients have the right to access is termed the **designated record set.** The types of information that HIPAA does not provide access to are:

- Oral information
- Psychotherapy notes
- Information compiled in anticipation of, or for use in, a civil, criminal, or administrative action or proceeding
- PHI the CE maintains that is subject to or exempted from the Clinical Laboratory Improvements Amendment (CLIA) of 1988

This right of access applies to all three categories of CEs that actually create or receive PHI other than as a business associate of another CE.

The patient's request can be denied without giving the patient an opportunity to request review of the denial. In addition to the PHI types noted above to which the patient is not given access, access can be denied in the following circumstances:

- When the CE is a correctional institution or a CE acting under the direction of the correctional institution and such access would jeopardize the health, safety, security, custody, or rehabilitation of the individual or others
- When PHI was created or obtained during research that includes treatment (access is suspended while the research is in progress as long as the patient agreed to the access denial when consenting to participate in the research and the patient had been advised that the right would be reinstated upon completion of the research)
- When the PHI is contained in records subject to the Privacy Act of 1974 and is also not available for access under the Privacy Act

The Privacy Rule gives patients a third right, which is to request that the CE *amend* the designated record set (45 CFR §164.526). It provides that this request also can be granted or denied. Grounds for denying an amendment request include the following:

- The PHI was not created by the CE, unless the patient indicates that the originator is no longer available.
- The PHI is not part of the designated record set.
- The PHI would not be available for the patient to inspect.
- The PHI is accurate and complete.

One of the most striking features of this legislation is found in Section 164.528(I) wherein it gives a patient the right to obtain an *accounting of disclosures* of PHI made by a CE in the six years or less prior to the request date (45 CFR 164.528 [HIPAA-n]). (See figure A.23 in appendix A.) An accounting does not need to include such disclosures as the following:

- To carry out treatment, payment, and healthcare operations
- To the patient who is the subject of the PHI
- Those that are incidental to treatment, payment, or healthcare operations
- Those pursuant to patient authorization
- For a facility directory or to family or caregivers
- For national security or intelligence purposes
- To correctional institutions or law enforcement under specific circumstances
- PHI included in a limited data set
- Those made prior to the compliance date for the CE

If disclosures have been made to an oversight agency or law enforcement official and the agency or official notifies the CE that including these disclosures in an accounting would likely impede the agency's activities, the CE must temporarily suspend the patient's right to receive the requested accounting. For each disclosure included in an accounting, the accounting report must include the disclosure date, the recipient's name and address, and a brief description of the PHI disclosed and of the purpose of the disclosure. The Privacy Rule provides a specific procedure for multiple disclosures to the same person or entity for a single purpose or for research purposes.

Another right is that of requesting the CE to *restrict the use of PHI* to carry out treatment, payment, or healthcare operations; to those involved in the patient care; and for notification purposes [45 CFR §164.522(a)]. Again, the CE is not required to agree to the requested restriction. If the CE agrees to the requested restriction, it must document the restriction and must maintain that documentation for six years. A patient also may request health plans and healthcare clearinghouses, which create or receive PHI other than as a business associate, to restrict uses and disclosures.

Moreover, patients are given the right to request that CEs communicate with them in a confidential manner or method

[45 CFR §164.522(b)]. Confidential communications may be either by an alternative means or at alternative locations. For example, a patient may request that any telephone contact be made only at work or that all written communication be sent to a post office box rather than to his or her home address. A CE that is a healthcare provider:

- Must accommodate reasonable requests
- May not require the patient to provide an explanation of the basis for the request
- May require the patient to place the request in writing

A CE that is a health plan also must accommodate reasonable requests. However, the health plan is permitted to require the patient to provide a statement that the disclosure of all or part of the information to which the request pertains could endanger the patient.

Check Your Understanding 10.3

Instructions: Answer the following questions on a separate piece of paper.

1. Who owns the physical health record?

2. Who owns the information contained in the health record, whether paper or computer based?

3. What is the primary focus of the HIPAA Privacy Rule?

4. Who are the covered entities covered by the HIPAA Privacy Rule?

5. Does HIPAA preempt all state laws addressing privacy? Discuss your answer.

6. What information must be described in the Notice of Privacy Practices?

7. When are healthcare providers who have a direct relationship with the patient required to provide the patient with a copy of the Notice of Privacy Practices?

8. What formats of information are protected under HIPAA?

9. To what types of information is the patient not provided access?

10. What is the most striking feature of the Privacy Rule?

11. List five types of disclosures that do not need to be included in an accounting.

12. Can the patient's request to access his or her own health information be denied? Explain your answer.

13. Under the Privacy Rule, who may sign an authorization for the disclosure of information?

14. Discuss the circumstances listed in the Privacy Rule under which a facility may deny a patient's request for access to his or her own health information without providing the patient the opportunity to have the denial reviewed.

15. Explain the access to health information available to the news media.

16. Under what circumstances does the Privacy Rule permit disclosure of health information to a patient's employer?

17. What, if any, circumstances might make a healthcare provider liable for breach of confidentiality when reporting public health information?

Types of Disclosures Requiring Opportunity to Agree or Object

The Privacy Rule provides patients an opportunity to agree or object to specific types of disclosures (45 CFR §164.510). These do not require a written authorization; verbal authorization is acceptable. However, communication with the patient regarding these types of disclosures and the patient's decision should be documented in the health record or other appropriate manner of documentation.

Absent the patient's objection, a covered healthcare provider may use specific PHI to maintain a directory of patients in its facility. This information includes the patient's:

- Name
- Location in the provider's facility, including the emergency room
- Condition in very general terms that do not include specific medial information about the patient
- Religious affiliation

The general terms that can be used to indicate the condition include undetermined, good, fair, serious, critical, stable, died, and treated and released. The patient is not required to provide information regarding religious affiliation. The covered provider may disclose the name, location, and condition to anyone asking for the patient by name, including the news media. The covered provider may disclose these elements plus the religious affiliation to members of the clergy even if they do not ask for the patient by name. If the patient does not specifically express an objection to being included in the facility's directory, the PHI may be released as noted without the patient's consent or authorization.

When a patient is incapacitated or in an emergency situation and cannot object to being included in the facility's directory, the covered provider may disclose the information as noted if the disclosure is:

- Consistent with any previously expressed preference that is known to the provider
- In the patient's best interest as determined by the provider using professional judgment

If, during the patient's stay in the facility, he or she regains the capacity to make his or her own decisions, the provider must advise the patient about the facility's directory policies and provide the patient the opportunity to object to being included in it.

The covered provider also may obtain the patient's verbal agreement or objection to disclose PHI for the following purposes (45 CFR §164.510):

- Disclosure to family, friends, or other caregivers identified by the patient relevant to their involvement with the patient's care. The requirement for patient authorization typically extends to a request by a patient's family members, including the spouse. However, healthcare providers may discuss general information about the patient's condition with family members without authorization unless the patient has instructed otherwise. If the patient is incapacitated, the physician and other caregivers may discuss health information and treatment plans with the next of kin or the patient's representative (however that is defined by a given state) to the extent necessary to make medical decisions on the incapacitated patient's behalf. The Privacy Rule permits the hospital to disclose to a family member, other relative, close personal friend, or any person identified by the patient health information directly relevant to that person's involvement in the patient's care or payment for healthcare [Section 164.510(b)(1)(i)]. (See further discussion under the section on use and disclosure with patient authorization.)

- The hospital may use or disclose health information to notify or assist in notifying (identifying or locating) a family member, a personal representative, or some other person responsible for the patient's care of the patient's location, general condition, or death [Section 164.510(b)(1)(ii)]. In such disclosures in situations of incapacity or emergency, the CE may exercise professional judgment to determine whether the disclosure is in the patient's best interest). State law defines who may serve as a personal representative.

- Disclosure to a public or private entity assisting in disaster relief efforts.

Check Your Understanding 10.4

Instructions: Answer the following questions on a separate piece of paper.

1. Does releasing information from the directory require the patient's written authorization? Explain your answer.

2. To whom can religious affiliation information be released?

3. Under what circumstances might the hospital disclose information from the directory if the patient is incapacitated or in an emergency situation?

4. Discuss whether the hospital can disclose information to family, friends, or other caregivers.

Use and Disclosure with Patient Authorization

Except as permitted or required under the HIPAA Privacy rule, a valid patient authorization is required for the use or disclosure of PHI [45 CFR §164.508(a)(1)]. This requirement typically extends to a request by a patient's family members, including the spouse. The hospital must have clear policies and procedures for releasing confidential health information with patient authorization. These policies must provide for careful review of each request. They must provide for a careful review of the authorization to ensure that it meets all requirements stated in applicable state and federal statutes and regulations, depending on which requirements are more stringent. As provided in the Privacy Rule, the procedure must permit the opportunity for the patient to revoke an authorization at any time in writing, except to the extent that the hospital has relied on the authorization and taken action as a result of it [Section 164.508(b)(5)(i)]. It is good practice to require a patient to sign an authorization for releasing confidential health information to the patient on whom the information is maintained. Finally, all policies and procedures for releasing confidential health information with patient authorization must follow the guidelines established in the Privacy Rule discussed next.

The Privacy Rule gives very detailed specifications for patient authorization to disclose confidential health information [Section 164.508(c)–(f)]. The authorization must include a specific description of the information to be used or disclosed. In addition, the name or other specific identification of the person(s) authorized to request and receive the requested information must be included. Further, the authorization must include the expiration date or event that relates to the individual or the purpose of the use or disclosure. The patient must be given the right to revoke the authorization in writing, the exceptions to this right, and a description of how he or she may revoke it. The authorization also must advise the patient that information released pursuant to the authorization may be subject to redisclosure by the recipient and no longer protected. Finally, the patient must sign and date the authorization.

If a personal representative signs the authorization, a description of his or her authority to act for the patient must be included in the authorization form. Further, the form must be written in plain language. The patient must be advised that the hospital will not condition treatment, payment, enrollment in a health plan, or eligibility for benefits on his or her providing authorization for the requested information. The authorization must include a description of each purpose for the requested information. Further, the authorization must contain a statement to the effect that the patient may inspect or copy the information and may refuse to sign it. The hospital must disclose to the patient whether disclosure of the information will result in direct or indirect remuneration to the facility from a third party. If there is remuneration, the authorization must state that such remuneration will result. Also, the patient is entitled to a copy of the signed authorization.

Authorizations for uses and disclosures of health information created for research that includes treatment of the patient must contain additional elements. For example, there must be a description of the extent to which the information will be used or disclosed to carry out treatment, payment, or healthcare operations. The authorization must further include a description of any health information that could be disclosed but will not be disclosed for facility directories or public health purposes. However, the facility may not include a limitation affecting its right to disclose information required by law.

If the facility has or intends to obtain a general consent or has provided or intends to provide the individual with a Notice of Privacy Practices, the authorization must refer to that consent or notice and state that the statements made are binding.

Pursuant to Section 164.508(b)(2), if any of the following circumstances pertain to the authorization, it is considered "defective":

- The expiration date has passed or the expiration event has occurred.

- The authorization is not completely filled out.

- The authorization has been revoked.
- Any required elements are missing.
- The authorization is combined with any other document to create a "compound authorization" except where permitted.
- The facility knows that material information included in the authorization is false.

For an unemancipated minor, the legal representative is the parent, guardian, or other person acting in *loco parentis*. For the incompetent adult, the conservator of the person (probate or psychiatric) or the attorney in-fact may serve as the legal representative. The patient's spouse or the person financially responsible for the patient may sign only for the limited purpose of enrolling the patient in a third-party payer plan. For a deceased patient, the executor, administrator, or other person with authority to act on behalf of the patient or of the patient's estate may sign an authorization for the disclosure of health information. In addition, there are many medical treatments for which a minor (whether or not emancipated) can self-refer under state and federal statutes and regulations. In most states, these treatments include outpatient mental health treatment, drug and alcohol testing and treatment, pregnancy counseling, and treatment for sexually transmitted diseases. In these circumstances, the minor, and not the minor's parent or guardian, controls the disclosure of health information.

To be valid, the written authorization must state the limitations, if any, on the types of health information to be disclosed. Further, it must state the specific uses and limitations, if any, on the use of the health information by the recipients.

The two categories of uses and disclosures that the Privacy Rule specifically refers to as requiring patient authorization are psychotherapy notes and marketing. Psychotherapy notes are those notes recorded in any medium by a mental health professional documenting or analyzing conversations from a private counseling session or a group, joint or family counseling session [45 CFR §164.508(a)(2)]. These notes are maintained separately from the rest of the patient's health record. Psychotherapy notes exclude medication prescription and monitoring, counseling session start and stop times, the modalities and frequencies of treatment furnished, results of clinical tests, and any summary of the diagnosis, functional status, treatment plan, symptoms, prognosis, and progress to date (45 CFR §164.501). However, HIPAA does provide an exception to the authorization requirements for psychotherapy notes; in these circumstances no patient authorization is required:

- In treatment, payment, or healthcare operations:
  - Use by the originator of the treatment notes
  - Use or disclosure by the CE in its own training programs in which students, trainees, or practitioners in mental health learn under supervision
  - Use or disclosure by the CE to defend itself in a legal action or other proceeding brought by the patient

- As required or permitted as part of oversight of the originator of the psychotherapy notes

As defined in the Privacy Rule, marketing requires an authorization that contains the above described elements and an additional statement regarding direct or indirect payment by a third party. HIPAA defines marketing as a communication about a product/service that encourages recipients of the communication to purchase or use the product/service or as an arrangement between a covered entity and any other entity where the covered entity discloses PHI to the other entity, in exchange for direct or indirect remuneration, to permit the other entity to encourage recipients to purchase or use its product/service.

Even in these circumstances classified as marketing, HIPAA provides exceptions that are discussed in the next section.

Check Your Understanding 10.5

Instructions: Answer the following questions on a separate piece of paper.

1. Does the requirement for a written authorization for use and disclosure apply to obtaining information about family members, including the spouse?

2. List five elements that must be included in a HIPAA-compliant authorization for use and disclosure.

3. Discuss the elements required in an authorization for use and disclosure when health information is created for research that includes treatment.

4. Who can sign an authorization for use and disclosure when the patient is a minor?

5. For what two categories of uses and disclosures does HIPAA specifically require an authorization for uses and disclosures?

Use and Disclosure without Patient Authorization

The basic rule under HIPAA is that the healthcare facility may use or disclose PHI without an authorization for treatment, payment, or healthcare operations purposes [45 CFR §164.506(a)]. Although health information can be released without patient authorization in these circumstances, such requests must be scrutinized carefully. Thus, healthcare facilities also must have clear policies and procedures for releasing confidential health information without patient authorization. For example, reporting required by statutes, whether federal or state, should be addressed. Information that can be released to the public without patient authorization should be specified. Typical mandatory disclosures that should be addressed in policies and procedures include those under court order and subpoena, whether served by a party to a suit or administrative proceeding, or by a government agency in the course of an investigation. Mandatory disclosure pursuant to orders by a board, commission, or administrative agency engaged in formal adjudication of a dispute should be included in policies and procedures. Further, policies should address releasing health information pursuant to an order by an arbitrator or arbitration panel carrying out arbitration under the law. Also disclosure without patient authorization can occur pursuant to a search warrant. This type of disclosure should be detailed very carefully in policies and procedures. Disclosure of health information in response to requests in workers' compensation cases is controlled by state law and should be included in hospital policies. Finally, policies also must identify the categories of internal staff needing confidential health information to carry out their job duties. Policies also should specify the types of information needed and the reasons for permitting access (First Guidance). Policies and procedures should permit the opportunity for the patient to restrict how health information is used and disclosed to carry out treatment, payment, or healthcare operations [Section 164.506(c)(4)(i)]. All policies and procedures for releasing confidential health information without patient authorization must also follow the guidelines set in the Privacy Rule.

As discussed in the patient's rights section of this chapter, patients and their representatives have access to PHI without signing an authorization form (45 CFR §164.524). In reality, many facilities may have the patient or patient's representative complete the authorization form as a means of documenting the request. Although care should be taken in releasing all health information to a patient, particular care should be taken in releasing specialized information such as information related to mental health, drug and alcohol abuse, and sexually transmitted diseases. Federal and some state statutes address some or all of these types of specialized information. The Privacy Rule in Section 164.524(a)(1) provides the patient's right of access to inspect and obtain a copy of health information, except for psychotherapy notes and information compiled in reasonable anticipation of, or for use in, a civil, criminal, or administrative action or proceeding.

Further, under the Privacy Rule, the hospital may deny access for other reasons, provided the patient is given a right to have such denials reviewed by a licensed healthcare professional designated by the hospital to act as a reviewing official and who did not participate in the original decision to deny. This reviewer must provide or deny access [Section 164.524(a)(3)].

Numerous other types of disclosures of confidential health information may be made without patient authorization. These include disclosure for direct patient care purposes, for payment purposes, for healthcare operations activities, as required by law, and several others.

Disclosure for *direct patient care (treatment) purposes* is among the most common and most important disclosures without patient authorization. Those involved with patient care must have timely access to health information. In sections 164.501 and 164.506(c)(1) and (2), the Privacy Rule permits the facility and healthcare providers to use or disclose confidential information for:

- Providing, coordinating, or managing healthcare and related services by one or more healthcare providers, including with a third party

- Consulting among healthcare providers relating to a patient
- Referring a patient for healthcare from one healthcare provider to another

Payment purposes is another important type of disclosure that may be made without patient authorization. The Privacy Rule permits the healthcare provider to use or disclose health information for payment purposes such as health plans obtaining premiums, determining coverage, and providing benefits. It also includes healthcare providers or health plans obtaining or providing reimbursement for services [45 CFR §164.501; §164.506(c)(1),(3)].

Healthcare operations consists of a number of activities carried out in a typical provider setting [45 CFR §164.501; §164.506 (c)(1),(4),(5)]. One activity that is important to a hospital is quality improvement (QI). Under HIPAA, QI is a standard healthcare operation and does not require the CE to obtain patient authorization to use confidential health information. Other healthcare operations functions include peer review; underwriting; medical review, legal services, and auditing; business planning, development, management, and administration; educational programs; and licensing and accreditation. Specifically, many organizations participate in educational activities for their medical staff members and their clinical and nonclinical staff members. Some also participate in formalized training programs for physicians, nurses, and allied health professionals. All these trainees require some level of access to confidential health information as part of their training. However, such access should be on a need-to-know basis. Typically, such use of confidential information does not require patient authorization.

Further, because health records are considered hospital business records, the information in them has many administrative uses that are considered healthcare operations. Hospital professional, technical, and administrative staff should have access to these records on a need-to-know basis. Administrative uses include, but are not limited to, auditing, billing, filing, replying to inquiries, and defending litigation.

PHI may be disclosed without an authorization as *required by law*. The use or disclosure is limited to the requirements of the particular law under which is it is used or disclosed [45 CFR §164.512(a)(1)]. In some cases, there is a common-law duty to disclose health information, for example, to warn persons of the presence of contagious disease. In many states, there also is a duty to warn an individual against whom a patient has made a credible threat to harm (*Tarasoff v. Board of Regents* 1976). In another case, a physician failed to warn his patient that she had contracted HIV through a blood transfusion. As a result, the hospital and the physician were sued three years later when the patient's sexual partner was exposed to the virus. The court held that the hospital was liable for the physician's failure to warn (Kadzielski 2004; *Reisner v. Regents of the University of California* 1995).

These cases should not be confused. Reisner involved failure to warn a patient of a serious condition; Tarasoff involved failure to warn a third party about potential harm from his patient.

No authorization is needed to use or disclose PHI for *public health activities* [45 CFR §164.512(b)]. Some health records contain information that is important to the public welfare. Such information must be reported to the state's public health service to ensure public safety. The Privacy Rule provides that the hospital or healthcare provider may disclose confidential health information to:

- A public health authority authorized to collect or receive information for preventing or controlling disease, injury, or disability
- A public health authority or other government authority authorized to receive reports of child abuse or neglect
- A person subject to the FDA
- A person who may have been exposed to a communicable disease or may be at risk of contracting or spreading a disease or condition (if the entity is authorized to notify such person [Section 164.512(b)(1)(i)–(iii)]. Activities that are reported include:
  –Disease and injury reporting
  –Vital statistics reporting (births and deaths)
  –Public health investigation, surveillance, or intervention
  –Child abuse/neglect reporting (HIPAA specifically stated to follow state law, 65 *Federal Register* 82527, December 18, 2000)
  –Product safety, quality, or effectiveness reporting to the FDA
  –Communicable disease reporting
  –Reporting to an employer in very limited circumstances regarding medical surveillance of the workplace or work-related illness/injury

The Privacy Rule addresses disclosure of health information in the last activity above in Section 164.512(b)(1)(v). The hospital may disclose information to an employer when one of the following conditions is met:

- The care provider is a member of the employer's workforce or provides healthcare to the patient at the employer's request.
- The care relates to a medical surveillance of the workplace or to a work-related illness or injury.
- The information that is disclosed consists of findings concerning a work-related illness or injury or a workplace-related medical surveillance.
- The employer needs the findings to comply with its obligations under federal and state laws.

The Privacy Rule also requires the hospital to provide written notice to the individual that health information relating to the workplace medical surveillance and work-related illnesses and injuries will be disclosed to the employer.

Reporting of other types of *abuse, neglect, or domestic violence* also is permitted under HIPAA [45 CFR §164.512(c); 65 *Federal Register* 82527, December 18, 2000] when required by law; when the patient agrees to the reporting; and when the CE, in its professional judgment, believes disclosure is necessary to prevent serious harm to the patient or other potential victims. Further, the CE may disclose in situations where the patient is incapacitated and law enforcement or some other public official authorized to receive such information indicates that the disclosure is not to be used against the patient and that immediate enforcement activity depends on the disclosure and would be adversely affected by waiting.

Persons complying with reporting statutes are not considered to be making an unauthorized disclosure. Although the disclosure of certain health information is statutorily mandated in these and other circumstances, a court could view disclosure to the wrong agency as a breach of confidentiality.

Health oversight agencies may receive PHI without authorization for their activities but must be authorized to oversee the healthcare system (public or private) or government programs in which health information is necessary to determine eligibility or compliance or to enforce civil rights laws for which health information is relevant. Health oversight agency activities include audits; civil, criminal, or administrative investigations or proceedings; licensure; disciplinary actions; inspections; or other activities necessary for appropriate oversight of any of the following entities:

- The healthcare system
- Government benefit programs for which health information is relevant to beneficiary eligibility
- Entities subject to government regulatory programs for which information is necessary for determining compliance with program standards
- Entities subject to civil rights laws for which health information is necessary for determining compliance [Section 164.412(d)]

A CE also may disclose PHI *in judicial and administrative proceedings*. Disclosing confidential health information in compliance with the legal process is typically provided for statutorily. Under the Privacy Rule in Section 164.512(e)(i)–(iv), a hospital may disclose health information in the course of any judicial or administrative proceeding in response to any of the following:

- Court or administrative tribunal order if the hospital discloses only the health information expressly authorized by such order
- Subpoena, discovery request, or other lawful process not accompanied by a court or administrative tribunal order if the hospital receives satisfactory assurance that reasonable efforts have been taken to give notice of the request to the person who is the subject of the requested

information or to secure a qualified protective order that meets specific requirements

A hospital can disclose health information in response to a lawful process without receiving the above-discussed satisfactory assurance when it makes reasonable efforts to provide notice to the individual or to seek a qualified protective order [Section 164.512(e)(v)].

Law enforcement agencies and officers may have a need to access health information. Records in a sealed envelope addressed to the court may be given to law enforcement officials for delivery to the court. This is not considered a direct disclosure to the law enforcement officer.

Pursuant to the Privacy Rule in Section 164.512(f), the hospital may disclose health information to law enforcement officials without authorization for law enforcement purposes when one of the following conditions is met:

- The disclosure is required by law, including laws that require the reporting of certain types of wounds or other physical injuries.
- The disclosure is made in compliance with a court order, court-ordered warrant, subpoena, summons, or grand jury subpoena.
- The disclosure is made in response to an administrative request, that is, a subpoena or summons, a civil demand or an authorized investigative demand, or a similar process authorized under law.
- The purpose of the request is to identify or locate a suspect, fugitive, material witness, or missing person (information related to the individual's DNA or DNA analysis, dental records, typing, samples or body fluids, or tissue analysis may not be released).
- The disclosure is made in response to a law enforcement official's request for such information about an individual who is, or is suspected to be, a victim of a crime.
- The purpose of the disclosure is to alert law enforcement of the suspicion that a patient's death may have resulted from criminal conduct.
- The hospital believes the health information is evidence of criminal conduct that occurred on its premises.

When providing healthcare in an emergency situation, other than such emergency on the premises of the healthcare provider, the provider may disclose health information to law enforcement officials when it appears necessary to alert law enforcement to any of the following:

- Commission and nature of a crime
- Location of the crime or of the victim(s)
- Identity, description, and location of the perpetrator of the crime [Section 164.512(f)(6)]

Coroners, medical examiners, and funeral directors may receive PHI as necessary to carry out their duties with respect to decedents. Such duties for a coroner or medical examiner include identifying a deceased person, determining a cause

of death, or other duties as authorized by law. If it is necessary for a funeral director to have PHI prior to, and in reasonable anticipation of, the individual's death, the CE may disclose that information necessary to carry out the funeral director's function.

Organ Procurement Organizations

An *organ procurement organization* or a tissue bank processing the tissue of a decedent for transplantation into the body of another person also may be given health information. Section 164.512(h) of the Privacy Rule provides that a hospital may disclose health information to organ procurement organizations.

Research is another activity for which confidential health information is important. Hospital policy often requires that researchers' access to health information be documented as bona fide research. Such documentation may be provided through a recognized institutional review board's approval of the research. Many states and the federal government have established regulations for the protection of human subjects, including protecting confidential information [45 CFR §46.111(a)(7)], protection of human subjects]. Any use of confidential health information for research purposes must comply with all such regulations, including those set forth in the Privacy Rule. Under the Privacy Rule in Section 164.512(i), researchers may use or disclose health information, as necessary, to prepare a research protocol or for research purposes. This section also provides that researchers may use or disclose health information for the purpose of research on such information for decedents. The facility that creates confidential health information for research that includes treatment of the patient must obtain an authorization for the use or disclosure of that information.

PHI may be disclosed to *avert a serious threat to health and safety* [45 CFR §164.512(j)]. To do so, the CE must, in good faith, believe the use or disclosure is necessary to prevent or lessen a serious and imminent threat to the health and safety of a person or the public and is reasonably able to prevent or lessen the threat. Moreover, the CE may disclose PHI if it believes in good faith that the disclosure is necessary for law enforcement to identify or apprehend an individual because of a statement by a person admitting participation in a violent crime that the CE believes may have caused serious physical harm to the victim. Further, the CE may disclose PHI in cases where the individual has escaped from a correctional institution or from lawful custody.

PHI can be disclosed for *specialized governmental functions* [45 CFR §164.512 (k)]. These functions include:

- Military and veterans activities
- National security and intelligence activities
- Protective services to the president and heads of state
- Medical suitability determination (for example, security clearance purposes)
- Correctional and law enforcement custodial facilities for the health and safety of the patient, other inmates, or officers or employees at the correctional facility

- Government programs providing public benefits
- Workers' compensation programs to comply with state laws for the provision of benefits for work-related injuries or illness [Section 164.512(l)]

With regard to workers' compensation cases, statutes in some states permit the disclosure of health information without patient authorization, but some states require patient authorization or a subpoena from an administrative agency or court for release. It is important to be familiar with a particular state's laws before disclosing any health information in workers' compensation cases.

Without the patient's authorization, an organization may use only demographic data (name, address, and other contact information, date of birth, gender, insurance status, and so on) and dates of service to carry out *fundraising* activities. Demographic data do not include information about diagnoses, procedures, or the nature of the patient's illness or services. The organization may disclose this demographic data to a philanthropic foundation that is a 501(c)(3) organization whose charter explicitly indicates it raises funds for the organization. The organization also may provide such data to a business associate that conducts fundraising on behalf of the organization. Any fundraising materials sent to a patient must include instructions on how to opt out of receiving future fundraising materials.

As stated in the Use and Disclosure with Patient Authorization section, there are *marketing exceptions to the requirement for an authorization.* When the communication is a face-to-face encounter with a patient or when it involves a promotional gift of nominal value, no authorization is required. Furthermore, the Privacy Rule describes specific circumstances that are not considered marketing, such as:

- The covered entity describing its own health-related products and services
- Communications about entities participating in a healthcare provider network or health plan network, replacement of or enhancements to a health plan, and health-related products or services available only to a health plan enrollee that adds value to the benefits
- Communications about products and services related to a patient's treatment
- Communications for case management or care coordination
- Recommendations to the patient about alternative treatments, therapies, healthcare providers, or care settings

The Privacy Rule establishes the requirement for verifying the identity of the person receiving the PHI and his or her authority to have access to the requested information.

Penalties

The penalties for violating the HIPAA provisions are found at Title 42 of the United States Code. These provisions provide both civil fines and criminal fines and punishments. The HHS Office of Civil Rights is charged with the investigation and enforcement of any violation of the HIPAA Privacy Rule. The Department of Justice also may choose to prosecute any violation determined to be criminal in nature.

The general civil monetary penalty for anyone violating the HIPAA rules is not more than $100 for each violation, with civil fines capped at $25,000 per calendar year for each provision violated (42 U.S.C. §1320d-5). Civil penalties may not be imposed when:

- The entity being held subject to the penalty can satisfy the secretary of HHS that the person violating the rule(s) did not know, and would not have known, that he or she violated them.
- The violation was not because of willful neglect and can be corrected within a 30-day period.
- The act is a violation of the criminal provisions [42 U.S.C. §1320d-6(a)] discussed below. This means both civil and criminal penalties may not be applied to a wrongdoer for the same violation.

Should the violation be classified as a criminal violation, penalties are assessed pursuant to 42 U.S.C. §1320d–6(a). The key to criminal violation is the concept of "knowingly" committing an act. This means purposefully committing an act or acting in willful disregard of the existence of the statutory scheme (Malone 2004). Any of the following actions are classified as criminal:

- Knowingly using or causing to be used a unique health identifier in violation of the rules
- Knowingly obtaining patient PHI in violation of the rules
- Knowingly disclosing patient PHI to another person in violation of the rules

Maximum penalties for criminal violations are set forth in 42 U.S.C. §1320d–6(b). The actual penalty imposed against someone convicted of a criminal violation is determined pursuant to the Federal Sentencing Guidelines (Malone 2004). The Sentencing Guidelines were established by the United States Sentencing Commission to establish "uniform punishment that is applied to similarly situated defendants upon conviction" (Malone 2004). The guidelines provide for the judge to consider the offense level and the defendant's criminal history in setting the sentence. They specify the following penalties:

- A fine of not more than $50,000, imprisonment for not more than one year, or both.
- If the violation is committed under false pretenses, the fine is not more than $100,000, imprisonment for not more than five years, or both.
- If the violation is committed with the intent to sell, transfer, or use PHI for commercial advantage, personal gain, or malicious harm, the fine is not more than $250,000, imprisonment for not more than ten years, or both.

Use of Health Records in Litigation

This section discusses how the health record is used in litigation. The health record serves as documentation of care provided when the patient alleges wrongdoing against the hospital and healthcare providers in a lawsuit or seeks damages from another party who caused an injury or illness.

Admissibility of the Health Record

The health record may be valuable evidence in a legal proceeding. To be admissible, the court must be confident that the record

- Is complete, accurate, and timely (recorded at the time the event occurred).
- Was documented in the normal course of business
- Was made by healthcare providers who have knowledge of the "acts, events, conditions, opinions, or diagnoses appearing in it." (Adair et al 2005, p. 64A).

The court must accept that the information was recorded as the result of treatment, not in anticipation of a legal proceeding. Further, to be admissible, the health record must be pertinent and proper. The health record is considered hearsay because the healthcare providers made the entries in the record and not in court under oath (McWay 2003, pp. 135–36). However, the judge or jury uses the exception to the hearsay rule of evidence codified in the Federal Rules of Evidence and the Uniform Rules of Evidence to determine what is pertinent and proper (McWay 2003, p. 135; Frawley and Thomas 2005).

To have an electronic health record admissible, the court must be confident that the system from which the record was produced is accurate and trustworthy. Characteristics used to support a system's accuracy and trustworthiness are:

- The type of computer used and that computer's acceptance as standard and efficient equipment
- The record's method of operation

- The method and circumstances of preparation of the record (Adair et al 2005, p. 64A)

Medical witnesses may refer to the health record to refresh their recollection. The custodian of records, typically the health information manager, may be called as a witness to identify the record as the one subpoenaed. He or she also may be called to testify as to policies and procedures relevant to the following:

- Creation of the record including the system or process used
- Maintenance of the record to prevent it from being altered
- Maintenance of the record to prevent it from being accessed without proper authorization

The actual admissibility as evidence depends on the facts and circumstances of the case and the applicable state and federal rules of evidence.

Privileges

Professional relationships between the patient and specific groups of caregivers further affect use of the record and its contents as evidence. These relationships are referred to as **privileges.** The information exchanged between patient and caregiver pursuant to a privilege is a confidential communication that the patient anticipates will be held confidential. One such widely recognized privilege is the physician–patient privilege. This privilege provides that the physician is not permitted to testify as a witness about certain information gained as a result of this relationship without the patient's consent.

The information included in the physician–patient privilege is insulated from the discovery process when there is no patient authorization, waiver, or an overriding law or public policy (Davis, McConnell, and Shaw 2004). The physician–patient relationship usually does not apply to court-ordered examinations or other examinations completed on behalf of other third parties, such as insurance companies (Miller 1986). Depending on the state, similar privileges exist between psychotherapist and patient, sexual assault victim and counselor, and domestic violence victim and counselor.

In states where these professional relationships are recognized, they apply when the caregiver is being compelled to testify as a witness concerning information obtained as a result of the relationship. However, these privileges do not preclude the caregiver from making reports as required by law.

Patient's Waiver of Privilege

The patient may release the caregiver from the privileges discussed through words or actions. This release is known as a waiver of the privilege. For example, a patient who placed his or her treatment at issue in a trial could not continue to claim a privilege to protect the information. The caregiver then could be compelled to testify regarding the information previously considered confidential.

Government's Right of Access to Health Records

The government, whether federal or state, has the right to access health information with or without patient authorization in certain circumstances. Healthcare providers must sign an agreement with HHS to receive payments for care provided to patients covered under the Medicare program (Miller 1986). Medicaid is a joint federal and state program to provide medical care to individuals unable to pay for care. Healthcare providers apply to the responsible state agency for a contract with the state to provide services to Medicaid recipients in return for payment for services provided (Miller 1986). Both HHS and the state Medicaid agency may request information from the health record to support the healthcare provider's bill submitted for payment. By signing up with Medicare or Medicaid, the patient gives permission for the healthcare provider to disclose confidential health information to the appropriate agency without further authorization.

The government also may require access to health information for other investigative purposes such as pursuant to the federal fraud and abuse statutes that require information-sharing arrangements to be undertaken in an arm's-length transaction and pursuant to a written agreement (Kadzielski 2004). An arm's-length transaction is a transaction in which "parties are dealing from equal bargaining positions, neither party is subject to the other's control or dominant influence, and the transaction is treated with fairness, integrity and legality" (Trautmann 2003).

Another important federal statute for which the government may need access to health information as part of an investigation is the Emergency Medical Treatment and Active Labor Act. This act involves the transfer of uninsured individuals from one hospital emergency department to another for financial reasons (Kadzielski and Kogan 1997).

Individuals are personally liable for their own acts of unauthorized disclosure of confidential health information. The individual's liability is based on fault because he or she did something wrong or failed to do something he or she should have done. Employers also may be held liable for any job-related acts of their employees or agents. It must be distinguished that the hospital is not liable for a breach of confidentiality by the members of its medical staff because they are not employees or agents of the hospital. However, the hospital may be liable for the consequences of any unauthorized disclosure, whether by employees, agents, or medical staff members, because of the breach of its duty to maintain information confidential. The injured person benefits from these concepts of fault because he or she can sue the employer, the employee, or both.

Unauthorized disclosure by various healthcare professionals also may be addressed in professional licensing and certifying laws or regulations. These provisions subject the professional to potential discipline by the licensing or certifying agency for breach of confidentiality because it is considered unprofessional conduct.

Check Your Understanding 10.7

Instructions: Answer the following questions on a separate piece of paper.

1. What are the three methods by which a physician–patient privilege may be created?

2. What actions or requirements can release the care provider from the applicable privilege?

3. Give two examples of government access to health information with or without patient authorization.

4. If the custodian of records is called to testify pursuant to a subpoena, what can she or he testify to?

Case Law since HIPAA

There are a number of areas of uncertainty in the HIPAA regulations. Interpretation of these areas requires one to make a judgment call, a good faith effort to follow the regulations, and then to take a wait-and-see approach to see if these areas are tested in the courts. Because at the time of this writing the final regulations have been effective for only a few years, case law since implementation of the Privacy Rule is still in flux.

Sample Cases

In *Law v. Zuckerman,* a federal court in Maryland ruled that HIPAA preempted a state law that would have required a plaintiff's current doctor to discuss the patient's condition with the defendants' lawyer without notice to, or consent of, the patient. The court held that Maryland's law was not more stringent than the HIPAA regulations. In *In re PPA Litigation*, a New Jersey state court ruled that HIPAA did not preempt the state-authorized practice of permitting defendants in personal injury cases to conduct information interviews with the plaintiff's treating physician where patient authorization requirements are not met. In this case, HIPAA-compliant authorization forms were not required by the court.

The first HIPAA privacy criminal prosecution occurred in *U.S. v. Gibson.* In this case, an employee of the Seattle Cancer Care Alliance was charged with illegal disclosure of a patient's PHI in order to fraudulently obtain and make purchases with credit cards in the patient's name. Pursuant to the penalties discussed above, this disclosure was for personal gain and potentially subjected the defendant to a fine of up to $250,000 and up to 10 years in prison. The defendant pleaded guilty and entered into a plea bargain with the federal government that recommends 10 to 16 months in prison and requires full restitution to the patient and the credit card companies. In November 2004, under the HIPAA Privacy

Rule, U.S. District Judge Ricardo Martinez sentenced the defendant to 16 months in prison, three years of supervised release, and more than $9,000 in restitution.

Of interest in this case is that the defendant is not a covered entity under HIPAA, but rather an employee of a CE that is subject to HIPAA. This case demonstrates that at least one U.S. attorney interprets the HIPAA criminal provisions as applying personally to members of the CE's workforce. There is still considerable debate as to whether the HIPAA criminal provisions apply to persons and/or organizations that are not CEs.

The Release of Information Process and Function

Managing the release (use and disclosure) of information (ROI) process and function requires an attention to detail and constant vigilance. The ROI manager must constantly stay current with changes in local, state, and federal laws and regulations affecting the use and disclosure of PHI. Further, the ROI manager must be cognizant of JCAHO and other regulatory agency requirements regarding protecting a patient's confidentiality and privacy by protecting health information. The manager must constantly ensure that policies and procedures reflect all current local, state, and federal statutes and regulations and regulatory agency requirements.

The ROI manager must provide education that reinforces the organization's policies and the importance of following them. Additionally, ROI staff must be provided with, and express an understanding of, the expectations for them to follow ROI policies and procedures.

The ROI manager must participate in the QI process. This can be used as one means of evaluating staff compliance with policies and procedures. Furthermore, the manager must gather statistics regarding performance (request turnaround time, number of requests processed per employee per month, number of subpoenas processed per employee per month, and so on). These statistics, among others, can be used as the basis for requesting additional staff or as part of the annual evaluation process. Completing requests according to departmental standards, which are based on regulations such as HIPAA and/or state law, demonstrates the individual employee's competence, or lack thereof, in his or her job.

In some organizations, the ROI functions are decentralized; that is, carried out in other areas in addition to the HIM department. Although having use and disclosure requests processed where the applicable record is maintained may seem the most efficient approach, such an organizational structure presents many management challenges. The ROI manager must ensure that all entities within the organization carrying out the ROI function are following standardized policies and procedures. This requires strong organizational and supervision skills.

The manager is responsible for participating with the organization's privacy officer to investigate any alleged violations of the HIPAA rules by ROI staff. The investigation should be conducted pursuant to the organization's investigation policy and may include involving the human resources (HR) department to impose disciplinary action pursuant to HR policies.

Finally, it is the manager's responsibility to establish an environment in which employees can be successful. Therefore, the ROI manager must develop and implement systems that support the employees' needs.

Check Your Understanding 10.8

Instructions: Answer the following questions on a separate piece of paper.

1. What uses can the ROI manager make of data collected?

2. In addition to the statistics mentioned above, list three other categories of statistics that would be useful to the ROI manager in managing this function.

3. What education should the ROI manager provide the ROI staff?

4. Does the ROI manager participate in investigating alleged HIPAA violations by ROI staff? Discuss your answer.

Medical Staff Appointments, Privileges, and Peer Review

Patients expect the physicians who treat them in hospitals to have been evaluated for competency in their selected area of medical practice. Patients expect to receive treatment at or above the acceptable standard of care. Hospitals use the medical staff appointment process to accomplish this evaluation.

Duty to Use Reasonable Care in Granting Staff Appointments

The hospital governing board typically is composed of members from the community and sometimes includes medical staff members. This body has final responsibility for the operation of the hospital. Because of its responsibility for managing the hospital and upholding a satisfactory standard of care, it has the legal duty to select medical staff members. The governing board must use reasonable care in approving a physician's application to be a staff member and grant clinical privileges before the physician can treat patients in the hospital. Typically, after the physician is granted initial medical staff membership, he or she must reapply for membership and privileging every year or every two years. It must be noted that medical staff members are not employees or agents of the hospital. However, even though they are independent of the hospital, they are accountable individually and collectively to the board for the quality of care they provide.

In *Darling v. Charleston Community Memorial Hospital,* the court specifically held that the governing board has the "duty to establish mechanisms for the medical staff to evaluate, counsel, and when necessary, take action against an unreasonable risk of harm to a patient arising from the patient's treatment by a personal physician" (Pozgar 2004, p. 175). Further, the *Darling* court held that based on the hospital's obligation to select high-quality physicians to be medical staff members, the hospital may be held liable for a patient's injury caused by a physician who does not meet those standards but was given medical staff membership and privileges.

Darling involved an 18-year-old college football player studying to be a teacher and coach who suffered a broken leg during a game. He was taken to a small, accredited community hospital where the only physician on duty in the emergency department was a general practitioner who had not treated a severe leg fracture for three years. The physician ordered x-rays that revealed fractures of both bones in the lower leg. The physician reduced the fractures and applied a full-leg plaster cast. The patient complained of pain, and the physician split the cast and visited the patient while in the hospital. However, the physician never called in a specialist because he thought it unnecessary. Two weeks later, the plaintiff was transferred to a larger hospital where he was treated by an orthopedic surgeon. The specialist found dead tissue in the fractured leg and removed dead tissue several times over the next two months. Ultimately, he was unable to save the leg and amputated it eight inches below the knee.

The plaintiff's father rejected any settlement and filed suit against the hospital and the physician. The physician was eventually able to settle, but the case against the hospital continued to trial. A judgment was returned against the hospital and upheld in the Illinois Supreme Court.

The hospital's governing board relies on the medical staff structure to conduct the actual evaluation of physicians applying for medical staff membership and to make recommendations regarding their suitability for membership. The mechanisms for selecting medical staff members pursuant to *Darling* and applicable state statutes indicate that peer review is the best system for monitoring physicians. Many states provide that peer review must be conducted in a reasonable and fair manner.

The Credentialing Process

The **credentialing process** is the screening process through which the medical staff evaluates a physician's application for medical staff membership. In this process, the medical staff validates the physician's credentials: medical education, including medical school, residencies, postdoctoral studies, and fellowships; license to practice; and medical practice experience. This process also includes reviewing and evaluating professional references and professional society membership. This process also applies to other licensed independent practitioners (for example, nurse practitioners and allied health practitioners).

One major step taken in this process is searching the **National Practitioner Data Bank** regarding judgments and settlements of claims of professional negligence regardless of the amount (Cohen 2004). Further, this process includes validating the physician's liability insurance. Having a license to practice medicine in a particular state does not give the physician the right to be a medical staff member in any hospital; rather, it is merely one required criterion. Credentialing criteria should be related directly to patient care and based on objective factors such as education, experience, and current competence (Kadzielski 2004, p. 198). To avoid the appearance of discrimination based on profession, credentialing criteria for different types of practitioners (radiologists, psychiatrists, orthopedists, and so on) should be objective and based on community standard of care (Kadzielski 2004, p. 198).

Federal laws in the form of the Medicare Conditions of Participation for Hospitals, home health agencies, and long-term care facilities, among others, set forth requirements for medical staff credentialing (Kadzielski 2004). Most states typically address medical staff appointments in licensing statutes or statutes specific for the selection of medical staff members or both. Further accreditation standards, such as those published by JCAHO, require physician credentialing prior to granting privileges to practice in a healthcare facility (Kadzielski 2004).

The Privileging Process

After a physician is determined to meet the criteria to be a medical staff member in a particular hospital, the medical staff must evaluate his or her quality of medical practice and determine the services and procedures he or she is qualified to provide. This is known as the **privileging process.** A physician's clinical privileges determine the services he or she may provide, such as what operations he or she may perform. The medical staff must have established a written definition of what it means to be granted the privilege to provide a particular service. Some hospitals grant privileges for specific procedures; others grant privileges for categories of procedures. Still other hospitals grant privileges based on levels of care, such as privileges to care for critical care patients. Another approach is to grant privileges by medical specialty based on the services a particular specialty is permitted to perform.

To evaluate a physician for privileging, a hospital may require the physician to obtain a consultation before performing specific procedures. Physicians also may be required to have operative procedures proctored by an observing or assisting physician. A hospital may require certification beyond a license, such as board certification in a particular medical specialty, before granting privileges for a physician to practice in that specialty.

As stated above, physicians must periodically reapply for medical staff membership. As part of the reapplication process, their privileges are reevaluated using established criteria. For example, the hospital may review, among other factors, the physician's blood usage patterns, lengths of stay, infection rates, complications and complication rates, health record documentation, and closed malpractice claims (Kurdwanowski and Schaedler 1997). The hospital also may review the outcome of focused studies, such as those discussed below. Moreover, physicians who have gained additional training since the last appointment may seek privileges not previously held. For any new privileges requested, the physician may be required to have consultation or proctoring performed. Most state statutes and the federal Health Care Quality Improvement Act require this collection and review of information in the privileging process (Davis, McConnell, and Shaw 2004).

The goal of privileging is to ensure that all physicians have the requisite training and experience to perform the requested services. This process also applies to other licensed independent practitioners (for example, nurse practitioners and allied health practitioners).

Accessibility and Confidentiality of Credentialing Files

In this discussion, *credentialing* is used as a collective term for the credentialing and privileging processes. In looking at accessibility to credentialing files, third parties, such as JCAHO, and state and federal regulatory organizations, may review credentialing files as part of their accrediting and licensing functions. Some states statutorily protect credentialing files from discovery in legal proceedings. However, when a plaintiff alleges negligent credentialing against a hospital, whether the protection will hold up comes into question (Davis, McConnell, and Shaw 2004). In such a circumstance, the hospital finds itself in the situation of attempting to protect the information in the credentialing files while at the same time needing those very same documents to defend it (Davis, McConnell, and Shaw 2004). Although statutory protections may be in place for credentialing information, facilities should be reluctant to share such information "because any subsequent disclosure of peer review committee records could result in a loss of this protection" (Kadzielski 2004, p. 205).

Confidentiality of QI and Concurrent Review Activities

As noted above, outcomes of focused studies may be used to evaluate a physician's application for continued medical staff membership and privileges to practice. These studies are usually conducted as part of the hospital's QI activities. QI is the process of improving medical care and potentially decreasing healthcare costs. (This process is discussed more fully in chapter 23.)

QI activities can be carried out on a concurrent review basis or on a retrospective basis. *Concurrent review* consists of evaluating medical care as it is being given. Concurrent review activities can be carried out in a variety of ways. One method is through case management (utilization review) that focuses on the appropriateness of the admission, the level of care, and length of stay (Miller 1986).

Retrospective review occurs after patient discharge. This review may take the form of a focused study based on a pattern of questionable care identified during concurrent review or other retrospective review activities. The questionable care leading to a focused study may be care provided by any caregiver, including physicians. The hospital has a responsibility to address any problems discovered through either review process. If a physician was the caregiver providing the questionable care and it is determined that he or she is not practicing at the expected level of care, an educational session may be conducted with the particular physician. If warranted, more stringent steps, such as suspension of the physician's medical staff privileges or medical staff membership termination, may be taken.

These review activities involve collecting outcomes and performance data on how a physician performed as a physician and may affect continued medical staff membership. Accordingly, the review files are considered confidential. Many states have statutes that specifically provide confidentiality to these types of files (Davis, McConnell, and Shaw 2004). California Evidence Code Section 1157 is an example of such a law. This statute protects from discovery the proceedings and records of organized peer review committees responsible for the evaluation and improvement of the quality of care.

Check Your Understanding 10.9

Instructions: Answer the following questions on a separate piece of paper.

1. After he or she completes an application, what is the process for granting a physician membership on the hospital medical staff?

2. What documentation is typically reviewed for the initial membership appointment?

3. What activities may a medical staff require of a physician in order to grant the physician privileges to provide a specific service?

4. As part of the reapplication process, what additional factors may the medical staff review in the privileges component?

5. Discuss circumstances in which confidential information in a credentialing file may be accessed.

6. Distinguish between concurrent and retrospective review activities.

7. What is the basis for maintaining QI and concurrent review files confidential?

Other Liability Issues

Hospitals and other healthcare providers face other liability issues. Hospital staff members have a duty to advise an appropriate member of administration when they become aware of any action or failure to act that is below the standard of care. The standard of care does not just apply to direct patient care. By definition, it applies to the safeguarding of patients' personal belongings whether or not they are placed in the direct care of the facility. For patient and staff personal belongings not placed in the direct care of the facility, the facility must have policies and procedures for addressing questions of theft by staff.

The standard of care also applies to the physical safety of the premises for patients, staff, visitors, vendors, and members of the general public who come onto the premises. Physical safety means being free from physical defects in buildings and grounds and from being harmed by patients, nonstaff members, or staff members. Moreover, the hospital must address staff safety as it relates to treatment of violent or uncontrolled patients (for example, a patient under the influence of drugs or alcohol while being treated in the emergency department).

Computerized Health Records

The move toward a fully computerized health record brings special liability issues with it. In particular, liability issues can be classified in two categories (McWay 2003, pp. 215–16):

- Those in which the information in the computerized health record serves as proof in a lawsuit of the quality of patient care provided
- Those that arise from unauthorized access to, or the careless handling or maintenance of, patient information in a computerized environment

The first issue focuses on whether the computerized health record can be admitted as evidence. This raises the hearsay rule and how it can be overcome for electronically stored medical records. Although admissibility of such records has been tested on a limited basis, federal courts have allowed a computer printout into evidence where the foundation, trustworthiness, and accuracy requirements were shown to have been met (McWay 2003, p. 218).

The second issue focuses on the legal requirements to keep the computerized health records safe and secure. The computerized health record must be subject to all three components of the HIPAA Security Rule: administrative safeguards (policies, procedures, risk assessment [45 CFR §164.308]); physical safeguards (facility access control [45 CFR §164.310]); and technical safeguards (access control [45 CFR §164.312]).

Incident Reports

A happening that is inconsistent with the standard of care is generally defined as an incident. As discussed above, standards of care are not related only to direct patient care. Therefore, incidents do not relate only to patient care. Anyone witnessing or involved in an incident should complete an incident report as soon as possible after the incident as a way to capture the details of what happened. The incident report is one tool staff can use to report unusual incidents to administration. Data should be collected from the incident reports and analyzed to determine whether trends are developing.

Because incident reports contain facts, hospitals strive to protect their confidentiality. In some states, incident reports are protected under statutes protecting QI studies and activities (Davis, McConnell, and Shaw 2004). They also may be protected under attorney–client privilege (Davis, McConnell, and Shaw 2004; McWay 2003). Protection under this doctrine may be based on whether the primary purpose of the incident report is to provide information to the hospital's attorney or liability insurer (Davis, McConnell, and Shaw 2004; McDonough 2004; McWay 2003).

To further ensure incident report confidentiality, no copies should be made and the original must not be filed in the health record nor removed from the files in the department responsible for maintaining them, typically risk management or QI (McDonough 2004; McWay 2003). Also no reference to the completion of an incident report should be made in the health record. Such a reference would likely render the incident report discoverable because it is mentioned in a document that is discoverable in legal proceedings.

Relationship to Risk Manager

The health information manager and the risk manager should work as a team. The risk manager depends on the health information manager to alert him or her to potentially compensible events. These are events that could result in a settlement or judgment against the facility, further resulting in a payout of funds whether through insurance or from facility internal funds. Such events can be identified through coding and abstracting, and various health record review activities conducted by HIM department staff. The health information manager also can advise the risk manager when an attorney requests a copy of a health record. The risk manager then can review records identified by any of these methods to determine whether further action is necessary from a risk management standpoint.

Check Your Understanding 10.10

Instructions: Answer the following questions on a separate piece of paper.

1. Define incident as it relates to the healthcare environment.
2. Discuss at least two doctrines under which incident reports may be protected.
3. Why should incident reports be protected?
4. Discuss the relationship between the health information manager and the risk manager.

Real-World Case

Adapted from a recent publication on the Internet discussing the subject of employers' practice of maintaining health information in the employees' personnel records. (Small Business, Medical Investigations, available at businessweek. findlaw.com/employmentbook/HFCHP5_e.html)

Mary Beth Jones, RHIA professional, is the new director of the HIM department at a midsized hospital in an eastern state. She has recently learned that the HR department maintains detailed medical information in its personnel files. Additionally, she has learned that her employer routinely uses this information when collecting health information for its group insurance plan, when employees request time off for a medical leave, and as part of its substance abuse assistance program.

State law recognizes a duty of confidentiality to protect this information and to avoid dissemination to nonessential third parties. Moreover, it requires that employers maintain health records separately from personnel files and recognize a claim for negligent maintenance of personnel files if they are not maintained separately. Further, employers in Mary Beth's state are prohibited from using or disclosing employee medical information unless (1) such disclosure is compelled by law, (2) the information is relevant to a lawsuit between employer and employee, or (3) disclosure is necessary to administer an employee benefit plan.

Summary

The basic court system is the same from one state to another. However, the health information management professional should become familiar with the differences that do exist for the state in which he or she works. This knowledge gives the HIM professional the ability to communicate effectively with legal counsel regarding health records and policies and procedures affecting health records when the inevitable lawsuit arises.

Knowledge that is more important and valuable to the HIM professional is of the statutes that control the use and disclosure of confidential health information. These statutes are both federal and state in nature. This area of law is constantly in flux and requires the HIM professional to constantly review the many available resources pertaining to such statutes, including publications and seminars. These resources also should address case law that may affect the ongoing applicability of federal and state statutes and regulations.

Another body of knowledge the HIM professional should develop is a clear understanding of licensure and accreditation standards that affect the creation, completion, maintenance, and protection of health records.

The HIM professional must ensure that health records policies and procedures are in place and enforced and that they reflect all statutes, regulations, and standards pertaining to health records, particularly those pertaining to the use and disclosure of confidential information.

Among the many members of the hospital staff with whom the HIM professional works, he or she must have a close relationship with the facility risk manager. The HIM professional can provide the risk manager tremendous assistance in identifying and addressing incidents that may place the facility at risk.

References

Adair, D., et al. 2005. Practice brief: Maintaining a legally sound health record: Paper and electronic (updated). *Journal of American Health Information Management Association.* Available online from ahima.org.

Administrative Procedures Act, 5 U.S.C.S. §500-576 (Law. Co-op. 1989).

Arizona Constitution, Section 8, Right to privacy. Available online from azleg.state.az.us/const/2/8.htm.

California Constitution, Article 1, Declaration of rights, Section 1. Available online from leginfo.ca.gov/.const/.article_1.

Cohen, M. 2004. Statutes, standards, and regulations. In *Risk Management Handbook for Health Care Organizations,* 4th ed., edited by R. Carroll. San Francisco: Jossey-Bass.

Darling v. Charleston Community Memorial Hospital, 33 Ill.2d 326, 211 N.E. 2d, 253 (1965).

Davis, K.S., J.C. McConnell, and E.D. Shaw. 2004. Data management. In *Risk Management Handbook for Health Care Organizations,* 4th ed., edited by R. Carroll. San Francisco: Jossey-Bass.

Florida Constitution, Article I, Section 23, Right of privacy. Available online from leg.state.fl.us/.

Frawley, K , and Thomas, A. 2005. Practice brief: The legal process and electronic health records. *Journal of American Health Information Management Association.* Available online from ahima.org.

Griswold v. Connecticut, 381 U.S. 479 (1965).

Health Insurance Portability and Accountability Act of 1996. Public Law 104-191.

Hughes, G. 2002. Practice brief: Laws and regulations governing the disclosure of health information (updated). *Journal of American Health Information Management Association.* Available online from ahima.org.

Hughes, G. 2003. Practice brief: Transfer of patient health information across the continuum (updated). *Journal of American Health Information Management Association.* Available online from ahima.org.

In re PPA Litigation, 2003 WL 22203834 (NJ Super L 2003).

Judge v. Rockford Memorial Hospital, 17 Ill. App. 2d 365, 150 N.E. 2d 202 (1958).

Kadzielski, M.A. 2004. Physician and allied health professional credentialing. In *Risk Management Handbook for Health Care Organizations,* 4th ed., edited by R. Carroll. San Francisco: Jossey-Bass.

Kadzielski, M.A., and E.I. Kogan. 1997. Physician and allied health professional credentialing. In *Risk Management Handbook for Health Care Organizations,* 2nd ed., edited by R. Carroll. Chicago: American Hospital Publishing.

Kurdwanowski, F., and P.A. Schaedler. 1997. Internal and external relationships. In *Risk Management Handbook for Health Care Organizations,* 2nd ed., edited by R. Carroll. Chicago: American Hospital Publishing.

Law v. Zuckerman, 307 F. Supp. 2d 705 (D. MD 2004).

Malone, E.F. 2004. *Who Goes to Jail? A Guide for HIPAA Privacy Officers.* Chicago: AHIMA.

McDonough, W.J. 2004. Systems for risk identification. In *Risk Management Handbook for Health Care Organizations,* 4th ed., edited by R. Carroll. San Francisco: Jossey-Bass.

McWay, D.C. 2003. *Legal Aspects of Health Information Management.* Clifton, NY: Delmar.

Miller, R.D. 1986. *Problems in Hospital Law.* Rockville, MD: Aspen.

Pozgar, G.D. 2004. *Legal Aspects of Health Care Administration.* Sudbury, MA: Jones and Bartlett.

Pub. Law 104-191, 110 Stat. 1936 (codified in scattered sections of 18, 26, 29, and 42 U.S.C.) (HIPAA-a).

Pub. Law 104-191, §261; 65 Fed. Reg. 82463 (Dec. 28, 2000) (HIPAA-d).

Pub. Law 104-191, §§263, 264 (codified at 42 U.S.C. 1320d-2 to 1320d-8); Carter at 1 (HIPAA-f).

Pub. Law No. 104-191, preface 110 Stat. at 1936; Carter, Patricia I. (2003). *HIPAA Compliance Handbook 2003.* Aspen Publishers, at 1 (HIPAA-b). 65 Fed. Reg. 82463 (Dec. 28, 2000). (HIPAA-e).

Reisner v. Regents of the University of California, 37 Cal. Rptr2d 518 (1995).

Rhodes, H., and Hughes, G. 2003. Practice brief: Redisclosure of patient health information. *Journal of American Health Information Management Association* 74(4): 56A–C.

Tarasoff v. Board of Regents, 17 Cal.3d 425, 551 P.2d 334 (Cal. 1976).

Trautmann, Carl O. 2003. Small Business Dictionary. Available from small-business-dictionary.org/default.asp?.

U.S. v. Gibson, CR 04-0374RFM (W.D. WA 2004).

Chapter 11
Ethical Issues in Health Information Management

Laurinda B. Harman, PhD, RHIA

Learning Objectives

- To recognize some core health information ethical problems, including those related to privacy and confidentiality; compliance, fraud, and abuse; clinical code selection and use; quality review; research and decision support; public health; managed care; clinical care; electronic health information systems; the management of sensitive information; and the roles of manager, entrepreneur, and advocate as well as business relationships with vendors
- To identify ethical principles and professional values that can guide health information management (HIM) professionals who must confront and respond to ethical problems
- To apply the AHIMA Code of Ethics in guiding behaviors such as protecting privacy, advancing HIM knowledge and practice, advocating for others, and refusing to participate in or conceal unethical behaviors
- To follow the steps in an ethical decision-making process that can be used to resolve complex ethical problems

Key Terms

Autonomy
Beneficence
Bioethics
Blanket authorization
Confidentiality
Ethical agent
Ethical decision making
Ethicist
Ethics
Justice
Moral values
Need-to-know principle
Nonmaleficence
Privacy
Secondary release of information
Security

Introduction

The responsibilities of the health information management (HIM) professional include a wide range of functions and activities. Regardless of the employer (healthcare facility, vendor, pharmaceutical company, or research firm), the HIM professional's core ethical obligation is to protect patient **privacy** and confidential communication. The documentation in the paper and electronic health information systems include many sacred stories that must be protected on behalf of the patient and the aggregate community of patients and consumers served by the healthcare system. The obligation to protect this information is at the center of the decisions made on behalf of patients, the healthcare team, peers, colleagues, the public, or the many other stakeholders who seek access to patient and consumer information.

The terms in this chapter describe ethical principles that most people already know, although the terms themselves may not be familiar. For example, recognizing the importance of individuals being able to decide what happens to them is **autonomy,** doing good is included in the ethical principle of **beneficence,** not harming others is **nonmaleficence,** and treating people fairly is **justice** (Beauchamp and Childress 2001). This chapter provides the language and framework for understanding more about **ethics** within the context of dealing with complex health information issues. It also offers a step-by-step process that HIM professionals can use to make appropriate ethical choices and to analyze what is and is not justified from an ethical perspective.

Theory into Practice

With regard to one of the HIM professional's primary functions, how might ethical principles apply in the case of deciding whether to release patient information?

- Autonomy would require the HIM professional to ensure that the patient, and not a spouse or third party, makes the decisions regarding access to his or her health information.
- Beneficence would require the HIM professional to ensure that the information is released only to individuals who need it to do something that will benefit the patient (for example, to an insurance company for payment of a claim).
- Nonmaleficence would require the HIM professional to ensure that the information is not released to someone who does not have authorization to access it and who might harm the patient if access were permitted (for example, a newspaper seeking information about a famous person).
- Justice would require the HIM professional to apply the rules fairly and consistently for all and not to make special exceptions based on personal or organizational perspectives.

Moral Values and Ethical Competencies

Although most people probably have never undertaken a formal study of ethics, everyone is exposed to ethical principles, moral perspectives, and values throughout a lifetime. Individuals learn about basic **moral values** from families, religious leaders, teachers, the government, community organizations, and other groups that influence our experiences and perspectives. Moral values are taught as "this is right and that is wrong." For example, some might consider it right to be nice to a neighbor and wrong to destroy the neighbor's property. However, these are not universal values. Others might consider it acceptable to be rude or mean to a neighbor they do not like and to destroy the neighbor's property. Applying this language to health information management, it is right—and a moral obligation—to protect the neighbor's privacy when you learn about diseases and conditions while working and it is wrong to share the neighbor's secrets with other neighbors, family, and friends.

HIM professionals should not make ethical decisions on behalf of others based solely on personal moral values or perspectives because not everyone shares the same moral perspectives or values. Professional responsibilities often require an individual to move beyond personal values. For example, an individual might demonstrate behaviors that are based on the values of honesty, providing service to others, or demonstrating loyalty. In addition to these, professional values might require promoting confidentiality, facilitating interdisciplinary collaboration, and refusing to participate or conceal unethical practices. Professional values could require a more comprehensive set of values than what an individual needs to be an **ethical agent** in his or her personal life. For example, an HIM professional who hears information about a friend at a party has a range of options. He or she can share the information, share only part of it, change it, or not confirm or share it with anyone. However, that same individual in his or her role as an HIM professional cannot share overheard information under any circumstances.

Ethics provides a language and a framework for formally discussing ethical issues, taking into account the values and obligations of others. Ethical discussion offers an opportunity to resolve conflicts when competing values are at stake. **Ethical decision making** requires people to explore choices beyond the perspective of simple right or wrong (moral) options. According to Glover, "ethics refers to the formal process of intentionally and critically analyzing the basis for one's moral judgments for clarity and consistency" (Glover 2006). When making health information decisions, HIM professionals must go beyond the personal right or wrong moral perspective and evaluate the many values and perspectives of others who are engaged in the decision to be made.

Ethical discussions outside the healthcare environment can be theoretical in nature, and the analysis of a problem does not necessarily result in an action. For example, **ethicists** could discuss whether to require all citizens living in a certain community to donate 10 hours a week to people in need as part of their civic duty. One ethicist might argue for a decision based on the ethical principle of beneficence, which would guide action to do good things for others. Another ethicist might argue for the same decision but base the decision on the principle of justice in which every citizen should contribute his or her fair share for the good of the whole. These discussions and decisions would not necessarily require an action but would help frame the ethical justification for a certain action.

In contrast, **bioethics** involves problems or issues regarding clinical care or the health information system that are never strictly theoretical in nature and must always result in a decision. HIM professionals cannot merely deliberate whether to release patient information, assign the correct code, or purchase a new software system. Rather, they must apply ethical principles and then perform an action. In short, ethics applied in the work environment cannot remain theoretical and must result in an action.

Ethical Foundations in Health Information Management

Ethical principles and values have been important to the HIM profession since its beginning in 1928. The first ethical pledge was presented in 1934 by Grace Whiting Myers, a visionary leader who recognized the importance of protecting information in medical records. The HIM profession was launched with recognition of the importance of privacy and the requirement of authorization for the release of health information:

> I pledge myself to give out no information from any clinical record placed in my charge, or from any other source to any person whatsoever, except upon order from the chief executive officer of the institution which I may be serving (Huffman 1972, p. 135).

Today, it is the patient who authorizes the release of information and not the chief executive officer (CEO) of the healthcare organization, as was stated in the original pledge. The most important values embedded in this pledge are to protect patient privacy and confidential information and to recognize the importance of the HIM professional as a moral agent in protecting patient information (Rinehart-Thompson and Harman 2006). The HIM professional has a clear ethical and professional obligation not to give any information to anyone unless its release has been authorized, regardless of employment site, including direct patient care, facilities that need access to health information, or vendors.

Protection of Privacy, Maintenance of Confidentiality, and Assurance of Data Security

The terms *privacy,* *confidentiality,* and *security* are often used interchangeably. However, there are some important distinctions, including:

- *Privacy* is "the right of an individual to be let alone. It includes freedom from observation or intrusion into one's private affairs and the right to maintain control over certain personal and health information" (Harman 2006, p. 634).
- *Confidentiality* carries "the responsibility for limiting disclosure of private matters. It includes the responsibility to use, disclose, or release such information only with the knowledge and consent of the individual" (Harman 2006, pp. 627–28). Confidential information may be written or verbal.
- *Security* includes "physical and electronic protection of the integrity, availability, and confidentiality of computer-based information and the resources used to enter, store, process, and communicate it. The means to control access and protect information from accidental or intentional disclosure" (Harman 2006, p. 635).

The HIM professional's responsibilities include ensuring that patient privacy and confidential information are protected and that data security measures are used to prevent unauthorized access to information. This responsibility includes ensuring that the release policies and procedures are accurate and up-to-date, that they are followed, and that all violations are reported to the proper authorities.

The Health Insurance Portability and Accountability Act (HIPAA) of 1996 establishes national standards for the privacy and security of health information. This law deals with privacy, information standards, data integrity, confidentiality, and data security (Rinehart-Thompson and Harman 2006). HIPAA was passed in 1996. It took five years before the Privacy Rule became effective on April 14, 2001, with an April 14, 2003, compliance date. Congress passed the statute and the U.S. Department of Health and Human Services (HHS) developed the regulations contained within the Privacy Rule (HHS 2003). The final HIPAA Security Rule regulations were published in the Federal Register on February 20, 2003, and became effective on April 21, 2005.

This legislation, which includes administrative simplification standards and security and privacy standards, has had—and will continue to have—a major impact on the collection and dissemination of information for years to come. This legislation has an enforcement program, and HIM professionals will play an important role in ensuring compliance. Although privacy is a right protected by the U.S. Constitution, each state can effect its own legislation regarding access to patient information. Preemptive federal legislation was needed so that all patient information would be protected regardless of where a patient lived or received healthcare. Moreover, this legislation protects individuals from losing their health insurance when leaving or changing jobs by providing insurance continuity (portability) and increases the federal government's authority over fraud and abuse in the healthcare arena (accountability) (Harman 2005).

Part of the impetus for HIPAA was the development of the electronic health record (EHR) (Amatayakul 2004; Dick et al. 1997; Hanken and Murphy 2006; Johns 2002; Murphy et al. 1999). As patient information was moved to the electronic medium, integrated systems across the continuum of care were developed and information was released and redisclosed to many people and agencies needing access to it. Thus, standardized federal legislation became an imperative. HIPAA was designed to guarantee that information transferred from one facility to the next would be protected. The National Committee on Vital and Health Statistics (NCVHS) supports a National Health Information Infrastructure (NHII) so that patient care information can be transferred and protected in our integrated healthcare systems. As a result, patients benefit from the continuity of care and can control their personal health information (NCVHS 2001; Gellman 2004).

In an electronic environment, protecting privacy has become extremely difficult and patients are becoming increasingly concerned about the loss of privacy and their inability to control the dissemination of information about them. As patients become more aware of the misuses of information, they may become reluctant to share information with their healthcare team. This may, in turn, result in problems with the healthcare that is provided and the information given to researchers, insurers, the government, and the many other stakeholders who legitimately need to access to the information. Increasingly, patients are seeking anonymity and responding to issues related to the use and disclosure of health information for directory purposes; to family and close personal friends; for notification purposes such as disasters; and for other disclosures required by law such as public health, employer medical surveillance, and funeral directors (Hughes 2002a; Hughes 2002b; Rhodes 2001; AHIMA 2002).

Ethical Responsibilities of the HIM Professional

In general, the HIM professional's primary responsibilities include those related to designing and implementing a system to ensure the completeness, accuracy, and timeliness of health information. In support of these responsibilities, the HIM professional is accountable for complying with laws, rules, regulations, standards, and policies from many sources, including the government, accreditation and licensure organizations, and the healthcare facility. Some of the HIM professional's core ethical responsibilities include the following (Harman 2006):

- Protecting patient privacy and confidential information (Rinehart-Thompson and Harman 2006)
- Making appropriate decisions regarding the selection and use of clinical diagnostic and procedural codes (Schraffenberger and Scichilone 2006)
- Developing policies and procedures that ensure coding accuracy that supports clinical care and research and meets the requirements for reimbursement, while avoiding fraud and abuse violations (Rinehart-Thompson 2006)

- Reporting quality review outcomes honestly and accurately, even when the results might create conflict for an individual or an institution (Spath 2006)
- Ensuring that research and decision support systems are reliable (Johns and Hardin 2006)
- Releasing accurate information for public health purposes for patients with communicable diseases, such as AIDS or venereal disease, and assisting with the complexities of information management in the context of bioterrorism and the threat or reality of global diseases, such as smallpox or avian flu (Neuberger 2006)
- Supporting managed care systems by providing accurate, reliable information about patients/consumers, clinicians, healthcare organizations, and patterns of care, with special care devoted to issues related to access to information (Schick 2006)
- Facilitating the exchange of information for patients, families, and providers of care, especially for those affected by chronic and terminal illness, that ensure patient autonomy and beneficence (Tischler 2006)
- Ensuring that the EHR meets the standards of privacy and security according to HIPAA and other federal and state laws (Hanken and Murphy 2006), the standards of information security (Czirr et al. 2006), and software development (Fenton 2006).
- Ensuring that clinical data repositories, data marts, data warehouses, and EHRs meet the standards of the best practices of health information and database management (Lee et al. 2006)
- Participating in the development of integrated delivery systems so that patients can move across the continuum of care and the right information can be provided to the right people at the right time (Olson and Grant 2006)
- Working in the context of e-health technologies that allow consumers, patients, and caregivers to search for health information and advice, create and maintain personal health records, and conduct virtual consultations with their care providers (Baur and Deering 2006)
- Ensuring that health information technology systems, including EHRs, electronic prescribing, bedside bar coding, computerized physician order entry (CPOE), and clinical decision support systems reduce errors and improve quality (Bloomrosen 2006)
- Managing the protection of sensitive information, including genetic information (Fuller and Hudson 2006); drug, alcohol, sexual, and behavioral information (Randolph and Rinehart-Thompson 2006); and adoption information (Jones 2006)
- Developing moral awareness and nurturing an ethical environment in the context of managing a health information system (Flite and Laquer 2006)
- Serving as entrepreneur and advocate for patients, the healthcare team, and others who have interests in the health information system (Gardenier 2006; Helbig 2006)

- Working with vendors in the development of business relationships that ensure ethical processes when selecting and communicating with vendors, managing vendor relationships, and dealing with the contract negotiation process (Olenik 2006)

Ethical Issues Related to Documentation and Privacy

Just a few decades ago, only a few people created documentation in patient health records and fewer still wanted access to patient information after the episode of care was completed. In today's healthcare system, many providers document their decision-making process and patient outcomes in the health information system and many more people want access to that information. The HIM professional plays a critical role in developing policies and procedures to ensure the integrity of patient information, including appropriate and authorized access.

In addition to writing policies and procedures to ensure compliance with federal and state laws, accrediting and licensing agencies, and the bylaws of the healthcare facility, the HIM professional can serve many functions that support the integrity of data and the protection of privacy. As a member of the HIM team, the HIM professional can design and deliver educational sessions to the healthcare team to make them aware of the documentation and access rules and regulations. Sometimes educational sessions address the issue of avoiding participation in fraudulent or retrospective documentation practices. Retrospective documentation practices are those where healthcare providers add documentation after care has been given for the purpose of increasing reimbursement or avoiding a medical legal action.

Unacceptable documentation practices include backdating progress notes or other documentation in the patient's record and changing the documentation to reflect the known outcomes of care (versus what was done at the time of the actual care). It is the HIM professional's responsibility to work with others to ensure that patient documentation is accurate, timely, and created by authorized parties. The professional Code of Ethics requires the HIM professional to assure accurate and timely documentation.

Ethical Issues Related to Release of Information

Three primary ethical problems are pertinent to the release of information (ROI):

- Violations of the **need-to-know principle**
- Misuse of **blanket authorizations**
- Violations of privacy that occur as a result of **secondary release of information** procedures

In the past, the standard for ROI was the need to know. If an insurance company had a patient request to pay for surgery, the request was sent to the healthcare facility and the HIM professional carefully examined it for legitimacy. He or she would:

- Compare the patient's signature to the one collected upon admission to the facility
- Check the date to ensure that the request was dated after the occurrence so that the patient was aware of what was being authorized and released
- Verify the insurance company as the one belonging to the patient
- Review the request for what was wanted and whether the requestor was entitled to the information

The HIM professional then reviewed the documentation and provided the information requested. For example, the admission and discharge dates, the diagnoses of cholecystitis and cholelithiasis, and the surgical procedure of cholecystectomy were provided to the insurance company so that the bill could be paid.

Today, the process of abstracting needed information is virtually nonexistent, except for disability cases, and documentation is copied above and beyond the criterion of need to know. For example, in response to the request to verify an admission for a cholecystectomy, the history and physical, the operative report, the discharge summary, and the laboratory report could be copied. That documentation could reveal social habits, genetic risks, and family history of disease that have nothing to do with the surgery. Patient privacy could be violated as a result of the release of the information through subsequent discrimination by insurers.

Another common ethical problem is misuse of blanket authorizations. Patients often sign a blanket authorization, which authorizes the release of information from that point forward, without understanding the implications. The requestor of the information then could use the authorization to receive health information for many years. The problem with the use of blanket authorizations is that there is no way for the patient to know that the information is being accessed. Patients cannot authorize the release of information in 1994 for diagnoses or care that has not yet been provided. For example, by 2005, the patient might have AIDS or cancer and might not want this information released.

A third problem is secondary release to others by the authorized recipient to an unauthorized party. This problem has increased in frequency since the computerization of health information. A legitimate request might be processed to pay for an insurance claim, but adequate safety and protections may not be in place for the information after it has been released. The initial requestor then could forward the information to others without patient authorization. An HIM professional cannot merely think about ROI within the context of the single request. The responsibility to "follow the information" is much more serious today than it was a few years ago. Does the HIM professional know who gains access to the information after it is released to an authorized requestor?

If not, he or she may be contributing to the violations of patient privacy and a subsequent instance of discrimination by employers or insurance companies based on the information that was released.

Patients have increasingly expressed concerns about the use of blanket authorizations and secondary ROI by the initial requestor or receiving party. They fear that more information is being given out than is necessary and that they do not know about the many people and agencies that are gaining access to this information.

HIPAA has been designed to address several issues related to patient privacy, including a return to the need-to-know principle. The HIM professional needs to participate in the development of computerized systems that can replicate the original human decisions regarding ROI to release what is needed but not more. Although it is easier to just photocopy the information, the HIM professional needs to carefully consider the implications of doing this within the context of patient privacy. This situation has created an opportunity for HIM professionals to participate with other HIM professionals in efforts to correct these problems.

Because the HIM professional works in many employment sites throughout the healthcare delivery system, the ethical obligations extend into a variety of areas, as noted above. In fulfilling the responsibilities of the position, the HIM professional must apply ethical values when making decisions wherever he or she is positioned within the organization.

Professional Code of Ethics

HIM professionals used the pledge as the basis for guiding ethical decision making until 1957, at which time the American Association of Medical Record Librarians' (AAMRL) House of Delegates passed the first Code of Ethics for the Practice of Medical Record Science. (See figure 11.1.) The first code of ethics combined ethical principles with a set of professional values to help support the decisions that HIM professionals had to make at work. The original Code of Ethics has been revised several times since 1957—in 1978, 1988, 1998, and 2004. (See figures 11.2, 11.3, and 11.4, respectively, and Appendix E for the 2004 Code).

Upon being awarded the credential of RHIA (registered health information administrator) by the American Health Information Management Association (AHIMA), the HIM professional agrees to follow the principles and values discussed in this chapter and to base all professional actions and decisions on those principles and values. Even if federal or state laws did not require the protection of patient privacy, the HIM professional would be responsible for protecting it according to the AHIMA's Code of Ethics.

Professional Values and Obligations

The ethical obligations of the health information management (HIM) professional include the protection of patient privacy and confidential information. Core health informa-

tion issues include what information should be collected; how the information should be handled, who should have access to the information, and under what conditions the information should be disclosed.

Ethical obligations are central to the professional's responsibility, regardless of the employment site or the method of collection, storage, and security of health information. Health information ethical and professional values are based on obligations to the patient, the healthcare team, the employer, the interests of the public, and oneself, one's peers, and one's professional associations (Harman 1999).

Figure 11.1.   1957 Code of Ethics for the Practice of Medical Record Science

[Note: Gender-neutral language was not used in the 1950s, so the male pronoun should be read as "he or she."]

As a member of one of the paramedical professions he shall:

1. Place service before material gain, the honor of the profession before personal advantage, the health and welfare of patients above all personal and financial interests, and conduct himself in the practice of this profession so as to bring honor to himself, his associates, and to the medical record profession.

2. Preserve and protect the medical records in his custody and hold inviolate the privileged contents of the records and any other information of a confidential nature obtained in his official capacity, taking due account of the applicable statutes and of regulations and policies of his employer.

3. Serve his employer loyally, honorably discharging the duties and responsibilities entrusted to him, and give due consideration to the nature of these responsibilities in giving his employer notice of intent to resign his position.

4. Refuse to participate in or conceal unethical practices or procedures.

5. Report to the proper authorities, but disclose to no one else, any evidence of conduct or practice revealed in the medical records in his custody that indicates possible violation of established rules and regulations of the employer or of professional practice.

6. Preserve the confidential nature of professional determinations made by the staff committee which he serves.

7. Accept only those fees that are customary and lawful in the area for services rendered in his official capacity.

8. Avoid encroachment on the professional responsibilities of the medical and other paramedical professions, and under no circumstances assume or give the appearance of assuming the right to make determinations in professional areas outside the scope of his assigned responsibilities.

9. Strive to advance the knowledge and practice of medical record science, including continued self-improvement, in order to contribute to the best possible medical care.

10. Participate appropriately in developing and strengthening professional manpower and in representing the profession to the public.

11. Discharge honorably the responsibilities of any Association post to which appointed or elected, and preserve the confidentiality of any privileged information made known to him in his official capacity.

12. State truthfully and accurately his credentials, professional education, and experiences in any official transaction with the American Association of Medical Record Librarians and with any employer or prospective employer.

Copyright ©1957 by the American Association of Medical Libraries

Figure 11.2.   1977 AMRA Bylaws and Code of Ethics

The medical record practitioner is concerned with the development, use, and maintenance of medical and health records for medical care, preventive medicine, quality assurance, professional education, administrative practices and study purposes with due consideration of patients' right to privacy. The American Medical Record Association believes that it is in the best interests of the medical record profession and the public which it serves that the principles of personal and professional accountability be reexamined and redefined to provide members of the Association, as well as medical record practitioners who are credentialed by the Association, with definitive and binding guidelines of conduct. To achieve this goal, the American Medical Record Association has adopted the following restated Code of Ethics:

1. Conduct yourself in the practice of this profession so as to bring honor and dignity to yourself, the medical record profession and the Association.

2. Place service before material gain and strive at all times to provide services consistent with the need for quality health care and treatment of all who are ill and injured.

3. Preserve and secure the medical and health records, the information contained therein, and the appropriate secondary records in your custody in accordance with professional management practices, employer's policies and existing legal provisions.

4. Uphold the doctrine of confidentiality and the individual's right to privacy in the disclosure of personally identifiable medical and social information.

5. Recognize the source of the authority and powers delegated to you and conscientiously discharge the duties and responsibilities thus entrusted.

6. Refuse to participate in or conceal unethical practices or procedures in your relationship with other individuals or organizations.

7. Disclose to no one but proper authorities any evidence of conduct or practice revealed in medical reports or observed that indicates possible violation of established rules and regulations of the employer or professional practice.

8. Safeguard the public and the profession by reporting to the Ethics Committee any breach of this Code of Ethics by fellow members of the profession.

9. Preserve the confidential nature of professional determinations made by official committees of health and health-service organizations.

10. Accept compensation only in accordance with services actually performed or negotiated with the health institution.

11. Cooperate with other health professions and organizations to promote the quality of health programs and advancement of medical care, ensuring respect and consideration for the responsibility and the dignity of medical and other health professions.

12. Strive to increase the profession's body of systematic knowledge and individual competency through continued self-improvement and application of current advancements in the conduct of medical record practices.

13. Participate in developing and strengthening professional manpower and appropriately represent the profession in public.

14. Discharge honorably the responsibilities of any Association position to which appointed or elected.

15. Represent truthfully and accurately professional credentials, education, and experience in any official transaction or notice, including other positions and duality of interests.

Based on an analysis of the AHIMA Code of Ethics for 1957, 1977, 1988, 1998 and 2004, the following themes and values were identified (Harman and Mullen 2006).

Obligations to the Patient and the Healthcare Team

With regard to the patient and the healthcare team, the HIM professional is obligated to:

- Protect health, medical, genetic, social, personal, financial, and adoption information: Clinical information (for example, diagnoses, procedures, pharmaceutical dosages, or genetic risk factors) must be protected as well as behavioral information (for example, use of drugs or alcohol, high-risk hobbies, sexual habits). It is increasingly important to protect genetic and social information so that patients will not be vulnerable to the risks of discrimination.

- Protect confidential information: This involves ensuring that the information collected and documented in the patient information system is protected by all members of the healthcare team and by anyone with access to the information. This responsibility also includes protection of verbal communications on behalf of a patient and can involve communication with those in the legal profession, the media or others who seek patient information.

Figure 11.3.   1988 AMRA Code of Ethics and Bylaws

The medical record professional abides by a set of ethical principles developed to safeguard the public and to contribute within the scope of the profession to quality and efficiency in health care. This code of ethics, adopted by the members of the American Medical Record Association, defines the standards of behavior which promote ethical conduct.

1. The Medical Record Professional demonstrates behavior that reflects integrity, supports objectivity, and fosters trust in professional activities.

2. The Medical Record Professional respects the dignity of each human being.

3. The Medical Record Professional strives to improve personal competence and quality of services.

4. The Medical Record Professional represents truthfully and accurately professional credentials, education, and experience.

5. The Medical Record Professional refuses to participate in illegal or unethical acts and also refuses to conceal the illegal, incompetent, or unethical acts of others.

6. The Medical Record Professional protects the confidentiality of primary and secondary health records as mandated by law, professional standards, and the employer's policies.

7. The Medical Record Professional promotes to others the tenets of confidentiality.

8. The Medical Record Professional adheres to pertinent laws and regulations while advocating changes which serve the best interest of the public.

9. The Medical Record Professional encourages appropriate use of health record information and advocates policies and systems that advance the management of health records and health information.

10. The Medical Record Professional recognizes and supports the association's mission.

Figure 11.4.   1998 AHIMA Code of Ethics and Bylaws

AHIMA's Mission

The American Health Information Management Association is committed to the quality of health information for the benefit of patients, providers, and other users of clinical data. Our professional organization:

- Provides leadership in HIM education and professional development
- Sets and promotes professional practice standards
- Advocates patient privacy rights and confidentiality of health information
- Influences public and private policies including educating the public regarding health information
- Advances health information technologies

Guiding Principles

We are committed to the:

- Creation and utilization of systems and standards to ensure quality health information
- Achievement of member excellence
- Development of a supportive environment and provision of the resources to advance the profession
- Provision of the highest-quality service to members and health care information users
- Investigation and application of new technology to advance the management of health information

We value:

- The balance of patients' privacy rights and confidentiality of health information with legitimate uses of data
- The quality of health information as evidenced by its integrity, accuracy, consistency, reliability, and validity
- The quality of health information as evidenced by its impact on the quality of health care delivery

This Code of Ethics sets forth ethical principles for the HIM profession. Members of this profession are responsible for maintaining and promoting ethical practices. This Code of Ethics, adopted by the American Health Information Management Association, shall be binding on health information management professionals who are members of the Association and all individuals who hold an AHIMA credential.

  I. Health information management professionals respect the rights and dignity of all individuals.

 II. Health information management professionals comply with all laws, regulations, and standards governing the practice of health information management.

III. Health information management professionals strive for professional excellence through self-assessment and continuing education.

IV. Health information management professionals truthfully and accurately represent their professional credentials, education, and experience.

 V. Health information management professionals adhere to the vision, mission, and values of the Association.

VI. Health information management professionals promote and protect the confidentiality and security of health records and health information.

VII. Health information management professionals strive to provide accurate and timely information.

VIII. Health information management professionals promote high standards for health information management practice, education, and research.

IX. Health information management professionals act with integrity and avoid conflicts of interest in the performance of their professional and AHIMA responsibilities.

- Provide service to those who seek access to patient information: Individuals who may request access to patient information include healthcare providers; insurance, research, or pharmaceutical companies; government agencies; and employers. Disclosure and redisclosure policies and procedures must be developed and followed. The HIM professional must ensure the honor of the profession before personal advantage and the health and welfare of patients before all other interests. He or she also must balance the many competing interests of all the stakeholders who want patient information, avoiding conflicts of interest.

- Preserve and secure health information: This includes obligations to maintain and protect the medium that stores the information, such as, paper documentation, computer, microfilm, CD-ROM and the EHR, including the protection all databases and detailed secondary records and registries.

- Promote the quality and advancement of healthcare: As an important member of the healthcare team, the HIM professional provides valuable expertise in the collection of health information that will help providers improve the quality of care they deliver. The HIM professional should develop expertise in clinical medicine, pharmacology, biostatistics, and quality improvement methodologies so as to interpret clinical information and support research.

- Function within the scope of responsibility and restrain from passing clinical judgment: Sometimes healthcare data may indicate a problem with a provider of care, the treatment of a diagnosis, or some other problem. The HIM professional's obligation is to provide the data; however, the obligation of evaluating the significance of the data rests with those held accountable for the review of the data. The HIM professional should repeatedly, consistently, and accurately report the results of studies, regardless of the volatility of the research outcomes.

Obligations to the Employer

With regard to the employer, the HIM professional is obligated to:

- Demonstrate loyalty to the employer: The HIM professional can do this by respecting and following the policies, rules, and regulations of employment unless they are illegal or unethical.

- Protect committee deliberations: The HIM professional should be as committed to protecting committee conversations and decisions as he or she is to protecting patient information. Examples of such committees include medical staff and employer committees.

- Comply with all laws, regulations, and policies that govern the health information system: The HIM professional should keep up-to-date with state and federal laws, accrediting and licensing standards, employer policies and procedures, and any other standards that affect the health information system.

- Recognize both the authority and the power associated with the job responsibility. The HIM professional is the expert on privacy and confidentiality and must be present at strategic meetings with clinical providers, administrative staff, and financial and operations management personnel to be sure that HIM expertise is presented and understood. Unethical behaviors would be to hide and not be at the top-level strategic meetings, wait for the outcomes and then complain about the decisions that were made, such as, inappropriately releasing information to an employer. For example, the HIM professional cannot remain quiet and let others have the power to decide what information is released, what software is installed, or other important HIM decisions. HIM professionals do have both the power and the authority to say, "No, that is not acceptable" or "This is appropriate action."

- Accept compensation only in relationship to work responsibilities. Increasingly, there are groups or individuals who could benefit by having access to patient information and are willing to pay for such information. Access to databases with patient information on certain diagnoses such as AIDS or cancer could be sought by employers, commercial vendors, or others. The HIM professional must avoid the temptation to accept money for disclosing patient information or proprietary vendor secrets.

Obligations to the Public

With regard to the public interest, the HIM professional is obligated to:

- Advocate change when patterns or system problems are not in the best interests of the patients. The HIM professional should be a change agent and lead initiatives to change laws, rules, and regulations that do not ensure the integrity of patient information, including the protection of privacy and confidentiality. Moreover, the HIM professional should be proactive about protecting patients, the healthcare team, the organization, the professional association, peers, and himself or herself. State and national policy and legislative advocacy activities support this ethical obligation.

- Report violations of practice standards to the proper authorities. The HIM professional should not share information learned at work with family or friends or discuss such information in public places. The HIM professional should report the results of audits to the proper authorities only and bring potential or actual problems to the attention of those individuals responsible for the delivery and assessment of care and services.

- Promote interdisciplinary cooperation and collaboration. As an important member of the healthcare team,

the HIM professional should work with others to analyze and address health information issues, facilitate conflict resolution, and recognize the expertise and dignity of his or her fellow team members.

Obligations to Self, Peers, and Professional Associations

With regard to self, peers, and professional associations, the HIM professional is obligated to:

- Be honest about degrees, credentials, and work experiences. The HIM professional should only report an acquired degree (such as a BS or MS) or successfully earned credentials (such as an RHIA or a CCS). Work experiences must be reported accurately and honestly.

- Bring honor to oneself, one's peers, and one's profession. This obligation refers to personal competency and professional behavior (for example, at professional meetings). The HIM professional should try to ensure that peers and colleagues are proud to have him or her on the health information team.

- Commit to continuing education and lifelong learning. The HIM professional's education should not stop when he or she has earned a degree or a credential. Rather, the HIM professional should continue to attend educational sessions to keep abreast of changing laws, rules, and regulations that affect the health information system. The HIM professional should be a lifelong learner and contribute to improving the quality of healthcare service delivery. HIM professionals can keep their credentials by meeting the ongoing certification requirements of the AHIMA. Maintaining competency through self-improvement is an important directive that ensures the continuance of the profession.

- Strengthen health information professional membership. This obligation includes belonging to professional associations, actively participating on committees, making presentations, writing for publications, and encouraging others to seek health information management as a career.

- Represent the health information profession to the public. The HIM professional has a responsibility to advocate for the public interest in areas related to the principles and values of HIM practice. For example, HIM professionals serve an important role when advocating for needed legislation to protect privacy and confidentiality, educational manpower funding, or appropriate electronic health record (EHR) applications.

- Promote and participate in health information research. For example, when problems are discovered with the health information system, the HIM professional should conduct studies to clarify their sources and potential solutions.

Instructions: On a separate piece of paper, match the HIM professional's obligations to the following groups with the professional values expressed in the AHIMA's 1998 Code of Ethics (figure 11.1).

a. Patients and the healthcare team
b. Employer
c. Public interest
d. Oneself and one's peers and professional associations

1. ____ Accept compensation only in relationship to responsibilities
2. ____ Advocate change
3. ____ Preserve and secure health information
4. ____ Be honest
5. ____ Commit to continuing education and lifelong learning
6. ____ Promote interdisciplinary cooperation and collaboration
7. ____ Promote and participate in research
8. ____ Demonstrate loyalty to employer
9. ____ Discharge association duties honorably
10. ____ Protect committee deliberations
11. ____ Stay within the scope of responsibility and restrain from passing clinical judgment
12. ____ Bring honor to self, peers, and profession
13. ____ Protect medical and social information
14. ____ Promote the quality and advancement of healthcare
15. ____ Represent the profession to the public
16. ____ Comply with laws, regulations, and policies
17. ____ Report violations of practice standards to the proper authorities
18. ____ Refuse to participate in or conceal unethical practices
19. ____ Provide service
20. ____ Strengthen professional membership
21. ____ Recognize authority and power
22. ____ Promote confidentiality

Ethical Decision-Making Matrix

HIM professionals must factor several criteria into their decision making, as illustrated in figure 11.5. These include, but are not limited to:

- Cost: Can the facility and the health information system afford the improvement in the system?
- Technological feasibility: Will the technological application provide accurate and reliable information for the decision-making process?
- Federal and state laws: Are there federal or state laws that must be considered before a change is made in the system?
- Medical staff bylaws: Are there rules or regulations unique to the facility that require or prohibit a decision?
- Accreditation and licensing standards: Which agencies have standards that are important to the decision being made? Do the standards allow or prohibit a certain action?
- Employer policies, rules, or regulations: Does the facility have policies, rules, or regulations that require or prohibit a decision?

Although these criteria must be assessed in the decision-making process, they cannot be used alone. Virtually every decision the HIM professional makes also must be based on ethical principles and professional values.

Ethicists provide assistance in this process. Glover (2006, pp. 35–38, 50) has proposed a seven-step process to guide ethical decision making. When faced with an ethical issue, the HIM professional should ask and answer all of the following questions. The questions represent the steps in the decision-making process.

1. What is the ethical question?
2. What facts do you know, and what do you need to find out?
3. Who are the different stakeholders, what values are at stake, and what are the different obligations and interests of each of the stakeholders?
4. What options for action do you have?
5. What decision should you make, and what core HIM values are at stake?
6. What justifies the choice, and what are the value-based reasons to support the decision? What choice or choices cannot be justified?
7. What prevention options can be put into place so that this issue will not come up again?

When a decision must be made about an issue and only one choice is identified, the decision most likely will be based on an individual's narrow moral perspective of right or

Figure 11.5.   Ethical decision-making matrix

ETHICAL PROBLEM		
Steps	**Information**	
1. What is the question?		
2. What are the facts?	**KNOWN**	**TO BE GATHERED**
3. What are the values? Examine the shared and competing values, obligations, and interests in order to fully understand the complexity of the ethical problem(s).	**Patient:** **HIM Professional:** **Healthcare professionals:** **Administrators:** **Society:** **Other, as appropriate:**	
4. What are my options?		
5. What should I do?		
6. What justifies my choice?	*JUSTIFIED*	*NOT JUSTIFIED*
7. What can I do to prevent this ethical problem?		

Source: Harman 2006.

wrong. If it is an ethical problem, the decision makers must take into account the perspectives of competing stakeholders and their values. Decisions made without this model will not benefit from an ethical decision-making process that considers multiple options.

Check Your Understanding 11.2

Instructions: Using a, b, c, and so on, rearrange the steps of the ethical decision-making process in the correct order on a separate piece of paper.

1. ___ What decision should you make, and what core HIM values are at stake?

2. ___ What facts do you know, and what do you need to find out?

3. ___ What options for action do you have?

4. ___ What is the ethical question?

5. ___ What justifies the choice, and what are the reasons to support the decision, based on values? What choice or choices cannot be justified?

6. ___ What prevention options can be put into place so that this issue will not happen again?

7. ___ Who are the different stakeholders, what values are at stake, and what are the different obligations and interests of each of the stakeholders?

Core Health Information Ethical Problems

Several problems face HIM professionals in today's complex world, including issues related to the use of information; computerized health information systems; the management of sensitive health information; process and strategies for decision making; and the HIM roles as manager, entrepreneur, and advocate. The business relationships with vendors can also create ethical tensions. There are issues raised because of the uses of information, including clinical code selection and use, quality review, research and decision support, public health, managed care and clinical care (Harman 2006).

Ethical Issues Related to Coding

In the past, coding was done almost exclusively for clinical studies and quality assurance review processes. Although codes were provided for reimbursement purposes, the healthcare facility was reimbursed on the basis of usual, customary, and reasonable costs. The codes that were assigned became the basis of retrieval for clinical studies and the reimbursement system. Over time, healthcare facilities have continued to use the coding systems to retrieve information in health records for clinical and administrative studies, but they also have begun to use the codes for reimbursement purposes. After the codes became the basis for reimbursement, there were inherent incentives to code so that the greatest amount of reimbursement could be given. This placed the importance of accurate coding at the forefront of the ethical issues facing HIM professionals.

Ethical problems have risen in the past few years as a result of the direct linkage between coding and payments for care. Increased pressure has been put on HIM professionals who are coding to transmit inaccurate information, creating problems that are legal and/or ethical in nature. Problems include pressure to code inappropriate levels of service, discovering misrepresentation in physician documentation, miscoding to avoid conflicts, discovering miscoding by other staff, lacking the tools and educational background to code accurately, and being required by employers to engage in negligent coding practices (Schraffenberger and Scichilone 2006). In response to these issues, the AHIMA passed standards that specifically address coding issues (figure 11.5, p. 278).

Failure to heed the complex rules of coding for reimbursement can lead to problems with compliance and with fraud and abuse for the HIM professional. If the HIM professional fails to establish adequate monitoring systems for accurate code assignment or submits a false claim, the consequences could include penalties, such as fees and prison. The HIM professional must know the laws and the penalties for failure to follow the laws and, most important, have the expertise to develop preventive programs to ensure that the false claim is a nonoccurrence. Fraud and abuse problems include documentation that does not justify the billed procedure, acceptance of money for information, fraudulent retrospective documentation on the part of the provider to avoid suspension, and code assignment without physician documentation. An important emerging role for the HIM professional is that of compliance officer (Rinehart-Thompson 2006).

Ethical Issues Related to Quality Management, Decision Support, Public Health, Managed Care, and Clinical Care

Many factors contribute to the ethical problems faced by quality management professionals, including the rising cost of healthcare, limited resources, and concerns with patient safety. Some of the common quality outcome problems include (Spath 2006):

- Inaccurate performance data that are inappropriately shared with the public
- Negative care outcomes, such as infections, that occur in the course of providing home health care
- Failure to check a physician's licensure status
- Incomplete health records hidden in preparation for accreditation or licensure surveys
- Patterns of inappropriate healthcare

The pressures to conceal information that could be potentially harmful to an employer and problems with patient safety require constant diligence and the courage to repeatedly report the truth. Research and decision support responsibilities include ensuring data integrity and confidentiality, assuring compliance with human subject research protocols, and maintaining and enhancing professional competence (Johns and Hardin 2006).

Career opportunities for the HIM professional are growing in public health systems. Careers in this area require an understanding of the government's role in the collection and use of health information. The government's responsibility to protect the health of the public sometimes competes with the need to protect patient privacy, such as in the case of reporting HIV status. State and local mandatory reporting requirements exist for certain conditions, including infectious and communicable diseases. The government needs this information to monitor, investigate, and implement interventions, when necessary. Sometimes problems arise when the public's right to know or duty to one's employer conflicts with patient privacy (Neuberger 2006). The HIM professional can provide invaluable assistance with public health initiatives that will contribute to environmental and personal health. This role requires constant advocacy so that the interests of both the public and the individual patient can be served. New threats of bioterrorism and global infections, such as, SARS or avian flu, pose new ethical dilemmas in the management of health information. There will need to be a balance between protecting privacy of those injured and providing information to the government and health care professionals so that the medical crisis can be resolved.

There are many important ethical issues faced by an HIM professional working on behalf of managed care organizations. Problems arise if high-quality information is not provided so that commitments to patients, clinicians, and communities cannot be met. As with other situations, access to information is key to the problems faced by the HIM professional as he or she helps with the organization's strategies regarding pricing, access to providers, and quality of care. Job responsibilities in this work context include providing information about provider practices, providing patient clinical and demographic information, and establishing policies and procedures that provide for patient privacy (Schick 2006).

As the baby boomers age, there is an increasing number of patients who will require information in order to make difficult end-of-life decisions. Problems dealing with aging, frailty, autonomy of those near death, physician bias and equity, treatment choices, treatment goals and beneficence, advance care planning, palliative care, and managing pain are a few of the difficult decisions that must be made, and ethical decision-making is imperative (Tischler 2006).

Ethical Issues Related to Sensitive Health Information

All health information must be protected, but additional ethical issues have emerged around the release of sensitive information such as genetic, drug, and alcohol treatment; communicable disease; and psychiatric and adoption information. At least two levels of genetic information can be reported in an information system: presence of a disease, such as cystic fibrosis, and presence of a risk of disease, such as a genetic risk for breast cancer. Various state laws govern the use and release of genetic information, and the HIM professional must be aware of them. In recent years, there have been growing concerns about discrimination in employment and insurance based on the misuse of genetic information (Fuller and Hudson 2006). According to Fuller and Hudson, the HIM professional must be aware of the following issues related to genetic information:

(1) Genetic research and testing can give researchers, clinicians, and patients a means to prevent, treat, or screen for a disease. Often, however, individuals are reluctant to participate in genetic research and testing because they believe they cannot be sure of the privacy of the genetic information that will be obtained from them and placed in their medical records or in research records.

(2) Insurers and employers may seek genetic information to identify at-risk individuals and deny them employment or insurance coverage, fire them, or raise their insurance premiums. Genetic information may also be sought in custody battles or in cases of third-party liability. Even when this information is not used to discriminate, individuals may be concerned about its disclosure because of its possibility of causing psychosocial harm, such as harm to family relationships.

(3) It is difficult to provide special protections for genetic information as a category because it cannot be clearly separated from other medical information. Therefore, the best way to protect genetic information is to strengthen privacy/confidentiality protections for medical information in general and to enact antidiscrimination legislation.

(4) The HIPAA Privacy Rule provides a basic level of privacy and confidentiality protection for protected health information. The Privacy Rule does not preempt state laws (including genetic antidiscrimination laws) that offer a higher level of privacy protection.

(5) The generation of experimental data by a research protocol is not specifically addressed by most state laws.

(6) HIM professionals have the responsibility to ensure that their practices are guided by state and federal laws and regulations to protect genetic information and by the ethical imperative to protect the privacy and confidentiality of patients.

One of the most important opportunities for an HIM professional is to become involved in resolving the above-stated issues on behalf of patients and the healthcare system.

Federal and state laws also govern the use of behavioral health information and special concerns with its use. The HIM professional must respond to the government, the police, and other agencies that seek drug, alcohol, sexual, or other behavioral information (Randolph and Rinehart-Thompson 2006). The inappropriate release of information can have serious discriminatory consequences, such as:

- The police officer presents an arrest warrant to a behavioral health facility. Do you confirm that the patient has been treated? What are the implications for patient privacy if you do?
- A patient with schizophrenia and assaultive behavior is about to be released from a healthcare facility. Do you have a responsibility to inform the girlfriend, who has been assaulted in the past? What are your obligations to protect the privacy of the patient being released?

The ROI dealing with substance abuse, sexually transmitted diseases, and mental health require extra caution on the part of the HIM professional when developing release policies and procedures. There are often competing interests between public safety and patient privacy. How does one deal with law enforcement officials within this context? Federal and state legislation can provide some guidance, but often additional legal counsel must be sought

The release of adoption information is another example of an issue in which laws are necessary, but insufficient, for solving the problems. Decisions cannot be made merely by following the legal rules. More and more often, access to adoption information is being requested by adopted children seeking their biological parents, and vice versa. Biological parents often look for children who could be organ donors or for other assistance. This issue reflects the complexities of releasing genetic and behavioral information because, increasingly, "self" is defined within genetic parameters and biological heritage is becoming more important in defining self. Access to adoption information raises the larger issue of familial access to information, regardless of adoptive status. If biological children can gain access to health information for their biological parent(s), why can't all children gain access to familial information? (Jones 2006). HIM professionals must be alert to these special needs and refrain from processing requests for adoption information without carefully considering the risks for violations of patient privacy, discrimination, or inappropriate access.

Ethical Issues Related to Electronic Health Record Systems

With a paper-based health record, access issues were relatively simple. Only one person at a time could access the information, and it was extremely difficult to collect and use data of an aggregate nature. With computerization, many requestors are allowed multiple, simultaneous access and it is relatively easy to share information across a continuum of care and with computerized systems well outside the boundaries of any individual care site. The advent of the electronic information system has presented complex challenges with regard to record integrity and information security, integrated linkage of information systems across a continuum of care, software development and implementation, and the protection of information in e-health systems (Harman 2006, chapters 11–17).

E-HIM affords information exchange that necessitate active participation on the part of HIM professionals, in both the public and private sectors. There are many ethical challenges, including developing and maintaining information and systems security, exchanging information within and across jurisdictions, executing technical and clinical services contracts, handling release of information, implementing and managing telehealth applications, maintaining and documenting compliance with HIPAA and state privacy rules, and maintaining the legal electronic medical record (Bloomrosen 2006).

As information systems became computerized and healthcare facilities began to link various health information systems, the temptation increased to sacrifice privacy and data integrity for the sake of business efficiency and timely access to information. There is an exponential increase in the risk to privacy and the protection of confidential information (Hanken and Murphy 2006). The HIM professional must do a thorough systems analysis of the independent systems and ensure that the merged systems meet the criteria of data integrity, information security, and ethical use of the information.

Information security carries additional burdens of ethical decision making. Many requestors, such as insurance companies, government agencies, managed care organizations, and employers, need health information to do their jobs. Unauthorized access to patient information becomes a constant challenge, given the need to balance the responsibility to protect information while giving others access to information within the context of job responsibilities. Internal requestors include, but are not limited to, patients, providers of care, financial agencies, and administrative and clinical personnel such as quality or risk management professionals. External stakeholders include other healthcare facilities, research institutes, accrediting and licensing agencies, and fiscal intermediaries (Czirr et al. 2006). The HIM professional must develop a comprehensive information security policy, including detailed audit trails of access and actions. Moreover, the policy must be monitored with consequences for violations. Increasingly, HIM professionals are being designated as the information security officers within a healthcare facility or healthcare system.

Development and implementation of software systems are inherently interdisciplinary in nature, and the process requires collaboration and conflict resolution. The physicians, the HIM professional, the information technology experts, and administrative personnel often have competing interests. The HIM professional is often in the position of carefully delineating the details of competing interests so that appropriate decisions can be made. This role of being able to see the systems implications within the context of protecting privacy is invaluable (Fenton 2006). The HIM professional's role as interdisciplinary facilitator is crucial, which is why educational sessions on organizational development, team building, and conflict resolution are often key components of the HIM professional's continuing education program.

The expertise of the HIM professional includes data resource management because computerized information systems generate data repositories and huge amounts of health information of interest to many people. A primary focus of the HIPAA legislation is to ensure that systems are developed that protect privacy, threats of violations of information integrity, and unauthorized access. Data resource managers must have both HIM technical expertise and information technology expertise so that they can design and monitor systems that ensure data security and patient privacy. These functions are accomplished through the use of many decision-making tools, including databases, clinical data repositories, and data-mining tools, among others. The primary ethical dilemma involves balancing the competing interests of access and appropriate use of information (Lee et al. 2006).

As HIM systems became computerized, the capacity for developing integrated delivery systems across a continuum of care became technologically possible. HIM systems relied on paper-based systems in which each facility had its own health record and the only way to transmit information from one site of care to another was through copying procedures. Now, information can follow the patient and be instantly and simultaneously shared and made available as needed. This is both good news and bad. The segregated, independent systems had some inherent protections of privacy. The integrated computerized systems require HIM professional diligence to ensure protection of information and access to only those who have a need to know. Information management policies, rules, and procedures for individual healthcare entities must be compatible with those of other facilities, and often the issues of competing interests can create major ethical conflicts as to the appropriate action.

The master patient index presents a major problem because there is often no consistency among facilities in terms of how and what information is collected. If the information is to follow the patient, the individual systems must be accurate and compatible. Data quality issues include accuracy, comprehensiveness, consistency, currency, granularity, precision, relevancy, and timeliness (AHIMA 1998). Negotiation and problem-solving skills are an inherent requirement for the HIM professional working in an integrated delivery system (Olson and Grant, 2006). The HIM professional must lead the organization in addressing data quality issues associated with implementing integrated information systems.

Last, but not least, the HIM professional's ethical expertise is needed in the burgeoning e-health systems. Some of the ethical issues the HIM professional faces in the work environment include the quality of online information, privacy protections, and equity and privacy. The issue of equity is important to e-health systems because not everyone has access to the information on the electronic systems. There cannot be equity when one patient instead of another can easily gain access to invaluable and voluminous information about symptoms, diseases, pharmaceutical interventions, and treatment options. Privacy can be an issue when patients reveal sensitive information to a Web site and have no idea what will happen to the information or who will have access to it. The opportunities for the HIM professional are unlimited given the problems of consumer access to information, quality of information provided, and access to information. This nontraditional advocacy role for HIM professionals is important in this emerging technological advancement (Baur and Deering 2006).

Roles of Manager, Entrepreneur and Advocate

The HIM professional deals with daily complexities that require the need for understanding ethics. Problems such as late and absent employees, temptations at conventions and meetings, employees who should be terminated and poor work performance, are a few of the many dilemmas facing the busy HIM manager (Flite and Laquer 2006). As an entrepreneur, the HIM professional must understand the complexities of business practices intersecting with professional values and ethical principles. Common ethical dilemmas occur when establishing contracts, clarifying the roles of intrapreneur and entrepreneur, or acting as an independent contractor. Difficulties may arise when consulting for competitors (having access to sensitive information that might be of value to the competition), dealing with advertising, confronting unrealistic client expectations, or confusing profit versus not-for-profit motivations for decisions (Gardenier 2006).

HIM professionals have always been advocates for patients and providers, and the advocate role is important in today's healthcare delivery system. For the HIM professional, advocacy "is ethics in action: choosing to take a stand for and speak out for the rights or needs of a person, group, organization, or community" (Helbig 2006). For example, HIM problems that require advocacy include:

- Protecting the privacy of prominent citizens because it is more tempting to want access to the information of prominent citizens, such as elected officials and famous actors
- Demonstrating compassion for drug-dependent peers
- Protecting the work environment for HIM employees
- Ensuring that consent forms are properly designed so that patients understand what they are signing and so that patient information is protected from unauthorized secondary disclosure

The advocacy role requires HIM expertise, ethical expertise, and an understanding of the patient's bill of rights (Helbig 2006).

Business relationships with vendors also pose ethical dilemmas. What issues are raised when vendors are also friends? What is the appropriate use of gifts? Should some vendors be "preferred" when dealing with requests for proposals? How can you assure ethical dealings when negotiating contracts? (Olenik 2006).

Check Your Understanding 11.3

Instructions: On a separate piece of paper, match the ethical principle with its definition.

1. ____ Autonomy
2. ____ Beneficence
3. ____ Nonmaleficence
4. ____ Justice

5. ___ Moral values

6. ___ Ethical decisions

7. ___ Privacy

8. ___ Confidentiality

9. ___ Data security

10. ___ HIPAA

a. Right or wrong
b. Reasoned discourse
c. Right to be let alone
d. Promote good
e. Self-determination
f. Healthcare communication
g. Do no harm
h. Fairness in applying rules
i. Establishes privacy and security standards
j. Electronic protection of information

Real-World Case

Carol Wright is an outstanding manager. She has worked for C&S Pharmaceuticals for 15 years. She has received five promotions and is currently responsible for abstracting and quality operations. Carol has been quick to identify personnel problems and provides educational and instructional support to her staff.

Carol supervises Joan, who is often absent or late for work. When she does come to work, she makes many mistakes, but she always seems to meet work standards prior to her performance reviews. Various forms of motivation, education, and administrative support have been offered to Joan in the past. This week, Joan failed to show up for three days without notifying the office. The company policy states that if an employee does not show up for work for three consecutive days without notifying the office by the end of the third business day (5 p.m.), the employee's employment shall be terminated.

On the third day, some managers may be anxiously waiting for the employee to call and explain the absence, but this was not the case with Carol. Carol had recognized that this employee was nonproductive, noncompliant, and met the criteria for job abandonment. Carol was prepared to terminate Joan, because she repeatedly demonstrated a clear disregard for the policy related to reporting to work. Carol no longer had any patience for Joan's behaviors. Carol was confident that the employee was not going to comply with the policy and that this would be an easy termination. She completed the termination paperwork based on job abandonment at 3 p.m. and left it on her desk for the 5 p.m. submission to the human resources department. At 4:30 p.m., Carol's secretary told her that Joan was on the telephone, but Carol did not accept the call. The paperwork was sent to the human resources department at 5 p.m. and Joan's employment was terminated the next day (Harman 2006, p. 510).

Summary

Ethical decision making is one of the health information professional's most challenging and rewarding job respon-

sibilities. It requires courage because there will always be people who choose not tell the truth or do the right thing. HIM professionals must discuss these issues with their peer professionals and seek the advice of the professional association when necessary.

The HIM professional's job responsibilities inherently require an understanding of ethical principles, professional values and obligations, and the importance of using an ethical decision-making matrix when confronting difficult challenges at work. With this knowledge, the informed HIM professional can move from understanding problems based on a moral perspective only to understanding the importance of applying an ethical decision-making process. Ethical decision making takes practice, and discussions with peers will help the HIM professional to build competency in this important area.

When making ethical decisions, the HIM professional should use the complete ethical decision-making matrix to consider all the stakeholders and their obligations and the important HIM professional values. More than one response can be given for any ethical issue as long as the complete matrix is applied. Just as there can be more than one "right" answer to a problem, there can be "wrong" answers, especially when an answer is based only on a moral value or the perspective of one individual or when the action violates ethical principles.

Bioethical decisions involving the use of health information require action, and such actions always require courage. The healthcare team, the patients, and the others who are served need to know that the HIM professional has the expertise and the courage to make appropriate ethical decisions.

References

Amatayakul, M.K. 2004. *Electronic Health Records: A Practical Guide for Professionals and Organizations,* 2nd ed. Chicago: AHIMA.

American Health Information Management Association. 2002 (October). Practice brief: Consent for uses and disclosures of information. Updated from *Journal of American Health Information Management Association* 72 (5):64E–64G. Available online from ahima.org.

Baur, C., and M.J. Deering. 2006. e-Health for consumers, patients and caregivers. Chapter 16 in *Ethical Challenges in the Management of Health Information: Process and Strategies for Decision-Making,* 2nd ed., edited by L.B. Harman. Sudbury, MA: Jones and Bartlett.

Beauchamp, T., and J. Childress. 2001. *Principles of Biomedical Ethics.* New York: Oxford University Press.

Bloomrosen, M. 2006. E-HIM: Information technology and information exchange. Chapter 17 in *Ethical Challenges in the Management of Health Information: Process and Strategies for Decision-Making,* 2nd ed., edited by L.B. Harman. Sudbury, MA: Jones and Bartlett.

Czirr, K., K. Rosendale, and E. West. 2006. Information security. Chapter 12 in *Ethical Challenges in the Management of Health Information: Process and Strategies for Decision-Making,* 2nd ed., edited by L.B. Harman. Sudbury, MA: Jones and Bartlett.

Department of Health and Human Services. 2003. Summary of the HIPAA Privacy Rule. *OCR Privacy Brief.* Available online from hhs.gov/ocr/privacysummary.pdf.

Dick, R.S., E.B. Steen, and D.E. Detmer, eds. 1997. *The Computer-Based Patient Record: An Essential Technology for Health Care,* rev. ed. Washington, DC: National Academy Press.

Fenton, S.H. 2006. Software development and implementation. Chapter 13 in *Ethical Challenges in the Management of Health Information: Process and Strategies for Decision-Making,* 2nd ed., edited by L.B. Harman. Sudbury, MA: Jones and Bartlett.

Flite, C., and S. Laquer. 2006. Management. Chapter 21 in *Ethical Challenges in the Management of Health Information: Process and Strategies for Decision-Making,* 2nd ed., edited by L.B. Harman. Sudbury, MA: Jones and Bartlett.

Fuller, B.P., and K.L. Hudson. 2006. Genetic information. Chapter 18 in *Ethical Challenges in the Management of Health Information: Process and Strategies for Decision-Making,* 2nd ed., edited by L.B. Harman. Sudbury, MA: Jones and Bartlett.

Gardenier, M. 2006. Entrepreneurship. Chapter 22 in *Ethical Challenges in the Management of Health Information: Process and Strategies for Decision-Making,* edited by L.B. Harman. Sudbury, MA: Jones and Bartlett.

Gellman R. 2004 (June 23). When HIPAA meets NHII: A new dimension for privacy. Presentation to U.S. Department of Health and Human Services Data Council Privacy Committee, Washington, DC.

Glover, J.J. 2006. Ethical decision-making guidelines and tools. Chapter 2 in *Ethical Challenges in the Management of Health Information: Process and Strategies for Decision-Making,* 2nd ed., edited by L.B. Harman. Sudbury, MA: Jones and Bartlett.

Hanken, M.A., and G. Murphy. 2006. Electronic patient record. Chapter 11 in *Ethical Challenges in the Management of Health Information: Process and Strategies for Decision-Making,* edited by L.B. Harman. Sudbury, MA: Jones and Bartlett.

Harman, L.B., ed. 2006. *Ethical Challenges in the Management of Health Information: Process and Strategies for Decision-Making.* 2nd ed., Sudbury, MA: Jones and Bartlett.

Harman, L. 2005. HIPAA: A few years later. *Online Journal of Issues in Nursing* 10(2). Available online from nursingworld.org/ojin/topic27/tpc27_2.htm.

Harman, L.B. 1999. HIM and ethics: Confronting ethical dilemmas on the job, an HIM professional's guide. *Journal of the American Health Information Management Association* 71(5):45–49.

Harman, L.B., and V.L. Mullen. 2006. Professional values and the code of ethics. In *Ethical Challenges in the Management of Health Information: Process and Strategies for Decision-Making,* 2nd ed., edited by L.B. Harman. Sudbury, MA: Jones and Bartlett.

Helbig, S. 2006. Advocate. Chapter 24 in *Ethical Challenges in the Management of Health Information: Process and Strategies for Decision-Making,* 2nd ed., edited by L.B. Harman. Sudbury, MA: Jones and Bartlett.

Huffman, E.K. 1972. *Manual for Medical Record Librarians,* 6th ed. Chicago: Physician's Record Company.

Hughes, G. 2002a (November). Practice brief: Laws and regulations governing the disclosure of health information. Updated from *Journal of American Health Information Management Association* 72(5):64A–64C. Proprietary content from ahima.org.

Hughes, G. 2002b (October). Practice brief: Required content for authorizations to disclose. Updated from *Journal of American Health Information Management Association* 72(10):72A–72D. Proprietary content from ahima.org.

Johns, M.L. 2002. *Information Management for Health Professions,* 2nd ed. Albany, NY: Delmar.

Johns, M.L., and J.M. Hardin. 2006. Research and decision support. Chapter 7 in *Ethical Challenges in the Management of Health Information: Process and Strategies for Decision-Making,* 2nd ed., edited by L.B. Harman. Sudbury, MA: Jones and Bartlett.

Jones, M.L. 2006. Adoption information. In *Ethical Challenges in the Management of Health Information: Process and Strategies for Decision-Making,* 2nd ed., edited by L.B. Harman. Sudbury, MA: Jones and Bartlett.

Lee, F.W., A.W. White, and K.A. Wager. 2006. Data resource management. Chapter 14 in *Ethical Challenges in the Management of Health Information: Process and Strategies for Decision-Making,* 2nd ed., edited by L.B. Harman. Sudbury, MA: Jones and Bartlett.

Murphy, G., M.A. Hanken, and K.A. Waters. 1999. *Electronic Health Records: Changing the Vision.* Philadelphia: W.B. Saunders.

National Committee on Vital and Health Statistics. 2001. Information for health: A strategy for building the national health information infrastructure. Available online from aspe.hhs.gov/sp/nhii/Documents/NHIIReport2001/report11.htm.

Neuberger, B.J. 2006. Public health. Chapter 8 in *Ethical Challenges in the Management of Health Information: Process and Strategies for Decision-Making,* 2nd ed., edited by L.B. Harman. Sudbury, MA: Jones and Bartlett.

Olenik, K. 2006. Vendor Relationships. Chapter 23 in *Ethical Challenges in the Management of Health Information: Process and Strategies for Decision-Making,* 2nd ed., edited by L.B. Harman. Sudbury, MA: Jones and Bartlett.

Olson, B., and K.G. Grant. 2006. Integrated delivery systems. Chapter 15 in *Ethical Challenges in the Management of Health Information: Process and Strategies for Decision-Making,* 2nd ed., edited by L.B. Harman. Sudbury, MA: Jones and Bartlett.

Randolph, S. J., and L.A. Rinehart-Thompson. 2006. Drug, alcohol, sexual, and behavioral health information. Chapter 20 in *Ethical Challenges in the Management of Health Information: Process and Strategies for Decision-Making,* 2nd ed., edited by L.B. Harman. Sudbury, MA: Jones and Bartlett.

Rhodes, H. 2001 (Updated). Practice brief: Patient anonymity. *Journal of American Health Information Management Association* 72(5):64O–64R.

Rinehart-Thompson, L.A. 2006. Compliance, fraud, and abuse. Chapter 4 in *Ethical Challenges in the Management of Health Information: Process and Strategies for Decision-Making,* 2nd ed., edited by L.B. Harman. Sudbury, MA: Jones and Bartlett.

Rinehart-Thompson, L.A., and L.B. Harman. 2006. Privacy and confidentiality. Chapter 3 in *Ethical Challenges in the Management of Health Information: Process and Strategies for Decision-Making,* 2nd ed., edited by L.B. Harman. Sudbury, MA: Jones and Bartlett.

Schick, I.C. 2006. Managed care: Lessons in integration. Chapter 9 in *Ethical Challenges in the Management of Health Information: Process and Strategies for Decision-Making,* 2nd ed., edited by L.B. Harman. Sudbury, MA: Jones and Bartlett.

Schraffenberger, L.A., and R.A. Scichilone. 2006. Clinical code selection and use. Chapter 5 in *Ethical Challenges in the Management of Health Information: Process and Strategies for Decision-Making,* 2nd ed., edited by L. B. Harman. Sudbury, MA: Jones and Bartlett.

Spath, P.L. 2006. Quality review. Chapter 6 in *Ethical Challenges in the Management of Health Information: Process and Strategies for Decision-Making,* 2nd ed., edited by L.B. Harman. Sudbury, MA: Jones and Bartlett.

Tischler, J.F. 2006. Clinical care: End of life. Chapter 10 in *Ethical Challenges in the Management of Health Information: Process and Strategies for Decision-Making,* 2nd ed., edited by L.B. Harman. Sudbury, MA: Jones and Bartlett.

Part III

Aggregate Healthcare Data

Chapter 12
Secondary Records and Healthcare Databases

Elizabeth Bowman, MPA, RHIA

Learning Objectives

- To distinguish between primary and secondary data and between patient-identifiable and aggregate data
- To identify the internal and external users of secondary data
- To compare the facility-specific indexes commonly found in hospitals
- To describe the registries used in hospitals according to purpose, methods of case definition and case finding, data collection methods, reporting and follow-up, and pertinent laws and regulations affecting registry operations
- To define the terms pertinent to each type of secondary record or database

- To discuss agencies for approval and education and certification for cancer, immunization, trauma, birth defects, diabetes, implant, transplant, and immunization registries
- To distinguish among healthcare databases in terms of purpose and content
- To compare manual and automated methods of data collection and vendor systems with facility-specific systems
- To assess data quality issues in secondary records
- To recognize appropriate methods for ensuring data security and the confidentiality of secondary records
- To identify the role of the health information management professional in creating and maintaining secondary records

Key Terms

Abbreviated Injury Scale (AIS)
Abstracting
Accession number
Accession registry
Activities of daily living
Agency for Healthcare Research and Quality (AHRQ)
Aggregate data
Audit trail
Autodialing system
Case definition
Case finding
Claim
Clinical trial
Collaborative Stage Data Set
Computer virus

Credentialing
Data confidentiality
Data security
Database
Demographic information
Disease index
Disease registry
Edit
Encryption
Facility-based registry
Facility-specific system
Food and Drug Administration (FDA)
Health services research
Healthcare Integrity and Protection Data Bank (HIPDB)

Histocompatibility
Incidence
Index
Injury Severity Score (ISS)
Interrater reliability
Master population/patient index (MPI)
Medical Literature, Analysis, and Retrieval System Online (MEDLINE)
Medicare Provider Analysis and Review (MEDPAR)
National Health Care Survey
National Practitioner Data Bank (NPDB)
National Vaccine Advisory Committee (NVAC)

Operation index
Patient-specific/identifiable data
Physician index
Population-based registry
Primary data source
Protocol
Public health
Secondary data source
Staging system
Traumatic injury
Unified Medical Language System (UMLS)
User groups
Vendor system
Vital statistics

Introduction

As a rich source of data about an individual patient, the health record fulfills the uses of patient care and reimbursement for individual encounters. However, it is not easy to see trends in a population of patients by looking at individual records. For this purpose, data must be extracted from individual records and entered into specialized **databases** that support analysis across individual records. These data may be used in a facility-specific or **population-based registry** for research and improvement in patient care. In addition, they may be reported to the state and become part of state- and federal-level databases that are used to set health policy and improve healthcare.

The health information management (HIM) professional can play a variety of roles in managing secondary records and databases. He or she plays a key role in helping to set up databases. This task includes determining the content of the database or registry and ensuring compliance with the laws, regulations, and accrediting standards that affect the content and use of the registry or database. All data elements included in the database or registry must be defined in a data dictionary. In this role, the HIM professional may oversee the completeness and accuracy of the data abstracted for inclusion in the database or registry.

This chapter explains the difference between primary and secondary data sources and their users. It also offers an in-depth look at the types of secondary databases, including **indexes** and registries, and their functions. Finally, the chapter discusses how secondary databases are processed and maintained.

Theory into Practice

A hospital with a level I trauma center serving a tri-state area had an ongoing problem. It was required to provide care to all major trauma cases from the three states within its service area regardless of the patients' ability to pay. However, one of the states (state X) was unwilling to pay for the care provided to its indigent patients. Because trauma care can be extremely intensive and costly, the hospital was losing a lot of money.

The American College of Surgeons (ACS) requires certified trauma centers to maintain a trauma registry. To demonstrate the extent of the problem, the hospital administrator asked the trauma registrar to gather data on patients from state X. The trauma registrar easily identified these patients and provided information by zip code on their location and the type and severity of their injuries. After the patients had been identified, the business office was able to calculate the cost to the hospital of providing their care. The administrator then presented this information to state X's legislature to obtain the money to pay for the care the trauma center provided to the state's indigent patients.

Primary versus Secondary Data Sources and Databases

The health record is considered a **primary data source** because it contains information about a patient that has been documented by the professionals who provided care or services to that patient. Data taken from the primary health record and entered into registries and databases are considered a **secondary data source.**

Data also are categorized as either **patient-specific/ identifiable data** or **aggregate data.** The health record consists entirely of patient-identifiable data. In other words, every fact recorded in the record relates to a particular patient identified by name. Secondary data also may be patient identifiable. In some instances, data are entered into a database, along with information such as the patient's name, maintained in an identifiable form. Registries are an example of patient-identifiable data on groups of patients.

More often, however, secondary data are considered aggregate data. Aggregate data include data on groups of people or patients without identifying any particular patient individually. Examples of aggregate data are statistics on the average length of stay (ALOS) for patients discharged within a particular diagnosis-related group (DRG).

Purposes and Users of Secondary Data Sources

Secondary data sources consist of facility-specific indexes; registries, either facility or population based; and other healthcare databases. Healthcare organizations maintain those indexes, registries, and databases that are relevant to their specific operations.

Secondary data sources provide information that is not easily available by looking at individual health records. For example, if the HIM director doing a research study wanted to find the health records of 25 patients who had the principal diagnosis of myocardial infarction, he or she would have to look at numerous individual records to locate the number needed. This would be a time-consuming and laborious project. With a diagnosis index, the task would involve simply looking at the list of diagnoses in numerical order and selecting those with the appropriate ICD-9-CM diagnosis code for inclusion in the study.

Data extracted from health records and entered into disease-oriented databases can, for example, help researchers determine the effectiveness of alternate treatment methods. They also can quickly demonstrate survival rates at different stages of disease.

Internal users of secondary data are individuals located within the healthcare facility. For example, internal users include medical staff and administrative and management staff. Secondary data enable these users to identify patterns and trends that are helpful in patient care, long-range planning, budgeting, and benchmarking with other facilities.

External users of patient data are individuals and institutions outside the facility. Examples of external users are state data banks and federal agencies. States have laws that cases of patients with diseases such as tuberculosis and AIDS must be reported to the state department of health. Moreover, the federal government collects data from the states on vital events such as births and deaths.

The secondary data provided to external users is generally aggregate data and not patient-identifiable data. Thus, these data can be used as needed without risking breaches of confidentiality.

Check Your Understanding 12.1

Instructions: Answer the following questions on a separate piece of paper.

1. What is the difference between a primary data source and a secondary data source?

2. What is the difference between patient-identifiable data and aggregate data?

3. Why are secondary data sources developed?

4. What are the differences between internal users and external users of secondary data sources?

Facility-Specific Indexes

The secondary data sources that have been in existence the longest are those that have been developed within facilities to meet their individual needs. These indexes enable health records to be located by diagnosis, procedure, or physician. Prior to extensive computerization in healthcare, these indexes were kept on cards. They now are usually computerized reports available from data included in databases routinely maintained in the healthcare facility. Most acute care facilities maintain indexes described in the following subsections.

Master Population/Patient Index

The **master population/patient index** (MPI), which is sometimes called the master person index, contains patient-identifiable data such as name, address, date of birth, dates of hospitalizations or encounters, name of attending physician, and health record number. Because health records are filed numerically in most facilities, the MPI is an important source of patient health record numbers. These numbers enable the facility to quickly retrieve health information for specific patients.

Hospitals with a unit numbering system also depend on the MPI to determine whether a patient has been seen in the facility before and therefore has an existing medical record number. Having this information in the MPI avoids issuance of duplicate record numbers. Most of the information in the MPI is entered into the facility database at the time of the admission/preadmission or registration process.

Disease and Operation Indexes

In an acute care setting, the **disease index** is a listing in diagnosis code number order for patients discharged from the facility during a particular time period. Each patient's diagnoses are converted from a verbal description to a numerical code, usually using a coding system such as the *International Classification of Diseases, Ninth Revision, Clinical Modification* (ICD-9-CM). In many cases, patient diagnosis codes are entered into the facility health information system as part of the discharge processing of the patient health record. The index always includes the patient's health record number as well as the diagnosis codes so that records can be retrieved by diagnosis. Because each patient is listed with the health record number, the disease index is considered patient-identifiable data. The disease index also may include other information such as the attending physician's name or the date of discharge. In nonacute settings, the disease index might be generated to reflect patients currently receiving services in the facility.

The **operation index** is similar to the disease index except that it is arranged in numerical order by the patient's procedure code(s) using ICD-9-CM or Current Procedural Terminology (CPT) codes. The other information listed in the operation index is generally the same as that listed in the disease index except that the surgeon may be listed in addition to, or instead of, the attending physician.

Physician Index

The **physician index** is a listing of cases in order by physician name or physician identification number. It also includes the patient's health record number and may include other information, such as date of discharge. The physician index enables users to retrieve information about a particular physician, including the number of cases seen during a particular time period.

Check Your Understanding 12.2

Instructions: Answer the following questions on a separate piece of paper.

1. How do HIM departments use facility-specific indexes?

2. What is the purpose of the master population/patient index? What types of information does it include?

3. What is the purpose of disease and operations indexes? What types of information do they include?

4. What is the purpose of the physician index? What types of information does it include?

Registries

Disease registries are collections of secondary data related to patients with a specific diagnosis, condition, or procedure. Registries are different from indexes in that they contain more extensive data. Index reports can usually be produced using data from the facility's existing databases. Registries often require more extensive data from the patient record. Each registry must define the cases that are to be included in it. This process is called **case definition.** In a trauma registry, for example, the case definition might be all patients admitted with a diagnosis falling into ICD-9-CM code numbers 800 through 959, the trauma diagnosis codes.

After the cases to be included have been determined through the case definition process described above, the next step in data acquisition is usually **case finding.** Case finding includes the methods used to identify the patients who have been seen and/or treated in the facility for the particular disease or condition of interest to the registry. After cases have been identified, extensive information is abstracted from the paper-based patient record into the registry database or extracted from other databases and entered into the registry database.

The sole purpose of some registries is to collect data from the patient health record and to make them available for users. Other registries take further steps to enter additional information in the registry database, such as routine follow-up of patients at specified intervals. Follow-up might include rate and duration of survival and quality of life issues over time.

Cancer Registries

Cancer registries have a long history in healthcare. According to the National Cancer Registrars Association (NCRA), the first hospital registry was founded in 1926 at Yale-New Haven Hospital. It has long been recognized that aggregate clinical information is needed to improve the diagnosis and treatment of cancer. Cancer registries were developed as an organized method to collect these data. The registry may be *facility based* (located within a facility such as a hospital or clinic) or *population based* (gathering information from more than one facility within a geographic area such as a state or region).

The data from **facility-based registries** are used to provide information for the improved understanding of cancer, including its causes and methods of diagnosis and treatment. The data collected also may provide comparisons in survival rates and quality of life for patients with different treatments and at different stages of cancer at the time of diagnosis. In population-based registries, emphasis is on identifying trends and changes in the **incidence** (new cases) of cancer within the area covered by the registry.

The Cancer Registries Amendment Act of 1992 provided funding for a national program of cancer registries with population-based registries in each state. According to the law, these registries were mandated to collect data such as:

- **Demographic information** about each case of cancer
- Information on the industrial or occupational history of the individuals with the cancers (to the extent such information is available from the same record)
- Administrative information, including date of diagnosis and source of information
- Pathological data characterizing the cancer, including site, stage of neoplasm, incidence, and type of treatment

Case Definition and Case Finding in the Cancer Registry

As defined previously, case definition is the process of deciding what cases should be entered in the registry. In a cancer registry, for example, all cancer cases except certain skin cancers might meet the definition for the cases to be included. Skin cancers such as basal cell carcinomas might be excluded because they do not metastasize and do not require the follow-up necessary for other cancers included in the registry. Data on benign and borderline brain/central nervous system tumors also must be collected by the National Program of Cancer Registries (Ringer and Cain 2004).

In the facility-based cancer registry, the first step is case finding. One way to find cases is through the discharge process in the HIM department. During the discharge procedure, coders and/or discharge analysts can easily earmark cases of patients with cancer for inclusion in the registry. Another case-finding method is to use the facility-specific disease indexes to identify patients with diagnoses of cancer. Additional methods may include reviews of pathology reports and lists of patients receiving radiation therapy or other cancer treatments to determine cases that have not been found by other methods.

Population-based registries usually depend on hospitals, physician offices, radiation facilities, ambulatory surgery centers (ASCs), and pathology laboratories to identify and report cases to the central registry. The population-based registry has a responsibility to ensure that all cases of cancer in the target area have been identified and reported to the central registry.

Data Collection for the Cancer Registry

Data collection methods vary between facility-based registries and population-based registries. When a case is first entered in the registry, an **accession number** is assigned. This number consists of the first digits of the year the patient was first seen at the facility, with the remaining digits assigned sequentially throughout the year. The first case in 2005, for example, might be 05-0001. The accession number may be assigned manually or by the automated cancer database used by the organization. An **accession registry** of all cases can be kept manually or provided as a report by the database software. This listing of patients in accession number order provides a way to monitor that all cases have been entered into the registry.

In a facility-based registry, data are initially obtained by reviewing and collecting them from the patient's health record. In addition to demographic information (such as name, health record number, address), patient data in a registry include:

- Type and site of the cancer
- Diagnostic methodologies
- Treatment methodologies
- Stage at the time of diagnosis

The stage provides information on the size and extent of spread of the tumor throughout the body. Historically, several different **staging systems** have been used. The American Joint Committee on Cancer (AJCC) has worked, through its Collaborative Stage Task Force, with other organizations with staging systems to develop a new standardized data set, the **Collaborative Stage Data Set,** which uses computer algorithms to describe how far a cancer has spread (AJCC 2005).

After the initial information is collected at the patient's first encounter, information in the registry is updated periodically through the follow-up process discussed in the following section.

Frequently, the population-based registry only collects information when the patient is diagnosed. Sometimes, however, it receives follow-up information from its reporting entities. These entities usually submit the information to the central registry electronically.

Reporting and Follow-up for Cancer Registry Data

Formal reporting of cancer registry data is done through an annual report. The annual report includes aggregate data on the number of cases in the past year by site and type of cancer. It also may include information on patients by gender, age, and ethnic group. Often a particular site or type of cancer is featured with more in-depth data provided.

Other reports are provided as needed. Data from the cancer registry are frequently used in the quality assessment process for a facility as well as in research. Data on survival rates by site of cancer and methods of treatment, for example, would be helpful in researching the most effective treatment for a type of cancer.

Another activity of the cancer registry is patient follow-up. On an annual basis, the registry attempts to obtain information about each patient in the registry, including whether he or she is still alive, status of the cancer, and treatment received during the period. Various methods are used to obtain this information. For a facility-based registry, the facility's patient health records may be checked for return hospitalizations or visits for treatment. The patient's physician also may be contacted to determine whether the patient is still living and to obtain information about the cancer.

When patient status cannot be determined through these methods, an attempt may be made to contact the patient directly, using information in the registry such as address and telephone number of the patient and other contacts. In addition, contact information from the patient's health record may be used to request information from the patient's relatives. Other methods used include reading newspaper obituaries for deaths and using the Internet to locate patients through sites such as the Social Security Death Index and online telephone books. The information obtained through follow-up is important to allow the registry to develop statistics on survival rates for particular cancers and different treatment methodologies.

Population-based registries do not always include follow-up information on the patients in their databases. Those that do, however, usually receive the information from the reporting entities such as hospitals, physician offices, and other organizations providing follow-up care.

Standards and Agencies in the Approval Processes

Several organizations have developed standards or approval processes for cancer programs. (See table 12.1.) The American College of Surgeons (ACS) Commission on Cancer has an approval process for cancer programs. One of the requirements of this process is the existence of a cancer registry as part of the program. The ACS standards are published in the Cancer Program Standards (ACS 2005a). When the ACS surveys the cancer program, part of the survey process is a review of cancer registry activities.

The North American Association of Central Cancer Registries (NAACCR) has a certification program for state population-based registries. Certification is based on the quality of data collected and reported by the state registry. The NAACCR has developed standards for data quality and format and works with other cancer organizations to align their various standards sets.

The Centers for Disease Control and Prevention (CDC) also has national standards regarding completeness, timeliness, and quality of cancer registry data from state registries through the National Program of Cancer Registries (NPCR). The NPCR was developed as a result of the Cancer Registries Amendment Act of 1992. The CDC collects data from the NPCR state registries.

Education and Certification for Cancer Registrars

Traditionally, cancer registrars have been trained through on-the-job training and professional workshops and seminars. The National Cancer Registrars Association (NCRA) has worked with colleges to develop formal educational programs for cancer registrars. A cancer registrar may become certified as a certified cancer registrar (CTR) by passing an examination provided by the National Board for Certification of Registrars (NBCR). Eligibility requirements for the certification examination include a combination of experience and education (NCRA 2005).

Trauma Registries

Trauma registries maintain databases on patients with severe traumatic injuries. A **traumatic injury** is a wound or other injury caused by an external physical force such as an automobile accident, a shooting, a stabbing, or a fall. Examples of such injuries would include fractures, burns, and lacerations.

Table 12.1.   Standard-setting or approval agencies for cancer registries

Agency	Type of Registry
American College of Surgeons (ACS)	Facility based
North American Association of Central Cancer Registries (NAACCR)	Population based
Centers for Disease Control and Prevention	Population based

Information collected by the trauma registry may be used for performance improvement and research in the area of trauma care. Trauma registries are usually facility based but may, in some cases, include data for a region or state.

Case Definition and Case Finding for Trauma Registries

The case definition for the trauma registry varies from registry to registry but frequently involves the inclusion of cases with diagnoses from ICD-9-CM sections 800 through 959, the trauma diagnosis codes. To find cases with trauma diagnoses, the trauma registrar may access the disease indexes looking for cases with codes in this section of ICD-9-CM. In addition, the registrar may look at deaths in services with frequent trauma diagnoses such as trauma, neurosurgery, orthopedics, and plastic surgery to find additional cases.

Data Collection for Trauma Registries

After the cases have been identified, information is abstracted from the health records of the injured patients and entered into the trauma registry database. The data elements collected in the abstracting process vary from registry to registry but usually include:

* Demographic information on the patient
* Information on the injury
* Care the patient received before hospitalization (such as care at another transferring hospital or care from an emergency medical technician who provided care at the scene of the accident and/or in transport from the accident site to the hospital)
* Status of the patient at the time of admission
* Patient's course in the hospital
* ICD-9-CM diagnosis and procedure codes
* **Abbreviated Injury Scale** (AIS)
* **Injury Severity Score** (ISS)

The AIS reflects the nature of the injury and the severity (threat to life) by body system. It may be assigned manually by the registrar or generated as part of the database from data entered by the registrar. The ISS is an overall severity measurement calculated from the AIS scores for the three most severe injuries of the patient (Trauma.org 2005).

Reporting and Follow-up for Trauma Registries

Reporting varies among trauma registries. An annual report is often developed to show the activity of the trauma registry. Other reports may be generated as part of the performance improvement process, such as self-extubation (patients removing their own tubes) and delays in abdominal surgery or patient complications. Some hospitals report data to the National Trauma Data Bank (ACS 2005b). An example of the use of such population data is the number of head injuries from motorcycle accidents in a state to encourage passage of a helmet law.

Trauma registries may or may not do follow-up of the patients entered in the registry. When follow-up is done, emphasis is frequently on the patient's quality of life after a period of time. Unlike cancer, where physician follow-up is crucial to detect recurrence, many traumatic injuries do not require continued patient care over time. Thus, follow-up is often not given the emphasis it receives in cancer registries.

Standards and Agencies for Approval of Trauma Registries

The ACS certifies levels I, II, III, and IV trauma centers. As part of its certification requirements, the ACS states that the level I trauma center must have a trauma registry (Garthe 1997, p. 26).

Education and Certification of Trauma Registrars

Trauma registrars may be registered health information technicians (RHITs), registered health information administrators (RHIAs), registered nurses (RNs), licensed practical nurses (LPNs), emergency medical technicians (EMTs), or other health professionals. Training for trauma registrars is accomplished through workshops and on-the-job training. The American Trauma Society (ATS), for example, provides core and advanced workshops for trauma registrars. It also provides a certification examination for trauma registrars through its Registrar Certification Board. Certified trauma registrars have earned the credential CSTR (certified specialist in trauma registry).

Birth Defects Registries

Birth defects registries collect information on newborns with birth defects. Often population based, these registries serve a variety of purposes. For example, they provide information on the incidence of birth defects to study causes and prevention of birth defects, to monitor trends in birth defects to improve medical care for children with birth defects, and to target interventions for preventable birth defects such as folic acid to prevent neural tube defects.

In some cases, registries have been developed after specific events have put a spotlight on birth defects. After the Persian Gulf War, for example, some feared an increased incidence of birth defects among the children of Gulf War veterans. The Department of Defense subsequently started a birth defects registry to collect data on the children of these veterans to determine whether any pattern could be detected.

Case Definition and Case Finding for Birth Defects Registries

Birth defects registries use a variety of criteria to determine which cases to include in the registry. Some registries limit cases to those found within the first year of life. Others include those with a major defect that occurred in the first year of life and was discovered within the first five years of life. Still other registries include only children who were liveborn or stillborn babies with discernible birth defects.

Cases may be detected in a variety of ways, including review of disease indexes, labor and delivery logs, pathology and autopsy reports, ultrasound reports, and cytogenetic reports. In addition to information from hospitals and physicians, cases may be identified from rehabilitation centers and children's hospitals and from vital records such as birth, death, and fetal death certificates.

Data Collection for Birth Defects Registries

A variety of information is abstracted for the birth defects registry, including:

- Demographic information
- Codes for diagnoses
- Birth weight
- Status at birth, including liveborn, stillborn, aborted
- Autopsy
- Cytogenetics results
- Whether the infant was a single or multiple birth
- Mother's use of alcohol, tobacco, or illicit drugs
- Father's use of drugs and alcohol
- Family history of birth defects

Diabetes Registries

Diabetes registries collect data about patients with diabetes for the purpose of assistance in managing care as well as for research. Patients whose diabetes is not kept under good control frequently have numerous complications. The diabetes registry can keep up with whether the patient has been seen by a physician in an effort to prevent complications.

Case Definition and Case Finding for Diabetes Registries

There are two types of diabetes mellitus: insulin-dependent diabetes (type I) and non-insulin-dependent diabetes (type II). Registries sometimes limit their cases by type of diabetes. In some instances, there may be further definition by age. Some diabetes registries, for example, only include children with diabetes.

Case finding includes the review of health records of patients with diabetes. Other case-finding methods include the reviews of the following types of information:

- ICD-9-CM diagnostic codes
- Billing data
- Medication lists
- Physician identification
- Health plans

Although facility-based registries for cancer and trauma are usually hospital based, facility-based diabetes registries are often maintained by physician offices and clinics. The office or clinic is the main location for diabetes care. Thus, the data about the patient to be entered into the registry are available at these sites rather than at the hospital. Patient health records of diabetes patients in the physician practice may be identified through ICD-9-CM code numbers for diabetes (code numbers in category 250), billing data for diabetes-related services, medication lists for patients on diabetic medications, or identification of patients as the physician sees them.

Health plans also are interested in optimal care for their enrollees because diabetes can have serious complications when not managed correctly. They may provide information to the office or clinic on enrollees in the health plan who are diabetics.

Data Collection for Diabetes Registries

In addition to demographic information about the cases, other data collected may include laboratory values such as HBA1c. This test is used to determine the patient's blood glucose for a period of approximately 60 days prior to the time of the test. Moreover, facility registries may track patient visits to follow up with patients who have not been seen in the past year.

Reporting and Follow-up for Diabetes Registries

A variety of reports may be developed from the diabetes registry. For facility-based registries, one report may keep up with laboratory monitoring of the patient's diabetes to allow intensive intervention with patients whose diabetes is not well controlled. Another report might be of patients who have not been tested within a year or who have not had a primary care provider visit within a year.

Population-based diabetes registries might provide reporting on the incidence of diabetes for the geographic area covered by the registry. Registry data also may be used to investigate risk factors for diabetes.

Follow-up is aimed primarily at ensuring that the diabetic is seen by the physician at appropriate intervals to prevent complications.

Implant Registries

An implant is a material or substance inserted in the body, such as breast implants, heart valves, and pacemakers. Implant registries have been developed for the purpose of tracking the performance of implants, including complications, deaths, and defects resulting from implants, as well as longevity.

In the recent past, the safety of implants has been questioned in a number of highly publicized cases. In some cases, implant registries have been developed in response to such events. For example, there have been questions about the safety of silicone breast implants and temporomandibular joint implants. When such cases arise, it has often been difficult to ensure that all patients with the implant have been notified of safety questions. At one time, there was a national implant registry, but it was halted after several years because of minimal participation (Shelton 2000). It was felt that the legal implications of problem implants have prevented more interest in implant registries.

A number of federal laws have been enacted to regulate medical devices, including implants. These devices were first covered under Section 15 of the Food, Drug and Cosmetic Act. The Safe Medical Devices Act of 1990 was passed and then amended through the Medical Device Amendments of 1995. These acts required facilities to report deaths and severe complications thought to be due to a device to the manufacturer and the **Food and Drug Administration** (FDA). Implant registries can help in complying with the legal requirement for reporting for the sample of facilities required to report.

Case Definition and Case Finding for Implant Registries

Implant registries sometimes include all types of implants but often are restricted to a specific type of implant such as cochlear, saline breast, or temporomandibular joint.

Data Collection for Implant Registries

Demographic data on patients receiving implants are included in the registry. The FDA requires that all reportable events involving medical devices include information on the following (CDRH 1996, p. 4):

- User facility report number
- Name and address of the device manufacturer
- Device brand name and common name
- Product model, catalog, and serial and lot number
- Brief description of the event reported to the manufacturer and/or the FDA
- Where the report was submitted (for example, to the FDA, manufacturer, or distributor)

Thus, these data items also should be included in the implant registry to facilitate reporting.

Reporting and Follow-up for Implant Registries

Data from the implant registry may be used to report to the FDA and the manufacturer when devices cause death or serious illness or injury. Follow-up is important to track the performance of the implant. When patients are tracked, they can be easily notified of product failures, recalls, or upgrades (Shelton 2000).

Transplant Registries

Transplant registries may have varied purposes. Some organ transplant registries maintain databases of patients who need organs. When an organ becomes available, a fair way then may be used to allocate the organ to the patient with the highest priority. In other cases, the purpose of the registry is to provide a database of potential donors for transplants using live donors, such as bone marrow transplants. Posttransplant information also is kept on organ recipients and donors.

Because transplant registries are used to try to match donor organs with recipients, they are often national or even international in scope. Examples of national registries include the Scientific Registry of the United Network for Organ Sharing (UNOS) and the registry of the National Marrow Donor Program (NMDP).

Data collected in the transplant registry also may be used for research, policy analysis, and quality control projects.

Case Definition and Case Finding for Transplant Registries

Physicians identify patients needing transplants. Information about the patient is provided to the registry. When an organ becomes available, information about it is matched with potential donors. For donor registries, donors are solicited through community information efforts similar to those carried out by blood banks to encourage blood donations.

Data Collection for Transplant Registries

The type of information collected varies according to the type of registry. Pretransplant data about the recipient include:

- Demographic data
- Patient's diagnosis
- Patient's status codes regarding medical urgency
- Patient's functional status
- Whether the patient is on life support
- Previous transplantations
- **Histocompatibility**

Information on donors varies according to whether the donor is living. For organs harvested from patients who have died, information is collected on:

- Cause and circumstances of the death
- Organ procurement and consent process
- Medications the donor was taking
- Other donor history

For a living donor, information includes:

- Relationship of the donor to the recipient (if any)
- Clinical information
- Information on organ recovery
- Histocompatibility

Reporting and Follow-up for Transplant Registries

Reporting includes information on donors and recipients as well as survival rates, length of time on the waiting list for an organ, and death rates. Follow-up information is collected for recipients as well as living donors. For living donors, the information collected might include complications of the procedure and length of stay (LOS) in the hospital. Follow-up on recipients includes information on status at the time of follow-up (for example, living, dead, lost to follow-up), functional status, graft status, and treatment, such as immunosuppressive drugs. Follow-up is carried out at intervals throughout the first year after the transplant and then annually after that.

Immunization Registries

Children are supposed to receive a large number of immunizations during the first six years of life. These immunizations are so important that the federal government has set several objectives related to immunizations in Healthy People 2010, a set of health goals for the nation. These include increasing the proportion of children and adolescents who are fully immunized (Objective 14–24) and increasing the proportion of children in population-based immunization registries (Objective 14–26).

Immunization registries usually have the purpose of increasing the number of infants and children who receive proper immunizations at the proper intervals. To accomplish this goal, they collect information within a particular geographic area on children and their immunization status. They also help by maintaining a central source of information for a particular child's immunization history, even when the child has received immunizations from a variety of providers. This central location for immunization data also relieves parents of the responsibility of maintaining immunization records for their own children.

Case Definition and Case Finding for Immunization Registries

All children in the population area served by the registry should be included in the registry. Some registries limit their inclusion of patients to those seen at public clinics, excluding those seen exclusively by private practitioners. Although children are usually targeted in immunization registries, some registries do include information on adults for influenza and pneumonia vaccines.

Children are often entered in the registry at birth. Registry personnel may review birth and death certificates and adoption records to determine what children to include and what children to exclude because they died after birth. In some cases, children are entered electronically through a connection with an electronic birth record system. Accuracy and completeness of the data in the registry are dependent on the thoroughness of the submitters in reporting immunizations.

Data Collection for Immunization Registries

The National Immunization Program at the CDC has worked with the **National Vaccine Advisory Committee** (NVAC) to develop a set of core immunization data elements to be included in all immunization registries. These data elements include (CDC 2005a):

- Patient's name (first, middle, and last)
- Patient's birth date
- Patient's sex
- Patient's birth state/country
- Mother's name (first, middle, last, and maiden)
- Vaccine type
- Vaccine manufacturer
- Vaccination date
- Vaccine lot number

Other items may be included, as needed, by the individual registry.

Reporting and Follow-up for Immunization Registries

Because the purpose of the immunization registry is to improve the number of children who receive immunizations in a timely manner, reporting should emphasize immunization rates, especially changes in rates in target areas. Immunization registries also can provide automatic reporting of children's immunization to schools to check the immunization status of their students.

Follow-up is directed toward reminding parents that it is time for immunizations as well as seeing whether the parents do not bring the child in for the immunization after a reminder. Reminders may include a letter or postcard or telephone calls. **Autodialing systems** may be used to call parents and deliver a prerecorded reminder. Moreover, registries must decide how frequently to follow up with parents who do not bring their children for immunization. Maintaining up-to-date addresses and telephone numbers is an important factor in providing follow-up. Registries may allow parents to opt out of the registry if they prefer not to be reminded.

Standards and Agencies for Approval of Immunization Registries

The CDC, through its National Immunization Program, provides funding for some population-based immunization registries. The CDC has identified 12 minimum functional standards for immunization registries (CDC 2005a), including:

- Electronically store data on all NVAC-approved core data elements.
- Establish a registry record within six weeks of birth for each newborn child born in the catchment area.
- Enable access to and retrieval of immunization information in the registry at the time of the encounter.
- Receive and process immunization information within one month of vaccine administration.
- Protect the confidentiality of healthcare information.
- Ensure the security of healthcare information.
- Exchange immunization records using Health Level Seven (HL7) standards.
- Automatically determine the routine childhood immunization(s) needed, in compliance with current ACIP (Advisory Committee on Immunization Practices) recommendations, when an individual presents for a scheduled immunization.
- Automatically identify individuals due/late for immunization(s) to enable the production of reminder/recall notifications.
- Automatically produce immunization coverage reports by providers, age groups, and geographic areas.
- Produce official immunization records.
- Promote the accuracy and completeness of registry data.

It has been proposed that CDC develop a certification program for immunization registries.

Other Registries

Registries may be developed for any type of disease or condition. Other types of registries that are commonly kept include HIV/AIDS and cardiac registries.

In addition, registries may be developed for administrative purposes. The National Provider Registry is an example of an administrative registry. Data collected for healthcare administrative purposes are discussed in the next subsection.

Instructions: Answer the following questions on a separate piece of paper.

1. What is the difference between an index and a registry?

2. How is case definition different from case finding?

3. What is the difference between a facility-based registry and a population-based registry?

Answer questions 4 through 10 for each of the following registries: cancer, trauma, birth defects, diabetes, implant, transplant, and immunization.

4. What methods are used for case definition and case finding?

5. What methods of data collection are used?

6. What methods of reporting are used?

7. What methods of follow-up are used?

8. What standards are applicable, and what agencies approve or accredit the registry?

9. What education is required for registrars?

10. What certification is available for registrars? What agency/organization provides certification? What are the certification requirements?

Healthcare Databases

Databases may be developed for a variety of purposes. The federal government, for example, has developed a wide variety of databases to enable it to carry out surveillance, improvement, and prevention duties. Health information managers may provide information for these databases through data abstraction or from data reported by a facility to state and local entities. They also may use these data to do research or work with other researchers on issues related to reimbursement and health status.

National and State Administrative Databases

Some databases are established for administrative rather than disease-oriented reasons. Data banks are developed, for example, for **claims** data submitted on Medicare. Other administrative databases assist in the **credentialing** and privileging of health practitioners.

Medicare Provider Analysis and Review File

The **Medicare Provider Analysis and Review** (MEDPAR) file is made up of acute care hospital and skilled nursing facility (SNF) claims data for all Medicare claims. It consists of the following types of data:

- Demographic data on the patient
- Data on the provider
- Information on Medicare coverage for the claim
- Total charges
- Charges broken down by specific types of services, such as operating room, physical therapy, and pharmacy charges
- ICD-9-CM diagnosis and procedure codes
- DRGs

The MEDPAR file is frequently used for research on topics such as charges for particular types of care and analysis by DRG. The limitation of the MEDPAR data for research purposes is that it only contains data about Medicare patients.

National Practitioner Data Bank

The **National Practitioner Data Bank** (NPDB) was mandated under the Health Care Quality Improvement Act of 1986 to provide a database of medical malpractice payments, sanctions taken by boards of medical examiners, and certain professional review actions (such as denial of medical staff privileges) taken by healthcare entities such as hospitals against physicians, dentists, and other healthcare providers. The problem that the NPDB was developed to alleviate was the lack of information on malpractice decisions, denial of medical staff privileges, or loss of medical license. Because these data were not widely available, physicians could move to another state or another facility and begin practicing again with the current state and/or facility unaware of the previous actions against the physician.

Information in the NPDB is provided through a required reporting mechanism. Entities making malpractice payments, including insurance companies, boards of medical examiners, and entities such as hospitals and professional societies must report to the NPDB. The information to be reported includes information on the practitioner, the reporting entity, and the judgment or settlement. Information on physicians must be reported, but information on other healthcare providers, though not mandatory, also will be accepted. Monetary penalties may be assessed for failure to report.

The law requires healthcare facilities to query the NPDB as part of the credentialing process when a physician initially applies for medical staff privileges and every two years thereafter.

Healthcare Integrity and Protection Data Bank

Part of the Health Insurance Portability and Accountability Act (HIPAA) of 1996 mandated the collection of information on healthcare fraud and abuse because there was no central place to obtain this information. As a result, the national **Healthcare Integrity and Protection Data Bank** (HIPDB) was developed. The types of items that must be reported to the data bank include reportable final adverse actions such as:

> Actions related to provider, supplier, and practitioner practices that are inconsistent with accepted sound fiscal, business or medical practices, directly or indirectly resulting in (OIG 1998, pp. 58341–58342):
>
> (1) unnecessary costs to the program;
>
> (2) improper payment;
>
> (3) services that fail to meet professionally recognized standards of care or that are medically unnecessary; or
>
> (4) adverse patient outcomes, failure to provide covered or needed care in violation of contractual arrangements, or delays in diagnosis or treatment.

These would include federal or state criminal convictions related to the delivery of healthcare, civil judgments related to the delivery of healthcare, exclusions from participation in federal or state healthcare programs such as Medicare and Medicaid, and other adjudicated actions or decisions. Civil judgments resulting in malpractice payments are not included because they are incorporated in the NPDB. There may be some overlap with the Healthcare Practitioner Data Bank, so a single report is made and then sorted to the appropriate data bank.

Information to be reported includes information on the healthcare provider, supplier, or practitioner that is the subject of the final adverse action, the nature of the act, and a description of the actions on which the decision was based. Only federal and state government agencies and health plans are required to report, and access to the data bank is limited to these organizations and to practitioners, providers, and suppliers who may only query about themselves.

States also frequently have health-related administrative databases. Many states, for example, collect either UHDDS or UB-92 data on patients discharged from hospitals located within their area. The Statewide Planning and Research Cooperative System (SPARCS) in New York state is an example of this type of administrative database. It combines UB-92 data with data required by the state of New York.

National, State, and County Public Health Databases

Public health is the area of healthcare dealing with the health of populations in geographic areas such as states or counties. One of the duties of public health agencies is the surveillance of health status within their jurisdiction.

Databases developed by public health departments provide information on the incidence and prevalence of diseases, possible high-risk populations, survival statistics, and trends over time. Data for these databases may be collected using a variety of methods including interviews, physical examination of individuals, and review of health records. At the national level, the National Center for Health Statistics (NCHS) has responsibility for these databases.

National Health Care Survey

One of the major national public health surveys is the **National Health Care Survey.** To a large extent, it relies on data from patient health records. It consists of a number of databases, including:

- The National Discharge Survey
- The National Ambulatory Medical Care Survey
- The National Nursing Home Survey
- The National Hospital Ambulatory Medical Care Survey
- The National Home and Hospice Care Survey

Table 12.2 lists the component databases of the National Health Care Survey, along with their corresponding data sources.

Data in the National Discharge Survey are abstracted manually from a sample of acute care hospitals or from discharged inpatient records or are obtained from state or other discharge databases. Items collected follow the Uniform Hospital Discharge Data Set (UHDDS), including demographic data, admission and discharge dates, and final diagnoses and procedures.

The National Ambulatory Medical Care Survey includes data collected by a sample of office-based physicians and their staffs from the records of patients seen in a one-week reporting period. Data included are demographic data, the patient's reason for visit, the diagnoses, diagnostic/screening services, therapeutic and preventive services, ambulatory surgical procedures, and medications/injections, in addition to information on the visit disposition and time spent with the physician.

The National Nursing Home Survey provides data on the facility, current residents, and discharged residents. Information is gathered through an interview process. The administrator or designee provides information about the facility. For information on the residents, the nursing staff member most familiar with the resident's care is interviewed. The staff member uses the resident's health record for reference

Table 12.2. National healthcare databases

Database	Type of Setting	Content	Data Source	Method of Data Collection
National Ambulatory Medical Care Survey	Office-based physician practice	Data on the patient and the visit	State discharge databases Office-based physician records	Abstract
National Nursing Home Survey	Nursing Home	Data on the facility and current and discharged residents	Administrator Nurse caregiver	Interview
National Hospital Ambulatory Medical Care Survey	Hospital Emergency Departments and Outpatient Clinics	Data on the patient, the visit, and the method of payment	Emergency Department and Outpatient Clinic Records	Abstract
National Home and Hospice Care Survey	Home Health and Hospice	Facility data and patient data	Administrator Caregiver	Interview
National Electronic Disease Surveillance System (NEDSS)	Public Health Departments	Possible bioterrorism incidents	Local and state public health departments	Electronic surveillance

in the interview. Data collected on the facility includes information on ownership, size, certification status, admissions, services, full-time equivalent employees, and basic charges. Both the current and discharged resident interviews provide demographic information on the resident as well as LOS, diagnoses, level of care received, **activities of daily living** (ADL), and charges.

Data for the National Hospital Ambulatory Medical Care Survey are collected on patient visits to hospital-based emergency departments and outpatient clinics. Information is obtained through an abstracting process from the patient health record. Different abstracting forms are used for the emergency department records and the outpatient clinics. The emergency department abstract includes demographic data on the patient, expected source of payment, how soon the patient should be seen, the patient's complaints or reason for visit, diagnoses, diagnostic/screening services, procedures, medications/injections, providers seen, and visit disposition. The outpatient department abstract includes similar information. Facility personnel do the abstracting.

For the National Home and Hospice Care Survey, data are collected on the home health or hospice agency as well as on its current and discharged patients. For the facility, data collected include the agency identifier, the number of current patients, type of ownership, certification status (for example, Medicare or Medicaid), number of staff, and services available. For current and discharged patients, data include patient demographic information, current living arrangements, source of referral, diagnoses, type of care received, primary caregiver, vision and hearing status, ADL, and expected sources of payment. Facility data are obtained through an interview with the administrator or designee. Patient information is obtained from the caregiver most familiar with the patient's care. The caregiver may use the patient's health record in answering the interview questions.

Because of the bioterrorism scares in recent years, the CDC is developing the National Electronic Disease Surveillance System (NEDSS). It will provide a national surveillance system by connecting the CDC with local and state public health partners. This integrated system will allow the CDC to monitor trends from disease reporting at the local and state level to look for possible bioterrorism incidents.

Other national public health databases include the National Health Interview Survey and the National Immunization Survey.

State and local public health departments also develop databases, as needed, to perform their duties of health surveillance, disease prevention, and research. An example of a state database is the infectious/notifiable disease database. Each state has a list of diseases that must be reported to the state, such as AIDS, measles, and syphilis, so that containment and prevention measures may be taken to avoid large outbreaks. As mentioned above, these state and local reporting systems will be connected with the CDC through NEDSS to evaluate trends in disease outbreaks. Statewide

databases/registries also may collect extensive information on particular diseases and conditions such as birth defects, immunization, and cancer registries.

Vital Statistics

Vital statistics include data on births, deaths, fetal deaths, marriages, and divorces. Responsibility for the collection of vital statistics rests with the states. The states share information with NCHS. The actual collection of the information is carried out at the local level. For example, birth certificates are completed at the facility where the birth occurred. They are then sent to the state. The state serves as the official repository for the certificates and provides vital statistics information to NCHS. From the vital statistics collected, states and the national government develop a variety of databases.

One vital statistics database at the national level is the Linked Birth and Infant Death Data Set. In this database, the information from birth certificates is compared to death certificates for infants under one year of age who die. This database provides data to conduct analyses for patterns of infant death. Other national programs that use vital statistics data include the National Maternal and Infant Health Survey, the National Mortality Followback Survey, the National Survey of Family Growth, and the National Death Index (CDC 2005b). In some of these databases, such as the National Maternal and Infant Health Survey and the National Mortality Followback Survey, additional information is collected on deaths originally identified through the vital statistics system.

Similar databases using vital statistics data as a basis are found at the state level. Birth defects registries, for example, frequently use vital records data with information on the birth defect as part of their data collection process.

Clinical Trials Databases

A **clinical trial** is a research project in which new treatments and tests are investigated to determine whether they are safe and effective. The trial proceeds according to a **protocol.** A protocol is the list of rules and procedures to be followed. Clinical trials databases have been developed to allow physicians and patients to find clinical trials. A patient with cancer or AIDS, for example, might be interested in participating in a clinical trial but not know how to locate one applicable to his or her type of disease. Clinical trials databases provide the data to enable patients and practitioners to determine what clinical trials are available and applicable to the patient.

The Food and Drug Administration Modernization Act of 1997 mandated that a clinical trials database be developed. The National Library of Medicine has developed the database, called ClinicalTrials.gov, which is available on the Internet for use by both patients and practitioners (NLM 2005). Information in the database includes:

- Study identification number
- Study sponsor

- Brief title
- Brief summary
- Location of trial
- Recruitment status
- Contact information
- Eligibility criteria
- Study type
- Study design
- Study phase
- Condition
- Intervention
- Data provider
- Date last modified

Each data element has been defined. For example, the study sponsor is the organization carrying out the clinical trial. The brief summary gives an overview of the treatments being studied and types of patients to be included. The location of the trial tells where the trial is being carried out so that patients can select trials in convenient locations. Recruitment status indicates whether subjects are currently being entered in the trial or will be in the future or whether the trial is closed to new subjects. Eligibility criteria include information on the type of condition to be studied, in some cases the stage of the disease, and what other treatments are allowed during the trial or must have been completed before entering the trial. Age is also a frequent eligibility criterion. Study types include diagnostic, genetic, monitoring, natural history, prevention, screening, supportive care, training, and treatment (McCray and Ide 2000, p. 316). Study design includes the research design being followed.

A clinical trial consists of four study phases. Phase I studies research the safety of the treatment in a small group of people. In phase II studies, emphasis is on determining the treatment's effectiveness and further investigating safety. Phase III studies look at effectiveness and side effects and make comparisons to other available treatments in larger populations. Phase IV studies look at the treatment after it has entered the market.

Some clinical trials databases concentrate on a particular disease. The Department of Health and Human Services, for example, has developed ACTIS, the AIDS Clinical Trials Information Service. The National Cancer Institute sponsors PDQ (Physician Data Query), a database for cancer clinical trials. These databases contain information similar to ClinicalTrials.gov.

Although ClinicalTrials.gov has been set up for use by both patients and health practitioners, some databases are more oriented to practitioners. Moreover, some efforts have been made to develop databases of published articles and proceedings from meetings on the subject of clinical trials. The Cochrane Central Register of Controlled Trials, for example, is a bibliographic database of literature on clinical trials developed by the Cochrane Library, an electronic library.

Health Services Research Databases

Health services research is research concerning healthcare delivery systems, including organization and delivery and care effectiveness and efficiency. Within the federal government, the organization most involved in health services research is the **Agency for Healthcare Research and Quality** (AHRQ). AHRQ looks at issues related to the efficiency and effectiveness of the healthcare delivery system, disease protocols, and guidelines for improved disease outcomes.

A major initiative for AHRQ has been the Healthcare Cost and Utilization Project (HCUP). HCUP uses data collected at the state level from either claims data from the UB-92 or discharge-abstracted data, including UHDDS items reported by individual hospitals and, in some cases, by freestanding ambulatory care centers. Which data are reported depends on the individual state. Data may be reported by the facilities to a state agency or to the state hospital association, depending on state regulations. The data are then reported from the state to AHRQ where they become part of the HCUP databases.

HCUP consists of a set of databases, including:

- The Nationwide Inpatient Sample (NIS), which consists of inpatient discharge data from a sample of approximately 1,000 hospitals throughout the United States
- The State Inpatient Database (SID), which includes data collected by states on hospital discharges
- The State Ambulatory Surgery Database (SASD), which includes information from a sample of states on hospital-affiliated ASCs and, from some states, data from freestanding surgery centers
- The Kids Inpatient Database (KID), which is made up of inpatient discharge data on children younger than 19 years old

These databases are unique because they include data on inpatients whose care is paid for by all types of payers including Medicare, Medicaid, and private insurance as well as by self-paying and/or uninsured patients. Data elements include demographic information, information on diagnoses and procedures, admission and discharge status, payment sources, total charges, LOS, and information on the hospital or freestanding ambulatory surgery center. Researchers may use these databases to look at issues such as those related to the costs of treating particular diseases, the extent to which treatments are used, and differences in outcomes and cost for alternative treatments.

National Library of Medicine

The National Library of Medicine produces two databases of special interest to the HIM professional: MEDLINE and UMLS.

Medical Literature, Analysis, and Retrieval System Online

Medical Literature, Analysis, and Retrieval System Online (MEDLINE) is the best-known database from the

National Library of Medicine. It includes bibliographic listings for publications in the areas of medicine, dentistry, nursing, pharmacy, allied health, and veterinary medicine. HIM professionals use MEDLINE to locate articles on HIM issues as well as articles on medical topics necessary to carry out quality improvement and medical research activities.

Unified Medical Language System

The **Unified Medical Language System** (UMLS) provides a way to integrate biomedical concepts from a variety of sources to show their relationships. This process allows links to be made between different information systems for purposes such as the electronic health record. UMLS is of particular interest to the HIM professional because medical classifications such as ICD-9-CM, CPT, and HCPCS (Healthcare Common Procedure Coding System) are among the items included. UMLS is covered extensively in chapter 13.

Check Your Understanding 12.4

Instructions: Answer the following questions on a separate piece of paper.

1. What information is included in the Medicare Provider Analysis and Review File?

2. What limitations are encountered when using MEDPAR data in research?

3. Why was the National Practitioner Data Bank developed? What law requires its use? Why was the Healthcare Integrity and Protection Data Bank developed? What law requires its use?

4. What types of information must be reported to the National Practitioner Data Bank and the Healthcare Integrity and Protection Data Bank? Do the two data banks overlap in any way?

5. How do healthcare organizations use the NPDB? Who may use the Healthcare Integrity and Protection Data Bank?

6. How can the health information manager contribute to public health databases?

7. Which of the eight National Health Care Survey databases use data from health records?

8. What is a clinical trial? Why are clinical trials databases developed? Which law mandated development of a national clinical trials database?

9. What is the source of data for the Healthcare Cost and Utilization Project?

10. Why is UMLS of interest to HIM professionals?

Processing and Maintenance of Secondary Databases

Several issues surround the processing and maintenance of secondary databases. HIM professionals are often involved in decisions concerning these issues.

Manual versus Automated Methods of Data Collection

Although registries and databases are almost universally computerized, data collection is commonly done manually. The most frequent method is **abstracting.** Abstracting is the process of reviewing the patient health record and entering the required data elements into the database. In some cases, the abstracting may initially be done on an abstract form. The data then would be entered into the database from the form. In many cases, it is done directly from the primary patient health record into a data collection screen in the computerized database system.

Not all data collection is done manually. In some cases, data can be downloaded directly from other electronic systems. Birth defects registries, for example, often download information on births and birth defects from the vital records system. In some cases, providers such as hospitals and physicians send information in electronic format to the registry or database. The National Discharge Survey from the National Center for Health Statistics uses information in electronic format from state databases.

Vendor Systems versus Facility-Specific Systems

A **vendor system** is an information system (IS) developed by an outside company and sold to a variety of organizations. A **facility-specific system** is an IS developed within the facility for its own use.

One clear advantage to using vendor systems is that they have been used at a variety of sites. Thus, the vendor likely has developed expertise in the system based on past experience. When investigating possible systems, purchasers can find out about the performance of vendor systems from other users. As changes in healthcare occur, such as the HIPAA privacy and security regulations, it is often easier for a vendor to make the necessary changes because its entire business is related to a limited number of products. In addition, **user groups** are often developed from organizations that have purchased the system and can be helpful in maximizing its performance.

One disadvantage to a vendor system is that the vendor may be unable to modify it to meet all the organization's needs. Moreover, the level of training and problem-solving support varies from vendor to vendor. In some cases, vendors are unavailable to help with system problems after the initial start-up period.

One advantage to a facility-specific system is that it can be developed to meet the specific information needs of the healthcare facility. Because the system's developers are on-site, training and problem solving are always available.

However, if the system is not well documented when it is developed, it will be difficult to sustain maintenance in the event the original developers leave the facility. Moreover, in-house developers may not have the broad experience in the type of product developed that a vendor is likely to have. The ability of facility personnel to undertake system development and maintenance should be considered very carefully before deciding to develop a system in house.

Data Quality Issues

Indexes, registries, and databases are only helpful when the data they contain are accurate. Decisions concerning new treatment methods, healthcare policy, and physician credentialing and privileging are made based on these databases. Incorrect data will likely result in serious errors in decision making.

Several factors must be addressed when assessing data quality, including data validity, reliability, completeness, and timeliness.

Validity of the Data

Validity refers to the accuracy of the data. For example, in a cancer registry, the stage of the neoplasm must be recorded accurately because statistical information on survival rates by stage is commonly reported.

Several methods may be used to ensure validity. One method is to incorporate **edits** in the database. An edit is a check on the accuracy of the data, such as setting data types. When a particular data element, such as admission date, is set up with a data type of date, the computer will not allow other types of data, such as name, to be entered in that field. Other edits may use comparisons between fields to ensure accuracy. For example, an edit might check to see that all patients with the diagnosis of prostate cancer are listed as males in the database.

Reliability of the Data

Another factor to be considered in looking at data quality is reliability. Reliability refers to the consistency of the data. For example, all patients in a trauma registry with the same level, severity, and site of injury should have the same Abbreviated Injury Scale. Reliability is frequently checked by having more than one person abstract data for the same case. The results are then compared to identify any discrepancies. This is called an **interrater reliability** method of checking. Several different people may be used to do the checking, for example, a supervisor within the area. In the cancer registry, physician members of the cancer committee are called on to check the reliability of the data.

The use of uniform terminology is an important way to improve data reliability. This has been evident in case definition for registries. The criteria for including a patient in a registry must have a clear definition. Definitions for terms such as race, for example, must include the categories to be used in determining race. When uniform terms are not used, the data will not be consistent. Also, it will be impossible to make comparisons between systems when uniform terms have not been used for all data. A data dictionary in which all data elements are defined helps ensure that uniform data definitions are being followed. An example would be the term *discharge time*. Discharge time could be the time the physician writes the discharge order, the time the information about the discharge is entered into the ADT system, or the time the patient leaves the floor. The data dictionary could define it as the time the information is entered in the ADT system, and then everyone recording discharge time would be using the same time for that data element.

Completeness of the Data

Completeness is another factor to be considered in data quality. Missing data may prevent the database from being useful for research or clinical decision making. To avoid missing data, some databases will not allow the user to move to the next field without making an entry in the current one, especially for fields considered crucial. Looking at a variety of sources in case finding is a way to avoid omitting patients who should be included in a registry.

Timeliness of the Data

Another concept important in data quality is timeliness. Data must be available within a time frame helpful to the user. Factors that influence decisions may change over time, so it is important that the data reflect up-to-date information.

Data Security and Confidentiality Issues

Data security usually refers to efforts to control access to health information. **Data confidentiality** usually refers to efforts to guarantee the privacy of personal health information. When looking at data security and confidentiality issues, it is important to consider the HIPAA regulations for privacy and security. Under HIPAA, the data collection done by registries is considered part of "healthcare operations." The patient does not, therefore, have to sign an authorization for release of protected health information (PHI) to the registry. Reporting of notifiable diseases to the state comes under "required reporting" and does not require patient authorization for release. (Handling Cancer Registry Requests 2003, p. 7) Release of information to requestors other than the state will depend on the requestor. Data may be released to internal users, such as physicians for research, without the patient's consent as well because research also comes under healthcare operations. External users, such as the American College of Surgeons, collect aggregate data from facilities, so individual patient authorization is not required.

HIPAA security regulations also apply to data in registries and indexes. These regulations require policies in the areas of administrative, technical, and physical security, which are discussed below. (See chapter 10 for further discussion of privacy, security, and confidentiality.)

Data Security

A number of methods may be used to ensure that only authorized people have access to patient data in the facility's computer system. An example of HIPAA security requirements in the administrative area include policies regarding access control. One common method is the use of passwords. Other methods may involve using retinal scans or fingerprints. Tokens such as identification badges also may be used.

Moreover, the facility may establish levels of access to the computer system. In this case, each user would be allowed access to only certain parts of the system. Only those parts of the system to which the users have access appear on the screen. In addition, a record of all transactions in the system, called an **audit trail,** should be maintained and reviewed for instances of unauthorized access.

Loss of data is another important consideration in data security. Although data sometimes are lost as a result of unauthorized access, more often they are lost in more routine ways. For example, a computer malfunction can cause data to be erased or lost. Backing up the data on electronic media such as tapes or disks is commonly done to avoid such losses. The backup must be done frequently, and the backup media must be kept away from the site where the main system is kept. When the backup is kept on site, it is vulnerable to the same destruction affecting the main system from sources such as fire and flood.

Computer viruses constitute yet another threat to data security. These are computer programs that attack systems and reproduce themselves. They may alter or destroy data. Facilities must use antivirus software to combat viruses. Moreover, they must keep the antivirus software up-to-date because new viruses appear regularly.

Physical security of the system is a consideration that is required under the HIPAA security regulations. Computer terminals must be kept in areas that are not physically accessible to unauthorized people. Reports and printouts from the system should not be left where they can be seen. When they are no longer needed, they should be destroyed.

Technical security under HIPAA involves issues such as whether sensitive data need to be encrypted. **Encryption** is a method of scrambling data so that they cannot be read without first being decoded. An AIDS registry, for example, might want to use an encryption method to protect patient-identifiable information.

Data Confidentiality

Maintaining the confidentiality of health data is a traditional role of HIM professionals. When looking at methods to protect secondary records, patient-specific information requires more control than aggregate data because individual patients cannot be identified in aggregate data. Policies on who may access the data provide the basic protection for confidentiality.

The type of data maintained also may affect policies on confidentiality. For many of the government databases discussed earlier, the information is aggregate and the data are readily available to any interested users. For example, public health data are frequently published in many formats, including printed reports, Internet access, and direct computer access.

As is true of all employees working with patient data, employees working with data in indexes, registries, and databases should receive training on confidentiality. Further, they should be required to sign a yearly statement indicating that they have received the training and understand the implications of failure to maintain confidentiality of the data.

Trends in the Collection of Secondary Data

The most significant trend in collecting secondary data is the increased use of automated data entry. Registries and data-bases are more commonly using data already available in electronic form rather than manually abstracting all data. As the computerized health record becomes more common, separate databases for various diseases and conditions such as cancer, diabetes, and trauma will become unnecessary. The patient health record itself will be a database that can be queried for information currently obtained from specialized registries.

Check Your Understanding 12.5

Instructions: Answer the following questions on a separate piece of paper.

1. What factors must be considered when determining the quality of data?
2. Which errors in registries and other secondary databases can cause serious problems?
3. What methods and systems can be used to ensure the quality of secondary healthcare data?
4. What is the difference between security and confidentiality?
5. What methods might be used to control access to a health information system?
6. How can a potential loss of data be avoided?
7. Which factors should be considered when developing a physical security program?
8. What types of data should be encrypted?
9. What methods can be used to ensure data confidentiality?
10. What trends are evident in the collection of secondary data?

Real-World Case

In an article entitled "Benchmarking with National ICD-9-CM Coded Data," Carol Osborn (1999, p. 59) stated that:

> As HIM professionals, we want to be assured that we are providing the highest quality data for reimbursement and research and research purposes. We can review coded data internally, but this does not give us a clear picture of the total information that is being submitted to the Health Care Financing Administration (HCFA) [now called the Centers for Medicare and Medicaid Services, CMS]. . . . Recently a new tool has come out that helps HIM professionals evaluate the quality of coded data. This tool, *DRG Resource Book: Data for Benchmarking and Analysis,* is published by the Center for Health-care Industry Performance Studies in Columbus, OH. The book contains comparative information for the top 50 medical and the top 25 surgical DRGs for the Medicare population, so HIM professionals can compare their coded data to a national database. The source of this information is the HCFA Medicare Provider and Review File (MEDPAR file) for the federal fiscal year 1995, which consists of data compiled from UB-92 data submitted by hospitals for inpatient Medicare discharges.

This resource reports DRG summary information, cost analysis information, state-specific profiles of charges per discharge and by department, utilization and quality indicators, and clinical coding analysis—all by DRG. This article [analyzes] the ICD-9-CM codes reported for the top 75 medical and surgical DRGs.

Summary

Health records contain extensive information about individual patients but are difficult to use when attempting to perceive trends in care or quality. For that reason, secondary records were developed. One type of secondary record is the index. An index is a report from a database that provides information on patients and supports retrieval by diagnosis, procedure, or physician. Health information management departments routinely produce indexes.

Disease registries are developed when extensive information is needed about specific diagnoses, procedures, or conditions. They are commonly used for research and to improve patient care and health status. From the database created through the data collection process, reports can be developed to answer questions regarding patient care or issues such as rates of immunization and birth defects. In some cases, patient follow-up is done to assess survival rates and quality of life after a disease or accident.

HIM professionals perform a variety of roles in relation to registries. In some cases, they work on setting up the registry. Moreover, they may work in data collection and management of registry functions. HIM professionals are well suited to such positions because of their background and education in management, health record content, regulatory and legal compliance, and medical science and terminology.

Today, organizations and institutions of all types commonly maintain databases pertaining to healthcare. At the federal level, some administrative databases provide data and information for decisions regarding claims and practitioner credentialing. Other databases focus on the public health area, using data collected at the local level and shared with states and the federal government. These databases assist in government surveillance of health status in the United States. Some databases, such as the clinical trials database, are mandated by law and help patients and providers locate clinical trials regardless of source or location.

Registries and databases raise a number of managerial issues. Data collection is often time-consuming, so some databases now use automated entry methods. In addition, decisions must be made between vendor and facility-specific products. Finally, the quality of the data is an important issue because the decisions made based on data in registries and databases depend on the data's validity, reliability, accuracy, and timeliness.

Another important issue related to registries and databases is data security. Facilities must adopt methods that will ensure controlled access to data as well as prevent the loss of data. Confidentiality is always of concern to the HIM professional, and steps must be taken to protect it.

In the future, separate registries and databases may become less common with the advent of the computer-based patient record. Essentially a large database, the electronic health record can be queried directly rather than having to first abstract data from the primary record into a secondary record.

References

American College of Surgeons. 2005a. Commission on cancer. Available online from facs.org/cancer/.

American College of Surgeons. 2005b. Trauma programs. Available online from facs.org/trauma/index.html.

American Joint Committee on Cancer. 2005. cancerstaging.org.

Center for Devices and Radiological Health. 1996. Medical device reporting for user facilities. Available online from fda.gov/cdrh/mdruf.pdf.

Centers for Disease Control. 2005a. National immunization program. Available online from cdc.gov/nip/registry/min-funct-stds2001.htm#1.

Centers for Disease Control. 2005b. National Center for Health Statistics. Available online from cdc.gov/nchs/nvss.htm.

Garthe, E. 1997. Overview of trauma registries in the United States. *Journal of American Health Information Management Association* 68(7):26,28,30–31.

Handling cancer registry requests for information. 2003. *In Confidence* 11(8):7.

McCray, A., and N.C. Ide. 2000. Design and implementation of a national clinical trials registry. *Journal of the American Medical Informatics Association* 7(3):313–23.

National Cancer Registrars Association. 2005. ncra-usa.org.

National Library of Medicine. 2005. clinicaltrials.gov.

Office of Inspector General. 1998. Health Care Fraud and Abuse Data Collection Program: Reporting of Final Adverse Actions, Notice of proposed rulemaking. *Federal Register* 63(210):58341–58342.

Osborn, C.E. 1999. Benchmarking with national ICD-9-CM coded data. *Journal of American Health Information Management Association* 70(4):59–69.

Ringer, D., and W. Cain. 2004. COC revises cancer standards, creates FORDS. *Advance for Health Information Professionals.* Available online from health-information.advanceweb.com/common/EditorialSearch/AViewer.aspx?CC=28947

Shelton, D.L. 2000. Retrieved implants could be a source of important data. *American Medical News* 43(6).

Trauma.org. 2005.

Chapter 13
Clinical Classifications and Terminologies

*Matthew J. Greene, RHIA, CCS,
and Susan H. Fenton, MBA, RHIA*

Learning Objectives

- To differentiate among, and to identify the correct uses of, classifications, nomenclatures, and terminologies
- To discuss the strengths and weaknesses of the classification systems currently required in the United States
- To differentiate between encoding and automated coding and to describe how each can be used in the coding process
- To discuss emerging healthcare terminologies
- To identify data retrieval needs and to select a terminology most likely to meet them
- To understand the need for a terminology in a computer-based patient record

Key Terms

ABC Codes
Alliance Standards Directory
Ambulatory Payment Classification (APC)
American National Standards Institute (ANSI)
American Nurses Association (ANA)
American Society for Testing and Materials (ASTM)
Breast Imaging Reporting and Data System Atlas (BI-RADS)
Center for Drug Evaluation and Research Data Standards (CDER) Manual
Clinical Care Classification (CCC)
Clinical Document Architecture (CDA)
Clinical Special Product Label (SPL)
Coding
Connecting For Health
Consolidated Health Informatics (CHI)
Context
Current Dental Terminology (CDT)
Diagnosis-Related Groups (DRG)
Digital Imaging and Communications in Medicine (DICOM)
EHR Collaborative

Encoder
Environmental Protection Agency (EPA) Substance Registry System (SRS)
Established Name for Active Ingredients and FDA Unique Ingredient Identifier (UNII) Codes
Food and Drug Administration (FDA)
Galen Common Reference Model (CRM)
Global Medical Device Nomenclature (GMDN)
Grouper
Health Information Standards Board (HISB)
Health Level Seven (HL7)
Human Genome Nomenclature (HUGN)
Institute of Electrical and Electronics Engineers (IEEE) 1073
Institute of Medicine (IOM)
International Classification of Diseases for Oncology (ICD-O)
International Classification on Functioning, Disability, and Health (ICF)
International Classification for Nursing Practice (ICNP)
International Classification of Primary Care (ICPC-2)
Lexicon

Logical Observation Identifier Names and Codes (LOINC)
Medical Subject Headings (MeSH)
National Alliance for Health Information Technology (NAHIT)
National Cancer Institute (NCI) Thesaurus
National Council for Prescription Drug Programs (NCPDP)
National Committee on Vital and Health Statistics (NCVHS)
National Drug Codes (NDC)
National Drug Code (NDC) Directory
National Drug File–Reference Terminology (NDF-RT)
National Library of Medicine (NLM)
Nomenclature
North American Nursing Diagnosis Association (NANDA II)
Nosology
Nursing Information and Data Set Evaluation Center (NIDSEC)
Nursing Interventions Classification (NIC)
Nursing Management Minimum Data Set (NMMDS)

Nursing Minimum Data Set (NMDS)
Nursing Outcomes Classification (NOC)
Omaha System
Patient Care Data Set (PCDS)
President's E-Gov Initiative
President's Information Technology Advisory Committee (PITAC)
Public Health Informatics Institute (PHII)
Reference terminology
Relationship
Semantic Clinical Drug (SCD) of RxNorm
Systemized Nomenclature of Medicine (SNOMED)
Systemized Nomenclature of Medicine Clinical Terms (SNOMED CT)
Systemized Nomenclature of Medicine Reference Terminology (SNOMED RT)
Terminology
UMLS Metathesaurus
UMLS Semantic Network
UMLS SPECIALIST Lexicon
Unified Medical Language System (UMLS)
Universal Medical Device Nomenclature System (UMDNS)
Vocabulary

Introduction

Healthcare is faced with many challenges, including an aging population, the need to conserve resources, medical knowledge that is increasing exponentially, and a consumer population with Internet access. To meet these challenges, healthcare organizations must have the ability to operate effectively and efficiently using the latest medical data and knowledge. Unfortunately, the healthcare industry in the United States has yet to agree on a common terminology that would allow healthcare facilities and practitioners throughout the country to exchange and use information reliably.

It is difficult to believe that the quest to classify morbidity and mortality is quite old. London parishes first began to keep death records in 1532. In 1662, John Graunt, a merchant, wrote *Natural and Political Observations . . . Made upon the Bills of Mortality.* His friend, Sir William Petty, was able to extrapolate from mortality rates an estimate of community economic loss caused by deaths. Two hundred years later, Florence Nightingale, in *Notes on a Hospital,* wrote, "In attempting to arrive at the truth, I have applied everywhere for information, but in scarcely an instance have I been able to obtain hospital records fit for any purposes of comparison. If they could be obtained . . . they would show subscribers how their money was being spent, what amount of good was really being done with it, or whether the money was not doing mischief rather than good" (Barnett et al. 1993, p. 1046).

Many of the same issues remain in healthcare today. It is vitally important to be able to compare data for outcomes measurement, quality assurance, resource utilization, best practices, and medical research. These tasks can be accomplished only when healthcare has a common terminology that is easily integrated into the computer-based patient record.

This chapter examines the history and current practices of classification in the healthcare industry. It also considers various emerging terminologies and the desired characteristics of a terminology.

Theory into Practice

Dr. French walks into his clinic in the morning and activates his personal digital assistant (PDA). It immediately connects to the organizational database via wireless technology and downloads all of his appointments for the day, as well as e-mail and other items requiring his attention. His schedule shows that his first appointment is a clinic patient. After accessing the organizational computer-based patient record (CPR), he downloads the patient information and begins reviewing it. As he reads, he has a question about one of the patient's conditions. He indicates on the screen that he would like more information on the specified condition, and within two minutes, the latest relevant abstracts have been downloaded into his PDA. Upon review, he finds an article that will answer his questions and downloads it.

When Dr. French meets with the patient, he recommends a particular course of treatment. The patient's first question is "How have other patients responded to this treatment?" Using recently developed software, Dr. French searches many healthcare organization databases to determine how patients with similar characteristics have responded to the recommended treatment and shares his findings with the patient. This gives the patient the information he needs to make an informed decision.

As Dr. French finishes documenting the patient's condition and the agreed-upon treatment, the administrative components of the system analyze the documentation. If necessary, it alerts Dr. French to any required components that may be missing or ambiguous. If the documentation is determined to be complete, the appropriate billing codes are assigned and the required data are instantly transmitted to the third-party payer.

Development of Classifications Systems for Healthcare Data

As the discussion of classification systems for healthcare data begins, it is important to have a common understanding of how classifications, nomenclatures, and terminologies are defined. Unfortunately, it is difficult to get complete agreement in even this area. The most widely accepted terminology standard is the International Standards Organization (ISO) Standard 1087 (Terminology-Vocabulary) (Hammond and Cimino 2000, p. 224). AHIMA's Coding Policy and Strategy Committee has defined the entity classification (AHIMA 1999, p. 72). Its definition is essentially equivalent to the ISO's definition of a **nomenclature:** a system of clinical terms of preferred terminology.

AHIMA's Coding Policy and Strategy Committee also defines a clinical **vocabulary** as a list or collection of clinical words or phrases with their meanings. In the committee's opinion, a clinical **terminology** provides for the proper use of clinical words as names or symbols. The committee equated a clinical terminology with a nomenclature (AHIMA 1999, p. 72). It is important to recognize that this problem of multiple definitions and names is endemic in the field of healthcare terminology. Standardized terms can be efficiently mapped to broader classifications for administrative, regulatory, oversight, and fiscal requirements (Chute 2000, p. 301).

Because all these definitions can be confusing, the illustration in figure 13.1 may be helpful. The terms *classification* and *nomenclature* are often used interchangeably. Chute (2000, p. 298) stated, "classifications and nomenclatures can be more helpfully regarded as lying along a continuum, where the first categorizes and aggregates while the second supports detailed descriptions." Further down from the apex of the pyramid is a terminology, which is the whole set of terms representing the system of concepts of a particular subject field. So, while a classification or nomenclature categorizes and aggregates, a terminology represents the whole of

Figure 13.1.   Comparative level of detail in nomenclatures, terminologies, and languages

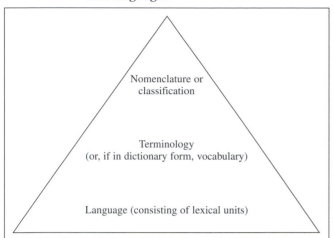

a subject field. The pyramid in figure 13.1 illustrates how a nomenclature can be less specific than a terminology, which is less specific than a language.

Check Your Understanding 13.1

Instructions: Answer the following questions on a separate piece of paper.

1. What are the general functions of classifications and nomenclatures? Give examples of each.

2. What is one of the most significant problems in the field of healthcare terminology and vocabulary standards today? Explain the problem's significance.

Current Systems of Classification and Nomenclature

Systems for classifying diseases have progressed through various stages since the first classification system was developed in the late 19th century. The following sections describe past, current, and near-future developments.

International Classification of Diseases

The International Classification of Diseases began as the Bertillon Classification of Diseases in 1893. In 1900, the French government convened an international meeting to update the Bertillon classification to the International List of Causes of Death. The goal was to develop a common system for describing the causes of mortality. The latest version of the International Classification of Diseases is the 10th edition (ICD-10), which was released in 1992. According to the Centers for Disease Control (CDC), the current purpose of ICD-10 is to promote international comparability in the collection, classification, processing, and presentation of mortality statistics.

In 1999, the United States began using ICD-10 to report mortality statistics under its agreement with the World Health

Organization (WHO). The U.S. Department of Health and Human Services (HHS) reports that WHO currently has no plans to issue an ICD-11. WHO has established a procedure for updating ICD-10 regularly. The National Center for Health Statistics (NCHS) is the WHO Collaborating Center for the Classification of Diseases for North America.

International Classification of Diseases, Ninth Edition, Clinical Modification

Developed by the NCHS, the International Classification of Diseases, Ninth Revision, Clinical Modification (ICD-9-CM) is a derivative work of the International Classification of Diseases, Ninth Revision, as developed by the WHO. ICD-9-CM is used in the United States only to code and classify diagnoses from inpatient and outpatient records, as well as inpatient procedures. Although diagnostic and procedural coding were the original functions of the system, ICD-9-CM also has been used to communicate provider reimbursement information on healthcare services since 1983. Today, coding for reimbursement is a vital part of healthcare operations. The official ICD-9-CM coding guidelines are published quarterly in Coding Clinic for ICD-9-CM by the Central Office on ICD-9-CM Coding of the American Hospital Association.

Changes and updates to ICD-9-CM are managed by the ICD-9-CM Coordination and Maintenance Committee, a federal committee co-chaired by representatives from the NCHS and the Centers for Medicare and Medicaid Services, or CMS. The NCHS is responsible for volumes 1 and 2 (diagnoses), and the CMS is responsible for volume 3 (procedures). Both the public and private sectors are invited to make suggestions for modifications to ICD-9-CM, and meetings are open to the public. Modifications are implemented on April 1 and October 1 of each year. Figure 13.2 (p. 308) is an example of a section of an entry in the Tabular Listing of Diseases (ICD-9-CM, volume 1).

International Classification of Diseases, 10th Revision, Clinical Modification

As with ICD-9, the U.S. government modified ICD-10 for the reporting of morbidity data. Between December 1997 and February 1998, the NCHS posted a draft of the ICD-10-CM Tabular List of Diseases on its Web site for public comment. Public comments were received, and the revised ICD-10-CM was rereleased in June 2003. The revised version can be downloaded from the NCHS Web site, cdc. gov.

ICD-10-CM contains substantial increases in content over ICD-9-CM. Improvements in the content and format of the draft include:

- Additional information relevant to ambulatory and managed care encounters
- Expanded injury codes
- New combination diagnosis/symptom codes to reduce the number of codes needed to fully describe a condition

- New six-digit codes
- Additional four- and five-digit subclassification codes
- Laterality (right and left)
- Greater specificity in code assignment

As of this writing, there is no anticipated implementation date for ICD-10-CM. Implementation will be based upon the process for adoption of standards under the HIPAA Act of

Figure 13.2.   Example of Volume 1 ICD-9-CM entry

TUBERCULOSIS (010–018)

Includes: infection by Mycobacterium tuberculosis (human) (bovine)

Excludes: | *congenital tuberculosis (771.2)*
late effects of tuberculosis (137.0–137.4)

The following fifth-digit subclassification is for use with categories 010–018:

0   unspecified
1   bacteriological or histological examination not done
2   bacteriological or histological examination unknown (at present)
3   tubercle bacilli found (in sputum) by microscopy
4   tubercle bacilli not found (in sputum) by microscopy, but found by bacterial culture
5   tubercle bacilli not found by bacteriological examination, but tuberculosis confirmed histologically
6   tubercle bacilli not found by bacteriological or histological examination but tuberculosis confirmed by other methods [inoculation of animals]

§ 010   Primary tuberculous infection
  010.0   Primary tuberculous infection

  Excludes: | *nonspecific reaction to tuberculin skin test without active tuberculosis (795.5)*
  positive:
  PPD (795.5)
  tuberculin skin test without active tuberculosis (795.5)

  010.1   Tuberculous pleurisy in primary progressive tuberculosis
  010.8   Other primary progressive tuberculosis

  Excludes: | *tuberculous erythema nodosum (017.1)*

  010.9   Primary tuberculous infection, unspecified
§ 011   Pulmonary tuberculosis
    Use additional code to identify any associated silicosis (502)
  011.0   Tuberculosis of lung, infiltrative
  011.1   Tuberculosis of lung, nodular
  011.2   Tuberculosis of lung with cavitation
  011.3   Tuberculosis of bronchus

  Excludes: | *isolated bronchial tuberculosis (012.2)*

  011.4   Tuberculous fibrosis of lung
  011.5   Tuberculous bronchiectasis
  011.6   Tuberculous pneumonia [any form]
  011.7   Tuberculous pneumothorax
  011.8   Other specified pulmonary tuberculosis
  011.9   Pulmonary tuberculosis, unspecified
    Respiratory tuberculosis NOS
    Tuberculosis of lung NOS

§ Requires fifth-digit. See codes and definitions.

1996. If and when the final notice for implementing ICD-10-CM is published in the Federal Register, there will be a two-year implementation window (NCVHS 2003).

ICD-10-CM Field Test Study
AHIMA and the American Hospital Association (AHA) collaborated on an ICD-10-CM Field Testing Project in 2003. There were a number of reasons why this test was conducted:

- ICD-9-CM outdated and obsolete
- ICD-9-CM unable to accommodate advances in technology and medical knowledge
- Increasing pressure to implement ICD-10
- Greater specificity required in reporting conditions and procedures

The goal of this project was to assess the functionality of ICD-10-CM and its ability to describe conditions better than ICD-9-CM. Volunteers with adequate coding knowledge and experience with ICD-9-CM were recruited to code 50 records using both ICD-9-CM and ICD-10-CM. Procedures were not included in this study. Volunteers selected for the study were required to undergo several hours of training in regards to ICD-10-CM coding guidelines and how to use the reporting tool developed by the Ohio State University. After training, the volunteers were advised to select 50 medical records from various care settings to code. They were then required to submit the codes from both systems, the amount of time required to code each case in both systems, and any difficulties that they experienced with the ICD-10-CM system. This information was tallied by the Ohio State University and AHIMA. The findings included the following key observations:

- Clinical descriptors were found to be 71.7 percent better in ICD-10-CM than ICD-9-CM
- 76.3 percent of the respondents reported that ICD-10-CM was an improvement over ICD-9-CM
- 78.6 percent of the respondents suggested that ICD-10-CM should be implemented for coding conditions in three years or less
- 60 percent of the respondents recommended that coders would require 16 hours or less of training before using ICD-10-CM
- Over 50 percent of the respondents reported that there was no time differences required to code in both systems
- The respondents also reported that coding in ICD-10-CM may require less time if adequate coding tools and training are provided and when the coders become familiar with ICD-10-CM
- No significant change in documentation practices by clinicians will be required

See table 13.1 for a comparison of ICD-9-CM and ICD-10-PCS using the NCVHS characteristics.

The study participants were also requested to submit ideas for making ICD-10-CM better. They noted:

151 diagnoses were identified that could not be coded because there was insufficient documentation, the diagnoses were not indexed under expected main terms or subterms, and no concept existed in ICD-10-CM.

The report findings were submitted to the **National Committee on Vital and Health Statistics** (NCVHS) for review and evaluation (AHIMA and AHA 2003).

International Classification of Diseases, 10th Revision, Procedural Coding System

In the mid-1990s, CMS awarded a contract to the 3M Health Information Systems group to develop a new procedural coding system to replace the Tabular List of Procedures, volume 3 of ICD-9-CM. The objectives of the project were to:

- Improve the accuracy and efficiency of coding
- Reduce training efforts
- Improve communication with physicians

The International Classification of Diseases, 10th Revision, Procedural Coding System (ICD-10-PCS), is based on a seven-character alphanumeric code with the following four essential characteristics:

- Completeness: All substantially different procedures have a unique code.
- Expandability: The structure of the system allows incorporation of new procedures as unique codes.
- Standardized terminology (or definitions): Each term is assigned a specific meaning.
- Multiaxial structure: Each code character has the same meaning with the specific procedure section and across procedure sections to the extent possible.

ICD-10-PCS is divided into 16 sections, each of which covers a specific diagnostic area (for example, medical and surgical, chiropractic, and so on). Depending on the requirements of each section, the seven characters are assigned different meanings. For example, in the medical and surgical section, the fourth character represents the body part or region involved in the procedure; in the placement section, it represents the body region or orifice; and in the chiropractic section, it represents the body region.

As of this writing, the CMS has not published information for an implementation timeline for ICD-10-PCS.

Table 13.1. Comparison of ICD-9-CM and ICD-10-PCS using NCVHS characteristics (select examples)

NCVHS Characteristics	ICD-9-CM	ICD-10-PCS
Hierarchical structure Each code has a unique definition forever, not reused.	Some codes do not have a unique definition because the codes have been reused.	All codes have a unique definition.
Expandability Flexibility to new procedures and technologies ("empty" code numbers).	Minimal flexibility. New procedures and technologies are difficult to incorporate. Virtually no empty code numbers.	Extensive flexibility. New procedures and technologies are easily incorporated. Unlimited empty code values are available.
Comprehensive Provides NOS and NEC categories so that all possible procedures can be classified somewhere.	Extensive use of NOS and NEC categories. All procedures can be categorized somewhere. Broad NOS and NEC categories result in procedure codes that are ambiguously defined.	Limited use of NOS and NEC categories. NEC and NOS categories are specific to each axis of code. All procedures can be categorized somewhere. Procedure codes are precisely defined even when NOS and NEC options are used.
Ease of use Adequate indexing and annotation for all users.	Full index, but specificity of index varies across codes.	Full index. Index is computer generated so specificity of index is consistent across all codes.
Setting and Provider Neutrality Same code regardless of who or where procedure is performed.	Codes are independent of who or where procedure is performed.	Codes are independent of who or where procedure is performed.
Multiaxial Technology used.	Limited and inconsistent specification of technology used.	Technology used is specified in the approach character of the code.

Source: Averill et al. 2005.

International Classification of Diseases for Oncology

The **International Classification of Diseases for Oncology** (ICD-O) is currently in its third edition. This classification is used for coding diagnoses of neoplasms in tumor and cancer registries and in pathology laboratories. The topography code describes the site of origin of the neoplasm and uses the same three- and four-character categories as in the neoplasm section of the second chapter of ICD-10. The morphology code describes the characteristics of the tumor itself, including cell type and biologic activity. The topography codes remain the same as in the previous edition, but the morphology codes have been thoroughly reviewed and revised where necessary.

To the greatest extent possible, ICD-O uses the nomenclature published in the WHO series, International Histological Classification of Tumors. ICD-O is under the purview of the heads of the WHO Collaborating Centres for Classification of Disease. The International Association of Cancer Registries (IACR) is an additional resource (WHO 2005).

International Classification on Functioning, Disability, and Health

The **International Classification of Functioning, Disability, and Health** (ICF) is a classification of health and health related domains that describe body functions and structures, activities and participation. Three lists exist within ICF:

- Body functions and structure
- Domains of activity and participation
- Environmental factors that interact with all these components

ICD-10 and ICF are complementary, and users are encouraged to use them together to create a broader and more meaningful picture of the experience of health of individuals and populations. See table 13.2 for examples of ICF self-care codes.

Current Procedural Terminology (CPT)

The American Medical Association (AMA) publishes the Current Procedural Terminology (CPT). According to the AMA, the purpose of CPT is "to provide a uniform language that accurately describes medical, surgical, and diagnostic services, and thereby serves as an effective means for reliable nationwide communication among physicians, patients, and third parties." CPT was first developed and published by the AMA in 1966. In 1983, the system was adopted by CMS as level I of the Healthcare Common Procedure Coding System (HCPCS). Since that time, CPT has become widely used as a standard for outpatient and ambulatory care procedural coding in contexts related to reimbursement.

CPT is updated every year on January 1. The codebook is organized into chapters by specialty, body system, or service provided. The codes themselves consist of five digits, and the descriptions of the codes are often accompanied by inclusion and exclusion notes. Modifiers to the five-digit codes also are used extensively.

CPT is maintained by the CPT Editorial Panel, which is authorized to revise, update, and modify CPT. The majority (11 of 16) of the panel's members are physicians, with the rest coming from industry and government. Supporting the

Table 13.2.   Examples of ICF self-care codes

Chapter	Description	Categories	Category Description	Subcategories
Self-Care	This chapter is about caring for oneself; washing and drying oneself; caring for one's body and body parts; dressing, eating, and drinking; and looking after one's health	d530 Toileting	Planning and carrying out the elimination of human waste (menstruation, urination, and defecation) and cleaning oneself afterwards.	**d5300** Regulating urination **d5301** Regulating defecation **d5302** Menstrual care **d5308** Toileting, other specified **d5309** Toileting, unspecified
		d540 Dressing	Carrying out the coordinated actions of putting on and taking off clothes and footwear in sequence and in keeping with climatic and social conditions, such as by putting on, adjusting, and removing shirts, skirts, blouses, pants, undergarments, saris, kimono, tights, hats, gloves, coats, shoes, boots, sandals, and slippers.	**d5400** Putting on clothes **d5401** Taking off clothes **d5402** Putting on footwear **d5403** Taking off footwear **d5404** Choosing appropriate clothing **d5408** Dressing, other specified **d5409** Dressing, unspecified

Source: WHO 2005.

work of the CPT Editorial Panel is the CPT Health Care Professionals Advisory Committee (HCPAC). The HCPAC includes participation in the CPT process from organizations representing limited-license medical practitioners and allied health professionals.

The AMA is responsible for developing and publishing the official guidelines for CPT. The association provides support in several ways. It publishes CPT Assistant, a monthly newsletter, and offers CPT Information Services, a telephone service that provides users with expert advice on code use. The association also conducts an annual CPT coding symposium.

The AMA is engaged in an effort to respond to emerging user needs and HIPAA confidentiality and security requirements. The AMA's stated intent is to "ensure that CPT meets all the requirements of, and is unambiguously selected by the Secretary of HHS as the standard for reporting physicians' services under HIPAA." All enhancements and modifications will occur gradually through the usual CPT editorial process. Some of the changes outlined on the AMA Web site include:

- The elimination of ambiguous terms
- Codes for home health services
- A new section for performance measurement codes
- A new section for investigational service codes
- Codes for evaluation and assessment services performed by health professionals who are not physicians
- Counseling or preventive medicine services codes/core concept extenders
- Code combinations for included and excluded services
- Web-based communication to enhance the editorial process, including code change requests
- Development of a terminology model
- XML-enabled, browser-based versions of CPT
- An annual list of deleted codes

It remains to be seen whether these changes will be enough for the secretary of HHS to determine that CPT should continue to be the coding standard for physician and ambulatory care services. For detailed information on CPT and the revision process, readers should refer to the AMA Web site at ama-assn.org.

Healthcare Common Procedure Coding System

The Healthcare Common Procedure Coding System (HCPCS) is used to report physicians' services provided to Medicare recipients. HCPCS is administered by the CMS and includes three levels of codes. Level I is made up entirely of CPT codes as published by the AMA. Level II includes alphanumeric procedure and modifier codes established by the CMS's Alphanumeric Editorial Panel. Level II codes primarily represent items, supplies, and nonphysician services not covered by the AMA's CPT codes. The codes are used in reimbursement claims processing.

Except for temporary codes (those beginning with G, K, or Q), HCPCS codes are updated every year on January 1. The HCPCS level II codes can be downloaded from the HCPCS Web site; however, the file does not include the **Current Dental Terminology** (CDT) codes (HCPCS codes beginning with D) as published by the American Dental Association. HCPCS level III codes (W to Z) are used by Medicare carriers and fiscal intermediaries as local procedure and modifier codes. Table 13.3 shows an example of HCPCS codes.

HCPCS was included in the HIPAA final rule on transaction and code sets, with the exception of the level III codes. The presence of level III codes is not consistent with HIPAA's national standards goal. The future of HCPCS beyond the first HIPAA implementation is unclear.

Diagnostic and Statistical Manual of Mental Diseases

The Diagnostic and Statistical Manual of Mental Diseases was first published by the American Psychiatric Association (APA) in 1952. The fourth and most recent complete revision was introduced in 1994. In 2000, the APA introduced DSM-IV-TR (Text Revision), which is the most current version available.

DSM is a multiaxial coding system with five axes. Axis I includes the mental disorders or illnesses comparable to general medical illnesses. Axis II includes personality disorders. Axis III includes general medical illnesses. Axis IV covers

Table 13.3.   Examples of HCPCS codes

Transportation Services Including Ambulance A0021–A0999	
Code	**Service**
A0428	AMBULANCE SERVICE, BASIC LIFE SUPPORT, NON-EMERGENCY TRANSPORT, (BLS)
A0429	AMBULANCE SERVICE, BASIC LIFE SUPPORT, EMERGENCY TRANSPORT (BLS-EMERGENCY)
A0430	AMBULANCE SERVICE, CONVENTIONAL AIR SERVICES, TRANSPORT, ONE WAY (FIXED WING)
A0431	AMBULANCE SERVICE, CONVENTIONAL AIR SERVICES, TRANSPORT, ONE WAY (ROTARY WING)
A0432	PARAMEDIC INTERCEPT (PI), RURAL AREA, TRANSPORT FURNISHED BY A VOLUNTEER
A0432	AMBULANCE COMPANY WHICH IS PROHIBITED BY STATE LAW FROM BILLING THIRD PARTY
A0432	PAYERS
A0433	ADVANCED LIFE SUPPORT, LEVEL 2 (ALS 2)
A0434	SPECIALTY CARE TRANSPORT (SCT)
A0435	FIXED WING AIR MILEAGE, PER STATUTE MILE
A0436	ROTARY WING AIR MILEAGE, PER STATUTE MILE

Source: CMS 2005.

life events or social problems that affect the patient. Axis V is the overall level of the patient's functioning, usually as determined by the Global Assessment of Functioning (GAF). Figure 13.3 provides an example of DSM-IV-TR codes and instructions.

The APA Web site states two general uses for DSM: as a source of diagnostic information that enhances clinical practice, research, and education and as a language for communicating diagnostic information to other parties, such as government agencies and insurance companies. Theoretically, DSM can be used for reimbursement purposes because all of the diagnostic codes in DSM-IV are also valid ICD-9-CM codes. The APA updates the DSM to correspond to ICD-9-CM each year. According to the APA Web site (psych.org), the DSM will be updated to ICD-10-CM when it is implemented in the United States.

Diagnosis-Related Groups

The **Diagnosis-Related Groups** (DRG) classification system is primarily used for healthcare organizations to bill for inpatient services rendered. It is based upon the ICD-9-CM diagnosis and procedure codes assigned during an inpatient stay. According to the 2003 DRG Expert, "A DRG is one of 520 currently valid groups that classify patients into clinically cohesive groups that demonstrate similar consumption of hospital resources and length-of-stay patterns." DRG assignment is based upon the following criteria:

- Principal and secondary diagnoses and procedure codes
- Sex
- Age
- Discharge status

Figure 13.3.   Example of DSM-IV-TR codes

Diagnostic Criteria for Mental Retardation

A. Significantly subaverage intellectual functioning: an IQ of approximately 70 or below on an individually administered IQ test (for infants, a clinical judgment of significantly subaverage intellectual functioning).

B. Concurrent deficits or impairments in present adaptive functioning (i.e., the person's effectiveness in meeting the standards expected for his or her age by his or her cultural group) in at least two of the following areas: communication, self-care, home living, social/interpersonal skills, use of community resources, self-direction, functional academic skills, work, leisure, health, and safety.

C. The onset is before age 18 years.

Code based on degree of severity reflecting level of intellectual impairment:

317 Mild Mental Retardation: IQ level 50–55 to approximately 70
318.0 Moderate Mental Retardation: IQ level 35–40 to 50–55
318.1 Severe Mental Retardation: IQ level 20–25 to 35–40
318.2 Profound Mental Retardation: IQ level below 20 or 25
319 Mental Retardation, Severity Unspecified: when there is strong presumption of Mental Retardation but the person's intelligence is untestable by standard tests

Copyright ©1994, American Psychiatric Association.

- Presence or absence of complications and comorbidities (CCs)
- Birthweight for neonates

Besides being used for reimbursement purposes, DRGs can also be used for utilization review reporting. For example, certain wards or units in a hospital may be interested in knowing their top DRGs and average length of stays. This provides them with critical data to plan the services provided to each patient and a target date for discharge. Also, the Joint Commission for Accreditation of Healthcare Organizations (JCAHO) routinely asks for a hospital's top 5 or 10 DRGs during surveys. They usually want to review some inpatient charts assigned these DRGs to assess provider documentation patterns, patient safety issues, etc. (Ingenix 2002).

The DRG changes for fiscal year 2005 include three new DRGs:

- 541: Tracheostomy and Mechanical Ventilation 96+ hours or Principal Diagnosis Excluding Face, Mouth, and Neck Diagnoses with Major OR Procedure
- 542: Tracheostomy with Mechanical Ventilation 96+ Hours or Principal Diagnosis Excluding Face, Mouth, and Neck Diagnoses without Major OR Procedure
- 543: Craniotomy with Implantation of Chemotherapeutic Agent or Acute Complex Central Nervous System Principal Diagnosis (Willard, Worthington, and Ashley 2004).

See table 13.4 for an example of the top 10 annual DRGs for a hospital.

Ambulatory Payment Classification

The **Ambulatory Payment Classification** (APC) System is the outpatient reimbursement equivalent to the inpatient DRG System. APCs are based on the grouping of procedures by CPT/HCPCS codes that have similar costs or resource inputs. APCs were created because the Balanced Budget Act of 1997 required the Department of Health and Human Services (HHS) to implement a prospective payment system (PPS) for hospital services. Each CPT code listed in the APC system has a status indicator that determines reimbursement:

- T—Surgical services subject to discounting. 100 percent of allowance is paid for the highest weight procedure, and 50 percent of the allowance is paid for all subsequent procedures.
- S—Significant procedures not subject to discounting. 100 percent of allowance is paid, even when performed with other procedures at the same time or on the same date of service.
- X—No discounting applies to these ancillary procedures.
- N—No separate payment is made for these procedures, since they are considered incidental to another procedure or service.

Table 13.4.   Example of top 10 annual DRGs for a hospital

DRG	DRG Description	National Arithmetic Mean Length of Stay	Hospital Average Length of Stay
133	Atherosclerosis w/o CC	2.3	3.2
127	Heart Failure & Shock	5.3	4.8
149	Major Small and Large Bowel Procedures w/o CC	6.5	7.6
132	Atherosclerosis w/CC	2.9	5.1
88	Chronic Obstructive Pulmonary Disease	5.1	3.9
75	Major Chest Procedures	10.1	8.9
89	Simple Pneumonia and Pleurisy, Age Greater than 17 w/CC	5.9	5.6
131	Peripheral Vascular Disorders w/o CC	4.1	4.2
106	Coronary Bypass w/PTCA	11.4	9.6
122	Circulatory Disorders w/Acute Myocardial Infarction w/o Major Complications, Discharged Alive	3.8	3.8

- V—Visit APCs where separate reimbursement is furnished for the X (ancillary) APCs in addition to the visit APC for emergency room or clinic visits (Scichilone 1999).

See table 13.5 for examples of APC impact on lesion measurement.

The International Classification of Primary Care

The **International Classification of Primary Care** (ICPC-2) is a coding terminology for the classification of primary care developed by the World Organization of National Colleges, Academies, and Academic Associations of General Practitioners/Family Physicians (WONCA) International Classification Committee (NAHIT 2005). According to WONCA, ICPC-2 has been developed as a tool for general practitioners and family doctors throughout the world. It has been mapped to ICD-10 so that conversion systems can be used. Extensive use has confirmed that it and ICD-10 are complementary rather than in competition. ICPC-2 includes a severity of illness checklist and functional status assessment charts (Jamoulle 1998). See table 13.6 for four categories of diagnosis in primary care in ICPC-2.

Current Dental Terminology (CDT-2005)

CDT-2005 contains the version of the Code on Dental Procedures and Nomenclature (the Code) that is effective for services provided on or after January 1, 2005. The Code has been designated as the national standard for reporting dental services by the Federal Government under HIPAA, and is recognized by third-party payers nationwide. CDT-2005 is published

Table 13.5.   Examples of APC impact on lesion measurement

CPT Code	Lesion Size	APC Assignment	Rate Proposed
11603	2.1–3.0 cm	161	$176.37
11604	3.1–4.0 cm	162	$287.44
11606	>4.0 cm	163	$538.88

Source: Scichilone 1999.

Table 13.6.   ICPC-2 four categories of diagnosis in primary care

Category	Description	Examples
1. Aetiological and pathological	The diagnosis has proven pathology or aetiology	Appendicitis, acute myocardial infarction
2. Pathophysiological	The diagnosis has a proven pathophysiological substrate	Presbycusis, hypertension
3. Nosolical	The diagnosis depends on a symptom complex based on consensus between physicians	Depression, irritable bowel syndrome
4. Symptom	A symptom or complaint is the best medical label for the episode	Fatigue, eye pain

by the American Dental Association (ada.org). The Code is organized into 12 categories of service, each with its own series of five-digit alphanumeric codes (see table 13.7). Each category of service is divided into subcategories of generally recognized related procedures (AMA 2004).

Galen Common Reference Model

The **Galen Common Reference Model** (CRM) is a computer-based clinical terminology developed in Europe for representing medical concepts. It is designed to support mappings to other coding systems and languages, data analysis, sharing information between applications and reuse (NAHIT 2005). It uses a formalism called the Structured Meta Knowledge (SMK). In SMK, terms are defined through relationships to other terms, and grammars are provided to allow combinations of terms into sensible phrases. It is intended to represent patient information in a way that is independent of the language being recorded and of the data model used by an electronic medical record system (Hammond and Cimino 2001).

National Drug Codes

The **Food and Drug Administration** (FDA) developed the **National Drug Codes** (NDC) codes to serve as a universal product identifier for human drugs. It identifies the labeler/vendor, product, and trade package size. In 2004, the NDC codes were adopted as a federal healthcare information interoperability standard to enable the federal healthcare sector to share information regarding drug products. It has been approved as a HIPAA billing/financial transaction code set (NAHIT 2005).

Table 13.7.   Examples of CDT 2005 codes

Category of Service	Code Series	Example Code	Nomenclature	Descriptor (if applicable)
I. Diagnostic	D0100–D0999	D0277	Vertical bitewings–7 to 8 films	This does not constitute a full mouth intraoral radiographic series.
II. Preventive	D1000–D1999	D1320	Tobacco counseling for the control and prevention of oral disease	Tobacco prevention and cessation services reduce patient risks of developing tobacco-related oral diseases and conditions and improves prognosis for certain dental therapies.
III. Restorative	D2000–D2999	D2390	Resin-based composite crown, anterior	Full resin-based composite coverage of tooth.
IV. Endodontics	D3000–D3999	D3410	Apicoectomy/periradicular surgery–anterior	For surgery on root of anterior tooth. Does not include placement of retrograde filling material.
V. Periodontics	D4000–D4999	D4355	Full mouth debridement to enable comprehensive evaluation and diagnosis	The gross removal of plaque and calculus that interfere with the ability of the dentist to perform a comprehensive oral evaluation. This preliminary procedure does not preclude the need for additional procedures.
VI. Prosthodontics, removable	D5000–D5899	D5110	Complete denture–maxillary	
VII. Maxillofacial Prosthetics	D5900–D5999	D5984	Radiation shield	Synonymous terminology: radiation stent, tongue protector, lead shield. An intraoral prosthesis designed to shield adjacent tissues from radiation during orthovoltage treatment of malignant lesions of the head and neck region.
VIII. Implant Services	D6000–D6199	D6010	Surgical placement of implant body: endosteal implant	Includes second-stage surgery and placement of healing cap.
IX. Prosthodontics, fixed	D6200–D6999	D6794	Crown–titanium	
X. Oral Surgery	D7000–D7999	D7220	Removal of impacted tooth–soft tissue	Occlusal surface of tooth covered by soft tissue; requires mucoperiosteal flap elevation.
XI. Orthodontics	D8000–D8999	D8691	Repair of orthodontic appliance	Does not include bracket and standard fixed ortho appliances. It does include functional appliances and palatal expanders.
XII. Adjunctive General Services	D9000–D9999	D9230	Analgesia, anxiolysis, inhalation of nitrous oxide	

Source: ADA 2004.

Each drug product is assigned a unique 10-digit, 3-segment number. This identifies the:

- First segment—labeler code, assigned by the FDA. A labeler is a firm that manufactures, repacks, or distributes a drug product
- Second segment—product code, identifies a specific strength, dose form, and formulation for a particular firm.
- Third segment—package code, identifies package sizes. Both the product and package codes are assigned by the firm.

The NDC will be in one of the following configurations: 4-4-2, 5-3-2, or 5-4-1 (see table 13.8).

Each manufacturer defines the specific codes for their own products. Therefore, there is no uniform class hierarchy for the codes, and codes may be reused at the manufacturer's discretion (Hammond and Cimino 2001).

ABC Codes

ABC codes are a terminology created by Alternative Link that describes alternative medicine, nursing and other integrative healthcare interventions. They work with and extend the value of CPT and HCPCS II codes. They also ensure the financing, administration and delivery of healthcare is legal and HIPAA compliant. In May 2004, the ABC codes were adopted as a federal healthcare information interoperability billing/financial code set standard allowed for use under a demonstration project for participants in a pilot. The code set may be used in other non-HIPAA commercial transactions, but with HIPAA transactions only under the demonstration project constraints (NAHIT 2005) (see table 13.9, p. 316).

Table 13.8.   Examples of NDC codes

Drug	NDC Code
Fluoxetine 100 mg Caps	00172-4363-70
Prenatal Plus Tab	0093-9111-01
Hydrocodone/APAP 7.5/500 mg Tab	00591-0385-05
Glycolax 3350 NF POW	62175-442-31
Flonase 0.05% Nasal Spray	00173-0453-01
Progesterone 600 mg Supp	51927-1046-00
Seraquel 100 mg Tab	00310-0271-10
Axert 12.5 mg Tab	00062-2085-06
Amitriptyline 25 mg Tab	00603-2213-32
Amoxicillin 400 mg/5 Susp	63304-0970-04

Check Your Understanding 13.2

Instructions: Answer the following questions on a separate piece of paper.

1. What was the original purpose of ICD-9-CM?
2. What are the four essential characteristics of ICD-10-PCS? Describe them.
3. What is the primary function of CPT?
4. What does the topography code in ICD-O describe?

Coding

Traditionally, health information management (HIM) professionals have been responsible for the process of **coding**, or clinical code assignment, in healthcare organizations. Historically, the coding function has served two primary purposes: to create secondary records (for example, diagnostic and procedural indexes) and to create documentation for reimbursement purposes.

Standards of Ethical Coding

In the U.S. healthcare system, the majority of expenses are reimbursed by third-party payers such as government programs and insurance companies rather than by the patients themselves. As healthcare costs have risen over the past 30 years, third-party payers have searched for ways to contain costs. With the implementation of prospective payment systems based on coded clinical data, procedural reviews of documentation to substantiate code assignment have become routine. In other words, accurate coding has become central to the financial survival of healthcare provider organizations.

The coding professional's first responsibility is to ensure the accuracy of coded data. To this end, AHIMA has established a code of professional ethics by which coders must abide. (See figure 13.4, p. 317.) Coders also need to balance the following three competing responsibilities:

- To perform their tasks using established guidelines and their best professional judgment
- To safeguard the viability of their hospitals in order to serve their communities
- To remain employed and able to support themselves and their families (Fox 1992, p. 34)

Elements of Coding Quality

The quality of coded clinical data depends on a number of factors, including:

- Adequate training for everyone involved in the coding process, including coders, coding supervisors, clinicians, and financial personnel
- Adequate references and support resources, including up-to-date coding books, as well as subscription publications that communicate official guidelines (namely, *Coding Clinic for ICD-9-CM* and *CPT Assistant*) and, in some cases, encoders or other support software

Table 13.9.   Example of ABC code hierarchy for practice specialties

Section	Subsection	Heading
C – Practice Specialties		
	A – Oriental Medicine	B – Common Procedures
		C – Modalities
		D – Therapies
		E - Anesthesia
	B – Somatic Practices and Massage	A – Body Mind
		B – Body Work
		C – Energy Work
		D – Ergonomics
		E – Massage
		G – Oriental Massage
		H – Somatic Education
	C – Chiropractic Services	A – Chiropractic Adjustments
		B – Closed Joint Adjustment
		C - Taping
	D – Mental Health Services	A – Counseling
		B – Testing, Evaluation & Interpretation
	E – Midwifery Services	A – Miscellaneous Services
		B – Prenatal
		C – Delivery
		D – Postpartum
		E – Newborn Care
		F – Family Planning
	F – Naturopathic Manipulation	A – Osseous
		B – Visceral
		C – Other Naturopathic Services
	G – Osteopathic Manipulation	A – Manipulation
	H – Indigenous Medicine	A – Ayurvedic Medicine
		B – Native American
		C – Curandera
	I – Spiritual Care	A – Christian Science
		B – Spiritual Care Nursing
		C – Multidenominational
	J – Distinct Practices	A – Naprapathic Manipulation
		F – Other Heart or Vascular Procedures

Source: Alternative Link 2005.

Figure 13.4.   Standards of ethical coding

In this era of payment based on diagnostic and procedural coding, the professional ethics of health information coding professionals continue to be challenged. A conscientious goal for coding and maintaining a quality database is accurate clinical and statistical data. The following standards of ethical coding, developed by AHIMA's Coding Policy and Strategy Committee and approved by AHIMA's Board of Directors, are offered to guide coding professionals in this process.

1. Coding professionals are expected to support the importance of accurate, complete, and consistent coding practices for the production of quality healthcare data.

2. Coding professionals in all healthcare settings should adhere to the ICD-9-CM (*International Classification of Diseases, Ninth Revision, Clinical Modification*) coding conventions, official coding guidelines approved by the Cooperating Parties,* the CPT (*Current Procedural Terminology*) rules established by the American Medical Association, and any other official coding rules and guidelines established for use with mandated standard code sets. Selection and sequencing of diagnoses and procedures must meet the definitions of required data sets for applicable healthcare settings.

3. Coding professionals should use their skills, their knowledge of currently mandated coding and classification systems, and official resources to select the appropriate diagnostic and procedural codes.

4. Coding professionals should only assign and report codes that are clearly and consistently supported by physician documentation in the health record.

5. Coding professionals should consult physicians for clarification and additional documentation prior to code assignment when there is conflicting or ambiguous data in the health record.

6. Coding professionals should not change codes or the narratives of codes on the billing abstract so that meanings are misrepresented. Diagnoses or procedures should not be inappropriately included or excluded because payment or insurance policy coverage requirements will be affected. When individual payer policies conflict with official coding rules and guidelines, these policies should be obtained in writing whenever possible. Reasonable efforts should be made to educate the payer on proper coding practices in order to influence a change in the payer's policy.

7. Coding professionals, as members of the healthcare team, should assist and educate physicians and other clinicians by advocating proper documentation practices, further specificity, and resequencing or inclusion of diagnoses or procedures when needed to more accurately reflect the acuity, severity, and occurrence of events.

8. Coding professionals should participate in the development of institutional coding policies and should ensure that coding policies complement, not conflict with, official coding rules and guidelines.

9. Coding professionals should maintain and continually enhance their coding skills, as they have a professional responsibility to stay abreast of changes in codes, coding guidelines, and regulations.

10. Coding professionals should strive for optimal payment to which the facility is legally entitled, remembering that it is unethical and illegal to maximize payment by means that contradict regulatory guidelines.

*The Cooperating Parties are the American Health Information Management Association, American Hospital Association, Health Care Financing Administration, and National Center for Health Statistics. All rights reserved. Reprint and quote only with proper reference to AHIMA's authorship.

Source: AHIMA 1999b.

- Accurate and complete clinical documentation that includes every pertinent condition and service provided to the patient
- The support of senior managers, who must understand how important the coding function is to the organization's continued existence
- A performance improvement plan for the coding function that ensures continuous quality improvement processes
- When all of these components are present, the quality of coded clinical data can be evaluated according to the following elements:
  —Reliability: The extent to which the data can be reproduced by subsequent measurements or tests (for example, coded clinical data are considered reliable when multiple coders assign the same codes to a record)
  —Validity: The extent to which the coded data accurately reflect the patient's diagnoses and procedures (Bowman 2001, p. 250)
  —Completeness: The extent to which the coded data represent all of the patient's relevant diagnoses or procedures
  —Timeliness: The extent to which the coded data are available within the time frames required for billing purposes, decision support, and other uses

Coding Policies and Procedures

As with other organizational policies and procedures, coding policies and procedures are needed to promote consistency. Items to be included in coding policies and procedures include:

- Directions for reviewing the record
- Instructions on how to address incomplete or conflicting documentation
- Instructions for communicating with physicians and developing physician queries and for clarification and recording health record addenda
- Instructions on the actions to be taken when an appropriate code cannot be located
- Use of codes not required for reimbursement (optional codes)
- Standardized definitions or codes sets (for example, HIPAA requirements)
- Use of reference materials and books and instructions for updating
- Computerized data entry or other processes (Bowman 2001, p. 251)

These items must be specified in policies and procedures so that coders know what is expected of them and so that the healthcare organization can ensure its compliance with government and payer requirements.

Steps in the Coding Process

Although the coding process may vary from organization to organization, or even within an organization between care settings, certain steps are usually followed when codes are assigned either manually or with an encoder. Initially, the coder should review the relevant documentation, whether it is a complete patient record for an inpatient stay or a short note for an ambulatory care encounter. Using their knowledge of the applicable definitions such as principal diagnosis, primary diagnoses, principal procedure, and so on, the coder then should select the conditions, treatment, and procedures that need to be coded. The definitions are important because they determine the order (or sequence) in which the codes are submitted to the third-party payer. After selecting the applicable conditions, treatments, or procedures, the coder should use the required coding system or nomenclature and select the most appropriate code, again, based on the guidelines.

After the code assignments and the order of the codes have been determined, it is imperative to use the correct reimbursement classification or grouping system. For example, in ambulatory care, APCs are used. (See chapter 14 for more information on reimbursement systems.) Services in each APC are similar clinically and in terms of the resources they require. A payment rate has been established for each APC. The APC is determined by a combination of ICD-9-CM diagnosis and CPT procedure codes. In most cases, a computerized software program called a **grouper** is used for this function. It is common for all of the coding and grouping data to be entered into and stored in a computerized information system. When the codes and other data provided by the coders are deemed complete, they are often transmitted or otherwise communicated to the billing personnel for reimbursement purposes. Figure 13.5 shows the steps in the coding process.

Quality Assessment for the Coding Process

Quality assessment for the coding process is also referred to as performance improvement for the coding process. It involves looking at more than just the assigned codes. As stated previously, accurate coding is essential to the economic survival of the healthcare organization; hence, ongoing efforts to improve the coding process should yield better economic benefits.

Most important to improving any coding process is to first document and understand the current coding process. The preceding section can be used as a guide for documenting that process, remembering that the actual process is different in every organization. One of the most important items in the coding process is the quality of the clinical documentation. Even though HIM professionals have little to no direct con-

trol over the documentation, they should work with the clinicians and other personnel to continue to improve its quality.

After the current coding process has been documented, quality measurement points should be established at specific stages in the process. Baseline measurements need to be taken, and benchmarks for improvement should be set up. For example, if the current process results in records being coded an average of 10 work-hours after arriving in the HIM department, a benchmark for improvement might be to code records in under 8 hours. To establish valid internal coding data monitors, comparative data will be necessary. Comparative data can be obtained from a variety of sources, including state data organizations, hospital associations, peer review organizations, and the Medicare MedPar data, which can be obtained from the CMS. The National Health Information Resource Center (nhirc.org) and the National Association of Health Data Organizations (nahdo.org) are additional sources of information on health data.

Quality assessment of a process is generally ongoing. Even when the most ambitious goals for the most important measures have been accomplished, the measures should continue to be monitored. In addition, management should continually search for ways to improve the coding process through computerization or other methods.

Check Your Understanding 13.3

Instructions: Answer the following questions on a separate piece of paper.

1. What is the coder's primary responsibility?
2. What is the main factor in ensuring the quality of clinical coding?
3. Why is it important for organizations to establish and follow specific coding policies and procedures?
4. Describe the quality assessment process for coding.

Application of Technology to the Coding Process

Recent technologies are having a considerable impact on the coding process, and new technologies hold promise for the future. Some of the most significant advances are discussed below.

Encoders

An **encoder** is a computer software program designed to assist coders in assigning appropriate clinical codes to words and phrases expressed in natural human language (Slee and Slee 1991). Initially developed during the era of paper-based health records, the principal purpose of encoders was to help ensure accurate reporting for reimbursement (Beinborn 1999).

Encoders come in two distinct categories: logic-based and automated codebook formats. A logic-based encoder prompts the user through a variety of questions and choices

Figure 13.5.   Steps in the coding process

1. Review relevant documentation.
2. Select conditions, treatments, and procedures to be coded.
3. Select most appropriate codes.
4. Enter or abstract data into the computer.
5. Utilize the appropriate reimbursement classification system.

based on the clinical terminology entered. The coder selects the most accurate code for a service or condition (and any possible complications or comorbidities).

An automated codebook provides screen views that resemble the actual format of the coding system. This allows the coder to review code selections, notes, look-up tables, edits, and various other automated notations that help him or her to choose the most accurate code for a condition or service. Although encoders can cite official coding guidelines and provide code optimization guidance, they require user interaction. Encoders promote accuracy as well as consistency in the coding of diagnoses and procedures.

A number of companies currently market encoder products. An up-to-date list of these products can be found in the annual coding issue of the *Journal of the American Health Information Management Association.*

Automated Code Assignment

Rather than prompting the user to make various selections on the basis of patient record documentation, automated code assignment uses data that have been entered into the computer to automatically assign codes (Beinborn 1999). Automated code assignment uses natural language processing (NLP) technology to read the data contained in a CPR. The natural language processing technology used might be algorithmic (rules based) or statistical. Schnitzer (2000) has stated that statistical approaches that can predict how an experienced coder might code a record and use machine learning techniques are superior to rigid rule sets. This opinion is congruent with the oft-heard argument that "coding is subjective."

According to Schnitzer, the advantages to using automated code assignment include:

- Consistency: Automated code assignment is consistently correct and consistently incorrect; thus, errors, once detected, are easier to locate and fix.
- Accuracy: As with medical knowledge, the amount of information that must be synthesized to correctly code patient records has increased substantially. Expert computer software programs can apply these rules and guidelines accurately.
- Speed: The computational power of computers can apply the many coding rules and guidelines efficiently.

It is important to note, however, that automated code assignment is not a magic bullet. For example, it cannot address the major obstacle facing today's human coder: the lack of accurate, complete clinical documentation. As Schnitzer (2000) put it, "If a service isn't appropriately documented, there's no way for NLP to find it, assume it, or infer it." In addition, automated code assignment has not developed to the point where it can operate without substantial human interaction (Warner 2000). Finally, the most effective automated code assignment system will need to accommodate any weaknesses and deficiencies in the classification and coding systems it uses (Beinborn 1999).

As automated code assignment continues to evolve, so, too, will the role of the coding professional. In its Vision 2006, the AHIMA (1996) pictures a clinical data specialist in the future and predicts that this individual will manage data in a number of areas, including clinical coding, outcomes measurement, specialty registries, and research databases. Beinborn (1999) stated that coders will be essential to the implementation and maintenance of automated code assignment systems as well as of decision support systems, data interpretation, and other evolving areas that rely on healthcare data.

Emerging Technologies

As is apparent from the preceding subsection, the status quo will not continue for coding. A number of emerging technologies will likely be used to support the coding function.

Speech recognition is one candidate for improving the coding process as well as coding accuracy. As speech recognition improves and has the ability to accurately document what the clinician is saying, the ease of completely documenting healthcare services also improves. Schwager (2000, p. 64) has maintained that "speech recognition, combined with technology designed to extract and structure medical information (natural language processing) contained in narrative text, can automate the coding process used in reimbursement." He also has discussed the possibility that the computerized patient record software could analyze the record in an interactive fashion, prompting the clinician for higher-quality documentation.

Handheld computers or personal digital assistants (PDAs) also are becoming commonplace. Many physicians and other healthcare professionals find them helpful. As computer systems continue to develop, it will only be a matter of time before these small units are used for data entry and other functions in healthcare organizations.

A discussion of emerging technologies to support coding would not be complete without a discussion of clinical terminologies. The currently emerging vocabularies and classifications, as well as the characteristics necessary in a clinical terminology and considerations when selecting a clinical terminology, are discussed later in this chapter.

Check Your Understanding 13.4

Instructions: Answer the following questions on a separate piece of paper.

1. What is the difference between encoders and automated code assignment?
2. Name two emerging technologies and describe their impact on classification and clinical terminologies.

Emerging Vocabulary and Classification Initiatives

A number of initiatives related to vocabularies and classifications have been developed in recent years, some of which may have a significant impact on the role of the HIM professional in the future. The following sections examine some of these recent and emerging initiatives.

President's Information Technology Advisory Committee

In President George W. Bush's 2004 State of the Union Address, he stated, "By computerizing health records, we can avoid dangerous medial mistakes, reduce costs and improve care." As a result, the **President's Information Technology Advisory Committee** (PITAC) was created in 2003 to address HIT issues. The committee's key goals are to:

- Accelerate the adoption of information technology in the healthcare sector
- Achieve substantial economic and social benefits
- Reduce medical errors
- Reduce unproductive healthcare expenditures
- Improve quality and consistency of care

One of the four essential elements of this plan is to have interoperable electronic information interchange. This includes specific standards for the capture of new data and tools for capturing nonstandards-compliant electronic information from legacy systems. One of the draft recommendations is to perform a study to reassess the cost-benefit of the planned conversion of diagnosis and procedure coding requirements for Federal programs from ICD-9-CM to ICD-10-CM, compared to the potential alternative of moving directly to reporting diagnoses and procedures coded for clinical purposes in the **Systemized Nomenclature of Medical Reference Terminology** (SNOMED CT). This might provide incentives for standardized EHR implementations. Another draft recommendation is to develop a single set of standards for EHR systems that can be implemented across all federally implemented EHRs and shared with the private sector. They further recommend increasing Federal support of pathfinder demonstrations that share appropriate Federal Health IT implementation knowledge across all departments of the government and to the private sector. Such demonstrations should use the standards analyses and recommendations of the **Consolidated Health Informatics** (CHI) eGovernment initiative as a foundation. The PITAC has also recommended devoting Federal research and development resources to the development of a single set of data standards for the most common forms of clinical information. This includes:

- An effort that should leverage efforts underway within federally implemented systems
- Examples of data to be included in the standard are vital signs, examination findings, and review of systems information
- These standards should be developed in the public domain in conjunction with voluntary, standards developing organizations such as HL7 and ASTM so that they may be implemented in proprietary EHR systems and also used as a fully interoperable transport standard between EHR systems (NITRD 2004)

President's E-Gov Initiative

In President's Bush's 2002 budget submission, he outlined a management agenda for making government more focused on citizens and results, which includes expanding Electronic Government, or E-Government (E-Gov). E-Gov uses improved Internet-based technology to make it easy for citizens and businesses to interact with the government, save taxpayer dollars, and streamline citizen to government communications. The E-Gov strategy has identified several high payoffs, governmentwide initiatives to integrate agency operations and information technology investments. The goal of these initiatives will be to eliminate redundant systems and significantly improve the government's quality of customer service for citizens and businesses. One of the new requirements of this initiative is to sponsor ongoing dialogue with state, local, and tribal governments, as well as the general public, private, and nonprofit sectors to find innovative ways to improve the performance of governments in collaborating on the use of information technology to improve the delivery of Government information and services (OMB 2005).

Consolidated Health Informatics (CHI)

One of the key E-Gov projects established so far is the CHI program. This initiative adopts a portfolio of existing health information interoperability standards (vocabulary and messaging) enabling all agencies in the federal health enterprise to "speak the same language" based on common enterprise-wide business and information technology architectures (NAHIT 2005). One of its goals is to use the same vocabulary to enable exchange of health information over secure electronic networks within the federal healthcare sector. The three leading partners in this project are the Departments of Health and Human Services, Defense, and Veterans Affairs. A number of other federal agencies provide a supporting role. An interagency council directs the initiative, and decisions are made on a consensus basis. Once CHI agrees on certain standards, they are presented to the NCVHS which communicates the CHI recommendations to the private sector and obtains their feedback. Workgroups consisting of clinical domain experts were formed to identify standards for 24 clinical domains. These workgroups analyzed all the standards that could possibly be used for each domain. Recommendations are then made on specific standards unless there is not one that is sufficient to meet the needs of a domain or no adequate standard exists at all. These recommended standards must then be review and approved by the NCVHS. Adoption of the first five standards occurred in March 2003 and another 15 were adopted in May 2004. Subsequent work involves facilitating the implementation of these standards in federal health information technology projects, working with industry standards organizations to improve the adopted standards, and addressing identified needs for new standards (Evans 2004) (see table 13.10).

Table 13.10.   CHI-adopted standards

Domain	Adopted Standard	Comments
Anatomy/Physiology	Anatomy: SNOMED-CT, NCI Thesaurus	No current standard meets the requirements for Physiology
Billing/Financial	HIPAA Medical Code Sets: ICD-9-CM, NDC, HCPCS, CPT-4, CDT, ABC Codes, DRGs	
Chemicals	EPA SRS	w/conditions
Clinical Encounters	SNOMED-CT w/gaps	
Clinical Laboratory Results	LOINC	
Demographics	HL7 Version 2.4 & Higher	
Diagnosis/Problem Lists	SNOMED-CT	SNOMED-Ct categories of Diseases & Findings
Disability	Deferred to Phase II	Recommend support for further research for one standard
Drug Ordering	NCDCP	
Genes & Proteins	HUGH for genes	No recommendation for proteins yet
History & Physical	Deferred to Phase II	More time needed to align efforts w/other Standards Development Organizations (SDOs)
Immunizations	HL7 CVX & MVX	
Interventions/Procedures Lab Test Order Names	LOINC	
Interventions/Procedures (Excluding Lab)	SNOMED-CT	Has some gaps including mappings between SNOMED-CT, CPT, HCPCS, ICD-9-CM Vol. 3, & ICD-10-PCS via UMLS
Lab Result Contents	SNOMED-CT	
Medical Devices & Supplies	Deferred to Phase II	
Medications	FDA Established Name, FDA UNII Codes, RxNorm SCD, FDA/CDER DSM, FDA NDC Product Name/Code, HL7 SPL, HL7 Vocab Tables, NDF-RT	FDA Established Name & UNII Codes Active Ingredients, RxNorm SCD Clinical Drug including Administered Dosage Form, FDA/CDER DSM Manufactured Dosage Form & Medication Package, FDA NDC Drug Product including Finished Dosage Form, HL7 SPL Labeling Section Headers, HL7—Special Populations (Race, Ethnicity & Gender), NDF-RT Drug Classification
Messaging Connectivity	IEEE	
Messaging Image Retrieval & Transfer	DICOM	
Messaging Nonpharmacy	HL7	
Messaging Pharmacy	NCPDP SCRIPT	
Multimedia	Deferred to Phase II	
Nursing	SNOMED-CT	HHCC, Omaha System, NIC, PNDS, NANDA, PNDS, NOC are included in SNOMED-CT. Discussions ongoing with the ICN and PCDS.
Population Health	Deferred to Phase II	No adequate standard currently
Supplies	GMDN & UMDNS	Wait for these two systems to merge and then adopt the resulting terminology
Text-Based Reports	HL7 CDA	
Units	HL7 Units Codes	

Source: OMB 2005.

National Committee on Vital and Health Statistics

The NCVHS is an advisory body on health data and statistics to the HHS. As part of their responsibilities under the HIPAA Act of 1996, they study, select and recommend new clinical data standards, in collaboration with CHI, to HHS. They encourage federal health programs to be early adopters of these standards. Instead of using mandates, the NCVHS is using incentives to encourage adoption. The NCVHS has four Guiding Principles regarding standards:

- Extent to which the standard enables interoperability between information systems
- Ability of the standard to facilitate comparability of data
- Aspects of the standard that support data quality, accountability, and integrity
- Degree of market acceptance of the standard

The NCVHS is also responsible for providing communication and outreach to consumer groups, the health industry, standard development organizations (SDOs), the research community, and state and local governments.

Institute of Medicine

The **Institute of Medicine** (IOM) has been very active in the last two decades in calling for the adoption of EHRs and interoperability standards. In 1991, they called for the elimination of paper-based record within 10 years. They have issued several reports on patient safety issues due to paper-based systems in the 1990s. In 2003, HHS asked the IOM to provide guidance on Key Capabilities of an EHR System. The IOM Data Standards for Patient Safety project is responsible developing a plan the development of standards applicable to the collection, coding and classification of patient safety information (Institute of Medicine 2005).

The IOM has identified a set of eight core care delivery functions that EHR systems should be capable of performing in order to promote greater safety, quality and efficiency in health care delivery. This will be used by HL7 to devise a common industry standard for EHR functionality that will guide the efforts of software developers. (NAHIT 2005).

National Library of Medicine

The **National Library of Medicine** (NLM) is the world's largest medical library. It collects materials in all aspects of biomedicine and healthcare, as well as works on biomedical aspects of technology, the humanities, and the physical, life, and social sciences. It is a standards-supporting/promoting organization that explores the uses of computer and communication technologies to improve organizations and the use of biomedical information. It is responsible for publishing **Medical Subject Headings** (MeSH), RxNorm, **Semantic Clinical Drug** (SDC) **of RxNorm** and the **Unified Medical Language Systems** (UMLS) (NAHIT 2005).

The Public Health Informatics Institute (PHII)

The **Public Health Informatics Institute** (PHII) brings together experts in public health, health information systems, and informatics established to develop health information systems. Its goal is to foster effective health information systems through collaboration, innovation, and action. The institute grew out of All Kids Count, a program funded by the Robert Wood Johnson Foundation. All Kids Count was instrumental in the development of immunization registries. It evolved into the PHII. The Institute has four key principles. Principle 3 is the Plan for Operability. Principle 3 states, "Data standards make possible interoperability of information systems, and major national initiatives [National Health Information Infrastructure (NHII) and PHIN] support the vision of electronic health records that enable timely response by providers at the point of care and by public health agencies in the community." The PHII assists health organizations to assess the compatibility of systems with current standards (PHII 2005).

The National Alliance for Health Information Technology

The **National Alliance for Health Information Technology** (NAHIT) was founded in 2002. It is a partnership of government and private sector leaders from various healthcare organizations working to use technology to achieve improvements in patient safety, quality of care, and operating performance. The NAHIT operates the **Alliance Standards Directory,** which includes 850 voluntary and mandatory standards and links to more than 200 standards development organizations (see figure 13.6). The directory was made available for public use in 2004. It also contains members-only access to detailed summaries and evaluations of standards. The directory is an excellent tool for learning more about specific standards, how they are used, their level of adoption, etc. It contains two ways to view standards: by SDO or by Standard Publication. Rod Piechowski, Alliance Program Manager, states, "For the first time, the healthcare community can locate and research pertinent standards as they plan information technology projects. The directory provides a centralized reference that also will help eliminate redundant standards development efforts by highlighting the relationships among the many organizations attempting to improve patient safety and the quality of care" (Healthcare IT News 2004).

The EHR Collaborative

The **EHR Collaborative** is a group of organizations representing key stakeholders in healthcare (eHealth Initiative 2004). The Collaborative's goal is to facilitate rapid input from the healthcare community in development initiatives that advance adoption of information standards for healthcare. It accomplishes this by offering open forums for end-user participation and input. The EHR Collaborate sponsored a number of open forums in 2003 and 2004 to gain feedback about HL7's Draft EHR Functional Model. As a result, they published the EHR Collaborative Report: HIMSS and Web Site Responses to HL7 EHR Ballot 2 on March 3, 2004 that provided private sector input feedback about this model. This organization ensures that federal government standards development initiatives receive important feedback from the private sector. The Collaborative is currently comprised of the following organizations (eHealth Initiative 2004):

- American Health Information Management Association (AHIMA)
- Healthcare Information and Management Systems Society (HIMSS)
- American Medical Association (AMA)
- American Medical Informatics Association (AMIA)
- College of Healthcare Information Management Executives (CHIME)
- eHealth Initiative (eHI)
- National Alliance for Health Information Technology (NAHIT)

Connecting For Health

Connecting for Health is a public-private collaborative designed to address the barriers to development of an interconnected health information infrastructure. The first phase of the Collaborative's work drove consensus on the adoption of an initial set of data standards, developed case studies on privacy and security, and helped define the electronic personal heath record (PHR). It is expected that an agreed-upon set of interoperability standards will improve decision making, reduce medications errors, accelerate research on patient outcomes and increase the effectiveness of public health efforts (Markle Foundation 2002). Connecting for Health was established by the Markle Foundation and receives additional funding and support from the Robert Wood Johnson Foundation. "Clinical data standards are critical to providing the best possible patient care," said Herbert Pardes, MD, President of New York–Presbyterian Hospital (Markle Foundation 2002).

The American National Standards Institute

The **American National Standards Institute** (ANSI) is an organization that promotes voluntary standardization and con-

Figure 13.6.   Example of Alliance Standards Directory page

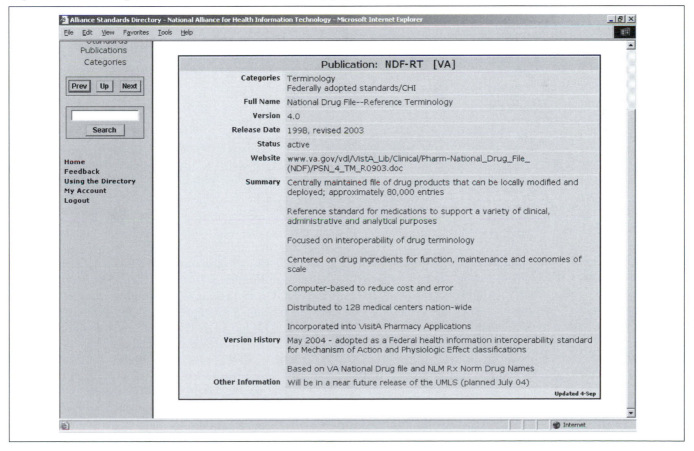

Source: NAHIT 2005.

formity assessment systems. It represents the United States in standards development internationally in the International Organization for Standardization (ISO) and the International Electrotechnical Commission (IEC). ANSI has a **Healthcare Informatics Standards Board** (HISB) that provides an environment that coordinates and harmonizes national and international healthcare standards. Every major developer of healthcare informatics standards participates in the ANSI HISB (NAHIT 2005). ANSI does not write standards; rather, it assists standards developers and users from the private sector and from government to reach consensus on the need for standards. It helps them to avoid duplication of work and provides a forum for resolution of differences (Hammond and Cimino 2001).

American Society for Testing and Materials

The **American Society for Testing and Materials** (ASTM) was founded in 1898. It is a scientific and technical organization for the development of standards for characteristics and performance of materials. Their original focus was on standard test methods, but has since been expanded to include products, systems, and services. ASTM technical committees serve as Technical Advisory Groups (TAGs) for developing U.S. positions on international standards. ASTM Committee E31 on Computerized Systems is responsible for the development of medical information standards (Hammond and Cimino 2001) (see table 13.11).

Check Your Understanding 13.5

1. Name two government agencies or committees involved in the development and deployment of vocabularies and terminologies in electronic health records.

2. Describe the actions of one nongovernmental organization involved in electronic health record activities.

3. Discuss why standards organizations are important for the electronic health record.

Emerging Vocabularies and Classifications

A number of vocabularies and classifications have been developed in recent years, some of which will have a significant impact on the role of the HIM professional in the future. The following sections examine some of these recent and emerging vocabularies and classifications.

Systematized Nomenclature of Medicine

The **Systematized Nomenclature of Medicine** (SNOMED) is developed, maintained, and distributed by the College of American Pathologists (CAP). SNOMED was originally built on the Systematized Nomenclature of Pathology (SNOP), which was introduced in 1965. Like SNOP, SNOMED uses an alphanumeric, multiaxial coding scheme (Kudla and Blakemore 2001).

Table 13.11. ASTM E31 committees

Subcommittee	Medical-Information Standard
E31.01	Controlled Vocabularies for Healthcare Informatics
E31.10	Pharmaco-Informatics Standards
E31.11	Electronic Health Record Portability
E31.13	Clinical Laboratory Information Management Systems
E31.14	Clinical Laboratory Instrument Interface
E31.16	Interchange of Electrophysiological Waveforms and Signals
E31.17	Access, Privacy, and Confidentiality of Medical Records
E31.19	Electronic Health Record Content and Structure
E31.20	Data and System Security for Health Information
E31.21	Health Information Networks
E31.22	Health Information Transcription and Documentation
E31.23	Modeling of Health Informatics
E31.24	Electronic Health Record System Functionality
E31.25	XML for Document Type Definitions in Healthcare

In 1997, the CAP worked with a team of physicians and nurses from Kaiser Permanente to begin development of the **Systematized Nomenclature of Medicine Reference Terminology** (SNOMED RT) (Kudla and Blakemore 2001). In 1997, Spackman, Campbell, and Cote defined a **reference terminology** for clinical data as "a set of concepts and relationships that provides a common reference point for comparison and aggregation of data about the entire health care process, recorded by multiple different individuals, systems or institutions." One of the ways that SNOMED RT did this was by including an elementary mapping to ICD-9-CM (Kudla and Blakemore 2001). SNOMED also worked with the **Digital Imaging and Communications in Medicine** (DICOM) community, the **Logical Observation Identifier Names and Codes** (LOINC) system, and the various nursing vocabularies to further expand its content.

In 2002, SNOMED-RT and Clinical Terms, Version 3 (CTV3), also known as the Read Codes, merged to create the SNOMED–Clinical Terminology (CT) system (NHS 1999). This merge more than doubled the content of the system to more than 300,000 unique clinical concepts and more than 900,000 descriptions to express these concepts. SNOMED-CT provides coverage of the following:

- Disease
- Procedure
- Body structure
- Organism
- Finding
- Observable entity
- Specimen
- Substance
- Pharmaceutical/biologic product
- Physical object
- Physical force
- Measurable
- Events
- Social context
- Environmentals and geographical locations
- Staging and scales

SNOMED-CT also provides cross mappings to:

- ICD-O topography
- ICD-9-CM
- ICD-10
- LOINC
- Nursing classifications PNDS, NANDA, and Omaha (Ryske and Imel 2003)

See tables 13.12 and 13.13 for SNOMED clinical detail comparisons.

U.S. License

In July 2003, the NLM, on behalf of the Department of Health and Human Services, signed a five-year contract to license and supply SNOMED-CT for use in healthcare information systems. Because of this agreement, any U.S. organization can freely acquire and use SNOMED-CT from NLM's UMLS Metathesaurus. (Bowie 2004).

The Department of Health and Human Services recommended SNOMED-CT as part of a core set of patient medical record information (PMRI) terminology in November 2003. Then in May 2004, SNOMED-CT was adopted as a federal information technology interoperability standard:

- To describe specific nonlaboratory interventions and procedures performed/delivered
- To exchange results of laboratory tests between facilities
- To describe anatomical locations for clinical, surgical, pathological, and research purposes
- For diagnosis and problem lists
- To define terminology of the delivery of nursing care

The SNOMED-CT Healthcare Terminology Structure is also ANSI-approved (NAHIT 2005).

Examples of Implementations of SNOMED-CT

Kaiser Permanente has based most of its terminology domains in SNOMED-CT, including Problem List. Other

Table 13.12. SNOMED ICD clinical detail comparison: Specimen adequacy

SNOMED	Description	ICD
112631006	Specimen unsatisfactory for diagnosis	799.9
77289001	Insufficient tissue for diagnosis	
67736002	Specimen poorly fixed	
54192004	Specimen obscured by foreign material	
63038006	Specimen obscured by inflammation	
84567002	Specimen obscured by blood	
7667005	Specimen shows excessive cytolysis	

Source: CAP n.d.

Table 13.13. SNOMED CPT clinical detail comparison: Procedures

SNOMED-CT	Description	CPT
	Total abdominal hysterectomy with or without removal of tubes, with or without removal of ovaries	58150
86477000	–with removal of tube and ovary	
27950001	–with unilateral removal of ovary	
31545000	–with unilateral removal of tube	

Source: CAP n.d.

healthcare organizations have implemented or planned to implement their problem lists on SNOMED-CT, for example, the University of Nebraska, Cedar-Sinai and the Department of Veterans Affairs (VA). The VA is also using SNOMED-CT to standardize some Allergy elements and anatomy coding in autopsy reports. Intermountain Health Care is also using SNOMED.

Logical Observation Identifier Names and Codes

The work on LOINC began in February 1994. Today, LOINC is generally accepted as the exchange standard for laboratory results, enabling standards to be developed and adopted relatively quickly to meet a desperate need. The Regenstrief Institute (regenstrief.org) maintains the LOINC database and its supporting documentation.

The goal for LOINC is not to replace the laboratory fields in facility databases but, rather, to provide a mapping mechanism. The LOINC committee hoped that laboratories would create fields in their master files for storing LOINC codes and names as attributes of their own data elements.

The LOINC committee first established a rule for creating LOINC names. "If a test has its own column on a clinical report, or has a reference range that is significantly different from other tests, or has clinical significance distinct from other closely related tests, it should be assigned a separate name" (Forrey et al. 1996, p. 82). Thus, each LOINC name identifies a distinct laboratory observation.

Each LOINC name is structured and can contain up to six parts, including:

- Analyte/component (for example, potassium, hemoglobin)
- Kind of property measured or observed (for example, mass, mass concentration, enzyme concentration)
- Time aspect of the measurement or observation (a point in time versus an observation integrated over time)
- System/sample type (for example, urine, blood, serum)
- Type of measurement or observation scale (quantitative [a number] versus qualitative [a trait such as cloudy])
- Type of measurement or observation method used (for example, clean catch or catheter)

After the names were established, unique codes were simply assigned to the names. The codes have no inherent meaning; they were designed for use by computers, not humans. LOINC has rules for using each part of the LOINC name. That detail can be accessed on the LOINC Web site at regenstrief.org/loinc. Table 13.14 provides an example of LOINC codes and names.

The LOINC database contains 23 fields in addition to the 6 named ones. Finally, records that should no longer be used are tagged as such rather than removed.

The primary disadvantage to LOINC is that it may require significant modifications to work with a current laboratory information system. As with SNOMED-RT and CTV3, LOINC is usable only in computerized systems.

A distinct advantage to using LOINC is that it enables the standardized communication of laboratory results. Large integrated delivery systems that have very diverse laboratory processing systems (the machines that perform the tests) will find it easier to maintain and use a CPR with valid laboratory results.

LOINC is divided into two major sections: Lab LOINC and Clinical LOINC. Clinical LOINC includes entries for vital signs, hemodynamics, intake/output, EKG, obstetric ultrasound, cardiac echo, urologic imaging, gastroendoscopic procedures, pulmonary ventilator management, selected survey instruments, and other clinical observations.

In March 2003, LOINC was adopted as a federal health information interoperability standard for the electronic exchange of laboratory test orders and drug label section headers (Structured Product Labeling Sections) (Regenstrief Institute 2005).

Examples of LOINC Implementations

LOINC has been implemented in a number of different healthcare settings. Intermountain Health Care uses Lab LOINC extensively to mediate with outside lab providers. They also use Clinical LOINC for ventilator management, prostate tumors, radiation oncology complications, nursing assessment measurements, etc. Representatives from IHC, Vanderbilt University and Columbia University have submitted new nursing content for inclusion into the LOINC database, primarily nursing goals. The Department of Veterans Affairs has implemented Lab LOINC as their primary coding system for laboratory tests and HL7 messages. They are also proposing to use Clinical LOINC to fully specify a text document naming nomenclature. It has also been discussed in regards to vital measurements and the Clinical Observations (Clio) project (for example, cardiac procedures, endoscopies, rheumatology procedures, etc.). Columbia University and Barnes Hospital at Washington University in St. Louis are using Lab LOINC to exchange laboratory data as part of the "Combining Laboratory Data Sets from Multiple Institutions Using the LOINC Names and Codes."

Nursing Classifications

The care delivered by nurses is very different from the care delivered by other healthcare professionals. In an effort to research, teach, practice, and create public policy for nursing, the nursing profession, under the leadership of the **American Nurses Association** (ANA), has developed nursing classifications. The purpose of these classifications is to describe the nursing process, document nursing care, and facilitate aggregation of data for comparisons at the local, regional, national, and international levels (Henry et al. 1998).

The ANA established the Steering Committee on Databases (SCD) to Support Clinical Nursing Practice to monitor and support the development and evolution of the use of multiple vocabularies and classification schemes (Henry et al. 1998). The **Nursing Information and Data Set Evaluation Center** (NIDSEC) arose from that initiative. The purpose of the NIDSEC is to review, evaluate against defined criteria, and recognize IS developers and manufacturers that support nursing care documentation with automated Nursing Information Systems (NIS) or within CPR systems (nursingworld.org/nidsec). Figure 13.7 lists the ANA criteria for recognition of nursing classifications (Henry et al. 1998). Through the NIDSEC, the ANA has recognized a total of 12 classifications for nursing.

Currently, nursing professionals are working with SNOMED-RT and other vocabulary system developers to

Table 13.14.   LOINC codes and names

Code	Name
11-7	AMIKACIN:SUSC:PT:ISLT:QN:MBC
2603-9	MALONATE:MCNC:PT:SER:QN
5874-3	RESPIRATORY SYNCYTIAL VIRUS
AG	:ACNC:PT:THRT:SQ:EIA

Source: Regenstrief Institute 2005.

create classifications that will meet the needs of nursing. As Henry states in the May 1998 Journal of the American Health Information Management Association, "In this era of numerous requests for data and information from multiple accrediting, governing, and quality monitoring agencies, it is vital that the HIM professional be aware of classification systems and related national efforts, beyond those that are typically physician-centric in nature (for example, ICD-9-CM and CPT). Without reliable and valid data concerning the contributions of the entire healthcare team, it is truly impossible to engage in the practice of evidence-based healthcare delivery."

North American Nursing Diagnosis Association

North American Nursing Diagnosis Association (NANDA II) is a nursing terminology used to develop and classify nursing diagnoses in a taxonomy. It was recognized by the ANA in 1991, added to NLM's Metathesaurus in 1993, registered by HL7 in 2000 and licensed by SNOMED in 2002 (NAHIT 2005).

Proposed diagnoses and revisions undergo a systematic review to determine consistency with the established criteria for a nursing diagnosis (NANDA International 2005).

Nursing Interventions Classification

Nursing Interventions Classification (NIC) is a terminology that describes the treatments that nurses perform. It contains a standardized list of 514 interventions. The classification is maintained by the Center for Nursing Classification & Clinical Effectiveness, The University of Iowa College of Nursing (Dochterman 2004).

Each intervention has a definition, a set of activities that the nurse performs to carry out the intervention, and a short list of background readings (see table 13.15). Interventions are organized in a three-level taxonomic structure that makes it easier to select an intervention and use on a computer. It is useful for clinical documentation, communication of care across settings, integration of data across systems, and curricular design. NIC was recognized by the ANA in 1990, included in the JCAHO's chapter management of information in 1994, was registered in 2000 by HL7 and licensed by SNOMED in 2002 (NAHIT 2005).

Nursing Outcomes Classification

Nursing Outcomes Classification (NOC) is a comprehensive standardized classification of patient/client outcomes

Figure 13.7. ANA criteria for the recognition of nursing classifications

1. The classification must be clinically useful for making diagnostic, intervention, and/or outcome decisions.
2. The classification must go beyond an application or synthesis/adaptation of vocabulary/classification schemes currently recognized by the ANA or present an explicit rationale why it should also be recognized.
3. The classification must be stated in clear and unambiguous terms, with the terms precisely defined.
4. The classification must have been tested for reliability of the vocabulary terms.
5. The classification must have been validated as useful for clinical purposes.
6. The classification must be accompanied by documentation of a systematic methodology for development.
7. The classification must be accompanied by evidence of process for periodic review and provision for addition, revision, and deletion of terms.
8. The classification must have a taxonomic structure that is conceptually coherent.
9. The classification must have terms that are associated with a unique identifier or code.
10. The classification must leave a machine-readable audit trail.
11. The classification must include defining characteristics, especially for nursing diagnoses.

Table 13.15.   Examples of NIC intervention labels and definitions

Code	Intervention	Definition
6400	Abuse Protection Support	Identification of high-risk dependent relationships and actions to prevent further infliction of physical or emotional harm
6402	Abuse Protection Support: Child	Identification of high-risk dependent relationships and actions to prevent further infliction of physical, sexual, or emotional harm or neglect of basic necessities of life
6403	Abuse Protection Support: Domestic Partner	Identification of high-risk dependent relationships and actions to prevent further infliction of physical, sexual, or emotional harm or exploitation of a domestic partner
6404	Abuse Protection Support: Elder	Identification of high-risk dependent relationships and actions to prevent further infliction of physical, sexual, or emotional harm; neglect of basic necessities of life or exploitation
1910	Acid-Base Management	Promotion of acid-base balance and prevention of complications resulting from acid-base imbalance
1911	Acid-Base Management: Metabolic Acidosis	Promotion of acid-base balance and prevention of complications resulting from serum HCO3 levels lower than desired
1912	Acid-Base Management: Metabolic Alkalosis	Promotion of acid-base balance and prevention of complications resulting from serum HCO3 levels higher than desired
1913	Acid-Base Management: Respiratory Acidosis	Promotion of acid-base balance and prevention of complications resulting from serum PCO3 levels higher than desired
1920	Acid-Base Monitoring	Collection and analysis of patient data to regulate acid-base balance
4920	Active Listening	Attending closely to and attaching significance to a patient's verbal and nonverbal messages

Source: The University of Iowa College of Nursing 2005.

developed to evaluate the effects of nursing interventions. It contains a list of 330 standardized outcomes, each with a definition, a list of indicators that can be used to evaluate patient status in relation to the outcome, a five-point Likert scale to measure patient status, and a short list of references used in development of the outcome (see table 13.16). The classification is also maintained by the Center for Nursing Classification & Clinical Effectiveness, The University of Iowa College of Nursing (Moorhead 2004).

This terminology may be used to follow patient outcomes throughout an illness episode or over an extended period of care. Each outcome has a unique code number that facilitates the use of outcomes in computerized clinical information systems and the manipulation of data to answer questions about healthcare quality and effectiveness. NOC is recognized by the ANA's Congress of Nursing Practice Steering Committee on Databases to Support Clinical Nursing Practice as a classification system useful for clinical nursing practice. It has been included in NLM's UMLS (NAHIT 2005).

Clinical Care Classification

This **Clinical Care Classification** (CCC), formerly known as the Home Health Care Classification (HHCC), consists of two interrelated taxonomies; the CCC of Nursing Diagnoses and Outcomes and the CCC of Nursing Interventions and Actions. Each provides a standardized framework for documenting patient care in hospitals, home health agencies, ambulatory care clinics, and other healthcare settings. It consists of 21 Care Components that serve as a framework for mapping and linking the two interrelated CCC taxonomies to each other and to other health-related classifications (see table 13.17). They are used to track and measure patient/client care holistically over time, across settings, population groups, and geographic locations. The system was developed from federally funded research. It was formally recognized

by the ANA in 1991. The CCC was developed and maintained by Sabacare (Saba 2005).

The Omaha System

The **Omaha System** is a research based comprehensive taxonomy designed to generate data following usual or routine client care. It consists of three components (NAHIT 2005) (see table 13.18, p. 330):

- Problem Classification Scheme
- Intervention Scheme
- Problem Rating Scale for Outcomes

It is a practice and documentation tool used by multidisciplinary health care practitioners from the time of admission to discharge. The Omaha System translates data into information for practice, education, and research. EHR systems based on the Omaha System provide an information management tool for data collection, aggregation, and analysis. Initial development and research began early in the 1970s. The most recent revision was published in 2005. The system is maintained by Martin Associates and a 12-member Omaha System Board (Martin 2005). The Omaha System was one of the first vocabularies recognized by the ANA. It is also included in the NLM's UMLS Metathesaurus, the ANSI HISB Inventory of Clinical Information Standards, SNOMED International, LOINC, HL7, and in the accreditation standards of the JCAHO and the Community Health Accreditation Program (Martin 2005).

Nursing Management Minimum Data Set

The **Nursing Management Minimum Data Set** (NMMDS) supports description, analysis, and comparisons of nursing care and nursing resources in light of the effects of context on complex health care outcomes. It was designed to complement the

Table 13.16.   Examples of NOC outcomes labels and definitions (330 outcomes)

Code	Label	Definition
2500	Abuse Cessation	Evidence that the victim is no longer hurt or exploited
1400	Abuse Behavior–Self-Restraint	Self-restraint of abusive or neglectful behaviors towards others
1300	Acceptance–Health Status	Reconciliation to significant change in health circumstances
0005	Activity Tolerance	Physiological response to energy-consuming movements with daily activities
1401	Aggression Self-Control	Self-restraint of assaultive, combative, or destructive behaviors towards others
0706	Allergic Response–Systemic	Severity of systemic hypersensitive immune response to a specific environmental (exogenous) antigen
0200	Ambulation	Ability to walk from place to place independently with or without assistive device
1211	Anxiety Level	Severity of manifested apprehension, tension, or uneasiness arising from an unidentifiable source
1918	Aspiration Prevention	Personal actions to prevent the passage of fluid and solid particles into the lung
0700	Blood Transfusion Reaction	Severity of complications with blood transfusion reaction

Source: The University of Iowa College of Nursing 2005.

Table 13.17.   Examples of CCC system nursing diagnoses

Code	Category	Diagnosis
A01	Activity Alteration	Change in or modification of energy used by the body
A01.1	Activity Intolerance	Incapacity to carry out physiological or psychological daily activities
A01.2	Activity Intolerance Risk	Increased chance of an incapacity to carry out physiological or psychological daily activities
O38.1	Activities of Daily Living (ADLs) Alteration	Change in modification of ability to maintain oneself
Q45.1	Acute Pain	Physical suffering or distress; to hurt
E12.1	Adjustment Impairment	Inadequate adaptation to condition or change in health status
U61.4	Adolescent Behavior Alteration	Change in or modification or normal standards of performing developmental skills and behavior of a typical adolescent from 12 years through 20 years of age
U61.5	Adult Behavior Alteration	Change in or modification or normal standards of performing developmental skills and behavior of a typical adult from 21 years through 64 years of age
L26.1	Airway Clearance Impairment	Inability to clear secretions/obstructions in airway
N58.2	Alcohol Abuse	Excessive use of distilled liquors

Source: Saba 2005.

clinical patient-oriented data designated in the **Nursing Minimum Data Set** (NMDS) (NAHIT 2005).

Nursing Minimum Data Set (NMDS)

The NMDS provides uniform definitions and categories concerning the specific dimensions of nursing, which meet the information needs of multiple data users in the healthcare system. It was built on the concept of the uniform minimum health data sets (UMHDSs) and includes the label and conceptual definition of the essential, specific elements that are used by nurses across all types of settings in the delivery of care. It also establishes comparability of nursing data across clinical populations, settings, geographic areas, and time. The NMDS was recognized by the ANA in 1999 (NAHIT 2005).

The NMDS includes three broad categories of elements (NMDS 2003) (see table 13.19, p. 331):

- Nursing care
- Patient or client demographics
- Service elements

Patient Care Data Set

The **Patient Care Data Set** (PCDS) (Version 4.0 1998) consists of a three-component dictionary of:

- Patient problems (363 terms)
- Patient care goals (311 terms)
- Patient care orders (1,357 terms)

The intent of this set is to serve as a set of standard terms to represent and capture clinical data for inclusion in patient care information systems. It was recognized in 1998 by the ANA as one of the vocabularies considered for use by nurses and is included in the NLM's Metathesaurus. The PCDS is owned and maintained by the Vanderbilt University Medical

Center. The terms of the PCDS are organized into 22 components (Ozbolt 1999):

- Activity (see table 13.20, p. 331)
- Circulation
- Cognition
- Coping and Mental Health
- Fluids and Electrolytes
- Gastrointestinal Function
- Health Knowledge and Behaviors
- Immunology
- Medications and Blood Products
- Metabolism
- Nutrition
- Physical Regulation
- Pre-, Intra, and Post-Procedure
- Respiration
- Role Relationships
- Safety
- Self Care
- Self Concept
- Sensation, Pain, and Comfort
- Tissue Integrity
- Tissue Perfusion
- Urinary Elimination

International Classification for Nursing Practice

The **International Classification for Nursing Practice** (ICNP) is a unified nursing language system into which existing terminologies can be cross-mapped (see table 13.21, p. 331). It was created in 1989 by ICN. ICNP Version 1 is scheduled for release in 2005 (NAHIT 2005). It was established as a common language for describing nursing practice in order to improve

Table 13.18.   The Omaha System concepts and ratings of the problem-rating scale for outcomes

Concepts	1	2	3	4	5
Knowledge: Ability of the client to remember and interpret information	No knowledge	Minimal knowledge	Basic knowledge	Adequate knowledge	Superior knowledge
Behavior: Observable responses, actions, or activities of the client fitting the occasion or purpose	Not appropriate behavior	Rarely appropriate behavior	Inconsistently appropriate behavior	Usually appropriate behavior	Consistently appropriate behavior
Status: Condition of the client in relation to objective and subjective defining characteristics	Extreme signs/ symptoms	Severe signs/ symptoms	Moderate signs/ symptoms	Minimal signs/ symptoms	No signs/symptoms

Domains and Problems of the Problem Classification Scheme

Domain	Description	Examples
Environmental	Material resources and physical surroundings both inside and outside the living area, neighborhood, and broader community	Income Sanitation Residence Neighborhood/workplace safety
Psychosocial	Patterns of behavior, emotion, communication, relationships, and development	Communication with community resources Social contact Role change Interpersonal relationship
Physiological	Functions and processes that maintain life	Hearing Vision Speech and language Oral health
Health-Related Behaviors	Patterns of activity that maintain or promote wellness, promote recovery, and decrease the risk of disease	Nutrition Sleep and rest patterns Physical activity Personal care

Categories of the Intervention Scheme

Categories	Description
Teaching, Guidance, and Counseling	Activities designed to provide information and materials, encourage action and responsibility for self-care and coping, and assist the individual/family/community to make decisions and solve problems
Treatments and Procedures	Technical activities such as wound care, specimen collection, resistive exercises, and medication prescriptions that are designed to prevent, decrease, or alleviate signs and symptoms of the individual/family/community
Case Management	Activities such as coordination, advocacy, and referral that facilitate service delivery, improve communication among health and human service providers, promote assertiveness, and guide the individual/family/community toward use of appropriate resources.
Surveillance	Activities such as detection, measurement, critical analysis, and monitoring intended to identify the individual/family/community's status in relation to a given condition or phenomenon.

Targets of the Intervention Scheme—Examples

	Anatomy/physiology	Bowel care
	Anger management	Cardiac care
	Behavior modification	Caretaking/parenting skills
	Bladder care	Cast care
	Bonding/attachment	Communication

Source: Martin 2005.

Table 13.19.   Examples of NMDS elements

Nursing Care Elements	Patient or Client Demographic Elements	Service Elements
Nursing Diagnosis	Personal Identification	Unique Facility or Service Agency Number
Nursing Intervention	Date of Birth	Unique Health Record Number or Patient or Client
Nursing Outcome	Sex	Unique Number of Principle Registered Nurse Provider
Intensity of Nursing Care	Race and Ethnicity Residence	Episode Admission or Encounter Date Discharge or Termination Date Disposition of Patient or Client Expected Payer for Most of This Bill (Anticipated Financial Guarantor for Services)

Source: The University of Iowa College of Nursing 2005.

Table 13.20.   PCDS elements on the goals axis and their values in the activity component

Subject	Performance	Level of Performance	Object	Equipment	Manifestations	Evaluation
Patient	Will achieve	Adequate	Activity	By use of appropriate equipment	Rest periods	Achieved
Spouse	Will adhere to	As prescribed for subject	Activity: Activity restrictions	By use of assistive devices	Uninterrupted 60–90 minute sleep cycles	Progressing ahead of schedule
Significant Other	Will conserve	Baseline	Activity: Activity tolerance	By use of orthotic devices	Usual sleep patterns	Progressing on schedule
Family	Will experience	Minimal or no	Activity: Ambulation	By use of wheelchair	Voluntary limitation of activities	Progressing behind schedule
Adult Child(ren)	Will express satisfaction with	Physically independent	Activity: Energy			Not progressing
Child(ren)	Will incorporate into daily activities	Verbally independent	Activity: Exercise			Regressing
Infant(s)	Will maintain	Within acceptable range for subject	Activity: Fatigue			Goal abandoned
Fetus(es)	Will progress beyond		Activity: Immobilization			

Source: Ozbolt 1999.

Table 13.21.   ICNP example displaying combining terms from select axes to compose nursing interventions

Select Axes	Select Terms	Select Terms	Select Terms	Select Terms
Action Type	Alleviating	Reducing	Teaching	Testing
Target	Pain	Anxiety	Exercising habits	Water supply
Beneficiary	Individual	Individual	Group (distributively)	Community (Collectively)
Means	Cold pack	Guided imagery technique	Instructional materials	Protocol

Interventions: Alleviating an individual's pain by applying a cold pack.
              Reducing anxiety using a guided imagery technique.
              Teaching group members about exercising habits using instructional materials.
              Testing the water supply for a community using an established protocol.				

Source: ICNP 2004.

communication among nurses, and between nurses and others. It can also be used to project trends in patient needs, provision of nursing treatments, resources, and outcomes of nursing care. ICNP is composed of the following elements:

- Nursing Phenomena (nursing diagnoses)
- Nursing Actions (nursing interventions)
- Nursing Outcomes

The ICNP is maintained by the ICNP Program Director, University of Wisconsin–Milwaukee College of Nursing (ICNP 2004).

LOINC

LOINC was recognized by the ANA in 2002 as a nursing terminology. A clinical LOINC nursing subcommittee has been formed to add nursing content to LOINC with a main focus on nursing goals. This committee was also formed to provide nursing content to LOINC at a faster rate. The mission of the subcommittee is to meet the needs for machine-readable clinical, administrative, and regulatory nursing data by providing LOINC codes for observations at key stages of the nursing process, including assessments, goals, and outcomes. The nursing subcommittee plans to fulfill the following responsibilities:

- Act as a point of entry for those who wish to submit nursing data to LOINC, assisting as needed with understanding LOINC methods and processes.
- Triage of all nursing content to LOINC.
- Identify gaps in the content and solicit input from experts who can assist in the creation of content for those gaps.
- Create task forces as needed to work on specific terminology areas.
- Submit content to the Clinical LOINC committee in a "fit" condition to use.
- Disseminate starter sets, such as vital signs assessment data, to nurses to review and critique.
- Disseminate new content in the literature

Some gaps that exist include nursing goals and assessments. Providing a comprehensive set of nursing measurements in LOINC requires a great deal of new LOINC content creation. (Matney, Ozbolt, Bakken 2003).

Unified Medical Language System

The **Unified Medical Language System** (UMLS) is a government-funded project from the NLM. The UMLS has been in development since 1986. According to the UMLS Fact Sheet, "The purpose of the UMLS is to aid the development of systems that help health professionals and researchers retrieve and integrate electronic biomedical information from a variety of sources and to make it easy for users to link disparate information systems, including computer-based patient records, bibliographic databases, factual databases, and expert systems." This goal is achieved through the three knowledge

sources found in the UMLS: (1) the UMLS Metathesaurus, (2) the SPECIALIST Lexicon, and (3) the UMLS Semantic Network. (More information on the UMLS can be obtained from the NLM Web site at nlm.nih.gov/research/umls.) When looking in-depth at the UMLS, it is important to keep in mind that it has been designed for computer use; its layouts and so on are meant for machines.

UMLS Metathesaurus

The **UMLS Metathesaurus** contains information on biomedical concepts and terms from more than 60 controlled vocabularies and classifications used in health records, administrative health data, bibliographic and full-text databases, and expert systems. It preserves the names, meanings, hierarchical contexts, attributes, and interterm relationships present in its source vocabularies; adds certain basic information to each concept; and establishes new relationships among terms from different source vocabularies. Its source vocabularies include terminologies designed for use in health record systems; large disease and procedure classifications used for statistical reporting and billing; more narrowly focused vocabularies used to record data related to psychiatry, nursing, medical devices, adverse drug reactions, and so on; disease and finding terminologies from expert diagnostic systems; and some thesauri used in information retrieval.

Computer programs can use information in the Metathesaurus to interpret user inquiries, interact with users to refine their questions, identify the databases that contain information relevant to particular inquiries, and convert the users' terms into the vocabulary used by relevant information sources. The scope of the Metathesaurus is determined by the combined scope of its source vocabularies.

The Metathesaurus is produced by the automated processing of machine-readable versions of its source vocabularies, followed by human review and editing by subject experts. It is intended primarily for use by system developers but also can be a useful reference tool for database builders, librarians, and other information professionals.

UMLS SPECIALIST Lexicon

The **UMLS SPECIALIST Lexicon** is an English-language **lexicon** containing many biomedical terms. It has been developed in the context of the SPECIALIST natural language processing project at the NLM. The current version includes some 108,000 lexical records, with more than 186,000 strings (concept names).

The lexicon entry for each word or term records syntactic, morphological, and orthographic information. (Syntactic refers to the formal properties of language; morphological refers to the study and description of word formation in a language, including inflection, derivation, and compounding; and orthographic refers to the correctness of spelling or the representation of the sounds of a language by written or printed symbols.) Lexical entries may be single-word or multiword terms. Entries that share their base form and spelling variants, if any, are collected into a single lexical record. The base form is the uninflected form of the lexical item—the singular form in the case of a noun, the infinitive form in the case of a verb, and the positive form in the case of an adjective or adverb.

UMLS Semantic Network

The **UMLS Semantic Network,** through its 134 semantic types, provides a consistent categorization of all concepts represented in the UMLS Metathesaurus. The 54 links between semantic types provide the structure for the network and represent important relationships in the biomedical domain. All information on specific concepts is found in the Metathesaurus; the network provides information on the basic semantic types assigned to these concepts and defines their possible relationships.

Medical Subject Headings

Medical Subject Headings (MeSH) is the NLM's controlled vocabulary thesaurus. It consists of terms naming descriptors in a hierarchical structure that permits searching at various levels of specificity (NAHIT 2005). The descriptors exist in both alphabetic and hierarchical structures. It contains very broad headings, such "Mental Disorders," and more specific levels, such as "Conduct Disorder." There are 22,568 descriptors in MeSH and more than 139,000 headings, called Supplementary Concept Records, within a separate thesaurus. Thousands of cross-references also exist. MeSH is used by the NLM for indexing articles from 4,600 of the world's leading biomedical journals for the MEDLINE/PubMed database. Each bibliographic reference is associated with a set of MeSH terms that describe the content of the item. Staff subject specialists are responsible for revising and updating the vocabulary on a continuous basis. MeSH is available in electronic format at no charge at nlm.nih.gov/mesh and a hard copy version is published each January (UMLS 2004).

Examples of UMLS Implementation

The VA has used the UMLS Metathesaurus as a lookup tool for finding concepts, synonyms and linkages to other terminologies in the data standardization of allergies data. They are also using the UMLS RxNorm for standardizing pharmacy data and are sharing that data with the Department of Defense as part of the Consolidated Health Data Repository (CHDR) interagency project. It has also been proposed to use UMLS as the mediation terminology for VA drug classes in the CHDR project. Vanderbilt University has used UMLS in their WizOrder order entry and decision support system.

Digital Imaging and Communications in Medicine

Through a cooperative effort between the American College of Radiology and the National Electronic Manufacturers Association, **Digital Imaging and Communications in Medicine** (DICOM) was originally created to permit the interchange of biomedical image waveforms and related information. These organizations define the health record to include not only textual, coded, and numeric information (linguistic), but also a detailed, structured record of image-related information (Bidgood 1997).

The information associated with each image is the standard administrative and billing information used today—patient name, procedure code, and so on. Combined with the open protocol, this only provides for data interchange, not data understanding. The developers of the exchange standard now have taken another step and suggested a mapping/terminology resource to index the content of biomedical images in a clinically relevant manner (Bidgood 1997).

DICOM is used by most medical professions that utilize imaging within the healthcare industry including cardiology, dentistry, endoscopy, mammography, ophthalmology, orthopedics, etc. DICOM was adopted as the federal health information interoperability messaging standard for imaging in March 2003 (NAHIT 2005).

Health Level Seven

Health Level 7 (HL7) is a not-for-profit, ANSI-accredited standards developing organization. It provides standards, guidelines and methodologies to enable healthcare information system interoperability and sharing of electronic health records. It focuses on the interface requirements of the entire health care organization. Technical Committees and Special Interest Groups made up of volunteers are responsible for defining the HL7 standard protocol. Its 2,000 members represent over 500 corporate members, including 90 percent of the largest information systems vendors serving healthcare. Membership is available to everyone interested in the development of a cost-effective approach to system connectivity (NAHIT 2005).

The HL7 **Clinical Document Architecture** (CDA) provides an exchange model for clinical documents (such as discharge summaries and progress notes), and brings the healthcare industry closer to the realization of an electronic health record. The CDA utilizes XML, the HL7 Reference Information Model (RIM), and coded vocabularies to make documents machine-readable so they can be easily parsed and processed electronically. It also makes documents human-readable so they can be easily retrieved and used by the people who need them. CDA documents can be displayed using XML-aware Web browsers or wireless applications such as cell phones. The CDA was adopted in May 2004 as the federal health information interoperability standard to identify standards and terminologies used to define the messaging architecture and syntax of clinical text documents (NAHIT 2005).

HL7 was adopted for Special Populations, specifically the fields "race and ethnicity" and "gender" as well as demographics. CHI is also adopting the HL7 codes for Units and their immunization registry for immunizations, specifically the CVX (clinical vaccine formulation) and MVX (manufacturer) codes.

National Council for Prescription Drug Programs

The **National Council for Prescription Drug Programs** (NCPDP) creates and promotes data interchange standards for the pharmacy services sector of healthcare. The NCPDP Provider Identification Number supplies 70,000 pharmacies with a unique identifying number for interactions with federal agencies and third-party processors. It was incorporated in 1977 and is a not-for-profit, ANSI-accredited standards development organization. Eleven working groups meet quarterly to develop and/or modify standards for the transmission of pharmacy data. NCPDP SCRIPT was developed for transmitting prescription information electronically between prescribers and providers. It covers the electronic transmission of new prescriptions, prescription refill requests, prescription fill status notifications, and prescription cancellations. NCPDP SCRIPT was adopted as the federal health information interoperability messaging standard for prescription data (NAHIT 2005).

Institute of Electrical and Electronics Engineers 1073

Institute of Electrical and Electronics Engineers (IEEE) 1073 provides for open systems communications in healthcare applications, primarily between bedside medical devices and patient care information systems, optimized for the acute care setting. The IEEE 1073 Series was adopted as a federal health information interoperability standard for electronic data exchange (NAHIT 2005).

Medication Standards

Medication use is an important method of treatment in healthcare. Because of the growing number of available medications and the potential for adverse effects, several organizations have developed standards to assist the healthcare industry with medication safety and administration.

Food and Drug Administration Established Name for Active Ingredients and FDA Unique Ingredient Identifier Codes

The FDA's **Unique Ingredient Identifier (UNII) Codes** were developed as a standard to enable the federal health care sector to share information regarding medication active ingredients. An active ingredient is a substance responsible for the effects of a medication. The UNII Codes were adopted in May 2004 as the federal healthcare information interoperability standard for active ingredients in medications (NAHIT 2005).

Semantic Clinical Drug of RxNorm

RxNorm provides standardized names for clinical drugs (active ingredient + strength + dose form) and for dose forms as administered. It provides links from clinical drugs to their active ingredients, drug components (active ingredient + strength) and some related brand names. RxNorm is produced in consultation with the FDA, the Department of Veterans Affairs (VA), and the HL7 standards development organizations. RxNorm is only released in the UMLS Metathesaurus (NAHIT 2005).

The Semantic Clinical Drug (SCD) is a subset of RxNorm for the ingredient plus strength and dose form. An example is: Fluoxetine 4MG/ML Oral Solution. The SCD of RxNorm was adopted as a federal healthcare information interoperability standard for clinical drug nomenclature (NAHIT 2005).

FDA Center for Drug Evaluation and Research Data Standards Manual

The **FDA Center for Drug Evaluation and Research Data Standards Manual** (CDER) is a compilation of standardized nomenclature monographs that have been reviewed and approved by the CDER Nomenclature Standards Committee (see table 13.22). The CDER standards are considered binding upon all existing automated databases when undergoing a major redesign. Use of the standards is strictly voluntary for static existing databases. In May 2004, the CDER Data Standards Manual was adopted as a federal healthcare information interoperability standard for sharing information regarding manufactured drug dosage forms (NAHIT 2005).

Some of the databases using the standards include the Centerwide Oracle Management Information System (COMIS), the Division Files System (DFS), and the Drug Product Reference File (DPRF), among others. (FDA n.d.).

FDA National Drug Code Directory

The FDA **National Drug Code** (NDC) Directory is a list of all drugs manufactured, prepared, propagated, compounded, or processed by a drug establishment registered under the Federal Food, Drug, and Cosmetic Act. The NDC serves as a universal product identifier for human drugs. It consists of prescription and selected over-the-counter, insulin, domestic, and foreign drug products that are in commercial distribution in the United States. It is updated quarterly within five working days after the end of March, June, September, and December (NAHIT 2005).

Table 13.22.   Examples of FDA CDER drug nomenclature monographs

Drug Nomenclature Monographs	Monograph Number
Drug Classification	C-DRG-00101
Dosage Form	C-DRG-00201
Route of Administration	C-DRG-00301
Ingredient Name	C-DRG-00401
Proprietary Name	C-DRG-00402
Animal Common Names	C-DRG-00403
Animal Cell Tissue Fluid Biomolecule	C-DRG-00404
Biotechnology Origin	C-DRG-00405
Potency	C-DRG-00501
Indications	C-DRG-00601

LOINC Clinical Special Product Label

The LOINC **Clinical Special Product Label** (SPL) standard provides information found in the approved FDA drug label or package insert in a computer readable format for use in electronic prescribing and decision support. It is intended to make drug labeling more accessible, easier to read, and standardized. It was approved as an official ANSI-approved standard in September 2004 and as the federal health information interoperability standard for medication product labeling. Pharmaceutical companies must start submitting labeling in SPL to the FDA in 2005. It was adopted as a CHI standard upon gaining approval status by HL7 for the SPL specification and upon incorporation of the terminology into LOINC (NAHIT 2005).

The SPL is a computer file standard for product information. It consists of three parts:

- Header: General information about the label and product
- Sections: Divide the label into blocks of text (for example, indications section, contraindications section, warnings section) and define a list of acceptable sections based on regulations and needs
- Data Elements: Specific information about the product (for example, active ingredient, dosage form, how supplied) and how new data elements can be added

The SPL is also extensible in that additions can be made to the standard based on the requirements for the product label (Levin 2004).

National Drug File–Reference Terminology

National Drug File–Reference Terminology (NDF-RT) is a centrally maintained file of drug products developed by the Department of Veterans Affairs (VA) that can be locally modified and deployed. It is a reference standard for medications to support a variety of clinical, administrative and analytical purposes. It is based on the VA Nation Drug file and NLM's RxNorm Drug Names. The NDF-RT is focused on the interoperability of drug terminology. It is centered on drug ingredients for function, maintenance and economies of scale. NDF-RT is computer-based to reduce cost and error. It is incorporated into the VA's VistA Pharmacy Applications in 128 medical centers nationwide. It contains approximately 80,000 entries (NAHIT 2005).

National Cancer Institute Thesaurus

The **National Cancer Institute** (NCI) Thesaurus contains the working vocabulary used in NCI data systems. It covers clinical, translational and basic research as well as administrative terminology (see figure 13.8). In May 2004, the NCI Thesaurus was adopted as a federal healthcare information interoperability standard to describe anatomical locations for clinical, surgical, pathological and research purposes (NAHIT 2005).

The NCI Terminology Browser displays the NCI Thesaurus. The Thesaurus is an open content vocabulary that is free to use with virtually no restrictions. It is built so that both humans and computers can interpret it (NCI 2004).

Figure 13.8. NCI thesaurus taxonomy concept details

Identifiers:	
Name	Pancreas
Code	C12393
Relationships to other concepts:	
Anatomic_Structure_Has_Location	Epigastric Region
Anatomic_Structure_is_Physical_Part-of	Gastrointestinal System
Information about this concept:	
Display_Name	Pancreas
Mitelman_Code	218
Preferred_Name	Pancreas
Semantic_Type	Body Part, Organ, or Organ Component
Subsource	ICD
Subsource	LASH
Subsource	Mitelman
Unified Medical Language System	C0030274

Source: NCI 2005.

Human Genome Nomenclature

The **Human Genome Nomenclature** (HUGN) provides data for all human genes which have approved symbols (see table 13.23, p. 336). It is managed by the HUGO Gene Nomenclature Committee (HGNC) as a confidential database containing over 16,000 records. Gene records can be searched on the Web by symbol or name to directly retrieve information on gene symbol, gene name, cytogenic location, OMIM number and PubMed ID. Data are integrated with other human gene databases and approved gene symbols are carefully coordinated with the Mouse Genome Database (MGD). The online version of the database is updated weekly. HUGN was adopted as a federal health information interoperability standard for exchanging information regarding the role of genes in biomedical research and healthcare (NAHIT 2005).

Global Medical Device Nomenclature

The **Global Medical Device Nomenclature** (GMDN) is a collection of internationally recognized terms used to accurately describe and catalogue medical devices. It describes the products used in the diagnosis, prevention, monitoring, treatment or alleviation of disease or injury in humans (see figure 13.9, p. 336). GMDN was developed through the harmonization of six established medical device terminologies including a previous version of the UMDNS owned by ECRI. It is a CEN/ISO standard, approved by the FDA and maintained by GMDN Maintenance Agency Policy Group

Table 13.23. Human genes with approved symbols: Single-letter amino acid codes

Amino Acid	Three-Letter Symbol	One-Letter Symbol
Alanine	Ala	A
Arginine	Arg	R
Asparagine	Asn	N
Aspartic Acid	Asp	D
Asn + Asp	Asx	B
Cysteine	Cys	C
Glutamine	Gln	Q
Glutamic Acid	Glu	E
Gln + Glu	Glx	Z
Glycine	Gly	G

Source: Wain et al. 2002

Figure 13.9. GMDN device categories

The Standard allocates codes for a possible 20 categories. For this version of the GMDN 13 device categories are now established. These are:	
01	Active implantable devices
02	Anaesthetic and respiratory devices
03	Dental devices
04	Electro mechanical medical devices
05	Hospital hardware
06	In vitro diagnostic devices (IVD)
07	Nonactive implantable devices
08	Ophthalmic and optical devices
09	Reusable instruments
10	Single use devices
11	Technical aids for disabled persons
12	Diagnostic and therapeutic radiation devices
13	Obsolete terms
14	Vacant
15	Vacant
16	Vacant
17	Vacant
18	Vacant
19	Vacant
20	Vacant

Source: BSI Group 2004.

(MAPG) with significant FDA representation. GMDN was adopted as a federal health information interoperability standard for exchanging information regarding medical devices (NAHIT 2005).

The GMDN contains nearly 7,000 terms plus more than 10,000 synonyms. GMDN is currently divided into 12 Categories of devices to encompass all of these products. As new product areas need to be included into this classification system, a new category will be allotted and that category developed.

Universal Medical Device Nomenclature System

The UMDNS is a standard international nomenclature and computer coding system for medical devices. It facilitates identifying, processing, filing, storing, retrieving, transferring, and communicating data about medical devices. It has been adopted by many nations, including the entire European Union (EU). It is used in applications ranging from hospital inventory and work-order controls to national agency medical device regulatory systems. It is incorporated into the UMLS. UMDNS is free to nonprofit organizations to government medical regulatory systems, but they must register with the ECRI and sign a standard license agreement. CHI proposed that HUGN and UMDNS merge into one system as the federally adopted health information interoperability standard for medical devices in May 2004 (NAHIT 2005).

Environmental Protection Agency Substance Registry System

The Environmental Protection Agency (EPA) **Substance Registry System** (SRS) provides information on substances and how they are represented in the EPA's regulations and information systems. It provides a common basis for identification of chemicals, biological organisms, and other substances listed in EPA regulations and data systems, as well as substances of interest from other sources, such as publications. The EPA SRS was adopted as the federal health information interoperability standard for chemicals in May 2004 (See table 13.24) (NAHIT 2005).

Breast Imaging Reporting and Data System Atlas

Breast Imaging Reporting and Data System Atlas (BI-RADS) was designed to serve as a comprehensive guide providing standardized breast imaging terminology, a report organization, assessment structure and a classification system for mammography, ultrasound and MRI of the breast (NAHIT 2005).

Bi-RADS is the product of a collaboration effort among members of various committees of the American College of Radiology with cooperation from the National Cancer Institute, the Centers for Disease Control and Prevention, the FDA, and the College of American Pathologists. Results are

Table 13.24. Example of an EPA SRS substance list

Name	Liquid Nitrogen (Containing)
Molecular Formula	[No Criteria Specified]
Type	All
Classification	All
Display Option	Substance Name
Sort Option	Name
Systematic Name	Nitrogen
EPA Registry Name	Nitrogen
Classification	Chemical
CAS number	7727-37-9
TSN	
ICTV	
EPA ID	
Compare?	

Source: EPA 2005.

compiled in a standardized manner that permits the maintenance and collection analysis of demographic, mammographic and outcome data. (See table 13.25) (ACR 2003).

Mapping Initiatives

There are a number of terminology mapping initiatives underway and in the planning stages in the United States. HL7 has issued a three-year contract with the NLM to:

- Develop and apply methods to ensure UMLS Metathesaurus is in step with HL7 Vocabulary Standards
- Conduct pilot transfer of EHR data using HL7 Messaging and Implementation guides

HL7 plans to provide data and services necessary to ensure the CHI approved vocabularies as distributed through NLM's UMLS Metathesaurus are usable with HL7. It also plans to create implementation guides for the use of HL7 to transmit EHR data and documents between two systems, independent of source and destination architectures (HL7 2005).

The NLM, within the framework of the UMLS, is pursuing mapping activities. In addition to distributing SNOMED CT under the national license, they have committed to incorporating SNOMED:ICD-9-CM maps as well as SNOMED:CPT maps. The ICD-9-CM maps will be created by SNOMED International. Kaiser Permanente and the Veterans Health Administration will collaborate on the CPT map. The American Health Information Management Association has received the contract to validate the maps for the NLM. These maps are extremely important as they

will enable electronic health record users to operate more efficiently, entering data for clinical purposes and mapping it to reimbursement classifications when possible. Because of the very different terminologies and classification systems being mapped, no one expects all reimbursement coding to be automated.

Mapping, or cross-mapping, is the process by which concepts and terms in one system are associated with concepts and terms in another system. This field is extremely new in healthcare and has almost no existing standard procedures. Many maps are created to support a specific use case. For example, the map created for a reimbursement use case might be very different from a public health use case. This is even if the two use cases were mapping between the same two systems.

Most often, the mapping is done using categories. Examples of these categories are:

- One-to-One: An exact match is made between the systems
- Narrow-to-Broad: A more granular term in the starting system maps to a more general term in the receiving system
- Broad-to-Narrow: A more general term in the starting system maps to a more granular term in the receiving system
- Unmappable: There is no match in the receiving system

Once the map has been created, issues of validation and maintenance are raised. There are no easy answers, again, because the field is to new.

Table 13.25. BI-RADS mammography assessment categories

Assessment	Category
a. Mammographic Assessment is Incomplete	0: Need Additional Imaging Evaluation and/or Prior Mammograms for Comparisons
b. Mammographic Assessment is Complete–Final Categories	1: Negative
	2: Benign Finding(s)
	3: Probably Benign Finding–Initial Short-Interval Follow-Up Suggested
	4: Suspicious Abnormality–Biopsy Should Be Considered
	5: Highly Suggestive of Malignancy–Appropriate Action Should Be Taken (Almost certainly malignant)
	6: Known Biopsy–Proven Malignancy–Appropriate Action Should Be Taken

Source: ACR 2003.

As electronic health records continue to evolve, the need for cross-system maps and for persons who understand map creation, validation and maintenance will increase.

Nosology

Nosology is the branch of medical science that deals with classification issues. Practically, nosology is different from coding in that it is about all classification issues, whether they are related to reimbursement or other purposes.

As the need grows to formalize (classify in some manner) all health record data in any medium (text, image, voice) for purposes of outcomes research, decision support, and knowledge management, HIM professionals will have to expand their coding classification horizons to become nosologists.

Check Your Understanding 13.6

Instructions: Answer the following questions on a separate piece of paper.

1. A connection between two terms is called a **relationship.** Explain some uses of relationships in a terminology?
2. What is the future goal of DICOM?
3. Name the three knowledge sources found in the UMLS.
4. Define the term nosology.
5. Name the main advantage and the main disadvantage to using the LOINC system.
6. Name a device classification system and give examples of three clinical situations in which it might be useful.
7. List and give a one-sentence description of three nursing classification systems.
8. Discuss how recent activities by the NLM are helping to meet the clinical vocabulary needs of the U.S. healthcare industry.

Evaluation of Clinical Terminologies and Classification Systems

As HIM professionals search for ways to formalize the myriad types of data contained in EHRs, it helps to be able to evaluate the different classifications and terminologies. Certain characteristics are desirable. The first 12 characteristics listed below are taken from Cimino (1998). The second six are taken from Campbell (Campbell et al. 1999), who presented additional requirements after his experience with implementing a terminology for Kaiser Permanente. The characteristics are:

1. Content: The content of clinical classifications and terminologies should be determined by their intended use. It is wise to assume that the first identified need will never be the last or only need. It is far better to have too much content initially than to have too little to meet subsequent needs.
2. Concept orientation: The content of terminologies and classifications should be oriented toward concepts rather than terms or code numbers. For example,

"cold" can either be a disease (Chronic Obstructive Lung Disease the Common Cold), or a feeling of temperature—these are three separate concepts.

3. Concept permanence: Terminologies and classifications must be permanent if they are to be useful for longitudinal reporting. Concepts may be inactivated but must never be deleted.
4. Nonsemantic concept identifier: No implicit or explicit meaning can be associated with the code numbers used in a classification system. Because primary healthcare systems are now computerized, the human ability to use a classification system without a computer is no longer necessary. For example, in ICD-9-CM code 250.xx is related to diabetes regardless of when the condition was put into ICD-9-CM. Thus, 250 has meaning.
5. Polyhierarchy: Multiple relationships should exist for every concept. For example, bacterial pneumonia is both a pulmonary disease and an infectious disease.
6. Formal definitions: Standardized definitions are necessary to ensure comparability among terminologies and classifications. They also reduce confusion.
7. Reject Not Elsewhere Classified (NEC): Not Elsewhere Classified is not the same as Not Otherwise Specified (NOS). NOS means that there is no additional information. NEC means you have more information but no place to put it. It also means that any additional information will be lost forever if it is assigned the NEC label (for example, assigning Pneumonia, NEC when you know the bacterial agent causing the pneumonia, but ICD-9-CM doesn't accommodate it).
8. Multiple granularities: Because classifications and terminologies must fulfill multiple purposes, the information in them may be specific or general so that all needs can be met.
9. Multiple consistent views: Classifications and terminologies must accommodate more than one viewpoint to allow them to be multipurpose as well as to ensure continuity of care. When caring for the same patient, nurses want to use nurse speak and physicians want to use physician speak.
10. Context representation: Words have different meanings when used in different contexts or as different grammatical parts of language. **Context** is determined by how the concepts relate to each other. For example, consider the term "cold." In the phrase "the patient is cold," cold is how the patient feels. In the phrase, "the patient has a cold," cold is a disease. The difference between the two phrases reflects the two different contexts of the word "cold."
11. Graceful evolution: The days of yearly updates need to end soon. Future updates will have to be made monthly or, more likely, weekly. The growth of medical knowledge is exponential; classification systems and terminologies must to be able to keep up.

12. Recognized redundancy: Classifications and terminologies need to accommodate redundancy.

13. Licensed and copyrighted: Terminologies and classifications need to be copyrighted and licensed to control local modifications, which result in semantic drift and produce incomparable data.

14. Vendor neutral: Classifications and terminologies must be vendor neutral so that they can be readily used as national standards by all vendors without conferring a competitive advantage to any one of them.

15. Scientifically valid: Terminologies and classifications should be understandable, reproducible, and useful and should reflect the current understanding of the science.

16. Adequate maintenance: A central authority that provides a rapid response to requests for new terms is essential to minimize the need for local enhancements and to keep terminologies and classifications current.

17. Self-sustaining: Classifications and terminologies should be supported by public or endowment funding. Alternatively, licensing fees should be proportional to the value the system provides to users.

18. Scalable infrastructure and process control: The tools and processes for maintaining a terminology or classification should be scalable, especially for a nationally standardized terminology.

ASTM Standard E 2087-00

In addition to following the preceding criteria, HIM professionals should use all of their system analysis and data management skills when evaluating the appropriateness of a clinical terminology for a particular function or need. Another helpful reference for evaluating the quality of a clinical terminology is the ASTM Standard E 2087-00: Standard Specification for Quality Indicators for Controlled Health Vocabularies. (ASTM International 2000) This standard covers the documentation of the principal notions necessary and sufficient to assign value to a controlled health vocabulary. (NAHIT 2005).

Following is a subsection of the ASTM E2087-00 evaluation criteria (ASTM 2000):

6. Evaluation

6.1 As we seek to understand quality in the controlled vocabularies that we create or use, we need standard criteria for the evaluation of these systems. All evaluations should reflect and specifically identify the purpose and scope of the vocabulary being evaluated.

6.2 Purpose and Scope: Important dimensions along which scope should be defined include:

6.2.1 Clinical Area of Use, Disease Area of Patients, and Expected Profession of Users—What parts of healthcare is it intended to be used in and by whom?

6.2.2 Primary Use—Includes: Reporting for remuneration, management planning, epidemiological research, indexing for bibliographic, Web-based retrieval, recording of clinical details for direct patient care, use for decision support, linking of record to decision support, etc.

6.2.3 Persistence and Extent of Use—Some vocabularies are intended, at least initially, primarily for a specific study or a specific site. If a vocabulary is intended to be persistent, there should be a means of updating or some kind of change management.

6.2.4 Degree of Automatic Inferencing Intended—Is it intended that classification be automatic? Is it intended that validation on input be possible and, if so, within what limits? If post-coordinated expressions are to be accepted, what can be inferred about them and what restrictions must be placed on them?

6.2.5 Transformations (Mappings) to Other Vocabularies—What transformations/mappings are supported for what intended purpose? For example, transformation for purposes of bibliographic retrieval may require less precision than transformation for clinical usage. What is the sensitivity and specificity of the mappings?

6.2.6 User/Developer Extensibility—Is it intended that the vocabulary be extended by users or applications developers? If so, within what limits? If not, what mechanisms are available for meeting new needs as they arise?

6.2.7 Natural Language Input or Output—Are they supported for analysis or input? To what level of competence are they supported, for example, stilted telegraphic presentation, idiomatic presentation, etc.?

6.2.8 Other Functions—What other functions are intended? Examples include linkage to specific decision support systems, linkage to post-marketing surveillance, etc.

6.2.9 Current Status—To what extent is the system intended to be finished or a work in progress? If different components of the terminology are at different stages of completion, how is this indicated?

Check Your Understanding 13.7

Instructions: Answer the following questions on a separate piece of paper.

1. Why is concept of permanence important in clinical terminologies and classifications?

2. What is another name for context representation? What does the term mean?

Real-World Case

Diane Parisian, RHIA, CCS, works at the National Aeronautics and Space Administration Johnson Space Center in Houston, Texas. Diane's official employer is Wyle Laboratories. She is working on a longitudinal study of astronaut health. The goal of this study is to investigate the incidence of morbidity and mortality of astronauts and to determine whether the occupational exposures are related to an increased risk of morbidity or mortality.

Diane's title is coder/analyst. This is a fairly generic job title and her duties go beyond what a coder/analyst performs in a hospital setting. Her official job description includes entering data from many different sources into a research database. The research project entails getting as much past and present health information as possible about the astronauts, from any and all sources. The data is then encoded and entered into the database.

Although they currently use both ICD-9-CM and SNOMED-CT, the researchers plan to eventually discontinue the ICD-9-CM coding. The researchers originally tried to used ICD-9-CM but found that it did not have enough detail. When they would search the database, they would retrieve irrelevant records. The researchers needed the data representation to be more accurate so they could be more efficient. NASA is hoping that, as the electronic health record (EHR) becomes more prevalent and providers start using SNOMED-CT, more information will be able to be shared electronically.

Diane received her Bachelor's in Health Information Management from the University of Texas Medical Branch (UTMB) in Galveston, TX. After graduation she worked as an area manager for a release of information company and was a coder at a hospital before the job at NASA. Diane found out about the job at NASA from a friend who saw the posting on the Internet. When they talked about the job Diane realized she lived close to NASA and even knew other health information managers who worked at NASA. She called her contact at NASA and, while she knows that didn't get her the job, she believes it helped get her in the door for the interview. Diane decided she was ready for a new challenge and accepted the position.

When asked to describe her training for the position, Diane says most of it was on-the-job training. There is another coder/analyst who had already received SNOMED training and she trained Diane. Diane said that her understanding of coding, communication skills and flexibility have been most useful in this position. The coding and classification skills learned for ICD-9-CM can be transferred to SNOMED-CT. The communication skills necessary include technical writing, presentation skills, and the ability to get along with others. Diane has had to work a lot in teams on different projects and says she can't image doing a job without these skills. The flexibility has been needed as Diane has had to take the lead on certain aspects of this project. Diane thinks she would have been better prepared for the job if she had had more training in database design and some basic programming.

The most unexpectedly frustrating part of the job has been coding with SNOMED-CT. There are no instructions for coding with SNOMED-CT as there are for ICD-9-CM so now the NASA team is working with other experts in the field on the best methods for coding in SNOMED-CT. The team was interested in making the data comparable but couldn't find anyone with an answer so they have decided to develop their own internal guidelines. To support these guidelines, they are developing their own software. This will assist the coders in getting the data in so the researchers can get information out. Diane is on the team developing the software and has been involved in writing technical requirement and use case documents. The most surprising thing about Diane's job is that she finds herself involved in many projects outside her normal duties. Both HIM and non-HIM related projects. She says that her HIM and organizational skills transfer to other projects.

Diane sees terminologies and vocabularies as a huge opportunity for the future of health information management. She says we shouldn't be afraid to venture into new territory. To quote her "If we don't step up and deal with it, someone else will." Diane encourages everyone to keep up with the developments in the field of classifications and vocabularies.

Summary

The coding and classification systems currently used in the healthcare industry are inadequate to support today's standards of patient care, but they are necessary for reimbursement. The technologies to support healthcare information needs will continue to develop at a phenomenal rate. As with other industries, healthcare requires information systems that cannot only facilitate its current work but also assist in managing the knowledge explosion. These systems are impossible to develop without a "language for healthcare." HIM professionals must participate in the development, implementation, and maintenance of information systems that use standard vocabularies, nomenclatures, and classification systems.

References

Alternative Link. The ABC Code Set. Available online from alternativelink. com/ali/abc_codes/wiify.asp.

American College of Radiology. 2003. BI-RADS Atlas. Available online from acr.org.

American Dental Association. 2004. *Current Dental Terminology, CDT-2005.* Chicago: ADA.

American Health Information Management Association. 1999a. Clarification of clinical data sets, vocabularies, terminologies, and classifications. *Journal of American Health Information Management Association* 70(2):72–73.

American Health Information Management Association. 1999b. Standards of Ethical Coding.

American Health Information Management Association and American Hospital Association. 2003 (Sept. 23). *ICD-10-CM Field Testing Project: Report on Findings.* Chicago: AHIMA and AHA.

American Medical Association. 2005. Current Procedural Terminology (CPT). Available online from ama-assn.org.

American National Standards Institute, n.d. ansi.org.

American Nurses Association, n.d. ana.org.

American Psychiatric Association, DSM-IV Questions and Answers. Available online from psych.org.

ASTM International. 2000. ASTM E2087-00: Standard specification for quality indicators for controlled health vocabularies. West Conshohocken, PA: ASTM.

Averill, R.F., R.L. Mullin, B.A. Steinbeck, N.I. Goldfield, T.M. Grant, and R.R. Butler. 2005. *Development of the ICD-10 Procedure Coding System (ICD-10-PCS).* 3M HIS Research Report 1-05. St. Paul, MN: 3M.

Barnett, O.G., et al. 1993. The computer-based clinical record: Where do we stand? *Annals of Internal Medicine* 119(10):1046-48.

Beinborn, J. 1999. Automated coding: The next step. *Journal of American Health Information Management Association* 70(7).

Bidgood, W.D., Jr. 1997. Documenting the information content of images. Proceedings of the AMIA Annual Fall Symposium, pp. 424–28.

Bowie, J. 2004. Four Options for Implementing SNOMED. *Journal of American Health Information Management Association* 75(7):30–33.

Bowman, E. 2001. Coding, classification, and reimbursement systems. In *Health Information: Management of a Strategic Resource,* 2nd ed., edited by M. Abdelhak et al. Philadelphia: W.B. Saunders Company.

BSI Group. 2004. Global Medical Device Nomenclature (GMDN). Available online from gmdn.org.

Campbell, K.E., B. Hochhalter, J. Slaughter, and J. Mattison. 1999. Enterprise issues pertaining to implementing controlled terminologies. IMIA Conference Proceedings. Edmonton, AB: IMIA.

Centers for Medicare and Medicaid Services. Available online from cms.gov.

Chute, C. G. 2000. Clinical classification and terminology: Some history and current observations. *Journal of the American Medical Informatics Association* 70(3):298–303.

Cimino, J.J. 1998. Desiderata for controlled medical vocabularies in the twenty-first century. *Methods of Information in Medicine* 37:394–403.

College of American Pathologists. n.d. cap.org.

Department of Agriculture. EGovernment Program, Consolidated Health Informatics. Available online from https://www.egov.usda.gov.

Department of Veterans Affairs. n.d. va.gov.

Dochterman, J.C., and G. M. Bulechek (Eds.). 2004 *Nursing Interventions Classification (NIC),* fourth edition. St. Louis, MO: Mosby.

Environmental Protection Agency Substance Registry System. (EPA SRS). 2005. Substance List. Available online from epa.gov/srs/.

eHealth Initiative. 2004. Who We Are: EHR Collaborative. Available online from ehealthinitiative.org.

Evans, K. 2004 (July 14). Statement to the subcommittee on technology, information policy, intergovernmental relations and the census. Washington, DC: U.S. House of Representatives.

Food and Drug Administration. n.d. fda.gov.

Forrey, A.W., C.J. McDonald, G. DeMoor, et al. 1996. Logical Observation Identifier Names and Codes (LOINC) Database: A public use set of codes and names for electronic reporting of clinical laboratory results. *Clinical Chemistry* 42:1:81–90.

Fox, L.A. 1992. An ethical dilemma: Coding medical records for reimbursement. *Journal of American Health Information Management Association* 63(1):34–37.

Hammond, W.E., and J.J. Cimino. 2001. Standards in medical informatics. In *Health Informatics,* edited by K.J. Hannah and M.J. Ball. New York: Springer-Verlag.

Hammond, W.E., and J.J. Cimino. 2000. Standards in medical informatics. In *Medical Informatics: Computer Applications in Health Care and Biomedicine,* 2nd ed., edited by E.H. Shortliffe and L.E. Perreault, pp. 212–56. New York: Springer.

Health and Human Services, Centers for Disease Control, National Center for Health Statistics. 2005. *International Classification of Diseases,* 10th Revision. Available online from hhs.gov.

Health and Human Services. 2005. Administrative simplification transaction and code sets, frequently asked questions. Available online from aspe.os.dhhs.gov.

Health Level Seven. 2005. HL7 NLM contract announcement. Available online from hl7.org.

Health Level Seven. 2005 (Oct. 13). HL7 Position Statement on CCR/CDA Harmonization. Available online from hl7.org.

Healthcare IT News. 2004 (June 7). NAHIT healthcare standards available. Available online from healthcareitnews.com.

Henry, S.B., et al. 1998. Nursing data, classification systems, and quality indicators: What every HIM professional needs to know. *Journal of American Health Information Management Association* 69(5):48–54.

ICD-9-CM Coordination and Maintenance Committee. 2001 (May 17). Meeting minutes. Available online from cms.gov.

Ingenix. 2006. *DRG Expert: A Comprehensive Guidebook to the DRG Classification System.* Reston, VA: Ingenix.

Institute of Medicine of the National Academies. 2005. IOM data standards for patient safety. Available online from iom.edu/project.asp?id=4629.

International Classification for Nursing Practice (ICNP). 2004. Available online from icn.ch/icnp.htm.

Jamoulle, M. 1998. ICPC-2: The international classification of primary care: An introduction. Available online from ulb.ac.be/esp/wicc/icpc2.html.

Kudla, K.M., and M. Blakemore. 2001. SNOMED takes the next step. *Journal of American Health Information Management Association* 72(7):62–68.

Levin, R. 2004 (June 14). FDA related activities: Structured product labeling project for the daily med initiative. Drug Information Association annual meeting. Available online from fda.gov/cder/present/DIA2004/Levin_DailyMed.PPT.

Markle Foundation. 2002. *Connecting For Health* press release. Available online from connectingforhealth.org.

Martin, K.S. 2005. Omaha System. Available online from omahasystem.org.

Matney, S., J.G. Ozbolt, and S. Bakken. 2003. Update on Logical Observation Identifier Name and Codes (LOINC). Available online from eaa-Knowledge.com.

NANDA International. 2005. NANDA International Taxonomy II. Available online from nanda.org/html/taxonomy.html.

National Alliance for Health Information Technology (NAHIT). 2005. Alliance Standards Directory. Available online from hitsdir.org.

National Cancer Institute. NCI DTS browser. Available online from ncit-erms.nci.nih.gov/NCI Browser.

National Center for Health Statistics. ICD-9. Available online from cdc.gov/nchs.

National Center for Health Statistics. ICD-10-CM. Available online from cdc.gov/nchs.

National Committee on Vital and Health Statistics. 2005. NCVHS Subcommittee on Standards and Security. Available online from ncvhs.hhs.gov/stdschrg.htm.

National Committee on Vital and Health Statistics. 2004. Consolidated Health Informatics initiative final recommendation information sheet. Available online from ncvhs.hhs.gov/040127p1.htm.

National Committee on Vital and Health Statistics. 2003 (Nov. 5). Letter to Tommy G. Thompson, Secretary, Department of Health and Human Services. Available online from ncvhs.hhs.gov/031105/t.htm.

National Coordination Office for Information Technology Research and Development (NITRD). 2004 (April 13). President's Information Technology Advisory Committee (PITAC). Health care delivery and information technology (HIT) subcommittee: Draft recommendations. Available online from nitrd.gov/pitac.

National Council for Prescription Drug Programs. 2005 (January). *NCPDP Basic Guide To Standards.* Scottsdale, AZ: NCPDP.

National Health Service Information Centre. 1999. *The READ Codes* demonstration CD. Birmingham, England: NHS Information Authority.

National Library of Medicine. 2005. Fact sheet: Medical subject headings. Available online from nlm.nih.gov/pubs/factsheets/mesh.html.

Nursing Information & Data Set Evaluation Center. 2005. Available online from nursingworld.org/nidsec.

Office of Management and Budget. 2005. E-Gov Background. Available online from whitehouse.gov/.

Ozbolt, J.G. 1999. *The Patient Care Data Set: Profile.* Nashville, TN: Vanderbilt University Medical Center.

Public Health Informatics Institute. 2005. Guiding principles for effective health information systems. Available online from phii.org.

Public Health Informatics Institute (PHII). 2005. Available online from phii.org.

Regenstrief Institute. 2005. LOINC. Available online from regenstrief.org.

Ryske, E., and M. Imel. 2003. SNOMED International: How SNOMED Will Affect Health Information Management. *AHIMA's 75th Anniversary National Convention and Exhibit Proceedings, October 2003.* Chicago: AHIMA.

Saba, V.K. 2005. Clinical Care Classification (CCC) System. Available online from sabacare.com.

Schnitzer, G.L. 2000. Natural language processing: A coding professional's perspective. *Journal of American Health Information Management Association* 71(9):95–98.

Schwager, R. 2000. Speech recognition propels transcription revolution. *Journal of American Health Information Management Association* 71(9):64–68.

Scichilone, R. 1999. Getting Ready for APCs. *Journal of American Health Information Management Association* 70(8):84–92.

Slee, V.N., and D.A. Slee. 1991. Health Care Terms, 2nd ed. St. Paul, MN: Tringa Press.

SNOMED. 2005. snomed.org.

Spackman, K.A., K.E. Campbell, and R.A. Cote. 1997. SNOMED RT: A reference terminology for health care. Proceedings of the American Medical Informatics Association Annual Symposium, pp. 640–44. Bethesda, MD: AMIA.

Unified Medical Language System. 2005. RxNorm. Available online from nlm.nih.gov/research/umls/rxnorm_main.html.

University of Iowa College of Nursing. 2005. nursing.uiowa.edu.

University of Iowa College of Nursing, Nursing Minimum Data Set Consortium. 2003. *USA Brief Synopsis of the Nursing Minimum Data Set (NMDS).* Adapted from Werley, H.H., and Lang, N.M., eds. 1988. *Identification of the Nursing Minimum Data Set.* New York: Springer.

Wain, H.M., E.A. Bruford, R.C. Lovering, M.J. Lush, M.W. Wright, and S. Povey. 2002. Guidelines for Human Gene Nomenclature. *Genomics* 79(4): 464–470. Available online from gene.ucl.ac.uk/nomenclature/guidelines.html.

Warner, H.R., Jr. 2000. Can natural language processing aid outpatient coders? *Journal of American Health Information Management Association* 71(8):78–81.

Willard, D., D. Worthington, and P. Ashley. 2004. 2005 ICD-9-CM codes and DRG changes. *Journal of American Health Information Management Association* 75(10):67–72.

World Health Organization. 2005. who.int.

Chapter 14
Reimbursement Methodologies

*Anita C. Hazelwood, MLS, RHIA, FAHIMA,
and Carol A. Venable, MPH, RHIA, FAHIMA*

Learning Objectives

- To understand the historical development of healthcare reimbursement in the United States
- To describe current reimbursement processes, forms, and support practices for healthcare reimbursement
- To understand the difference between commercial health insurance and employer self-insurance
- To describe the purpose and basic benefits of the following government-sponsored health programs: Medicare Part A, Medicare Part B, Medicare Advantage, Medicaid, CHAMPVA, TRICARE, HIS, TANF, PACE, SCHIP, workers' compensation, and FECA

- To understand the concept of managed care and to provide examples of different types of managed care organizations
- To identify the different types of fee-for-service reimbursement methods
- To understand ambulatory surgery center rates
- To describe prospective payment systems
- To understand the purpose of the fee schedules, chargemasters, and auditing procedures that support the reimbursement process

Key Terms

Accept assignment
Accounts receivable
Acute care prospective payment system (PPS)
Administrative services only (ASO) contracts
Advance Beneficiary Notice (ABN)
All patient DRGs (AP-DRGs)
All patient refined DRGs (APR-DRGs)
Ambulatory payment classification (APC) system
Ambulatory surgery center (ASC)
American National Standards Institute (ANSI)
Attending Physician Statement (APS) (or COMB-1)
Auditing
Balance billing
Balanced Budget Refinement Act (BBRA)
Blue Cross and Blue Shield (BC/BS)
Blue Cross and Blue Shield Federal Employee Program (FEP)
Bundled payments
Capitation
Case-mix group
Case-mix group (CMG) relative weights
Case-mix index
Categorically needy eligibility groups (Medicaid)
Chargemaster

Civilian Health and Medical Program of the Uniformed Services (CHAMPUS)
Civilian Health and Medical Program–Veterans Administration (CHAMPVA)
Claim
CMS-1500
Coinsurance
Comorbidity
Compliance
Compliance program guidance
Complication
Coordination of benefits (COB) transaction
Cost outlier
Cost outlier adjustment
CPT (Current Procedural Terminology)
Department of Health and Human Services (HHS)
Diagnosis-related groups (DRGs)
Discharge planning
Discounting
DRG grouper
Electronic remittance advice (ERA)
Emergency Maternal and Infant Care Program (EMIC)
Employer-based self-insurance

Episode-of-care (EOC) reimbursement
Exclusive provider organization (EPO)
Explanation of Benefits (EOB)
External reviews (audits)
Federal Employees' Compensation Act (FECA)
Fee schedule
Fee-for-service basis
Fiscal intermediary (FI)
Fraud and abuse
Geographic practice cost index (GPCI)
Global payment
Global surgery payment
Group health insurance
Group model health maintenance organization
Group practice without walls (GPWW)
Hard-coding
Health maintenance organization (HMO)
Health Plan Employer Data and Information Set (HEDIS)
Healthcare Common Procedure Coding System (HCPCS)
Healthcare provider
Home Assessment Validation and Entry (HAVEN)
Home health agency (HHA)
Home health prospective payment system (HH PPS)
Home health resource group (HHRG)
Hospice
Hospitalization insurance (HI) (Medicare Part A)
ICD-9-CM (International Classification of Diseases, Ninth
    Revision, Clinical Modification)
Indemnity plans
Independent practice association (IPA)
Indian Health Service (IHS)
Inpatient psychiatric facility (IPF)
Inpatient rehabilitation facility (IRF)
Inpatient Rehabilitation Validation and Entry System (IRVEN)
Insured
Insurer
Integrated delivery system (IDS)
Integrated provider organization (IPO)
Long-term care hospital (LTCH)
Low-utilization payment adjustment (LUPA)
Major diagnostic category (MDC)
Major medical insurance (catastrophic coverage)
Managed care
Management service organization (MSO)
Medicaid
Medical foundation
Medical Group Management Association (MGMA)
Medically needy option (Medicaid)
Medicare
Medicare Advantage
Medicare carrier
Medicare fee schedule (MFS)
Medicare Summary Notice (MSN)
Medigap
Minimum Data Set 2.0 (MDS)
National Committee for Quality Assurance (NCQA)
National conversion factor (CF)
National Correct Coding Initiative (NCCI)
National Uniform Billing Committee (NUBC)
National Uniform Claim Committee (NUCC)

Network model health maintenance organization
Network provider
Nonparticipating providers
Omnibus Budget Reconciliation Act (OBRA)
Outcome and Assessment Information Set (OASIS)
Out-of-pocket expenses
Outpatient code editor (OCE)
Outpatient prospective payment system (OPPS)
Packaging
Partial hospitalization
Payer of last resort (Medicaid)
Payment status indicator (PSI)
Per member per month (PMPM)
Per patient per month (PPPM)
Physician–hospital organization (PHO)
Point-of-service (POS) plan
Policyholder
Preferred provider organization (PPO)
Premium
Primary care manager (PCM)
Primary care physician (PCP)
Principal diagnosis
Principal procedure
Professional component (PC)
Programs of All-Inclusive Care for the Elderly (PACE)
Prospective payment system (PPS)
Public assistance
Relative value unit (RVU)
Remittance advice (RA)
Resident Assessment Instrument (RAI)
Resident Assessment Validation and Entry (RAVEN)
Resource Utilization Groups, Version III (RUG-III)
Resource-based relative value scale (RBRVS)
Respite care
Retrospective payment system
Revenue codes
Skilled nursing facility prospective payment system (SNF PPS)
Social Security Act
Staff model health maintenance organization
State Children's Health Insurance Program (SCHIP)
State workers' compensation insurance funds
Supplemental medical insurance (SMI) (Medicare Part B)
Tax Equity and Fiscal Responsibility Act of 1982 (TEFRA)
Technical component (TC)
Temporary Assistance for Needy Families (TANF)
Third-party payer
Traditional fee-for-service reimbursement
TRICARE
TRICARE Extra
TRICARE Prime
TRICARE Prime Remote
TRICARE Senior Prime
TRICARE Standard
UB-04
UB-92 (CMS-1450)
Unbundling
Upcoding
Usual, customary, and reasonable (UCR) charges
Voluntary Disclosure Program
Workers' compensation

Introduction

In the United States, the systems used to pay healthcare organizations and individual healthcare professionals for the services they provide are very complex. This complexity is due in part to the variety of reimbursement methods in use today as well as to strict requirements for detailed documentation to support medical **claims.** The government and other third-party payers also are concerned about potential **fraud and abuse** in claims processing. Therefore, ensuring that bills and claims are accurate and correctly presented is an important focus of healthcare **compliance.**

A reimbursement claim is a statement of services submitted by a **healthcare provider** (for example, a physician or a hospital) to a **third-party payer** (for example, an insurance company or **Medicare**). The claim documents the medical and/or surgical services that were provided to a specific patient during a specific episode of care. Accurate reimbursement is critical to the operational and financial health of healthcare organizations. In most healthcare organizations, health insurance specialists process reimbursement claims. Health information management (HIM) professionals also play an important role in healthcare reimbursement by:

- Ensuring that health record documentation supports services billed
- Assigning diagnostic and procedural codes according to patient record documentation
- Applying coding guidelines and edits when assigning codes or **auditing** for coding quality and accuracy
- Appealing insurance claims denials

This chapter reviews the history of healthcare reimbursement in the United States and explains the different reimbursement systems commonly used since the advent of the various types of **prospective payment systems.** It then discusses a variety of healthcare reimbursement methodologies with a focus on Medicare prospective payment systems. Finally, it explains how reimbursement claims are processed and the support processes involved.

Theory into Practice

It is not uncommon to hear the phrase "if it wasn't documented, it wasn't done" in reference to health record documentation. In the context of reimbursement, this phrase means that when a healthcare provider (for example, a hospital) provides a service to a patient but fails to document the service in the patient's health record, that provider has no documentation to support a claim for the service. As a result, the third-party payer may deny the claim.

For example, a hospital submitted a claim for outpatient services totaling $1,950. When the third-party payer reviewed the claim, it might disallow $200 in charges for which there was no health record documentation. The payer then would recalculate the claim for a total payment of $1,750. The hospital would have lost $200 in revenue on this one case. If the hospital were underpaid $200 on every case because of incomplete documentation and there were 36,500 patient encounters per year, the potential revenue loss for one year would be $7,300,000!

History of Healthcare Reimbursement in the United States

Healthcare reimbursement in the United States has a long and complex history. Until the late 1800s, Americans paid their own healthcare expenses. Many people without the means to pay for care received charity care or no care at all. Over the past 100 years, a number of groups have attempted to develop systems that would ensure adequate healthcare for every American. But the development of prepaid insurance plans and third-party reimbursement systems did not follow a straight path. The result is the complicated reimbursement system in place today.

Campaigns for National Health Insurance

The American Association of Labor Legislation (AALL) began the campaign for health insurance in the United States with the creation of a committee on social welfare. The committee held its first national conference in 1913 and drafted model health insurance legislation in 1915. The proposed legislation limited coverage to the working class and others who earned less than $1,200 a year, including their dependents. Coverage included the services of physicians, nurses, and hospitals; sick pay; maternity benefits; and a death benefit of $50 to pay for funeral expenses. Although the plan was supported by the American Medical Association (AMA), it was never passed into law.

During the 1930s, expanding access to medical care services became the focus of healthcare reforms. Hospital costs increased as the middle class used more hospital services. Medical care, especially hospital care, became a bigger item in family budgets. The Committee on the Cost of Medical Care (CCMC) was formed to address concerns about the cost and distribution of medical care. It was funded by eight philanthropic organizations, including the Rockefeller, Millbank, and Rosenwald foundations. It first met in 1926 and stopped meeting in 1932. The CCMC's published research findings demonstrated the need for additional healthcare services. The committee recommended that national resources be allocated for healthcare and that voluntary health insurance be provided as a means of covering medical costs. Like the AALL's earlier efforts, however, nothing came of the CCMC initiative.

In 1937, the Tactical Committee on Medical Care was formed. It drafted the Wagner National Health Act of 1939. The act supported a federally funded national health program to be administered by states and localities. The Wagner Act evolved from a proposal for federal grants-in-aid to a plan for national health insurance. The proposal called for compulsory national health insurance and a payroll tax. Although the proposed legislation generated extensive national debate, it was not passed into law by Congress.

In 1945, the healthcare issue received the support of an American president for the first time when Harry Truman introduced a plan for universal comprehensive national health insurance. Proposed compromises included a system of private insurance for those who could afford it and public welfare services for the poor. Truman's plan died in a congressional committee in 1946.

After the Second World War, private insurance systems expanded and union-negotiated healthcare benefits served to protect workers from the impact of unforeseen healthcare expenses. The Hill-Burton Act (formally called the Hospital Survey and Construction Act) was passed in 1946. This health facility construction program was instituted under Title VI of the Public Health Service Act. The program was designed to provide federal grants for modernizing hospitals that had become obsolete due to a lack of capital investment during the Great Depression and the Second World War (1929 to 1945). The program later evolved to address other types of infrastructure needs. In return for federal funds, facilities agreed to provide medical services free or at reduced rates to patients who were unable to pay for their own care.

Congress first introduced a bill to fund coverage of hospital costs for Social Security beneficiaries in 1948. In response to criticism from the AMA, the proposed legislation was expanded to cover physician services. The concept of federal health insurance programs for the aged and the poor was highly controversial. It was not until 1965 that President Lyndon Johnson signed the law that created federal healthcare programs for the elderly and poor as part of his Great Society legislation (also called the War on Poverty).

Title XVIII of the **Social Security Act,** or Health Insurance for the Aged and Disabled, is commonly known as Medicare. Medicare legislation was enacted as one element of the 1965 amendments to the Social Security Act. Medicare is a health insurance program designed to complement the retirement, survivors, and disability insurance benefits enacted under Title II of the Social Security Act. It covered most Americans over the age of 65 when it was first implemented in 1966. In 1973, several additional groups became eligible for Medicare benefits, including those entitled to Social Security or Railroad Retirement disability cash benefits for at least 24 months, most persons with end-stage renal disease (ESRD), and certain individuals over 65 who were not eligible for paid coverage but elected to pay for Medicare benefits.

Medicaid was designed as a cost-sharing program between the federal and state governments. It pays for the healthcare services provided to many low-income Americans. The program became effective in 1966 under Title XIX of the Social Security Act. It allowed states to add health coverage to their **public assistance** programs for low-income groups, families with dependent children, the aged, and the disabled. Because Medicaid eligibility is based on meeting criteria other than income, today the program covers only about 40 percent of the population living in poverty.

The Medicare and Medicaid programs were originally the responsibility of the Department of Health, Education, and Welfare (predecessor to the **Department of Health and Human Services** [HHS]). The Social Security Administration (SSA) administered the Medicare program, and the Social and Rehabilitation Service (SRS) administered the Medicaid Program. In 1977, administration of Medicare and Medicaid was transferred to a newly created administrative agency within HHS, the Health Care Financing Administration (HCFA). HCFA's name was changed in 2001, and the agency is now called the Centers for Medicare and Medicaid Services (CMS).

The demand for medical services grew tremendously during the 1970s and early 1980s. As a result, health insurance premiums and the cost of funding Medicare and Medicaid programs skyrocketed. By the mid-1980s, both private and government-sponsored healthcare programs had instituted cost-cutting programs.

Since 1983, CMS has developed prospective payment systems (PPSs) to manage the costs of the Medicare and Medicaid programs. The PPS for inpatient acute care was the first to be implemented, followed by numerous others ranging from home health services to outpatient facility services. The most recently implemented system is the inpatient psychiatric facilities. Medicare and Medicaid reimbursement is discussed in more detail later in the chapter.

Private and self-insured health insurance plans also have implemented a number of cost-containing measures, most notably, **managed care** delivery and reimbursement systems. Managed care has virtually eliminated **traditional fee-for-service reimbursement** systems in just two decades. The implementation of managed care systems has had far-reaching effects on healthcare organizations and providers in every setting. However, hospitals have experienced the greatest financial pressure. Managed care is discussed in detail later in this chapter.

Development of Prepaid Health Plans

In 1860, Franklin Health Assurance Company of Massachusetts became the first commercial insurance company in the United States to provide private healthcare coverage for injuries that did not result in death. Within 20 years, 60 other insurance companies offered health insurance policies. By 1900, both accident insurance companies and life insurance companies were offering policies. These early policies covered loss of income and provided benefits for a limited number of illnesses (such as typhus, typhoid, scarlet fever, and smallpox).

Modern health insurance was born in 1929 when Baylor University Hospital in Dallas, Texas, agreed to provide healthcare services to Dallas schoolteachers. The hospital agreed to provide room, board, and certain ancillary services to the teachers for a set monthly fee of 50 cents. This plan is generally considered to be the first Blue Cross plan. Such plans were attractive to consumers and hospitals alike because they provided a way to ensure that patients would be able to pay for hospital services when they needed them. Payment was made directly to the hospital, not to the patient. In addition, coverage usually included a hospital stay for a specified number of days or for specific hospital services.

The Blue Cross plans contrasted with standard **indemnity plans** (insurance benefits provided in the form of cash payments) offered by private insurance companies that reimbursed (or indemnified) the patient for covered services up to a specified dollar limit. It was then the responsibility of the hospital to collect the money from the patient. Blue Shield plans were eventually developed by physicians. The plans were similar to Blue Cross plans except that they offered coverage for physicians' services.

Starting in the 1930s and continuing through the Second World War, traditional insurance companies added health insurance coverage for hospital, surgical, and medical expenses to their accident and life insurance plans. During the Second World War, **group health insurance** was offered as a way to attract scarce wartime labor. Group health insurance plans provide healthcare benefits to full-time employees of a company. This trend was strengthened by the favorable tax treatment for fringe benefits. Unlike monetary wages, fringe benefits were not subject to income or Social Security taxes. Therefore, a pretax dollar spent on health insurance coverage was worth more than an after-tax dollar spent directly on medical services. After the war, the Supreme Court ruled that employee benefits, including health insurance, were a legitimate part of the labor–management bargaining process. Health insurance quickly became a popular employee benefit.

Although early health insurance policies covered expenses associated with common accidents and illnesses, they were inadequate for coverage of extended illnesses and lengthy hospital stays. To correct this deficiency, insurance companies began offering **major medical insurance** coverage for catastrophic illnesses and injuries during the early 1950s. Major medical insurance provides benefits up to a high-dollar limit for most types of medical expenses. However, it usually requires patients to pay large deductibles. It also may place limits on charges (for example, room and board) and may require patients to pay a portion of the expenses. **Blue Cross and Blue Shield** soon followed by offering similar plans.

Typically, the major medical insurance **policyholder** (or **insured**) paid a specified deductible (the amount the insured pays before the **insurer** assumes liability for any remaining costs of covered services). After the deductible had been paid, insured and insurer (third-party payer) shared covered losses according to a specified ratio, and the insured paid a

coinsurance amount. Coinsurance refers to the amount the insured pays as a requirement of the insurance policy. For example, an insurance company may require the insured to pay a percentage of the daily costs for inpatient care.

According to the Washington Insurance Council (a nonprofit association of insurance companies and insurance professionals), by 1955, health insurance coverage continued to expand, and eventually 77 million Americans were covered by either an indemnity plan or a major medical plan. In subsequent years, insurance companies introduced high-benefit-level major medical plans, which limited out-of-pocket expenses. **Out-of-pocket expenses** are the healthcare expenses the insured is responsible for paying. After the insured has paid an amount specified in the insurance plan (that is, the deductible plus any copayments), the plan pays 100 percent of covered expenses. Such health insurance plans are common today and have been expanded to include coverage for advanced medical technology.

According to the U.S. Census Bureau, the percentage of people covered by health insurance in 2003 was 84.4 percent, lower than in previous years. (See table 14.1.)

Table 14.1. Health insurance coverage status: 1987–2003

Year	Total U.S. Population (000)	Number Covered (000)	Percentage Covered
2003	288,280	243,320	84.4
2002	285,933	242,360	84.8
2001	282,082	240,875	85.4
2000	279,517	239,714	85.8
1999	274,087	231,533	84.5
1998	271,743	227,462	83.7
1997	269,094	225,646	83.9
1996	266,792	225,077	84.4
1995	264,314	223,733	84.6
1994	262,105	222,387	84.8
1993	259,753	220,040	84.7
1992	256,830	218,189	85.0
1991	251,447	216,003	85.9
1990	248,886	214,167	86.1
1989	246,191	212,807	86.4
1988	243,685	211,005	86.6
1987	241,187	210,161	87.1

Source: Based on U.S. Census Bureau information (www.census.gov/hhes/www/hlthins/reports.html).

The lack of health insurance for so many Americans continues to be a serious concern. Because of the financial constraints brought about by changes in Medicare/Medicaid and managed care reimbursement, many hospitals are no longer able to provide charitable services. As a result, underfunded and overcrowded public hospitals are struggling to provide services to uninsured patients who cannot pay for their own care. In addition, many uninsured patients delay seeking medical treatment until they are extremely ill, with long-term consequences for their own health and for the healthcare system. Thousands of patients with chronic diseases such as diabetes and asthma are brought to hospital emergency departments every day because they do not have access to basic healthcare services.

One solution to the problem may be to expand government-sponsored healthcare programs. Another may be to create tax incentives to help individuals and small employers purchase private health insurance. For example, tax deductions could be offered to low-income people who buy their own insurance, or tax credits could be offered to small employers that offer health insurance coverage to employees.

Check Your Understanding 14.1

Instructions: Answer the following questions on a separate piece of paper.

1. How did the uninsured pay for healthcare services prior to implementation of government programs (for example, Medicare)?
2. Why did the Centers for Medicare and Medicaid Services develop prospective payment systems?
3. Using table 14.1, calculate the percentage change in health insurance coverage status from 2002 to 2003.
4. Which government agency administers the Medicaid and Medicare programs?
5. During the Second World War, what did employers do to try to increase wartime labor?

Healthcare Reimbursement Systems

Before the widespread availability of health insurance coverage, individuals were assured access to healthcare only when they were able to pay for the services themselves. They paid cash for services on a retrospective **fee-for-service basis,** in which the patient was expected to pay the healthcare provider after a service was rendered. Until the advent of managed care, **capitation,** and other PPSs, private insurance plans and government-sponsored programs also reimbursed providers on a retrospective fee-for-service basis.

Fee-for-service reimbursement is now rare for most types of medical services. Today, most Americans are covered by some form of health insurance and most health insurance plans compensate providers according to predetermined discounted rates rather than fee-for-service charges. However, some types of care are not covered by most health insurance plans and are still paid for directly by patients on a fee-for-service basis. Cosmetic surgery is one example of a medical service that is not considered medically necessary and so is not covered by most insurance plans. Many insurance plans also limit coverage for psychiatric services, substance abuse treatment, and the testing and correction of vision and hearing.

Commercial Insurance

Most Americans are covered by private group insurance plans tied to their employment. Typically, employers and employees share the cost of such plans. Two types of commercial insurance are commonly available: private insurance and **employer-based self-insurance.**

Private Health Insurance Plans

Private commercial insurance plans are financed through the payment of **premiums.** Each covered individual or family pays a preestablished amount (usually monthly), and the insurance company sets aside the premiums from all the people covered by the plan in a special fund. When a claim for medical care is submitted to the insurance company, the claim is paid out of the fund's reserves.

Before payment is made, the insurance company reviews every claim to determine whether the services described on the claim are covered by the patient's policy. The company also reviews the diagnosis codes provided on the claim to ensure that the services provided were medically necessary. Payment then is made to either the provider or the policyholder.

When purchasing an insurance policy, the policyholder receives written confirmation from the insurance company when the insurance goes into effect. This confirmation document usually includes a policy number and a telephone number to be called in case of medical emergency. An insurance policy represents a legal contract for services between the insured and the insurance company.

Most insurance policies include the following information:

- What medical services the company will cover
- When the company will pay for medical services
- How much and for how long the company will pay for covered services
- What process is to be followed to ensure that covered medical expenses are paid

Employer-Based Self-Insurance Plans

During the 1970s, a number of large companies discovered that they could save money by self-insuring their employee health plans rather than purchasing coverage from private insurers. Large companies have large workforces, and so aggregate (total) employee medical experiences and associated expenses vary only slightly from one year to the next. The exception to this is during periods of rapid inflation in healthcare charges. The companies understood that it was in their best interest to self-insure their health plans because yearly expenses could be predicted relatively accurately.

The cost of self-insurance funding is lower than the cost of paying premiums to private insurers because the premiums reflect more than the actual cost of the services provided to beneficiaries. Private insurers build additional fees into premiums to compensate them for assuming the risk of providing insurance coverage. In self-insured plans, the employer assumes the risk. By budgeting a certain amount to pay its employees' medical claims, the employer retains control over the funds until such time as medical claims need to be paid.

Employer-based self-insurance has become a common form of group health insurance coverage. Many employers enter into **administrative services only (ASO) contracts** with private insurers and fund the plans themselves. The private insurers administer self-insurance plans on behalf of the employers.

Blue Cross and Blue Shield Plans

Blue Cross and Blue Shield (BC/BS) plans, also known as the Blues, were the first prepaid health plans in the United States. Originally, Blue Cross plans covered hospital care and Blue Shield plans covered physicians' services.

The first Blue Cross plan was created in 1929. In 1939, a commission of the American Hospital Association (AHA) adopted the Blue Cross national emblem for plans that met specific guidelines. The Blue Cross Association was created in 1960, and the relationship with the AHA ended in 1972.

The first Blue Shield plan was created in 1939, and the Associated Medical Care Plans (later known as the National Association of Blue Shield Plans) adopted the Blue Shield symbol in 1948. In 1982, the Blue Cross Association and the National Association of Blue Shield Plans merged to create the Blue Cross and Blue Shield Association.

Today, the Blue Cross and Blue Shield Association includes over 60 independent, locally operated companies with plans in 50 states, the District of Columbia, and Puerto Rico. The Blues offer health insurance to individuals, small businesses, seniors, and large employer groups. In addition, federal employees are eligible to enroll in the **BC/BS Federal Employee Program (FEP)** (also called the BC/BS Service Benefit Plan). The plan offers the two products to federal employees:

- A **preferred provider organization** (PPO) plan, in which healthcare providers provide healthcare services to members of the plan at a discounted rate
- A **point-of-service (POS) plan,** in which subscribers are encouraged to select providers from a prescribed network but are allowed to seek healthcare services from providers outside the network at a higher level of copayment

Government-Sponsored Healthcare Programs

The federal government administers several healthcare programs. The best known are Medicare and Medicaid. The Medicare program pays for the healthcare services provided to Social Security beneficiaries 65 years old and older as well as permanently disabled people, people with end-stage renal disease, and certain other groups of individuals. State governments work with the federal Medicaid program to provide healthcare coverage to low-income individuals and families

In addition, the federal government offers three health programs to address the needs of military personnel and their dependents as well as native Americans. The **Civilian Health and Medical Program–Veterans Administration (CHAMPVA)** provides healthcare services for dependents and survivors of disabled veterans, survivors of veterans who died from service-related conditions, and survivors of military personnel who died in the line of duty. **TRICARE** (formerly CHAMPUS, the Civilian Health and Medical Program–Uniformed Services) provides coverage for the dependents of armed forces personnel and retirees receiving care outside a military treatment facility. The **Indian Health Service** (IHS) provides federal health services to American Indians and Alaska natives.

Medicare
The original Medicare program was implemented on July 1, 1966. In 1973, Medicare benefits were expanded to include individuals of any age who suffered from a permanent disability or end-stage renal disease.

For Americans receiving Social Security benefits, Medicare automatically provides **hospitalization insurance (HI) (Medicare Part A).** It also offers voluntary **supplemental medical insurance** (SMI) (Medicare Part B) to help pay for physicians' services, medical services, and medical–surgical supplies not covered by the hospitalization plan. Enrollees pay extra for Part B benefits. To fill gaps in Medicare coverage, most Medicare enrollees also supplement their benefits with private insurance policies. These private policies are referred to as **Medigap** insurance. **Medicare Advantage** (formerly Medicare+Choice) was established by the Balanced Budget Act (BBA) of 1997 to expand the options for participation in private healthcare plans.

According to CMS, approximately 19 million Americans were enrolled in the Medicare program in 1966. In 2005, approximately 40 million people were enrolled in Parts A and/or B of the Medicare program, and 6.4 million of the enrollees participated in a Medicare Advantage plan.

Medicare Part A
Medicare Part A is generally provided free of charge to individuals age 65 and over who are eligible for Social Security or Railroad Retirement benefits. Individuals who do not claim their monthly cash benefits are still eligible for Medicare. In addition, workers (and their spouses) who have been employed in federal, state, or local government for a sufficient period of time qualify for Medicare coverage beginning at age 65.

Similarly, individuals who have been entitled to Social Security or Railroad Retirement disability benefits for at least 24 months and government employees with Medicare coverage who have been disabled for more than 29 months are entitled to Part A benefits. This coverage also is provided to insured workers (and their spouses) with end-stage renal disease as well as to children with end-stage renal disease. In addition, some otherwise-ineligible aged and disabled beneficiaries who voluntarily pay a monthly premium for their coverage are eligible for Medicare Part A.

The following healthcare services are covered under Medicare Part A: inpatient hospital care, long-term care, skilled nursing facility (SNF) care, home health care, and **hospice** care. (See table 14.2.) Inpatient hospital care and long-term care are paid for under Medicare Part A when such care is medically necessary. An initial deductible payment is required for each hospital admission, plus copayments for all hospital days following day 60 within a benefit period.

Each benefit period begins the day the Medicare beneficiary is admitted to the hospital and ends when he or she has not been hospitalized for a period of 60 consecutive days. Inpatient hospital care is usually limited to 90 days during each benefit period. There is no limit to the number of benefit periods covered by Medicare hospital insurance during a beneficiary's lifetime. However, copayment requirements apply to days 61 through 90. When a beneficiary exhausts the 90 days of inpatient hospital care available during a benefit period, a nonrenewable lifetime reserve of up to a total of 60 additional days of inpatient hospital care can be used. Copayments are required for such additional days.

SNF care is covered when it occurs within 30 days of a three-day-long or longer hospitalization and is certified as medically necessary. The number of SNF days provided under Medicare is limited to 100 days per benefit period, with a copayment required for days 21 through 100. Medicare Part A does not cover SNF care when the patient does not require skilled nursing care or skilled rehabilitation services.

Care provided by a **home health agency** (HHA) may be furnished part-time in the residence of a homebound beneficiary when intermittent or part-time skilled nursing and/or certain other therapy or rehabilitation care is needed. Certain medical supplies and durable medical equipment (DME) also may be paid for under the Medicare home health benefit.

The Medicare program requires the HHA to develop a treatment plan that is periodically reviewed by a physician. Home health care under Medicare Part A has no limitations on duration, no copayments, and no deductibles. For DME, beneficiaries must pay 20 percent coinsurance, as required under Medicare Part B.

Terminally ill persons whose life expectancies are six months or less may elect to receive hospice services. To qualify for Medicare reimbursement for hospice care, patients must elect to forgo standard Medicare benefits for treatment of their illnesses and agree to receive only hospice care. When a hospice patient requires treatment for a condition that is not related to his or her terminal illness, however, Medicare does pay for all covered services necessary for that condition. The Medicare beneficiary pays no deductible for hospice coverage but does pay coinsurance amounts for drugs and inpatient **respite care.**

Table 14.2   Medicare Part A benefit period, beneficiary deductibles and copayments, and Medicare payment responsibilities according to healthcare setting

Healthcare Setting	Benefit Period	Patient's Responsibility	Medicare Payments
Hospital (Inpatient)	First 60 days	$912 annual deductible	All but $912
	Days 61–90	$228 per day	All but $228/day
	Days 91–150 (these reserve days can be used only once in the patient's lifetime)	$456 per day	All but $456/day
	Beyond 150 days	All costs	Nothing
Skilled Nursing Facility	First 20 days	Nothing	100% approved amount
	Days 21–100	$114 per day	All but $114 per day
	Beyond 100 days	All costs	Nothing
Home Health Care	For as long as patient meets Medicare medical necessity criteria	Nothing for services, but 20% of approved amount for durable medical equipment (DME)	100% of the approved amount and 80% of the approved amount for DME
Hospice Care	For as long as physician certifies need for care	Limited costs for outpatient drugs and inpatient respite care	All but limited costs for outpatient drugs and inpatient respite care
Blood	Unlimited if medical necessity criteria are met	First 3 pints unless you or someone else donates blood to replace what you use	All but first 3 pints per calendar year

Source: Adapted from *Medicare and You* 2005.

(Respite care is any inpatient care provided to the hospice patient for the purpose of providing primary caregivers a break from their caregiving responsibilities.)

Medicare Part B

Medicare Part B (supplemental medical insurance) covers the following services and supplies:

- Physicians' and surgeons' services, including some covered services furnished by chiropractors, podiatrists, dentists, and optometrists; and services provided by the following Medicare-approved practitioners who are not physicians: certified registered nurse anesthetists, clinical psychologists, clinical social workers (other than those employed by a hospital or an SNF), physician assistants, and nurse practitioners and clinical nurse specialists working in collaboration with a physician
- Services in an emergency department or outpatient clinic, including same-day surgery and ambulance services
- Home health care not covered under Medicare Part A
- Laboratory tests, x-rays, and other diagnostic radiology services, as well as certain preventive care screening tests
- Ambulatory surgery center (ASC) services in Medicare-approved facilities
- Most physical and occupational therapy and speech pathology services
- Comprehensive outpatient rehabilitation facility services and mental healthcare provided as part of a partial hospitalization psychiatric program when a physician certifies that inpatient treatment would be required without the partial hospitalization services. (A partial hospitalization program offers intensive psychiatric treatment on an outpatient basis to psychiatric patients, with an expectation that the patient's psychiatric condition and level of functioning will improve and that relapse will be prevented so that rehospitalization can be avoided.)
- Radiation therapy, renal dialysis and kidney transplants, and heart and liver transplants under certain limited conditions
- DME approved for home use, such as oxygen equipment, wheelchairs, prosthetic devices, surgical dressings, splints, and casts, walkers, and hospital beds needed for use in the home
- Drugs and biologicals that cannot be self-administered, such as hepatitis B vaccines and immunosuppressive drugs (plus certain self-administered anticancer drugs)
- Preventive services such as bone mass measurements, cardiovascular screening blood tests, colorectal cancer screening, diabetes services, glaucoma testing, Pap test and pelvic exam, prostate cancer screening, screening mammograms, and vaccinations (flu, pneumococcal, hepatitis B)

To be covered, all Medicare Part B services must be either documented as medically necessary or covered as one of several prescribed preventive benefits. Part B services also are generally subject to deductibles and coinsurance payments. (See table 14.3, p. 352.) Certain medical services and related care are subject to special payment rules, for example:

- Deductibles for administration of blood and blood products
- Maximum approved amounts for Medicare-approved physical or occupational therapy services performed in settings other than hospitals
- Higher cost-sharing requirements, such as those for outpatient psychiatric care

It should be noted that the following healthcare services are usually not covered by Medicare Part A or B and are only covered by private health plans under the Medicare Advantage program:

- Long-term nursing care
- Custodial care
- Dentures and dental care
- Eyeglasses
- Hearing aids
- Most prescription drugs

Medicare Advantage

Medicare Advantage provides expanded coverage of many healthcare services. Although any Medicare beneficiary may receive benefits through the original fee-for-service program, most beneficiaries enrolled in both Parts A and B can choose to participate in a Medicare Advantage plan instead. Organizations that offer Medicare Advantage plans must meet specific requirements as determined by CMS.

Primary Medicare Advantage products include the following types of plans:

- *Managed care plans:* In a managed care plan, patients can only go to doctors, specialists, or hospitals on the plan's list, which is referred to as a network, except in an emergency. Patients also may have to choose a primary care doctor and be referred to see a specialist, but they pay lower copayments and receive extra benefits.
- *PPO plans:* In a PPO plan, patients use doctors, specialists, and hospitals in the plan's network and can go to doctors and hospitals not on the list, usually at an additional cost. Patients do not need referrals to see doctors or go to hospitals that are not part of the plan's network and may pay lower copayments and receive extra benefits.
- *Private fee-for-service plans:* These plans allow beneficiaries to go to any doctor or hospital that accepts the terms of the plan's payment. The private company, rather than the Medicare program, decides how much it will pay and how much patients pay for services rendered.
- *Medical specialty plans:* Medical specialty plans provide more focused healthcare for specific people.

Table 14.3.   Medicare Part B benefit deductibles and copayments and Medicare payment responsibilities according to type of service

Type of Service	Benefit	Deductible and Copayment	Medicare Payment
Medical Expenses	Physicians' services, inpatient and outpatient medical and surgical services and supplies, and durable medical equipment (DME)	$110 annual deductible, plus 20% of approved amount after deductible has been met, except in outpatient setting	80% of approved amount (after patient has paid $110 deductible)
	Mental health care	50% of most outpatient care	50% of most outpatient care
	Occupational, physical, and speech therapy	20% of the first $1500 and all charges thereafter	80% of first $1500
Clinical Laboratory Services	Blood tests, urinalysis, and more	Nothing	100% of approved amount
Home Health Care	Intermittent skilled care, home health aide services, DME and supplies, and other services	Nothing for home care service	100% of approved amount
		20% of approved amount for DME	80% of approved amount for DME
Outpatient Hospital Services	Services for diagnosis and/or treatment of an illness or injury	$110 annual deductible, plus a coinsurance amount for *each service* received during an outpatient visit. For *each* outpatient service received, the coinsurance amount cannot be greater than the Medicare Part A inpatient hospital deductible. The coinsurance amount is based on 20% of the national median charge for services in the ambulatory payment classification associated with the service. Charges for items or services that Medicare does not cover	Payment based on ambulatory patient classifications/outpatient prospective payment system
Blood	Unlimited if medical necessity criteria are met	First 3 pints (if met under Part B, does not have to be met again under Part A)	All but first 3 pints

Source: Adapted from *Medicare & You* 2005.

Medicare Prescription Drug, Improvement and Modernization Act

The Medicare Prescription Drug, Improvement and Modernization Act, also known as the Medicare Reform Bill, was signed into law by President George W. Bush on December 8, 2003. This legislation provides seniors and individuals with disabilities with a prescription drug benefit, more choices, and better benefits under Medicare.

Out-of-Pocket Expenses and Medigap Insurance

Medicare beneficiaries who elect the fee-for-service option are responsible for charges not covered by the Medicare program and for various cost-sharing aspects of Parts A and B. These liabilities may be paid by the Medicare beneficiary; by a third party, such as an employer-sponsored health plan or private Medigap insurance; or by Medicaid, when the person is eligible.

Medigap is private health insurance that pays, within limits, most of the healthcare service charges not covered by Medicare Parts A and/or B. These policies must meet federal and state laws.

The payment share for beneficiaries enrolled in Medicare Advantage plans is based on the cost-sharing structure of the specific plan they select. Most plans have lower deductibles and coinsurance than are required of Medicare fee-for-service

beneficiaries. Such beneficiaries pay the monthly Part B premium and may pay an additional plan premium, depending on the plan.

For hospital care covered under Medicare Part A, a fee-for-service beneficiary's payment share includes a one-time deductible amount payable at the beginning of each benefit period. For 2005, the deductible is $912. This deductible covers the beneficiary's part of the first 60 days of each inpatient hospital stay. When continued inpatient care is needed beyond the 60 days, additional coinsurance payments ($228 per day in 2005) are required through the 90th day of a benefit period. Each Part A beneficiary also has a lifetime reserve of 60 additional hospital days that may be used when the covered days within a benefit period have been exhausted. Lifetime reserve days may be used only once, and coinsurance payments ($456 per day in 2005) are required.

For SNF care covered under Part A, Medicare fully covers the first 20 days in a benefit period. For days 21 through 100, a copayment ($114 per day in 2005) is required. Medicare benefits expire after the first 100 days of SNF care during a benefit period.

Home health care services require no deductible or coinsurance payment by the beneficiary. For any Part A service, the beneficiary is responsible for paying fees to cover the first three pints or units of nonreplaced blood per calendar year. The beneficiary has the option of paying the fee or arranging for the blood to be replaced by family and friends.

Most beneficiaries covered by Medicare Part A pay no premiums. Eligibility is generally earned through the work experience of the beneficiary or of his or her spouse. In addition, most individuals over 65 who are otherwise ineligible for Medicare Part A coverage can enroll voluntarily by paying a monthly premium when they also enroll in Part B.

For Part B (table 14.3), the beneficiary's payment share includes:

- One annual deductible ($110 in 2005)
- Monthly premiums ($78.20 per month in 2005)
- Coinsurance payments for Part B services (usually 20 percent of medically allowable charges)
- Any deductibles for blood products
- Certain charges above approved charges (for claims not on assignment)
- Payment for any services that are not covered by Medicare

Medicaid

Title XIX of the Social Security Act enacted Medicaid in 1965. The Medicaid program pays for medical assistance provided to individuals and families with low incomes and limited financial resources. Individual states must meet broad national guidelines established by federal statutes, regulations, and policies to qualify for federal matching grants under the Medicaid program. Individual state medical assistance agencies, however, establish the Medicaid eligibility standards for residents of their states. The states also determine the type, amount, duration, and scope of covered services; calculate the rate of payment for covered services; and administer local programs.

Medicaid policies on eligibility, services, and payment are complex and vary considerably among states, even among states of similar size or geographic proximity. Therefore, an individual who is eligible for Medicaid in one state may not be eligible in another. In addition, the amount, duration, and scope of care provided vary considerably from state to state. Moreover, Medicaid eligibility and/or services within a state can change from year to year.

Medicaid Eligibility Criteria

Low income is only one test for Medicaid eligibility. Other financial resources also are compared against eligibility standards. These standards are determined by each state according to federal guidelines.

Generally, each state is allowed to determine which groups Medicaid will cover. Each state also establishes its own financial criteria for Medicaid eligibility. However, to be eligible for federal funds, states are required to provide Medicaid coverage to certain individuals. These individuals include recipients of federally assisted income maintenance payments, as well as related groups of individuals who do not receive cash payments. The federal **categorically needy eligibility groups** include:

- Individuals eligible for Medicaid when they meet requirements for **Temporary Assistance for Needy Families** (TANF)
- Children below age six whose family income is at or below 133 percent of the federal poverty level (FPL) (the income threshold established by the federal government)
- Pregnant women whose family income is below 133 percent of the FPL (services are limited to those related to pregnancy-related medical care)
- Supplemental Security Income (SSI) recipients in most states
- Recipients of adoption or foster care assistance under Title IV-E of the Social Security Act
- Specially protected groups (typically individuals who lose their cash assistance due to earnings from work or from increased Social Security benefits, but who may keep Medicaid for a period of time)
- Infants born to Medicaid-eligible pregnant women
- Certain low-income Medicare beneficiaries

States also have the option of providing Medicaid coverage to other categorically related groups. Categorically related groups share the characteristics of the eligible groups (that is, they fall within defined categories), but the eligibility criteria are somewhat more liberally defined. A **medically needy option** also allows states to extend Medicaid eligibility to persons who would be eligible for Medicaid under one of the mandatory or optional groups except that their income and/or resources are above the eligibility level set by their state. Individuals may qualify immediately or may "spend down" by incurring medical expenses that reduce their income to or below their state's income level for the medically needy.

In 1996, Congress passed the Personal Responsibility and Work Opportunity Reconciliation Act (also known as welfare reform). The act made restrictive changes in the eligibility requirements for SSI coverage. These changes also affected eligibility for participation in the Medicaid program.

The welfare reform act also affected a number of disabled children. Many lost their SSI benefits as a result of the restrictive changes. However, their eligibility for Medicaid was reinstituted by the BBA.

In addition, the welfare reform act repealed the open-ended federal entitlement program known as Aid to Families with Dependent Children (AFDC). TANF, which replaced AFDC, provides states with grant money to be used for time-limited cash assistance. A family's lifetime cash welfare benefits are generally limited to a maximum of five years. Individual states also are allowed to impose other eligibility restrictions.

Medicaid Services

To be eligible for federal matching funds, each state's Medicaid program must offer medical assistance for the following basic services:

- Inpatient hospital services
- Outpatient hospital services
- Emergency services
- Prenatal care
- Vaccines for children
- Physicians' services
- SNF services for persons aged 21 or older
- Family planning services and supplies
- Rural health clinic services
- Home health care for persons eligible for skilled nursing services
- Laboratory and x-ray services
- Pediatric and family nurse practitioner services
- Nurse-midwife services
- Federally qualified health center (FQHC) services and ambulatory services performed at an FQHC that would be available in other settings
- Early and periodic screening and diagnostic and therapeutic services for children under age 21
- States also may receive federal matching funds to provide some of the optional services, the most common being:
- Diagnostic services
- Clinic services
- Prescription drugs and prosthetic devices
- Transportation services
- Rehabilitation and physical therapy services
- Prosthetic devices
- Home care and community-based care services for persons with chronic impairments

The BBA also called for implementation of a state option called **Programs of All-Inclusive Care for the Elderly** (PACE). PACE provides an alternative to institutional care for individuals 55 years old or older who require a level of care usually provided at nursing facilities. It offers and manages all of the health, medical, and social services needed by a beneficiary and mobilizes other services, as needed, to provide preventive, rehabilitative, curative, and supportive care.

PACE services can be provided in day healthcare centers, homes, hospitals, and nursing homes. The program helps its beneficiaries to maintain their independence, dignity, and quality of life. PACE also functions within the Medicare program. Individuals enrolled in PACE receive benefits solely through the PACE program.

Medicaid–Medicare Relationship

Medicare beneficiaries who have low incomes and limited financial resources also may receive help from the Medicaid program. For persons eligible for full Medicaid coverage, Medicare coverage is supplemented by services that are available under their state's Medicaid program according to their eligibility category. Additional services may include, for example, nursing facility care beyond the 100-day limit covered by Medicare, prescription drugs, eyeglasses, and hearing aids. For those enrolled in both programs, any services covered by Medicare are paid for by the Medicare program before any payments are made by the Medicaid program because Medicaid is always the **payer of last resort.** Table 14.4 provides a comparison of the Medicare and Medicaid programs.

State Children's Health Insurance Program

The **State Children's Health Insurance Program** (SCHIP) (Title XXI of the Social Security Act) is a program initiated by the BBA. SCHIP (sometimes referred to as the Children's Health Insurance Program, or CHIP) allows states to expand existing insurance programs to cover children up to age 19. It provides additional federal funds to states so that Medicaid eligibility can be expanded to include a greater number of children.

SCHIP became available on October 1, 1997, and is jointly funded by the federal government and the states. Following broad federal guidelines, states establish eligibility and coverage

Table 14.4.   Comparison of Medicare and Medicaid programs

Medicare	Medicaid
Health insurance for people age 65 and older, or people under 65 who are entitled to Medicare because of disability or are receiving dialysis for permanent kidney failure	Health assistance for people of any age
Administered through fiscal intermediaries, insurance companies under contract to the government to process Medicare claims	Administered by the federal government through state and local governments following federal and state guidelines
Medicare regulations are the same in all states	Medicaid regulations vary from state to state
Financed by monthly premiums paid by the beneficiary and by payroll tax deductions	Financed by federal, state, and county tax dollars
For people age 65 and over, eligibility is based on Social Security or Railroad Retirement participation. For people under age 65, eligibility is based on disability. For people who undergo kidney dialysis, eligibility is not dependent on age	Eligibility based on financial need
Beneficiary responsible for paying deductibles, coinsurance or copayments, and Part B premiums	Medicaid can help pay Medicare deductible, coinsurance or copayment, and premiums
Hospital and medical benefits; preventive care and long-term care benefits are limited	Comprehensive benefits include hospital, preventive care, long-term care, and other services not covered under Medicare such as dental work, prescriptions, transportation, eyeglasses, and hearing aids

guidelines and have flexibility in the way they provide services. Recipients in all states must meet three eligibility criteria:

- They must come from low-income families.
- They must be otherwise ineligible for Medicaid.
- They must be uninsured.

States are required to offer the following services:

- Inpatient hospital services
- Outpatient hospital services
- Physicians' surgical and medical services
- Laboratory and x-ray services
- Well-baby/child care services, including age-appropriate immunizations

TRICARE

TRICARE is a healthcare program for active-duty members of the military and other qualified family members. CHAMPUS-eligible retirees and their family members, as well as eligible survivors of members of the uniformed services, also are eligible for TRICARE.

The idea of medical care for the families of active-duty members of the uniformed military services dates back to the late 1700s. It was not until 1884, however, that Congress directed Army medical officers and contract surgeons to care for the families of military personnel free of charge.

There was very little change in the provision of medical care to members of the military and their families until the Second World War, when the military was made up mostly of young men who had wives of childbearing age. The military medical care system could not handle the large number of births or the care of young children. So, in 1943, Congress authorized the **Emergency Maternal and Infant Care Program** (EMIC). The program provided maternity and infant care to dependents of service members in the lowest four pay grades.

During the early 1950s, the Korean conflict also strained the capabilities of the military healthcare system. As a result, the Dependents Medical Care Act was signed into law in 1956. Amendments to the act created the **Civilian Health and Medical Program of the Uniformed Services** (CHAMPUS) in 1966.

During the 1980s, the search for ways to improve access to top-quality medical care and at the same time control costs led to implementation of CHAMPUS demonstration projects in various parts of the country. The most successful of these projects was the CHAMPUS Reform Initiative (CRI) in California and Hawaii. Initiated in 1988, the CRI offered military service families a choice in the way their military healthcare benefits could be used. Five years of successful operation and high levels of patient satisfaction persuaded Department of Defense officials that they should extend and improve the CRI concepts as a uniform program nationwide.

The new program, known as TRICARE, was phased in nationally by 1998. Expansion to overseas military bases will soon be complete. TRICARE offers three options: **TRICARE Prime, TRICARE Extra,** and **TRICARE Standard.**

TRICARE Prime

Of the three options, TRICARE Prime provides the most comprehensive healthcare benefits at the lowest cost. Military treatment facilities, such as military base hospitals, serve as the principal source of healthcare, and a **primary care manager** (PCM) is assigned to each enrollee.

Two specialized programs supplement TRICARE Prime. **TRICARE Prime Remote** provides healthcare services to active-duty military personnel stationed in the United States in areas not served by the traditional military healthcare system. (Active-duty personnel include members of the Army, Navy, Marine Corps, Air Force, Coast Guard, and active National Guard.) **TRICARE Senior Prime** is a managed care demonstration program designed to serve the medical needs of military retirees who are 65 years old or over and their dependents and survivors.

TRICARE Extra

TRICARE Extra is a cost-effective preferred provider network (PPN) option. Healthcare costs in TRICARE Extra are lower than for TRICARE Standard because beneficiaries must select physicians and medical specialists from a network of civilian healthcare professionals working under contract with TRICARE. The healthcare professionals who participate in TRICARE Extra agree to charge a preestablished discounted rate for the medical treatments and procedures provided to participants in the plan.

TRICARE Standard

TRICARE Standard incorporates the services previously provided by CHAMPUS. TRICARE Standard allows eligible beneficiaries to choose any physician or healthcare provider. It pays a set percentage of the providers' fees, and the enrollee pays the rest. This option permits the most flexibility but may be the most expensive for the enrollee, particularly when the provider's charges are higher than the amounts allowed by the program.

CHAMPVA

The Civilian Health and Medical Program–Veterans Administration (CHAMPVA) is a healthcare program for dependents and survivors of permanently and totally disabled veterans, survivors of veterans who died from service-related conditions, and survivors of military personnel who died in the line of duty. CHAMPVA is a voluntary program that allows beneficiaries to be treated for free at participating VA healthcare facilities, with the VA sharing the cost of covered healthcare services and supplies. Because of the similarity between CHAMPVA and TRICARE (which replaced CHAMPUS), people sometimes confuse the two programs. However, CHAMPVA is separate from TRICARE and there are distinct differences between them.

Indian Health Service

The provision of health services to native Americans originally developed from the relationship between the federal government and federally recognized Indian tribes. This relationship was established in 1787. It is based on Article I, Section 8, of the U.S. Constitution. It has been given form and substance by numerous treaties, laws, Supreme Court decisions, and executive orders.

The IHS is an agency within the HHS. It is responsible for providing healthcare services to American Indians and Alaska natives. The American Indians and Alaska natives served by the IHS receive preventive healthcare services, primary medical services (hospital and ambulatory care), community health services, substance abuse treatment services, and rehabilitative services. Secondary medical care, highly specialized medical services, and other rehabilitative care are provided by IHS staff or by private healthcare professionals working under contract with the IHS.

A system of acute and ambulatory care facilities operates on Indian reservations and in Indian and Alaska native communities. In locations where the IHS does not have its own facilities or is not equipped to provide a needed service, it contracts with local hospitals, state and local healthcare agencies, tribal health institutions, and individual healthcare providers.

Workers' Compensation

Most employees are eligible for some type of **workers' compensation** insurance. Workers' compensation programs cover healthcare costs and lost income associated with work-related injuries and illnesses. Federal government employees are covered by the **Federal Employees' Compensation Act** (FECA). Individual states pass legislation that addresses workers' compensation coverage for nonfederal government employees. Some states exclude certain workers, for example, business owners, independent contractors, farm workers, and so on. Texas employers are not required to provide workers' compensation coverage.

Federal Workers' Compensation Funds

In 1908, President Theodore Roosevelt signed legislation to provide workers' compensation for certain federal employees in unusually hazardous jobs. The scope of the law was narrow, and its benefits were limited. The 1908 law represented the first workers' compensation program to pass the test of constitutionality applied by the U.S. Supreme Court.

FECA replaced the 1908 statute in 1916. Under FECA, civilian employees of the federal government are provided medical care, survivors' benefits, and compensation for lost wages. The Office of Workers' Compensation Programs (OWCP) administers FECA as well as the Longshore and Harbor Workers' Compensation Act of 1927 and the Black Lung Benefits Reform Act of 1977.

FECA also provides vocational rehabilitation services to partially disabled employees. Employees who fully or partially recover from their injuries are expected to return to work. FECA does not provide retirement benefits.

State Workers' Compensation Funds

According to the American Association of State Compensation Insurance Funds (AASCIF), state workers' compensation insurance was developed in response to the concerns of employers. Before state workers' compensation programs became widely available, employers faced the possibility of going out of business when insurance companies refused to provide coverage or charged excessive premiums. Legislators in most states have addressed these concerns by establishing **state workers' compensation insurance funds** that provide a stable source of insurance coverage and serve to protect employers from uncertainties about the continuing availability of coverage. Because state funds are provided on a nonprofit basis, the premiums can be kept low. In addition, the funds provide only one type of insurance: workers' compensation. This specialization allows the funds to concentrate resources, knowledge, and expertise in a single field of insurance.

State workers' compensation insurance funds do not operate at taxpayer expense because, by law, the funds support themselves through income derived from premiums and investments. As nonprofit departments of the state or as independent nonprofit companies, they return surplus assets to policyholders as dividends or safety refunds. This system reduces the overall cost of state-level workers' compensation insurance. Numerous court decisions have determined that the assets, reserves, and surplus of the funds are not public funds but, instead, the property of the employers insured by the funds.

In states where state funds have not been mandated, employers purchase workers' compensation coverage from private carriers or provide self-insurance coverage.

Managed Care

Healthcare costs in the United States rose dramatically during the 1970s and 1980s. As a result, the federal government, employers, and other third-party payers began investigating more cost-effective healthcare delivery systems. The federal government decided to move toward PPSs for the Medicare program in the mid-1980s. Prospective payment as a reimbursement methodology is discussed later in this chapter. Commercial insurance providers looked to managed care.

Managed care is the generic term for prepaid health plans that integrate the financial and delivery aspects of healthcare services. In other words, managed care organizations work to control the cost of, and access to, healthcare services at the same time that they strive to meet high-quality standards. They manage healthcare costs by negotiating discounted providers' fees and controlling patients' access to expensive healthcare services. In managed care plans, services are carefully coordinated to ensure that they are medically appropriate and needed.

The cost of providing appropriate services also is monitored continuously to determine whether the services are being delivered in the most efficient and cost-effective way possible.

Since 1973, several pieces of federal legislation have been passed with the goal of encouraging the development of managed healthcare systems. (See table 14.5.) The Health Maintenance Organization Assistance Act of 1973 authorized federal grants and loans to private organizations that wished to develop **health maintenance organizations** (HMOs). Another important advancement in managed care was development of the **Health Plan Employer Data and Information Set** (HEDIS) by the **National Committee for Quality Assurance** (NCQA).

The NCQA is a private, not-for-profit organization that accredits, assesses, and reports on the quality of managed care plans in the United States. It worked with public and private healthcare purchasers, health plans, researchers, and consumer advocates to develop HEDIS in 1989. HEDIS is a set of standardized measures used to compare managed care plans in terms of the quality of services they provide. The standards cover areas such as plan membership, utilization of and access to services, and financial indicators. The goals of the program include:

- To help beneficiaries make informed choices among the numerous managed care plans available
- To improve the quality of care provided by managed care plans

- To help the government and other third-party payers make informed purchasing decisions

CMS offers several managed care options to Medicare and Medicaid enrollees. It began collecting HEDIS data from Medicare managed care plans in 1996.

Several kinds of managed care plans are available in the United States, including:

- Health maintenance organizations (HMOs)
- Preferred provider organizations (PPOs)
- Point-of-service (POS) plans
- **Exclusive provider organizations** (EPOs)
- **Integrated delivery systems** (IDSs)

Health Maintenance Organizations

An HMO is a prepaid voluntary health plan that provides healthcare services in return for the payment of a monthly membership premium. HMO premiums are based on a projection of the costs that are likely to be involved in treating the plan's average enrollee over a specified period of time. If the actual cost per enrollee were to exceed the projected cost, the HMO would experience a financial loss. If the actual cost per enrollee turned out to be lower than the projection, the HMO

Table 14.5. Federal legislation relevant to managed care

Year	Legislative Title	Legislative Summary
1973	Federal Health Maintenance Organization Assistance Act of 1973 (HMO Act of 1973)	• Authorized grants and loans to develop HMOs under private sponsorship • Defined a federally qualified HMO (certified to provide healthcare services to Medicare and Medicaid enrollees) as one that has applied for and met federal standards established in the HMO Act of 1973 • Required most employers with more than 25 employees to offer HMO coverage when local plans were available
1974	Employee Retirement Income Security Act of 1974 (ERISA)	• Mandated reporting and disclosure requirements for group life and health plans (including managed care plans) • Permitted large employers to self-insure employee healthcare benefits • Exempted large employers from taxes on health insurance premium
1982	Tax Equity and Fiscal Responsibility Act of 1982 (TEFRA)	• Modified the HMO Act of 1973 • Created Medicare risk programs, which allowed federally qualified HMOs and competitive medical plans that met specified Medicare requirements to provide Medicare-covered services under a risk contract • Defined risk contract as an arrangement among providers to provide capitated (fixed, prepaid basis) healthcare services to Medicare beneficiaries • Defined competitive medical plan (CMP) as an HMO that meets federal eligibility requirements for a Medicare risk contract but is not licensed as a federally qualified plan
1981	Omnibus Budget Reconciliation Act of 1981 (OBRA)	• Provided states with flexibility to establish HMOs for Medicare and Medicaid programs • Resulted in increased enrollment
1985	Preferred Provider Health Care Act of 1985	• Eased restrictions on preferred provider organizations • Allowed subscribers to seek healthcare from providers outside the PPO
1985	Consolidated Omnibus Budget Reconciliation Act of 1985 (COBRA)	• Established an employee's right to continue healthcare coverage beyond scheduled benefit termination date (including HMO coverage)
1988	Amendment to the HMO Act of 1973	• Allowed federally qualified HMOs to permit members to occasionally use non-HMO physicians and be partially reimbursed
1989	Health Plan Employer Data and Information Set (HEDIS)—developed by National Committee for Quality Assurance (NCQA)	• Created standards to assess managed care systems in terms of membership, utilization of services, quality, access, health plan management and activities, and financial indicators
1994	HCFA's Office of Managed Care established	• Facilitated innovation and competition among Medicare HMOs

would show a profit. Because most HMOs are for-profit organizations, they emphasize cost control and preventive medicine.

Today, most employers and insurance companies offer enrollees some type of HMO option. The benefit to third-party payers and enrollees alike is cost savings. Most HMO enrollees have significantly lower out-of-pocket expenses than enrollees of traditional fee-for-service and other types of managed care plans. The HMO premiums shared by employers and enrollees also are lower than the premiums for other types of healthcare plans.

HMOs can be organized in several different ways, including the **group model HMO,** the **independent practice association** (IPA), the **network model HMO,** and the **staff model HMO.**

Group Model HMOs

In the group model HMO, the HMO enters into a contract with an independent multispecialty physician group to provide medical services to members of the plan. The providers usually agree to devote a fixed percentage of their practice time to the HMO. Alternatively, the HMO may own or directly manage the physician group, in which case the physicians and their support staff would be considered its employees.

Group model HMOs are closed-panel arrangements. In other words, the physicians are not allowed to treat patients from other managed care plans. Enrollees of group model HMOs are required to seek services from the designated physician group.

Independent Practice Associations

IPAs are sometimes called individual practice associations. In the IPA model, the HMO enters into a contract with an organized group of physicians who join together for purposes of fulfilling the HMO contract but retain their individual practices. The IPA serves as an intermediary during contract negotiations. It also manages the premiums from the HMO and pays individual physicians as appropriate. The physicians are not considered employees of the HMO. They work from their own private offices and continue to see other patients. The HMO usually pays the IPA according to a prenegotiated list of discounted fees. Alternatively, physicians may agree to provide services to HMO members for a set prepaid capitated payment for a specified period of time. Capitation is discussed later in this chapter.

The IPA is an open-panel HMO, which means that the physicians are free to treat patients from other plans. Enrollees of such HMOs are required to seek services from the designated physician group.

Network Model HMOs

Network model HMOs are similar to group model HMOs except that the HMO contracts for services with two or more multispecialty group practices instead of just one practice. Members of network model HMOs receive a list of all the physicians on the approved panel and are required to select providers from the list.

Staff Model HMOs

Staff model HMOs directly employ physicians and other healthcare professionals to provide medical services to members. Members of the salaried medical staff are considered employees of the HMO rather than independent practitioners. Premiums are paid directly to the HMO, and ambulatory care services are usually provided within the HMO's corporate facilities. The staff model HMO is a closed-panel arrangement.

Preferred Provider Organizations

PPOs represent contractual agreements between healthcare providers and a self-insured employer or a health insurance carrier. Beneficiaries of PPOs select providers such as physicians or hospitals, from a list of participating providers who have agreed to furnish healthcare services to the covered population. Beneficiaries may elect to receive services from nonparticipating providers but must pay a greater portion of the cost (in other words, higher deductibles and copayments). Providers are usually reimbursed on a discounted fee-for-service basis.

Point-of-Service Plans

POS plans are similar to HMOs in that subscribers must select a **primary care physician** (PCP) from a network of participating physicians. (The PCP is usually a family or general practice physician or an internal medicine specialist.) The PCP acts as a service gatekeeper to control the patient's access to specialty, surgical, and hospital care as well as expensive diagnostic services.

POS plans are different from HMOs in that subscribers are allowed to seek care from providers outside the network. However, the subscribers must pay a greater share of the charges for out-of-network services. POS plans were created to increase the flexibility of managed care plans and to allow patients more choice in providers.

Exclusive Provider Organizations

EPOs are similar to PPOs except that EPOs provide benefits to enrollees only when the enrollees receive healthcare services from **network providers.** In other words, EPO beneficiaries do not receive reimbursement for services furnished by nonparticipating providers. In addition, healthcare services must be coordinated by a PCP. EPOs are regulated by state insurance departments. (In contrast, HMOs are regulated by state departments of commerce or departments of incorporation.)

Integrated Delivery Systems

An IDS is a healthcare provider made up of a number of associated medical facilities that furnish coordinated healthcare services. Most IDSs include a number of facilities that provide services along the continuum of care, for example, ambulatory surgery centers, physicians' office practices, outpatient clinics, acute care hospitals, SNFs, and so on.

Integrated delivery systems can be structured according to several different models, including:

- **Group practices without walls** (GPWWs)
- **Integrated provider organizations** (IPOs)
- **Management service organizations** (MSOs)
- **Medical foundations**
- **Physician–hospital organizations** (PHOs)

Group Practices without Walls

A GPWW is an arrangement that allows physicians to maintain their own offices but to share administrative, management, and marketing services (for example, medical transcription and billing) for the purpose of fulfilling contracts with managed care organizations.

Integrated Provider Organizations

An IPO manages and coordinates the delivery of healthcare services performed by a number of healthcare professionals and facilities. IPOs typically provide acute care (hospital) services, physicians' services, ambulatory care services, and skilled nursing services. The physicians working in an IPO are salaried employees. IPOs are sometimes referred to as delivery systems, horizontally integrated systems, health delivery networks, accountable health plans, integrated service networks (ISNs), vertically integrated plans (VIPs), and vertically integrated systems.

Management Service Organizations

MSOs provide practice management (administrative and support) services to individual physicians' practices. They are usually owned by a group of physicians or a hospital.

Medical Foundations

Medical foundations are nonprofit organizations that enter into contracts with physicians to manage the physicians' practices. The typical medical foundation owns clinical and business resources and makes them available to the participating physicians. Clinical assets include medical equipment and supplies, and treatment facilities. Business assets include billing and administrative support systems.

Physician-Hospital Organizations

PHOs, previously known as medical staff–hospital organizations, provide healthcare services through a contractual arrangement between physicians and hospital(s). PHO arrangements make it possible for the managed care market to view the hospital(s) and physicians as a single entity for the purpose of establishing a contract for services.

Check Your Understanding 14.2

Instructions: Answer the following questions on a separate piece of paper.

1. What is fee-for-service reimbursement? Why is it rarely used today as a reimbursement method?

2. How are private commercial insurance plans financed?

3. What process do most insurance companies use to reimburse healthcare services?

4. What are administrative services only contracts?

5. What federal program pays for healthcare services provided to financially needy individuals?

6. For which populations of individuals do TRICARE (formerly CHAMPUS) and CHAMPVA reimburse healthcare services?

7. Why is Medicare Part B referred to as supplemental medical insurance?

8. What federal legislation expanded Medicare options by creating Medicare Advantage?

9. What private health insurance pays (within limits) for most healthcare services not covered by Medicare Part A?

10. How did the Medicare and Medicaid programs come into effect? How are the two programs different?

11. How are Medicaid eligibility standards established?

12. What is the difference between a preferred provider organization and a point-of-service plan?

13. What is the purpose of the State Children's Health Insurance Program?

14. What type of Medicare coverage applies to inpatient hospitalization? To prescription eyeglasses? To emergency department visits? To dental care? To ambulatory surgery center service? To hospice care?

15. What is the difference between TRICARE Extra and TRICARE Prime?

16. How does state workers' compensation coverage differ from federal workers' compensation coverage?

17. What type of HMO model employs physicians and other healthcare professionals to provide healthcare services to members?

18. What is the difference between an independent practice association and a staff model HMO?

19. Define managed care and describe the various types of managed care programs available in the United States?

20. What do management service organizations do?

Healthcare Reimbursement Methodologies

As mentioned earlier in this chapter, about 85 percent of Americans are covered by some type of private prepaid health plan or federal healthcare program. Therefore, most healthcare expenses in the United States are reimbursed through third-party payers rather than by the actual recipients of the services. The recipients can be considered the "first parties" and the providers the "second parties." Third-party payers include commercial for-profit insurance companies, nonprofit Blue Cross and Blue Shield organizations, self-insured employers, federal programs (Medicare, Medicaid, SCHIP, TRICARE, CHAMPVA, and IHS), and workers' compensation programs.

Providers charge their own determined amounts for services rendered. However, providers are rarely reimbursed this full amount because third-party payers may have a unique reimbursement methodology. For example, commercial insurance plans usually reimburse healthcare providers under some type of **retrospective payment system.** The federal Medicare program uses PPSs. In retrospective payment systems, the exact amount of the payment is determined after the service has been delivered. In a PPS, the exact amount of the payment is determined before the service is delivered.

Fee-for-Service Reimbursement Methodologies

Fee-for-service reimbursement methodologies issue payments to healthcare providers on the basis of the charges assigned to each of the separate services that were performed for the patient. The total bill for an episode of care represents the sum of all the itemized charges for every element of care provided. Independent clinical professionals such as physicians and psychologists who are not employees of the facility issue separate itemized bills to cover their services after the services are completed or on a monthly basis when the services are ongoing.

Before prepaid insurance plans became common in the 1950s and the Medicare and Medicaid programs were developed in the 1960s, healthcare providers sent itemized bills directly to their patients. Patients were held responsible for paying their own medical bills. When prepaid health plans and the Medicare/Medicaid programs were originally developed, they also based reimbursement on itemized fees.

Traditional Fee-for-Service Reimbursement

In traditional fee-for-service (FFS) reimbursement systems, third-party payers and/or patients issue payments to healthcare providers after healthcare services have been provided (for example, after the patient has been discharged from the hospital). Payments are based on the specific services delivered. The fees charged for services vary considerably by the type of services provided, the resources required, and the type and number of healthcare professionals involved.

Payments can be calculated on the basis of actual billed charges, discounted charges, prenegotiated rate schedules, or the usual or customary charges in a specific community.

For example, some third-party payers pay only the maximum allowable charges as determined by the plan. Maximum allowable charges may be significantly lower than the provider's billed charges. Some payers issue payments on the basis of **usual, customary, and reasonable (UCR)** charges. Commercial insurance and Blue Cross/Blue Shield plans often issue payments based on prenegotiated discount rates and contractual cost-sharing arrangements with the patient.

For many plans, the health plan and the patient share costs on an 80:20 percent arrangement. The portion of the claim covered by the patient's insurance plan would be 80 percent of allowable charges. After the third-party payer transmits its payment to the provider, the provider's billing department issues a final statement to the patient. The statement shows the amount for which the patient is responsible (in this example, 20 percent of allowable charges).

The traditional FFS reimbursement methodology is still used by many commercial insurance companies for visits to physicians' offices.

Managed Fee-for-Service Reimbursement

Managed FFS reimbursement is similar to traditional FFS reimbursement except that managed care plans control costs primarily by managing their members' use of healthcare services. Most managed care plans also negotiate with providers to develop discounted **fee schedules.** Managed FFS reimbursement is common for inpatient hospital care. In some areas of the country, however, it also is applied to outpatient and ambulatory services, surgical procedures, high-cost diagnostic procedures, and physicians' services.

Utilization controls include the prospective and retrospective review of the healthcare services planned for, or provided to, patients. For example, a prospective utilization review of a plan to hospitalize a patient for minor surgery might determine that the surgery could be safely performed less expensively in an outpatient setting. Prospective utilization review is sometimes called precertification.

In a retrospective utilization review, the plan might determine that part or all of the services provided to a patient were not medically necessary or were not covered by the plan. In such cases, the plan would disallow part or all of the provider's charges and the patient would be responsible for paying the provider's outstanding charges.

Discharge planning also can be considered a type of utilization control. The managed care plan may be able to move the patient to a less intensive, and therefore less expensive, care setting as soon as possible by coordinating his or her discharge from inpatient care.

Episode-of-Care Reimbursement Methodologies

Plans that use **episode-of-care (EOC) reimbursement** methods issue lump-sum payments to providers to compensate them for all the healthcare services delivered to a patient for a specific illness and/or over a specific period of time. EOC payments also are called **bundled payments.** Bundled payments cover multiple services and also may involve multiple providers of care. EOC reimbursement methods include capitated payments, global payments, global surgery payments, Medicare ambulatory surgery center rates, and Medicare PPSs.

Capitation

Capitation is based on per-person premiums or membership fees rather than on itemized per-procedure or per-service charges. The capitated managed care plan negotiates a contract with an employer or government agency representing a specific group of individuals. According to the contract, the managed care organization agrees to provide all the contracted healthcare services that the covered individuals need over a specified period of time (usually one year). In exchange, the individual enrollee and/or third-party payer agrees to pay a fixed premium for the covered group. Like other insurance plans, a capitated insurance contract stipulates as part of the contract exactly which healthcare services are covered and which ones are not.

Capitated premiums are calculated on the projected cost of providing covered services **per patient per month** or **per member per month** (PPPM or PMPM). The capitated premium for an individual member of a plan includes all the services covered by the plan, regardless of the number of services actually provided during the period or their cost. If the average member of the plan actually used more services than originally assumed in the PPPM calculation, the plan would show a loss for the period. If the average member actually used fewer services, the plan would show a profit.

The purchasers of capitated coverage (usually the member's employer) pay monthly premiums to the managed care plan. The individual enrollees usually pay part of the premium as well. The plan then compensates the providers who actually furnished the services. In some arrangements, the managed care plan accepts all the risk involved in the contract. In others, some of the risk is passed on to the PCPs who agreed to act as gatekeepers for the plan.

The capitated managed care organization may own or operate some or all of the healthcare facilities that provide care to members and directly employ clinical professionals. Staff model HMOs operate in this way. Alternatively, the capitated managed care organization may purchase services from independent physicians and facilities, as do group model HMOs. For example:

> The ABC HMO awarded a capitated contract to the XYZ Medical Center for a total compensation of $3,600,000 in the year 2004. According to the terms of the contract, the medical center agreed to provide comprehensive healthcare services to all 500 enrollees covered under the contract for 12 months. The medical center received lump-sum payments of $300,000 per month over the 12-month period. A large, multispecialty PHO owned by the hospital acted as primary care gatekeepers and provided medical services to the enrollees. Inpatient and outpatient services were provided directly by the medical center.

Global Payment

Global payment methodology is sometimes applied to radiological and similar types of procedures that involve professional and technical components. Global payments are lump-sum payments distributed among the physicians who performed the procedure or interpreted its results and the healthcare facility that provided the equipment, supplies, and technical support required. The procedure's **professional component** is supplied by physicians (for example, radiologists), and its **technical component** (for example, radiological supplies, equipment, and support services) is supplied by a hospital or freestanding diagnostic or surgical center. For example:

> Larry Timber underwent a scheduled carotid angiogram as a hospital outpatient. He had complained of ringing in his ears and dizziness, and his physician scheduled the procedure to determine whether there was a blockage in one of Larry's carotid arteries. The procedure required a surgeon to inject radiopaque contrast material through a catheter into Larry's left carotid artery. A radiological technician then took an x-ray of Larry's neck. The technician was supervised by a radiologist, and both were employees of the hospital.

> *Professional component:* Injection of radiopaque contrast material by the surgeon

> *Technical component:* X-ray of the neck region

> *Global payment:* The facility received a lump-sum payment for the procedure and paid for the services of the surgeon from that payment.

Global Surgery Payments

A single **global surgery payment** covers all the healthcare services entailed in planning and completing a specific surgical procedure. In other words, every element of the procedure from the treatment decision through normal postoperative patient care is covered by a single bundled payment. For example:

> Tammy Murdock received all the prenatal, perinatal, and postnatal care involved in the birth of her daughter from Dr. Thomas Michaels. She received one bill from the physician for a total of $2,200. The bill represented the total charges for the obstetrical services associated with her pregnancy. However, the two-day inpatient hospital stay for the normal delivery was not included in the global payment nor were the laboratory services she received during her hospital stay. Tammy received a separate bill for these services. In addition, if she had suffered a postdelivery complication (for example, a wound infection) or an unrelated medical problem, the physician and hospital services required to treat the complications would not have been covered by the global surgical payment.

Medicare Ambulatory Surgery

CMS defines an **ambulatory surgery center** (ASC) as a state-licensed, Medicare-certified supplier (not a provider) of surgical healthcare services. ASCs must **accept assignment** on Medicare claims, which means the supplier accepts as payment in full whatever Medicare reimburses. Because payments are subject to Medicare Part B deductible and coinsurance requirements, reimbursement is 80 percent of the prospectively determined rate (adjusted for regional wage variations). CMS replaced the ASC rates (which categorized approximately 2,500 surgical procedures into what were then eight payment groups) with the **ambulatory payment classification** (APC) **system** and the **outpatient prospective payment system** (OPPS) in 2000 for hospital-based outpatient services and procedures.

To qualify as a Medicare-certified ASC, the surgery center must be a separate entity distinguishable from any other entity or type of facility. This means that the ASC must be separate from any other organization with respect to licensure, accreditation, governance, professional supervision, administrative functions, clinical services, record keeping, financial and accounting systems, and national identifier or supplier number. The ASC can be physically located within the space of another entity and still be considered separate for Medicare payment purposes when the preceding criteria are met.

Medicare pays a prospectively determined fee for ASC services that are included on the approved list. The services that fall within the scope of ASC services include, but are not limited to, services performed by nurses and technicians, supplies, drugs and biologicals, surgical dressings, housekeeping services, and use of the facility.

The professional services of physicians and other practitioners do not fall within the scope of ASC facility services. Therefore, the ASC facility fee does not include payment for the professional services of physicians and other practitioners. ASCs should not bill for the following physicians' services: anesthesiology, surgery, or assistance at surgery services. The anesthesiologist, surgeon, and assistant surgeon submit separate claims.

CMS's ASC rates are now categorized into nine separate payment groups. (See table 14.6.) The payment groups are based on the complexity of the surgical procedures involved. CMS also updates and publishes the rate-setting methodology and establishes wage index (WI) tables for use in urban and rural areas.

Special rules apply when more than one surgical procedure is performed during the same operative session. The ASC is reimbursed at 100 percent for the procedure classified in the highest payment group, and any other procedure performed during the same session is reimbursed at 50 percent of the procedure's applicable group rate. Bilateral procedures are reimbursed at 150 percent of the applicable rate. The reimbursement of physicians for ASC-approved procedures is subject to 20 percent coinsurance and deductible provisions. Payment is made at 80 percent of the Medicare physician fee schedule, which is discussed in more detail later in this chapter. Fees for approved procedures in an ASC setting are noted on the fee schedule as a facility fee.

Prospective Payment

In 1983, CMS implemented a PPS for inpatient hospital care provided to Medicare beneficiaries. This PPS methodology is called **diagnosis-related groups** (DRGs). The DRG system was implemented as a way to control Medicare spending. It reimburses hospitals a predetermined amount for each Medicare inpatient stay. Payments are determined by the DRG to which each case is assigned according to the patient's **princi-**

pal diagnosis, which is defined as the condition which, after study, is determined to have occasioned the admission of the patient to the hospital for care.

After DRG implementation in 1983, expenditures for Medicare post-acute care benefits quickly escalated. According to the HHS, post-acute expenditures totaled approximately $2.5 billion in 1986 but more than $30 billion in 1996. This drastic increase in spending alarmed Medicare policy makers. In response, the BBA mandated PPS implementation for nonacute care services, including care in SNFs, outpatient services and procedures, home health care, and rehabilitation care. In addition, the act included a legislative proposal on a PPS for long-term care.

Check Your Understanding 14.3

Instructions: Answer the following questions on a separate piece of paper.

1. What type of payment system is in place when the amount of payment is determined before the service is delivered?

2. What is a chargemaster, and why do healthcare facilities develop chargemasters?

3. What are usual, customary, and reasonable (UCR) charges based on?

4. Many insurance plans require patients to share costs for healthcare services. What is the most typical cost share ratio?

5. Which utilization control is most closely associated with managed fee-for-service reimbursement?

6. What would a managed care plan likely show when a group of patients uses more services than the plan originally calculated in its contract with the group?

7. What are bundled payments? What is another name for bundled payments?

8. Describe the concept of capitation and explain how capitated payments are calculated.

9. How are ambulatory surgery center rates calculated?

10. How is reimbursement limited when multiple ambulatory surgery center procedures are performed on the same patient during the same visit?

11. How did the first prospective payment system implemented by CMS affect inpatient reimbursement?

12. What are diagnosis-related groups? What was the effect of DRG implementation in 1983 on Medicare expenditures?

13. What are the general steps taken by the billing department after codes have been assigned?

Medicare's Prospective Payment Systems

As discussed briefly in the preceding section, Congress enacted the first Medicare PPS in 1983 as a cost-cutting measure. Implementation of the **acute care prospective payment system** resulted in a shift of clinical services and expenditures away from the inpatient hospital setting to outpatient settings. As a result, spending on nonacute care exploded.

Congress responded by passing the **Omnibus Budget Reconciliation Act** (OBRA) of 1986, which mandated that HCFA develop a prospective system for hospital-based out-

Table 14.6.   ASC payment groups and rates for 2005

ASC Group	Reimbursement Rate
Group 1 Procedure	$333
Group 2 Procedure	$446
Group 3 Procedure	$510
Group 4 Procedure	$630
Group 5 Procedure	$717
Group 6 Procedure	$826 ($676 + $150 for intraocular lenses)
Group 7 Procedure	$995
Group 8 Procedure	$973 ($823 + $150 for intraocular lenses)
Group 9 Procedure	$1,339

Source: CMS 2005b.

patient services provided to Medicare beneficiaries. In subsequent years, Congress mandated the development of PPSs for other healthcare providers.

Medicare's Acute Care Prospective Payment System

As mentioned previously, prior to 1983, Medicare Part A payments to hospitals were determined on a traditional FFS reimbursement methodology. Payment was based on the cost of services provided, and reasonable cost and/or per-diem costs were used to determine payment.

During the late 1960s, just a few years after the Medicare and Medicaid health programs were implemented, Congress authorized a group at Yale University to develop a system for monitoring quality of care and utilization of services. This system was known as diagnosis-related groups (DRGs). DRGs were implemented on an experimental basis by the New Jersey Department of Health in the late 1970s as a way to predetermine reimbursement for hospital inpatient stays.

At the conclusion of the New Jersey DRG experiment, Congress passed the **Tax Equity and Fiscal Responsibility Act of 1982** (TEFRA). TEFRA modified Medicare's retrospective reimbursement system for inpatient hospital stays by requiring implementation of the DRG PPS in 1983. Medicare now pays most hospitals for inpatient hospital services according to a predetermined rate for each discharge under DRGs.

At this time, several types of hospitals are excluded from Medicare acute care PPS. The following facilities are still paid on the basis of reasonable cost, subject to payment limits per discharge or under a separate PPS:

- Psychiatric and rehabilitation hospitals and psychiatric and rehabilitation units within larger medical facilities
- **Long-term care hospitals** (LTCH), which are defined as hospitals with an average length of stay of 25 days or more
- Children's hospitals
- Cancer hospitals
- Critical access hospitals

To determine the appropriate DRG, a claim for a healthcare encounter is first classified into one of 25 **major diagnostic categories,** or MDCs. Most MDCs are based on body systems and include diseases and disorders relating to a particular system. However, some MDCs include disorders and diseases involving multiple organ systems (for example, burns). The number of DRGs within a particular MDC varies.

The principal diagnosis determines the MDC assignment. Within each MDC, decision trees are used to determine the correct DRG. (See figure 14.1, p. 364.) Within most MDCs, cases are divided into surgical DRGs (based on a surgical hierarchy that orders individual procedures or groups of procedures by resource intensity) and medical DRGs. Medical DRGs generally are differentiated on the basis of diagnosis and age. Some surgical and medical DRGs are further differentiated on the basis of the presence or absence of **complications** or **comorbidities.**

Under the **acute care prospective payment system** (PPS), a predetermined rate based on the DRG (only one is assigned per case) assigned to each case is used to reimburse hospitals for inpatient care provided to Medicare beneficiaries. Hospitals determine DRGs by assigning **ICD-9-CM** codes to each patient's principal diagnosis, comorbidities, complications, **principal procedure,** and/or secondary procedures. These code numbers and other information on the patient (age, gender, and discharge status) are entered into a **DRG grouper.** A DRG grouper is a computer software program that assigns appropriate DRGs according to the information provided for each episode of care.

Reimbursement for each episode of care is based on the DRG assigned. Different diagnoses require different levels of care and expenditures of resources. Therefore, each DRG is assigned a different level of payment that reflects the average amount of resources required to treat a patient assigned to that DRG. Each DRG is associated with a description, a relative weight, a geometric mean length of stay (LOS), and an arithmetic mean LOS. The relative weight represents the average resources required to care for cases in that particular DRG relative to the national average of resources used to treat all Medicare patients. A DRG with a relative weight of 2.000, on average, requires twice as many resources as a DRG with a relative weight of 1.000. The geometric mean LOS is defined as the total days of service, excluding any outliers or transfers, divided by the total number of patients; the arithmetic mean LOS is defined as the total days of service divided by the total number of patients.

For example, DRG 1, organized within MDC 01, is described as SURG CRANIOTOMY AGE >17 WCC and has a relative weight of 3.3344, a geometric mean LOS of 7.5 and an arithmetic mean LOS of 10.0.

CMS adjusts the Medicare DRG list and reimbursement rates every fiscal year (October 1 through September 30). For fiscal year 2004–2005, the list includes 543 DRGs (approximately 20 of which are invalid).

In some cases, the DRG payment received by the hospital may be lower than the actual cost of providing Medicare Part A inpatient services. In such cases, the hospital must absorb the loss. In other cases, the hospital may receive a payment for more than its actual cost and, therefore, makes a profit. It is expected that, on average, hospitals will be reimbursed for their total costs in providing services to Medicare patients.

Special circumstances also can apply to inpatient cases and result in an outlier payment to the hospital. An outlier case results in exceptionally high costs when compared with other cases in the same DRG. For fiscal year (FY) 2005, to qualify for a **cost outlier,** a hospital's charges for a case (adjusted to cost) must exceed the payment rate for the DRG by $25,800. The additional payment amount is equal to 80 percent of the difference between the hospital's entire cost for the stay and the threshold amount.

Figure 14.1.   Portion of major diagnostic category: Diseases and disorders of the digestive system

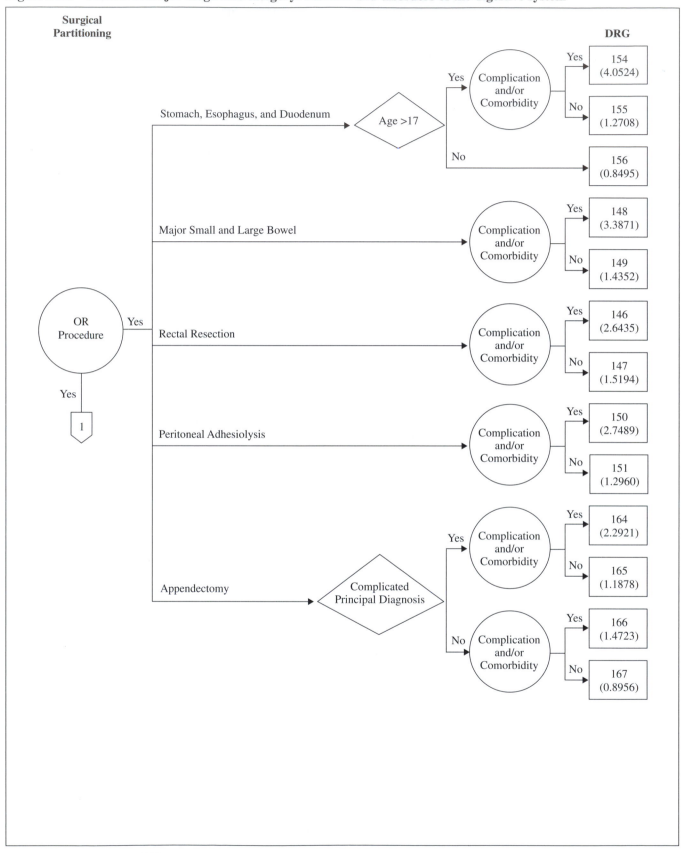

The DRG system creates a hospital's **case-mix index** (types or categories of patients treated by the hospital) based on the relative weights of the DRG. The case-mix index can be figured by multiplying the relative weight of each DRG by the number of discharges within that DRG. This provides the total weight for each DRG. The sum of all total weights divided by the sum of total patient discharges equals the case-mix index. A hospital may relate its case-mix index to the costs incurred for inpatient care. This information allows the hospital to make administrative decisions about services to be offered to its patient population. For example:

> The hospital's case-mix report indicated that a small population of patients was receiving obstetrical services, but that the costs associated with providing such services was disproportionately high. This report along with other data might result in the hospital's administrative decision to discontinue its obstetrical services department.

An **all patient DRG** (AP-DRG) system was developed in 1988 by 3M Health Information Systems as the basis for New York's hospital reimbursement program for non-Medicare discharges. AP-DRGs are still used in a number of states as a basis for payment of non-Medicare claims. AP-DRGs use the patient's age, sex, discharge status, and ICD-9-CM diagnoses and procedure codes to determine a DRG that, in turn, determines reimbursement. 3M also has developed **all patient refined DRGs** (APR-DRGs) as an extension of the DRG concept. APR-DRGs adjust patient data for severity of illness and risk of mortality, help to develop clinical pathways, are used as a basis for quality assurance programs, and are used in comparative profiling and setting capitation rates (3M HIS 2002).

Resource-Based Relative Value Scale (RBRVS) System

In 1992, CMS implemented the **resource-based relative value scale** (RBRVS) system for physician's services such as office visits covered under Medicare Part B. The system reimburses physicians according to a fee schedule based on predetermined values assigned to specific services.

The **Medicare fee schedule** (MFS) is the listing of allowed charges that are reimbursable to physicians under Medicare. Each year's MFS is published by CMS in the *Federal Register.*

To calculate fee schedule amounts, Medicare uses a formula that incorporates the following factors:

- **Relative value units** for physician work (RVUw)
- Practice expenses (RVUpe)
- Malpractice costs (RVUm)

Sample 2005 RVUs for selected HCPCS codes are shown in table 14.7.

Payment localities are adjusted according to three **geographic practice cost indices** (GPCIs):

- Physician work (GPCIw)
- Practice expenses (GPCIpe)
- Malpractice costs (GPCIm)

Sample GPCIs for selected U.S. cities are shown in table 14.8, p. 366.

A geographic cost index is a number used to multiply each RVU so that it better reflects a geographical area's relative costs. For example, costs of office rental prices, local taxes, average salaries, and malpractice costs are all affected by geography.

A **national conversion factor** (CF) converts the RVUs into payments. In 2005, the CF was $37.8975.

The RBRVS fee schedule uses the following formula:

$$[(RVUw \times GPCIw) + (RVUpe \times GPCIpe) + (RVUm \times GPCIm)] \times CF = Payment$$

As an example, payment for performing a drainage of a skin abscess in Birmingham, Alabama, in 2005, can be calculated. RVU values include:

- Work RVU (RVUw) = 1.17
- Practice expense RVU (RVUpe) = 0.93
- Malpractice RVU (RVUm) = 0.12

GPCI values include:

- Work GPCI (GPCIw) = 1.00
- Practice expense GPCI (GPCIpe) = 0.858
- Malpractice GPCI (GPCIm) = 0.752
- National CF = $37.8975

The calculation is as follows:

$$(1.17 \times 1.00) + (0.93 \times 0.858) + (0.12 \times 0.752) \times \$37.8975$$
$$1.17 + 0.80 + 0.09 \times \$37.8975$$
$$2.06 \times \$37.8975$$
$$Fee\ schedule\ payment = \$78.00$$

Table 14.7.   Sample 2005 RVUs for selected HCPCS codes

HCPCS Code	Description	Work RVU	Practice Expense RVU	Malpractice Expense RVU
99203	Office visit	1.34	.48	.09
99204	Office visit	2.00	.71	.12
10080	I&D of pilonidal cyst, simple	1.17	1.11	.11
45380	Colonoscopy with biopsy	4.43	1.73	.35
52601	TURP, complete	12.35	5.1	.87

Table 14.8.   Sample GPCIs for selected U.S. cities

City	Work GPCI	Practice Expense GPCI	Malpractice Expense GPCI
St. Louis	1.000	.946	.941
Dallas	1.010	1.063	1.061
Seattle	1.010	1.115	.819
Philadelphia	1.020	1.098	1.386

Medicare Skilled Nursing Facility Prospective Payment System

The BBA mandated implementation of a **skilled nursing facility prospective payment system** (SNF PPS). The system was to cover all costs (routine, ancillary, and capital) associated with covered SNF services furnished to Medicare Part A beneficiaries. Certain educational activities were exempt from the new system.

The SNF PPS was implemented on July 1, 1998. Under the PPS, SNFs are no longer paid under a system based on reasonable costs. Instead, they are paid according to a per-diem PPS based on case mix–adjusted payment rates.

Medicare Part A covers posthospital SNF services and all items and services paid under Medicare Part B before July 1, 1998 (other than physician and certain other services specifically excluded under the BBA). Major elements of the SNF PPS include rates, coverage, transition, and consolidated billing. OBRA required CMS to develop an assessment instrument to standardize the collection of SNF patient data. That instrument is known as the **Resident Assessment Instrument** (RAI) and includes the **Minimum Data Set 2.0** (MDS). A draft of MDS 3.0 is under review.

The MDS is the minimum core of defined and categorized patient assessment questions that serves as the basis for documentation and reimbursement in an SNF. The MDS form contains a face sheet for documentation of resident identification information, demographic information, and the patient's customary routine.

Resource Utilization Groups

SNF reimbursement rates are paid according to **Resource Utilization Groups, Version III** (RUG-III) (a resident classification system) based on the MDS resident assessments.

The RUG-III classification system uses resident assessment data from the MDS collected by SNFs to assign residents to one of 44 groups. SNFs complete MDS assessments according to a schedule specifically designed for Medicare payment (that is, on the 5th, 14th, 30th, 60th, and 90th days after admission to the SNF). For Medicare billing purposes, specific codes are associated with each of the 44 RUG-III groups, and each assessment applies to specific days within a resident's SNF stay. SNFs that fail to perform timely assess-

ments are paid a default payment for the days they are not in compliance with this schedule.

Resident Assessment Validation and Entry

HCFA (now called CMS) developed a computerized data-entry system for long-term care facilities that offers users the ability to collect MDS assessments in a database and transmit them in CMS-standard format to their state database. The data-entry software is entitled **Resident Assessment Validation and Entry** (RAVEN). RAVEN imports and exports data in standard MDS record format; maintains facility, resident, and employee information; enforces data integrity via rigorous edit checks; and provides comprehensive online help. It includes a data dictionary and a RUG calculator.

Consolidated Billing Provision

The BBA includes a billing provision that requires an SNF to submit consolidated Medicare bills for its residents for services covered under either Part A or Part B except for a limited number of specifically excluded services. For example, when a physician provides a diagnostic radiology service to an SNF patient, the SNF must bill for the technical component of the radiology service because this is included in the SNF consolidated billing payment. The rendering physician must develop a business relationship with the SNF in order to receive payment from the SNF for the services he or she rendered. The professional component of the physician services is excluded from SNF consolidated billing and must be billed separately to the **Medicare carrier.** There are, of course, other exclusions to this provision, including physician assistant services, nurse practitioner services, and clinical nurse specialists when these individuals are working under the supervision of, or in collaboration with, a physician, certified midwife services, qualified psychologist services, and certified registered nurse anesthetist services. Other exclusions include hospice care, maintenance dialysis, selected services furnished on an outpatient basis such as cardiac catheterization services, CAT scans and MRIs, radiation therapy, and ambulance services. In addition, SNFs report **Healthcare Common Procedure Coding System** (HCPCS) codes on all Part B bills.

Medicare/Medicaid Outpatient Prospective Payment System

The BBA authorized implementation of a Medicare PPS for outpatient services. The OPPS, implemented in October 2001, applies to the following services:

- Services provided by hospital outpatient departments, including **partial hospitalization** services
- Certain Part B services provided to hospital inpatients who have no Part A coverage
- Partial hospitalization services provided by community mental health centers (CMHCs)
- Vaccines, splints, casts, and antigens provided by HHAs that provide medical and health-related services

- Vaccines provided by comprehensive outpatient rehabilitation facilities (CORFs)
- Splints, casts, and antigens provided to hospice patients for the treatment of nonterminal illnesses

The OPPS does not apply to critical access hospitals (CAHs) or hospitals in Maryland that are excluded because they qualify under the Social Security Act for payment under the state's payment system. In addition, IHS hospitals and hospitals located outside the 50 states, the District of Columbia, and Puerto Rico are excluded.

Implementation of the OPPS resulted in the discontinuation of the blended payment method for radiology and other diagnostic services and for ASC services provided in hospital-based outpatient departments. In addition, the following provisions are associated with the OPPS:

- Payments are established in a budget-neutral manner.
- OPPS payment weights, rates, payment adjustments and groups, and annual consultation are reviewed and updated annually by an expert provider advisory panel.
- Budget-neutral outlier adjustments are based on charges, adjusted to costs, for all OPPS services included on outpatient bills submitted before January 1, 2002, and, thereafter, based on individual services billed.
- Provisions for transitional pass-through are related to additional costs of new and current medical devices, drugs, and biologicals.
- Provisions are in place for OPPS payment for implantable devices, including DME, prosthetics, and implantable devices used in diagnostic testing.

The OPPS is not applicable to clinical diagnostic laboratory services, orthotics, prosthetics, and take-home surgical dressings. These services are paid on the basis of a fee schedule. Chronic dialysis is reimbursed under the composite rate, but acute dialysis (for example, for treatment of poisonings) is paid under the OPPS. Reimbursement for screening mammographies is based on the Medicare physician fee schedule. Outpatient rehabilitation services (physical, speech-language-pathology, and occupational therapy) are reimbursed under the Medicare physician fee schedule.

The calculation of payment for services under the OPPS is based on the categorization of outpatient services into APC groups according to **CPT**/HCPCS codes. ICD-9-CM coding is not utilized in the selection of APCs. The more than 700 APCs are categorized into significant procedure APCs, radiology and other diagnostic APCs, medical visit APCs, and a partial hospitalization APC. Services within an APC are similar, both clinically and with regard to resource consumption, and each APC is assigned a fixed payment rate for the facility fee or technical component of the outpatient visit. Payment rates then are adjusted according to the hospital's wage index. Multiple APCs may be appropriate for a single episode of care as the patient may receive various types of services such as radiology or surgical procedures.

Medicare has assigned **payment status indicators** (PSIs) (table 14.9) to HCPCS/CPT codes to indicate whether a service/procedure is to be reimbursed under the OPPS.

OPPS payments will be made for clinical diagnostic laboratory tests and radiology and other diagnostic services in addition to the payment for a surgical procedure or medical visit performed on the same day. However, the OPPS also incorporates the **packaging** of certain items, such as anesthesia, supplies, certain drugs, and the use of recovery and observation rooms.

Table 14.9.   OPPS payment status indicators and description of payment under OPPS

Status Indicator	Description of Payment under OPPS
SI A	Services paid under some other method (such as a fee schedule): • Ambulance services • Clinical diagnostic laboratory services • Nonimplantable prosthetic and orthotic devices • EPO for ESRD patients • Physical, occupation, and speech therapy • Routine dialysis services for ESRD patients provided in a certified dialysis unit of a hospital • Diagnostic mammography • Screening mammography
SI B	Codes that are not recognized by OPPS when submitted on an outpatient hospital Part B bill type
SI C	Inpatient procedures
SI D	Discontinued codes
SI E	Items, codes, and services not covered by Medicare
SI F	Corneal tissue acquisition; certain CRNA services
SI G	Pass-through drugs, biologicals, and radiopharmaceutical agents
SI H	Pass-through device categories; brachytherapy sources
SI K	Non-pass-through drugs, biologicals, and radiopharmaceutical agents
SI L	Influenza vaccine; Pneumococcal pneumonia vaccine
SI N	Items and services packaged into APC rates
SI P	Partial hospitalization
SI S	Significant procedure, not discounted when multiple
SI T	Significant procedure, multiple reduction applies
SI V	Clinic or emergency department visit
SI Y	Nonimplantable durable medical equipment
SI X	Ancillary services

Discounting applies to multiple surgical procedures furnished during the same operative session. For discounted procedures, the full APC rate is paid for the surgical procedure with the highest rate and other surgical procedures performed at the same time are reimbursed at 50 percent of the APC rate. Similar discounting occurs under the physician fee schedule and the payment system for ASCs.

Surgical procedures terminated after a patient is prepared for surgery, but before induction of anesthesia, are paid for at 50 percent of the APC rate. In addition, when multiple surgical procedures are performed during the same operative session, the beneficiary's coinsurance is discounted in proportion to the APC payment.

Note: Services that Medicare has identified as "inpatient only" are not reimbursed by Medicare when they are provided on an outpatient basis.

Home Health Prospective Payment System

The BBA called for the development and implementation of a **home health prospective payment system** (HH PPS) for reimbursement of services provided to Medicare beneficiaries. The PPS for HHAs was implemented on October 1, 2000.

OASIS and HAVEN

HHAs use the OASIS data set and HAVEN data-entry software to conduct all patient assessments, not just the assessments for Medicare beneficiaries. OASIS stands for **Outcome and Assessment Information Set.** It consists of data elements that (1) represent core items for the comprehensive assessment of an adult home care patient and (2) form the basis for measuring patient outcomes for the purpose of outcome-based quality improvement (OBQI). OASIS is a key component of Medicare's partnership with the home care industry to foster and monitor improved home health care outcomes. The Conditions of Participation for HHAs require that HHAs electronically report all OASIS data.

CMS also developed the OASIS data-entry system called HAVEN (**Home Assessment Validation and Entry**). HAVEN is available to HHAs at no charge through CMS's Web site or on CD-ROM. HAVEN offers users the ability to collect OASIS data in a database and transmit them in a standard format to state databases. The data-entry software imports and exports data in standard OASIS record format; maintains agency, patient, and employee information; maintains data integrity through rigorous edit checks; and provides comprehensive online help.

Home Health Resource Groups

Home health resource groups (HHRGs) represent the classification system established for the prospective reimbursement of covered home care services to Medicare beneficiaries during a 60-day episode of care. Covered services include skilled nursing visits, home health aide visits, therapy services (for example, physical, occupational, and speech therapy), medical social services, and nonroutine medical supplies. DME is excluded from the episode-of-care payment. DME is reimbursed under the DME fee schedule.

The classification of a patient into one of 80 HHRGs is based on OASIS data, which establish the severity of clinical and functional needs and services utilized. Grouper software is used to establish the appropriate HHRG. The HHRG is a six-character alphanumeric code that represents severity levels in three domains: clinical, functional, and service utilization. (See table 14.10.) For example:

OASIS data collected on a 76-year-old male home care patient resulted in an HHRG of C3F4S3. This HHRG is interpreted as a clinical domain of high severity, a functional domain of high severity, and a service utilization domain of high utilization.

EOC reimbursements vary from $1,000 to almost $6,000 and are affected by treatment level and regional wage differentials. The initial episode is reimbursed under a 60:40 split, with 60 percent paid at the start of treatment and the remainder paid at the end of the episode. Additional episodes are paid under a 50:50 split. There is no limit to the number of 60-day episodes of care that a patient may receive as long as Medicare coverage criteria are met.

Low Utilization and Outlier Payments

When a patient receives fewer than four home care visits during a 60-day episode, an alternate (reduced) payment, or **low-utilization payment adjustment** (LUPA), is made instead of the full HHRG reimbursement rate. HHAs are eligible for a **cost outlier adjustment,** which is a payment for certain high-cost home care patients whose costs are in excess of a threshold amount for each HHRG. The threshold is the 60-day episode payment plus a fixed-dollar loss that is constant across the HHRGs.

Ambulance Fee Schedule

A new Medicare payment system for medically necessary transports effective for services provided on or after April 1,

Table 14.10. HHRG severity levels in three domains: Clinical, functional, and service utilization

Domain	Score	Points	Severity Level
Clinical	C0	0–7	Minimal severity
	C1	8–19	Low severity
	C2	20–40	Moderate severity
	C3	41+	High severity
Functional	F0	0–2	Minimal severity
	F1	3–15	Low severity
	F2	16–23	Moderate severity
	F3	24–29	High severity
	F4	30+	Maximum severity
Service utilization	S0	0–2	Minimum utilization
	S1	3	Low utilization
	S2	4–6	Moderate utilization
	S3	7	High utilization

2002, was included as part of the BBA. The final rule established a five-year transition period during which time payment will be based on a blended amount, based in part on the ambulance fee schedule and in part on reasonable cost or reasonable charge. By year five (CY 2006), the fee schedule will be fully implemented with 100 percent of payment based on the schedule. The new payment system applies to all ambulance services, including volunteer, municipal, private, independent, and institutional providers (hospitals, critical access hospitals, SNFs, and HHAs).

Ambulance services are reported on claims using HCPCS codes that reflect the seven categories of ground service and two categories of air service. Mandatory assignment is required for all ambulance service providers.

The seven categories of ground (land and water) ambulance services include:

- Basic life support
- Basic life support—emergency
- Advanced life support, level 1
- Advanced life support, level 1—emergency
- Advanced life support, level 2
- Specialty care transport
- Paramedic intercept

The air service categories include fixed-wing air ambulance (airplane) and rotary-wing air ambulance (helicopter).

Inpatient Rehabilitation Facility (IRF) Prospective Payment System

The BBA (as amended by the **Balanced Budget Refinement Act of 1999**) authorized implementation of a per-discharge PPS for care provided to Medicare beneficiaries by inpatient rehabilitation hospitals and rehabilitation units, referred to as **inpatient rehabilitation facilities** (IRFs). The PPS for IRFs became effective on January 1, 2002.

IRFs must meet the regulatory requirements to be classified as a rehabilitation hospital or rehabilitation unit that is excluded from the PPS for inpatient acute care services. To meet the criteria, an IRF must operate as a hospital. Requirements state that during the most recent, consecutive, and appropriate 12-month time period, the hospital will have treated an inpatient population that met or exceeded the following percentages:

1. For cost reporting periods beginning on or after July 1, 2004, and before July 1, 2005, the hospital must have served an inpatient population of whom at least 50 percent required intensive rehabilitative services for treatment of one or more of the medical conditions specified in figure 14.2.
2. For cost reporting periods beginning on or after July 1, 2005, and before July 1, 2006, the hospital must have served an inpatient population of whom at least 60 percent required intensive rehabilitative services for treatment of one or more of the medical conditions specified in figure 14.2.

Figure 14.2.   Medical conditions that are criteria for classification as inpatient rehabilitation facility

1. Stroke
2. Spinal cord injury
3. Congenital deformity
4. Amputation
5. Major multiple trauma
6. Fracture of femur (hip fracture)
7. Brain injury
8. Neurological disorders including multiple sclerosis, motor neuron diseases, polyneuropathy, muscular dystrophy, and Parkinson's disease
9. Burns
10. Active, polyarticular rheumatoid arthritis, psoriatic arthritis, and seronegative arthropathies
11. Systemic vaculidities with joint inflammation
12. Severe or advanced osteoarthritis involving two or more weight-bearing joints
13. Knee or hip joint replacement or both

Source: CMS 2005a.

3. For cost reporting periods beginning on or after July 1, 2006, and before July 1, 2007, the hospital must have served an inpatient population of whom at least 65 percent required intensive rehabilitative services for treatment of one or more of the medical conditions specified in figure 14.2.
4. For cost reporting periods beginning on or after July 1, 2007, the hospital must have served an inpatient population of whom at least 75 percent required intensive rehabilitative services for treatment of one or more of the medical conditions specified in figure 14.2.

Patient Assessment Instrument

IRFs are required to complete a patient assessment instrument (PAI) upon each patient's admission and also discharge from the facility. CMS provides facilities with IRVEN **(Inpatient Rehabilitation Validation and Entry)** System to collect the IRF-PAI in a database that can be transmitted electronically to the IRF-PAI national database. These data are used in assessing clinical characteristics of patients in rehabilitation settings. Ultimately, they can be used to provide survey agencies with a means to objectively measure and compare facility performance and quality and to allow researchers to develop improved standards of care.

The IRF PPS uses information from the IRF-PAI to classify patients into distinct groups on the basis of clinical characteristics and expected resource needs. Data used to construct these groups, called **case-mix groups** (CMGs), include rehabilitation impairment categories (RICs), functional status (both motor and cognitive), age, comorbidities, and other factors deemed appropriate to improve the explanatory power of the groups. There are currently 100 CMGs into which patients are classified.

CMG Relative Weight

An appropriate weight, called the **CMG relative weight,** which measures the relative difference in facility resource intensity among the various groups, is assigned to each case-mix group. Separate payments are calculated for each group, including the application of case- and facility-level adjustments. Facility-level adjustments include wage-index adjustments, low-income patient adjustments, and rural facility adjustments. Case-level adjustments include transfer adjustments, interrupted-stay adjustments, and cost outlier adjustments.

Long-Term Care Hospitals (LTCHs) Prospective Payment System

The Balanced Budget Refinement Act of 1999 amended by the Benefits Improvement Act of 2000 mandated the establishment of a per discharge, DRG-based PPS for longer-term care hospitals beginning on October 1, 2002. There is a five-year transition period with full implementation by October 1, 2006. This transition period is applicable only to existing hospitals and replaces the cost-based payment system previously used. New facilities are paid 100 percent of the LTC-DRG.

LTCHs are defined as having an average inpatient LOS greater than 25 days.

LTC-DRGs

Patients are classified into distinct diagnosis groups based on clinical characteristics and expected resource use. These groups are based on the current inpatient DRGs. There are approximately 170 LTC-DRGs. The payment system includes the following three primary elements:

1. Patient classification into a LTC-DRG weight.
2. Relative weight of the LTC-DRG. The weights reflect the variation in cost per discharge as they take into account the utilization for each diagnosis.
3. Federal payment rate. Payment is made at a predetermined per discharge amount for each LTC-DRG.

Adjustments

The PPS does provide for case-(patient)-level adjustments such as short-stay outlier, interrupted stays, and high-cost outliers. Facility-wide adjustments include area wage index and cost of living adjustments.

A short-stay outlier is an adjustment to the payment rate for stays that are considerably shorter than the average length of stay (ALOS) for a particular LTC-DRG. A case would qualify for short-stay outlier status when the LOS is between one day and up to and including five-sixths of the ALOS for the LTC-DRG. Both the ALOS and the five-sixths of the ALOS periods are published in the *Federal Register.* Payment under the short-stay outlier is made using different payment methodologies. (See table 14.11 for examples of LTC-DRGs and the ALOS for each.)

An interrupted stay occurs when a patient is discharged from the long-term care hospital and then is readmitted to the same facility for further treatment after a specific number of days away from the facility. There are different policies if the patient is readmitted to the facility within three days (called three-day or less interrupted-stay policy) or if the patient is away from the facility more than three days (called the greater than three-day interrupted-stay policy).

A high-cost outlier is an adjustment to the payment rate for a patient when the costs are unusually high and exceed the typical costs associated with a LTC-DRG. High-cost outlier payments reduce the facility's potential financial losses that can result from treating patients who require more costly care than is normal. A case qualifies for a high-cost outlier payment when the estimated cost of care exceeds the high-cost outlier threshold, which, for example, in 2005 was $17,864.

Inpatient Psychiatric Facilities (IPFs) Prospective Payment System

The Balanced Budget Refinement Act of 1999 mandated the development of a per diem PPS for inpatient psychiatric services furnished in hospitals and exempt units. The PPS became effective on January 1, 2005, establishing a stan-

Table 14.11.   Examples of LTC-DRGs, relative weights, geometric ALOS, and five-sixths of the geometric ALOS

LTC-DRG	Description	Relative Weight	Geometric ALOS	Five-sixths of the Geometric ALOS
2	Craniotomy age >17 w/o CC	1.1899	28.5	23.8
3	Craniotomy age 0–17	1.1899	28.5	23.8
6	Carpal tunnel release	0.6064	21.1	17.6
26	Seizure and headache age 0–17	0.6064	21.1	17.6
30	Traumatic stupor and coma less than 1 hour age 0–17	0.8508	24.3	20.3
32	Concussion age >17 w/o CC	0.6064	21.1	17.6
36	Retinal procedures	0.4586	16.9	14.1
195	Cholecystectomy w/ CDE w/ CC	1.8658	38.6	32.2

dardized per diem rate to **inpatient psychiatric facilities** (IPFs) based on the national average of operating, ancillary, and capital costs for each patient day of care in the IPF. The system uses the same DRGs as the acute care hospital inpatient system.

CMS is phasing in the PPS for existing facilities over a three-year period with full payments under the PPS beginning in the fourth year. The per diem payment is adjusted to reflect both patient and facility characteristics that cause significant cost increases.

Adjustments

Patient-level or case-level adjustments are provided for age, specified DRGs, and certain comorbidity categories. Payment adjustments are made for eight age categories beginning with age 45 at which point, statistically, costs are increased as the patient ages.

The IPF receives a DRG payment adjustment for a principal diagnosis that groups to one of 15 psychiatric DRGs. (See table 14.12.) Seventeen comorbidity categories that require comparatively more costly treatment during an inpatient stay also generate a payment adjustment. The list of comorbidity categories and their associated ICD-9-CM diagnosis codes can be found in table 14.13, p. 372.

There also is a variable per diem adjustment to recognize higher costs in the early days of a psychiatric stay.

The IPF PPS also includes an outlier policy for those patients who require more expensive care than expected in an effort to minimize the financial risk to the IPF. Although the basis of the system is a per diem rate, outlier payments are made on a per case basis rather than on the per diem basis.

The PPS also includes regulations on payments when there is an interrupted stay, meaning the patient is discharged from an IPF and returns to the same or another facility before midnight on the third consecutive day. The intent of the policy is to prevent a facility from prematurely discharging a patient after the maximum payment is received and subsequently readmitting the patient.

Facility adjustments include a wage-index adjustment, a rural location adjustment, and a teaching status adjustment.

Check Your Understanding 14.4

Instructions: Answer the following questions on a separate piece of paper.

1. When did Congress enact the first Medicare prospective payment system?
2. What were Medicare Part A payments to hospitals based on prior to implementation of the diagnosis-related group PPS?
3. What type of diagnosis is the DRG prospective payment rate based on?
4. What is the name of the computer software program that assigns appropriate DRGs according to information provided for each episode of care?
5. What kinds of hospitals are excluded from the Medicare acute care PPS?
6. How are diagnosis-related groups organized?
7. What does case mix refer to? What is the relationship between DRGs and case mix?
8. What act mandated implementation of the skilled nursing facility PPS?
9. What are resident assessment data? From what are they collected?
10. What is the purpose of the resource-based relative value scale?
11. What types of hospitals are not reimbursed according to the outpatient prospective payment system?
12. What concept is applied when multiple surgical procedures are furnished during the same operative session?
13. Which data set for patient assessments is used by the home health PPS?
14. What types of services are covered by the home health resource group classification system?
15. What PPS uses a Patient Assessment Instrument to gather data on patients?
16. What is the purpose of the IRVEN software?
17. To meet the definition of a long-term care hospital, what must the average length of stay be?
18. What is a short-stay outlier in relation to the LTCH PPS, and how is it calculated?
19. What other PPSs use the DRGs currently used for inpatient hospitals?
20. The IPF prospective payment system identifies comorbidities that generate a payment adjustment. What are some of the other factors that generate adjustments with the IPF PPS?

Table 14.12.   Psychiatric DRGs

DRG	DRG Description
424	Procedure with principal diagnosis of mental illness
425	Acute adjustment reaction
426	Depressive neurosis
427	Neurosis, except depressive
428	Disorders of personality
429	Organic disturbances
430	Psychosis
431	Childhood disorders
432	Other mental disorders
433	Alcohol/Drug use, left against medical advice
521	Alcohol/Drug use, w/ CC
522	Alcohol/Drug use, w/o CC
523	Alcohol/Drug use, w/o rehab
12	Degenerative nervous system disorders
23	Nontraumatic stupor and coma

Table 14.13.   Comorbidity categories affecting IPS payment

Category	ICD-9-CM Diagnosis Codes
Developmental disabilities	317, 318.0, 318.1, 318.2, and 319
Coagulation factor deficit	286.0 through 286.4
Tracheostomy	519.00 through 519.09; V44.0
Renal failure, acute	584.5 through 584.9, 636.3, 637.3, 638.3, 639.3, 669.32, 669.34, 958.5
Renal failure, chronic	403.01, 403.11, 403.91, 404.02, 404.03, 404.12, 404.13, 404.92, 404.93, 585, 586, V45.1, V56.0, V56.1, V56.2
Oncology treatment	140.0 through 239.9 with either 99.25 or a code from 92.21 through 92.29
Uncontrolled Type I diabetes mellitus with or without complications	250.02, 250.03, 250.12, 250.13, 250.22, 250.23, 250.32, 250.33, 250.42, 250.43, 250.52, 250.53, 250.62, 250.63, 250.72, 250.73, 250.82, 250.83, 250.92, 250.93
Severe protein calorie malnutrition	260 through 262
Eating and conduct disorders	307.1, 307.50, 312.03, 312.33, 312.34
Infectious diseases	010.01 through 041.10, 042, 045.00 through 053.19, 054.40 through 054.49, 055.0 through 077.0, 078.2 through 078.89, 079.50 through 079.59
Drug and/or alcohol-induced mental disorders	291.0, 292.0, 292.12, 292.2, 303.00, 304.00
Cardiac conditions	391.0, 391.1, 391.2, 402.01, 404.03, 416.0, 421.0, 421.1, 421.9
Gangrene	440.24, 785.4
Chronic obstructive pulmonary disease	491.21, 494.1, 510.0, 518.83, 518.84, V46.1
Artificial openings—digestive and urinary	569.60 through 569.69, 997.5, V44.1 through V44.6
Severe musculoskeletal and connective tissue disorders	696.0, 710.0, 730.00 through 730.09, 730.10 through 730.19, 730.20 through 730.29
Poisoning	965.00 through 965.09, 965.4, 967.0 through 969.9, 977.0, 980.0 through 980.9, 983.0 through 983.9, 986, 989.0 through 989.7

Processing of Reimbursement Claims

Understanding payment mechanisms is an important foundation for accurately processing claims forms. However, it is not enough just to understand payment mechanisms.

A facility's patient accounts department is responsible for billing third-party payers, processing **accounts receivable,** monitoring payments from third-party payers, and verifying insurance coverage. Medicare carriers and **fiscal intermediaries** (FIs) contract with CMS to serve as the financial agent between providers and the federal government to locally administer Medicare's Part A and Part B.

Coordination of Benefits

In many instances, patients have more than one insurance policy and the determination of which policy is primary and which is secondary is necessary so that there is no duplication of benefits paid. This process is called the coordination of Benefits (COB) or the **coordination of benefits transaction.** The monies collected from third-party payers cannot be greater than the amount of the provider's charges.

Explanation of Benefits/ Remittance Advice

An **Explanation of Benefits** (EOB) is a statement sent to the patient to explain services provided, amounts billed and payments made by the health plan. Medicare replaced its Explanation of Medicare Benefits (EOMB) with the **Medicare Summary Notice** (MSN). (See figure 14.3 for a sample Part B MSN.)

A **remittance advice** (RA) is sent to the provider to explain payments made by third-party payers. Prior to the availability of the ANSI ASC X12 835, commonly known as the **electronic remittance advice** (ERA), providers used either paper or tape transmissions to post payments to their accounts; however, tape transmissions are no longer an option. (See figure 14.4, p. 375, for a sample RA.)

Figure 14.3. Sample Medicare summary notice

		Page 1 of 2
CMS CENTERS for MEDICARE & MEDICAID SERVICES	**Medicare Summary Notice**	July 1, 2004

CUSTOMER SERVICE INFORMATION

BENEFICIARY NAME
STREET ADDRESS
CITY, STATE   ZIP CODE

Your Medicare Number: 111-11-1111A

If you have questions, write or call:
Medicare
555 Medicare Blvd., Suite 200
Medicare Building
Medicare, US XXXXX-XXXX

Local: (XXX) XXX-XXXX
Toll-free: 1-800-XXX-XXXX
TTY for Hearing Impaired: 1-800-XXX-XXXX

BE INFORMED: Beware of "free" medical services or products. If it sounds too good to be true, it probably is.

This is a summary of claims processed from 05/15/2004 through 06/10/2004.

PART A HOSPITAL INSURANCE – INPATIENT CLAIMS

Dates of Service	Benefit Days Used	Non-Covered Charges	Deductible and Coinsurance	You May Be Billed	See Notes Section
Claim Number: 12435-84956-84556-45621					a
Cure Hospital, 213 Sick Lane,					
** Dallas, TX 75555**					
Referred by: Paul Jones, M.D.					
04/25/04 – 05/09/04	14 days	$0.00	$876.00	$776.00	b, c
Claim Number: 12435-84956-845556-45622					
Continued Care Hospital, 124 Sick Lane,					
** Dallas, TX 75555**					
Referred by: Paul Jones, M.D.					
05/09/04 – 06/20/04	11 days	$0.00	$0.00	$0.00	

PART B MEDICAL INSURANCE – OUTPATIENT FACILITY CLAIMS

Dates of Service	Services Provided	Amount Charged	Non-Covered Charges	Deductible and Coinsurance	You May Be Billed	See Notes Section
Claim Number: 12435-8956-8458						d
Medicare Hospital, 123 Medicare Lane,						
** Dallas, TX 75209**						
Referred by: Paul Jones, M.D.						
04/02/04	L.V. Therapy (Q0081)	$33.00	$0.00	$6.60	$6.60	
	Lab (3810)	1,140.50	0.00	228.10	228.10	
	Operating Room (31628)	786.50	0.00	157.30	157.30	
	Observation Room (99201)	293.00	0.00	58.60	58.60	
	Claim Total	**$2,253.00**	**$0.00**	**$450.60**	**$450.60**	
					(continued)	

THIS IS NOT A BILL – Keep this notice for your records.

(Continued on next page)

Figure 7.3.   (Continued)

> **Notes Section:**
>
> a The amount Medicare paid the provider for this claim is $XXXX.XX.
>
> b $776.00 was applied to your inpatient deductible.
>
> c $30.00 was applied to your blood deductible.
>
> d The amount Medicare paid the provider for this claim is $XXXX.XX.

Deductible Information:

You have met the Part A deductible for this benefit period.

You have met the Part B deductible for 2004.

You have met the blood deductible for 2004.

General Information:

You have the right to make a request in writing for an itemized statement that details each Medicare item or service you have received from your physician, hospital, or any other health supplier or health professional. Please contact them directly, in writing, if you would like an itemized statement.

Compare the services you receive with those that appear on your Medicare Summary Notice. If you have questions, call your doctor or provider. If you feel further investigation is needed due to possible fraud and abuse, call the phone number in the Customer Service Information Box.

Appeals Information—Part A (Inpatient) and Part B (Outpatient)

If you disagree with any claims decision on either Part A or Part B of this notice, you can request an appeal by November 1, 2004. Follow the instructions below:

1) Circle the item(s) you disagree with and explain why you disagree.

2) Send this notice or a copy, to the address in the "Customer Service Information" box on Page 1. (You may also send any additional information you may have about your appeal.)

3) Sign here _____   Phone number _____

Revised 02/04

Figure 7.4. Sample single-claim remittance advice

```
Medicare National Standard Intermediary Remittance Advice
FPE:                                    07/30/04
PAID:                                   01/25/04
CLM#                                    2
TOB:                                    111
-------------------------------------------------------------------
PATIENT:     JOHN DOE                                    PCN:   235617
HIC:         123456            SVC FROM:    01/05/04     MRN:   124767
PAT STAT:    01    CLAIM STAT:    1    THRU:    01/06/04 ICN:   987654
-------------------------------------------------------------------
CHARGES:              PAYMENT DATA: 140=DRG         0.000    =REIM RATE
1939.90  =REPORTED    2741.69 =DRG AMOUNT   0.00    =MSP PRIM PAYER
0.00     =NONCOVERED  2497.26 =DRG/OPER     0.00    =PROF COMPONENT
0.00     =DENIED      244.43  =DRG/CAPITAL  0.00    =ESRD AMOUNT
1939.90  =COVERED     0.00    =OUTLIER      0.00    =HCPCS AMOUNT
DAYS/VISITS:          0.00    =CAP OUTLIER  0.00    =ALLOWED AMOUNT
1        =COST REPT   768.00  =CASH DEDUCT  0.00    =G/R AMOUNT
1        =COVD/UTIL   0.00    =BLOOD DEDUCT 0.00    =INTEREST
0        =NONCOVERED  0.00    =COINSURANCE  -801.79 =CONTRACT ADJ
0        =COVD VISITS 0.00    =PAT REFUND   675.00  =PER DIEM AMT
0        =NCOV VISITS 0.00    =MSP LIAB MET 1973.69 =NET REIM AMT
ADJ REASON CODES:  CO  A2 -801.79
                   PR     1
                   768
REMARK CODES:    MA02
```

Third-Party Payers

Depending on the services provided to patients, either the **CMS-1500** or the **UB-92** (CMS-1450) claim form is submitted to the third-party payer for reimbursement purposes. The CMS-1500 is used to bill third-party payers for provider services (for example, physician's office visit), and the UB-92 is submitted for inpatient, outpatient, home health care, hospice, and long-term care services. Health claims data are frequently transmitted electronically between a healthcare organization and a third-party payer using electronic data interchange (EDI), which is addressed in chapter 7.

CMS-1500

In 1958, the Health Insurance Association of America (HIAA) and the American Medical Association (AMA) originally created a standardized insurance claim form called the **Attending Physician Statement** (APS) (or COMB-1). However, some third-party payers did not accept its use. In April 1975, the AMA and CMS cochaired the Uniform Claim Form Task Force, which approved a universal claim form now known as CMS-1500. (See figure 14.5, p. 376.) CMS-1500 is used for processing both group and individual

healthcare claims. It has specific form locators (FLs) that must be completed according to third-party payer guidelines. (See table 14.14, p. 377.)

In 1995, the Uniform Claim Form Task Force was replaced by the **National Uniform Claim Committee** (NUCC). The NUCC developed a standard data set to be used in the transmission of noninstitutional provider claims to and from third-party payers. NUCC membership includes representation from the following organizations:

- Alliance for Managed Care
- American Association of Health Plans
- AMA
- ANSI ASC X12N
- Blue Cross and Blue Shield Association
- CMS (formerly HCFA)
- Health Insurance Association of America
- **Medical Group Management Association**
- National Association of Insurance Commissioners
- National Association of Medical Equipment Services
- National Association of State Medicaid Directors
- **National Uniform Billing Committee** (NUBC)

Figure 14.5.   CMS-1500 claim form

PLEASE
DO NOT
STAPLE
IN THIS
AREA

CARRIER →

HEALTH INSURANCE CLAIM FORM

| | PICA | | | | | | | PICA | | |

1. MEDICARE   MEDICAID   CHAMPUS   CHAMPVA   GROUP HEALTH PLAN   FECA BLK LUNG   OTHER
   (Medicare #)   (Medicaid #)   (Sponsor's SSN)   (VA File #)   (SSN or ID)   (SSN)   (ID)

1a. INSURED'S I.D. NUMBER   (FOR PROGRAM IN ITEM 1)

2. PATIENT'S NAME (Last Name, First Name, Middle Initial)

3. PATIENT'S BIRTH DATE   MM   DD   YY   SEX   M   F

4. INSURED'S NAME (Last Name, First Name, Middle Initial)

5. PATIENT'S ADDRESS (No., Street)

6. PATIENT RELATIONSHIP TO INSURED   Self   Spouse   Child   Other

7. INSURED'S ADDRESS (No., Street)

CITY   STATE

8. PATIENT STATUS   Single   Married   Other

CITY   STATE

ZIP CODE   TELEPHONE (Include Area Code)   (   )

Employed   Full-Time Student   Part-Time Student

ZIP CODE   TELEPHONE (INCLUDE AREA CODE)   (   )

9. OTHER INSURED'S NAME (Last Name, First Name, Middle Initial)

10. IS PATIENT'S CONDITION RELATED TO:

11. INSURED'S POLICY GROUP OR FECA NUMBER

a. OTHER INSURED'S POLICY OR GROUP NUMBER

a. EMPLOYMENT? (CURRENT OR PREVIOUS)   YES   NO

a. INSURED'S DATE OF BIRTH   MM   DD   YY   SEX   M   F

b. OTHER INSURED'S DATE OF BIRTH   MM   DD   YY   SEX   M   F

b. AUTO ACCIDENT?   PLACE (State)   YES   NO

b. EMPLOYER'S NAME OR SCHOOL NAME

c. EMPLOYER'S NAME OR SCHOOL NAME

c. OTHER ACCIDENT?   YES   NO

c. INSURANCE PLAN NAME OR PROGRAM NAME

d. INSURANCE PLAN NAME OR PROGRAM NAME

10d. RESERVED FOR LOCAL USE

d. IS THERE ANOTHER HEALTH BENEFIT PLAN?   YES   NO   *If yes*, return to and complete item 9 a-d.

READ BACK OF FORM BEFORE COMPLETING & SIGNING THIS FORM.

12. PATIENT'S OR AUTHORIZED PERSON'S SIGNATURE I authorize the release of any medical or other information necessary to process this claim. I also request payment of government benefits either to myself or to the party who accepts assignment below.

SIGNED _____   DATE _____

13. INSURED'S OR AUTHORIZED PERSON'S SIGNATURE I authorize payment of medical benefits to the undersigned physician or supplier for services described below.

SIGNED _____

14. DATE OF CURRENT: ILLNESS (First symptom) OR   MM   DD   YY   INJURY (Accident) OR   PREGNANCY(LMP)

15. IF PATIENT HAS HAD SAME OR SIMILAR ILLNESS. GIVE FIRST DATE   MM   DD   YY

16. DATES PATIENT UNABLE TO WORK IN CURRENT OCCUPATION   MM   DD   YY   FROM   TO   MM   DD   YY

17. NAME OF REFERRING PHYSICIAN OR OTHER SOURCE

17a. I.D. NUMBER OF REFERRING PHYSICIAN

18. HOSPITALIZATION DATES RELATED TO CURRENT SERVICES   MM   DD   YY   FROM   TO   MM   DD   YY

19. RESERVED FOR LOCAL USE

20. OUTSIDE LAB?   YES   NO $ CHARGES

21. DIAGNOSIS OR NATURE OF ILLNESS OR INJURY. (RELATE ITEMS 1,2,3 OR 4 TO ITEM 24E BY LINE)

1. |___.__   3. |___.__

2. |___.__   4. |___.__

22. MEDICAID RESUBMISSION CODE   ORIGINAL REF. NO.

23. PRIOR AUTHORIZATION NUMBER

24. A						B	C	D		E	F	G	H	I	J	K
DATE(S) OF SERVICE						Place of Service	Type of Service	PROCEDURES, SERVICES, OR SUPPLIES (Explain Unusual Circumstances)		DIAGNOSIS CODE	$ CHARGES	DAYS OR UNITS	EPSDT Family Plan	EMG	COB	RESERVED FOR LOCAL USE
From			To					CPT/HCPCS	MODIFIER							
MM	DD	YY	MM	DD	YY											
1																
2																
3																
4																
5																
6																

25. FEDERAL TAX I.D. NUMBER   SSN   EIN

26. PATIENT'S ACCOUNT NO.

27. ACCEPT ASSIGNMENT? (For govt. claims, see back)   YES   NO

28. TOTAL CHARGE $

29. AMOUNT PAID $

30. BALANCE DUE $

31. SIGNATURE OF PHYSICIAN OR SUPPLIER INCLUDING DEGREES OR CREDENTIALS (I certify that the statements on the reverse apply to this bill and are made a part thereof.)

32. NAME AND ADDRESS OF FACILITY WHERE SERVICES WERE RENDERED (If other than home or office)

33. PHYSICIAN'S, SUPPLIER'S BILLING NAME, ADDRESS, ZIP CODE & PHONE #

SIGNED _____   DATE _____

PIN#   GRP#

PATIENT AND INSURED INFORMATION

PHYSICIAN OR SUPPLIER INFORMATION

(APPROVED BY AMA COUNCIL ON MEDICAL SERVICE 8/88)   **PLEASE PRINT OR TYPE**   APPROVED OMB-0938-0008 FORM CMS-1500 (12-90),   FORM RRB-1500,
APPROVED OMB-1215-0055 FORM OWCP-1500,   APPROVED OMB-0720-0001 (CHAMPUS)

Table 14.14.   CMS-1500 form locators and brief description of information to be entered into each

Form Locator	Brief Description	Form Locator	Brief Description
1	Type of insurance	17a	ID Number of referring physician
1a	Insured's ID number	18	Hospitalization dates related to current services
2	Patient's name	19	Reserved for local use
3	Patient's birth date/sex	20	Outside lab
4	Insured's name	21	Diagnosis or nature of illness or injury
5	Patient's address	22	Medicaid resubmission
6	Patient's relationship to insured	23	Prior authorization number
7	Insured's address	24A	Dates of service
8	Patient's marital status/employment status	24B	Place of service
9	Other insured's name	24C	Type of service
9a	Other insured's policy or group number	24D	Procedures, services, or supplies
9b	Other insured's date of birth/sex	24E	Diagnosis code
9c	Employer's name or school name	24F	Charges
9d	Insurance plan name or program name	24G	Days or units
10a–10c	Indicate whether patient's condition is related to a work injury, an automobile accident, or another type of accident	24H	EPSDT family plan
10d	Reserved for local use	24I	Emergency
11	Insured's policy group or FECA number	24J	Coordination of benefits
11a	Insured's date of birth/sex	24K	Reserved for local use
11b	Employer's name or school name	25	Federal tax ID number
11c	Insurance plan name or program name of insured	26	Patient's account number
11d	Indicate whether there is another health benefit plan	27	Accept assignment or not
12	Patient's or authorized person's signature	28	Total charge
13	Insured or authorized person's signature	29	Amount paid
14	Date of current illness or injury or pregnancy	30	Balance due
15	Date when patient first consulted provider for treatment of the same or similar condition	31	Signature of physician or supplier
16	Dates patient unable to work in current occupation	32	Name and address of facility where services were rendered
17	Name of referring physician or other source	33	Physician/supplier's billing name, address, ZIP code, and telephone number

CMS-1500 was revised in 1990 and printed in red ink to meet optical scanning guidelines. In May 1992, Medicare required that all services delivered to patients by physicians and suppliers except for ambulance services be billed on this scannable form. CMS-1500 contains 33 blocks that are completed according to third-party payer guidelines. Noninstitutional providers and suppliers submit it in accordance with these guidelines. It is important to follow payer guidelines when completing the claim form; otherwise, reimbursement will be delayed until the form is corrected.

UB-92 (CMS-1450)

Healthcare facilities, such as hospitals, currently submit the UB-92 (figure 14.6), or Uniform Bill, to third-party payers for reimbursement of patient services. The data elements and design of the UB-92 are the responsibility of the NUBC, which includes representation from the following organizations:

- American Association of Health Plans
- American Health Care Association
- American Hospital Association
- AHA's state hospital association representatives
- Alliance for Managed Care
- **American National Standards Institute** Accredited Standards
- Committee X12N-Insurance Subcommittee (ANSI ASC X12N)
- Blue Cross and Blue Shield Association
- Center for Healthcare Information Management
- Federation of American Health Systems
- CMS: Medicare
- CMS: Medicaid
- Health Insurance Association of America–National Association for Home Care
- National Association of State Medicaid Directors
- National Uniform Claim Committee
- Public Health/Health Services Research (national)
- Public Health/Health Services Research (state)
- TRICARE (CHAMPUS)

The UB-92 form and instructions are used by institutional and other selected providers to complete a Medicare, Part A, claim for submission to Medicare FIs (and other third-party payers). UB-92 contains 86 FLs, which are completed according to third-party payer guidelines. (See table 14.15, p. 380.) FLs of particular importance are those that require entry of **revenue codes,** which identify services provided to patients as reported on the UB-92. The types of organizations that submit the UB-92 include:

- Ambulance companies
- Ambulatory surgery centers
- HHAs
- Hospice organizations
- Hospitals (emergency department and inpatient and outpatient services)
- Psychiatric and drug/alcohol treatment facilities (inpatient and outpatient services)

- SNFs
- Subacute facilities
- Stand-alone clinical/laboratory facilities
- Walk-in clinics

UB-04

The NUBC began work to replace the UB-92 in 2001. The intent was to make the new form more HIPAA compliant, to improve the denial rate, and to reduce the need for resubmittals. The **UB-04** data set includes a number of improvements and enhancements resulting from nearly four years of surveys and study.

One of the most significant changes is in the number of diagnosis and procedure code fields available. The newly designed form will include nine additional diagnosis fields and more fields for E codes. The anticipated UB-04 will include 80 FLs.

In addition, the UB-04 anticipates the move to ICD-10-CM with expanded code fields. It also provides a space for national provider identifiers and national health plan identifiers.

January 2007 is the targeted implementation date for the new UB-04. (See figure 14.7, p. 381, and table 14.16, p. 382.)

Medicare Carriers

Medicare carriers process Part B claims for services by physicians and medical suppliers. Examples of carriers might include a state Blue Shield plan or commercial insurance companies or other organizations under contract with Medicare. Carriers are responsible for performing the following functions:

- Determining the charges allowed by Medicare
- Maintaining the quality of performance records
- Assisting in fraud and abuse investigations
- Providing education to providers, suppliers, and beneficiaries as necessary.
- Making payments to physicians and suppliers for Part B–covered services

Medicare Fiscal Intermediaries

Medicare FIs process Part A claims and hospital-based Part B claims for institutional services, including inpatient hospital claims, SNFs, HHAs, and hospice services. They also process outpatient claims for supplemental medical insurance (Medicare Part B). Examples of FIs include Blue Cross and Blue Shield organizations and commercial insurance companies under contract with Medicare.

FIs are responsible for performing the following functions:

- Determining costs and reimbursement amounts
- Maintaining records
- Establishing controls
- Safeguarding against fraud and abuse or excess use
- Conducting reviews and audits
- Making payments to providers for covered services
- Providing education to facilities and beneficiaries as necessary

Figure 14.6.   UB-92 (CMS-1450) claim form

APPROVED OMB NO. 0938-0279

Table 14.15.   UB-92 form locators and brief description of information to be entered into each

Form Locator	Brief Description	Form Locator	Brief Description
1	Provider's Name, Address, and Telephone Number	46	Units of Service
2	Unlabeled Field—State Use	47	Total Charges (by Revenue Code Category)
3	Patient's Control Number (Account Number)	48	Noncovered Charges
4	Type of Bill	49	Unlabeled Field—National Use
5	Federal Tax Number	50A–C	Payer Identification
6	Statement Covers Period	51A–C	Provider Number
7	Covered Days	52A–C	Release of Information Certification Indicator
8	Noncovered days	53A–C	Assignment of Benefits Certification Indicator
9	Coinsurance Days	54A–C, P	Prior Payments—Payers and Patient
10	Lifetime Reserve Days	55A–C, P	Estimated Amount Due
11	Unlabeled Field—State Use	56	DRG Number and Grouper ID
12	Patient Name	57	Unlabeled Field—National Use
13	Patient Address	58A–C	Insured's Name
14	Patient Birthdate	59A–C	Patient's Relationship to Insured
15	Patient Sex	60A–C	Health Insurance Claim Identification Number
16	Patient Marital Status	61A–C	Insured Group Name
17	Admission Date	62A–C	Insurance Group Number
18	Admission Hour	63A–C	Treatment Authorization Code
19	Type of Admission	64A–C	Employment Status Code
20	Source of Admission	65A–C	Employer Name
21	Discharge Hour	66A–C	Employer Location
22	Patient Status	67	Principal Diagnosis Code
23	Medical/Health Record Number	68–75	Other Diagnosis Codes
24–30	Condition Codes	76	Admitting Diagnosis
31	Unlabeled Field—National Use	77	External Cause of Injury Code (E-Code)
32–35a,b	Occurrence Codes and Dates	78	Not Titled
36a,b	Occurrence Span Codes and Dates	79	Procedure Coding Method Used
37	Internal Control Number (ICN)	80	Principal Procedure Code and Date
38	Responsible Party Name and Address	81A–E	Other Procedure Codes and Dates
39–41a–d	Value Codes and Amounts	82	Attending Physician ID
42	Revenue Code	83a–b	Other Physician ID
43	Revenue Description	84a–d	Remarks
44	HCPCS/Rates	85	Provider Representative Signature
45	Service Date	86	Date Bill Submitted

Figure 14.7. UB-04 (CMS-1450) claim form

Table 14.16. UB-04 form locators and brief description of information to be entered into each

Form Locator	Brief Description	Form Locator	Brief Description
1	Provider's name, address, and telephone number	49	Payer identification
2	Pay to provider name, address, and identification number	50	Health plan ID
3	Patient control number, medical record number	51	Release of information (primary, secondary)
4	Type of bill	52	Assignment of benefits
5	Federal tax number	53	Prior payments—Payers and patients
6	Statement covers period	54	Estimated amount due
7	Unlabeled—National use	55	NPI
8	Patient name	56a–c	Other provider ID
9	Patient address	57a–c	Insured's name
10	Patient birth date	58	Patient's relationship to insured
11	Patient sex	59	Insured's identifier
12	Admission date	60	Insurance group name (primary, secondary, tertiary)
13	Admission hour	61	Insured group number (primary, secondary, tertiary)
14	Type of admission/visit	62	Treatment authorization code
15	Source of admission	63	ICD/DCN
16	Discharge hour	64	Employer name
17	Patient status/discharge code	65	ICD/DX version qualifier
18–28	Condition codes	66a–q	Principal diagnosis code, other diagnosis codes
29a–c	Accident code, date, and location	67	Unlabeled
30–33a,b	Occurrence codes	68	Admitting diagnosis code
34–35a,b	Occurrence span codes	69	Patient reason for visit code
36	Unlabeled	70	PPS/DRG code
37	Responsible party name and address	71	External cause of injury code
38–40a,d	Value codes	72	Unlabeled
41	Revenue code	73a–e	Principal procedure code and dates, other procedure codes
42	Revenue code description	74	Unlabeled—National use
43	HCPCS/rates	75	Attending physician ID
44	Service date	76	Operating physician ID
45	Units of service	77	Other physician ID
46	Total charges (by revenue code)	78	Other ID
47	Noncovered charges	79	Remarks
48	Unlabeled	80	Code-Code-value

National Correct Coding Initiative (NCCI)

CMS implemented the **National Correct Coding Initiative** (NCCI) in 1996 to develop correct coding methodologies to improve the appropriate payment of Medicare Part B claims.

NCCI policies are based on:

- Coding conventions defined in the CPT codebooks
- National and local policies and coding edits
- Analysis of standard medical and surgical practice
- Review of current coding practices

The NCCI edits explain what procedures and services cannot be billed together on the same day of service for a patient. The mutually exclusive edit applies to improbable or impossible combinations of codes. For example, code 58940, Oophorectomy, partial or total, unilateral or bilateral, would never be used with code 58150, Total abdominal hysterectomy (corpus and cervix), with or without removal of tube(s), with or without removal of ovary(s). Modifiers may be used to indicate circumstances in which the NCCI edits should not be applied and payment should be made as requested. Modifier –59, for example, is used when circumstances require that certain procedures or services be reported together even though they usually are not.

Portions of the NCCI are incorporated into the **outpatient code editor** (OCE) against which all ambulatory claims are reviewed. The OCE also applies a set of logical rules to determine whether various combinations of codes are correct and appropriately represent services provided. Billing issues result from these CCI/OCE edits that often result in claim denials.

Check Your Understanding 14.5

Instructions: Answer the following questions on a separate piece of paper.

1. What is a COB transaction and what is its purpose?
2. What purpose does the remittance advice serve?
3. What is CMS-1500 used for? What is another name for this form?
4. What entity is responsible for the data elements and design of CMS-1450?
5. What types of organizations submit UB-92 (or the anticipated UB-04) form?
6. What kinds of codes are associated with CMS-1450?
7. What is the difference between a Medicare carrier and a fiscal intermediary? What functions is each responsible for performing?
8. What does the electronic data interchange (EDI) allow entities within healthcare organizations to do?
9. What is the purpose of the NCCI edits?
10. What are the NCCI policies implemented in 1996 to develop correct coding methodologies to improve appropriate payment of Medicare Part B claims based on?

Reimbursement Support Processes

Reimbursement support processes are routinely reviewed and revised by third-party payers to control payments to providers. Healthcare facilities also implement reimbursement support processes to make sure that they are receiving the level of reimbursement to which they are entitled. Third-party payers revise fee schedules, and healthcare facilities revise charge-masters, evaluate the quality of documentation and coding, conduct internal audits, and implement compliance programs.

Management of the Fee Schedules

Third-party payers that reimburse providers on a fee-for-service basis generally update fee schedules on an annual basis. A fee schedule is a list of healthcare services and procedures (usually CPT/HCPCS codes) and charges associated with each. (See table 14.17.) The fee schedule (sometimes referred to as a table of allowances) represents the approved payment levels for a given insurance plan (for example, Medicare, Medicaid, and BC/BS).

Physicians, practitioners, and suppliers must notify Medicare by December 31 of each year whether they intend to participate in the Medicare program during the coming year. Medicare participation means that the provider or supplier agrees to accept assignment for all covered services provided to Medicare patients. To accept assignment means the provider or supplier accepts, as payment in full, the allowed

Table 14.17. Partial 2005 Medicare physician fee schedule payment amounts for western New York state

Carrier Number	Locality Code	CPT Code	Nonfacility Fee Schedule Amount	Facility Fee Schedule Amount
00801	99	10040	81.86	74.10
00801	99	10060	90.06	80.20
00801	99	10061	161.77	150.49
00801	99	10080	156.42	86.28
00801	99	10081	242.71	152.13
00801	99	10120	125.79	83.50
00801	99	10121	233.86	172.89

charge (from the fee schedule). The provider or supplier is prohibited from **balance billing,** which means the patient cannot be held responsible for charges in excess of the Medicare fee schedule.

However, participating providers may bill patients for services that are not covered by Medicare. Physicians must notify a patient that the service will not be paid for by giving the patient a Notice of Exclusions from Medicare Benefits.

If a provider believes that a service may be denied by Medicare because it could be considered unnecessary, he must notify the patient before the treatment begins using an **Advance Beneficiary Notice** (ABN). (See figure 14.8.)

Nonparticipating providers (NonPAR) do not sign a participation agreement with Medicare but may or may not accept assignment. If the nonPAR physician elects to accept assignment, he or she is paid 95 percent (5 percent less than participating physicians) of the MFS. For example, if the MFS amount is $200, the PAR provider receives $160 (80 percent of $200), but the nonPAR provider receives only $152 (95 percent of $160).

NonPAR providers who choose not to accept assignment are subject to Medicare's limiting charge rule, which states that a physician may not charge a patient more than 115 percent of the nonparticipating fee schedule. The provider collects the full amount from the patient, and Medicare reimburses the patient. Figure 14.9, p. 386, illustrates the various fee schedules by type of provider.

Management of the Chargemaster

The **chargemaster** (table 14.18, p. 386), also called the charge description master (CDM), contains information about healthcare services (and transactions) provided to a patient. Its primary purpose is to allow the provider to accurately charge routine services and supplies to the patient. Services, supplies, and procedures included on the chargemaster generate reimbursement for almost 75 percent of UB-92 claims submitted for outpatient services alone.

The information that makes up a chargemaster line item may vary from one facility to another. There are, however, some common elements found in a typical chargemaster (Shraffenberger 2005, pp. 135–36). These include:

- *Description of service:* Examples might be the evaluation and management visit, observation, or emergency room visit.
- *CPT/HCPCS code:* This code must correspond to the description of the service.
- *Revenue code (also called the UB-92 code):* The revenue code is a three-digit code that describes a classification of a product or service provided to the patient. These revenue or UB-92 codes are required by CMS for reporting services. (See table 14.19, p. 387, for examples of revenue codes.)
- *Charge amount:* This is the amount the facility charges for the procedure or service. It is not necessarily what the facility will be reimbursed by the third-party payer.

- *Charge or service code:* The charge or service code is an internally assigned number that is unique to the facility. It identifies each procedure listed on the chargemaster and identifies the department or revenue center that initiated the charge. The charge code can be very useful for revenue tracking and budget analysis.
- *General ledger key:* The general ledger key is a two- or three-digit number that assigns a line item to a section of the general ledger in the hospital's accounting system.
- *Activity/status date:* The activity/status date indicates the most recent activity of an item.

Chargemasters may allow more than one CPT/HCPCS code per item to differentiate between payment schedules for different payers.

The CDM also can be used as a tool for collecting workload statistics that can be used to monitor production and compile budgets. It is often used as a decision support tool to evaluate costs related to resources and to prepare for contract negotiations with managed care organizations.

The CDM relieves coders from coding repetitive services and supplies that require little, if any, formal documentation analysis. In these circumstances, the patient is billed automatically by linking the service to the appropriate CPT/HCPCS code (referred to as **hard-coding**). The advantage of hard-coding is that the code for the procedure will be reproduced accurately each time that a test, service, or procedure is ordered. Services in the following areas are typically hard-coded: radiology, laboratory, EEG and EKG, rehabilitative services, and respiratory therapy (Schraffenberger 2005, p. 134).

Maintenance of the Chargemaster

The chargemaster must be updated routinely. Maintenance of the chargemaster is best accomplished by representatives from health information management, clinical services, finance, the business office/patient financial services, compliance, and information systems. The HIM professionals are generally consulted regarding the update of CPT codes. The CDM is updated when new CPT codes become available, when departments request a new item, and when the medical fee schedules/PPS rates are updated.

Some of the basic responsibilities of the CDM committee include (Rhodes 1999):

- Developing policies and procedures for the chargemaster review process
- Performing an annual chargemaster review when new CPT/HCPCS codes are available
- Reviewing key elements of the annual chargemaster review, including all CPT codes for accuracy, validity, and relationship to the CDM
- Reviewing all procedures and service descriptions for accuracy and clinical appropriateness
- Reviewing all revenue codes for accuracy and linkage to charge description numbers

Figure 14.8.   Advance beneficiary notice (ABN)

Patient's Name: Medicare # (HICN):

ADVANCE BENEFICIARY NOTICE (ABN)

NOTE: You need to make a choice about receiving these health care items or services.

We expect that Medicare will not pay for the item(s) or service(s) that are described below. Medicare does not pay for all of your health care costs. Medicare only pays for covered items and services when Medicare rules are met. The fact that Medicare may not pay for a particular item or service does not mean that you should not receive it. There may be a good reason your doctor recommended it. Right now, in your case, **Medicare probably will not pay for –**

Items or Services:
Because:

The purpose of this form is to help you make an informed choice about whether or not you want to receive these items or services, knowing that you might have to pay for them yourself. Before you make a decision about your options, you should **read this entire notice carefully.**
- x Ask us to explain, if you don't understand why Medicare probably won't pay.
- x Ask us how much these items or services will cost you (**Estimated Cost: $**_____),
     in case you have to pay for them yourself or through other insurance.

PLEASE CHOOSE **ONE** OPTION. CHECK **ONE** BOX. **SIGN & DATE** YOUR CHOICE.

Option 1. YES.   **I want to receive these items or services.**

I understand that Medicare will not decide whether to pay unless I receive these items or services. Please submit my claim to Medicare. I understand that you may bill me for items or services and that I may have to pay the bill while Medicare is making its decision. If Medicare does pay, you will refund to me any payments I made to you that are due to me. If Medicare denies payment, I agree to be personally and fully responsible for payment. That is, I will pay personally, either out of pocket or through any other insurance that I have. I understand I can appeal Medicare's decision.

Option 2. NO.   **I have decided not to receive these items or services.**

I will not receive these items or services. I understand that you will not be able to submit a claim to Medicare and that I will not be able to appeal your opinion that Medicare won't pay.

_____   _____
        Date   **Signature of patient or person acting on patient's behalf**

NOTE: Your health information will be kept confidential. Any information that we collect about you on this form will be kept confidential in our offices. If a claim is submitted to Medicare, your health information on this form may be shared with Medicare. Your health information which Medicare sees will be kept confidential by Medicare.

OMB Approval No. 0938-0566   Form No. CMS-R-131-G   (June 2002)

- Ensuring that the usage of all HCPCS, CPT, and revenue codes is in compliance with Medicare guidelines or other existing payer contracts
- Reviewing all charge dollar amounts for appropriateness by payer
- Reviewing all charge description numbers for uniqueness and validity

Figure 14.9.   Examples of physician reimbursement methodologies

Participating Provider	
Physician's fee	$180.00
MFS	$105.00
Medicare pays 80% of MFS or	$ 84.00
Patient pays 20% of MFS or	$ 21.00
Physician write-off ($180–$105)	$ 75.00
Nonparticipating provider who accepts assignment	
Physician's fee	$180.00
MFS	$105.00
Medicare nonPAR fee (95% of $105)	$ 99.75
Medicare pays 80% of nonPAR fee	$ 79.80
Patient pays 20% of nonPAR fee	$ 19.95
Physician write-off ($180–$99.75)	$ 80.25
Nonparticipating provider who does not accept assignment	
Physician's normal fee	$180.00
MFS	$105.00
Medicare nonPAR fee (95% of $105)	$ 99.75
Limiting charge (115% of $99.75)	$114.71
Patient billed	$114.71
Medicare pays patient (80% of nonPAR fee)	$ 79.80
Patient out of pocket ($114.71–$79.80)	$ 34.91

- Reviewing all department code numbers for uniqueness and validity
- Performing ongoing chargemaster maintenance as the facility adds or deletes new procedures, updates technology, or changes services provided
- Establishing a procedure to allow clinical department directors to submit chargemaster change requests for new, deleted, or revised procedures or services
- Making sure there is no duplication of code assignment by coders and chargemaster-assigned codes in any department
- Reviewing all charge ticket and order-entry screens for accuracy against the chargemaster and appropriate mapping to CPT/HCPCS codes, when required
- Reviewing and complying with directives in Medicare bulletins, transmittals, Medicare manual updates, and official coding guidelines
- Complying with guidelines in the NCCI or other known coding or bundling edits
- Carefully considering any application that involves one charge description number "exploding" into more than one CPT/HCPCS code to prevent inadvertent **unbundling** and unearned reimbursement for services
- Reviewing and taking action on all RA denials involving HCPCS/CPT coding or HCFA (now CMS) coding guidelines

An inaccurate chargemaster adversely affects facility reimbursement, compliance, and data quality. According to a 1999 AHIMA practice brief (Rhodes 1999), negative effects

Table 14.18.   Sample section from a chargemaster

Charge Code	Item Description	CPT/HCPCS Code			Revenue Code	G/L Key	Activity Date
		Insurance Code A	Insurance Code B	Insurance Code C			
2110410000	ECHO ENCEPHALOGRAM	76506	76506	Y7030	320	15	12/2/2004
2110410090	F/U ECHO ENCEPHALOGRAM	76506	76506	Y7040	320	15	12/2/2004
2110413000	PORT US ECHO ENCEPHALOGRAM	76506	76506	Y7050	320	15	12/2/2004
2120411000	ULTRASOUND SPINAL CONTENTS	76800	76800	Y7060	320	15	12/2/2004
2130401000	THYROID SONOGRAM	76536	76536	Y7070	320	15	1/1/2006
2151111000	TM JOINTS BILATERAL	70330	70330	Y7080	320	15	8/12/2005
2161111000	NECK LAT ONLY	70360	70360	Y7090	320	15	10/1/2004
2162111000	LARYNX AP & LATERAL	70360	70360	Y7100	320	15	10/1/2004
2201111000	LONG BONE CHLD AP	76061	76061	Y7110	320	15	8/12/2005
2201401000	NON-VASCULAR EXTREM SONO	76880	76880	Y7120	320	15	10/1/2004
2210111000	SKULL 1 VIEW	70250	70250	Y7130	320	15	1/1/2006
2210112000	SKULL 2 VIEWS	70250	70250	Y7140	320	15	8/12/2005
2210114000	SKULL 4 VIEWS	70260	70260	Y7150	320	15	8/12/2005
2211111000	MASTOIDS	70130	70130	Y7160	320	15	1/1/2006
2212111000	MANDIBLE	70110	70110	Y7170	320	15	12/2/2004
2213111000	FACIAL BONES	70140	70140	Y7180	320	15	12/2/2004
2213114000	FACIAL BONES MIN 4	70150	70150	Y7190	320	15	12/2/2004
2214111000	NASAL BONES	70160	70160	Y7200	320	15	1/1/2006
2215111000	ORBITS	70200	70200	Y7210	320	15	1/1/2006
2217111000	PARANASAL SINUSES	70220	70220	Y7220	320	15	1/1/2006

Table 14.19. Examples of UB-92 revenue codes

Revenue Code	Description
250	Pharmacy—General
251	Pharmacy—Generic Drugs
252	Pharmacy—Nongeneric Drugs
253	Pharmacy—Take-Home Drugs
260	IV Therapy—General
261	IV Therapy—Infusion Pump
262	IV Therapy—IV Therapy/Pharmacy Services
263	IV Therapy—IV Therapy/Drug/Supply Delivery
270	Medical/Surgical Supplies and Devices—General
271	Medical/Surgical Supplies and Devices—Nonsterile Supply
272	Medical/Surgical Supplies and Devices—Sterile Supply
273	Medical/Surgical Supplies and Devices—Take-Home Supplies
280	Oncology—General
289	Oncology—Other
290	DME—General
291	DME—Rental
292	DME—Purchase of New DME
293	DME—Purchase of Used DME
300	Laboratory—General
301	Laboratory—Chemistry
302	Laboratory—Immunology
303	Laboratory—Renal Patient (Home)
310	Laboratory Pathological—General
311	Laboratory Pathological—Cytology
312	Laboratory Pathological—Histology
320	Radiology—Diagnostic—General
321	Radiology—Diagnostic—Angiocardiography
322	Radiology—Diagnostic—Arthrography
360	Operating Room Services—General
361	Operating Room Services—Minor Surgery
362	Operating Room Services—Organ Transplant—Other Than Kidney
370	Anesthesia—General
371	Anesthesia—Incident to Radiology
372	Anesthesia—Incident to Other Diagnostic Services
410	Respiratory Services—General
411	Respiratory Services—Inhalation Services
412	Respiratory Services—Hyperbaric Oxygen Therapy

that may result from an inaccurate chargemaster include overpayment, underpayment, undercharging for delivery of healthcare services, claims rejections, and fines/penalties. Chargemaster programs are automated and involve the billing of numerous services for high volumes of patients, often without human intervention. Therefore, it is highly likely that a single error on the chargemaster could result in multiple errors before it is identified and corrected, resulting in a serious financial impact.

Management of the Revenue Cycle

Revenue cycle management involves many different processes and people, all working to make sure that the healthcare facility is properly reimbursed for the services provided. Effectively managing the revenue cycle is paramount to improving the revenues received by the facility. Delays in payment, denied claims, and other lost revenues impact tremendously on the facility's financial health.

The revenue cycle involves many functions in addition to the process of billing. According to an AHIMA practice brief (Youmans 2004), the major functions typically include:

- Admitting, patient access management
- Case management
- Charge capture
- Health information management
- Patient financial services, business office
- Finance
- Compliance
- Information technology

Revenue Cycle Management Committee

An effective method for managing the revenue cycle is through a revenue cycle management committee or team composed of individuals from all the departments involved in the revenue cycle. The HIM professional is an important player on this team. Various team members should analyze the revenue cycle indicators, which include:

- Value and volume of discharged, not final billed encounters
- Number of accounts receivable (AR) days
- Number of bill-hold days
- Percentage and amount of write-offs
- Percentage of clean claims
- Percentage of claims returned to provider
- Percentage of denials
- Percentage of accounts-missing documents
- Number of query forms
- Percentage of late charges
- Percentage of accurate registrations
- Percentage of increased point-of-service collections for elective procedures
- Percentage of increased DRG payments due to improved documentation and coding (Youmans 2004)

The HIM professional's area of expertise is varied and will be extremely useful in denials management, data analysis and presentation, write-off preparation, policy development, response to patient financial services requests, and review of OCEs and groupers.

Chapter 26 of this text also addresses revenue cycle management in relation to the financial management of the facility.

Management of Documentation and Coding Quality

According to Deborah Elder, manager of inpatient and outpatient coding services, Medical Management Plus, Inc., in Birmingham, Alabama:

> The importance of complete and accurate coding cannot be underestimated. ICD-9-CM and CPT-4 coding drives reimbursement and also presents a mechanism by which external and internal agents evaluate utilization of services, quality of care, and the hospital's patient acuity level. This numerically abbreviated medical information is only as complete as the physician documentation and is only as accurate as the coder's translation. Coders have a monumental impact on the hospital and this impact will broaden as other health care services are converted to a prospective payment method of reimbursement, including Outpatient Services, Extended Care Facilities and Home Health Agencies (Elder 2000).

The cornerstone of accurate coding is physician documentation. According to an AHIMA practice brief (Prophet 2001), ensuring the accuracy of coded data is a shared responsibility between coding professionals and physicians. Accurate diagnostic and procedural coded data originate from collaboration between physicians, who have a clinical background, and coding professionals, who have an understanding of classification systems.

Complete, accurate, legible, and timely documentation should:

- address the clinical significance of abnormal test results
- support the intensity of patient evaluation and treatment and describe the thought processes and complexity of decision making
- include all diagnostic and therapeutic procedures, treatments, and tests performed, in addition to their results
- include any changes in the patient's condition, including psychosocial and physical symptoms
- include all conditions that coexist at the time of admission, that subsequently develop, or that affect the treatment received and the length of stay. This encompasses all conditions that affect patient care in terms of requiring clinical evaluation, therapeutic treatment, diagnostic procedures, extended length of hospital stay, or increased nursing care and monitoring
- be updated as necessary to reflect all diagnoses relevant to the care or services provided
- be consistent and discuss and reconcile any discrepancies (this reconciliation should be documented in the medical record)

- be legible and written in ink, typewritten, or electronically signed, stored and printed (Prophet 2001, 88I)

Physician Query Process

There are instances, however, when it is necessary to query the physician for clarification of data that may influence proper code assignment. This might include instances when there is conflicting or incomplete information in the record. Query forms have proved to be an effective means of communication with physicians. AHIMA cautions coders that these forms are used to improve documentation and understanding of the clinical situation, but not to increase reimbursement (Prophet 2001).

The facility should develop a standard form to be used in communicating with physicians. Characteristics of a good query form are noted in figure 14.10.

Coding and Corporate Compliance

The federal government has initiated efforts to investigate healthcare fraud and to establish guidelines to ensure corporate compliance with the government guidelines. Part of the initiative involved providing healthcare organizations with guidelines for developing comprehensive compliance programs with specific policies and procedures.

History of Fraud and Abuse and Corporate Compliance in Healthcare

Probably the most pertinent fact in the history of corporate compliance related to healthcare organizations is that the federal government, specifically the HHS, is the largest purchaser of healthcare in the United States. Because one

Figure 14.10.   Characteristics of a good query form

The query form should:

- Be clearly and concisely written
- Contain precise language
- Present the facts from the medical record and identify why clarification is needed
- Present the scenario and state a question that asks the physician to make a clinical interpretation of a given diagnosis or condition based on treatment, evaluation, monitoring, and/or services provided. "Open-ended" questions that allow the physician to document the specific diagnosis are preferable to multiple-choice questions or questions requiring only a "yes" or "no" response. Queries that appear to lead the physician to provide a particular response could lead to allegations of inappropriate upcoding
- Be phrased such that the physician is allowed to specify the correct diagnosis. It should not indicate the financial impact of the response to the query. The form should not be designed so that all that is required is a physician signature
- Include patient name, admission date, medical record number, name and contact information (phone number and e-mail address) of the coding professional, specific questions and rationale, place for the physician to document his or her response, place for the physician to sign and date his or her response

Source: Prophet 2001, pp. 88I–88M.

of the federal government's duties is to use the taxpayers' monies wisely, federal agencies must ensure that the healthcare provided to enrollees in federal healthcare programs is appropriate and is actually provided.

Several federal initiatives and pieces of legislation related to investigating, identifying, and preventing healthcare fraud and abuse have been passed. Interestingly, the basis of these initiatives and laws lies within the Civil False Claims Act, which was passed during the Civil War to prevent government contractors from overbilling for services provided. The original law was updated and reinforced in subsequent legislation and is still used to prosecute offenders.

Several government agencies are involved in detecting, prosecuting, and preventing fraud and abuse. Among them are the HHS, the Office of the Inspector General (OIG), the Department of Justice (the attorney general), the Federal Bureau of Investigation (FBI), CMS, the Drug Enforcement Agency (DEA), the Internal Revenue Service (IRS), and state attorney generals.

Many initiatives are joint efforts among the agencies. For example, Operation Restore Trust, which began in 1995, is a joint effort of HHS, OIG, CMS, and the Administration on Aging. Operation Restore Trust spent only $7.9 million in the first two years to identify $188 million in overpayments to providers. It also led to implementation of special fraud alerts notifying providers of current investigative findings and to the **Voluntary Disclosure Program.**

The federal government began to actively investigate fraud in the Medicare program in 1977 with passage of the Anti-Fraud and Abuse Amendments of 1977 to Title XIX of the Social Security Act (SSA). However, detecting, preventing, and prosecuting fraud and abuse did not reach true prominence until the Health Insurance Portability and Accountability Act (HIPAA) of 1996 established Sections 1128C and 1128D of the SSA. Sections 1128C and 1128D authorized the OIG to conduct investigations, audits, and evaluations related to healthcare fraud. The BBA focused on fraud and abuse issues specifically relating to penalties.

The BBA also required that physicians and practitioners provide diagnostic information (to show medical necessity) prior to a facility performing lab or radiology services for a patient.

As previously mentioned, HIPAA expanded the OIG's duties to include:

- Coordination of federal, state, and local enforcement efforts targeting healthcare fraud
- Provision of industry guidance concerning fraudulent healthcare practices
- Establishment of a national data bank for reporting final adverse actions against healthcare providers

Significantly, HIPAA authorizes the OIG to investigate cases of healthcare fraud that involve private healthcare plans as well as federally funded programs, although, according to information on the OIG Web site, present policies restrict the OIG's investigative focus to cases of fraud that affect federally funded programs.

A major portion of HIPAA focused on identifying medically unnecessary services, **upcoding,** unbundling, and billing for services not provided. Upcoding is the practice of assigning a diagnosis or procedure code specifically for the purpose of obtaining a higher level of payment. It is most often found when reimbursement-grouping systems are used.

Unbundling is the practice of using multiple codes that describe individual components of a procedure rather than an appropriate single code that describes all steps of the procedure performed. Unbundling is a component of the NCCI.

HIPAA also expanded sanctions related to mandatory exclusion from Medicare, length of exclusion, failure to comply with statutory obligations, and antikickback penalties (Schraffenberger 2005).

From February 1998 until the present, the OIG continues to issue **compliance program guidance** for various types of healthcare organizations. The OIG Web site (oig.hhs.gov) posts the documents that most healthcare organizations need to develop fraud and abuse compliance plans. The goal of compliance programs is to prevent accusations of fraud and abuse, make operations run more smoothly, improve services, and contain costs (Anderson 2000).

Elements of Corporate Compliance

In the February 23, 1998 *Federal Register* (p. 8989), the OIG outlined the following seven elements as the minimum necessary for a comprehensive compliance program:

1. The development and distribution of written standards of conduct, as well as written policies and procedures that promote the hospital's commitment to compliance and that address specific areas of potential fraud, such as claims development and submission processes, code gaming, and financial relationships with physicians and other healthcare professionals
2. The designation of a chief compliance officer and other appropriate bodies, for example, a corporate compliance committee, charged with the responsibility for operating and monitoring the compliance program, and who report directly to the CEO and the governing body
3. The development and implementation of regular, effective education and training programs for all affected employees
4. The maintenance of a process, such as a hotline, to receive complaints and the adoption of procedures to protect the anonymity of complainants and to protect whistleblowers from retaliation
5. The development of a system to respond to allegations of improper/illegal activities and the enforcement of appropriate disciplinary action against employees who have violated internal compliance policies, applicable

statutes, regulations, or federal healthcare program requirements

6. The use of audits and/or other evaluation techniques to monitor compliance and assist in the reduction of identified problem areas

7. The investigation and remediation of identified systemic problems and the development of policies addressing the nonemployment or retention of sanctioned individuals

The OIG believes that a compliance program conforming to these elements above will not only "fulfill the organization's legal duty to ensure that it is not submitting false or inaccurate claims to government and private payers," but will also result in additional potential benefits, including, among others:

- Demonstration of the organization's commitment to responsible conduct toward employees and the community
- Provision of a more accurate view of behavior relating to fraud and abuse
- Identification and prevention of criminal and unethical conduct
- Improvements in the quality of patient care

In the January 31, 2005 *Federal Register,* the supplemental compliance program guidance for hospitals was published. This document supplements rather than replaces the 1998 compliance program guidance (CPG) document. The supplemental CPG contains new compliance recommendations and an expanded discussion of risk areas, current enforcement priorities, and lessons learned in the area of corporate compliance.

(For additional resources on compliance and fraud and abuse, see figure 14.11.)

Relationship between Coding Practice and Corporate Compliance

Any corporate compliance program must contain references to complete and accurate coding. Many of the documented fraud and abuse convictions have centered on the coding function.

OIG Work Plan

At the beginning of each fiscal year, the OIG publishes guidance on its "special areas of concern" for the upcoming year.

Figure 14.11.   Online compliance resources

Department of Health and Human Services, Office of the Inspector General	www.oig.hhs.gov
American Health Information Management Association	www.ahima.org
Health Care Compliance Association	www.hcca-info.org
National Health Care Anti-Fraud Association	www.nhcaa.org
Centers for Medicare and Medicaid Services	www.cms.hhs.gov
CMS Fraud Page	www.medicare.gov

The OIG refers to this as its work plan. The table of contents for the 2005 Work Plan is shown in figure 14.12; the full plan can be found on the OIG Web site.

The HIM Compliance Program

As mentioned above, one element of the corporate compliance program addresses the coding function. Because the accuracy and completeness of ICD-9-CM and CPT code assignment determine the provider payment, the reference to coding is not surprising. Thus, it is important that healthcare organizations have a strong coding compliance program. This coding compliance plan should be based on the same principles as that of the corporatewide program. The basic elements of a coding plan should include:

- Code of conduct
- Policies and procedures
- Education and training
- Communication
- Auditing
- Corrective action
- Reporting

Code of Conduct

The HIM department should develop a code of conduct or perhaps adopt AHIMA's Standards of Ethical Coding.

Policies and Procedures

Policies and procedures that describe the facility's coding standards and functions should be documented. This should be done through a coding compliance manual. Some of the items that should be included in this manual include policies on the following: ambiguous or incomplete documentation, rebilling of problem claims, use of official coding guidelines, issues where no official guidelines exist, and clarification of new or confusing coding issues.

Education and Training

Periodic and staff-appropriate education of staff is a key factor in a successful coding compliance program. Education for coders should be provided monthly (Schraffenberger 2005).

Areas that could be covered at training sessions include:

- The OIG work plan
- Clinical information related to problematic body systems, diagnoses, and procedures
- Changes to the PPSs
- Changes to ICD-9-CM, HCPCS Level II, and CPT codes
- Application of the Official Coding Guidelines
- Issues in *Coding Clinic for ICD-9-CM*
- Issues in *CPT Assistant*

All newly hired coding personnel should receive extensive training on the facility's and HIM department's compliance programs.

Figure 14.12. HHS/OIG fiscal year 2005 work plan table of contents

Medicare Hospitals
Quality Improvement Organization Mediation of Beneficiary Complaints
Medical Education Payments for Dental and Podiatry Residents
Nursing and Allied Health Education Payments
Graduate Medical Education Voluntary Supervision in Nonhospital Settings
Postacute Care Transfers
Diagnosis-Related Group Coding
Inpatient Prospective Payment System Wage Indices
Inpatient Outlier and Other Charge-Related Issues
Inpatient Rehabilitation Facilities Payments
Inpatient Rehabilitation Payments–Late Assessments
Medical Necessity of Inpatient Psychiatric Stays
Consecutive Inpatient Stays
Long-Term Care Hospital Payments
Level of Care in Long-Term Care Hospitals
Critical Access Hospitals
Organ Acquisition Costs
Rebates Paid to Hospitals
Coronary Artery Stents
Outpatient Cardiac Rehabilitation Services
Outpatient Outlier and Other Charge-Related Issues
Lifetime Reserve Days
Hospital Reporting of Restraint-Related Deaths

Medicare Home Health
Beneficiary Access to Home Health Agencies
Effect of Prospective Payment System on Quality of Home Health Care
Home Health Outlier Payments
Enhanced Payments for Home Health Therapy

Medicare Nursing Homes
Access to Skilled Nursing Facilities under the Prospective Payment System
Use of Additional Funds Provided to Skilled Nursing Facilities
Nurse Aide Registries
Nursing Home Deficiency Trends
Nursing Home Compliance with Minimum Data Set Reporting Requirements
Nursing Home Resident Assessment and Care Planning
Enforcement Actions against Noncompliant Nursing Homes
Nursing Home Informal Dispute Resolution
Nursing Home Residents' Rights
Skilled Nursing Facilities' Involvement in Consecutive Inpatient Stays
Imaging and Laboratory Services in Nursing Homes
Skilled Nursing Facility Rehabilitation and Infusion Therapy Services
State Compliance with Complaint Investigation Guidelines

Medicare Physicians and Other Health Professionals
Billing Service Companies
Medicare Payments to VA Physicians
Care Plan Oversight
Ordering Physicians Excluded from Medicare
Physician Services at Skilled Nursing Facilities
Physician Pathology Services
Cardiography and Echocardiography Services
Physical and Occupational Therapy Services
Part B Mental Health Services
Wound Care Services
Coding of Evaluation and Management Services
Use of Modifier –25
Use of Modifiers with National Correct Coding Initiative Edits
"Long Distance" Physician Claims
Provider-Based Entities

Medicare Medical Equipment and Supplies
Medical Necessity of Durable Medical Equipment
Medicare Pricing of Equipment and Supplies

Medicare Drug Reimbursement
Prescription Drug Cards
Employer Subsidies for Drug Coverage
Beneficiary Understanding of Drug Discount Card Program
Computation of Average Sales Price
Collecting and Maintaining Average Sales Price Data
Adequacy of Reimbursement Rate for Drugs under ASP
Payments for Non-End-Stage Renal Disease Epoetin Alfa

Other Medicare Services
Laboratory Services Rendered during an Inpatient Stay
Laboratory Proficiency Testing
Independent Diagnostic Testing Facilities
Therapy Services Provided by Comprehensive Outpatient Rehabilitation Facilities
New Payment Provisions for Ambulance Services
Air Ambulance Services
Quality of Care in Dialysis Facilities
Monitoring of Market Prices for Part B Drugs
Follow-up on Medicare Part B Payments for Ambulance Services
Follow-up on Medicare Part B Payments for Radiology Services
Emergency Health Services for Undocumented Aliens

Medicare Managed Care
Benefit Stabilization Fund
Adjusted Community Rate Proposals
Follow-up on Adjusted Community Rate Proposals
Administrative Costs
Managed Care Encounter Data
Enhanced Managed Care Payments
Enhanced Payments under the Risk Adjustment Model
Managed Care Excessive Medical Costs
Duplicate Medicare Payments to Cost-Based Plans
Prompt Payment
Marketing Practices of MCOs
Managed Care "Deeming" Organizations

Medicare Contractor Operations
Preaward Reviews of Contract Proposals
CMS Oversight of Contractor Performance
Program Safeguard Contractor Performance
Accuracy of the Provider Enrollment, Chain, and Ownership System
Handling of Beneficiary Inquiries
Carrier Medical Review: Progressive Corrective Action
Duplicate Medicare Part B Payments
Contractors' Administrative Costs
Pension Segmentation
Pension Costs Claimed
Unfunded Pension Costs
Pension Segment Closing
Postretirement Benefits and Supplemental Employee Retirement Plan Costs

Medicaid Hospitals
Medicaid Graduate Medical Education Payments
Hospital Outlier Payments
Medicaid Diagnosis-Related Group Payment Window
Disproportionate Share Hospital Payments
Hospital Eligibility for Disproportionate Share Hospital Payments

Medicaid Long-Term and Community Care
Payments to Public Nursing Facilities
Community Residence Claims
Assisted Living Facilities
Medicaid Home Health Care Services
Targeted Case Management
Personal Care Services
Home- and Community-Based Services Administrative Costs
Medicaid Eligibility and the Working Disabled

(Continued on next page)

Figure 14.12.   (Continued)

Medicaid Mental Health Services
Nursing Home Residents with Mental Illness and Mental Retardation
Claims for Residents of Institutions for Mental Diseases
Medicaid Services for Mentally Disabled Persons
Rehabilitation Services for Persons with Mental Illnesses
Community Mental Health Centers
Medicaid Reimbursement for Intermediate Care Facilities
Restraint and Seclusion in Children's Psychiatric Residential Treatment
    Facilities

Medicaid/State Children's Health Insurance Program
Duplicate Claims for Medicaid and State Children's Health Insurance
    Program
Enrollment of Medicaid Eligibles in SCHIP
State Evaluations of SCHIP Programs
Detecting and Investigating Fraud and Abuse in SCHIP

Medicaid Drug Reimbursement
Average Manufacturer Price and Average Wholesale Price
Medicaid Drug Rebates—Computation of AMP and Best Price
Oversight of Drug Manufacturer Recalculations for Medicaid Drug
    Rebates
Indexing the Generic Drug Rebate
Drug Rebate Impact from Drugs Incorrectly Classified as Generic
Dispute Resolution in the Medicaid Prescription Drug Rebate Program
Medicaid Drug Rebate Collections
Overprescribing of OxyContin and Other Psychotropic Drugs
Accuracy of Pricing Drugs in the Federal Upper-Limit Program
Medicaid Drug Utilization Review Program

Other Medicaid Services
Family Planning Services
School-Based Health Services
Adult Rehabilitative Services
Controls over the Vaccine for Children Program
Outpatient Alcoholism Services
Claims Paid for Clinical Diagnostic Laboratory Services
Payments for Services Provided after Beneficiaries' Deaths
Marketing and Enrollment Practices by Medicaid Managed Care
    Entities
Factors Affecting the Development, Referral, and Disposition of
    Medicaid Fraud Cases: State Agency and Medicaid Fraud Control
    Unit Experiences

Medicaid Administration
Contingency Fee Payment Arrangements
Upper Payment Limits
Calculation of Upper Payment Limits for Transition States
State Match for Medicaid Upper-Payment Limit Reimbursement
Medicaid Provider Tax Issues
State-Employed Physicians and Other Practitioners

Skilled Professional Medical Personnel
Physician Assistant Reimbursement
Medicaid Claims for Excluded Providers
Administrative Costs of Other Public Agencies
Administrative Costs for Medicaid Managed Care Contracts
University-Contributed Indirect Costs
Federal Financial Participation for Medicaid Cost Allocation Plans
Medicaid Accounts Receivable
Section 1115 Demonstration Waiver
Medicaid Management Information System Expenditures
Appropriateness of Medicaid Payments
Medicaid FFS Payments for Beneficiaries Enrolled in Managed Care
CMS Oversight of Home- and Community-Based Waivers

Information Systems Controls
Security Planning for CMS Systems under Development
Accuracy of the Fraud Investigation Database
Medicaid Statistical Information System
State Controls over Medicaid Payments and Program Eligibility
Replacement State Medicaid System
Smart Card Technology
Compliance with the Health Insurance Portability and Accountability
    Act Privacy Final Rule–University Hospital
MCO's Compliance With HIPAA

General Administration
FY 2004 Medicare Error Rate Estimate
FY 2005 Medicare Error Rate Estimate
Group Purchasing Organizations
Contractual Arrangements with Suppliers
Corporate Integrity Agreements
State Medical Boards as a Source of Patient Safety Data
Payments for Services to Dually Eligible Beneficiaries
Nursing Home Quality of Care: Promising Approaches
Payments to Psychiatric Facilities Improperly Certified as Nursing
    Facilities

Investigations
Health Care Fraud
Provider Self-Disclosure

Legal Counsel
Compliance Program Guidance to the Healthcare Industry
Resolution of False Claims Act Cases and Negotiation of Corporate
    Integrity Agreements
Providers' Compliance with Corporate Integrity Agreements
Advisory Opinions and Fraud Alerts
Antikickback Safe Harbors
Patient Antidumping Statute Enforcement
Program Exclusions
Civil Monetary Penalties

Education of the medical staff on documentation is likewise important to the success of any coding compliance program. Documentation education may be provided monthly, bimonthly, or quarterly depending on the importance of the issues covered (Schraffenberger 2005).

Examples of documentation problems that may need to be addressed with physicians include:

- Inconsistent documentation
- Incomplete progress notes
- Undocumented care
- Test results not addressed in physician documentation
- Historical diagnoses being documented as current diagnoses
- Long-standing, chronic conditions that are not documented
- Lack of documentation of postoperative complications
- Illegibility
- Documentation not completed on time (Bowman 2004)

Communication
Communication between the coding supervisor and the coding professionals is vital to ensure consistency in following coding policies and issues.

Internal Audits

Ongoing evaluation is critical to successful coding and billing for third-party payer reimbursement. In the past, the goal of internal audit programs was to increase revenues for the provider. Today, the goal is to protect providers from sanctions or fines. Healthcare organizations can implement monitoring programs by conducting regular, periodic audits of (1) ICD-9-CM and CPT/HCPCS coding and (2) claims development and submission. In addition, audits should be conducted to follow up on previous reviews that resulted in the identification of problems (for example, poor coding quality or errors in claims submission).

Auditing involves the performance of internal and/or **external reviews** to identify variations from established baselines (for example, review outpatient coding as compared with CMS outpatient coding guidelines). Internal reviews are conducted by facility-based staff (for example, HIM professionals), and external reviews are conducted by either consultants hired for this purpose (for example, corporations that specialize in such reviews and independent health information consultants) or third-party payers.

The scope and frequency of audits and the size of the sample depend on the size of the organization, available resources, the number of coding professionals, the history of noncompliance, risk factors, case complexity, and the results of initial assessments (Bowman 2004).

One of the elements of the auditing process is identification of risk areas. Some major risk areas include:

- DRG coding accuracy
- Variations in case mix
- Discharge status (transfers versus discharges)
- Services provided under arrangement
- Three-day payment window, formerly called the 72-hour rule (Under this rule, diagnostic services provided within three days of admission should be included (bundled) in the DRG, whether or not they are related to the admission. Non-diagnostic services provided within three days of admission should be included in the DRG only if they are related to the admission.)
- All nondiagnostic services that are unrelated to the admission can be billed separately.)
- Medical necessity
- Evaluation and management services
- Chargemaster description

Selecting types of cases to review also is important. Some examples of various case selection possibilities are found in figure 14.13.

The frequency of audits depends on the individual facility; daily, weekly, monthly or quarterly audits may be considered.

The results of the audits must be analyzed to determine the reason(s) for the coding errors. Focused reviews in one particular area may be necessary to review a higher volume of cases in which there were frequent errors. Certainly, focused reviews aimed at OIG target areas would be appro-

Figure 14.13. Examples of various case selections for auditing

Simple random sample
Medical DRGs by high dollar and high volume
Surgical DRGs by high dollar and high volume
Medical DRGs without comorbid conditions or complications
Surgical DRGs without comorbid conditions or complications
Major diagnostic category by high dollar and high volume
Most common diagnosis codes
Most common procedure codes
Significant procedure APCs by high dollar and high volume
Unlisted CPT codes
"Separate procedure" CPT codes reported in conjunction with related CPT codes
Unusual modifier usage patterns
Not elsewhere classified (NEC) and not otherwise specified (NOS) codes
Highest-level evaluation and management (E/M) codes
Consultation E/M codes
Critical Care E/M codes
Chargemaster review by service
Superbill, encounter form, and charge sheet review by specialty

priate. Significant variations from baselines should prompt an investigation to determine cause(s).

Feedback on the results of audits should be presented to interested parties such as coding staff, supervisors, and physicians.

Corrective Action

Certainly, the goal of corrective action activities is the prevention of the same or a similar problem in the future. Typical corrective actions for resolving problems identified during coding audits include:

- revisions to policies and procedures
- development of additional policies and procedures
- process improvements
- education of coders, physicians, and/or other organizational staff depending on the nature of the identified problem
- revision or addition of routine monitoring activities
- revisions to the chargemaster
- additions, deletions, or revisions to systems edits
- documentation improvement strategies
- disciplinary action (Bowman 2004, 73–4)

Reporting

Documentation on coding compliance activities should be maintained and reported as stated in the policies and procedures. Certainly, adverse findings should be reviewed with the corporate compliance officer and steps taken as necessary to report these findings.

Check Your Understanding 14.6

Instructions: Answer the following questions on a separate piece of paper.

1. How often do third-party payers update fee schedules?
2. What does the term *accept assignment* mean?
3. Explain the difference between a participating provider, a nonparticipating provider who accepts assignment, and a nonparticipating provider who does not accept assignment.
4. What is the limiting charge policy?
5. How might an inaccurate chargemaster affect facility reimbursement?
6. What are the typical items on the charge description master?
7. Who is responsible for maintaining the charge description master?
8. Who and what are involved in revenue cycle management?
9. What are some characteristics of a good physician query form?
10. What do coding compliance programs concentrate on preventing? Which federal agency has established the precise steps that each healthcare facility must follow in establishing its compliance program?
11. What do the terms *upcoding* and *unbundling* mean in relation to coding?
12. What items might be covered during educational programs for the medical staff?
13. What major risk areas are related to coding and billing?
14. Describe some of the benefits of effective corporate compliance programs for healthcare organizations.

Real-World Case

Itemized charges on the UB-92 that are not supported by patient record documentation are unlikely to be reimbursed by a third-party payer. Examples of charges that would not be paid upon review of the patient record in comparison to the UB-92 include the following:

- Duplicate charges for services rendered one time only (for example, multiple charges for same service, such as surgery)
- Laboratory panel tests for which there should be a single charge
- Medications and diagnostic tests not prescribed by a physician
- Medications that a patient did not receive
- Tests repeated because of hospital error
- Services listed for dates after the patient was discharged from the facility
- Professional services performed by nurses or technicians (for example, equipment monitoring)

Summary

From its very beginnings, financial reimbursement for healthcare services has followed several paths. Among these are private pay, commercial insurance, employer self-insurance, and various government programs. The mixture of payment mechanisms has made healthcare reimbursement in the United States very complex.

As a consequence, the processing of medical claims can be complicated. How a claim is processed, what documentation is required, and how much reimbursement will be paid depend on the payer and the type of claim. Many attempts have been made to create a uniform healthcare claim that would accommodate all payment mechanisms. Claims processed for payment under Medicare have been consolidated into a uniform bill.

Healthcare organizations have developed several tools to help manage the billing and reimbursement process, including development of fee schedules and chargemasters. The HIM professional is frequently called on to provide expertise in the development, management, and auditing of these tools. In addition, organizations have recognized that ongoing evaluation of the entire billing process is essential to ensure accurate payment as well as to avoid fraud and abuse sanctions or fines. The HIM professional's work is likely to involve helping to develop such audit programs in addition to conducting the audits themselves.

Over the past two decades, the billing and reimbursement process has become an integral part of the job functions of many HIM professionals. The expertise brought to bear on the process to ensure accurate and timely claims submission is critical to the operations of any healthcare organization.

Payments for the delivery of healthcare services increased from $27 billion in 1960 to more than $1.1 trillion in 1998. In response, private insurers introduced managed care programs and the federal government implemented prospective payment systems to replace the costly per diem (or traditional fee-for-service) reimbursement methods. The federal government also incorporated managed care into its healthcare programs.

Health claims reimbursement processing has evolved from the submission of handwritten CMS-1500 and UB-92 forms to specially designed forms to be used for optical scanning purposes to electronic data interchange. EDI was greatly affected by HIPAA legislation passed in 1996. Of recently enacted federal legislation affecting claims reimbursement processing, the NCCI and the OIG coding compliance programs have had the most effect on HIM professionals.

References

Abraham, P.R. 2001. *Documentation and Reimbursement for Home Health and Hospice Programs.* Chicago: AHIMA.

American Medical Association. 2004. *Current Procedural Terminology,* 2005 ed. Chicago: AMA.

Anderson, S. 2000. Audit outpatient bills to get all the money you deserve. *Medical Records Briefing* 15(12):6.

Averill, R.F. 1999. Honest mistake or fraud? Meeting the coding compliance challenge. *Journal of American Health Information Management Association* 70(5):16–21.

Bowman, S. 2004. *Health Information Management Compliance: A Model Program for Healthcare Organizations,* 3rd ed. Chicago: AHIMA.

Campbell, C., H. Schmitz, and L. Waller. 1998. *Financial Management in a Managed Care Environment.* Albany, NY: Delmar Thomson Learning.

Campbell, T. Opportunities for HIM in revenue cycle management. *Journal of American Health Information Management Association* 74(10):62–63.

Centers for Medicare and Medicaid Services. 2005a. IRVEN: CMS's IRF-PAI data entry software. Available online from cms.hhs.gov.

Centers for Medicare and Medicaid Services. 2005b. Transmittal 288: CMS manual system, pub. 100-04, Medicare claims processing. Effective date: Oct. 1, 2005.

Centers for Medicare and Medicaid Services. 2004. Transmittal 347: Inpatient rehabilitation facility (IRF) classification requirements. Oct. 29, 2004.

Centers for Medicare and Medicaid Services. 2002. Transmittal AB-02-131: Implementation of the ambulance fee schedule. Sept. 27, 2002.

Coder's Desk Reference. 2005. Salt Lake City: Ingenix.

Davis, J.B. 2000. *Reimbursement Manual for the Medical Office: A Comprehensive Guide to Coding, Billing and Fee Management.* Los Angeles: Practice Management Information Corporation.

Davison, J., and M. Lewis. 2000. *Working with Insurance and Managed Care Plans: A Guide for Getting Paid.* Los Angeles: Practice Management Information Corporation.

Dougherty, M. 2000. New home care PPS brings major changes. *Journal of American Health Information Management Association* 7110):78–82.

Elder, D. 2000. Coding: The key to compliance. Birmingham, AL: Medical Management Plus. Available online from mmplusinc.com.

Gannon, E.J. HCFA outlines new PPS for rehabilitation facilities. Available online from mxcity.com.

Green, M.A., and J.C. Rowell. 2004. *Understanding Health Insurance: A Guide to Professional Billing.* Albany, NY: Delmar Thomson Learning.

Harkins, P.D. 2000 (Oct. 16). The alphabet soup of Medicare reimbursement. *Advance for Health Information Professionals,* p. 25.

Health Care Financing Administration. 2000. HHS announces electronic standards to simplify health care transactions.Available online from aspe.hhs.gov/admnsimp/final/txfin00.htm.

Johnson, S.L. 2000. *Understanding Medical Coding: A Comprehensive Guide.* Albany, NY: Delmar Thomson Learning.

Jones, J., ed. 2001. *Reimbursement Methodologies for Healthcare Services.* Chicago: AHIMA.

Kuehn, L., and L. Wieland. 2005. *CPT/HCPCS Coding and Reimbursement for Physician Services.* Chicago: AHIMA.

Lewis, M. 2003. *Medicare Rules and Regulations.* Los Angeles: Practice Management Information Corporation.

Medical Records Briefing. 2000. Make sure that your APC claim makes it through the OCE. *Medical Records Briefing* 15(9):1.

Medicare and You. 2005. Baltimore: CMS. Available online from cms.hhs.gov/partnerships/2005medandyou.asp.

Medicare Hospital Outpatient Payment System Quick Reference Guide. 2004. Baltimore: CMS. Available online at cms.hhs.gov.

National Committee for Quality Assurance. ncqa.org.

Newby, C. 2005. *From Patient to Payment.* New York: McGraw-Hill.

Palmer, K. 1999. A brief history: Universal health care efforts in the U.S.: Late 1800s to Medicare. Available online from pnhp.org.

Prophet, S. 2001. Practice brief: Developing a physician query process. *Journal of American Health Information Management Association* 72(9):88I–88M.

Rhodes, H. 1999. Practice brief: The care and management of charge masters. *Journal of American Health Information Management Association* 70(7):supplement 2.

Rizzo, C.D. 2000. *Uniform Billing: A Guide to Claims Processing.* Albany, NY: Delmar Thomson Learning.

Role of the physician in the home health prospective payment system. 2000 (Nov. 7). Medicare Newsroom. Available online from hgsa.com.

Schraffenberger, L. 2004. *Basic ICD-9-CM Coding.* Chicago: AHIMA.

Schraffenberger, L. 2005. *Effective Management of Coding Services.* Chicago: AHIMA.

Smith, G. 2005. *Basic CPT/HCPCS Coding.* Chicago: AHIMA.

Stewart, M. 2001. *Coding and Reimbursement under the Outpatient Prospective Payment.* Chicago: AHIMA.

3M Health Information Systems. 2002. 3Mhis.com.

Valerius, J., N. Bayes, and C. Newby. 2005. *Medical Insurance: A Guide to Coding and Reimbursement.* New York: McGraw-Hill.

Youmans, K. 2004. Practice brief: An HIM spin on the revenue cycle. *Journal of American Health Information Management Association* 75(3):32–36.

Part IV

Comparative Data

Chapter 15
Healthcare Statistics

Carol E. Osborn, PhD, RHIA

Learning Objectives

- To identify various ways in which statistics are used in healthcare
- To differentiate between descriptive and inferential statistics
- To define hospital-related statistical terms
- To calculate hospital-related inpatient and outpatient statistics
- To define community-based morbidity and mortality rates
- To calculate community-based morbidity and mortality rates
- To define and calculate measures of central tendency and variability
- To describe the characteristics of the normal distribution
- To identify the relationships of measures of central tendency and variation to the normal distribution
- To display healthcare data using tables, charts, and graphs, as appropriate
- To calculate the case-mix index
- To locate healthcare-related state and federal databases on the Internet
- To use healthcare data collected from online databases in comparative statistical reports

Key Terms

Acute care
Ambulatory surgery center (ASC)
Average daily census
Average length of stay (ALOS)
Bar chart
Bed count (complement)
Bed count day
Bed turnover rate
Boxplot
Bubble charts
Case fatality rate
Case mix
Case-mix index (CMI)
Cause-specific death rate
Census
Consultation rate
Continuous variables
Crude birth rate
Crude death rate
Daily inpatient census
Descriptive statistics
Discrete variables
Encounter

Fetal autopsy rate
Fetal death (stillborn)
Fetal death rate
Frequency distribution
Frequency polygon
Gross autopsy rate
Gross death rate
Histogram
Hospital-acquired infection rate
Hospital autopsy
Hospital autopsy rate
Hospital death rate
Hospital inpatient autopsy
Hospital newborn inpatient
Incidence rate
Infant mortality rate
Inferential statistics
Inpatient bed occupancy rate (percentage of occupancy)
Inpatient service day (IPSD)
Interval scale
Length of stay (LOS)
Line graph

Maternal death rate (hospital based)
Maternal mortality rate (community based)
Mean
Measures of central tendency
Median
Mode
National Vital Statistics System (NVSS)
Neonatal mortality rate
Net autopsy rate
Net death rate
Newborn (NB)
Newborn autopsy rate
Newborn death rate
Nominal-level data
Normal distribution
Nosocomial (hospital-acquired) infection
Notifiable disease
Occasion of service
Ordinal scale of measurement
Outpatient visit

Pie chart
Population-based statistics
Postneonatal mortality rate
Postoperative infection rate
Prevalence rate
Proportion
Proportionate mortality ratio (PMR)
Range
Rate
Ratio
Ratio scale
Referred outpatient
Scales of measurement
Scatter chart
Standard deviation
Stem and leaf plots
Total length of stay (discharge days)
Variability
Variance
Vital statistics

Introduction

Complete and accurate information is at the heart of good decision making. The health information management (HIM) professional has responsibility for ensuring that the data collected are accurate and organized into information that is useful to healthcare decision makers.

The primary source of clinical data in a healthcare facility is the health record. To be useful in decision making, data taken from the health record must be as complete and accurate as possible. Data are compiled in various ways to help in making decisions about patient care, the facility's financial status, and/or facility planning, to name a few.

This chapter discusses common statistical measures and types of data used by organizations in different healthcare settings and data collection and reporting on a community, regional, and national basis. Methods and tools for graphically displaying data are then presented. The chapter concludes with a discussion of **normal distribution** and **descriptive statistics.**

Theory into Practice

The Department of Quality Improvement at Community Hospital asks the HIM director to provide the hospital's complication rate for DRG 209, Major Joint and Limb Reattachment Procedures of Lower Extremity, for the previous year for benchmarking purposes. It is recommended that the complication rate for any hospital not exceed 5 percent. For the previous year, the hospital had 556 cases that fell into DRG 209; 25 of these cases had complications following surgery. Its complication rate is 4.5 percent ([25/556] $\times$ 100). The quality improvement coordinator is pleased that the hospital's complication rate for DRG 209 falls within national benchmarks.

In another hospital, the administration is evaluating the appropriateness of an expansion program. The associate administrator in charge of facility planning asks the HIM director for the bed occupancy rate for the hospital and its major services for the past five years and the number of outpatient and emergency department visits for the same time period. The director's findings are displayed in table 15.1 and figure 15.1. The display

Table 15.1.   Bed occupancy rates, Community Hospital, 2000–2004

Hospital Service	2000	2001	2002	2003	2004
Total	85%	88%	90%	92%	95%
Medicine	90%	90%	92%	92%	95%
Surgery	80%	85%	85%	88%	90%
Obstetrics	65%	70%	72%	77%	79%
Pediatrics	85%	88%	88%	86%	89%

Figure 15.1.   Bed occupancy rate, community hospital, 2000–2004

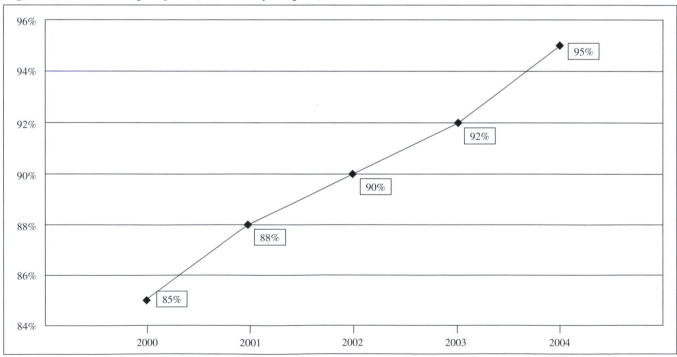

indicates that the bed occupancy rate for Community Hospital and its service lines has steadily increased over the five-year period. The data provide support for the associate administrator's plans for expansion.

Introduction to Measurement

Before discussing statistical measures used in healthcare, it is important to understand how the data collected are classified. Data collected falls on one of four **scales of measurement:** nominal, ordinal, interval, or ratio. Furthermore, the data collected is described as either continuous or discrete. These characteristics influence the type of graphic technique that can be used to display the data and the types of statistical analyses that can be performed.

Nominal-level data fall into groups or categories. The groups or categories are mutually exclusive, that is, a data element cannot be classified to more than one group. Some examples of nominal data collected in healthcare are related to patient demographics such as third-party payer, race, and sex. There is no order to the data collected within these categories.

Data that fall on the ordinal scale have some inherent order, and higher numbers are usually associated with higher values. On the **ordinal scale of measurement,** the order of the numbers is meaningful, not the number itself. Staging of a decubitus ulcer is an example of a variable that has order. A pressure ulcer has four stages, with stage I being the least severe ulcer and stage IV being the most severe. In this example, the higher number is associated with the most severe type of pressure ulcer.

Data that are nominal or ordinal are also considered discrete. **Discrete variables** are variables that fall into categories. For example, the variable "gender" has two categories: male and female. The variable "third-party payer" has a number of categories, depending on the healthcare facility. Examples include Medicare, Medicaid, commercial insurance, and private or self-pay.

Discrete variables can only take on a limited number of values and have gaps between successive values. In the above pressure ulcer example, the ulcer can be a stage I, II, III, or IV (limited number of values). It cannot be staged as 2.5 or 3.2 as there are "gaps" between each stage. This is an example of a discrete variable that has order to its categories.

The **ratio scale** is the highest level of measurement. On the ratio scale there is a defined unit of measure, a real zero point, and the intervals between successive values are equal. For example, consider the variable "length of stay." **Length of stay** (LOS) has defined units of measurement, day, and a real zero point, 0 days. Because there is a true zero point, we can state that an LOS of six days is twice as long as an LOS of three days. Multiplication on the ratio scale by a constant does not change its ratio character, but addition of a constant to a ratio measure does. For example, if we add two days to each LOS so that the stays are 8 and 5 days respectively, the

ratio of their stays is no longer 2:1. However, if we multiply the respective lengths of stay by 2 (e.g., 6×2 and 3×2), the ratio between the two lengths of stay remains 2:1.

The difference between the ratio and interval scales of measurement is that there is no true zero point on the **interval scale.** The most important characteristic of the interval scale is that the intervals between successive values are equal. On the Fahrenheit scale, the interval between 20°F and 21°F is the same as between 21°F and 22°F. But because there is no true zero on this scale, we cannot say that 40°F is twice as warm as 20°F.

Data that fall on the interval and ratio scales of measurement are continuous. With **continuous variables** there are no gaps in the measurement data. For example, an individual's weight may be 120 or 121 or any weight between 120 and 121. Continuous variables include fractions. Arithmetic operations—addition, subtraction, multiplication, and division—may be performed on continuous variables.

Check Your Understanding 15.1

Instructions: On a separate piece of paper, identify the scale of measurement for each of the following variables and indicate whether each variable is discrete or continuous.

1. ___ Zip code
2. ___ Blood pressure
3. ___ Heart Failure Classification I, II, III, IV
4. ___ Age
5. ___ Ethnicity
6. ___ Marital status
7. ___ Length of stay
8. ___ Discharge disposition (home, SNF and so on)
9. ___ Weight
10. ___ Level of education

Common Statistical Measures Used in Healthcare

Healthcare data are collected to describe the health status of groups or populations. The data reported about healthcare facilities and communities describe the occurrence of illnesses, births, and deaths for specific periods of time. Data that are collected may be either facility based or population based. The sources of facility-based statistics are **acute care** facilities, long-term care facilities, and other types of healthcare organizations. The population-based statistics are gathered from cities, counties, states, or specific groups within the population, such as individuals affected by arthritis.

Reporting statistics for a healthcare facility is similar to reporting statistics for a community. Rates for healthcare facilities are reported as per 100 cases or percent; a community rate is reported as per 1,000, 10,000, or 100,000 people. For example, if a hospital experienced two deaths in a given month and 100 patients were discharged in the same month, the death rate would be 2 percent ($[2 \times 100]/100$). If there were 200 deaths in a community of 80,000 for a given period of time, the death rate would be reported as 25 deaths per 10,000 population ([200 × 10,000]/80,000) for the same period of time.

Ratios, Proportions, and Rates

Many healthcare statistics are reported in the form of a **ratio**, **proportion**, or **rate**. These measures are used to report morbidity (illness), mortality (death), and natality (birthrate) at the local, state, and national levels. Basically, these measures indicate the number of times something happened relative to the number of times it could have happened. All three measures are based on formula 15.1. In this formula, x and y are the quantities being compared and x is divided by y. Further, 10^n is 10 to the nth power. The size of 10^n may equal 10, 100, 1,000, 10,000, and so on, depending on the value of n:

$$10^0 = 1$$
$$10^1 = 10$$
$$10^2 = 10 \times 10 = 100$$
$$10^3 = 10 \times 10 \times 10 = 1,000$$

Ratios

In a ratio, the quantities being compared, such as patient discharge status (x = alive, y = dead), may be expressed so that x and y are completely independent of each other, or x may be included in y. For example, the outcome of patients discharged from Community Hospital could be compared in one of two ways:

Alive/dead, or x/y
Alive/(alive + dead), or $x/(x + y)$

In the first example, x is completely independent of y. The ratio represents the number of patients discharged alive compared to the number of patients who died. In the second example, x is part of the whole ($x + y$). The ratio represents the number of patients discharged alive compared to all patients discharged. Both expressions are considered ratios.

Proportions

A proportion is a particular type of ratio in which x is a portion of the whole ($x + y$). In a proportion, the numerator is always included in the denominator. Figures 15.2 and 15.3 describe the procedures for calculating ratios and proportions.

Rates

Rates are often used to measure events over a period of time. Sometimes they also are used in performance improvement studies. Like ratios and proportions, rates may be reported daily, weekly, monthly, or yearly. This allows for trend analysis and comparisons over time. The basic formula for calculating a rate is shown in formula 15.2.

Healthcare facilities calculate many types of morbidity and mortality rates. For example, the cesarean section (C-section) rate is a measure of the proportion, or percentage, of C-sections performed during a given period of time. C-section rates are closely monitored because they present

more risk to the mother and baby and because they are more expensive than vaginal deliveries. In calculating the C-section rate, the number of C-sections performed during the specified period of time is counted and this value is placed in the numerator. The number of cases, or the population at risk, is the number of women who delivered during the same time period. This number is placed in the denominator. By convention, inpatient hospital rates are reported as the rate per 100 cases ($10^n = 10^2 = 10 \times 10 = 100$) and are expressed as percentages.

Formula 15.1.   General formula for calculating rates, proportions, and ratios

Ratio, proportion, rate = $x/y \times 10^n$

Figure 15.2.   Calculation of a ratio, discharge status of patients discharged in a month

1. Define x and y:

   x = number of patients discharged alive
   y = number of patients who died

2. Identify x and y:

   $x = 235$
   $y = 22$

3. *Set up the ratio x/y:*

   235/22

4. Reduce the fraction so that either x or y equals 1:

   10.68/1

There were 10.68 live discharges for every patient who died.

Figure 15.3.   Calculation of a proportion, discharge status of patients discharged in a month

1. Define x and y:

   x = number of patients discharged alive
   y = number of patients who died

2. Identify x and y:

   $x = 235$
   $y = 22$

3. Set up the proportion $x/x + y$:

   235/(235 + 22) = 235/257

4. Reduce the fraction so that either x or y equals 1:

   0.91/1

The proportion of patients discharged alive was 0.91.

Formula 15.2.   Formula for calculating risk for contracting a disease

$$\text{Risk rate} = \frac{\text{Number of cases occurring during a given time period}}{\text{Total number of cases or population at risk during the same time period}}$$

Figure 15.4 shows the procedure for calculating a rate. In the example, 33 of the 263 deliveries at Community Hospital during the month of May were C-sections. In the formula, the numerator is the number of C-sections performed in May (given period of time) and the denominator is the total number of deliveries including C-sections (the population at risk) performed within the same time frame. In calculating the rate, the numerator is always included in the denominator. Also, when calculating a facility-based rate, the numerator is first multiplied by 100 and then divided by the denominator.

Because hospital rates rarely result in a whole number, they usually must be rounded. The hospital should set a policy on whether rates are to be reported to one or two decimal places. The division should be carried out to at least one more decimal place than desired.

When rounding, if the last number is five or greater, the preceding number should be increased one digit. In contrast, if the last number is less than five, the preceding number remains the same. For example, when rounding 25.56 percent to one decimal place, the rate becomes 25.6 percent because the last number is greater than five. When rounding 1.563 percent to two places, the rate becomes 1.56 percent because the last digit is less than five. Rates of less than 1 percent are usually carried out to three decimal places and rounded to two. For rates less than 1 percent, a zero should precede the decimal to emphasize that the rate is less than 1 percent, for example, 0.56 percent.

Check Your Understanding 15.2

Instructions: on a separate piece of paper, identify the following statements as a rate, a ratio, or a proportion.

1. ____ Female discharges outnumber male discharges 3 to 1.

2. ____ Of the 100 discharges on October 1, 60 were female and 40 were male. Therefore, 0.60 of the discharges were women.

3. ____ Of the 100 patients discharged on October 1, 99 percent were discharged alive.

Figure 15.4.   Calculation of a rate, C-section rate for May 20xx

During May, 263 women delivered; of these, 33 deliveries were by C-section. What is the C-section rate for May?

1. Define the numerator (number of times an event occurred) and the denominator (number of times an event could have occurred):

    Numerator = total number of C-sections performed during the time period

    Denominator = total number of deliveries, including C-sections, in the same time period

2. Identify the numerator and the denominator:

    Numerator = 33
    Denominator = 263

3. Set up the rate:

    33/263

4. Multiply the numerator by 100 and then divide by the denominator:

    ([33 × 100]/263) = 12.5%

The C-section rate for May is 12.5 percent.

Basic Statistical Data Used in Acute Care Facilities

In the daily operations of any organization, whether in business, manufacturing, or healthcare, data are collected for decision making. To be effective, the decision makers must have confidence in the data collected. Confidence requires that the data collected be accurate, reliable, and timely. The types of data collected in the acute care setting are discussed in the following section.

Administrative Statistical Data

Hospitals collect data on both inpatients and outpatients on a daily basis. They use these statistics to monitor the volume of patients treated daily, weekly, monthly, or within some other specified time frame. The statistics give healthcare decision makers the information they need to plan facilities and to monitor inpatient and outpatient revenue streams. For these reasons, the HIM professional must be well versed in data collection and reporting methods.

Standard definitions have been developed to ensure that all healthcare providers collect and report data in a consistent manner. The *Glossary of Healthcare Terms,* developed by the American Health Information Management Association (AHIMA), is a resource commonly used to describe the types of healthcare events for which data are collected. (The glossary is currently published as an appendix in *Calculating and Reporting Healthcare Statistics* [Horton 2004].) It includes definitions of terms related to healthcare corporations, health maintenance organizations (HMOs), and other health-related programs and facilities. Some basic terms that HIM professionals should be familiar with include:

- *Hospital inpatient:* A patient who is provided with room, board, and continuous general nursing service in an area of the hospital where patients generally stay at least overnight.

- *Hospital newborn inpatient:* A patient who is born in the hospital at the beginning of the current inpatient hospitalization. **Newborns** are usually counted separately because their care is so different from that of other inpatients. Infants born on the way to the hospital or at home are considered hospital inpatients, not hospital newborn inpatients.

- *Inpatient hospitalization:* A period in a person's life during which he or she is an inpatient in a single hospital without interruption, except by possible intervening leaves of absence.

- *Inpatient admission:* The formal acceptance by a hospital of a patient who is to be provided with room, board, and continuous nursing service in an area of the hospital where patients generally stay overnight.

- *Inpatient discharge:* The termination of a period of inpatient hospitalization through the formal release of the inpatient by the hospital. The term includes patients who are discharged alive (by physician's order), who are discharged against medical advice (AMA), or who died while hospitalized. Unless otherwise indicated, inpatient discharges include deaths.

- *Hospital outpatient:* A hospital patient who receives services in one or more of the outpatient facilities when he or she is not currently an inpatient or home care patient. An outpatient may be classified as either an emergency outpatient or a clinic outpatient. An emergency outpatient is admitted to the emergency department of a hospital for diagnosis and treatment of a condition that requires immediate medical, dental, or other emergency services. A clinic outpatient is admitted to a clinical service of the clinic or hospital for diagnosis and treatment on an ambulatory basis.

Inpatient Census Data

Even though much of the data collection process has been automated, an ongoing responsibility of the HIM professional is to verify the **census** data that are collected daily. The census reports patient activity for a 24-hour reporting period. Included in the census report is the number of inpatients admitted and discharged for the previous 24-hour period as well as the number of intra-hospital transfers. An intra-hospital transfer is a patient who is moved from one patient care unit (for example, the intensive care unit) to another (for example, the surgical unit). The usual 24-hour reporting period begins at 12:01 a.m. and ends at 12:00 midnight. In the census count, adults and children (A&C) are reported separately from newborns.

Before compiling census data, however, it is important to understand their related terminology. The census is the number of hospital inpatients present at any one time. For example, the census in a 300-bed hospital may be 250 patients at 2:00 p.m. on May 1, but 245 an hour later. Because the census may change throughout the day as admissions and discharges occur, hospitals designate an official census-taking time. In most facilities, the official count takes place at midnight.

The result of the official count taken at midnight is called the **daily inpatient census.** This is the number of inpatients present at the official census-taking time each day. Also included in the daily inpatient census are any patients who were admitted and discharged that same day. For example, if a patient were admitted to the cardiac care unit (CCU) at 1:00 p.m. on May 1 and died at 4.00 p.m. on May 1, he would be counted as a patient who was both admitted and discharged the same day.

Because patients admitted and discharged the same day are not present at the census-taking time, the hospital must account for them separately. If it did not, credit for the services provided these patients would be lost. The daily inpatient census reflects the total number of patients treated during the 24-hour period. Figure 15.5 displays a sample daily inpatient census report.

Figure 15.5.   Daily inpatient census report, adults and children

May 2	
Number of patients in hospital at midnight, May 1	230
+ Number of patients admitted May 2	+ 35
− Number of patients discharged, including deaths, May 2	− 40
Number of patients in hospital at midnight, May 2	225
+ Number of patients both admitted and discharged, including deaths	+5
Daily inpatient census at midnight, May 2	230
Total inpatient service days, May 2	230

A unit of measure that reflects the services received by one inpatient during a 24-hour period is called an **inpatient service day** (IPSD). The number of IPSDs for a 24-hour period is equal to the daily inpatient census, that is, one service day for each patient treated. In figure 15.5, the total number of inpatient service days for May 2 is 230.

IPSDs are compiled daily, weekly, monthly, and annually. They reflect the volume of services provided by the healthcare facility: the greater the volume of services, the greater the revenues to the facility. Daily reporting of the number of IPSDs is an indicator of the hospital's financial condition.

As previously mentioned, the daily inpatient census is equal to the number of IPSDs provided for that day as shown below:

Day	Daily Inpatient Census	Inpatient Service Days
Day 1	240	240
Day 2	253	253
Day 3	237	237
Total		730

Thus, the total number of IPSDs for a week, a month, and so on can be divided by the total number of days in the period of interest to obtain the **average daily census.** In the preceding example, 730 IPSDs is divided by three days to obtain an average daily census of 243.3. The average daily census is the average number of inpatients treated during a given period of time. The general formula for calculating the average daily census is shown in formula 15.3.

In calculating the average daily census for adults and children (A&C), the average daily census for newborns is reported separately. This is because the intensity of services provided to adults and children is greater than it is for newborns. To calculate the A&C average daily census, the general formula is modified as shown in formula 15.4.

The formula for the average daily census for newborns is shown in formula 15.5. For example, the total number of IPSDs provided to adults and children for the week of May 1 is 1,729, and the total for newborns is 119. Using the formulas, the average daily census for adults and children is 247 (1,729/7) and for newborns it is 17 (119/7). The average daily census for all hospital inpatients for the week of May 1 is 264 ([1,729 + 119]/7). Table 15.2 compares the various formulas for calculating the average daily census.

Instructions: Answer the following questions on a separate piece of paper.

1. The inpatient census for Community Hospital at midnight on August 1 was 268; the daily inpatient census for August 1 was 270. On August 2, 16 patients were admitted, 9 were discharged, and 2 were admitted and discharged on the same day. Calculate the following statistics for August 2.

   a. ___ Inpatient census

   b. ___ Daily inpatient census

   c. ___ Inpatient service days

   d. ___ Total inpatient service days for August 1 and 2

2. Nine patients were in the intensive care unit (ICU) at midnight on August 1. On August 2, two patients were admitted, one was transferred from 3N to the ICU, one died, one was transferred from the ICU to the cardiology service, and two who were admitted on August 2 died on August 2. Calculate the following statistics for the ICU on August 2.

   a. ___ Inpatient census

   b. ___ Daily inpatient census

Formula 15.3. Formula for calculating average daily census

$$\text{Average daily census} = \frac{\text{Total number of inpatient service days for a given period}}{\text{Total number of days in the same period}}$$

Formula 15.4. Formula for calculating average daily census for adults and children

$$\text{Average daily census for A\&C} = \frac{\text{Total number of inpatient service days for A\&C for a given period}}{\text{Total number of days for the same period}}$$

Formula 15.5. Formula for calculating average daily census for newborns

$$\text{Average daily census for NBs} = \frac{\text{Total number of inpatient service days for NBs for a given period}}{\text{Total number of days for the same period}}$$

Inpatient Bed Occupancy Rate

Another indicator of the hospital's financial position is the **inpatient bed occupancy rate,** also called the percentage of occupancy. The inpatient bed occupancy rate is the percentage of official beds occupied by hospital inpatients for a given period of time. In general, the greater the occupancy rate, the greater the revenues for the hospital. For a bed to be included in the official count, it must be set up, staffed, equipped, and available for patient care. The total number of inpatient service days is used in the numerator because it is equal to the daily inpatient census or the number of patients treated daily. The occupancy rate compares the number of patients treated over a given period of time to the total number of beds available for the same period of time.

For example, if 200 patients occupied 280 beds on May 2, the inpatient bed occupancy rate would be 71.4 percent ($[200/\{280 \times 1\}] \times 100$). If the rate were for more than one day, the number of beds would be multiplied by the number of days within that particular time frame. For example, if 1,729 IPSDs were provided during the week of May 1, the inpatient bed occupancy rate for that week would be 88.2 percent ($[1,729/\{280 \times 7\}] \times 100$).

The denominator in this formula is actually the total possible number of IPSDs. That is, if every available bed in the hospital were occupied every single day, this would be the maximum number of IPSDs that could be provided. This is an important concept, especially when the official **bed count** changes for a given reporting period. For example, if the bed count changed from 280 beds to 300, the bed occupancy rate would reflect the change. The total number of inpatient beds times the total number of days in the period is called the total number of **bed count days.** The general formula for the inpatient bed occupancy rate is shown in formula 15.6 (p. 407).

For example, in May the total number of inpatient service days provided was 7,582. The bed count for the month of May changed from 280 beds to 300 on May 20. To calculate the inpatient bed occupancy rate for May, the total number of bed count days must be determined. There are 31 days in May; therefore, the total number of bed count days is calculated as:

Number of beds, May 1–May 19 = 280×19 days = 5,320 bed count days
Number of beds, May 20–May 31 = 300×12 days = 3,600 bed count days
5,320 + 3,600 = 8,920 bed count days

The inpatient bed occupancy rate for the month of May is 85.0 percent ($[7,582/8,920] \times 100$).

Table 15.2. Calculation of census statistics

Indicator	Numerator	Denominator
Average daily inpatient census	Total number of inpatient service days for a given period	Total number of days for the same period
Average daily inpatient census for adults and children (A&C)	Total number of inpatient service days for A&C for a given period	Total number of days for the same period
Average daily inpatient census for newborns (NBs)	Total number of inpatient services days for NBs for a given period	Total number of days for the same period

As with the average daily census, the inpatient bed occupancy rate for adults and children is reported separately from that of newborns. To calculate the total number of bed count days for newborns, the official count for newborn bassinets is used. Table 15.3 reviews the formulas for calculating inpatient bed occupancy rates.

It is possible for the inpatient bed occupancy rate to be greater than 100 percent. This occurs when the hospital faces an epidemic or disaster. In this type of situation, hospitals set up temporary beds that usually are not included in the official bed count. As an example, Community Hospital experienced an excessive number of admissions in January because of an outbreak of influenza. In January, the official bed count was 150 beds. On January 5, the daily inpatient census was 156. Therefore, the inpatient bed occupancy rate for January 5 was 104 percent ([156/150] × 100).

Bed Turnover Rate

The **bed turnover rate** is a measure of hospital utilization. It includes the number of times each hospital bed changed occupants. The formula for the bed turnover rate is shown in formula 15.7. For example, Community Hospital experienced 2,060 discharges and deaths for the month of April. Its bed count for April averaged 677. The bed turnover rate is 3.0 (2,060/677). The interpretation is that, on average, each hospital bed had three occupants during April.

Check Your Understanding 15.4

Instructions: Answer the following questions on a separate piece of paper.

1. What is the inpatient bed occupancy rate for each of the following patient care units for the month of August?

Inpatient Unit	Service Days	Bed Count	Occupancy Rate
Medical	2,850	100	_____
Surgical	988	34	_____
Pediatric	422	15	_____
Orthopedic	502	18	_____
Obstetric	544	20	_____
Newborn	524	18	_____
Total	_____	___	_____

2. In 2004, Community Hospital had 67,120 inpatient service days for adults and children and 4,850 inpatient service days for newborns. The bed count for adults and children was 220, and the bed count for newborn bassinets was 22.

   a. ___ What was the average daily inpatient census for adults and children?

   b. ___ What was the average daily inpatient census for newborns?

   c. ___ What was the inpatient bed occupancy rate for adults and children?

   d. ___ What was the inpatient bed occupancy rate for newborns?

Length of Stay Data

LOS is calculated for each patient after he or she is discharged from the hospital. It is the number of calendar days from the day of patient admission to the day of patient discharge. When the patient is admitted and discharged in the same month, the LOS is determined by subtracting the date of admission from the date of discharge. For example, the LOS for a patient admitted on May 12 and discharged on May 17 is five days (17 − 12 = 5)

When the patient is admitted in one month and discharged in another, the calculations must be adjusted. One way to calculate the LOS in this case is to subtract the date of admission from the total number of days in the month the patient was admitted and then to add the total number of hospitalized days for the month in which the patient was discharged. For example, the LOS for a patient admitted on May 28 and discharged on June 6 is nine days ([May 31–May 28 = 3 days] + [June 1–June 6 = 6 days]; LOS = 9 days)

When a patient is admitted and discharged on the same day, the LOS is one day. A partial day's stay is never reported as a fraction of a day. The LOS for a patient discharged the day after admission also is one day. Thus, the LOS for a patient who was admitted to the ICU on May 10 at 9:00 a.m. and died at 3:00 p.m. on the same day is one day. Likewise, the LOS for a patient admitted on May 12 and discharged on May 13 is one day.

When the LOS for all patients discharged for a given period of time is summed, the result is the **total length of stay.** As an example, five patients were discharged from the pediatric unit on May 9. The LOS for each patient was as follows:

Patient	LOS
1	5
2	3
3	1
4	8
5	10
Total LOS	27

In the preceding example, the total LOS is 27 days (5 + 3 + 1 + 8 + 10). The total LOS is also referred to as the number of days of care provided to patients who were discharged or died (discharge days) during a given period of time.

The **average length of stay** (ALOS) is calculated from the total LOS. The total LOS divided by the number of patients discharged is the ALOS. Using the data in the preceding example, the ALOS for the five patients discharged from the pediatric unit is 5.4 days (27/5)

The general formula for calculating ALOS is shown in formula 15.8. As with the measures already discussed, the ALOS for adults and children is reported separately from the ALOS for newborns. Table 15.4 reviews the formulas for ALOS. Table 15.5 (p. 408) displays an example of a hospital statistical summary prepared by the HIM department using census and discharge data.

Check Your Understanding 15.5

Instructions: Complete the following exercise on a separate piece of paper.

1. Calculate the total length of stay for all patient discharges and the average length of stay.

Number of Patients Discharged	Total Length of Stay	Discharge Days
10	2	_____
7	3	_____
2	4	_____
1	7	_____
1	9	_____
1	10	_____
1	16	_____

a. Total length of stay   _____

b. Average length of stay   _____

Patient Care/Clinical Statistical Data

Thus far, this chapter has discussed statistical measures that are indicators of volume of services and utilization of services. The collection of data related to morbidity and mortality also is an important aspect of evaluating the quality of hospital services. Morbidity/mortality rates are reported for all patient discharges within a certain time frame. They also may be reported by service or by physician or other variable of interest in order to identify trends or problems that require corrective action. The most frequently collected morbidity/mortality rates are presented in this section.

Hospital Death (Mortality) Rates

The **hospital death rate** is based on the number of patients discharged, alive and dead, from the hospital. Deaths are

Formula 15.6. Formula for calculating inpatient bed occupancy rate

$$\text{Inpatient bed occupancy} = \frac{\text{Total number of inpatient service days for a given period}}{\text{Total number of inpatient bed count days for the same period}} \times 100$$

Table 15.3. Calculation of inpatient bed occupancy rates

Rate	Numerator	Denominator
Inpatient bed occupancy rate	Total number of inpatient service days for a given period × 100	Total number of inpatient bed count days for the same period
Inpatient bed occupancy rate for adults and children (A&C)	Total number of inpatient service days for A&C for a given period × 100	Total number of inpatient bed count days for A&C for the same period
Newborn (NB) bed occupancy rate	Total number of NB inpatient service days for a given period × 100	Total number of bassinet bed count days for the same period

Formula 15.7. Formula for calculating bed turnover rate

$$\text{Bed turnover rate} = \frac{\text{Total number of discharges, including deaths, for a given time period}}{\text{Average bed count for the same time period}}$$

Formula 15.8. Formula for calculating average length of stay

$$\text{Average length of stay} = \frac{\text{Total length of stay for a given period}}{\text{Total number of discharges, including deaths, for the same period}}$$

Table 15.4. Calculation of LOS statistics

Indicator	Numerator	Denominator
Average LOS	Total LOS (discharge days) for a given period	Total number of discharges, including deaths, for the same period
Average LOS for adults and children (A&C)	Total LOS for A&C (discharge days) for a given period	Total number of discharges, including deaths, for A&C for the same period
Average LOS for newborns (NB)	Total LOS for all NB discharges and deaths (discharge days) for a given period	Total number of NB discharges, including deaths, for the same period

Table 15.5.   Statistical summary, Community Hospital for the period ending July 20xx

Admissions	July 20xx		Year-to-Date 20xx	
	Actual	Budget	Actual	Budget
Medical	728	769	5,075	5,082
Surgical	578	583	3,964	3,964
OB/GYN	402	440	2,839	3,027
Psychiatry	113	99	818	711
Physical Medicine & Rehab	48	57	380	384
Other Adult	191	178	1,209	1,212
Total Adult	2,060	2,126	14,285	14,380
Newborn	294	312	2,143	2,195
Total Admissions	2,354	2,438	16,428	16,575

Average Length of Stay	July 20xx		Year-to-Date 20xx	
	Actual	Budget	Actual	Budget
Medical	6.1	6.4	6.0	6.1
Surgical	7.0	7.2	7.7	7.7
OB/GYN	2.9	3.2	3.5	3.1
Psychiatry	10.8	11.6	10.4	11.6
Physical Medicine & Rehab	27.5	23.0	28.1	24.3
Other Adult	3.6	3.9	4.0	4.1
Total Adult	6.3	6.4	6.7	6.5
Newborn	5.6	5.0	5.6	5.0
Total ALOS	6.2	6.3	6.5	6.3

Patient Days	June 20xx		Year-to-Date 20xx	
	Actual	Budget	Actual	Budget
Medical	4,436	4,915	30,654	30,762
Surgical	4,036	4,215	30,381	30,331
OB/GYN	1,170	1,417	10,051	9,442
Psychiatry	1,223	1,144	8,524	8,242
Physical Medicine & Rehab	1,318	1,310	10,672	9,338
Other Adult	688	699	4,858	4,921
Total Adult	12,871	13,700	95,140	93,036
Newborn	1,633	1,552	12,015	10,963
Total Patient Days	14,504	15,252	107,155	103,999

Other Key Statistics	June 20xx		Year-to-Date 20xx	
	Actual	Budget	Actual	Budget
Average Daily Census	485	492	498	486
Average Beds Available	677	660	677	660
Clinic Visits	21,621	18,975	144,271	136,513
Emergency Visits	3,822	3,688	26,262	25,604
Inpatient Surgery Patients	657	583	4,546	4,093
Outpatient Surgery Patients	603	554	4,457	3,987

considered discharges because they are the end point of a period of hospitalization. In contrast to the rates discussed in the preceding section, newborns are not counted separately from adults and children.

Gross Death Rate

The **gross death rate** is the proportion of all hospital discharges that ended in death. It is the basic indicator of mortality in a healthcare facility. The gross death rate is calculated by dividing the total number of deaths occurring in a given time period by the total number of discharges, including deaths, for the same time period. The formula for calculating the gross death rate is shown in formula 15.9.

As an example, Community Hospital experienced 21 deaths (A&C and NBs) during the month of May. There were 633 total discharges, including deaths. The gross death rate is 3.3 percent ([21/633] × 100).

Net Death Rate

The **net death rate** is an adjusted death rate. It is calculated in the belief that certain deaths should not "count against the hospital." The net death rate is an adjusted rate because it does not include patients who die within 48 hours of admission. The reason for excluding these deaths is that 48 hours is not enough time to positively affect patient outcome. In other words, the patient was not admitted to the hospital in a manner timely enough for treatment to have an effect on his or her outcome. The formula for calculating the net death rate is shown in formula 15.10.

Continuing with the preceding example of the 21 patients who died at Community Hospital, three died within 48 hours of admission. Therefore, the net death rate is 2.9 percent ([{21 − 3}/{633 − 3}] × 100 = 2.9%). The fact that the net death rate is less than the gross death rate is favorable to Community Hospital because lower death rates may be an indicator of better care.

Newborn Death Rate

Even though newborn deaths are included in the hospital's gross and net death rates, the **newborn death rate** can be calculated separately. Newborns include only infants born alive in the hospital. The newborn death rate is the number of newborns who died in comparison to the total number of newborns discharged, alive and dead. To qualify as a newborn death, the newborn must have been delivered alive. A stillborn infant is not included in either the newborn death rate or the gross or net death rate. The formula for calculating the newborn death rate is shown in formula 15.11.

Fetal Death Rate

In healthcare terminology, the death of a stillborn baby is called a **fetal death.** A fetal death is a death prior to the fetus's complete expulsion or extraction from the mother in a hospital facility, regardless of the length of the pregnancy. Thus, stillborns are neither admitted nor discharged from the hospital. A fetal death occurs when the fetus fails to breathe or show any other evidence of life, such as a heartbeat, a pulsation of the umbilical cord, or a movement of the voluntary muscles.

Fetal deaths also are classified into categories based on length of gestation or weight. (See table 15.6, p. 410.) To calculate the **fetal death rate,** divide the total number of intermediate and late fetal deaths for the period by the total number of live births and intermediate and late fetal deaths for the same period. The formula for calculating the fetal death rate is shown in formula 15.12 (p. 410). For example, during the month of May, Community Hospital experienced 269 live births and 13 intermediate and late fetal deaths. The fetal death rate is 4.6 percent ([13/{269 + 13}] × 100).

Maternal Death Rate

Hospitals also calculate the **maternal death rate.** A maternal death is the death of any woman from any cause related to,

---

Formula 15.9. Formula for calculating gross death rate

$$\text{Gross death rate} = \frac{\text{Total number of inpatient deaths (including NBs) for a given period}}{\text{Total number of discharges, including A\&C and NB deaths, for the same period}} \times 100$$

Formula 15.10. Formula for calculating net death rate

$$\text{Net death rate} = \frac{\text{Total number of inpatient deaths (including NBs) minus deaths} < 48 \text{ hours for a given period}}{\text{Total number of discharges (including A\&C and NB deaths) minus deaths} < 48 \text{ hours for the same period}} \times 100$$

Formula 15.11. Formula for calculating newborn death rate

$$\text{Newborn death rate} = \frac{\text{Total number of NB deaths for a given period}}{\text{Total number of NB discharges (including deaths) for the same period}} \times 100$$

or aggravated by, pregnancy or its management, regardless of the duration or site of the pregnancy. Maternal deaths that result from accidental or incidental causes are not included in the maternal death rate.

Maternal deaths are classified as either direct or indirect. A direct maternal death is the death of a woman resulting from obstetrical (OB) complications of the pregnancy state, labor, or puerperium (the period including the six weeks after delivery). Direct maternal deaths are included in the maternal death rate. An indirect maternal death is the death of a woman from a previously existing disease or a disease that developed during pregnancy, labor, or the puerperium that was not due to obstetric causes, although the physiologic effects of pregnancy were partially responsible.

The maternal death rate may be an indicator of the availability of prenatal care in a community. The hospital also may use it to help identify conditions that could lead to a maternal death. The formula for calculating the maternal death rate is shown in formula 15.13. For example, during the month of May, Community Hospital experienced 275 maternal discharges. Two of these patients died. The maternal death rate for May is 0.73 percent ([2/275] × 100). Table 15.7 summarizes hospital-based mortality rates.

Check Your Understanding 15.6

Instructions: Using the data provided on deaths and discharges at Community Hospital for the past calendar year, answer the following questions on a separate sheet of paper.

Total discharges, including deaths (A&C)	754
Total deaths (A&C)	14
Deaths less than 48 hours after admission (A&C)	6
Fetal deaths	3
Live births	140
Newborn deaths	3
Newborn discharges, including deaths	122
Maternal deaths (direct)	2
OB discharges, including deaths	133

1. ____   What is the gross death rate for adults and children?

2. ____   What is the net death rate for adults and children?

3. ____   What is the fetal death rate?

4. ____   What is the newborn death rate?

5. ____   What is the gross death rate for adults and children and newborns combined?

6. ____   What is the maternal death rate (direct)?

Table 15.6. Classifications of fetal death

Classification	Length of Gestation	Weight
Early fetal death	Less than 20 weeks' gestation	500 grams or less
Intermediate fetal death	20 weeks' completed gestation, but less than 28 weeks	501 to 1,000 grams
Late fetal death	28 weeks' completed gestation	Over 1,000 grams

Formula 15.12. Formula for calculating fetal death rate

$$\text{Fetal death rate} = \frac{\text{Total number of intermediate and late fetal deaths for a given period}}{\text{Total number of live births plus total number of intermediate and late fetal deaths for the same period}} \times 100$$

Formula 15.13. Formula for calculating maternal death rate

$$\text{Maternal death rate} = \frac{\text{Total number of direct maternal deaths for a given period}}{\text{Total number of maternal (OB) discharges, including deaths, for the same period}} \times 100$$

Table 15.7. Calculation of hospital-based mortality rates

Rate	Numerator (x)	Denominator (y)
Gross death rate	Total number of inpatient deaths, including NBs, for a given period × 100	Total number of discharges, including A&C and NB deaths, for the same period
Net death rate (institutional death rate)	Total number of inpatient deaths, including NBs, minus deaths < 48 hours for a given period × 100	Total number of discharges, including A&C and NB deaths, minus deaths < 48 hours for the same period
Newborn death rate	Total number of NB deaths for a given period × 100	Total number of NB discharges, including deaths, for the same period
Fetal death rate	Total number of intermediate and late fetal deaths for a given period × 100	Total number of live births plus total number of intermediate and fetal deaths for the same period
Maternal death rate	Total number of direct maternal deaths for a given period × 100	Total number of maternal (obstetric) discharges, including deaths, for the same period
Infant death rate	Number of deaths under one year of age during a given time period	Number of live births during the same time period

Autopsy Rates

An autopsy is an examination of a dead body to determine the cause of death. Autopsies are very useful in the education of medical students and residents. In addition, they can alert family members to conditions or diseases for which they may be at risk.

Two categories of hospital autopsies are conducted in acute care facilities: hospital inpatient autopsies and hospital autopsies. A **hospital inpatient autopsy** is an examination of the body of a patient who died while being treated in the hospital. The patient's death marked the end of his or her stay in the hospital. A pathologist or some other physician on the medical staff performs this type of autopsy in the facility.

A **hospital autopsy** is an examination of the body of an individual who at some time in the past had been a hospital patient and was not a hospital inpatient at the time of death. A pathologist or some other physician on the medical staff performs this type of autopsy.

The following sections describe the different types of autopsy rates calculated by acute care hospitals.

Gross Autopsy Rates

A **gross autopsy rate** is the proportion or percentage of deaths that are followed by the performance of autopsy. The formula for calculating the gross autopsy rate is shown in formula 15.14. For example, during the month of May, Community Hospital experienced 21 deaths. Autopsies were performed on four of these patients. The gross autopsy rate is 19.0 percent ([4/21] × 100).

Net Autopsy Rates

The bodies of patients who have died are not always available for autopsy. For example, a coroner or medical examiner may claim a body for an autopsy for legal reasons. In these situations, the hospital calculates a **net autopsy rate.** In cal-culating the net autopsy rate, bodies that have been removed by the coroner or medical examiner are excluded from the denominator. The formula for calculating the net autopsy rate is shown in formula 15.15. Continuing with the example in the preceding section, the medical examiner claimed three of the patients for autopsy. The numerator remains the same because four autopsies were performed by the hospital pathologist. However, because three of the deaths were identified as medical examiner's cases and removed from the hospital, three is subtracted from 21. The net autopsy rate is 22.2 percent ([4/{21 − 3}] × 100).

Hospital Autopsy Rates

A third type of autopsy rate is called the **hospital autopsy rate.** This is an adjusted rate that includes autopsies on anyone who may have once been a hospital patient. The formula for calculating the hospital autopsy rate is shown in formula 15.16. The hospital autopsy rate includes autopsies performed on any of the following:

- Bodies of inpatients, except those removed by the coroner or medical examiner. When the hospital pathologist or other designated physician acts as an agent in the performance of an autopsy on an inpatient, the death and the autopsy are included in the percentage.
- Bodies of other hospital patients, including ambulatory care patients, hospital home care patients, and former hospital patients who died elsewhere, but whose bodies have been made available for autopsy to be performed by the hospital pathologist or other designated physician. These autopsies and deaths are included in computations of the percentage.

Generally, it is impossible to determine the number of bodies of former hospital patients who may have died in a

---

Formula 15.14.   Formula for calculating gross autopsy rate

$$\text{Gross autopsy rate} = \frac{\text{Total inpatient autopsies for a given period}}{\text{Total number of inpatient deaths for the same period}} \times 100$$

Formula 15.15.   Formula for calculating net autopsy rate

$$\text{Net autopsy rate} = \frac{\text{Total number of autopsies on inpatient deaths for a period}}{\text{Total number of inpatient deaths minus unautopsied coroners' or medical examiners' cases for the same period}} \times 100$$

Formula 15.16.   Formula for calculating hospital autopsy rate

$$\text{Hospital autopsy rate} = \frac{\text{Total number of hospital autopsies for a given period}}{\text{Total number of deaths of hospital patients whose bodies were available for autopsy for the same period}} \times 100$$

given time period. In the formula, the phrase available for **hospital autopsy** involves several conditions, including:

- The autopsy must be performed by the hospital pathologist or a designated physician on the body of a patient treated at some time at the hospital.
- The report of the autopsy must be filed in the patient's health record and in the hospital laboratory or pathology department.
- The tissue specimens must be maintained in the hospital laboratory.

Figure 15.6 explains how to calculate the hospital autopsy rate.

Newborn Autopsy Rates

Autopsy rates usually include autopsies performed on newborn infants unless a separate rate is requested. The formula for calculating the **newborn autopsy rate** is shown in formula 15.17.

Fetal Autopsy Rates

Hospitals sometimes also calculate the **fetal autopsy rate.** Fetal autopsies are performed on stillborn infants who have been classified as either intermediate or late fetal deaths. This is the proportion or percentage of autopsies done on intermediate or late fetal deaths out of the total number of intermediate or late fetal deaths. The formula for calculating the fetal autopsy rate is shown in formula 15.18. Table 15.8 summarizes the different hospital autopsy rates.

Check Your Understanding 15.7

Instructions: Read the scenario below and answer the questions that follow.

In October, Community Hospital experienced 44 deaths. Three of them were coroner's cases and one was autopsied by the hospital pathologist. Twenty-one autopsies were performed on the remaining deaths.

1. ___ What is the gross autopsy rate for Community Hospital for the month of October?

2. ___ What is the net autopsy rate for Community Hospital for the month of October?

Figure 15.6.   Calculation of the hospital autopsy rate

In June, 33 inpatient deaths occurred. Three of these were medical examiner's cases. Two of the bodies were removed from the hospital and so were not available for hospital autopsy. One of the medical examiner's cases was autopsied by the hospital pathologist. Fourteen other autopsies were performed on hospital inpatients who died during the month of June. In addition, autopsies were performed in the hospital on:

- A child with congenital heart disease who died in the emergency department
- A former hospital inpatient who died in an extended care facility and whose body was brought to the hospital for autopsy
- A former hospital inpatient who died at home and whose body was brought to the hospital for autopsy
- A hospital outpatient who died while receiving chemotherapy for cancer
- A hospital home care patient whose body was brought to the hospital for autopsy
- A former hospital inpatient who died in an emergency vehicle on the way to the hospital

Calculation of total hospital autopsies:

   1 autopsy on medical examiner's case
+14 autopsies on hospital inpatients
+ 6 autopsies on hospital patients whose bodies were available for autopsy
_____
 21 autopsies performed by the hospital pathologist

Calculation of number of deaths of hospital patients whose bodies were available for autopsy:

 33 inpatient deaths
− 2 medical examiner's cases
+ 6 deaths of hospital patients
_____
 37 total bodies available for autopsy

Calculation of the hospital autopsy rate:

$$\frac{\text{Total number of hospital autopsies for the period}}{\text{Total number of deaths of hospital patients with bodies available for hospital autopsy for the period}} \times 100$$

$$(21 \times 100)/37 = 56.8\%$$

Formula 15.17.   Formula for calculating newborn autopsy rate

$$\text{Newborn autopsy rate} = \frac{\text{Total number of autopsies on NB deaths for a given time period}}{\text{Total number of NB deaths for the same period}} \times 100$$

Formula 15.18.   Formula for calculating fetal autopsy rate

$$\text{Fetal autopsy rate} = \frac{\text{Total number of autopsies on intermediate and late fetal deaths for a given period}}{\text{Total number of intermediate and late fetal deaths for the same period}} \times 100$$

Hospital Infection Rates

The most common morbidity rates calculated for hospitals are related to hospital-acquired infections, or **nosocomial infections.** The hospital must continuously monitor the number of infections that occur in its various patient care units. Infection can adversely affect the course of a patient's treatment and possibly result in death. The Joint Commission on Accreditation of Healthcare Organizations (JCAHO) requires hospitals to follow written guidelines for reporting all types of infections. Examples of the different types of infections are respiratory, gastrointestinal, surgical wound, skin, urinary tract, septicemias, and infections related to intravascular catheters.

Hospital-Acquired Infection Rates

Hospital-acquired infection rates may be calculated for the entire hospital or for a specific unit in the hospital. They also may be calculated for the specific types of infections. Ideally, the hospital should strive for an infection rate of 0.0 percent. The formula for calculating the hospital-acquired infection rate is shown in formula 15.19. For example, Community Hospital discharged 725 patients during the month of June. Thirty-two of these patients experienced hospital-acquired infections. The hospital-acquired infection rate is 4.4 percent ([32/725] × 100).

Postoperative Infection Rates

Hospitals often track their **postoperative infection rate.** The postoperative infection rate is the proportion or percentage of infections in clean surgical cases out of the total number of surgical operations performed. A clean surgical case is one in which no infection existed prior to surgery. The postoperative infection rate may be an indicator of a problem in the hospital environment or of some type of surgical contamination.

The individual calculating the postoperative infection rate must know the difference between a surgical procedure and a surgical operation. A surgical procedure is any separate, systematic process on or within the body that can be complete in itself. A physician, dentist, or some other licensed practitioner performs a surgical procedure, with or without instruments, to:

- Restore disunited or deficient parts
- Remove diseased or injured tissues
- Extract foreign matter
- Assist in obstetrical delivery
- Aid in diagnosis

A surgical operation involves one or more surgical procedures that are performed on one patient at one time using one approach to achieve a common purpose. An example of a surgical operation is the resection of a portion of both the intestine and the liver in a cancer patient. This involves two procedures, removal of a portion of the liver and removal of a portion of the colon; but it is considered only one operation because there is only one operative approach or incision. In contrast, an esophagoduodenoscopy (EGD) and a colonoscopy performed at the same time are two procedures with two different approaches. In the former, the approach is the upper gastrointestinal tract; in the latter, the approach is the lower gastrointestinal tract. In this case, the two procedures do not have a common approach or purpose. The formula for calculating the postoperative infection rate is shown in formula 15.20 (p. 414).

Table 15.8.   Calculation of hospital autopsy rates

Rate	Numerator	Denominator
Gross autopsy rate	Total number of autopsies on inpatient deaths for a given period × 100	Total number of inpatient deaths for the same period
Net autopsy rate	Total number of autopsies on inpatient deaths for a given period × 100	Total number of inpatient deaths minus unautopsied coroner or medical examiner cases for the same period
Hospital autopsy rate	Total number of hospital autopsies for a given period × 100	Total number of deaths of hospital patients whose bodies are available for hospital autopsy for the same period
Newborn (NB) autopsy rate	Total number of autopsies on NB deaths for a given period × 100	Total number of NB deaths for the same period
Fetal autopsy rate	Total number of autopsies on intermediate and late fetal deaths for a given period × 100	Total number of intermediate and late fetal deaths for the same period

Formula 15.19.   Formula for calculating nosocomial infection rate

$$\text{Hospital-acquired infection rate} = \frac{\text{Total number of hospital-acquired infections for a given period}}{\text{Total number of discharges, including deaths, for the same period}} \times 100$$

Formula 15.20.   Formula for calculating postoperative infection rate

$$\text{Postoperative infection rate} = \frac{\text{Number of infections in clean surgical cases for a given period}}{\text{Total number of surgical operations for the same period}} \times 100$$

Consultation Rates

A consultation occurs when two or more physicians collaborate on a particular patient's diagnosis or treatment. The attending physician requests the consultation and explains his or her reason for doing so. The consultant then examines the patient and the patient's health record and makes recommendations in a written report. The formula for calculating the **consultation rate** is shown in formula 15.21.

Case-Mix Statistical Data

Case mix is a method of grouping patients according to a predefined set of characteristics. Diagnosis-related groups (DRGs) are often used to determine case mix in hospitals.

When calculating case mix using DRGs, the **case-mix index** (CMI) is the average DRG weight for patients discharged from the hospital. The CMI is a measure of the resources used in treating the patients in each hospital or group of hospitals. It may be calculated for all patients discharged, discharges by payer (table 15.9), and/or the discharges of a particular physician (table 15.10).

Table 15.11 provides an example of a case-mix calculation for 10 DRGs at Community Hospital. The CMI is calculated by multiplying the number of cases for each DRG by the relative weight of the DRG, summing the result (1511.2332) and dividing by the total number of cases (484). By convention, the CMI is calculated to five decimal points and rounded to four.

The CMI can be used to indicate the average reimbursement for the hospital. From table 15.9, the reimbursement is approximately 1.567 times the hospital's base rate. It also is a measure of the severity of illness of Medicare patients. In table 15.9, we can see that Medicare patients, as expected, have the highest CMI at 2.0059.

Other data analyzed by DRG include LOS and mortality rates. LOS and mortality data are benchmarked against the hospital's peer group and national data. The process of benchmarking is comparing the hospital's performance against an external standard or benchmark. An excellent source of information for benchmarking purposes is the Healthcare Cost Utilization Project database (HCUPnet), which is available online at http://hcup.ahrq.gov. A comparison of hospital and national data for DRG 127 appears in table 15.12.

Gross analysis of the data indicates that Community Hospital's ALOS and mortality rate are better than the national average. But, at the same time, the average charges are somewhat higher than the national average.

Check Your Understanding 15.8

Instructions: Using the table below, answer the following questions on a separate piece of paper.

1. ___ Twenty patients were discharged from the medical ICU during the week of January 1. Five of these patients had a hospital-acquired infection. What is the hospital-acquired infection rate for the week of January 1?

2. ___ During the month of April, 822 patients were discharged from Community Hospital. One hundred twenty-two (122) patients had consults from specialty physicians. What is the consultation rate for the month of April?

3. ___ Dr. Green discharged 21 patients from Medicine Service during the month of August. The table below presents the number of patients discharged by DRG. Calculate the CMI for Dr. Green.

DRG	DRG Title	RW	N	N*DRG
079	Respiratory Infections & Inflammations Age >17 w/ CC	1.6238	2	
085	Pleural Effusion w/ CC	1.2405	1	
087	Pulmonary Edema	1.3654	3	
089	Simple Pneumonia & Pleurisy Age >17 w/ CC	1.0320	1	
121	Circulatory Disorders w/ AMI & Major Complications, Discharged Alive	1.6136	1	
130	Peripheral Vascular Disorders w/ CC	0.9425	1	
143	Chest Pain	0.5659	1	
174	GI Hemorrhage w/ CC	1.0060	2	
182	Esophagitis, Gastroenteritis, & Miscellaneous Digestive Disorders Age >17 w/ CC	0.8413	2	
240	Connective Tissue Disorder w/ CC	1.4051	1	
243	Medical Back Problems	0.7658	1	
316	Renal Failure	1.2692	1	
395	Red Blood Cell Disorders Age >17	0.8328	1	
416	Septicemia Age >17	1.6774	1	
450	Poisoning & Toxic Effects of Drugs Age >17 w/o CC	0.4282	1	
475	Respiratory System Diagnosis w/ Ventilator Support	3.6091	1	
Total			**21**	

Formula 15.21.   Formula for calculating consultation rate

$$\text{Consultation rate} = \frac{\text{Total number of patients receiving consultations for a given period}}{\text{Total number of discharges and deaths for the same period}}$$

Table 15.9.   Case-mix index by payer, Community Hospital, 2004

Payor	CMI	N
Commercial	1.8830	283
Government Managed Care	.9880	470
Managed Care	1.4703	2336
Medicaid	1.3400	962
Medicare	2.0059	1776
Other	1.3251	148
Self-Pay	1.3462	528
Total	1.5670	6503

Table 15.10.   Case-mix index of one physician, 2004

Physician	CMI	N
A	1.0235	71
B	1.6397	71
C	1.1114	86
Total	1.2501	228

Table 15.11.   Calculation of case-mix index for ten DRGs, Community Hospital, 2004

DRG	Number (N)	DRG Weight	N × DRG Weight
124	84	1.4367	120.6828
125	41	1.0947	44.8827
127	61	1.0265	62.6165
174	41	1.0025	41.1025
182	43	0.8223	35.3589
202	45	1.3120	59.0400
320	26	0.8853	23.0178
416	31	1.5918	49.3458
475	61	3.6000	219.6000
483	51	16.7762	855.5862
Total	484		1511.2332
CMI			3.1224

Table 15.12.   Benchmark data, Community Hospital vs. national average for DRG 127, heart failure and shock

	ALOS	Mortality Rate	Average Charges
Community Hospital	4.6	0.3%	$12,042
National Average	5.4	5.0%	$9,694

Statistical Data Used in Ambulatory Care Facilities

Ambulatory care includes healthcare services provided to patients who are not hospitalized (that is, who are not considered inpatients or residents and do not stay in the healthcare facility overnight). Such patients are referred to as outpatients. Most ambulatory care services today are provided in freestanding physicians' offices, emergency care centers, and ambulatory surgery centers that are not owned or operated by acute care organizations. Hospitals do, however, provide many hospital-based healthcare services to outpatients. Hospital outpatients receive services in one or more areas within the hospital, including clinics, same-day surgery departments, diagnostic departments, and emergency departments.

Outpatient statistics include records of the number of patient visits and the types of services provided. Many different terms are used to describe outpatients and ambulatory care services, including:

- *Hospital ambulatory care:* Hospital-directed preventive, therapeutic, and rehabilitative services provided by physicians and their surrogates to patients who are not hospital inpatients or home care patients
- *Outpatient:* A patient who receives care without being admitted for inpatient or residential care
- *Hospital outpatient:* A patient who receives services in one or more of the facilities owned and operated by a hospital
- *Emergency outpatient:* A patient who is admitted to the emergency department or equivalent service of a hospital for diagnosis and treatment of a condition that requires immediate medical services, dental services, or related healthcare services
- *Clinic outpatient:* A patient who is admitted to a clinical service of a clinic or hospital for diagnosis or treatment on an ambulatory basis
- ***Referred outpatient:*** A patient who is provided special hospital-based diagnostic or therapeutic services on an ambulatory basis; the services are ordered by a referring

physician and the responsibility for medical care remains with that physician rather than with the hospital

- *Outpatient visit:* A provision of services to an outpatient in one or more units or facilities located in or directed by the provider maintaining the outpatient healthcare services
- *Encounter:* A contact between a patient and a health-care professional who has primary responsibility for assessing and treating the patient at a given contact and for exercising independent medical judgment
- *Occasion of service:* A specified, identifiable service involved in the care of a patient or consumer that is not an encounter; occasions of service may be the result of an encounter, for example, to fulfill physicians' orders for tests or procedures ordered as part of an encounter
- *Ambulatory surgery centers:* Hospital-based or free-standing surgical facilities that perform elective surgical procedures on patients who are classified as outpatients and who are typically released from the facility on the same day the surgery was performed; also referred to as short-stay surgery, one-day surgery, same-day surgery, or come-and-go surgery services

Public Health Statistics and Epidemiological Information

Just as statistics are collected in the healthcare organizational setting, they also are collected on a community, regional, and national basis. **Vital statistics** are an example of data collected and reported at these levels. The term *vital statistics* refers to the collection and analysis of data related to the crucial events in life: birth, death, marriage, divorce, fetal death, and induced terminations of pregnancy. These statistics are used to identify trends. For example, a higher-than-expected death rate among newborns may be an indication of the lack of prenatal services in a community. A number of deaths in a region due to the same cause may indicate an environmental problem.

These types of data are used as part of the effort to preserve and improve the health of a defined population—the public health. The study of factors that influence the health status of a population is called epidemiology.

National Vital Statistics System

The **National Vital Statistics System** (NVSS) is responsible for maintaining the official vital statistics of the United States. These statistics are provided to the federal government by state-operated registration systems. The NVSS is housed in the National Center for Health Statistics (NCHS) of the Centers for Disease Control and Prevention (CDC).

To facilitate data collection, standard forms and model procedures for the uniform registration of events are developed and recommended for state use through cooperative activities of the individual states and the NCHS. The standard certificates represent the minimum basic data set

necessary for the collection and publication of comparable national, state, and local vital statistics data. The standard forms are revised about every 10 years, with the last revision completed in 2003. To effectively implement these new certificates, the NCHS is working with its state partners to improve the timeliness, quality, and sustainability of the vital statistics system, along with collection of the revised and new content of the 2003 certificates. These revisions can be viewed online at cdc.gov.

The certificate of live birth is used for registration purposes and is composed of two parts. The first part contains the information related to the child and the parents. The second part is used to collect data about the mother's pregnancy. This information is used for the collection of aggregate data only. No identification information appears on this portion of the certificate nor does it ever appear on the official certificate of birth. Pregnancy-related information includes complications of pregnancy, concurrent illnesses or conditions affecting pregnancy, and abnormal conditions and/or congenital anomalies of the newborn. Lifestyle factors such as use of alcohol and tobacco also are collected. Thus, the birth certificate is the major source of maternal and natality statistics. A listing of pregnancy-related information appears in figure 15.7.

Data collected from death certificates are used to compile causes of death in the United States. The certificate of death contains decedent information, place of death information, medical certification, and disposition information. Data on causes of death are classified and coded using the International Classification of Diseases (ICD). Beginning in 1999, the United States implemented ICD-10 for the coding of causes of death. Examples of the content of death certificates appear in figure 15.8.

A report of fetal death is completed when a pregnancy results in a stillbirth. This report contains information on the parents, the history of the pregnancy, and the cause of the fetal death. Information collected on the pregnancy is the same as that recorded on the birth certificate. To assess the effects of environmental exposures on the fetus, the parents' occupational data are collected. Data items related to the fetus include:

- Cause of fetal death, whether fetal or maternal
- Other significant conditions of the fetus or mother
- When fetus died (before labor, during labor or delivery, or unknown)
- Risk factors related to pregnancy

The report of induced termination of pregnancy records information on the place of the induced termination of pregnancy, the type of termination procedure, and the patient. (See figure 15.9.)

A tool for monitoring and exploring the interrelationships between infant death and risk factors at birth is the linked birth and infant death data set. This is a service provided by the NCHS. In this data set, the information from the death

Figure 15.7. Content of U.S. certificate of live birth, 2003

Child's Information
Child's name
Time of birth
Sex
Date of birth
Facility (hospital) Name
    (if not an institution, give
    street address)
City
County

Mother's Information
Current legal name
Date of birth
Mother's name prior to first
    marriage
Birthplace
Residence (state)
County
City
Street number
Zip code
Inside city limits?
Mother married?
If no, has paternity
    acknowledgment been
    signed in the hospital?
Social Security number (SSN)
    requested for child?
Mother's SSN
Father's SSN
Education
Hispanic origin?
Race

Father
Current legal name
Date of birth
Birthplace
Education
Hispanic origin?
Race

Pregnancy History
Date of first prenatal care
    visit
Date of last prenatal care visit

Total number of prenatal visits
    for this pregnancy
Number of previous live births
Mother's height
Mother's pregnancy weight
Mother's weight at delivery
Did mother get WIC food for
    herself during this pregnancy?
Number of previous live births
Number of other pregnancy
    outcomes
Cigarette smoking before and
    during pregnancy
Principal source of payment for
    this delivery
Date of last live birth
Date of last other pregnancy
    outcome
Date last normal menses began
Risk factors in this pregnancy
Infections present and/or
    treated during this pregnancy
Obstetric procedures
Onset of labor
Characteristics of labor and
    delivery
Method of delivery
Maternal mortality

Newborn Information
Birth weight
Obstetric estimate of gestation
Apgar score (1 and 5 minutes)
Plurality
If not born first (born first,
    second, third, etc.)
Abnormal conditions of
    newborn
Congenital anomalies of the
    newborn
Was infant transferred within
    24 hours of delivery?
Is infant living at time of
    report?
Is infant being breast fed at
    discharge?

Source: NVSS 2005.

Figure 15.8. Content of U.S. certificate of death, 2003

Decedent Information
Name
Sex
Social Security number
Age
Date of birth
Birthplace
Residence (state)
County
City or town
Street and number
Zip code
Inside city limit?
Ever in U.S. armed forces?
Marital status at time of death
Surviving spouse's name (If
    wife, give name prior to
    first marriage)
Father's name
Mother's name (prior to first
    marriage)
Decedent's education
Hispanic origin?
Race
Informant's name
Relationship to decedent
Mailing address

Disposition Information
Method of disposition
Place of disposition
    (cemetery, crematory, other)
Location
Name and address of funeral
    facility

Place of Death Information
Place of death
If hospital, indicate inpatient,
    emergency room/outpatient,
    dead on arrival
If somewhere other than
    hospital, indicate hospice,
    nursing home/long-term
    care facility, decedent's
    home, other

Facility name
City, state, zip code
County

Medical Certification
Date pronounced dead
Time pronounced dead
Signature of person
    pronouncing death
Date signed
Actual or presumed date
    of death
Actual or presumed time
    of death
Was medical examiner
    contacted?
Immediate cause of death
Due to _____
Due to _____
Due to _____
Other significant conditions
    contributing to death
Was an autopsy performed?
Were autopsy findings available
    to complete the cause
    of death?
Did tobacco use contribute
    to death?
If female, indicate pregnancy
    status
Manner of death
For deaths due to injury:
    Date of injury
    Time of injury
    Place of injury
    Injury at work?
    Location of injury
    Describe how injury occurred
    If transportation injury,
        specify if driver/operator,
        passenger, pedestrian, other

Source: NVSS 2005.

certificate (such as age and underlying or multiple causes of death) is linked to the information in the birth certificate (such as age, race, birth weight, prenatal care usage, maternal education, and so on) for each infant who dies in the United States, Puerto Rico, the Virgin Islands, and Guam. The purpose of the data set is to use the many additional variables available from the birth certificate to conduct a detailed analysis of infant mortality patterns.

Birth, death, fetal death, and termination of pregnancy certificates provide vital information for use in medical research, epidemiological studies, and other public health programs. In addition, they are the source of data for compiling morbidity, birth, and mortality rates that describe the health of a given population at the local, state, or national level. Because of their many uses, the data on these certificates must be complete and accurate.

Figure 15.9. Content of U.S. standard report of induced termination of pregnancy, 1997

Place of Induced Termination
Facility name
Address (city, town, state,
    county)

Patient Information
Patient Identification
Age at last birthday
Marital status
Date or pregnancy termination
Residence (city, town, state,
    county

Inside city limits?
Zip code
Hispanic origin?
Race
Education
Date last normal menses began
Clinical estimate of gestation
Previous pregnancies
    Live births
    Other terminations
Type of termination procedure

Source: NVSS 2005.

Population-Based Statistics

Population-based statistics are based on the mortality and morbidity rates from which the health of a population can be inferred. The entire defined population is used in the collection and reporting of these statistics. The size of the defined population serves as the denominator in the calculation of these rates.

Birth Rates and Measures of Infant Mortality

Two community-based rates that are commonly used to describe a community's health are the **crude birth rate** and measures of infant mortality. The official international definition of a live birth is the delivery of a product of conception that shows any sign of life after complete removal from the mother. A sign of life may consist of a breath or cry, any spontaneous movement, a pulse or heartbeat, or pulsation of the umbilical cord.

Rates that describe infant mortality are based on age. Therefore, the definitions for the various age groups must be strictly followed. Table 15.13 summarizes the calculations for community-based birth and **infant mortality rates.** These mortality or death rates are broken down as follows:

- *Crude birth rate:* As shown in formula 15.22, the crude birth rate is the number of live births divided by the population at risk. As the formula shows, community rates are calculated using the multiplier 1,000, 10,000, or 100,000. The purpose is to bring the rate to a whole number, as discussed earlier in the chapter. The result of the formula would be stated as the number of live births per 1,000 population. For example, if there were 7,532 live births in a community of 600,000 in 1999, the crude birth rate for that year would be 12.6 per 1,000 population ([7,532/600,000] × 1000 = 1000).
- *Neonatal mortality rate:* The neonatal mortality rate can be used as an indirect measure of the quality of

prenatal care and/or the mother's prenatal behavior (for example, alcohol, drug, or tobacco use). The neonatal period is the period from birth up to, but not including, 28 days of age. In the formula for calculating the neonatal mortality rate, the numerator is the number of deaths of infants under 28 days of age during a given time period and the denominator is the total number of live births during the same time period.

- *Postneonatal mortality rate:* The postneonatal mortality rate is often used as an indicator of the quality of the home or community environment of infants. The postneonatal period is the period from 28 days up to, but not including, one year of age. In the formula for calculating the postneonatal mortality rate, the numerator is the number of deaths among infants from age 28 days up to but not including one year during a given time period and the denominator is the total number of live births less the number of neonatal deaths during the same time period.
- *Infant mortality rate:* The infant mortality rate is the summary of the neonatal and postneonatal mortality rates. In the formula for calculating the infant mortality rate, the numerator is the number of deaths among infants under one year of age and the denominator is the number of live births during the same period. The infant mortality rate is the most commonly used measure for comparing health status among nations. All the rates are expressed in terms of the number of deaths per 1,000.

Death (Mortality) Rates

Other measures of mortality with which the HIM professional should be familiar include the following:

- *Crude death rate:* The crude death rate is a measure of the actual or observed mortality in a given population. Crude death rates apply to a population without regard

Table 15.13.   Calculation of community-based birth and infant death (mortality) rates

Measure	Numerator (x)	Denominator (y)	10^n
Crude birth rate	Number of live births for a given community for a specified time period	Estimated population for the same community and the same time period	1,000
Neonatal death rate	Number of deaths under 28 days up to, but not including, one year of age during a given time period	Number of live births during the same time period	1,000
Postneonatal death rate	Number of deaths from 28 days up to, but not including, one year of age during a given time period	Number of live births during the same time period less neonatal deaths	1,000
Infant death rate	Number of deaths under one year of age during a given time period	Number of live births during the same time period	1,000

Formula 15.22.   Formula for calculating crude birth rate

$$\text{Crude birth rate} = \frac{\text{Number of live births for a given community for a specified time period}}{\text{Estimated population for the same community and the same time period}} \times 10^n$$

to characteristics such as age, race, and sex. They measure the proportion of the population that has died during a given period of time (usually one year) or the number of deaths in a community per 1,000 for a given period of time. The formula for calculating the crude death rate is shown in formula 15.23.

- *Cause-specific death rate:* As its name indicates, the cause-specific death rate is the rate of death due to a specified cause. It may be calculated for an entire population or for any age, sex, or race. In the formula, the numerator is the number of deaths due to a specified cause for a given time period and the denominator is the estimated population for the same time period. Table 15.14 displays cause-specific death rates for men and women due to influenza and pneumonia for the year 2001. The cause-specific death rates for each age group are consistently higher for men than for women. This information could lead to an investigation of why men are more susceptible to death from pneumonia than women.

- *Case fatality rate:* The case fatality rate measures the probability of death among the diagnosed cases of a disease, most often acute illness. In the formula for calculating the case fatality rate, the numerator is the number of deaths due to a specific disease that occurred during a specific time period and the denominator is the number of diagnosed cases during the same time period. The higher the case fatality rate, the more virulent the infection.

- *Proportionate mortality rate:* The proportionate mortality ratio (PMR) is a measure of mortality due to a specific cause for a specific time period. In the formula for calculating the PMR, the numerator is the number of deaths due to a specific disease for a specific time period and the denominator is the number of deaths from all causes for the same time period. Table 15.15 (p. 420) displays the PMRs for influenza pneumonia in the United States in 2001.

- *Maternal mortality rate:* The maternal mortality rate measures the deaths associated with pregnancy for a specific community for a specific period of time. It is calculated only for deaths that are directly related to pregnancy. In the formula for calculating the maternal mortality rate, the numerator is the number of deaths attributed to causes related to pregnancy during a specific time period for a given community and the denominator is the number of live births reported during the same time period for the same community. Because the maternal mortality rate is very small, it is usually expressed as the number of deaths per 100,000 live births.

Table 15.16 (p. 420) summarizes the calculations for these rates.

Check Your Understanding 15.9

Instructions: Review the mortality data in table 15.17 and then answer the following questions on a separate piece of paper.

1. ___ What is the crude death rate per 10,000 for men?
2. ___ What is the crude death rate per 10,000 for women?
3. ___ What is the crude death rate per 10,000 for the entire group?
4. ___ What is the crude death rate per 10,000 for men ages 35–44?
5. ___ What is the crude death rate per 10,000 for women ages 35–55?

Formula 15.23.   Formula for calculating crude death rate

$$\text{Crude death rate} = \frac{\text{Total number of deaths for a population during a specified time period}}{\text{Estimated population for the same time period}} \times 10^n$$

Table 15.14.   Cause-specific mortality rates, by sex, due to influenza and pneumonia (ICD-10 codes J10–J18.9) age 45+, United States, 2001

Age Group	Women			Men		
	Population	Deaths	Rate/100,000	Population	Deaths	Rate/100,000
45–54	19,971,971	702	3.51	19,256,395	1,009	5.71
55–64	13,160,005	1,117	8.49	12,155,918	1,587	13.06
65–74	10,020,545	2,918	29.12	8,301,935	3,732	44.95
75–84	7,585,929	9,383	123.69	4,996,556	9,294	148.44
85+	3,127,729	19,689	6229.50	1,320,580	10,502	795.26
Total	53,866,179	33,809	62.76	46,031,384	26,124	60.08

Source: CDC 2005a.

Measures of Morbidity

Two measures are commonly used to describe the presence of disease in a community or specific location (for example, a nursing home): **incidence** and **prevalence rates.** Disease is defined as any illness, injury, or disability. Incidence and prevalence measures can be broken down by race, sex, age, or other characteristics of a population.

An *incidence rate* is used to compare the frequency of disease in populations. Populations are compared using rates instead of raw numbers because rates adjust for differences in population size. The incidence rate is the probability or risk of illness in a population over a period of time. The formula for calculating the incidence rate is shown in formula 15.24. The denominator represents the population from which the case in the numerator arose, such as a nursing home, school, or organization. For 10^n, a value is selected so that the smallest rate calculated results in a whole number. The *prevalence rate* is the proportion of persons in a population who have a particular disease at a specific point in time or over a specified period of time. The formula for calculating the prevalence rate is shown in formula 15.25. The prevalence rate describes the magnitude of an epidemic and can be an indicator of the medical resources needed in a community for the duration of the epidemic.

Table 15.15.   Proportionate mortality ratios for influenza and pneumonia (ICD-10 codes J10–J18.9) age 45+, United States, 2001

Age Group	Influenza and Pneumonia Deaths	Total Deaths	PMR/100
0–4	411	32,675	1.26
5–9	46	3,093	1.49
10–14	46	4,002	1.15
15–19	66	13,555	0.49
20–24	115	18,697	0.62
25–34	339	41,683	0.81
35–44	983	91,674	1.07
45–54	1,801	168,065	1.07
55–64	2,704	244,139	1.11
65–74	6,650	430,960	1.54
75–84	18,677	701,929	2.66
85+	30,191	665,531	4.54

Source: CDC 2005a.

Table 15.16.   Calculation of community-based death (mortality) rates

Rate	Numerator (x)	Denominator (y)	10^n
Crude death rate	Total number of deaths for a population during a specified time period	Estimated population for the same time period	1,000 or 10,000 or 100,000
Cause-specific death rate	Total number of deaths due to a specific cause during a specified time period	Estimated population for the same time period	100,000
Case fatality rate	Total number of deaths due to a specific disease during a specified time period	Total number of cases due to a specific disease during the same time period	100
Proportionate mortality (ratio)	Total number of deaths due to a specific cause during a specified time period	Total number of deaths from all causes during the same time period	NA
Maternal mortality rate	Total number of deaths due to pregnancy-related conditions during a specified time period	Total number of live births during the same time period	100,000

It is easy to confuse incidence and prevalence rates. The distinction is in the numerators of their formulas. The numerator in the formula for the incidence rate is the number of new cases occurring in a given time period. The numerator in the formula for the prevalence rate is all cases present during a given time period. In addition, the incidence rate includes only patients whose illness began during a specified time period whereas the prevalence rate includes all patients from a specified cause regardless of when the illness began. Moreover, the prevalence rate includes a patient until he or she recovers.

Table 15.17.   Data for Check Your Understanding 15.9

Sex-Specific Death Rates, United States, 2001				
	Women		Men	
Age Group	Population	Deaths	Population	Deaths
Under 1 Year	1,968,011	12,091	2,057,922	15,477
1–4	7,491,412	2,208	7,841,553	2,899
5–9	9,861,089	1,366	10,347,035	1,727
10–14	10,199,195	1,561	10,711,245	2,441
15–19	9,847,662	3,789	10,423,650	9,766
20–24	9,630,499	4,500	10,080,924	14,197
25–34	19,698,788	12,926	20,116,087	28,757
35–44	22,675,474	33,510	22,464,812	58,164
45–54	19,971,971	63,217	19,256,395	104,848
55–64	13,160,005	99,181	12,155,918	144,958
65–74	10,020,545	189,379	8,301,935	241,581
75–84	7,585,929	361,187	4,996,556	340,742
85+	3,127,729	447,998	1,320,580	217,533
Total	145,238,309	1,232,913	140,074,612	1,183,090

Source: CDC 2005a.

National Notifiable Diseases Surveillance System

In 1878, Congress authorized the U.S. Marine Hospital Service to collect morbidity reports on cholera, smallpox, plague, and yellow fever from U.S. consuls overseas. This information was used to implement quarantine measures to prevent the spread of these diseases to the United States. In 1879, Congress provided for the weekly collection and publication of reports of these diseases. In 1893, Congress expanded the scope to include weekly reporting from states and municipalities. To provide for more uniformity in data collection, Congress enacted a law in 1902 that directed the surgeon general to provide standard forms for the collection, compilation, and publication of reports at the national level. In 1912, the states and U.S. territories recommended that infectious disease be immediately reported by telegraph. By 1928, all states, the District of Columbia, Hawaii, and Puerto Rico were participating in the national reporting of 29 specified diseases. In 1961, the CDC assumed responsibility for the collection and publication of data concerning nationally notifiable diseases.

A **notifiable disease** is one for which regular, frequent, and timely information on individual cases is considered necessary to prevent and control disease. The list of notifiable diseases varies over time and by state. The Council of State and Territorial Epidemiologists (CSTE) collaborates with the CDC to determine which diseases should be reported. State reporting to the CDC is voluntary. However, all states generally report the internationally quarantinable diseases in accordance with the World Health Organization's International Health Regulations. Completeness of reporting varies by state and type of disease and may be influenced by any of the following factors:

- The type and severity of the illness
- Whether treatment in a healthcare facility was sought
- The diagnosis of an illness
- The availability of diagnostic services
- The disease-control measures in effect
- Public awareness of the disease
- The resources, priorities, and interests of state and local public health officials

Information that is reported includes date, county, age, sex, race/ethnicity, and disease-specific epidemiologic information;

Formula 15.24.   Formula for calculating incidence rate

$$\text{Incidence rate} = \frac{\text{Total number of new cases of a specific disease during a given time period}}{\text{Total population at risk during the same time period}} \times 10^n$$

Formula 15.25.   Formula for calculating prevalence rate

$$\text{Prevalence rate} = \frac{\text{All new and preexisting cases of a specific disease during a given time period}}{\text{Total population during the same time period}} \times 10^n$$

personal identifiers are not included. A strict CSTE Data Release Policy regulates dissemination of the data. A list of nationally notifiable infectious diseases appears in figure 15.10. The list is updated annually.

National morbidity data are reported weekly. Public health managers and providers use the reports to rapidly identify disease epidemics and to understand patterns of disease occurrence. Case-specific information is included in the reports. Changes in age, sex, race/ethnicity, and geographic distributions can be monitored and investigated as necessary.

Figure 15.10.   Nationally notifiable infectious diseases, United States, 2005

Acquired Immunodeficiency Syndrome (AIDS)	Malaria
Anthrax	Measles
Arboviral neuroinvasive and non-neuroinvasive diseases	Meningococcal disease
California serogroup virus disease	Mumps
	Pertusis
Eastern equine encephalitis virus disease	Plague
	Poliomyelitis, paralytic
Powassan virus disease	Psittacosis
St. Louis encephalitis virus disease	Q fever
	Rabies (animal and human)
West Nile virus disease	Rocky Mountain spotted fever
Western equine encephalitis virus disease	Rubella
	Rubella, congenital syndrome
Botulism	Salmonellosis
Brucellosis	Severe Acute Respiratory Syndrome–associated Coronavirus (SARS-CoV) disease
Charcroid	
Chlamydia trachomatis, genital	Shigellosis
Cholera	Smallpox
Coccidioidomycosis	Streptococcal disease, invasive, Group A
Cryptosporidiosis	
Cyclosporiasis	Streptococcal toxic-shock syndrome
Diphtheria	
Ehrlichiosis	*Streptococcus pneumoniae,* drug resistant, invasive disease
Enterohemorrhagic *Escherichia coli*	*Streptococcus pneumoniae,* invasive in children <5 years
Giardiasis	
Gonorrhea	Syphilis
Haemophilus influenzae, invasive disease	Syphilis, primary
	Syphilis, secondary
Hansen disease	Syphilis, latent
Hantavirus pulmonary syndrome	Syphilis, late latent
Hemolytic uremic syndrome, post-diarrheal	Syphilis, latent unknown duration
	Neurosyphilis
Hepatitis, viral, acute	Syphilis, late, non-neurological
Hepatitis A, acute	Syphilis, congenital
Hepatitis B, acute	Syphilitic stillbirth
Hepatitis B virus, perinatal infection	Tetanus
	Toxic-shock syndrome
Hepatitis C, acute	Trichinellosis (Trichinosis)
Hepatitis, viral, chronic	Tuberculosis
Chronic Hepatitis B	Tularemia
Hepatitis C virus infection (past or present)	Typhoid fever
	Vancomycin–intermediate *Staphylococcus aureus* (VISA)
HIV infection	
Influenza-associated pediatric mortality	Vancomycin–resistant *Staphylococcus aureus* (VRSA)
Legionellosis	Varicella (morbidity)
Listeriosis	Varicella (deaths only)
Lyme disease	Yellow fever

Presentation of Statistical Data

Collected data are often more meaningful when presented in graphic form. Tables, charts, and graphs offer the opportunity to analyze data sets and to explore, understand, and present frequency distributions, trends, and relationships in the data. The purpose of tables, charts, and graphs is to communicate information about the data to the user of the data.

Whatever type of graphic form is used, it should:

- Display the data
- Allow the user to think about the meaning of the data
- Avoid distortion of the data
- Encourage the user to make comparisons
- Reveal data at several levels, from a broad overview to the fine detail

Methods of displaying the data in graphic form are discussed in the following subsections.

Tables

A table is an orderly arrangement of values that groups data into rows and columns. Almost any type of quantitative information can be organized into a table. Tables are useful for demonstrating patterns and other kinds of relationships. In addition, they may serve as the basis for more visual displays of data, such as charts and graphs, where some of the detail may be lost. However, because tables are not very interesting, they should be used sparingly.

A useful first step is to prepare a table shell that shows how the data will be organized and displayed. A table shell is the outline of a table with everything in place except for the data. (See table 15.18.) A table should contain all the information the reader needs to understand the data in it. It should have the following characteristics:

- It is a logical unit.
- It is self-explanatory and can stand on its own when photocopied and/or removed from its context.
- All sources are specified.
- Specific, understandable headings are provided for every column and row.
- Row and column totals are checked for accuracy.
- Blank cells are not left empty. When no information is available for a particular cell, the cell should contain a zero or a dash.
- Categories are mutually exclusive and exhaustive.

Table 15.18. Table shell

		Sex				Total	
		Male		Female			
Box Head	Age	Number	%	Number	%	Number	%
Stub	Row Variable	→→→→→	→→→→→	→→→→→	→→→→→	→→→→→	→→→→→
	< 45			Column Variable			
↓	45–54			↓			
↓	55–64			↓			
↓	65–74			↓			
↓	75+			↓			

Source: HHS 1994.

The data contained in tables should be aligned. Guidelines for aligning text and numbers include:

- Text in the table should be aligned at left.
- Text that serves as a column label may be centered.
- Numeric values should be aligned at right.
- When numeric values contain decimals, the decimals should be aligned.

The essential components of a table are summarized in figure 15.11.

Tables may contain information on one, two, or three variables. Tables 15.19 (p. 424) and 15.20 (p. 424) are examples of one- and two-variable tables, respectively.

Charts and Graphs

Charts and graphs of various types are the best means for presenting data for quick visualization of relationships. They emphasize the main points and analyze and clarify relationships among variables.

Several principles are involved in the construction of charts and graphs. When constructing charts and graphs, the following points should be considered:

- *Distortion:* To avoid distorting the data, the representation of the numbers should be proportional to the numerical quantities represented.
- *Proportion and scale:* Graphs should emphasize the horizontal. It is easier for the eye to read along the horizontal axis from left to right. Also, graphs should be greater in length than height. A useful guideline is to follow the three-quarter-high rule. This rule states that the height (*y*-axis) of the graph should be three-fourths the length (*x*-axis) of the graph.
- *Abbreviations:* Any abbreviations should be spelled out in notes.

Figure 15.11. Essential components of a table

Title	The title should be as complete as possible and should clearly relate to the content of the table. It should answer the following questions: • What are the data (e.g., counts, percentages)? • Who (e.g., white females with breast cancer; black males with lung cancer)? • Where are the data from (e.g., hospital, state, community)? • When (e.g., year, month)? A sample title might be: Site Distribution by Age and Sex of Cancer Patients upon First Admission to Community Hospital, 2000–2004
Box Head	The box head contains the captions or column headings. The heading of each column should contain as few words as possible but should explain exactly what the data in the column represent.
Stub	The row captions are knows as the stub. Items in the stub should be grouped to make it easy to interpret the data, for example, ages grouped into five-year intervals.
Cell	The cell is the box formed by the intersection of a column and a row.
Optional Items:	
Note	Notes are used to explain anything in the table that the reader cannot understand from the title, box head, or stub. They contain numbers, preliminary or revised numbers, or explanations of any unusual numbers. Definitions, abbreviations, and/or qualifications for captions or cell names should be footnoted. A note usually applies to a specific cell(s) within the table, and a symbol (e.g., ** or #) may be used to key the cell to the note. If several notes are used, it is better to use small letters than symbols or numbers. Note any numbers that may be confused with the numbers within the table.
Source	If data are used from a source outside the research, the exact reference to the source should be given. The source lends authenticity to the data and allows the reader to locate the original information if he or she needs it.

Source: HHS 1994.

Table 15.19. One-variable table, Community Hospital admissions by gender, 2004

Gender	Number	%
Male	3,141	46.0%
Female	3,683	54.0%
Total	6,824	100.0%

Table 15.20. Two-variable table, Community Hospital admissions by race and gender, 2004

Race	Gender Male	Gender Female	Total
White	2,607	2,946	5,553
Non-white	534	737	1,271
Total	3,141	3,683	6,824

- *Color:* Color may be used to highlight groupings that appear in the graph.
- *Print:* Both upper- and lowercase letters should be used in titles; the use of all capital letters can be difficult to read.

Bar Charts

Bar charts are used to display data from one or more variables. The bars may be drawn vertically or horizontally. The simplest bar chart is the one-variable bar chart. In this type of chart, a bar represents each category of the variable. For example, if the data in table 15.19 were displayed in a bar chart, "gender" would be the variable and "male and female" would be the variable categories. Figure 15.12 displays the data from table 15.19 as a bar chart. The length or height of each bar is proportional to the number of males and females discharged. Presentation of the data in a bar chart makes it easy to see that more males than females were admitted to Community Hospital in 2004.

Figure 15.13 displays the two-variable data from table 15.20 as a two-variable or grouped-variable bar chart in a three-dimensional format. Computer software makes it easy to present data in this way. However, presenting data in a three-dimensional format can be tricky. The reader may not always be able to estimate the true height of the bar. In a three-dimensional bar chart, the back edges of the bar appear higher than the front edge, as in figure 15.13. To make sure the reader correctly interprets the chart, the bars should include the actual values for each category.

Figure 15.14 presents guidelines for constructing bar charts.

Pie Charts

A **pie chart** is an easily understood chart in which the sizes of the slices of the pie show the proportional contribution of each part. Pie charts can be used to show the component parts of a single group or variable.

Figure 15.12. One-variable bar chart, Community Hospital admissions by gender, 2004

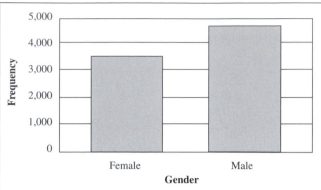

Figure 15.13. Two-variable bar chart, Community Hospital admissions by race and sex, 2004

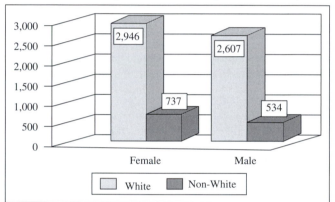

Figure 15.14. Guidelines for constructing a bar chart

When constructing a bar chart, keep the following points in mind:
- Arrange the bar categories in a natural order, such as alphabetical order, order by increasing age, or an order that will produce increasing or decreasing bar lengths.
- The bars may be positioned vertically or horizontally.
- The length of the bars should be proportional to the frequency of the event.
- Avoid using more than three bars (categories) within a group of bars.
- Leave a space between adjacent groups of bars, but not between bars within a group.
- Code different categories of variables by differences in bar color, shading, and/or cross-hatching. Include a legend that explains the coding system.

To calculate the size of each slice of the pie, first determine the proportion that each slice is to represent. Multiplying the proportion by 360 (the total number of degrees in a circle) will give the size of each slice of the pie in degrees.

Figure 15.15 shows payer data collected on admissions to Community Hospital. The summary data for one year show that managed care was the payer for 40.1 percent of the patients, Medicare was the payer for 30.5 percent, Medicaid was the payer for 16.5 percent, government-managed care was the payer for 8.19 percent of the patients, and 4.9 percent of the patients had commercial insurance.

With 40.1 percent of the pie chart, the managed care category equals approximately 144° (360° × 0.401 ≈ 144°). The Medicare category equals 30.5° (360° × 0.305 = 110°). The Medicaid category equals 59.4° (360 × 0.165 = 59.4°). The government-managed care category equals approximately 29° (360° × 0.081 ≈ 29°). And commercial insurance equals 17.6° (360° × 0.049 = 17.6°) Taken together, the slices equal 360° (144° + 110° + 59.4° + 29° + 17.6° = 360°).

The slices of the pie should be arranged in some logical order. By convention, the largest slices begin at twelve o'clock. Computer software is available to make the construction of pie charts easy. The pie chart in figure 15.15 was prepared using SPSS™.

Line Graphs

A **line graph** may be used to display time trends. The x-axis shows the unit of time from left to right, and the y-axis measures the values of the variable being plotted. A line graph does not represent a **frequency distribution.**

A line graph consists of a line connecting a series of points. Like all graphs, a line graph should be constructed so that it is easy to read. Selection of the proper scale, a complete and accurate title, and an informative legend is important. When a graph is too long and narrow, either vertically or horizontally, it has an awkward appearance and may exaggerate one aspect of the data.

A line graph is especially useful for plotting a large number of observations. It also allows several sets of data to be presented on one graph.

Either actual numbers or percentages may be used on the y-axis of the graph. Percentages should be used on the y-axis when more than one distribution is to be shown. A percentage distribution allows comparisons among groups where the actual totals are different.

When two or more sets of data are plotted on the same graph, the lines should be made different—solid or broken—for each set. However, the number of lines should be kept to a minimum to avoid confusion. Each line then should be identified in a legend located on the graph.

There are two kinds of time-trend data: point data and period data. Point data reflect an instant in time. Figure 15.16 displays point data—the total number of admissions for

Figure 15.15. Pie chart, Community Hospital admission by payer, 2004*

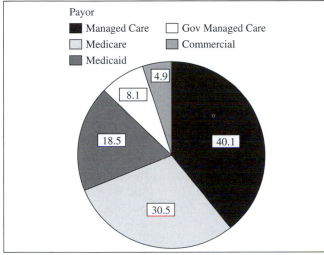

*rounded

Figure 15.16. Line graph with point data, Community Hospital admissions, 2000–2004

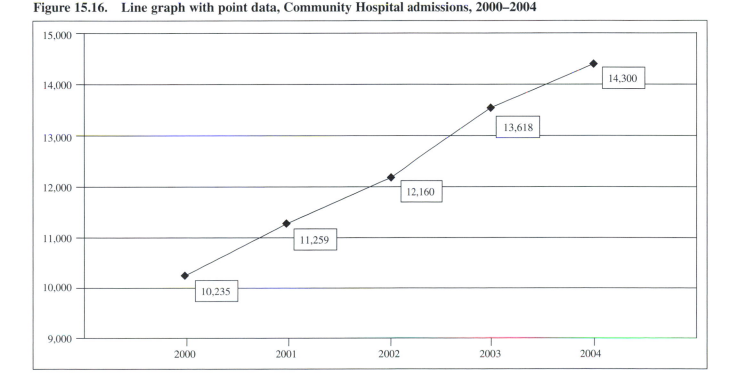

each year represented in the graph. Period data are averages or totals over a specified period of time, such as a five-year time frame. Table 15.21 summarizes period data for survival rates of patients diagnosed with kidney cancer. Figure 15.17 displays these period data in a line graph.

Histograms

A **histogram** is used to display a frequency distribution. It is different from a bar graph in that a bar graph is used to display data that fall into groups or categories. The categories are noncontinuous, or discrete. In a bar chart, the bars representing the different categories are separated. (See figures 15.12 and 15.13.) On the other hand, histograms are used to illustrate frequency distributions of continuous variables, such as age or LOS. A continuous variable can take on a fractional value (for example, 75.345°F). With continuous variables, there are no gaps between values because the values progress fractionally.

Table 15.21. Sample five-year survival rates for kidney cancer by stage, for patients diagnosed between 1996 and 2004

Year of Diagnosis	Midpoint of Interval	Survival Rate (%)		
		Localized	Regional	Distant
1996–1998	1997	80	71	28
1999–2001	2000	84	71	29
2002–2004	2003	85	74	31

In a histogram, the frequency distribution may be displayed as a number or a percentage. The histogram consists of a series of bars. Each bar has one class interval as its base and the number (frequency) or percentage of cases in that class interval as its height. A class interval is a type of category. It can represent one value in a frequency distribution (for example, three years of age) or a group of values (for example, ages three to five).

In histograms, there are no spaces between the bars. (See figure 15.18.) The lack of spaces between bars depicts the continuous nature of the distribution. The sum of the heights of the bars represents the total number, or 100 percent, of the cases. Histograms should be used when the distribution of the data needs to be emphasized more than the values of the distribution.

Frequency Polygons

A **frequency polygon** is an alternative to a histogram. Like a histogram, it is a graph of a frequency distribution, but in line form rather than bar form. The advantage of frequency polygons is that several of them can be placed on the same graph to make comparisons. Another advantage is that frequency polygons are easy to interpret.

When constructing a frequency polygon, the x-axis should be made longer than the y-axis to avoid distorting the data. The frequency of observations is always placed on the y-axis and the scale of the variable on the x-axis. The frequency polygon in figure 15.19 plots the same data that appear in the histogram in figure 15.18. Because the x-axis represents the entire frequency distribution, the line starts at zero cases and ends with zero cases.

Figure 15.17.   Period data trend line: Survival rates for kidney cancer by stage for patients diagnosed, 1996–2004

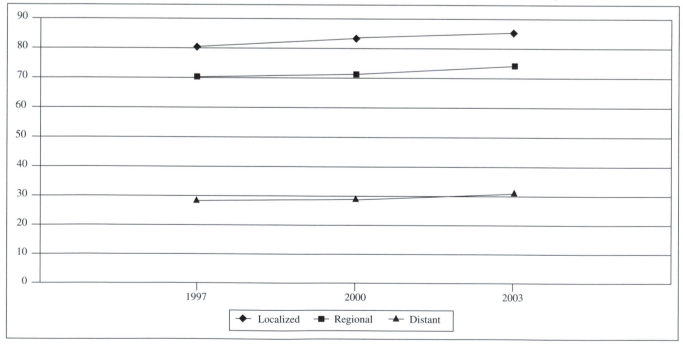

Scatter Charts

Scatter charts, also called scatter plots or scatter diagrams, are used when one wants to determine if there is a relationship between two variables, such as charges and LOS. Data collected for scatter charts must be at the interval or ratio level of measurement. The data for the two variables are arranged in pairs; one of the two variables is plotted on the *x*-axis and the other variable is plotted on the *y*-axis. The closer the data points come to making a straight line, the stronger the relationship between the two variables. If the data points form a straight line from the lower left of the *x*-axis to the upper right on the *y*-axis, the relationship is positive. (See figure 15.20, p. 428.) If the line begins at a high value on the *y*-axis and descends to a low value on the *x*-axis, the relationship is negative. (See figure 15.21, p. 428.) If the data points are widely scattered, there is no relationship between the two variables. (See figure 15.22, p. 428.)

Bubble Charts

A **bubble chart** is a type of scatter plot with circular symbols used to compare three variables; the size of the symbol indicates the value of a third variable. In developing the chart, one variable is displayed on the vertical or *y*-axis, and two variables are displayed on the horizontal or *x*-axis. Data must be at the interval or ratio-level of measurement.

As an example, an administrator is interested in displaying the average charges for the five highest volume DRGs in the organization. The number of discharges will be displayed on the *x*-axis, and average charges will be displayed on the *y*-axis. The size of the bubble indicates the percentage of total discharges for each DRG. The data are displayed in table 15.22, p. 428, and the corresponding bubble chart is displayed in figure 15.23, p. 429. It can easily be seen that DRG 391, Normal Newborn, has the highest proportion of overall discharges and the lowest average charges among the top-volume DRGs.

Stem and Leaf Plots

In **stem and leaf plots,** data can be organized so that the shape of a frequency distribution is revealed. As an example, a stem and leaf plot will be constructed on the age of 12 patients discharged from DRG 15, Nonspecific Cerebrovascular and Precerebral Occlusion without Infarction. The ages are ranked in order from lowest to highest:

44 51 52 52 62 65 65 66 68 72 76 82

Figure 15.18.   Histogram, Community Hospital LOS of patients discharged from DRG 127, 2004

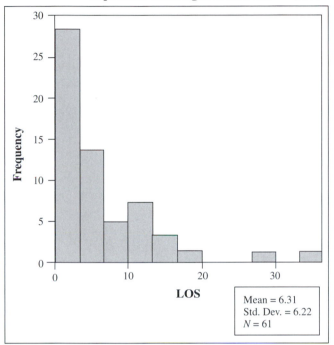

Mean = 6.31
Std. Dev. = 6.22
N = 61

Figure 15.19.   Frequency polygon, Community Hospital LOS of patients discharged from DRG 127, 2004

To develop the plot, break each number into two parts. The last number is called the leaf and the rest of the number is called the stem. Thus, for the number 51, 1 is the leaf and 5 is the stem, and for the number 125, 5 is the leaf and 12 is the stem. The data are then arranged in a table that looks somewhat like a T, with the stem portion in the first column and the leaf portion in the second column. For our data set, the stems are 4, 5, 6, 7 and 8. The leaf portion is then filled in with the last digits that correspond to each stem as shown below:

The completed plot reveals the distribution of the data set. It can immediately be seen that the lowest value in the distribution is 44 and the highest is 82 and that there are five observations in the 60s age group. Turning the table on its side shows a fairly normal bell-shaped distribution.

Figure 15.20.   Scatter chart, perfect positive relationship

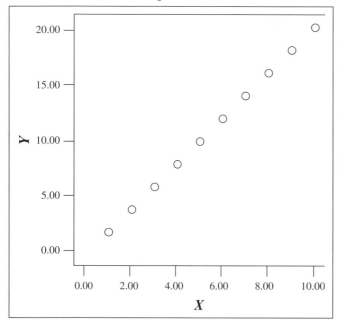

Figure 15.21.   Scatter chart, perfect negative relationship

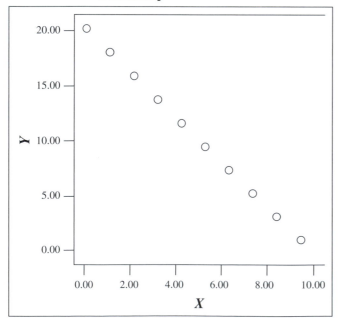

Figure 15.22.   Scatter chart, no relationship

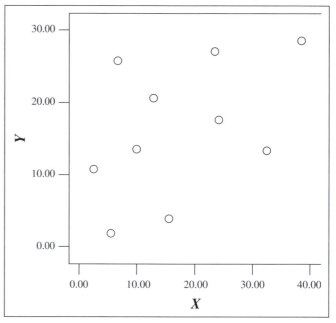

Table 15.22.   Top five high-volume discharges, average charges, and percent of total discharges, Community Hospital, 2004

DRG	Number of Discharges	Average Charges	Percent of Total Discharges
391—Normal Newborn	637	$1,239	9.8%
462—Rehabilitation	542	$21,517	8.4%
373—Vaginal Delivery w/o CC	505	$5,576	7.8%
127—Heart Failure and Shock	287	$12,043	4.4%
371—Cesarean Section w/o CC	189	$7,626	2.9%

Figure 15.23.   Bubble chart, top five high-volume discharges, average charges, and percent of total discharges, Community Hospital, 2004

Boxplots

Boxplots are useful in summarizing a data set. In a boxplot, a single variable in two categories can be compared. The boxplot reveals the **range, median,** and the 25th and 75th percentiles for the distribution. To illustrate, patients discharged from DRGs 14, Intracranial Hemorrhage or Cerebral Infarction, and 15, Nonspecific Cerebrovascular and Precerebral Occlusion without Infarction, are compared with age as the variable.

The frequency distributions appear in figures 15.24 and 15.25 (p. 430). Twelve patients were discharged from DRG 15 ranging in age from 44 to 82; 38 patients were discharged from DRG 14 ranging in age from 22 to 86. The boxplot, shown in figure 15.26 (p. 430), displays these data side by side. Even though there are more discharges from DRG 14 with a wider range in age, the median age for both DRGs is similar, 62 and 65 respectively. The interquartile range (25th to 75th quartile) for both groups is age 52 to 72 for DRG 14 and age 51 to 73 for DRG 15.

Spreadsheets and Statistical Packages

Electronic spreadsheets, such as Microsoft Excel, and statistical packages, such as SPSS or SAS, can be used to facilitate the data collection and analysis processes. The advantage of using one of these tools is that charts and graphs can be formulated at the time the data are being analyzed. Instruction on the use of these tools is beyond the scope of this chapter; however, they are available on the market and readers are encouraged to learn how to use them.

Figure 15.24.   Frequency distribution for age, DRG 15, nonspecific cerebrovascular and precerebral occlusion without infarction*

Age

N	Valid	12
	Missing	0
Median		65.00
Percentiles	25	52.00
	50	65.00
	75	71.00

Age

		Frequency	Percent	Valid Percent	Cumulative Percent
Valid	44	1	8.3	8.3	8.3
	51	1	8.3	8.3	16.7
	52	2	16.7	16.7	33.3
	62	1	8.3	8.3	41.7
	65	2	16.7	16.7	58.3
	66	1	8.3	8.3	66.7
	68	1	8.3	8.3	75.0
	72	1	8.3	8.3	83.3
	76	1	8.3	8.3	91.7
	82	1	8.3	8.3	100.0
	Total	12	100.0	100.0	

*rounded

Figure 15.25. **Frequency distribution for age, DRG 14, intracranial hemorrhage and stroke with infarction***

Statistics

Age

N	Valid	38
	Missing	0
Median		62.00
Percentiles	25	51.50
	50	62.00
	75	73.50

Age

		Frequency	Percent	Valid Percent	Cumulative Percent
Valid	22	1	2.6	2.6	2.6
	23	1	2.6	2.6	5.3
	26	1	2.6	2.6	7.9
	39	1	2.6	2.6	10.5
	44	1	2.6	2.6	13.2
	46	1	2.6	2.6	15.8
	47	1	2.6	2.6	18.4
	49	1	2.6	2.6	21.1
	50	1	2.6	2.6	23.7
	52	1	2.6	2.6	26.3
	55	1	2.6	2.6	28.9
	56	1	2.6	2.6	31.6
	57	3	7.9	7.9	39.5
	58	2	5.3	5.3	44.7
	60	2	5.3	5.3	50.0
	64	1	2.6	2.6	52.6
	68	2	5.3	5.3	57.9
	70	2	5.3	5.3	63.2
	71	2	5.3	5.3	68.4
	72	2	5.3	5.3	73.7
	73	1	2.6	2.6	76.3
	75	1	2.6	2.6	78.9
	76	1	2.6	2.6	81.6
	77	2	5.3	5.3	86.8
	78	1	2.6	2.6	89.5
	83	1	2.6	2.6	92.1
	84	1	2.6	2.6	94.7
	86	2	5.3	5.3	100.0*
	Total	38	100.0*	100.0*	

*rounded

Figure 15.26. **Boxplot of age, DRGs 14 and 15**

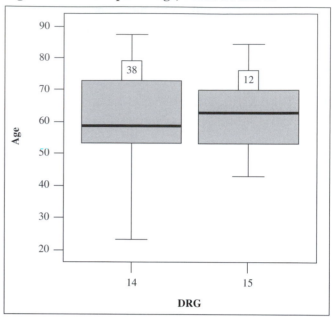

Check Your Understanding 15.11

Instructions: Complete the following sentences on a separate sheet of paper.

1. A presentation of data in rows and columns is a ___.
2. A graphic display technique used to display parts of a whole is a ___.
3. A graphic display technique used to show trends over time is a ___.
4. A graphic display technique used to display categories of a variable is a ___.
5. A graphic display technique that may be used to show the age distribution of a population is a ___.
6. A graphic technique that can visually compare the range of a variable between two categories is a ___.

Normal Distribution

Measures of central tendency and variation are interpreted as they relate to the normal distribution. The normal distribution is actually a theoretical family of distributions that may have any **mean** or any **standard deviation.** It is bell-shaped and symmetrical about the mean. Because it is symmetrical, 50 percent of the observations fall above the mean and 50 percent fall below it. In a normal distribution, the mean, median, and **mode** are equal. The values of the normal distribution range from minus infinity ($-\infty$) to plus infinity ($+\infty$).

In the normal distribution, the standard deviation indicates how many observations fall within a certain range of the mean. Typically, 68 percent of the observations fall within one standard deviation of the mean, 95 percent fall within two standard deviations, and 99.7 percent fall within three standard deviations.

Figure 15.27 shows an example of a normal distribution superimposed on a histogram. The center of the distribution, or mean, is 6. (The median and the mode also are 6.) The standard deviation is 2.45. This means that 68 percent of the ob servations in the frequency distribution fall within 2.45 standard deviations of 6 (6 ± 2.45). Thus, 68 percent fall between 3.55 and 8.45; 95 percent fall between 1.1 and 10.9; and 99.7 percent fall between 21.35 and 13.35.

As shown in the figure, a characteristic of the normal distribution is that each tail of the curve approaches the x-axis but never touches it, no matter how far from center the line is.

A histogram of the frequency distribution for the LOS data in table 15.23 is shown in figure 15.28 (p. 432). The distribution is more peaked than the normal distribution and so is considered kurtotic. Kurtosis is the vertical stretching of a distribution.

A skewed distribution is asymmetrical. Skewness is the horizontal stretching of a frequency distribution to one side or the other so that one tail is longer than the other. The longer tail has more observations. Because the mean is sensitive to extreme observations, it moves in the direction of the long tail when a distribution is skewed. When the direction of the tail is off to the right, the distribution is positively skewed, or skewed to the right. When the direction of the tail is off to the left, the distribution is negatively skewed, or skewed to the left. When the mean and the median approximate one another (as with the LOS data), the distribution is not significantly skewed.

Check Your Understanding 15.12

Instructions: Answer the following questions on a separate piece of paper.

1. What are the characteristics of a normal distribution?

2. What is the definition of the term *skewness*?

Figure 15.27.   Histogram of normal distribution

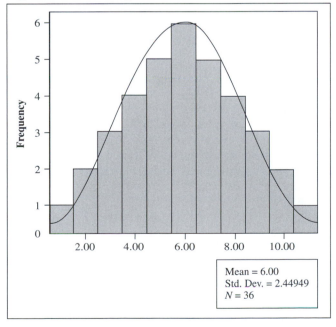

Mean = 6.00
Std. Dev. = 2.44949
N = 36

Table 15.23.   Calculation of the variance, LOS data

LOS	LOS − Mean (5.8) (X − $\overline{X}$)	(LOS − Mean)² (X − $\overline{X}$)²
1	−4.8	23.04
1	−4.8	23.04
2	−3.8	14.44
2	−3.8	14.44
4	−1.8	3.24
4	−1.8	3.24
4	−1.8	3.24
4	−1.8	3.24
4	−1.8	3.24
4	−1.8	3.24
5	−0.8	0.64
5	−0.8	0.64
5	−0.8	0.64
5	−0.8	0.64
5	−0.8	0.64
5	−0.8	0.64
6	0.2	0.04
6	0.2	0.04
6	0.2	0.04
6	0.2	0.04
6	0.2	0.04
6	0.2	0.04
6	0.2	0.04
6	0.2	0.04
6	0.2	0.04
6	0.2	0.04
6	0.2	0.04
7	1.2	1.44
7	1.2	1.44
7	1.2	1.44
7	1.2	1.44
7	1.2	1.44
7	1.2	1.44
8	2.2	4.84
8	2.2	4.84
8	2.2	4.84
8	2.2	4.84
8	2.2	4.84
9	3.2	10.24
9	3.2	10.24
9	3.2	10.24
10	4.2	17.64
Total	0*	179.88

*rounded

$$s^2 = \sum_{i}^{n} (X_i - \overline{X})^2 / N - 1$$
$$= 179.88/41$$
$$= 4.39$$

Figure 15.28.   Histogram of LOS with superimposed normal curve

Mean = 5.8333
Std. Dev. = 2.09432
N = 42

Descriptive Statistics

Measures of central tendency and measures of **variability** are used to describe frequency distributions. Measures of central tendency are measures of location; they indicate the typical value of a frequency distribution. Variation emphasizes differences and/or scattering around the typical value of a data set. Inferences about populations from samples are based on the variation of the observations in the data set.

Descriptive measures are computed from both populations and samples. A population is a group of persons or objects about which an investigator wishes to draw a conclusion. A sample is a subset of a population. Measures that result from a compilation of data from populations are called parameters. Measures that result from samples are called statistics. For example, if we are interested in the average age of undergraduates enrolled at City University, all registered undergraduates would be the defined population. If we calculate the average age of the entire population of undergraduate students, the resultant average is a population parameter. However, if we draw a sample from the registered undergraduate students and then calculate the average age, the resultant average is a sample statistic.

Measures of Central Tendency

Measures of central tendency and variability also can be used to describe populations. Measures of central tendency discussed in this subsection are the mean, the median, and the mode. The measures of variability discussed in the next subsection are the range, the **variance,** and the standard deviation.

A frequency distribution shows the values that a variable can take and the number of observations associated with each value. For example, using LOS as the variable, five patients were discharged with the following lengths of stay:

Patient	LOS
1	2 days
2	3 days
3	4 days
4	2 days
5	3 days

The data displayed in the table above are referred to as a frequency distribution. A frequency distribution displays the number of times a particular observation occurs for the variable being measured. In this example, the number of times a certain LOS occurs is the variable of interest. The frequency distribution for LOS, in ascending order, is 2, 2, 3, 3, and 4 days.

Frequency distributions may be constructed for both discrete and continuous data. As an example, Community Hospital wants to construct a frequency distribution showing the LOS of patients who were discharged on May 10. LOS is a continuous variable falling on the ratio scale of measurement. The hospital wants to see how many of these patients were in the hospital for a particular LOS (for example, four days). The variable is the LOS, and the frequency is the number of times a particular LOS occurred among the patients discharged on May 10.

To construct the frequency distribution, list all the values that the particular LOS can take, from the lowest observed value to the highest. Then enter the number of times a discharged patient had that particular LOS. Table 15.23 shows a frequency distribution for LOS on May 10. Notice that the frequency distribution lists all the values for LOS between the lowest and the highest, even when there are no observations for some of the values. For example, there are no observations of patients spending three days in the hospital. Six patients have LOS of four days. The data in table 15.23 can be used to calculate measures of both central tendency and variability.

The Mean

The mean is the arithmetic average of a frequency distribution. To calculate a mean, the data must fall on the interval or ratio scales of measurement. The mean is the sum of all scores in a frequency distribution divided by the number of scores. The symbol for the mean is $\overline{X}_i$ (pronounced x-bar). The formula for calculating the mean in a frequency distribution is:

$$X = \sum X_i / N$$

where $\sum$ is summation, X_i is each successive observation from the first one in the frequency distribution, $i = 1$, to the last observation (n), and N is the total number of observations.

To calculate the ALOS for the data in table 15.23, substitute the appropriate figures into the following formula:

$$X = \sum X_i / N$$
$$= 245/42$$
$$= 5.8$$

The ALOS for patients discharged from Community Hospital on May 10 is 5.8 days (rounded).

Two disadvantages are associated with using the mean as the most typical value in a frequency distribution. First, in this example, the LOS for the 42 patients are integers (whole numbers). However, the ALOS is fractional (5.8), even though there is no fractional LOS. Fractional values are considered more a problem of interpretation than a result that is not meaningful. In this case, the ALOS is interpreted as, "On average, the ALOS for the patients discharged from the Community Hospital on May 10 is between 5 and 6 days."

Second, the mean is sensitive to extreme measures. That is, it is strongly influenced by outliers. For example, if the 10-day LOS were actually a 25-day LOS, the ALOS would increase to 6.2 days.

Thus, the average or arithmetic mean may not always be the most appropriate way to summarize the most typical value of a frequency distribution. The measure of central tendency selected to describe the typical value of a frequency distribution should be based on the characteristics of that particular frequency distribution.

The Median

The median is the midpoint of a frequency distribution. It is the point at which 50 percent of the observations fall above and 50 percent fall below. If an odd number of observations is in the frequency distribution, the median is the middle number. In the following frequency distribution, the median is 13. Three observations fall above the value of 13, and three fall below it:

10   11   12   13   14   15   16

If an even number of observations is in the frequency distribution, the median is the midpoint between the two middle observations. It is found by averaging the two middle scores ($[x + y]/2$). In the following example, the median is 13.5 ($[13 + 14]/2$):

10   11   12   13   14   15   16   17

If the two middle observations take on the same value, the median is that value. When determining the median, it does not matter whether there are duplicate observations in the frequency distribution. Consider the following frequency distribution:

10 11 11 12 13 13 14 15 16 17

In this frequency distribution, the median falls between the fifth and sixth observations. Therefore, the median is 13 ($[13 + 13]/2$).

Table 15.23 records LOS data for 42 patients. In this example, the median falls between the 21st and 22nd observations. Placed in order from lowest to highest, the distribution is as follows:

1 1 2 2 4 4 4 4 4 5 5 5 5 5 5 6 6 6 6 6 6
6 6 6 6 7 7 7 7 7 7 8 8 8 8 9 9 9 10

The median is 6 ($[6 + 6]/2$).
The median offers the following three advantages:

- It is relatively easy to calculate.
- It is based on the whole distribution and not just a portion of it, as is the case with the mode.
- Unlike the mean, it is not influenced by extreme values or unusual outliers in the frequency distribution.

The Mode

The mode is the simplest measure of central tendency. It is used to indicate the most frequent observation in a frequency distribution. The mode offers several advantages, including:

- It is easy to obtain and interpret.
- It is not sensitive to extreme observations in the frequency distribution.
- It is easy to communicate and explain to others.
- It can be used with nominal-level data.

However, there are also disadvantages, including:

- It may not be descriptive of the distribution when the most frequent observation does not occur very often, especially when the number of observations is large.
- It may not be unique. That is, more than one mode may be in a distribution. A frequency distribution may be unimodal, bimodal, or multimodal. When each observation occurs an equal number of times, the distribution does not have a mode.
- It does not provide information about the entire distribution, only the observation that occurs most frequently.

In table 15.23, the mode is 6 because 11 patients had lengths of stay of 6 days. To summarize, for the LOS data in table 15.23, the measures of central tendency are similar. The mean is 5.8 days, the median is 6 days, and the mode is 6 days. These statistics are summarized in table 15.24.

Table 15.24. Descriptive statistics for LOS data

N	Valid	42
	Missing	0
Mean		5.8333
Median		6.0000
Mode		6.00
Standard deviation		2.09432
Variance		4.386
Range		9.00
Minimum		1.00
Maximum		10.00

Measures of Variability

In addition to measures of central tendency, the hospital can use measures of variability to describe frequency distributions. These measures indicate how widely the observations are spread out around the measures of central tendency. The measures of spread increase with greater variation in the frequency distribution. The spread is equal to zero when there is no variation. This subsection discusses the following measures of spread: the range, the variance, and the standard deviation.

The Range

The range is the simplest measure of spread. It is the difference between the smallest and largest values in a frequency distribution:

$$\text{Range} = X_{max} - X_{min}$$

The range for the LOS data in table 15.23 is 9 (10 − 1 = 9).

One disadvantage of the range is that it can be affected by extreme values, or outliers, in the distribution. Also, the range varies widely from sample to sample. Only the two most extreme observations affect its value, so it is not sensitive to other observations in the distribution.

Two frequency distributions may have the same range but differ greatly in variation. For example, the range for the following frequency distributions is 9 (10 − 1 = 9):

Distribution 1: 1   2   3   4   5   6   7   8   9   10

Distribution 2: 1   1.5   3   3.5   3.7   7   8   8.26   10   10

However, when the two distributions are compared, the second distribution has more variation than the first distribution. This is demonstrated when the variance is calculated. The variance for the first distribution is 9.1, and the variance for the second distribution is 11.8.

The Variance

The variance of a frequency distribution is the average of the squared deviations from the mean. The variance of a sample is symbolized by s^2. The variance of a distribution is larger when the observations are widely spread. The formula for calculating the variance is:

$$s^2 = \frac{\sum (X - \overline{X})^2}{N - 1}$$

The squared deviations of the mean are calculated by subtracting the mean of the frequency distribution from each value in the distribution. The difference between the two values is squared, $(X - X)^2$. The squared differences are summed and divided by $N - 1$. The calculations for the variance for the LOS data are shown in table 15.23.

In the calculations for the variance, the sum of $(X - \overline{X})$ is equal to zero. This is because the mean is the balance point in the distribution. When a value is less than the mean, the difference is negative (1 − 5.8 = −4.8); when the value is greater than the mean, the difference is positive (6 − 5.8 = 0.2). Therefore, the sum of the differences from the mean is equal to zero. In this example, the sum approximates zero

because the actual mean of 5.8333 was rounded to 5.8 for ease in calculation.

The Standard Deviation

The variance for the LOS data in table 15.23 is 4.39, but what does this mean? The interpretation of the variance is not meaningful at the descriptive level because the original units of measure—the lengths of stay—are squared to arrive at the variance. By calculating the square root of the variance, the data are returned to the original units of measurement. This is called the standard deviation, which is symbolized by s. The formula for the standard deviation is:

$$s = \sqrt{\frac{\sum (X - \overline{X})}{N - 1}}$$

The standard deviation for the LOS data is 2.1.

The standard deviation is the most widely used measure of variability in descriptive statistics. Because it is easy to interpret, it is the preferred measure of dispersion for frequency distributions. Most handheld calculators include features for calculating the variance and the standard deviation.

The measures of central tendency and variation may be calculated using a handheld calculator. Also, statistical packages such as SPSS are available for performing these and other descriptive and **inferential statistics.** The histograms were prepared using SPSS. The SPSS output for the LOS data appears in table 15.24. The slight differences between the handheld calculator results and the SPSS results in the mean, variance, and standard deviation are because of rounding.

Check Your Understanding 15.13

Instructions: Fifteen infants were born at Community Hospital during the week of December 1. Using a handheld calculator, determine the measures of central tendency and variability for the following infant birth weights (in grams):

2,450	2,750	2,600
2,540	2,815	2,540
2,300	1,735	1,720
2,715	1,800	2,780
2,400	2,485	2,640

1. ___ Mean
2. ___ Median
3. ___ Mode
4. ___ Range
5. ___ Variance
6. ___ Standard deviation

Real-World Case

The quality improvement committee of Community Hospital wanted to study DRG 320, Kidney and Urinary Tract Infections Age >17 with CC, because of wide variations in LOS and total charges. The committee asked the HIM director to prepare a profile of patients discharged from DRG 320. A summary of the patients discharged from DRG 320 at Community Hospital was prepared using information found in the hospital's online database.

Summary

Rates, ratios, proportions, and statistics are commonly used to describe community and hospital populations. They are considered to be descriptive statistics because they portray the characteristics of a group or population. Public health officials use community-based rates, ratios, and proportions to evaluate the general health status of a community. Morbidity and mortality rates are used as indicators of the accessibility and availability of healthcare services in a community.

Hospital-based rates are used for a variety of purposes. First, they describe the general characteristics of the patients treated at the facility. Hospital administrators use the data to monitor the volume of patients treated monthly, weekly, or within some other specified time frame. The statistics give healthcare decision makers the information they need to plan facilities and to monitor inpatient and outpatient revenue streams.

Graphic techniques are often used to summarize and clarify data. Data may be displayed in a variety of ways, for example, as charts, graphs, and/or tables. Graphic forms are effective ways to present large quantities of information.

The health information management professional is in a position to serve as a data broker for the healthcare organization. To do this, he or she must fully understand the clinical data that are collected and their application to the decision-making process. In addition, he or she must know what information is needed and how to provide it in a timely manner. With this knowledge, the HIM professional can become an invaluable member of the healthcare team.

References

Agency for Healthcare Research and Quality. 2000. AHRQ Profile: Quality research for quality healthcare. AHRQ publication no. 00-P005. Rockville, MD: AHRQ. Available online from ahrq.gov/about/profile.htm.

Agency for Health Care Policy and Research. 2000. HCUPnet: Healthcare cost and utilization project. Rockville, MD: AHRQ. Available online from hcup.ahrq.gov/HCUPnet.asp.

Centers for Disease Control and Prevention. 2005a. CDC Wonder Data Base. Available online from wonder.cdc.gov.

Centers for Disease Control and Prevention. 2005b. Division of Public Health Surveillance and Informatics. Nationally notifiable infectious diseases, United States, 2005. Available online from cdc.gov/epo/dphsi/phs/infdis2005.htm.

Department of Health and Human Services, Public Health Service. 1994. *Self-Instructional Manual for Cancer Registries, Book 7: Statistics and Epidemiology for Cancer Registries.* NIH Publication No. 94-3766. Washington, DC: HHS.

Ellerbruch, L. 2005. Department of Mathematics/Computer Science. Northern Michigan University, CS255 Computers in Elementary Education. Stem-and-Leaf Plot. Available online from ellerbruch.nmu.edu/cs255/jnord/stemplot.html.

Horton, L.A. 2004. *Calculating and Reporting Healthcare Statistics.* Chicago: AHIMA.

Microsoft Corporation. 2005. Creating a Bubble Chart. Available online from office.microsoft.com/en-us/assistance/HA011170761033.aspx.

National Center for Health Statistics. 2005. Centers for Disease Control and Prevention. Available online from cdc.gov/nchs.

National Vital Statistics System. 2005. Centers for Disease Control and Prevention. Available online from cdc.gov/nchs/nvss.htm.

Osborn, C.E. 2005. *Statistical Applications for Health Information Management.* Sudbury, MA: Jones and Bartlett.

Oswego City School District Regents Exam Prep Center. 2005. Box-and-Whisker Plots. Available online from regentsprep.org/Regents/math/data/boxwhisk.htm.

Chapter 16
Research Methods

Elizabeth Layman, PhD, RHIA, CCS, FAHIMA

Learning Objectives

- To describe basic research designs and methods used in the practice of health information management
- To formulate research problems in terms of research questions
- To search knowledge bases such as bibliographic databases
- To plan research projects appropriate to the research questions
- To ensure adherence to institutional review board policies and processes in the protection of human subjects
- To conduct research projects using standard and suitable tools and techniques
- To present research findings in formats consistent with the purpose of the research
- To critically evaluate research studies in health-related fields

Key Terms

Abstract
Alternative hypothesis
Applied research
Basic research
Bivariate
Case-control (retrospective) study
Case study
Categorical data
Causal-comparative research
Causal relationship
Census survey
Cluster sampling
Confounding (extraneous, secondary) variable
Construct validity
Content analysis
Content validity
Continuous data
Control group
Convenience sampling
Correlational research
Cross-sectional
Deductive reasoning
Dependent variable
Descriptive research
Descriptive statistics
Discrete data
Double-blind study
Empiricism
Ethnography
Evaluation research

Experimental (study) group
Experimental research
External validity
Focused studies
Generalizability
Heterogeneity
Historical research
Hypothesis
Independent variable
Inductive reasoning
Inferential statistics
Institutional review board (IRB)
Instrument
Internal validity
Interrater reliability
Interval data
Intervention
Interview guide
Interview survey
Intrarater reliability
Level of significance
Likert scale
Literature review
Longitudinal
Meta-analysis
Model
Mortality (attrition)
Multivariate
Naturalism
Naturalistic observation
Negative (inverse) relationship
Nominal data

Nonparametric (distribution-free) technique
Nonparticipant observation
Nonrandom sampling
Null hypothesis
Observational research
One-tailed hypothesis
Ordinal data
Paradigm
Parametric technique
Participant observation
Peer review
Peer-reviewed (refereed) journal
Pilot study
Placebo
Positive (direct) relationship
Positivism
Primary analysis
Primary source
Protocol
Purposive sampling
Qualitative approach
Quantitative approach
Questionnaire survey
Random sampling
Randomization
Randomized clinical trial (RCT)
Ratio data
Reliability
Research
Research method

Research methodology
Retrospective
Sample
Sample size
Sample size calculation
Sample survey
Scale
Scientific inquiry
Secondary analysis
Secondary source
Semantic differential scale
Semistructured question
Simple random sampling
Simulation observation
Stratified random sampling
Structured (close-ended) question
Survey
Systematic literature review
Systematic sampling
Target population
Test statistics
Theory
Treatment
Two-tailed hypothesis
Type I error
Type II error
Univariate
Unstructured (open-ended) question
Validity
Variable

Introduction

Health information management (HIM) is an intersection of many different fields of study, and health information managers are businesspeople in a health-related profession. Thus, health information managers draw on theories from the many fields associated with both business and healthcare, including management, organizational behavior, sociology, psychology, medical sciences, computer science, and decision support. In this chapter, **research** concepts are applied to healthcare settings and the role of the HIM professional in research is explored.

Research is a way to create knowledge. It answers questions and provides solutions to everyday problems. Research is not some vague, mysterious activity for geniuses, as some people believe; rather, it is a step-by-step method that ordinary people can use to collect reliable and accurate facts in order to generate valuable information.

Generally, there are two types of research: **basic research** and **applied research.** These two types are ends of a continuum, not separate entities. Therefore, the distinction between them is sometimes unclear. In essence, basic research focuses on the development of theories and their refinement whereas applied research focuses on the implementation of the theories in practice. For example, as applied researchers, some HIM professionals study questions they believe will improve health information practices in the continuum of care. Another way to differentiate basic and applied research is that basic research answers the question "why" and applied research answers the questions "what" and "how" (Gay and Airasian 2003).

Research into medicine and healthcare has greatly enhanced the quality and length of people's lives. For example, antibiotics, endoscopic surgery, and the Medicare inpatient prospective payment system, among many others, all are the result of research. Moreover, continued advances in effective treatments and efficient methods of healthcare delivery depend on future research.

This chapter overviews the role of research in medicine and healthcare and the development of **theories** and **models.** It also presents a step-by-step process for conducting research. Finally, the chapter addresses how HIM professionals can use the techniques of research to improve HIM practice and data quality.

Theory into Practice

Paul Bell is an HIM professional and researcher. He has used his knowledge of the content of health records in his research. This knowledge has made him a valuable member of research teams.

Bell participated on two research teams that investigated treatment of chest pain. The teams wanted to find out whether different patients received different care during their initial diagnosis of chest pain. The first team investigated emergency department treatment of chest pain at three hospitals in the Mid-

west (Bell, Micke, and Kasa 1998). The team reviewed 1,013 health records, extracting data on patient gender, age, race, diagnosis, comorbidities, procedures, and institutional size. The study revealed that men received more diagnostic procedures than women. The second study also investigated emergency department treatment of chest pain, but in a different geographic area, the mid-Atlantic. In this study, 379 records from two hospitals were analyzed, taking into account the effects of age, institutional size, comorbidities, and insurance status (Bell and Hudson 2001). This study found that, when compared to whites, African Americans waited longer to receive their first electrocardiogram, were less likely to receive cardiac catheterizations, and were more likely to receive echocardiography.

The research endeavor began at a midwestern university when Bell was approached by a research team in the field of clinical laboratory science. Included on the team were a senior faculty member and a faculty member with a strong statistical background.

He was invited to join the research team because its members believed that his health information background highly qualified him to collect and abstract data retrospectively from health records. In turn, Bell agreed to work with the team because the topic was timely and interesting. Moreover, as a junior faculty member, he needed to become involved in an area of research. He continued the research at a university in a Mid-Atlantic state.

Each researcher brought specific skills to the team. The senior faculty member interpreted serum enzyme studies used in the evaluation of chest pain. The faculty member with the statistics background conducted various statistical tests on the data in order to produce specific output and interpreted that output into readable language. Bell contributed his knowledge of health record content and health information practices.

Because Bell was the team member with the most expertise in reading hospital records, data collection became his responsibility. Skills in forms design allowed Bell to develop the data capture sheet. As the only member of the team with knowledge of coding, Bell developed an algorithm for selecting patient records based on admitting diagnoses related to ischemic causes of chest pain and on principal diagnoses of ischemic chest pain, myocardial infarction, or angina. His professional network with HIM practitioners facilitated the team's access to the hospitals in order to conduct record review. The HIM administrators and directors were comfortable allowing record access to another registered health information administrator (RHIA). It was understood that a fellow RHIA would recognize the importance of patient confidentiality and privacy. Finally, Bell collected data by manual abstraction from paper charts.

Bell used several skills related to the steps of research, including:

- Performing the **literature review.** The literature review influenced the course of the research project by identifying gaps in the body of knowledge and in the literature. These gaps became areas of focus for the team's research studies. For example, most research studies at that time argued that the difference between male and female rates of cardiac catheterization was due to the higher comorbidity for female patients because they tended to be older and sicker when chest pain was diagnosed. To address this issue, the research team's study controlled for the presence of comorbidities as potential mitigating factors. The literature review then helped to define and refine the research objective.

- Recommending **protocols** for the research, including designs and methods.
- Creating the data collection **instrument.**
- Devising a step-by-step plan for data gathering. This plan included: developing the schema for identifying records to be reviewed for the study, securing the approval of the appropriate **institutional review boards** (IRBs), and conducting the data collection. When Bell worked on these studies, the hospitals' HIS departments served as the conduits for IRB approval. He submitted the study proposal and protocol to the administrators or directors of the hospitals' HIS departments, who then forwarded the proposal and protocol to their IRBs.
- Disseminating findings and building body of knowledge. Bell wrote two articles and published them in a peer-reviewed journal. He also presented findings at the national conference of the American Health Information Management Association (AHIMA).

As an HIM professional, Bell demonstrated values that members of the profession share. These values include appreciation for accuracy and attention to detail, respect for patient rights and confidentiality of their health information, and commitment to protecting health data privacy and security. These HIM values are supportive of successful research projects.

Bell stated that the greatest obstacles to his research were working with manual records and collecting data from each case. Finding time and support for this labor-intensive task was daunting. However, the greatest rewards of conducting research were:

- Realizing that he and his fellow researchers had contributed to the body of knowledge related to the emergency treatment of chest pain

- Succeeding as an HIM professional in the research genre
- Being published

Bell still receives requests from healthcare researchers for permission to use the study in their research. These requests confirm the importance of shedding light on the accessibility and equity of the U.S. healthcare system.

As this case demonstrates, HIM professionals are contributors to research studies. (See table 16.1.) They are experts on health data; the data's location, accuracy, and format; and other aspects of HIM practice. Their training and education provide specific research skills; and their professional values are supportive of research.

Knowledge of research also supports HIM practice. Understanding **research methods** aids HIM professionals whenever they use data or information to answer a question or to make a decision. This chapter expands on the steps of research that Bell conducted and explains the entire process.

Research in Medicine and Healthcare

The history of research in medicine and healthcare parallels the history of civilization. The tradition of proposing rational explanations for the causes of disease dates back to 3500 BC. The Egyptians recorded symptoms and cures for illnesses, and the Greeks continued the tradition. Indeed, Hippocrates, practicing medicine in about 400 BC, wrote more than 50 books on health and disease. Similar advances occurred in India and China. Scientists and philosophers continued to advance knowledge about medicine and health throughout the Middle Ages and the Renaissance.

In the United States, research in medicine and healthcare and interest in the research university evolved together. The present form of the research university emerged in the 1860s (Rudolph 1990). Yale awarded the first doctoral degrees in the United States in 1861 (Rudolph 1990). Cornell University was chartered in 1865; the Johns Hopkins University was founded in 1867. In the 1890s, national learned societies and journals were established (Jencks and Riesman 1977). The university structure of departments, such as biology, philosophy, and history, also was established in the 1890s.

Table 16.1. HIM contributions to research teams

HIM-Specific Skills	Research-Specific Skills	HIM Values
Knowledge of health record content	Ability to conduct literature reviews	Accuracy
Form and view design	Knowledge of research protocols	Attention to detail
Expertise in classifications and nomenclatures	Capability to devise case-based algorithms	Respect for patient rights and confidentiality
Database query skills	Understanding of procedures of institutional review boards	Commitment to protecting health data privacy and security
Professional collegiality	Knowledge of data collection protocols	
	Written and oral communication of data, information, and knowledge	

By 1914, the two dozen leading U.S. universities had been established (Jencks and Riesman 1977).

During the early 1900s, Flexner (1910) investigated the quality of medical education and recommended that many shoddy medical schools be closed. He also described the ideal organization of medical education. Flexner recommended that medical schools be located in leading universities with associated hospitals. He identified outstanding examples such as the Johns Hopkins University, the University of Michigan, and the University of Minnesota. Today's, academic health center was born from the union of medical schools, hospitals, and research universities.

Academic health centers became especially important after the federal government increased its funding for research in the 1950s. These federal research grants became important sources of revenue for universities. As conduits for federal dollars, academic health centers became increasingly prominent in their universities. One major source of federal funding for medical research is the National Institutes of Health (NIH). Today, the NIH supports 35,000 grants related to medical research. Thus, research, as means to raise funds, became an integral part of the academic enterprise. (See chapter 18 for a discussion of clinical (medical) research, including clinical trials.)

Theory and Research

A theory is the systematic organization of knowledge that predicts or explains behavior or events. Theories and research have a chicken-and-egg relationship. Theories are both the result and the foundation of research. Researchers begin with informed predictions or raw theories of what they believe will happen. As they collect observations and data, they refine their theories. Over time, the refined theories become more predictive of subsequent events than their previous embryonic versions.

Theories are practical and efficient. They help people understand their world. Without theories, people are merely speculating. Although speculation may be informed by experiences and some facts, it is nevertheless speculation.

Apparent in all fields of study, theories explain what people have observed. In addition, they provide definitions, relationships, and boundaries. In other words, theories systematically organize everything people know about a concept. Amatayakul and Shah (1992) formally defined theories as:

- Concepts that are abstract ideas generalized from particular instances
- Interrelationships that are assumed to exist among these concepts
- Consequences that are assumed to follow logically from the relationships proposed in the theory

The best theories simplify the situation, explain the most facts in the broadest range of circumstances, and most accurately predict behavior (Singleton and Straits 1999). Thus, research theories are practical and efficient because they help

researchers explain and predict many events in simple and precise terms. In other words, theories organize knowledge. When knowledge is organized, ordinary people can access and use it. Everyone benefits.

Health Record Data in Research

Just as the history of medicine follows the history of civilization, so too does the use of the data in health records. With the development of writing, ancient physicians and scribes could record diseases and their treatments. For example, as early as 3000 BC, scribes recorded on papyrus the medical and surgical treatments of Egyptian physicians (Haas 1999). In the Ebers papyrus, the treatment of urinary retention and excessive urination with myrrh and other herbs is recorded (Nickels 2005). The Edwin Smith papyrus is a surgical textbook describing 48 surgical cases (Feldman and Goodrich 1999.) (See figure 16.1.)

More recently, medical records became an integral part of the hospital standardization program of the American College of Surgeons (ACS). In 1918, the ACS began to evaluate the quality of care that a hospital provided by evaluating its patient records. Since then, researchers have used patient records as a way to both log data during research and access existing data for their research.

Recently published studies demonstrate the use of medical records in research. These studies used both paper-based and computer-based patient records and were conducted in physician offices and hospitals.

Bedell and colleagues (2000) wanted to investigate whether patients used medications as prescribed by their physicians. The researchers compared what the patients said about their medications in interviews with what their physicians recorded in the outpatient records. In 76 percent of patients, there were discrepancies between patient-reported and physician-recorded medications. In another study, inpatient records were reviewed to investigate the incidence and types of preventable adverse events (medically induced injuries) (Thomas and Brennan 2000). The medical records of 15,000 inpatient discharges were reviewed. Preventable adverse events were more common in elderly patients than in nonelderly patients. However, the researchers concluded

Figure 16.1.   Sample of Egyptian surgical treatment

Examination
If thou examinest a man having a gaping wound in his head, penetrating to the bone, smashing his skull, and rending open the brain of his skull, thou shouldst palpate his wound.

Diagnosis
Thou shouldst say concerning him: "An ailment not to be treated."

Treatment
Thou shouldst anoint that wound with grease. Thou shalt not bind it; thou shalt not apply two strips upon it: until thou knowest that he has reached a decisive point.

Source: Feldman and Goodrich 1999, p. 282.

that this incidence was associated with the complexity of their care rather than age-based discrimination. An HIM professional participated in a study using computer-based patient records (Ornstein et al. 1999). The purpose of the study was to determine the impact of drug cost information on the prescribing patterns of family physicians. The study revealed that the presence of computerized drug cost information did not affect patients' overall drug costs. In another study, researchers at a tertiary hospital investigated which method of identifying adverse drug events was most efficient: computer-based monitor, chart review, or voluntary report (Jha et al. 1998). Although the most labor-intensive, chart review identified 65 percent of detected adverse drug events. Computer monitor identifed 45 percent and voluntary report 4 percent.

Although retrospective review of health records is a common method of research in healthcare, problems with this method have been identified. Researchers found that key data were not documented. For example, health information researchers found that data such as occupation, menopausal status, estrogen receptor and progesterone receptor values, and other items were not always documented in the health record or cancer registry abstract for African-American women diagnosed with breast cancer (Watzlaf, Katoh, and D'Amico 1996). Other researchers found that health records contained inadequate documentation to explain the cause of pediatric fractures and, thereby, to rule out abuse (Oral, Blum, and Johnson 2003). Thus, there are obstacles in the use of health records as a primary data source in research.

Despite the problems identified, however, thousands of studies have followed methods similar to these studies. They demonstrate the importance of health record data in research and their potential for improving the quality of patient care.

Research Models

A model is a representation of a theory in a visual format. Models can portray theories with objects, can be smaller-scaled versions, or can be graphic representations. A popular synonym for model is **paradigm.**

A model includes all of a theory's known properties. AHIMA, for example, has a theory about what defines data quality. Experts at AHIMA have identified collection, analysis, application, and warehousing as the functions of data quality management and hypothesize that data quality will result if practitioners follow proper procedures within these activities. (See figure 16.2 for a model of the AHIMA theory.)

Research methodology is the study and analysis of research methods and theories. At a higher and more general level, researchers in research methodology have described two overarching approaches to research: the **quantitative approach** and the **qualitative approach.**

The quantitative approach is the explanation of phenomena through **scientific inquiry** and **empiricism.** Scientific

Figure 16.2. AHIMA's model of data quality

Source: AHIMA 1998.

inquiry involves making predictions, collecting and analyzing evidence, testing alternative theories, and choosing the best theory. Empiricism means "based on observed and validated evidence." For example, research based on experiments is empirical. Objective knowledge is the desired end result. As the word *quantitative* implies, the data often can be quantified and result in statistical or numerical results. Another name for the quantitative approach is **positivism.** A classic example of quantitative research is the human genome project.

Researchers in the qualitative approach interpret non-numerical observations. These nonnumerical observations include words, gestures, activities, time, space, images, and perceptions. These observations are placed in context. Another term for the qualitative approach is **naturalism.** A classic example of qualitative research is Margaret Mead's anthropological study of the Polynesian culture of American Samoa in the early 1920s. Examples in medicine involve studies of near-death experiences, dying, and being a patient. Without qualitative research, healthcare personnel would not have learned that elderly, married patients cut their pills in half in order to share their prescriptions when they run out of money.

These two approaches to research are models on a grand scale. Within both approaches, researchers make certain basic assumptions. (See table 16.2, p. 442.) Some large topics require both approaches with many researchers conducting complementary studies. An emerging third approach is called mixed methods research (Johnson and Onwuegbuzie 2004). Mixed methods research combines quantitative and qualitative techniques within a single study and across related studies. An example is a study of the role of computerized physician order-entry (CPOE) systems in introducing the risk of medication errors (Koppel et al. 2005). The researchers conducted a qualitative and quantitative study of the interaction between house staff and the CPOE system at a tertiary-care teaching hospital. They found that CPOE systems facilitated 22 types of medication error risks.

Table 16.2.   Comparison of assumptions in quantitative and qualitative research approaches

Quantitative	Qualitative
Single truth exists	Multiple truths exist simultaneously
Single truth applies across time and place	Truths are bound to place and time (contextual)
Researchers can adopt neutral, unbiased stances	Neutrality is impossible because researchers choose their topics of investigation
Chronological sequence of causes can be identified	Influences interact with one another to color researchers' views of the past, present, and future

The purpose of the research determines the approach. Research that is exploratory and preliminary often begins with a qualitative investigation; research that investigates numerically measurable observations or tests a **hypothesis** is often quantitative.

Most advances in medicine have been the result of quantitative research. Quantitative research, with its scientific and evidence-based approach, is also the approach that HIM researchers often select.

Within both the quantitative and the qualitative approaches, researchers use **inductive reasoning** and **deductive reasoning.** Inductive reasoning, or induction, involves drawing conclusions based on a limited number of observations. For example, during his professional practice experience, a student might observe that all coders in the coding department at XYZ hospital had the RHIT credential. Thus, he might conclude that all coders have the RHIT credential. Deductive reasoning, or deduction, involves drawing conclusions based on generalizations. For example, all coders have the RHIT credential. Jane Doe is a coder. Therefore, Jane Doe must have the RHIT credential.

As the examples demonstrate, neither induction nor deduction alone is completely satisfactory. Used together, however, they are very effective and are the basis of the research.

Check Your Understanding 16.1

Instructions: Answer the following questions on a separate piece of paper.

1. What is research?
2. Why is the research conducted by HIM professionals considered applied research?
3. What are the three characteristics of a theory?
4. How does the phrase "keep it simple" apply to theories?
5. Why are health records important in research?
6. What are the advantages of models?
7. How do inductive reasoning and deductive reasoning differ?
8. Why is knowing their purpose so important for researchers?

Research Process

Conceptually, researchers participate in the following major activities:

1. Defining the research question (problem)
2. Summarizing prior pertinent knowledge
3. Gathering data
4. Analyzing the data
5. Interpreting and presenting findings

However, because these major activities are so broad, most researchers divide them into more manageable components. Thus, the research process becomes orderly problem solving. In the verbal shorthand of researchers, these basic components are:

1. Defining the research question (problem)
2. Performing a literature review
3. Determining a research design and method
4. Selecting an instrument
5. Gathering data
6. Analyzing the data
7. Presenting results

Defining the Research Question (Problem)

Research begins with defining the problem. Other language for defining the problem is specifying the research question. Whichever phrase is used, both mean that researchers must be crystal clear about what they are investigating. Vague notions lead to shoddy research, which is a waste of time, effort, and energy for both researchers and participants.

The importance of investing time and effort in developing the research question cannot be overstated. Experts "agree that the key element, the starting point and the most important issue in developing research, is the research question" (Metz 2001, p. 13).

According to Metz, the criteria for a well-developed research question are:

- The question is clearly and exactly stated.
- The question has theoretical significance, practical worth, or both.
- The question has obvious and explicit links to a larger body of knowledge, such as a theory or a research model.
- The research's results advance knowledge in a definable way.
- The answer to the question or the solution to the problem is worthwhile.

The first step in developing the research question is to identify a general problem in an area of interest and expertise. Three excellent sources of meaningful problems exist:

- *Research models:* Research models show all the factors and relationships in a theory. Researchers can select one or two factors that other researchers have raised questions about or have found problematic. An added benefit is that the model suggests the relationships among the factors. For example, researchers in health information management could use AHIMA's Model of Data Quality to develop a research problem. (See figure 16.2.) These hypothetical researchers could investigate the relationship between collection and data quality. Finally, research models explicitly link to a larger body of knowledge, one of the criteria for a well-developed research question.

- *Recommendations of earlier researchers:* In journal articles, researchers specifically make recommendations for future research. Their research raises yet more questions that later researchers can answer.
- *Gaps in the body of knowledge:* A comprehensive review of the literature related to the problem or question will identify gaps or problematic areas. (See next subsection on performing a literature review.) For example, in journal articles, researchers often identify unintentional flaws in their own study that later researchers could correct in a replication study. Correcting the flaw in the subsequent study could produce more accurate and predictive results than were found in the original study. In health information management and other fields, entire articles have been dedicated to reviewing the literature. These literature review articles can be examined for research questions. The literature review articles related to health information management have covered a wide range of subjects, including:
—Case mix and data quality (Siemon 1982)
—Legal aspects of patient records (Kennedy and Jacobs 1981)
—Quality management (Grove 1980)
—Cost containment in the management of departments of health information services (Lewis 1980)
—Use of computer-aided system engineering tools in the development of healthcare information systems (Lee 1996)
—Hospital information systems (Abdelhak 1982; Abelhak, Firouzan, and Ullman 1993)

In addition, researchers make recommendations for future research in master's theses and doctoral dissertations. Therefore, a careful and thoughtful reading of journal articles, literature review articles, master's theses, and doctoral dissertations can identify meaningful research problems.

The next step is to narrow the focus of the question to a manageable and researchable issue. Researchers clearly state the research problem or question in their article or paper in order to draw the reader into the topic. A helpful metaphor is the funnel. Researchers begin with a broad, general question and then gradually pinpoint the topic to their precise problem or question.

Moreover, an effective problem statement delimits or sets the boundaries of the problem. By clearly stating the study's area of investigation, researchers also specify the aspects of the problem that are beyond or outside the scope of their research. For example, the researcher might begin the problem statement with a general societal concern. Supporting citations would come from the popular literature, opinion articles, and journal articles. Then, he or she would concentrate the discussion by explaining how this problem or question affects the field of health information management. Finally, he or she would state the research problem or question succinctly and accurately.

Clearly delineating the problem helps the researcher later in the research process when he or she is writing the hypothesis. The hypothetis is written after the researcher completes the literature review. (See next section.) In the hypothesis, the researcher operationalizes his or her research question. (See later subsection on statement of hypothesis.)

The last step in developing the research question or problem is to ensure that the issue has merit. Similar to shoddy research, research on a trite issue that no one cares about is a waste of time, effort, and energy. Therefore, the key to defining the problem statement is to find a meaningful problem that needs a solution or a significant question that needs an answer.

Performing a Literature Review

A literature review is a systematic and critical investigation of the important information about a topic. After completing this orderly and organized approach to the literature, researchers know the following about a topic:

- Mainstream and lesser-known theories, theorists, and factors
- Key turning points in the development of ideas about the topic
- Typical research methods
- Major research instruments
- Appropriate analytical approaches

From the literature review, researchers are able to assess the competency of research studies and to identify gaps or holes in the field's body of knowledge. Because overviews identify gaps or discrepancies in a field's knowledge, they are both sources of problems or research questions that researchers can investigate and an excellent means to refine and focus a research question into a previously unexplored issue.

Literature review has three meanings. (See table 16.3, p. 444.) In the first meaning, it is the process of identifying, reading, analyzing, summarizing, and synthesizing the writings of other researchers and thinkers. In the second and third meanings, the literature review is a product. It is the portion of a manuscript or an article in which researchers record their analysis and summary of the literature they have read. A literature review article is a separate and independent peer-reviewed article. In a literature review article, the previously mentioned "portion" is expanded and refined into an entire article.

Table 16.3. Three meanings of the phrase "literature review"

Meaning	General Description	Example
One	Process	Identifying, reading, analyzing, summarizing, and synthesizing the works of researchers and experts
Two	Product—Portion of study's presentation	Excerpt from research article, Kesh, Someswar, and Wullianallur Raghupathi. 2004. Critical issues in bioinformatics and computing. *Perspectives in Health Information Management* 1(9):1–8. Bioinformatics is defined by the National Institutes of Health as the "research, development, or application of computational tools and approaches for expanding the use of biological, medical, behavioral or health data, including those to acquire, store, organize, archive, analyze, or visualize such data." The exponential growth in the amount of such data has necessitated the use of computers for information cataloging and retrieval; a more global perspective in the quest for new insights into health and disease and the resulting data mining also underscore the need for bioinformatics. Both sophisticated hardware and complex software play an increasingly critical role in the analysis of genomic data, and the accelerated maturation of the field of bioinformatics has implications for computing and life sciences professionals as well as the general public. Like computational biology, bioinformatics is anchored in the life sciences as well as computer and information sciences and technologies. Its interdisciplinary and integrative approach draws from fields such as mathematics, physics, computer science and engineering, biology, and behavioral science. The generally accepted subdisciplines include (1) development of new algorithms and statistics with which to assess relationships among members of large data sets; 2) analyses and interpretation of various types of sequences, domains, and structures; and (3) development and implementation of tools that enable efficient access and management of different types of information.
Three	Product—Entire research article or book	Citation in bibliographic databases includes publication type of "review" and number of references Mendonça, E.A., J.J. Cimino, S.B. Johnson, and Y.H. Seol. 2001 (April). Accessing heterogeneous sources of evidence to answer clinical questions. [Review] [92 refs] *Journal of Biomedical Informatics.* 34(2):85–98. Barrows, R.C., Jr., and P.D. Clayton. 1996 (March–April). Privacy, confidentiality, and electronic medical records. [Review] [42 refs] *Journal of the American Medical Informatics Association* 3(2):139–48. Systematic (integrative) review Meta-analysis

Both as a process and as a product, these overviews identify gaps or discrepancies in the body of knowledge for researchers.

Purpose of the Literature Review

The purpose of a literature review is to develop and present a strong knowledge base. The strong knowledge base can be used to:

- Conduct research
- Generate and analyze theories
- Develop evidence-based practice guidelines
- Develop curriculum
- Perform strategic planning
- Develop white (position) papers

The researcher comes to a complete understanding of the topic. This means that he or she can:

- Determine applicable theories, pertinent factors, and appropriate research designs and methods
- Outline a historical overview of a topic

- Explain the development and evolution of relevant theories
- Assess the thoroughness of literature reviews in published studies
- Relate theorists and researchers with their ideas and findings
- Differentiate between accepted theories and those outside the mainstream
- Discriminate between relevant and irrelevant factors
- Clarify concepts, recognize trends, explain debates, and identify confounding factors
- State advantages and disadvantages of various research methods
- Cite the strengths and weaknesses of various instruments
- Select appropriate techniques for analysis
- Identify competently conducted research and inadequately conducted research
- Detect the holes in the body of knowledge that his or her research can fill

Thus, the literature review results in the researcher "owning" this particular slice of the body of knowledge. He or she knows the theories; the names of the researchers, theorists, and collaborators; the sources of the data; common research designs; and gaps in the body of knowledge.

Process of the Literature Review

Researchers conducting a literature review identify, read, analyze, summarize, and synthesize knowledge and research on a topic and closely related topics. The process of a literature review is a systematic plan consisting of four steps:

1. Determine the literature to review.
2. Identify, categorize, organize, and obtain the literature.
3. Analyze the research questions, methods, and results presented in the literature.
4. Synthesize the information in the literature.

Sources of Information

In the first step, the researcher determines the literature to review. Sources of information include journals; periodicals; books, brochures, and book chapters; technical and research reports; proceedings of conferences; doctoral dissertations and master's theses; unpublished works; reviews; audiovisual media; and electronic media. (See figure 16.3.) These sources can be found in many bibliographic databases that index them. Because health information management combines theories from many academic fields, HIM researchers need to search a wide variety of databases that include sources related to management, organizational behavior, sociology, psychology, medical sciences, computer science, and decision support. Particularly helpful are databases that access the articles in journals related to medicine, health, health information management, health services administration, and bioinformatics. (See table 16.4, p. 446.)

The literature comprises **primary** and **secondary sources.** Primary sources are the original works of the researchers who conducted the investigation. Bell's articles described earlier in this chapter are primary sources. Research-based articles in the *New England Journal of Medicine* or *Science* are other examples of primary sources. Secondary sources are summaries of the original works. Encyclopedias and textbooks are familiar secondary sources. Other examples of secondary sources are annual reviews (also sometimes called tertiary sources). Annual reviews summarize and synthesize current

Figure 16.3.   Sources of information

Periodicals	Books, Brochures, and Book Chapters	Technical and Research Reports
Abstract	Book	Government bulletin
Annual review	Book chapter	Government report
Cartoon	Brochure	Industry report
Journal	Dictionary	Issue brief
Magazine	Encyclopedia	Monograph
Monograph	Legal citation	Nongovernment agency report
Newsletter	Manual	Position paper
Newspaper	Map or chart	Reference report
Press release	Pamphlet	University report
	Product insert	White paper
	Published or archived letter	Working paper
Proceedings of Meetings	**Doctoral Dissertations and Master's Theses**	**Unpublished Works**
Conference	Abstract of dissertation	Submitted manuscript
Meeting	Abstract of thesis	Unpublished letter
Poster session	Dissertation	Unpublished manuscript
Symposium	Thesis	Unpublished raw data
Unpublished proceeding paper		
Reviews	**Audiovisual Media**	**Electronic Media**
Book	Address	Abstract on CD-ROM
Film	Audiotape	CD-ROM
Video	Chart	Computer program
	Film	Computer software
	Lecture	Electronic database
	Music recording	Internet Web site
	Performance	Online abstract
	Published interview	Online book
	Recorded interview	Online journal
	Slide	Software manual
	Speech	
	Television broadcast and transcript	
	Television series and transcript	
	Unpublished interview	
	Work of art	

Table 16.4.   Selected bibliographic databases with emphases in medicine, health, HIM, health services administration, and bioinformatics

Bibliographic Database	Description
Alt-Health Watch	More than 170 international peer-reviewed and professional journals, many full text from 1990; also includes magazines, reports, proceedings, association and consumer newsletters, pamphlets, booklets, special reports, original research, and book excerpts
Allied and Complementary Medicine (AMED)	Indexes approximately 400 biomedical journals focused on alternative and complementary medicine with relevant articles taken from other journals plus newspapers and books; includes English-language and European sources
Applied Science & Technology Abstracts and Index (AppSciTechInd)	Indexes and abstracts articles from more than 410 periodicals, including publications and journals of trade, industry, and professional and technical societies, as well as buyers' guides, directories, and conference proceedings
BioMed Central	Peer-reviewed research of biology and medicine with immediate, barrier-free access from 1997
BioMedical FullTEXT Central	Almost 550 full journals including clinical medicine, psychiatry, psychology, nursing, and allied health
CANCERLIT	More than 4,000 sources of information about cancer therapy
CINAHL (Cumulative Index of Nursing and Allied Health Literature)	Journals and publications in nursing, biomedicine, health sciences librarianship, consumer health, and 17 allied health disciplines
Computer Source	Indexing and abstracting for more than 400 publications and full text for more than 300 publications with topics in computer science, programming, artificial intelligence, cybernetics, information systems, robotics, and software; full text from 1985
Health Business FullTEXT Elite	More than 410 full-text journals on health care administration and other nonclinical aspects of healthcare management
Health Reference Center—Academic	General-interest articles from a variety of health periodicals
Health Services Technology/Assessment Texts (HSTAT)	Free, Web-based, full-text documents on health information for healthcare decision making
Health Source: Consumer	Full text for more than 280 periodicals, almost 1,200 health pamphlets, and 20 health reference books; covers general health, nutrition, and professional healthcare
Health Source: Nursing/Academic	More than 500 scholarly full-text journals, many focused on nursing and allied health; indexing, 1984 to present; full text, 1990 to present
Library Literature and Information Science	Indexes periodicals, state journals, conference proceedings, pamphlets, books, and theses, includes full text for over 100 journals; index from 1984, full text from 1997
MD Consult	Collection of 49 leading medical reference books, over 71 medical journals with many articles in pdf, comprehensive drug information, and more than 1,000 clinical practice guidelines
MDXHealth	Records from thousands of health publications including newsletters, general magazines, medical journals, medical school and hospital publications, and bulletins; 1988 through present indexed, many full text
MEDLINE	Authoritative source of information on medicine, nursing, allied health, dentistry, veterinary medicine, healthcare system, and preclinical sciences
OVID	More than 90 databases including BIOSIS; CINAHL; EBM Reviews–ACP Journal Club, Cochrane, & Dare; EMBASE; HealthSTAR; and MEDLINE
OVID HealthSTAR (HSTR)	More than 3 million citations addressing health services, technology, administration, and research, published from 1975 to present, from the National Library of Medicine; includes both clinical and nonclinical topics in journal articles, government documents, newspaper articles, monographs, book chapters, technical reports, and meeting abstracts and papers
PubMed Central	NIH repository for peer-reviewed primary research reports in life science

and recent knowledge on a topic. They may be special issues of print or electronic journals or entire books. (Examples of annual reviews can be found at www.annualreviews.org.) For literature reviews, primary sources are preferable to secondary sources.

The gold standard for a literature review is primary research in **peer-reviewed journals. Peer review** is the process that ensures that the information reported in the journal is of the highest quality (Colaianni 1994). Journals may be peer reviewed (also called research, refereed, academic, and professional) or nonpeer-reviewed (also called popular). In peer-reviewed journals, the articles are evaluated in manuscript form by experts in the field (peers) for quality prior to publication.

Both print and electronic journals are peer reviewed. Examples of peer-reviewed journals are the *Journal of the American Medical Association,* the *New England Journal of Medicine, Science,* and the *Journal of the American Medical Informatics Association.* In the field of health information management, the major peer-reviewed journals are the *Journal of American Health Information Management Association* and *Perspectives in Health Information Management.* Thus, researchers must make a distinction between research (professional) literature and popular literature. Properly conducted and written literature reviews focus on primary sources in peer-reviewed journals.

Search Techniques

In the second step, researchers identify, categorize, organize, and obtain the literature. A systematic plan identifies the databases to search as well as all the terms used to query the databases. Categorizing includes listing all types of sources of information on the topic. Although traditional literature may constitute the major portion of the plan, other sources (such as videos, newscasts, and the Internet) can contribute and should be considered. Tables and lists are essential tools. The plan also includes organizing the documentation of the queries, the search terms, the results of the queries for each database, and the literature itself as it is received. This section focuses on the search techniques.

Procedure

The following steps describe the search procedure for refereed journal articles. Researchers can use similar tactics in other media and for popular literature.

1. Generate a list of key terms and synonyms (in the databases of medical literature these are medical subject headings or MeSH headings). Include synonyms and alternative formats and spellings (quality management, continuous quality improvement, performance improvement; manage, management; **meta-analysis,** metaanalysis).

2. Generate a list of target databases (such as Ovid Healthstar, MedLine, CINAHL). An excellent database for health-related research is PubMed from the National Library of Medicine. Fenton and Williams (2005) provide detailed instructions on how to query this database.

3. Search each database with each term. Use an advanced "All Fields" search and document each search.

4. Use the "Limit" function to narrow the searches to refereed journals (also sometimes called academic journals). Can also "limit" to human subjects, English language, and time periods.

5. Scan the **abstracts** of the articles to determine whether the articles are applicable. Abstracts summarize research studies' major parts: context; objective; design, setting, and participants; **interventions;** main outcome measures; results; and conclusions.

6. Print articles from online journals and from print journals.

7. Copy articles from print journals (bring an adequate supply of change or purchase a copy card). Note that although it may be convenient or expedient to only use online articles, the resulting literature review will be incomplete and biased. In some cases, academic libraries offer document delivery in which the library staff scan the articles and send the articles electronically to the requester. Be sure to investigate the costs of this procedure as it may be expensive.

8. Read and analyze the literature obtained to date.

9. Identify key journal articles.

10. Obtain the references cited at the end of the key articles. Track their order and receipt.

11. Note the medical subject headings (MeSH headings) of the key articles. If the original list missed these terms, rerun the searches of the databases on the new terms.

12. Identify key researchers in the topic. Run advanced searches on "author." Obtain every researcher's articles and books on the topic.

13. Alphabetize all the copies of the articles by author. This strategy avoids duplication and allows prompt access.

To avoid rework during the manuscript's composition, researchers should capture all data about the source when they first obtain it. The various style manuals have different requirements. To meet all the requirements, researchers should be sure to note the following information about their sources:

- Full name of the author, including first name and middle initial or name (be aware that some entries in Web sites have authors)
- Full title of the journal, book, video, or Internet site
- Complete information about dates of publication, including the year, month, and season (be aware that some entries in Web sites are dated)
- Complete name and address of the publisher (for books and videos)

- Inclusive page numbers
- Volume number and issue number (sometimes these data are only on the front of the publication)
- Accurate URL and access date (for the Internet)

As a means to organize the literature review, researchers are strongly encouraged to invest in a bibliographic software package at the beginning of their research. Bibliographic software packages greatly assist researchers. Helpful features of these packages allow researchers to:

- Create their own personal bibliographic databases
- Utilize the packages' search engines that directly download citations into the researchers' personal bibliographic databases
- Import the contents of databases into word-processing software
- Transform bibliographic entries into the required style of the journal (styles editor)

Commonly used bibliographic packages include Reference Manager, EndNote, and ProCite.

Library Research

Students and instructors have access to sources of information and bibliographic databases through the holdings of their educational institutions' libraries. Libraries have extensive holdings that include books, reference manuals, maps, videotapes, audiotapes, and literary and other databases. Many libraries list their holdings on the Internet. Book holdings can typically be accessed through the library's catalog. The databases and online journals usually can be found under electronic resources. Libraries purchase licenses that allow their users access to the various databases. Just as different libraries have purchased different books, different libraries have purchased different licenses.

In addition, AHIMA members have access to the holdings of the Foundation for Research and Education (FORE) Library in the Body of Knowledge (BoK) of the Communities of Practice (CoP). These holdings include:

- Full-text articles from the *Journal of the American Health Information Management Association* since 1998
- One hundred and twenty-five leading journals in healthcare and health information management
- A thousand books related to healthcare and health information management
- Limited access to some propriety bibliographic databases

There is also document delivery for a fee that varies by availability. Recent white papers about e-HIM, the transition from paper health records to electronic health records, also are available at the AHIMA Web site (http://www.ahima.org/infocenter/ehim/).

Practitioners also may access sources of information and databases through their workplaces. Healthcare organizations have libraries or some arrangement to access to libraries. As employees, practitioners may access these resources.

Although Web sites may have information that has not been peer reviewed, they may have valuable government reports and other documents. Some libraries have developed online tutorials on their Web sites that explain the features of various Internet search engines. Providing tutorials on search engines are the Web sites of the following two libraries: the University of South Carolina Beaufort Library (sc.edu/beaufort/library), and the Kansas City Public Library (kclibrary.org/guides/searchengines/).

In the steps of the search procedure, this brief statement is made: "Read and analyze the literature obtained to date." The brevity of this statement in no way represents the task of reading and analyzing the literature. In this analytical task, researchers should be noting:

- Major theories and theorists
- Trends
- Concepts, factors, and **variables**
- Research designs and methods
- Populations and sampling techniques
- Accepted and commonly used instruments
- Appropriate statistical techniques
- Controversial issues within the topic

Researchers can record the key features of each article in a table. (See table 16.5.) From this tool, they can identify trends, common characteristics, and gaps.

Development of Literature Review

The development of the literature review is the synthesis of the data and information captured in the process of the literature review. The word *synthesize* cannot be emphasized enough. In today's world of data and information overload, mere narrative reviews, which are long summaries of previous studies, are not adequate. Readers require the knowledge that comes from the analysis and synthesis of the literature.

After completing the literature review, researchers develop its products. These products are written and may be either a portion of a journal article, paper, or presentation or an entire article or paper. However, in both forms, the well-developed literature review concisely and logically states what is known and unknown about a topic.

For both forms, the characteristics of a good literature review are:

- A comprehensiveness that is also relevant and focused
- A critique that includes strengths, weaknesses, limitations, and gaps
- An analysis
- A summary that is succinct and logical and comprises mainly primary sources
- A synthesis

Several common conventions guide the development of both forms of literature reviews. These conventions are

Table 16.5.   Summary of the literature

Author	Year	Design & Method	Time Frame	Sample & Response Rate	Statistical Techniques	Key Findings, Limitations, & Recommendations
X and Y	1980	Descriptive	One-shot	20 patients, convenience 100%	Means and percentages	• More smokers in dermatology clinic • Small convenience sample limits generalizability • Recommends larger random sample
A and B	1995	Correlational	One-shot	70 random subjects, 30%	Bivariate correlation	• Relationship between smoking and skin tone • Limitations of self-report and one-shot approach • Recommend longitudinal, experimental research
L, M, and N	2001	Quasi-experimental	1 year	40 subjects, 100%	ANOVA	• Skin tone of nonsmokers significantly more toned than skin tone of smokers • Generalizability limited because subjects from one socioeconomic class and one clinic • Recommend larger and more heterogeneous sample

detailed in the following paragraphs. Unique aspects of each form conclude this subsection.

In a complex or broad topic, researchers should briefly describe the strategy they used to identify literature. In addition, they should explain the scope of the literature review by explicitly stating both their inclusion and exclusion criteria. For example, a researcher could state, "The topic of health information systems is broad. This literature review focused on research articles related to mental health."

Researchers should make a conscious effort to identify, consider, and use an organizing function or factor for the literature review. Using the research model is one organizing function; chronology is another. Explicitly stating the order helps to guide and direct the reader. A coherent and logical order clarifies the topic.

In the literature review, the researcher identifies the key points or turning points in the development of knowledge about a topic. The literature included should be the research studies that either moved the topic forward or added new factors to the topic. However, important studies with contradictory findings also should be included. Otherwise, readers could interpret the absence of contradictory studies as bias. Evidence of bias detracts from the credibility of the literature review. Explanations of the contradictory findings, based on evaluation and analysis, might be suggested.

Moreover, the studies included in the research study should be pertinent. When tangential studies are included, their relevance should be explicitly stated. Generally, the least-related studies should be discussed first and the most-related studies discussed last.

Research studies that either were conducted inadequately or resulted in gaps or conflicting results should be included, especially if the researcher is rectifying the errors. Again, the researcher should specifically point out the inadequacies, gaps, or conflicting results.

Key research studies or turning-point studies should be described in greater detail than replication or duplicative studies. Enough information about the key studies (design, time frame, method, **sample,** response rate, statistical techniques, and findings) should be included so that the reader can evaluate their quality. Research that has the same findings with the same factors should be bundled. For example, the author could state, "Research (citation one, citation two, citation three, and so on) has shown that smoking is bad for skin tone."

Tradition and logic demand that researchers pay close attention to verb tense when they write the literature review. The tense of the verb situates the event or idea in time. Present tense expresses truths, accepted theories, and facts. Recent, valid studies also are explained in the present tense. For example:

- *Accepted theory:* Specific goals motivate employees more than vague goals.
- *Recent study:* Johnson's results illustrate the importance of specific goals.

Past studies with continued historical value can be described in the past tense. Including the date to situate the study is a common practice. For example:

- *Study of historical importance:* In 1972, the study of Smith et al. showed the importance of expectancy in motivation.

However, the easiest and safest rule is to use present tense for published studies and theories.

A table that briefly highlights the important features of the studies in the literature review is an effective tool. Readers can quickly see trends and gaps in the literature. Bell (1999) created a table in his review of the literature on the use of computer-assisted instruction. His table listed each study in a row, with columns displaying its summary, advantages, and disadvantages. Another possible structure for the table is to use rows for the studies but substitute features of the studies in the columns. (See table 16.5.)

As a portion of a journal article, paper, or presentation, the purpose of the literature review is to persuade the reader or audience of the necessity of the research study. The literature review should guide the reader and audience to reach the same conclusions that the researchers reached and the same question or problem. Moreover, the reader and audience should conclude that the logical and necessary next step is the research proposed by the researchers. A secondary purpose is to assure the reader or audience that the researcher has conducted a thorough and diligent review of all aspects of the topic. The thoroughness of the literature review lends credibility to both the researcher and the entire investigation. Finally, the literature review should conclude with a clear and exact statement of the hypothesis.

As an entire article, the literature review is a specialized type of research. Terms for this type of research are **systematic literature review,** integrative review, or meta-analysis. The systematic literature review is a methodical approach to literature review that reduces the possibility of bias. It is characterized by:

- Explicit search criteria to identify literature
- Inclusion and exclusion criteria to select articles and information sources
- Evaluation against consistent methodological standards

This analytical summary of the literature is an amplified and enhanced version of the paragraphs that form the literature review in other research articles.

The meta-analysis is a specialized kind of systematic review that introduces statistical techniques to combine the results of several studies. This type of review is discussed in greater detail in the subsection on research methods.

The literature review article is a distillation and synthesis of the current status of knowledge on a topic. "Systematic reviews establish whether scientific findings are consistent and can be generalized across populations, settings, and **treatment** variations" (Mulrow 1994, p. 597). Annual reviews are examples of analytic summaries of the literature. Examples of annual reviews can be found in journal articles or entire books.

More information on performing literature reviews is available in *Health Sciences Literature Review Made Easy* (Garrard 2004), which focuses on literature reviews in the health sciences.

Check Your Understanding 16.2

Instructions: Answer the following questions on a separate piece of paper.

1. What are the seven basic steps of research?
2. What are five characteristics of a well-developed research question?
3. What are three rich sources of meaningful research questions?
4. Why is conducting a literature review important for a researcher?
5. List five data sources, other than journal articles, that a researcher should consider when doing a comprehensive search.
6. Why would a researcher limit the search of journal articles to refereed journals?
7. Why would the director of health information services select the productivity standard recommended in a peer-reviewed journal rather than the productivity standard recommended in a popular magazine?
8. How do researchers use key terms (MeSH headings)?
9. Why would a researcher use bibliographic software?
10. Why should studies with contradictory results be included in the review of the literature?
11. In the review of the literature, what information about key studies should readers expect?

Determining a Research Design and Method

Researchers can investigate the same broad question or problem using several different research designs. The design chosen depends on the purpose of the research. An important point to remember is that how the problem or question is defined in the problem statement indicates the appropriate research design.

Researchers can choose from among many research designs. Moreover, different disciplines, such as history, medicine, and anthropology, tend to emphasize and use different designs. Certain designs are better suited to answer certain types of questions or to solve certain types of problems than other designs are. (See table 16.6.)

Similarly, certain research methods are more associated with one design than another. However, there is considerable overlap among the methods and their designs. Again, the purpose of the research determines the appropriate research method. Thus, the choice of both the research design and the research method depends on the research question or problem.

Research Designs

There are six common research designs: **historical, descriptive, correlational, evaluation, experimental,** and **causal-comparative** (Gay and Airasian 2003). These designs are particularly well suited to research in topics related to healthcare and, specifically, health information management. Which design is appropriate depends on the problem and the researcher's definition of the problem.

Historical Research

Historical research investigates the past. Researchers examine primary and secondary sources such as wills, charters, reports, minutes, eyewitness accounts, letters, and e-mail records. Primary sources are superior to secondary sources. An example of historical research in healthcare would be an investigation of the development of health insurance in the United States. Examining both primary and secondary sources, researchers in health information management could explore the founding of the professional association, the development of the code of ethics, or the establishment of the technical-level and the various specialty credentials.

Descriptive Research

Descriptive research determines and reports the current status of topics and subjects. Common tools used to collect

Table 16.6   Designs of research and their applications

Design	Application	Method	Example in Healthcare
Historical	Understand past events	• Case study • Bibliography	• What factors led to the enactment of Medicare legislation? • How did events in the history of the American College of Surgeons affect the development of the field of health information management?
Descriptive	Describe current status	• Survey • Observation	• What barriers prevent healthcare personnel from using computers during the delivery of patient care? • How do coders use references and help screens when they code?
Correlational	Determine existence and degree of relationship	• Survey • Secondary analysis	• How are credential and performance related? • What is the relationship between provider satisfaction and EMR systems?
Evaluation	Evaluate effectiveness	• Case study	• How has implementation of an EMR system affected the enterprise's ability to deliver healthcare to underserved populations? • How has EDI reduced the costs of delivery of healthcare to Medicare patients?
Experimental	Establish cause and effect	• Randomized, double-blind, clinical trial • Pretest-posttest control group method • Solomon four-group method • Posttest-only control group	• Which group of molecules with innate immunity affects the risk and severity of invasive Blastomycosis dermatitidis infection? • Which dosage level of the medication is more efficacious and safer for immunocompromised patients with uncomplicated herpes zoster?
Causal-Comparative (Quasi-Experimental)	Detect causal relationship	• One-shot case study • One-group pretest-posttest • Static group comparison • Nonparticipant observation	• What is the effect of a coder training program on the case mix index? • What is the effect of having a working mother on childhood obesity?

descriptive data are **surveys,** interviews, and observations. The shortcomings of descriptive research include the lack of standardized questions, trained observers, and high-response rates. Examples of descriptive studies include polls of Americans' opinions concerning abortion, the patient's bill of rights, stem-cell research, and bioengineering.

In health information management, researchers also conduct descriptive studies. A very limited list of examples includes studies on the status of the composition of the HIM work force, employee morale in HIS departments, coding accuracy, the extent of electronic medical record (EMR) implementation, and the types of tasks that HIM technicians and administrators perform.

Correlational Research
Correlational research determines the existence and degree of relationships among factors. For example, HIM professionals have conducted correlational studies on factors related to burnout among directors of HIM departments (Brodnik 1993; Layman and Guyden 1999). Other correlational studies in health information management might investigate relationships between credential and coding accuracy, job satisfaction and educational level, and increased patient volumes and the level of organizational computerization.

The factors in correlational research and other research designs are called variables. The degree or strength of the relationship can range from .00 to 1.00 (or −1.00). A strength of .00 means absolutely no relationship; a strength of 1.00 (or −1.00) means a perfect relationship. For example, a **positive (direct) relationship** (.5332) exists between confidence and feelings of personal accomplishment (Layman and Guyden 1999). A positive relationship means that the more confident the person, the higher his or her feelings of personal accomplishment. Conversely, a **negative (inverse) relationship** (−.3993) exists between confidence and emotional exhaustion (Layman and Guyden 1999). An inverse relationship means that the more confident the person, the lower his or her emotional exhaustion. Strongly related variables allow researchers to make predictions. In prediction studies, the predictor variables suggest scores on criterion variables. For example, the predictor variable of a mother's smoking predicts a low birth weight (criterion variable) in her baby.

However, correlational research can only detect the existence and degree of relationship. For example, in the Layman and Guyden study mentioned above, the researchers could not state whether confidence causes feelings of personal accomplishment or whether feelings of personal accomplishment cause confidence. Adding to the researchers' difficulties, a third unlisted factor, such as self-esteem, could produce feelings of both personal accomplishment and confidence. This third, unlisted factor is called a **confounding (extraneous, secondary) variable** because it confounds (confuses) interpretation of the data.

Researchers conducting correlational studies use surveys, standardized tests, observations, and secondary data. The important point to remember is that correlational research never establishes **causal relationships.**

Evaluation Research

Evaluation research examines the effectiveness of policies, programs, or organizations. Researchers examine several aspects of programs or organizations, such as conceptualization, design, implementation, impact, and **generalizability** (Shi 1997). For example, researchers might investigate the effectiveness of a new agency for rehabilitation services. Educational programs also are often the focus of evaluation research. Often grants supporting public services require an evaluation of a service's effectiveness. Case studies are often associated with evaluation research.

In health information management, leaders of an integrated health delivery system could evaluate the effectiveness of aspects of different information systems (IS). For example, leaders of the health systems of the Veterans Administration (VA) evaluated the effectiveness of both the different IS designs and the results of different encoding software applications (Lloyd and Layman 1997). Eight VA medical centers tested encoding software applications from three vendors. The research found that the IS design was the crucial element in increasing coding speed.

Experimental Research

Experimental research establishes causal relationships. A causal relationship shows cause and effect. For example, smoking (the cause) results in lung cancer (the effect). Characteristics of experimental research are:

- Control
- Manipulation of treatment
- Random assignment of subjects to groups

The key and defining characteristic of experimental research is control. Experimental research is the gold standard.

Researchers conducting experimental research select both **independent variables** and **dependent variables.** Independent variables are the factors that researchers manipulate directly; independent variables are antecedent or prior factors. Dependent variables are the measured variables; they depend on the independent variables. The dependent variables reflect the results that the researcher theorizes. They occur subsequently or after the independent variables. Therefore, the independent variable causes an effect in the dependent variable.

The independent variables that researchers manipulate are also called interventions or treatments. Researchers use the term *treatment* generically or broadly, beyond its usual mean-

ing of therapy. Therefore, treatment could mean a physical conditioning program, a computer training program, a particular laboratory medium, or the timing of prophylactic medications.

In experimental research, researchers select subjects for comparison groups. The **experimental group** comprises the research subjects. Another group, the **control group,** comprises the control subjects. The experimental subjects undergo the intervention of the research study. For comparison, the control subjects do not.

Important elements of experimental research are **random sampling** and **randomization.** Although the terms are similar, they represent two different procedures. Random sampling is the unbiased selection of subjects from the population of interest. (Random sampling is discussed in greater detail in a subsection on gathering data.) Randomization is the random allocation of subjects between experimental groups and control groups. Thus, step one is to select subjects from the population using random sampling and step two is to randomly assign the randomly selected subjects to experimental or control groups.

Random sampling and randomization characterize **double-blind studies.** A double-blind study is an extremely rigorous form of experimental research in which neither the researcher nor the subject knows to which group the subject belongs. Random selection and random allocation eliminate the effects of expectations and perceptions. For instance, a participant receiving a new heart medication may expect to have more energy and actually believe that he or she does have more energy. In addition, the researcher who knows the participant is receiving the new heart medication may perceive that the participant's color has improved. Thus, double-blind studies control bias because of false expectations and perceptions.

Double-blind studies are often used in the investigation of new drugs. When experimental and control groups are created, neither the participants nor the researchers know to which group the individual participants belong. In order to receive what appears to be the new drug, the participants in the control group are given a **placebo.** A placebo looks exactly like the new drug but, instead, contains harmless ingredients (sometimes called a sugar pill). Therefore, the expectations of the researchers and the participants do not bias the results.

Causal-Comparative Research

Causal-comparative research is a type of quasi-experimental design. *Quasi* means resembling or having some of the characteristics. Therefore, causal-comparative research resembles experimental research by having many, but not all, of the characteristics of experimental research. However, causal-comparative research lacks two key characteristics of experimental research: manipulation of treatment and random assignment to a group.

Choosing causal-comparative research is correct when one of the three following situations exist:

- The variables cannot be manipulated (gender, age, race, birthplace).
- The variables should not be manipulated (accidental death or injury, child abuse).
- The variables represent different conditions that have already occurred (medication error, heart catheterization performed, smoking).

This research design is also called "ex post facto," meaning **retrospective.** Examples of quasi-experimental research are **case-control (retrospective) studies,** field experiments, and natural experiments.

Epidemiologists investigating the development of disease often use case-control (retrospective) studies. In case-control studies, the epidemiologists look for characteristics and occurrences that are related to the subsequent development of a disease. In these studies, epidemiologists collect masses of data from health records and through interviews with both persons with the disease (cases) and persons without it (controls). HIM professionals are often involved with case-control studies because they are experts on the content of health records and at finding cases and controls using various clinical and administrative classification systems, such as ICD-9-CM, ICD-10, DSM, and SNOMED CT.

Researchers investigating the sociology of medicine often conduct field experiments by going into the site (field) and observing activities. The strength of this type of research is that participants tend to act more naturally in their real setting. An outstanding example of field research is the research on health practitioners' conversations overheard in elevators. Researchers rode hospital elevators all day listening and recording conversations. They found that patient confidentiality was severely breached.

Researchers conducting natural experiments wait for the event to occur naturally. For example, researchers interested in the effectiveness of triage in emergencies would wait for a disaster. Prior to the disaster, they would establish baseline data and tools for data collection. When the disaster occurs, they would record their observations of the actions and results.

In case-control studies, field experiments, and natural experiments, researchers relinquish control of the situations. For purists, however, the lack of randomization and control of treatment lessens the value of causal-comparative (quasi-experimental) research. The research only weakly determines causation. However, as the examples illustrate, in some situations, causal-comparative research is the only design that is logistically and ethically feasible. Causal-comparative research, then, determines the possibility of causal relationships.

Time Frame as an Element of Research Design
Another element of design cuts across all six types of design. This element is the time frame of the study. The three time frames are retrospective, **cross-sectional,** and **longitudinal.**

Studies within a retrospective time frame look back in time. For example, many early research studies of stress were

retrospective. In these retrospective studies, the researchers measured the participant's level of stress and then asked the participant to reconstruct events that had occurred in a past period of time. Leadership studies in which the researcher asked the leader to list factors that led to his or her success are another example of a retrospective time frame. For some types of questions, such as those related to historic events, a retrospective design is the only possible design.

Research studies with a cross-sectional design collect data at one point in time. Cross-sectional studies are snapshots and, as such, may collect data at an entirely unrepresentative point in time. The great advantage of cross-sectional studies is that they are efficient.

Longitudinal studies collect data from the same participants at multiple points in time. Cancer registries that collect data on cancer patients throughout their lifetimes are prime examples of longitudinal studies. Other longitudinal studies include studies of breast cancer and cardiovascular disease. For example, the Nurses' Health Study has followed the health of more than 120,000 nurses for more than 20 years (Giovannucci et al. 1998).

The six types of research designs are not rigid boxes. Researchers often combine designs to address their particular research questions or problems. For instance, many studies include both descriptive and correlational findings. In describing their study, researchers also often state its time frame. Thus, a researcher would state that the study was descriptive, correlational, and cross-sectional. However, the key to classifying the design is to understand the purpose of the research.

Check Your Understanding 16.3

Instructions: Answer the following questions on a separate piece of paper.

1. What determines a researcher's choice of a research design?

2. Which research design would a researcher use to investigate the relationship between a supervisor's level of stress and the number of his or her subordinates?

3. What would be a direct relationship between the supervisor's level of stress and the number of his or her subordinates?

4. What is the key characteristic of experimental research?

5. How does quasi-experimental research differ from experimental research?

6. How do independent variables and dependent variables differ?

7. In a double-blind study, who knows which subjects are in the study group and which subjects are in the control group?

8. Why would a researcher choose a longitudinal study rather than a cross-sectional study?

Research Methods
A research method is the particular strategy that a researcher uses to collect, analyze, and present data. Particular methods are associated with certain designs, although considerable overlap exists. (See table 16.6.) For example, researchers can use surveys in both descriptive and correlational designs.

Surveys

A survey is a common research method. Surveys are a form of self-report research in which the individuals themselves are the source of data. Surveys collect data about a population to determine its current status with regard to certain factors (Gay and Airasian 2003). Surveys that collect data from all the members of the population are **census surveys;** surveys that collect data from representative members of the population are **sample surveys.**

HIM professionals conduct both types of surveys. For example, when surveying the members of the local HIM association, the past president of the association surveyed every member (Garvin 2001). On the other hand, when information about the members of the national association (a population of more than 40,000) is needed, researchers conduct only a sample survey. A census survey of a large population is generally beyond the resources of a solitary researcher or a small research team. For example, Brodnik (1993) surveyed a representative group of 700 directors of HIM departments to ascertain their level of burnout and then estimated the level of burnout for all directors of HIM departments.

Survey research is further categorized as interview or questionnaire. Researchers conduct **interview surveys** by personally questioning the members of the **target population.** In **questionnaire surveys,** researchers create electronic or paper forms that include the questions.

In both categories, questions may be structured, semistructured, or unstructured. **Structured (closed-ended) questions** list all the possible responses; **unstructured (open-ended) questions** allow free-form responses. In **semistructured questions,** researchers first ask structured questions and then follow with open-ended questions to clarify. The disadvantage of unstructured questions is that they are more difficult to quantify, tabulate, and analyze than structured questions are. The advantages of unstructured questions are that they allow in-depth questions and may uncover aspects of a problem unknown to the researcher.

For example, Lippin et al. (2000) investigated the effect of a training program on safety practices. They conducted a semistructured, telephone interview with 362 workers and managers using both structured questions from a written list and unstructured questions. For the analysis of the structured questions, the researchers calculated percentages to compare responses across the various job classes, such as hospital manager of public-sector blue-collar workers. However, in order to analyze the responses to the open-ended questions, the researchers first had to transcribe them verbatim and code them. The greater time commitment for open-ended questions is demonstrated.

Interviews

In interview surveys, researchers orally question the members of the population. Examples of interview surveys are telephone surveys, exit polls, and **focused studies.** Researchers can question members of the population individually or

as a group using a written list of questions called an **interview guide.** Use of an interview guide ensures that all members of the group are asked the same questions. In focused studies, the researcher and the group members have a group discussion. Researchers can strictly control the questions and responses or can allow a free-flowing conversation. They often record sessions and then transcribe the comments.

For example, Monsen (1999) conducted a study in which she asked the mothers of children with spina bifida to describe their experiences. She audiotaped the interviews, transcribed them, and then analyzed the texts using a specialized software program and multiple readings of the text to interpret the mothers' comments. The data revealed themes that helped nurses to understand the lives of mothers of children with disabilities.

Questionnaires

Questionnaire surveys also query members of the population. Rather than asking questions orally, researchers mail participants an electronic or print form to complete and return. Questionnaire studies are efficient because they require less time and money than interview studies do and because they allow the researchers to collect data from many more members of the target population. Moreover, questionnaire studies that are Internet based further enhance efficiency because the subjects' answers are entered directly into the database, which eliminates a step for the researchers.

For example, Garvin (2001) used a questionnaire to conduct a census survey of the members of the local HIM association. This research study explored the readiness of health information practitioners to assume the role of clinical data specialist. The leadership of the local association used this study to investigate its members' current knowledge of coding skills. Then, from the information the questionnaire provided, the leadership could project the future educational needs of the local members and plan appropriate workshops and seminars to meet those needs. In another example, Osborn (2000a) investigated managerial practices in HIM departments. She randomly selected 1,000 directors of acute care facilities from the membership roster of AHIMA and mailed them questionnaires; 200 directors responded. The questionnaire collected data about record turnaround time; discharge analysis procedures; inpatient coding productivity; assembly, analysis, and electronic storage; outsourcing; and other electronic functions. The data from this study describe current practices in health information management. Health information managers can use its findings to assess their own practices.

Observational Research

In **observational research,** researchers obtain data by observing rather than by asking. Observational research is used in many designs. For example, sociologists used a descriptive design to describe the culture of medical students (Becker et al. 1961). There are three common types of observational research: **nonparticipant observation, participant observation,** and **ethnography.**

Nonparticipant Observation

In nonparticipant observation, researchers act as neutral observers who neither intentionally interact with nor affect the actions of the population being observed. Of the three types of observational research, HIM professionals are more likely to encounter nonparticipant observation. This method takes three common forms: **naturalistic observation, simulation observation,** and **case study.**

Researchers use naturalistic observation for certain behaviors and events that are best observed as they occur naturally. The researchers observe, record, and analyze the behaviors and events. To record the behaviors and events, they typically use check sheets, audiotapes, or videotapes. For the audiotapes and videotapes, they must insert the additional step of transcription. Then, the researchers use coding systems to transform all the recorded observations into analyzable data. For example, researchers investigated the language development of children with compensatory articulation disorder (CAD), a common condition associated with cleft palate (Pamplona et al. 2000). The researchers observed and videotaped 58 children as they played and read stories over a two-week period. They coded the transcribed videotapes using the Situational-Discourse-Semantic Model. Using naturalistic observation, the researchers found that, in all contexts, the children with CAD had delays in language development. Thus, the researchers were able to improve the treatment of patients.

Simulation observation is very similar to naturalistic observation except that the researchers stage the events rather than allowing them to occur naturally. Researchers can invent their own simulations or use standardized vignettes to stage the events. For example, researchers in occupational therapy (Brown et al. 1996) investigated the congruence among therapists' assessments of patients' independence. Measures of independence are achievements of activities of daily living, such as making a purchase in a store and taking a bus. The researchers compared therapists' assessments on simulations and their assessments on tasks in the natural setting. They found that the assessments in the natural setting were more accurate. Therefore, this research assisted occupational therapists in their practice.

The case study is another type of nonparticipant observation. Case studies are in-depth investigations of one person, one group, or one institution. Researchers conduct case studies to determine characteristics associated with a person, group, or institution. The characteristics then can shed light on similar persons, groups, or institutions. Often case studies suggest hypotheses that researchers subsequently investigate using other methods. Case studies are intensive, and researchers amass extensive details. Sources of data include administrative records, financial records, policy and procedure manuals, legal documents, government documents, surveys, and interviews. These many sources result in layer upon layer of detailed data, often called rich data.

Sigmund Freud conducted case studies at the individual person level (Gall, Borg, and Gall 2003). This type of case study is called a clinical case study. Early research in medicine comprised clinical case studies. From a physician's presentation of detailed information about an individual patient, other physicians learned about similar patients.

Other case studies are at the group level and the institutional level. For example, at the group level researchers could investigate the influence that AIDS action groups have had on funding practices of the National Institutes of Health. At the institutional level, Meyer and Blumenthal (1996) investigated the effects of changes in Medicaid policies on two academic medical centers in Tennessee.

Participant Observation

In participant observation, researchers are also participants in the observed actions. They can participate overtly (openly) or covertly (secretly). For example, researchers in Australia (van de Mortel and Heyman 1995) wanted to know the incidence of hand washing postpatient contact. The researchers covertly observed the incidence of hand washing to establish a baseline and overtly observed the action to assess the effect of their intervention. On the positive side, participant observation presents the insiders' perspectives. On the negative side, the deception of covert observation undermines human relationships and breaches ethics (Johnson 1992). Moreover, as participants, researchers can reflect the biases and narrow view of insiders. Therefore, in participant observation, researchers attempt to maintain neutrality while in the "thick of the action."

Ethnography

Ethnography is observational research that came to the life sciences from anthropology. It includes both qualitative and quantitative approaches and both participant and nonparticipant observation. Ethnographers typically investigate aspects of culture in naturalistic settings. For example, an HIM professional could choose ethnography to investigate how the culture of a nursing unit or clinic affects the timeliness and comprehensiveness of provider documentation. Are areas of the unit or clinic set aside for documentation, indicating that the culture of the unit or clinic values accurate and comprehensive documentation? Or, do providers attempt to document in health records in corners or on ledges of the unit or clinic, indicating less attention to documentation?

Two key differences exist between ethnography and other types of research. First, in ethnography, the literature review results in working or tentative hypotheses rather than testable hypotheses (Gay and Airasian 2003). Second, ethnography is iterative, or cyclical (Byrne 2001). As ethnographers collect data, they analyze them, revising their working hypotheses and creating new working hypotheses. Therefore, ethnographers work in a cycle beginning with working hypotheses, collecting data, revising hypotheses and creating new working hypotheses, and then collecting more data about those hypotheses. This cyclical process contrasts with the linear processes of other research methods discussed in this chapter.

In order to understand cultures, ethnographers amass great volumes of detailed data while on studies in the field. Therefore, another characteristic of ethnography is that the researchers live or work with the population they are studying. For example, Hill and Tyson (1997) investigated the culture of clinical teaching conferences. They attended 52 sessions of morning report with the faculty physicians, house officers, and medical students and timed the length of people's comments, the commentator's status, and the content of the comments. In addition to the sessions of morning report, the researchers conducted 34 interviews lasting between 30 and 60 minutes with people from the three groups. The quantitative aspect of this study is that the researchers tabulated the minutes and averaged the time that members of each group spoke. The qualitative aspect of this study is that the researchers analyzed the comments for themes.

Ethnography has other unique characteristics, such as the attention that ethnographers pay to the environment (furniture, instruments, space, lighting, schedules, brochures, and clothing). For example, Hill and Tyson (1997) recorded data on x-ray equipment and the placement of a table and a sign-in sheet. In general, ethnographers also record details about members of the population, including jargon, feelings, points of view, beliefs, practices, and goals. In conclusion, the strength of ethnography is that researchers obtain insights not discoverable in other methods. Its weaknesses include volumes of data that are difficult to analyze, large investments of money and time, and the lack of generalizability and replicability.

Experimental Research

Experiments are another major category of research methods. These methods classify into two subcategories: experimental studies and quasi-experimental studies. Both subcategories involve treatments using the broad meaning of the term as some sort of intervention. The level of control that researchers establish differentiates experiments between experimental studies and quasi-experimental studies.

Campbell and Stanley (1963) wrote the classic text on experiments. They defined and described six major types of experiments, with three in the subcategory of experimental and three in the subcategory of quasi-experimental. Experimental studies include:

- Pretest–posttest control group method
- Solomon four-group method
- Posttest-only control group method

Quasi-experimental studies include:

- One-shot case study
- One-group pretest–posttest method
- Static group comparison

The key elements in the descriptions of these experiments are:

- Randomization
- Observation (pretest or posttest)
- Control group
- Treatment

Readers should be aware that, similar to the treatment, researchers use the terms *pretest, posttest,* and *observation* broadly. They simply mean that they have measured the variable in some way.

To demonstrate the differences among these six subcategories, descriptions of research studies conducted in each of the six subcategories will be described. (See table 16.7.) The description will include how the studies representing the subcategories conform with or deviate from the four key elements. To highlight the differences, the research studies all involve the same research topic. This topic is the medical students' utilization of voice recognition software.

Experimental Studies

Researchers conducted a pretest–posttest control group method to investigate medical students' utilization of voice recognition software. The researchers randomly assigned the first-year medical students to experimental and control groups. The researchers performed a pretest in which they established both groups' levels of utilization of voice recognition software. The researchers then conducted a two-hour training session (treatment). At the end of the academic year, the researchers measured both groups' utilization of voice recognition software. They could reasonably attribute differences in utilization to their "treatment." However, the researchers should be cautious because the possibility exists that the students' higher level of utilization of the software is a function of their exposure during the pretest observation. Familiarity with the software from exposure could predispose the students to use it.

The key elements of this study include:

- Randomization (randomly assigned medical students to groups)
- Pre- and posttest observation (levels of utilization of voice recognition software before and after the training session)
- Control group
- Treatment (two-hour training session)

The Solomon four-group method is a complex variation of the pretest–posttest control group method. The purpose of the Solomon four-group method is to provide a way to control for the potential effect of exposure. For example, as noted in the previous study, taking a pretest may affect performance on a posttest. In the previous study of utilization of voice recognition software, how much of the utilization is due to mere familiarity with the software related to the original exposure? Using the Solomon four-group method, researchers create two experimental groups and two control groups rather than only one of each. They then administer the pretest to only one of the experimental groups and to only one of the control groups. However, they administer the posttest to *all* four groups. The

Table 16.7.   Key elements of experimental and quasi-experimental studies*

Category/ Subcategory	Study Features	Elements			
		Randomization	Observation	Control Group	Treatment
Experimental					
Pretest–Posttest Control Group Method	Investigation of medical students' utilization of voice recognition software	X	X	X	X
	Random assignment to experimental and control groups				
	Observation to establish initial level of utilization (pretest)				
	Two-hour training session (treatment)				
	Observation to determine posttreatment utilization (posttest)				
	Potential that pretests exposure affected posttreatment performance				
Solomon Four-Group Method	Investigation of medical students' utilization of voice recognition software	X	X	X	X
	Random assignment to two experimental and two control groups				
	Observation to establish initial level of utilization (pretest)				
	Two-hour training session (treatment)				
	Observation to determine posttreatment utilization (posttest)				
	Controls for pretest exposure, but at the cost of double work because of double groups				
Posttest-Only Control Group Method	Investigation of medical students' utilization of voice recognition software	X	P	X	X
	Random assignment to experimental and control groups				
	Two-hour training session (treatment)				
	Observation to determine posttreatment utilization (posttest)				
	Controls for pretest exposure by eliminating pretest, but at cost of establishment of initial utilization level				
Quasi-Experimental					
One-Shot Case Study	Investigation of medical students' utilization of voice recognition software	0	P	0	X
	Two-hour training session (treatment)				
	Observation to determine posttreatment utilization (posttest)				
	Flaws of no pretest, no randomization, and no control group				
One-Group Pretest–Posttest Method	Investigation of medical students' utilization of voice recognition software	0	X	0	X
	Observation to establish initial level of utilization (pretest)				
	Two-hour training session (treatment)				
	Observation to determine posttreatment utilization (posttest)				
	Flaws of no control group and no randomization				
Static Group Comparison	Investigation of medical students' utilization of voice recognition software	0	P	X	X
	Assignment to experimental and control groups				
	Two-hour training session (treatment)				
	Observation to determine posttreatment utilization (posttest)				
	Flaws of no pretest and no randomization				

*X = Fully met; P = Partially met; 0 = Absent

difference in level of utilization between the two experimental groups would be the effect of the familiarity from pretesting. Therefore, the Solomon four-group method provides a valuable additional control. However, this additional control comes at a very high price: Everything is doubled.

The key elements of the Solomon four-group method are the same as those for the pretest–posttest control group method.

The posttest-only control group method is another method to offset the potential effect of familiarity related to exposure through pretesting. The posttest-only control group method is similar to the pretest–posttest control group method except that there is no pretest. In the research on utilization of voice recognition software, the researchers randomly assign half the first-year medical students to the experimental group and half to the control group. The researchers do not observe an initial level of utilization through a pretest. The experimental group receives the treatment of the training session, and the control group does not. Then, at the end of the academic year, the researchers measure the students' level of utilization of the software. This fairly simple method eliminates the potential bias introduced by pretesting.

The key elements of the posttest-only control group are randomization, posttest observation, control group, and treatment. HIM professionals also encounter the posttest-only control group method in clinical trials. For example, parasitologists used this method to observe the effects of drug regimens on multidrug-resistant malaria (Van Vugt et al. 1999). Patients with malaria presenting at the clinical trial sites were randomly and blindly assigned to study groups or control groups. Two study groups were given the experimental drug regimen, and the control group was given the currently recommended regimen. Laboratory results demonstrated the effects of various drug regimens on the disease.

Quasi-Experimental Studies

In the one-shot case study, researchers study one group only once following the treatment. For example, in the study of utilization of voice recognition software, researchers provide a two-hour training session on utilization of voice recognition software to all the first-year medical students at some point in the academic year. Then, at the end of the academic year, the researchers measure the students' level of utilization of the software. The researchers can make no credible statement about the effect of the training session on the utilization of voice recognition software because they (1) have not established with an observation (pretest) the level of utilization prior to the training (treatment) to use as a comparison and (2) have no other group of medical students (control group) to use as a comparison.

The key elements in this case are posttest observation and treatment.

The one-group pretest–posttest method corrects one flaw of the one-shot case study with the addition of the pretest. Therefore, the researchers investigating utilization of voice recognition software improve their experiment by adding some measurement, or pretest, that establishes the medical students' level of utilization prior to the training session. However, adding the pretest only minimally improves their investigation. Statements made by the researchers about the utilization of voice recognition software still are highly suspect because the researchers included no control group. Therefore, readers of this research could reasonably wonder whether other factors in the hospital or in society "caused" the level of utilization.

The key elements of this method are pre- and posttest observation and treatment.

The static group comparison corrects for the lack of a control group. Therefore, the static group comparison is similar to the one-shot case study except that researchers using the static group comparison add a second group, the control group. In the research on utilization of voice recognition software, the researchers allow half the students to choose to attend the training session. This group is the experimental group, and the half who choose not to receive the training are the control group. Then, at the end of the academic year, the researchers measure the students' level of utilization of the software. Unfortunately, a flaw of this study is that there is no random assignment to the groups. Perhaps all the technophiles joined the experimental group and all the technophobes joined the control group. In that case, the increased level of utilization of the experimental group could just be an effect of the group's inherent love of computers and not of the training session.

The key elements of the static group comparison are posttest observation, control group, and treatment.

Experimental research is important because this major category of research allows researchers to investigate cause and effect. It should be clear from these examples of research studies that true experimental studies are very difficult to conduct. Nevertheless, experimental research studies are extremely powerful research methods because only they can establish cause and effect (causal relationship). The types classified as quasi-experimental studies begin to determine that a causal relationship could exist. Some experts state that very large quasi-experimental studies weakly determine a causal relationship. However, to truly establish causal relationships, researchers must use one of the types classified as an experimental study.

Secondary Analysis

Secondary analysis is the analysis of the original work of another person or organization. Researchers make the distinction between **primary analysis** and **secondary analysis.** Primary analysis refers to analysis of original research data by the researchers who collected them. There are three types of secondary analysis:

- Secondary analysis of data sets
- Meta-analysis
- Content analysis

In *secondary analysis of data sets,* researchers reanalyze original data by combining data sets to answer new questions or by using more sophisticated statistical techniques (Cohen 1992). In the field of health information management, Osborn (1999, 2001) reanalyzed data sets to evaluate data quality. For example, she reanalyzed clinical databases to identify problems in specific diagnosis-related groups in order to reveal variations in charges and lengths of stay and to detect trends (2001). Reanalysis of secondary data is a powerful tool for health information managers because it allows them to compare their data with local, regional, state, and national benchmarks.

Meta-analysis is the integrative analysis of findings from many studies that examined the same question. Studies that are included in a meta-analysis have common underlying characteristics (Cohen 1992). Glass (1976) coined the term *meta-analysis,* defining it as "the statistical analysis of a large collection of results from individual studies for the purpose of integrating findings" (1976, p. 3). Meta-analysis began as a sophisticated way to present a literature review but has become a research method in its own right.

The advantage of meta-analysis is that it weighs findings from many studies, some of which are contradictory. Researchers who use meta-analysis must specify their inclusion criteria; explain how they searched and found articles; code the studies' designs, methods, and outcomes; and analyze the coded data (Cohen 1992).

For example, Lan, Colford, and Colford (2000) conducted a meta-analysis that analyzed studies of antibiotic treatment for streptococcal tonsillopharyngitis. First, they specified their inclusion criteria. To be included, the study must possess the following four characteristics: (1) it had to be a **randomized clinical trial** (RCT) that compared the efficacy of different dosing frequencies of 10-day oral penicillin or amoxicillin in the treatment of acute streptococcal tonsillopharyngitis; (2) diagnosis had to be based on both symptoms and positive clinical findings; (3) antibiotic treatment had to be initiated upon diagnosis; and (4) it had to be the most recent publication, if multiple publications arose from the same study. Second, the researchers explained their strategies to find all the studies. They searched Medline, dissertation abstracts, and abstracts of the annual Interscience Conference on Antimicrobial Agents and Chemotherapy. They used combinations of key words, such as tonsillopharyngitis, pharyngitis, penicillin, amoxicillin, clinical trial, streptococcus, and streptococcal. These search strategies yielded 30 potential documents. After review, only 6 met the inclusion criteria. The researchers then coded the studies' designs, methods, and outcomes. Finally, they conducted the meta-analysis statistical procedure called effect size analysis. "Effect size" is the strength of the impact of one factor on another (Shi 1997). Integrating the results of these studies revealed that two doses of penicillin per day are as efficacious as more frequent doses per day. Thus, using meta-analysis, the researchers synthesized the results from multiple studies in order to make an overall conclusion.

Content analysis is the systematic and objective analysis of communication. Most often, researchers analyze written documentation. However, they may analyze other modes of communication, such as speech, body language, music, television shows, commercials, and movies. The purpose of content analysis is to study and predict behaviors.

For example, consumer groups who notify the public about the "most violent" or the "most sexually graphic" shows on television have used content analysis to compile their reports. Healthcare personnel also use content analysis. For example, Wilson et al. (2000) evaluated the readability and cultural sensitivity of information on the National Cancer Institute's Web site. They used standardized tools to conduct this evaluation. From their analysis of 49 documents, they established that the reading level was the 12th grade. Because most newspapers are written at the 4th-grade level, this level would be too advanced for many patients. Thus, content analysis was valuable to oncology nurses who use various means to educate their patients about cancer.

Several key points are important to remember about research design and methods. Research is the systematic, orderly set of procedures that individuals choose to expand their knowledge or to answer their question. They can investigate the same broad question or problem using several of the research designs. (See table 16.8.) Preliminary, exploratory investigations are often descriptive or correlational. As researchers

Table 16.8.   Research designs in a progression of studies within one topic

Design	Example of Progression of Studies
Historical	The factors leading to the creation and expansion of The Medical Record (TMR) and the Regenstrief Medical Record System (RMRS) between 1970 and 1990
Descriptive	A survey of physicians to determine how and to what degree they use the computer-based patient record
Correlational	A study to determine the relationship among physicians' attributes, the setting, and use of the computer-based patient record
Evaluation	A study to evaluate the efficacy of the implementation of the computer-based patient record in an academic health center
Causal-Comparative (Quasi-Experimental)	A study to compare the use of the computer-based patient record of a group of physicians in a setting classified as low barrier and a group of physicians in a setting classified as high barrier
Experimental	A study to compare use of the computer-based patient record of two matched physician groups; one group trained in a low-barrier experimental computer laboratory and one group trained in a high-barrier experimental computer laboratory

refine these investigations, they conduct causal-comparative and experimental studies. The research design chosen depends on the purpose of the research. Certain methods, such as surveys and laboratory experiments, are associated with particular designs. However, methods can be associated with more than one design and overlap occurs. The key point is that how the problem or question is defined indicates the appropriate research design and method.

Check Your Understanding 16.4

Instructions: Answer the following questions on a separate piece of paper.

1. Which research method uses self-report data?

2. What type of question is question 1?

3. Why would researchers choose to conduct a structured interview using an interview guide?

4. If researchers wanted to investigate the impact of the Hill-Burton Act on a region's healthcare, which method would they choose?

5. Why would researchers choose to conduct a questionnaire survey?

6. If researchers wanted to establish that a new drug caused a reduction in blood pressure, which research method would they choose?

7. When would researchers choose to conduct a meta-analysis?

8. In questions 3 through 7, what common characteristic determined the researchers' choice of method?

Statement of Hypothesis

Formulation of precise and accurate hypotheses is a difficult task. In the statement of hypothesis, the researcher states the research question in measurable terms. Therefore, the statement of the hypothesis is more specific than the research question. Some experts explain that the statement of the hypothesis operationalizes the research question. Moreover, the statement of the hypothesis becomes the basis of the statistical tests. Therefore, there are two errors to avoid in the statement of the hypothesis: writing an ambiguous hypothesis and writing an untestable hypothesis. Finally, researchers should take care that the hypothesis actually reflects the intent of the research.

Researchers write **null hypotheses** and **alternative hypotheses.** The null hypothesis states that there is no association between the independent and dependent variables. (The word *null* means none.) The alternative hypothesis states that there is an association between the independent and dependent variables. Alternative hypotheses are **one-tailed** or **two-tailed.** If the researcher states that the association is more or less, the alternative hypothesis is a one-tailed hypothesis. If the researcher makes no prediction about the direction of the results (more or less), the alternative hypothesis is a two-tailed hypothesis. These hypotheses are matched pairs. For example:

- *Null hypothesis:* There is no difference in the levels of utilization of voice recognition software between the group of physicians receiving the training and the group not receiving it.

- *Alternative hypothesis (one-tailed):* The level of utilization of the group receiving the training is 10 percent higher than the level of the group not receiving it.

- *Alternative hypothesis (two-tailed):* There is a 10 percent difference in the levels of utilization of voice recognition software between the group of physicians receiving the training and the group not receiving it.

Researchers state what they believe in alternative hypotheses. Unfortunately, the properties of statistical techniques do not allow them to directly test the accuracy of the alternative hypotheses. Instead, statistical techniques test null hypotheses. Therefore, researchers also must write null hypotheses in order to conduct statistical analysis. If the null hypothesis is rejected, the alternative hypothesis is accepted.

Associated with the statement of the hypothesis is establishing the appropriate **level of significance,** known as the alpha (a) level. The level of significance is the criterion used for rejecting the null hypothesis. Common alpha levels are 0.05 and 0.01. Researchers set the lower alpha level when they want to minimize the chance that they might erroneously reject the null hypothesis when it is actually true.

Researchers can make two types of errors associated with rejecting or failing to reject null hypotheses. A **type I error** occurs when the researcher erroneously rejects the null hypothesis when it is true; in actuality, there is no difference. A **type II error** occurs when the researcher erroneously fails to reject the null hypothesis when it is false; in actuality, there is a difference. For example:

- *Null hypothesis:* There is no difference in blood pressure levels between the group of patients receiving the new drug and the group receiving the placebo.

- *Alternative hypothesis (one-tailed):* The blood pressure of the group of patients receiving the new drug is 15 percent lower than the blood pressure of the group receiving the placebo.

A researcher committing a type I error would reject the null hypothesis. Continuing in the error, he or she would report the efficacy of the new drug. Unfortunately, the fact is that there is no difference between the blood pressures of the two groups of patients; the new drug does not work as predicted. Researchers who set the alpha level at 0.05 have a 5 percent chance of making this error whereas those who set the alpha level at 0.01 have a 1 percent chance of making the error. Thus, an alpha level of 0.01 is stricter than an alpha level of 0.05.

Beta (b) designates the probability of making a type II error. In the previous example, the researcher would make a type II error if he or she failed to reject the null hypothesis and it was indeed false. The researcher would erroneously state that there was no difference between the blood pressure of the group taking the new drug and the blood pressure of the group taking the placebo. In fact, there was a difference and the new drug was working as predicted.

The level of significance is established prior to conducting statistical techniques. Statistical tests for significance result in a ρ value. A ρ value indicates the probability of obtaining the result by chance if the null hypothesis is true. Therefore, if the ρ value is 0.05, the probability that the difference occurred by pure chance is 5 percent. If the ρ value obtained from the statistical test is less than or equal to the level of predetermined alpha value, the study's results are considered unlikely to be mere chance and the null hypothesis is rejected.

The statement of the hypothesis is a crucial step in the development of the research plan. It leads to the establishment of the appropriate statistical techniques and the determination of the level of significance. These two actions, in turn, affect the interpretation of the consequences of the treatment.

Selection of a Research Method

In selecting a research method, researchers first and foremost should consider their purpose as reflected in their research question. If they want to establish a causal relationship, they should conduct one of the experimental studies. If they are breaking new ground in a poorly understood area of practice, they may want to consider an exploratory study in a qualitative design.

Other factors are associated with the researchers' expertise and resources. Researchers should establish a match between the method and the following factors:

- *Expertise:* Can the researcher conduct, interpret, and explain sophisticated statistical techniques, or are more basic statistical techniques within the researcher's comfort zone?
- *Skills:* Can the researcher conduct the laboratory experiments necessary for research? For example, to investigate physicians' utilization of clinical guidelines, is the researcher able to insert codes into a computer-based patient record? Is the researcher able to insert a time clock into the software and design a query mechanism?
- *Personal attributes:* If the researcher is considering interviewing people, is he or she able to easily establish rapport with people? Or do conversations with strangers make the researcher feel awkward?
- *Time:* Does the researcher have the time to devote to conduct the research plan well? For example, investigating the change in attitude of students in HIM programs from the freshman year through graduation is a meritorious idea. However, graduate programs have time frames within which students must complete their studies. A four-year research study may not fit the time frame.
- *Money:* Can the researcher afford the postage for a census survey of all 40,000 AHIMA members?
- *Potential subjects:* The Solomon four-group method is excellent and beautifully controlled; however, it requires double the number of subjects. If subjects are in short supply, would this method be feasible?

Finally, researchers should strive for parsimony or elegance. *Parsimony* means that the researcher has eliminated extraneous, unnecessary complications. Just as the best theory is the simplest, so too is the best method.

Validity and Reliability

There are three types of **validity. Internal validity** and **external validity** involve the integrity of the research plan. Validity without a modifier refers to an attribute of measurement instruments. **Reliability** involves the consistency of measurements.

Validity

Internal validity and external validity are key issues when implementing a research plan. Campbell and Stanley (1963) identified eight threats to internal validity. (See figure 16.4.) Internal validity is an attribute of a study's design that contributes to the accuracy of its findings. Threats to internal validity are potential sources of error that contaminate the study's results. These sources of error come from factors outside the study (confounding variables). Therefore, if internal validity is breached, researchers cannot state for certain that the independent variable caused the effect. External validity refers to the extent to which the findings can be generalized to other people or groups. *Generalizability* is the term that researchers use to mean the ability to apply the results to other groups, such as hospitals, patients, and states. Are the findings representative of many people or groups? Internal validity represents the bare minimum; internal validity combined with external validity is the ideal.

For example, researchers within the Department of Veterans Affairs (VA) evaluated the use of automated encoders in the VA system (Lloyd and Layman 1997). Eight VA medical centers tested encoding software programs from three vendors. During the course of the study, an earthquake badly damaged one of the VA medical centers, which never reopened. Therefore, no final data on the software program were available from that center. This event represents the

Figure 16.4.   Threats to internal validity

History:	Unplanned events occur during the research and affect the results
Maturation:	Subjects grow or mature during the period of the study
Testing:	Taking the first test affects subsequent tests; "practice effect"
Instrumentation:	Lack of consistency in data collection
Statistical Regression:	Subjects selected because of their extreme scores
Differential Selection:	Control group and experimental group differ and the difference could affect the study's findings
Experimental Mortality:	Loss of subjects during the study
Diffusion of Treatment:	Members of the control group learn about the treatment of the experimental group

threat to internal validity of **mortality (attrition),** meaning the loss of subjects. In addition, the VA centers were not covered by Medicare's inpatient prospective payment system (PPS) at the time. This uniqueness represents a threat to external validity because most hospitals are covered by the PPS. Thus, the findings lacked generalizability. Therefore, both internal validity and external validity are important considerations for researchers.

In terms of an instrument, validity means the extent to which the instrument measures what it is intended to measure. Multiple aspects of an instrument's validity are assessed. Two important aspects are **content validity** and **construct validity.** Content validity concerns whether the instrument's items relate to the topic (content). For example, an ICD-9-CM coding test with content validity would have items related to key aspects of coding, such as the definition of principle diagnosis, fifth digits, complications and comorbidities, V codes, E codes, and the neoplasm table. Construct validity is the instrument's ability to measure hypothetical, nonobservable traits called constructs. Classic examples of constructs are psychological concepts, such as intelligence, motivation, and anxiety. Although intelligence itself is not visible, its effects are. Therefore, if an instrument is intended to measure patient satisfaction, it should include issues associated with patient satisfaction. Researchers state in their journal articles the validity of the instruments they used. References about instruments also provide the validity of instruments.

Reliability

Reliability represents consistency. Instruments that have reliability are stable. Repeated administrations will result in reasonably similar findings. **Intrarater reliability** means that the same person repeating the test will have reasonably similar findings. **Interrater reliability** means that different persons taking the test will have reasonably similar findings. Thus, reliability means that, over time, a test or observation dependably measures whatever it was intended to measure.

Check Your Understanding 16.5

Instructions: Answer the following questions on a separate piece of paper.

1. In which hypothesis does the researcher state what he or she believes?

2. If the researcher believes that the treatment increases output, would he or she write a one-tailed or a two-tailed hypothesis?

3. What is the difference between a type I error and a type II error?

4. What does the value represent?

5. What issues are involved in internal validity?

6. Why is reliability important in tests?

Selecting an Instrument

An instrument is a standardized, uniform way to collect data. Common examples of instruments are interview guides and questionnaires, although many other types exist. (See figure 16.5.) Researchers can find standardized instruments

in several reference books (figure 16.6) and in electronic databases. Of particular interest to HIM professionals are three electronic databases: Health and Psychosocial Instruments (HAPI), Buros Institute of Mental Measurements, and ERIC/AE Test Locator. These databases provide descriptions and critiques of instruments.

Factors in Selection

Factors that determine the selection of an instrument include:

- Purpose
- Satisfactory ratings for reliability and validity
- Clarity of language
- Brevity and attractiveness
- Match between the theories underpinning the instrument and the researcher's investigation
- Match between the level of measurement (**nominal, ordinal, interval,** or **ratio** scales of data) and the proposed statistical analyses
- Public domain or proprietary
- Cost

Of these factors, purpose is the most important. Researchers should match their purpose and the instrument's purpose. They should obtain the instrument and then read it in its entirety to be sure that it is collecting what they want to collect and that the terms in it match their meaning for the

Figure 16.5.   Types of measurement instruments

Checklists	Projective techniques
Clinical screenings and assessments	Psychological tests
Coding schemes and manuals	Questionnaires
Educational tests	Rating scales
Index measures	Scenarios
Interview guides (schedules)	Vignettes
Personality tests	

Figure 16.6.   Print sources of measurement instruments

Buros Institute. 1938–2003. *The Mental Measurements Yearbook: The Yearbook 1938–2003.* Highland Park, NJ: Buros Institute.

Chun, K., S. Cobb, and J.R.P. French, Jr. 1975. *Measures for Psychological Assessment: A Guide to 3,000 Original Sources and Their Applications.* Ann Arbor, MI: Survey Research Center, Institute for Social Research.

Herndon, R.M., ed. 1997. *Handbook of Neurologic Rating Scales.* New York: Demos Vermande.

Keyser, D.J., and R.C. Sweetland, eds. 1991. *Test Critiques.* Kansas City, MO: Test Corporation of America.

Maddox, T., ed. 2003. *Tests: A Comprehensive Reference for Assessments in Psychology, Education, and Business,* 5th ed. Austin, TX: Pro-Ed.

McDowell, I., and C. Newell. 1996. *Measuring Health: A Guide to Rating Scales and Questionnaires,* 2nd ed. New York: Oxford University Press.

Redman, B.K., ed. 2003. *Measurement Tools in Patient Education,* 2nd ed. New York: Springer.

Spreen, O., and E. Strauss. 1997. *A Compendium of Neuropsychological Tests: Administration, Norms, and Commentary,* 2nd ed. New York: Oxford University Press.

terms. For example, if the instrument is measuring social support, does it mean social support in the workplace or social support in the family and home? A researcher studying the effect of social support from colleagues and coworkers in the workplace should select an instrument about social support in thc workplace. Selecting an instrument about social support in the family would be a grave error with negative consequences for the validity of the research. Thus, merely reading the description and critique in the reference database is insufficient.

Researchers should select instruments that other researchers have already developed and refined. The reliability and validity of these instruments are established. Construction of a reliable and valid measure is a research project in and of itself. Osborn (1998) explained that the construction of a questionnaire includes deciding on the content, considering the audience, determining the level of measurement, pilot testing, analyzing the validity and reliability, and confirming the scales. Researchers should undertake the difficult task of developing an instrument only after they have investigated and verified that one does not already exist.

Instruments may be in the public domain or proprietary. Instruments in the public domain can be copied and used freely. Instruments that are proprietary must be purchased and cannot be copied. However, researchers can often obtain samples of instruments for review at little or no cost. In addition, researchers must consider the quality of the research. Of what use is an instrument that collects inaccurate data only tangentially related to the researcher's topic? The instrument must match the purpose and contribute to the collection of accurate data that build knowledge.

Features of Instruments

Questions on instruments may be structured or unstructured. Structured (closed-ended) questions list all the possible responses. Unstructured (open-ended) questions allow free-form responses. The advantages of structured questions is that they are easier for the participant to complete and for the researcher to tabulate and analyze than unstructured questions. The advantages of unstructured questions are that they allow in-depth questions and may uncover aspects of a problem unknown to the researcher.

Structured questions may be numeric items or categorical items. Numeric items request the respondent to enter a number. When feasible, numeric items are preferable to categorical items (Alreck and Settle 2004). In writing a numeric item, researchers must be careful to be clear and to specify the unit of measure. For example, the question How long ago was your last visit to the dentist? does not give the respondent an explicit unit of measure. The respondent may write 365 days, 52 weeks, or 1 year.

Categorical items classify respondents into groupings. It is important to construct categories that:

- *Are all-inclusive:* All respondents must fit into a category, even if it is "other."

- *Are mutually exclusive:* Categories should not overlap and, thereby, confuse the respondents.
- *Form meaningful clusters:* Categories should make sense and be meaningfully distinct. The following set of categories does not form a reasonable, balanced progression: kindegarten to 12th grade, freshman, sophomore, junior, senior, and graduate school. A more meaningful set of categories is: high school education, associate degree, baccalaureate degree, and graduate degree.
- *Are sufficiently narrow or broad:* The number of categories for a question may range from two (yes or no, true or false) to six or eight. Respondents have difficulty seeing meaningful shades of meaning beyond eight categories. Alreck and Settle (2004) recommend that, when in doubt, use the narrower (greater number) categories. Researchers can always combine categories, but cannot disaggregate broad categories into fine-grained categories if the detailed data were not collected. On the other hand, requesting participants to respond to many, and unnecessarily narrow, categories may depress the response rate and introduce inaccuracy.

A type of categorical item is a scaled item. **Scales** are progressive categories such as size, amount, importance, rank, or agreement. (See table 16.9.) For example, Garvin (2001) used a scale on her questionnaire that allowed respondents to categorize their feelings of capability regarding various skills related to coding. (See figure 16.7, p. 464.)

Table 16.9.   Common scales

Scale	Purpose	Example
Two-Point	Dichotomous question	Yes, no Favor, oppose True, false
Three-Point	Importance, interest, or satisfaction	Very, fairly, not at all
	Satisfaction with amounts	Too much (many), just (about) right, not enough (too few)
Four-Point	Generic	Excellent, good, fair, poor
	Measurement of amounts	Very much, quite a bit, some, very little
Likert (Five-Point)	Indication of agreement or disagreement	Strongly agree, agree, neutral, disagree, strongly disagree
Verbal Frequency (Five-Point)	Frequency	Always, often, sometimes, rarely (seldom), never
Expanded Likert (Seven-Point)	Extra discrimination desirable	Very strongly agree, strongly agree, agree, neutral, disagree, strongly disagree, very strongly disagree

A commonly used scale is the **Likert scale,** named for its developer, Rensis Likert. A Likert scale records the respondents' level of agreement or disagreement. On a Likert scale, the categories are along a range: strongly agree, agree, neutral, disagree, strongly disagree. Each category is also called a point. Therefore, a scale with five categories is a five-point scale.

Researchers, marketers, and others use a **semantic differential scale** to ascertain a group's perspective or image of a product, healthcare organization, or program. (See figure 16.8.) A semantic differential scale uses adjectives to rate the product, organization, or program. Adjectives that are polar opposites are placed on the ends of the continua. Up to 20 adjective pairs may be used. Half the items should begin with the positive adjective of the pair and the other half with the negative adjective. Identifying polar opposite adjectives and capturing the major attributes make this scale difficult to construct. However, a well-constructed semantic differential scale can provide a valuable profile of a product, organization, or program's image (Alreck and Settle 2004).

Availability of an Internet format is another important feature. Internet-based instruments have been developed for many paper-based instruments. Researchers are evaluating whether Internet-based instruments have similar reliability to their paper-based versions. Ritter et al. (2004) found that, for 16 existing self-report instruments, their Internet and paper-based versions had similar reliabilities. Moreover, the Internet-based version achieved slightly higher completion rates with less follow-up that the paper-based version.

In summary, obtaining or developing the proper instrument is a key step. Researchers should carefully consider the various factors as they review and select instruments. Carelessness or haste during this step can lead to unusable, unanalyzable data. Purpose should drive the decision.

Gathering the Data

All too often, researchers fail to plan how to gather data. Researchers who make mistakes during this phase of the research violate one of the factors of internal validity: instrumentation. They have contaminated data and may have compromised their ability to analyze their data. Researchers must write a step-by-step, day-by-day plan for gathering data prior to implementation.

Data Sampling Methods

A sample is a set of units selected for study. It is a subset of a target population, which is the large group that is the focus of the study. For example, researchers cannot poll all U.S. citizens for their opinions on storing their health data on the Internet, but they can identify a sample, meaning a group of citizens representative of the entire population. Individuals are one set of units. In other studies, the sets of units could be bacteria, mice, families, schools, television shows, historical documents, Web sites, and so on. There are two major types of samples: random and nonrandom.

Random Samples
Random sampling underpins many statistical techniques that HIM professionals encounter. To generate random samples, researchers can use either a feature of spreadsheet applications called the random number generator, an option of statistical packages called select cases, or a table of random numbers from a basic statistics textbook. The four types of random sampling are **simple random sampling, stratified random sampling, systematic sampling,** and **cluster sampling.** (See table 16.10.) Researchers using these methods attempt to make the sample as representative of the population as possible.

Nonrandom Samples
Two common types of **nonrandom sampling** are **convenience sampling** and **purposive sampling.** Convenience samples cast doubt on the generalizability and usefulness of the research. Purposive sampling, on the other hand, serves a valuable function in qualitative research.

Researchers use convenience samples when they "conveniently" use any unit that is at hand. For example, HIM professionals investigating physician satisfaction with departmental services could interview physicians who came to the

Figure 16.7.   Excerpt from survey questionnaire

Questionnaire on Coding Skills
Contained in AHIMA's Vision 2006

On a scale of 1 to 5, 5 being the most capable, please designate how capable you feel in the following areas:

1. Understanding the current clinical coding systems relevant to the organization:
   A. ICD-9-CM   5 4 3 2 1
   B. CPT   5 4 3 2 1
   C. DSM-IV   5 4 3 2 1
   D. SNOMED   5 4 3 2 1
   E. ICD-O   5 4 3 2 1
   F. ICD-10   5 4 3 2 1

2. Ability to gather clinical data from primary data sources   5 4 3 2 1

3. Understanding of the elements required for research and outcomes   5 4 3 2 1

4. Ability to participate in the design of studies   5 4 3 2 1

Source: Garvin 2001.

Figure 16.8.   Semantic differential scale

Please mark with an "X" the space on each line below to show your opinion of the education received in your academic program.

Up-to-Date ___:___:___:___:___:___:___ Outdated
           1 2 3 4 5 6 7

Low-Tech ___:___:___:___:___:___:___ High-Tech
           1 2 3 4 5 6 7

Expensive ___:___:___:___:___:___:___ Economical
           1 2 3 4 5 6 7

Easy ___:___:___:___:___:___:___ Hard
      1 2 3 4 5 6 7

Table 16.10.   Types of random sampling

Type of Sampling	Description
Simple	The selection of units from a population so that every unit has exactly the same chance of being included in the sample. When a unit has been selected, it is returned to the population so that the other units' chances remain identical.
Stratified	Some populations have characteristics that divide them. For example, the human population is male and female. The male and female subgroups are called strata (singular, stratum). The percentage of the stratum in the population should equal the percentage of the stratum in the sample. Therefore, the sample should be 50% male and 50% female. Other percentages would cast doubt on the results.
Systematic	Units of the sample are selected from a list by drawing every nth unit. For example, health information professionals could choose every fourth surgery on the surgical schedule for surgical case review.
Cluster	The sample is clusters of units. The population is first divided into clusters of units, such as family, school, or community.

department. Unfortunately, this convenience sample ignores the opinions of all the physicians who did not come to the department and these physicians may find services substandard. Therefore, use of a convenience sample diminishes the credibility of the research.

Purposive sampling is a strategy of qualitative research. In purposive sampling, researchers use their expertise to select both representative units and unrepresentative units. This strategy reflects the qualitative view that there are many truths. For example, Freud's work is purposive sampling because it focuses on unusual cases. Psychiatrists investigating the psychopathology of mass murderers would use purposive sampling because mass murder is not generalizable (Chadwick, Bahr, and Albrecht 1984). Thus, purposive sampling has very specific applications.

Adequacy of the Sample Size

Sample size is the number of subjects the researcher determines should be included in the study in order to represent the population. The adequacy of the sample's size is a common concern. The size of the sample depends on the purpose of the study, the nature of the population, and the researchers' resources (Chadwick, Bahr, and Albrecht 1984). Some experts state that the general rule is to use the largest sample possible (Gall, Borg, and Gall 2003; Gay and Airasian 2003). However, Kish (1965) factored in utility to arrive at economic samples. An economic sample provides the level of detail needed to answer the question. Overall, although no absolute rule dictates the size of the sample, researchers should strive for a level of accuracy that makes the study worth conducting.

If a researcher's purpose was to explore areas of inconsistency between paper and electronic records, 90 randomly selected records at one academic health center may be sufficient (Mikkelsen and Aasly 2001). However, a study comparing the efficacy of various treatment protocols for breast cancer warrants a sample size in the thousands. If the researcher's purpose includes many variables, the sample size needs to be larger. Thus, purpose is a critical concern.

The nature of the population includes **heterogeneity** and typical response and attrition rates. Heterogeneity means variation or diversity. The more heterogeneous a population, the larger the sample. The sample needs to be larger to ensure that it includes all the diverse units in the population. Typical response rate is a factor for surveys. In the literature, other researchers report their response rates. The response rate is the number of people who returned the questionnaire or were reached for interview. If the typical response rate is 50 percent, the researcher will need to distribute twice as many surveys to achieve an adequate response. Attrition (mortality) rates are the numbers of subjects lost during the course of the study. Attrition is a threat to internal validity. High attrition rates also require a larger sample. Understanding the nature of the population contributes to the accuracy of the research.

Resources, namely time and money, also can affect sample size. Sometimes researchers must provide answers within a short time frame. For example, to respond in a timely fashion to a legislative initiative regarding photocopy charges, HIM professionals may conduct a quick survey of a small sample. Individual researchers often face financial constraints. These constraints sometimes result in smaller samples than purists would prefer.

Sample size calculation refers to the qualitative and quantitative procedures used to determine the appropriate sample size. Some experts have offered rules of thumb to calculate sample size. (See table 16.11, p. 466.) These rules of thumb try to account for frequency of the behavior, numbers of variables, and statistical technique. Other experts (Khan 1997; Osborn 2000b) offer statistical formulae to calculate adequate sample sizes. Formulae depend upon the sampling method used, such as simple random sampling or stratified random sample, and on the amount of information the researcher has about the population. For health information managers, Osborn's text offers excellent examples and step-by-step procedures. Finally, however, specific considerations should override reliance on these rules of thumb and formulae.

The following example outlines the procedure for arriving at an optimal sample size. (See figure 16.9, p. 466.) Suppose the HIS director at a large academic health center wanted to determine the sample size for a study on the medical staff's opinion of electronic medical records. One commonly used formula for determining sample size requires the researcher to know or decide on the size of the population, the proportion of subjects needed, and an acceptable amount of error.

Table 16.11.   Rules of thumb for sample size

Rule	Source
General: Minimum of 30 cases or responses	Bailey 1994
Pilot study: 20 to 50 cases	Sudman 1976
Descriptive study: Minimum 10 percent of population	Gay and Airasian 2003
Descriptive study: Minimum 20 percent of small population	Gay and Airasian 2003
Correlational study: Minimum of 30 cases or responses	Gall, Borg, and Gall 2003
Causal-comparative and experimental research: 15 to 30 cases per comparison group	Gall, Borg, and Gall 2003; Gay and Airasian 2003
Major subgroup: Minimum of 100 each Minor subgroups: Minimum of 20 to 50 each per subgroup	Sudman 1976
General: 200 cases or responses	Chadwick, Bahr, and Albrecht 1984

Figure 16.9.   Basic example of sample size calculation

Sample size = n
Size of the population = N

Proportion of subjects needed = p
Acceptable amount of error = B

Formula

$$n = \frac{Np(1-p)}{(N-1)\frac{(B^2)}{4} + (p)(1-p)}$$

Data from the Case
$N = 800$
$p = .5$
$B = .05$

Calculations

$$n = \frac{(800)(.5)(1-.5)}{(800-1)\frac{(.05^2)}{4} + (.5)(1-.5)}$$

$$n = \frac{200}{(799)(.000625) + .25}$$

$$n = \frac{200}{.75}$$

$$n = 267$$

In this instance, the director knows that the number of attending physicians on the medical staff is 800 but has little other information. Therefore, $p = .5$ and $B = .05$. Using the basic formula, the director calculates that, in this situation, a sample of 267 is needed if he or she is willing to accept 5 percent error due to variability in the sampling.

Data Collection Procedures

The research plan should consider every logistical detail of the collection of the data from start to finish. Lack of attention to detail at this point will breach factors of internal validity. Some issues related to data collection affect many of the methods; other issues are unique to the method. Data collection issues include:

- Obtaining approvals of oversight committees
- Listing each data element required to perform the appropriate statistical techniques
- Training for data collection procedures
- Performing a **pilot study**
- Considering the response rate
- Conducting the treatment
- Collecting the data
- Assembling the data for analysis

Federal regulations govern research on human subjects (Penslar 2001). The purpose of the regulations is to protect humans from researchers' abuses, such as those that occurred in the Tuskegee Syphilis Study. (See figure 16.10.) To comply with federal regulations, organizations have institutional review boards (IRBs). IRBs (sometimes called human subjects committees) are administrative bodies established to protect the rights and welfare of human subjects recruited to participate in research activities associated with institutions. IRBs provide oversight for the research studies conducted within their institutions. As specified by both federal regulations and institutional policies, IRBs have the authority to review and to approve or reject research studies within their jurisdictions. They also may require modifications in research protocols. As human health and life are at stake, the federal government imposes severe penalties on institutions and individuals who fail to comply.

Prior to conducting studies, researchers must obtain written approvals from the IRB and other oversight entities of their organizations. To obtain approvals, researchers complete the organization's documentation, providing descriptions of their research plan and copies of their informed consent forms. Sufficient time must be allowed in their plan for the board to review the research, meet, and respond.

Researchers should compile a list of each data element required for each statistical analysis they plan to conduct. Prior to beginning data collection, researchers should ensure that their data collection strategies will obtain all the data. Therefore, it is advisable to conduct mock statistical analyses on fabricated

Figure 16.10.   Tuskegee syphilis study

The Tuskegee Syphilis Study is a notorious chapter in medical research in the United States. From 1932 to 1972, the U.S. Public Health Service conducted research that had the stated purpose of obtaining more information about the clinical course of syphilis. The medical researchers from the U.S. Public Health Service experimented on 399 African American males in Macon County, Alabama. The medical researchers told the men that they were being treated for "bad blood." In fact, the researchers were deceiving the men and were denying them treatment for syphilis. Many of the men's wives were infected, and their children were subsequently born with congenital syphilis. The U.S. Public Health Service continued the study despite the advent of penicillin in 1947. The Tuskegee Syphilis Study is a symbol of unethical research.

data and to create tables and figures for the manuscript early in the planning of the research. For example, suppose researchers were investigating whether the time from heart transplant to the first rejection episode differed by ABO blood type and Rh factor. The blood types and Rh factors are not evenly distributed in the general population nor are they evenly distributed by national origin. Running mock statistical analyses would reveal that the researchers need a large sample size. Too often, graduate students have had to write in their theses or dissertations, "I did not have sufficient cases to run the statistical analysis." Planning can avoid this embarrassment.

Researchers and those they employ to assist them may require special training. For example, publishers of some psychological tests require verification of training to administer the tests. The researchers must obtain this verification (or select another instrument). To effectively conduct interviews or to observe vignettes, researchers and their assistants also need training.

Performing a pilot study (trial run) enhances the likelihood of its successful completion. When researchers conduct pilot studies, they work out the details of their research plan. The maxim, "The devil is in the details," is only too true. Pilot studies can reveal the following information:

- Biases in sample selection
- Volumes required
- Associated costs
- Performance features of equipment
- Defects, such as poorly worded cover letters, unclear questionnaire items, and leading questions in interviews
- Possible log jams (gridlock) in the mailing method
- Errors in the scoring key
- Discrepancies between the order of items on the data collection instrument and the order on the computer screen

Pilot studies demonstrate that the research study is logistically feasible. Even researchers conducting naturalistic studies perform simulations that test their instruments prior to the event. Pilot studies are as necessary as disaster drills.

Ensuring an adequate response rate is of particular concern for surveys. Low response rates jeopardize study accuracy and generalizability. Therefore, researchers strive to increase their response rates. To increase response rates, researchers can use the findings of Berdie and Anderson (1974). These researchers conducted the classic research study on the process of questionnaire surveys. Their research revealed many strategies to increase the response rate. (See figure 16.11.) Their primary recommendation was that researchers know their topic and their target population. This knowledge underpins decisions about the strategies and techniques to increase response rates.

Strategies to increase the response rate for questionnaire research include using a brief cover letter and multiple mailings. The cover letter should explain the purpose of the study and its benefits for the participants. Obtaining the sponsor-

Figure 16.11.   Summary of Berdie and Anderson's strategies to increase the response rate in questionnaire surveys

General
1. Physical attractiveness of cover letter, postcard, and questionnaire
2. Quality of printing and paper
3. Pleasingly colored paper
4. Error-free documents
5. Incentives, such as an offer of the study's results or money ($0.25 maximum)

Cover Letter
1. Salutation's formality is tailored to the target population.
2. Prestigious sponsor
3. Time frame for response is exact (10 days) or "as soon as possible," depending on the population.
4. Tone of sincerity and honesty
5. Assurance of confidentiality

Questionnaire
1. Title
2. Easy to complete
3. Clear instructions included in the body of the questionnaire
4. Reasonable length
5. Contact information and return mailing address at the bottom

Mailing
1. Initial contact (postcard) that is an appeal for participation
2. Self-addressed, stamped return envelope
3. Properly timed follow-up

ship of a professional association or officials is desirable. Moreover, the letter should thank the responder, provide a deadline, and offer the study results. In the field of health information management, ensuring the confidentiality of the response also is particularly important. Key characteristics of effective cover letters are shown in figure 16.12, p. 468. Multiple mailings in a timed sequence can significantly improve the response rate. For example, the tailored (total) design method routinely achieves response rates of 74 percent (Dillman 2000; Salant and Dillman 1994).

Internet surveys are becoming more prevalent because they are able to gather data from large samples directly and relatively inexpensively (Bethell et al. 2004). They are now being used to gather data on health status, access to care, and other health outcomes. Bethell and colleagues administered surveys both via the Internet and by telephone. The uncorrected response rate for the 13,400 e-mails surveys was 17.3 percent. Taking into account that, on average, 10 to 15 percent of e-mails are nonworking or dormant, the researchers concluded that the true response rate for the online survey was about 20 percent. The adjusted response rate for the telephone survey was 9.3 percent. In spite of six follow-up telephone calls, the one-time contact of the e-mail survey resulted in a higher response rate. Survey administration, statistical sampling, and weighted approaches to ensure representativeness were similar for the two survey strategies. The researchers concluded that, with the increasing resistance to telephone solicitations, Internet surveys represent an efficient, real-time strategy for data collection (Bethell et al. 2004).

Figure 16.12. Sample cover letter

Letterhead	ZHIMA 1800 Carriage Oxford, ZB 31002 October 1, 2002 Dear Colleague:
Purpose	The healthcare system and our field are rapidly changing. These changes place increasing demands on health information practitioners. Little research exists that explores stress and the buffers in directors of hospital health information management departments.
Study's Importance Participant's Importance	Therefore, you have been randomly selected to participate in a national survey on stress in the workplace. Please take the time to complete and return the survey. The accuracy of the results and the possible benefits for the profession depend on your participation.
Sponsor Time to Complete	This research is being sponsored by the AHIMA. The entire survey should take 15 to 20 minutes of your time. A detailed, personalized report on your coping resources is available. Should you wish to receive it, please write your name and address at the bottom of the pink Demographic Form.

Offer of Results

Time Frame	Please return the survey within 10 days in the postage-paid envelope.

SASE

Confidentiality

A vital concern of the health information management profession is confidentiality in research. The code number on your questionnaire is for mailing and follow-up purposes only. Only aggregate data will be reported, and at no time will the questionnaires be identified by respondent.

Appreciation Contact Instruction	I truly appreciate your participation, and I think the findings of the survey will benefit many members of our profession in these stressful times. If you have any questions about the survey, please write or call me. Sincerely Jane Edwards, PhD 123 Anyplace Street Anytown, IL 12345 (123) 456-7890 Enclosures

Researchers also must be on guard for bias in response. For example, do persons who volunteer to participate in the research differ from those who do not volunteer? Do the persons who responded to the survey (responders) differ from those who did not (nonresponders)? Finally, how similar are the participants, nonparticipants, responders, and nonresponders to the population?

In conducting the study, researchers must be careful to follow the plan they have written. Deviations from the protocol result in potential bias and inaccurate data. For example, in questionnaire research, the Dillman (2000) method depends on a strictly timed series of mailings. Does the researcher have staff to track the responses and to physically assemble the mailings?

Researchers must include a mechanism in the plan for compiling their data. If videotapes are involved, where will they be stored? Because sensitive data may be on personality tests, how will confidentiality be maintained? If the research includes measurement instruments, who will score them?

After researchers have collected the data, they must organize them in a way that allows analysis. In this step, the researchers must decide how they will enter the data into a software package. Who will enter the data? How will they ensure accuracy of data entry? Who will transcribe the contents of videotapes or audiotapes?

Data collection is a systematic, planned procedure that results in internal validity. Conducting a pilot study is a key step in ensuring a thorough and carefully conceived plan. The methods section of the study report documents the plan's execution. The methods section is also a recipe that other researchers can use to replicate the study. Therefore, careful attention to documentation and vigilant adherence to procedures are demanded.

Sources of Secondary Data

Researchers may choose to analyze data that other researchers or agencies have gathered. As noted in the subsection on research methods, analysis of secondary data is a powerful tool because it allows researchers to mine large databases at the regional, state, and national level. For example, Zhan and Miller (2003) analyzed 7.45 million uniform hospital discharge abstracts. The source of these data was the 2000 Healthcare Cost and Utilization Project Nationwide Inpatient Sample developed by the Agency for Healthcare Research and Quality. In this study, one finding among several was that excess length of stay attributable to medical injuries ranged from 0 days to 10.89 days.

Health information researchers used data from the 1994 Health Care Cost Utilization Project-3 (HCUP-3) study (Rudman and Davey 2000). The HCUP-3 data are medical record data from inpatient hospital discharges. The researchers were investigating the type of injury or illness and medical cost of domestic violence. The researchers reported that for females, mental disorder, trauma, and pregnancy complications accounted for over two-thirds the admissions and that for all victims the average cost of the hospitalization was $8,159.81.

Several other sources of data are available to researchers. For example, several states post Medicaid data on the Internet. Specific examples of available data include:

- Labor force, earnings, and prices (Bureau of Labor Statistics)
- Crime, demographics, education, and health (Social Statistics Briefing Room)
- Statistics and information from 70 federal agencies (FedStats)
- Behavorial health (Behavioral Risk Factor Surveillance System [BRFSS] of the Centers for Disease Control and Mental Health Inventories [MHIs] from the National Institute of Mental Health in the Alcohol, Drug Abuse, and Mental Health Administration)
- Health statistics (National Center for Health Statistics, FASTATS A–Z)
- Health statistics, social indicators, and population health research (Area Resource File [ARF] of the Bureau of Health Statistics)
- Medicare data (Medicare Provider Analysis and Review [MEDPAR] of Short-Stay Hospitals and Medicare Beneficiary Health Status Registry [MBHSR])
- Demographic data on U.S. population (Population Reference Bureau)
- Business, economic, and trade data from the federal government (STAT-USA)
- Hundreds of files from various governments (Statistical Resources on the Web)
- U.S. census data (U.S. Census Bureau)

The problem is that in order to transform the data into information, researchers must understand the underlying structure of the data and how they were collected. Each data source has unique characteristics.

For example, one hospital database contained a field related to death, which is typically a discharge status. However, with its death field (Field 342), the hospital could track the number of intraoperative deaths, postoperative deaths, autopsied deaths, and medical examiner's cases. The death field was a multiple-entry field, with each category having a number (intra-operative deaths = 1; postoperative death = 2; autopsied death = 3; and medical examiner's case = 4). A surgeon requested a report on the number of intra-operative deaths. The worker who usually ran reports was on vacation and another worker attempted to run the query. This worker wrote the query as Field 342 = "1." As a multiple-entry field, the query should have been written as Field 342 contains "1." The erroneously written query excluded all intra-operative deaths that were also postoperative deaths (2), autopsied deaths (3), and medical examiner's cases (4). Some cases are all four. The case of a multiple stabbing victim illustrates the point. From the emergency room, the patient is initially brought to the operating room (OR). His wounds are explored and sutured. Postoperatively, the patient is sent to the intensive care unit. While in the ICU, he begins to bleed internally again and is brought back to the OR. While in the OR the second time, the patient dies. This patient is both a postoperative death and an intra-operative death (2 and 1). In addition, the body was sent for autopsy, and as a crime victim, the patient is a medical examiner's case (3 and 4). Therefore, researchers must either learn the underlying structure of the database and query it directly or download the data into a database or spreadsheet with which they are familiar.

Similar to the approach to literary databases, researchers must take a systematic and orderly approach. HIM professionals, such as Osborn (2001), have queried Medicare's large databases to analyze reimbursement data. Secondary analysis is a productive research method for HIM professionals.

Check Your Understanding 16.6

Instructions: Answer the following questions on a separate piece of paper.

1. Why would a researcher choose to use an instrument that someone else has created?
2. What is an adequate sample?
3. Would directors of departments of health information services be considered a heterogeneous population or a homogenous population?
4. Why are IRBs important?
5. What is a pilot study?
6. Why are survey researchers concerned about their response rates?
7. What common mistake do researchers make in data collection?

Analyzing the Data

In this phase of the research process, researchers try to determine what they have found or what the data reveal. Many researchers fall into the common error of allowing too little time for analysis. Researchers should be sure to allocate sufficient time in their research plan to analyze and interpret the data.

Before conducting their study, researchers should determine which statistical techniques they will use. These techniques are specified in the methods section of the manuscript. The description of the statistical techniques should be clear so that other researchers can duplicate them.

Techniques for Data Analysis

This subsection briefly describes a few common statistical techniques. For a detailed discussion, see a standard statistical text, such as *Statistical Applications for Health Information Management* (Osborn 2000b). The purpose of this subsection is to suggest appropriate statistical techniques for general situations. The following three broad categories of statistical analysis are addressed:

- **Descriptive (summary) statistics** describe the data. Generally, researchers should begin with descriptive techniques to verify the accuracy of their data entry and to provide an overview of their respondents. Exploratory data analysis looks at the raw data. The raw data are presented in graphic displays. Two techniques of exploratory data analysis are box and whisker plots and stem and leaf diagrams. The stem and leaf diagram shows all the individual scores on a particular measure (Gall, Borg, and Gall 2003). Box and whisker plots are especially useful when the sets of data have hundreds or thousands of scores or the sets of data have unequal numbers of values. (See figure 16.13.) The shapes of these graphic displays allow researchers to see the range and distribution of scores. (See chapter 15, p. 399.) Outliers become visible. Descriptive techniques include means, frequency distributions, and standard deviations. These statistical techniques are also called **univariate** because they involve one variable.

- **Inferential statistics** allow the researchers to make inferences about the population characteristics (parameters) from the sample's characteristics. Examples of inferential statistics include the paired *t* test and the analysis of variance (ANOVA). Researchers investigating the differences between groups would use these statistical techniques.

- **Test statistics** examine the psychometric properties of measurement instruments. They describe and explore the validity and reliability of tests. Researchers conducting test statistics calculate the validity coefficient (correlation coefficient) and each item's validity. They also could perform factor analysis. Examples of approaches to verify reliability include test–retest and Kuder–Richardson formulae. Finally, test statistics include an index of difficulty, which is the percentage of persons correctly answering each item.

Most research data can be subjected to more than one statistical technique. Table 16.12 shows potential statistical tests for various combinations of data characteristics. The suggested statistical tests in the table are merely a starting point. Researchers should maximize the use of their data by using a variety of techniques to look at their data from multiple views. Multiple views of the data shed light on different aspects of the issue and expand the body of knowledge.

Appropriate statistical techniques vary by:

- Purpose of the research (research design)
- Number of variables

Table 16.12.   Statistical test by characteristics of data

No. of Variables	Characteristics	Test
1	One group, normal*	Mean and standard deviation
	One group, nonnormal	Binomial test
	Two groups, normal	*t*-test
	Two groups, nonnormal	Chi-square
	Three+ groups, normal	ANOVA
	Three+ groups, nonnormal	Nonparametric
2	Both continuous	Correlation
	1 continuous, 1 discrete	ANOVA
	Both categorical	Chi-square
3+	One group	Multiple regression, factor analysis, repeated measures ANOVA, analysis of covariance
	Two+ groups	Multivariate ANOVA, discriminant function

*Normal distribution

Figure 16.13.   Box and whisker plot

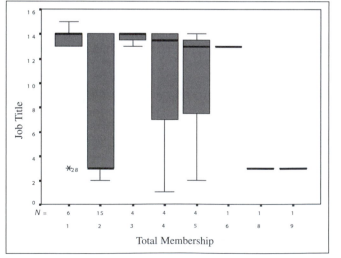

- Type of data
- Nature of the target population
- Number, size, and independence of the groups

Purpose of the Research

Researchers should match their purpose and their statistical technique. Researchers whose purpose is to investigate the differences between groups would use statistical techniques of the paired t test and the analysis of variance (ANOVA). On the other hand, researchers might be looking for relationships, such as in a correlational design. These researchers would want to know how the variables relate to one another. Therefore, these researchers would use correlational statistics. One correlational technique is the **bivariate** correlational coefficient. The bivariate correlational coefficient allows the researcher to describe the strength of the relationship between two variables in mathematical terms.

Number of Variables

The number of variables also affects the choice of statistical technique. **Multivariate** correlational methods involve many variables. For example, multiple linear regression examines the strength of relationship between several independent variables and one dependent variable. Other, more complex forms of regression exist.

Type of Data

Another factor in the choice of statistical technique is the type of data. There are five types of data:

- **Discrete data** are separate and distinct values or observations. Patients in the hospital represent discrete data because each patient can be counted.
- **Categorical data** are values or observations that can be sorted into a category (for example, gender).
- Nominal data are values or observations that can be labeled or named (nom = name). Therefore, the data can be coded (for example, Married = Y and Single = N or Male = 0 and Female = 1). Nominal data cannot be ranked or measured.
- Ordinal data represent values or observations that can be ranked (ordered). Ranking scales are common examples of ordinal data. For example, physicians often ask patients to evaluate the severity of their pain on a scale from 1 to 10. HIM professionals could use ordinal data when investigating customer satisfaction. For example, a health information manager could ask physicians how satisfied they are with the department's service on a scale from 1 to 5. However, because these rankings are subjective, the difference in satisfaction between 2 and 3 may be much less than the difference between 4 and 5.
- Metric data can be measured on some scale. Two subtypes are interval and ratio. The scale for interval data does not begin with a true zero. Time, as humans measure it, does not begin with a true zero. Interval data represent values or observations that occur on an evenly distributed scale. Time in years is an evenly distributed

scale. The interval between 1985 and 1990 is the same as the interval between 1991 and 1996. On the other hand, the scale for ratio data does begin at a true zero. Height, weight, and temperature are examples of ratio data.

Metric data are **continuous data.** They represent values or observations that have an indefinite number of points along a continuum. For example, measurements made with a ruler can be a foot, an inch, a half-inch, a quarter, an eighth, to infinity. Continuous data also exhibit characteristics of the other types of data; they can be counted (discrete) and ordered (ordinal) and can be grouped.

The type of data depends on the way the variable is measured, not some inherent attribute of the variable. For example, height can be measured in inches or categorized as short or tall. Therefore, researchers should be careful to collect data in the form that matches their intended statistical technique.

Nature of the Target Population

The nature of the target population also affects the choice of statistical technique. For example, some statistical techniques are based on the assumption that the variable is normally distributed in the population. **Parametric techniques,** such as the t-test, ANOVA, and Pearson r correlation efficient, are used in these cases. However, this assumption is not always true. In some cases, researchers use **nonparametric** or **distribution-free techniques** (for example, chi square and Spearman rho). Nonparametric techniques also are used for nominal and ordinal data. Osborn (2000b) provides a powerful discussion on the use of parametric and nonparametric statistical tests by type of data (level of measurement, nominal to metric).

Number, Size, and Independence of Groups

The selection of statistical test also depends on the number of samples or groups. In many instances, researchers want to compare two groups, the control group and the study group. However, in other types of studies, researchers may want to compare results from 10 different communities or all 50 states. The number of groups affects the choice of statistical test. Disparate sizes of groups also sometimes affect the choice of statistical test. Some statistical tests, however, are quite robust and can handle differences in sizes. For example, in many instances analysis of variance (ANOVA) can handle unequal group sizes. Researchers must take into account the inequality of sizes. For example, the smallest group size determines the precisions of estimates. The independence of the samples is also an issue. For instances, matched pairs of graduates and supervisors are used when an academic program wants to know the graduates' perspectives on the quality of the education and the supervisors' perspectives on the graduates' capabilities.

Statistical Software Packages

Many software packages are available to assist researchers in the analysis of data. For basic descriptive statistics, researchers can use spreadsheet software, such as Excel™. However, most researchers will choose to use dedicated statistical packages because these packages require less manipulation of the data than spreadsheet packages and because they perform many more statistical procedures. Other factors that influence the choice of software are type of data, planned analytical techniques, and cost.

Several software packages are commonly used in research projects. For example, Code-A-Text is used to code and analyze documents, transcripts, and sound files. Coding is the labeling of words or word groups (segments) with annotations or scales. These labels are characteristics of the segments. This software allows researchers to specify labels and easily insert them into the document or sound file. When the researcher has coded what the subjects said, the researcher can analyze the content of the document or sound file also using this software. The software produces descriptive statistics and tables and charts that support analysis. The software also assists researchers in categorizing the segments into themes, known as content analysis. Code-A-Text can be applied to field notes, open-ended questionnaires, and interviews. A multimedia version codes video and pictures.

Epi-Info is freeware from the Centers for Disease Control. This integrated package, which includes word processing, database, and statistics, is designed for public health. The software allows the handling of epidemiological data in questionnaire format, calculating the required sample size, analyzing data, and presenting results.

LISREL is a software package that conducts factor analysis. Factor analysis is used to evaluate the psychometric properties of measurement instruments. LISREL generates test statistics. For example, Aish and Wasserman (2001) used LISREL to evaluate the properties of a psychological test that predicts suicidal behavior.

Qualitative Solutions and Research Non-numerical Unstructured Data Indexing Searching and Theorizing (QSR NUD*IST) 4.0 is a software package used to analyze qualitative data. NUD*IST searches text to generate categories and indexes. This software assists qualitative researchers to generate themes and theory. Mechanic and Meyer (2000) used NUD*IST to analyze transcripts from audiotapes. The software broke responses down into individual phrases that expressed a single theme.

Statistical Analysis System (SAS) is a powerful software package that integrates data access, data management, data analysis, and data presentation. Researchers use SAS to enter data, retrieve and manage data, analyze data with statistical and mathematical techniques, write reports, and generate graphics.

Statistical Package for Social Sciences (SPSS) offers a broad array of analytical and graphic software. Its many components range from basic statistical techniques to advanced, specialized techniques. Basic statistics performs counts and cross-tabs. Advanced techniques include factor, regression, cluster analysis, binomial and multinomial logistic regression, and correspondence analysis.

Presenting Results

Researchers follow a two-step process when presenting their results. In the first step, they report their research findings with no commentary, explanation, or interpretation. This section of a manuscript is called research findings. In the second step, the researchers comment on, explain, and interpret their findings. This section of the manuscript is called discussion. Also included in the discussion are conclusions and recommendations for future research.

Researchers describe their results in the past tense; general truths are stated in the present tense. The style of writing for scientific manuscripts is objective, precise, and factual. Researchers avoid subjective interjections and emotional hyperbole. In the research findings, researchers must be very careful to maintain a neutral tone. They are merely recording their findings in narrative form.

In research findings, researchers describe the results for each hypothesis. Restating the hypothesis aids the readers. Researchers state whether or not the results support the hypotheses. They also record characteristics about the sample and describe the results of the statistical analyses that investigate whether the sample is similar to or different from the population. Supplemental statistical analyses also are described.

For research findings, researchers generate tables and graphs to support the readers' understanding of their findings. (See chapter 15 for more detailed descriptions of some common tables and graphs.) Day's (1988) rule of thumb is that data should be presented in only one way or mode. Researchers should present the particular data element in narrative text, in a table, or in a figure, but not in multiple modes. Graphics should clarify the data, not confuse the readers. Figure 16.14 lists 10 important points to remember when constructing graphics. Researchers must carefully consider which mode of communication is most effective for the particular data element. For example:

- *Tables* summarize data in a grid or matrix. The elements and numbers should be in the columns, not in the rows.
- *Pie charts* with their segments visually show the relationships among variables and the whole. They also can represent categorical data.
- *Bar charts* show comparisons between and among items. They often illustrate major characteristics in the distribution of data (male or female, age ranges). They

Figure 16.14. Considerations for effective graphics

1. Tables, graphs, and figures have titles.
2. Tables have subheads, spanner heads, and column heads for clarification.
3. Sources are cited.
4. Time frames and dates are noted.
5. Multiple tables, charts, graphs, and figures are numbered.
6. Both axes of graphs are labeled (bar titles, legends, scale captions).
7. Keys show the meaning of shadings and colors.
8. Scales start at zero.
9. Wedges (slices) of a pie chart represent percentages, and the percentages convert to 360 degrees.
10. Graphics are for emphasis; do not dilute the effect with clutter.

can be used to represent categorical, nominal, or ordinal data.

- *Line charts* show comparisons over time.
- *Histograms* are similar to bar charts. They show major characteristics in the distribution of data and summarize data about variables whose values are numerical and measured on an interval scale. Histograms are used for large data sets.

Writing the discussion section requires energy and creativity. Too often, researchers shortchange this section. The discussion section is not a superficial repetition of the findings section. Rather, it is where researchers create new knowledge.

In the discussion section, researchers should compare their findings to the findings in the literature, explaining similarities and discrepancies. More important, they should provide some rationale to explain why their findings were the same or different. In writing this section, researchers should return to why they conducted the study in the first place. They should answer the following questions:

- What theoretical significance or practical worth do their findings have?
- How do their findings explicitly link to the larger body of knowledge?
- How have their findings improved the field's research model?
- How have their findings expanded the body of knowledge?
- What new definitions have they added to the field's area of practice?
- How do their findings support practitioners in the workplace?
- What problems do their findings solve?
- What valid conclusions can the researchers and the readers draw?

Researchers also state their assumptions and the limitations of their research. A researcher describing a questionnaire study might state that one assumption is that people are honest and that one limitation is that the study only reflects one point in time. Also, research always raises new questions. These new questions become the recommendations for further research.

The discussion section closes the presentation of the findings. To accurately represent the time and effort that went into the research study, the discussion section should be rich and insightful. Sufficient time for reflection and contemplation should be scheduled into the research plan. The researchers' goal should be to put usable information into the hands of practitioners in the workplace.

Disseminating Research

Knowledge is disseminated and examined through poster sessions, presentations at professional meetings, and journal articles. Researchers have an ethical obligation to disseminate their research because this new knowledge advances the health information profession and helps practitioners in the workplace. It is only common sense that in order for the researchers' information to be useful, it must be available and accessible to practitioners.

Poster sessions and presentations occur at professional meetings, conferences, and symposia. Often these events have been planned far in advance. Up to 12 months before a professional meeting, professional associations will issue a call for session proposals. (See figure 16.15, p. 474.) In response to the call, researchers send brief descriptions of their proposed session. The meeting planners determine which proposals to accept based on the quality, number, and relevance of the topic to the theme of the conference.

Poster Sessions

Researchers must conform to poster guidelines when participating in a poster session. Prior to the event, meeting planners send out the requirements for the poster. These requirements state the size of the poster. Common size requirements are often 39 3 59 or 49 3 69. Meeting planners will also state the session's time slot on the meeting agenda. Typically, poster sessions last three to five hours on one day. During that time, the researcher stands near the poster and answers questions about the poster.

Institutional printing departments offer services that enhance posters. Commercial printing companies with staffs of commercial artists and graphic designers also will print the posters. Researchers need to submit word documents or PowerPoint slides. Posters typically include:

- A banner (header) with title of study, names of researchers, and institutional affiliation
- An abstract
- The purpose
- The method
- Results
- Discussion and conclusions

Posters should be colorful and readable at 10 feet. Charts and graphics are particularly striking. The posters can be laminated or mounted on poster board. Moreover, the researcher should take the time necessary to create a poster that looks professional.

Figure 16.15. Sample call for proposals

Call for Research Abstracts

Deadline for Abstracts: January 1, 20XX

Abstracts for the Summer Symposium are being solicited.

Topics:
• Workforce initiatives
• Innovations in service delivery
• Organizational or administrative issues in healthcare enterprises
• HIM best practices or performance improvement
• e-health implementations

Content of the research abstract should include:

• Title of presentation
• Name(s) of author(s) with title, credentials, and organization
• Method
• Brief results

Abstracts should be limited to 250 words. To be considered, abstracts must be submitted by January 1, 20XX. E-mail, regular mail, and fax submissions are all acceptable. (See addresses at bottom of message.)

Selection of abstracts will be made through a peer-reviewed process.

Authors of accepted abstracts will then be asked to submit the complete scholarly paper by February 15, 20XX. Scholarly papers will be published in *Symposium Proceedings*. Content for the scholarly paper includes: (a) abstract; (b) title; (c) name(s) of author(s) with title; credentials, and organization; (d) literature review; (e) purpose or problem statement; (f) methods including analytical technique; (g) results; (h) discussion; and (i) conclusions and recommendations for future research.

Authors of accepted papers will also be asked to submit handouts for their presentation. The deadline for handouts is April 15. Presentations will be limited to 12 minutes, inclusive of questions. Due to the time constraints, authors are asked to focus their presentation and corresponding handouts on the sections of Results, Discussion, and Conclusions. For reference, interested parties will have the entire scholarly paper in the *Symposium Proceedings*.

For authors of accepted abstracts, half the registration will be waived.

Address to submit Research Abstracts:

Liz Qualef, PhD, RHIA
Professor and Chair
Blank University
Department of Health Information Management
School of Allied Health Sciences
City, ST 12345
School Fax: 252.428.4070
E-Mail: qualefl@mail.blu.edu

Presentation

Professional presentations occur during sessions of regional, state, national, and international meetings. As described previously, researchers submit proposals in response to a call. Linking the response to the theme of the meeting increases the likelihood that the proposal will be accepted.

Presenters should remember their audience as they create and present their papers and PowerPoint slides. One researcher conducted research on the delivery of research papers (Edirisooriya 1996). Over seven years, she attended 126 sessions and viewed 748 presenters. Most presenters were allowed 12 minutes and found this limit inadequate. She found that 42 percent of presenters had not synthesized their data into information and, thus, wasted their time on unnecessary and trivial details. These presenters never reached the important points of their research. Edirisooriya recommended that presenters prepare for oral presentations by:

- Practicing their presentation
- Bringing all their materials
- Distilling their paper to four or five pages
- Showing eye-catching graphics (not tables with miniscule numbers)
- Focusing on results, discussion, and implications rather than background, theoretical framework, and rationales for analytical techniques

A more recent article reiterated these same ideas for effective presentations (Wineburg 2004). Generally, presenters should be prepared to talk about their research. Merely reading the notes is inadequate. Rather, presenters should try to be animated and talk to the people in the room. Other details regarding the mechanics of creating an effective PowerPoint presentation are listed in figure 16.16.

Publication

Scientific manuscripts follow the structure of known as IMRAD (Sollaci and Pereira 2004). IMRAD stands for introduction, methods, results, and discussion. Publication is important because it makes knowledge public. Practitioners, other researchers, and professionals in related fields can examine and critically analyze the research. Through publication, the HIM body of knowledge and the expertise of its professionals become available to the world.

This chapter has moved through the steps of research. In each step, the associated documentation was described. This documentation correlates with many sections of a research paper or journal article, including:

- Problem statement (introduction)
- Literature review
- Statement of hypothesis
- Method
- Results (including discussion)

Figure 16.16.   Guidelines for effective PowerPoint presentations

High contrast for visibility (black text on white background or dark blue background with white text and yellow highlights)
Lots of white space
Six by six rule (six words per line, six lines per slide)
Upper- and lowercase (all caps hard to read)
Eighteen minimum point size (24 recommended and 28 to 36 preferable)
Two inches character height for every 20 ft between visual and audience
Clear, simple fonts (Helvetica or Ariel)
Colors limited to 2 or 3
Colors' subliminal messages ("in the red")
Red-green color blindness
Color opposites on color wheel create "shimmer"
Transitions limited to 1 or 2 and nondistracting
Overuse of sounds annoying
Bullets are points of the outline
No paragraphs
Consistent verb tenses
Consistent tense of first words of parallel lines
Simple graphs
Proofread for spelling, math, grammar, numbering
Handouts should have three slides and room for notes

At this time, the researcher must complete the documentation by writing the abstract and expanding and detailing the sections already written.

It seems strange that the abstract, the first section of a journal article, is written last. However, the abstract is written last because it encompasses the entire study, including the study's findings.

An abstract is a brief summary of the major parts of a research study. It only reports the contents of the research; no additional information is included. An abstract is important because it is used in bibliographic databases to index and retrieve an article. Readers use it to decide whether the article contains valuable information and whether they should read the entire article. In writing an abstract, an author should focus on the research's important information, objectives, results, and conclusions. Brevity and directness are keys to a good abstract.

Table 16.13 (p. 476) serves as a final checklist for the composition and revision of the manuscript. Authors submitting manuscripts to journals in the field of health information management should take note that the peer reviewers highly value the following characteristics of manuscripts: (1) accuracy, (2) potential for contribution, (3) reasonableness of conclusions, (4) readability and style, and (5) organization (Layman and Watzlaf 2003). Common pitfalls are listed in figure 16.17 (p. 477). Careful attention to detail at this point has a high return on investment in terms of having journals accept the manuscripts. In preparing their manuscript for publication, researchers face two major remaining tasks: selecting the appropriate journal and following its submission guidelines.

Table 16.13. Organization of research publications

Section	Contents
Title Page	Concise and descriptive title, author, author's affiliation, grant information, disclaimer, corresponding author's address, telephone, fax, and e-mail
Abstract	Background, purpose, methods, results, conclusions or Context; objective; design, setting, and participants; interventions; main outcome measures; results, conclusions 45 to 250 words dependent upon call for papers or journal instructions 3 to 10 key words using medical subject headings (MeSH)
Introduction	Background; pertinent literature review that provides rationale for research; brief statement of research plan; purpose, objectives, or research question
Methods	Protocol with detail for replication Design, setting, and participants Definition of variables Reference established methods Sampling strategy Collection of data Statement about approval of IRB or other oversight entity Analytical strategy
Results	Core Important results followed by less important results Neutral reporting
Discussion	Relationship between results and purpose, objectives, or research question Evidence of relationship Similarities to and differences from previous research New knowledge in terms of theoretical framework Limitations Conclusions as related to purpose, objectives, or research question Implications for future research Recommendations as warranted Summary
Acknowledgment	Contributors whose level of involvement does not justify authorship
References	Citations per format in instructions
Tables	Consistent with narrative Expand abbreviations Format per instructions
Figures	Consistent with narrative Expand abbreviations Legend Format per instructions

Figure 16.17.   Pitfalls in presenting research

1. Allowing insufficient time to write the results or to develop the presentation
2. Interjecting subjective commentary and emotional hyperbole
3. Duplicating information in narrative and graphic forms
4. Creating confusing or inconsistent graphics
5. Believing that verbosity and inflated statements substitute for clarity and accuracy

Selecting the Appropriate Journal

As mentioned earlier, in health information management, research is published in two journals: the *Journal of the American Health Information Management Association* (JAHIMA) and *Perspectives in Health Information Management* (PHIM). However, depending on the topic, researchers should consider journals in other disciplines, such as informatics, public health, epidemiology, healthcare management, allied health, nursing, bioethics, health services, health policy, and health education. Researchers can obtain lists of journals from a library.

Selecting the appropriate journal requires thought and investigation, and researchers should take the time to skim through a number of journals. This investigation allows them to match their purpose, topic, research design, and style to the journal's scope, content, and audience.

First, researchers should determine their purpose. Is it altruism, service, or promotion and tenure? Certain journals are better suited to one purpose than another. For example, some journals have a practice orientation and others have a research orientation.

For altruism and service, researchers may send their manuscripts to journals oriented to practice, such as the *JAHIMA*. The researchers want to help their profession by putting effective techniques into the hands of practitioners. For example, if the researcher found that a particular graphical interface increased coder accuracy by 10 percent, he or she may decide to send that manuscript to the *JAHIMA*.

In addition to altruism and service, some researchers must meet work standards for promotion and tenure and publish as a condition of employment. Sometimes the work standards for publication specify quantity and quality. Quantity is the number of articles. Quality is less easily evaluated than quantity. One indirect measure is the prestige of the journal as indicated by its status as refereed or nonrefereed and its rejection rate. Another measure is the journal's impact factor. The impact factor reflects generally how often articles in the journal have been cited in a particular year. Researchers publishing to meet work standards should consider the refereed journals that have high rejection rates or high impact factors.

Second, researchers should match the content of their manuscript with the focus of the journal. For example, they should send manuscripts about research on the management of health information services to journals in the field of health information management. If their results have an impact on reimbursement or health policy, the researchers should consider journals with a broader base.

Third, researchers must match the design and method of their research to the types of designs and methods in the journal. Some journals include mostly experimental and quasi-experimental research; others include ethnographies, case studies, and personal histories. Researchers who match the design and method of their study with the types of typical designs and methods in the journal increase the likelihood of their manuscripts being accepted.

Fourth, researchers should strive for a match between their writing style and the preferences of the journal's audience. Journals that are oriented toward practice prefer brief articles written in simple, direct sentences. On the other hand, journals oriented toward scholarly work prefer a more formal and pedantic tone.

Finally, understanding the journal's audience combines the issues of topic and design. Researchers should submit their manuscripts to journals with audiences that would be interested in the topic. If the intended audience includes a broad range of fields, researchers should write manuscripts that are of interest to all potential readers. Moreover, researchers should clearly state how their manuscript affects and benefits the journal's intended audience.

Following the Journal's Submission Guidelines

Journals have rules for the format of manuscripts. The rules are both explicit and implicit. Explicit rules are openly stated; implicit rules are unwritten, but important. Editors and peer reviewers assume that researchers will naturally know and follow them. Different fields tend to have their own unique sets of implicit rules.

Journal editors state their explicit requirements for manuscripts in their style manual and submission guidelines. There are four major style manuals. (See figure 16.18.) Selection of style manual relates to the field. For example, journals in education generally require APA style whereas biomedical journals require AMA style. Journals in health information management use an adapted University of Chicago style. The variance in style manuals is illustrated in table 16.14 (p. 478).

The journal's submission guidelines include details such as the word-processing package, width of margins, length,

Figure 16.18.   Common style manuals

American Psychological Association. 2001. *Publication Manual of the American Psychological Association*, 5th ed. Washington, DC: APA. [Referred to as **APA Style**.]

Gibaldi, J. 2003. *MLA Handbook for Writers of Research Papers*, 6th ed. New York: Modern Language Association of America. [Referred to as **MLA Style**.]

Iverson, C. 1998. *American Medical Association Manual of Style: A Guide for Authors and Editors*, 9th ed. Baltimore, MD: Williams & Wilkins. [Referred to as **AMA Style**.]

University of Chicago Press. 2003. *Chicago Manual of Style*, 15th ed. Chicago: University of Chicago Press. [Referred to as **Chicago Style**.]

Table 16.14.   Variation in style manuals

Organization	Book	Journal
AMA	Jencks C, Riesman D. *The Academic Revolution.* Chicago: University of Chicago Press; 1977.	Lloyd SC, Layman E. The effects of automated encoders on coding accuracy and coding speed. *Top Health Inf Manage* February 1997; 17(3):72–79.
APA	Jencks, C., & Riesman, D. (1977). *The academic revolution.* Chicago: University of Chicago Press.	Lloyd, S. C., & Layman, E. (1997, February). The effects of automated encoders on coding accuracy and coding speed. Topics in *Health Information Management, 17*(3), 72–79.
Chicago	Jencks, Christopher, and David Riesman. 1977. *The Academic Revolution.* Chicago: University of Chicago Press.	Lloyd, Susan C., and Elizabeth Layman. 1997 (February). The effects of automated encoders on coding accuracy and coding speed. *Topics in Health Information Management* 17(3):72–79.
MLA	Jencks, Christopher, and David Riesman. *The Academic Revolution.* Chicago: University of Chicago Press, 1977.	Lloyd, Susan C., and Elizabeth Layman. "The Effects of Automated Encoders on Coding Accuracy and Coding Speed." *Topics in Health Information Management* 17.3 (1997): 72–79.

and organizational structure. (See figure 16.19.) For instance, the editors of *PHIM* prefer an organizational structure that generally includes the following elements:

- Abstract (105 words or less and up to 10 key words)
- Introduction
- Background (literature review)
- Research question or hypothesis
- Methods
- Results
- Discussion
- Conclusion
- References

However, most editors state that the organizational structure is flexible and that researchers should adapt the structure to suit their research. Researchers can find guidelines in journals or on the publishers' Web sites.

A journal's implicit rules reflect the culture of its audience. Culture is reflected in the use of the first person, anthropomorphism, passive voice, and tone. For example, an audience of qualitative researchers would accept use of the first person whereas its use probably would cause an audience of experimental researchers to doubt the article's credibility. Purists reject anthropomorphism as giving human traits to inanimate objects. Audiences that reject first person and anthropomorphism also tend to prefer passive voice and a detached, neutral tone. Time spent skimming journals would provide insight into their implicit rules.

Some editors and peer reviewers assume that sloppy writing indicates sloppy research. Moreover, some editors and peer reviewers believe that the inability to follow submission guidelines indicates the inability to follow research protocols. Therefore, attention to detail is important. Researchers seeking more information about writing and publishing manuscripts should read the style manuals and review samples of submission guidelines. For grammar and clarity, Strunk and

Figure 16.19.   Content of submission guidelines

Information needed about the author and contact
Style manual
Length and representativeness of title
Length of abstract in words
Length of manuscript in maximum number of pages or number of words
Font and font size
Line spacing
Justification
Margins
Pagination
Inclusive (nonsexist) language
Blinding (names of authors on separate page)
Format of charts and tables
Format of citations in text
Format of references (sometimes vary slightly from style manual)
General organizational structure of manuscript
Word-processing software
Number of paper copies
Diskette or electronic submission

White's book on writing is a classic (2000). First published in 1959 and periodically revised, its succinct discussions and precise examples provide clear guidance. Finally, researchers should carefully read Day's book (1988), which is dedicated to research writing and publishing.

Check Your Understanding 16.8

Instructions: Answer the following questions on a separate piece of paper.

1. How do the research findings and discussion sections differ?

2. What two factors should researchers consider when determining how to present a particular data element?

3. What three questions should a researcher answer when writing the discussion section?

4. What three factors should researchers consider when selecting a journal for manuscript submission?

Data Access and Confidentiality

When they access data, researchers pledge that they will keep them confidential. In their code of ethics, HIM professionals affirm that they will "uphold and defend the individual's right to privacy and the doctrine of confidentiality in the use and disclosure of information." This section describes the intersection of data access and protection of confidentiality.

Practical Considerations

Access to data depends on the type of data and their location. Data can range from totally uncontrolled to highly secured. For example, data on the Internet are easily accessed whereas data in health records require approvals from IRBs.

Data can be public or proprietary. Public data are often accessible under the Freedom of Information Act; some have been posted on the Internet. State registry data also are often accessible. Proprietary data require permission of the owner of the database.

Data can be individual or aggregate. Data that identify one individual are less accessible than aggregate data. Protections exist for identifiable data. In research using patient records, Bell and Hudson (2001) obtained approvals from three different IRBs. One approval was from the IRB of the university where they worked and the other two were from the IRBs of the two hospitals in which they reviewed patient records. Some organizations may require informed consents to review data. In addition, access to personally identifiable data has become more complex with the implementation of the regulations of the Health Insurance Portability and Accountability Act (HIPAA) of 1996.

After approvals or permissions are obtained, the location of data also affects ease of access. For data in databases, researchers can transfer the files over the Internet. For paper records, researchers must physically go to the site of storage where they must abide by the hours of operation and rules for security. In addition, they must arrange in some way to collect their data, for example, by entering them into a laptop.

Access to data becomes critical for researchers who conduct secondary analyses or combine their primary research with public databases. The key points for researchers who want to mine these rich resources are obtaining the approvals and allowing sufficient time.

Confidentiality

Confidentiality and anonymity are closely related concepts. *Confidentiality* pertains to the handling and maintenance of data so that the data are not divulged to others without the research participant's permission or divulged in ways contrary to the participant's understanding of the original disclosure. *Anonymity* pertains to data that have no identifiers linked to them and that cannot be traced back to the research participant.

Thus, confidentiality and anonymity are not synonymous and cannot be used interchangeably. Researchers must be careful in their use of the terms and not promise the more stringent concept of anonymity when they mean confidentiality.

The HIPAA regulations and its clauses related to de-identified data revolve around the concepts of confidentiality and anonymity.

Medical research, and by extension many other types of research in the United States, is covered under the Common Rule. The Common Rule is the set of regulations regarding research that 17 federal agencies share (HHS 2002). These agencies fund research at institutions that provide written assurance to the funding agency that the institutions will comply with the requirements of the Common Rule.

At a minimum, the Common Rule requires the following:

- An institutional statement of principles regarding the institution's responsibilities in the protection of human subjects involved in its research studies
- An IRB with sufficient staff
- A list of IRB members that demonstrates representative capacity to contribute to IRB deliberations
- Written procedures that the IRB follows for reviewing proposed research and ongoing oversight
- Written procedures that ensure prompt reporting of unanticipated problems, serious or continuing noncompliance, and suspension or termination of IRB approval (Burrington-Brown and Wagg 2003)

Institutions that are covered entities under HIPAA and that conduct federally funded research must comply with the regulations of both HIPAA and the Common Rule. The regulations of HIPAA articulate with the Common Rule. For example, under the Common Rule, researchers must obtain informed consent. HIPAA adds that the researcher also must obtain a signed authorization before protected health information may be used or disclosed for research. Further, HIPAA expands the role of the IRB by giving it authority, under specific stipulations, to approve waivers or alterations to the requirement to obtain authorization.

Health data that have been de-identified may be used without restriction for research purposes. However, the IRB must ensure that the data have been de-identified in the correct manner, that is, de-identified using statistical verification or all of the following identifiers removed: names, addresses (except state), date (except year), telephone and fax numbers, e-mail addresses, Social Security numbers, medical record numbers, health plan numbers, account numbers, certificate and license numbers, vehicle identifiers and serial numbers, device identifiers and serial numbers, URLs, IP addresses, biometric identfiers, full-face photographic images, and any other unique identifying number, characteristic, or code unless permitted by the privacy rule for re-identification (Gilles 2004).

A disadvantage to using de-identified data is that contacting the patient or client to improve the response rate or to notify the patient about some malfunction of a device or side effect of a drug is impossible.

Researchers who are preparing to conduct research with health information are encouraged to read the in-depth discussions provided by Burrington-Brown and Wagg (2003), Gilles (2004), and Roth (2004a, 2004b, 2004c). Finally, researchers should familiarize themselves with state laws protecting privacy. Some state laws are more restrictive than HIPAA. Researchers must comply with the more restrictive regulations.

Research and the Practitioner

Some HIM professionals have roles that are specifically related to research. These roles sort into three types: researcher, support staff to researchers in healthcare settings, and employee of a research company or agency. Other HIM professionals are users of research as they continue their education or attempt to implement best practices in their workplace.

First, many HIM professionals are researchers. They conduct research for several reasons, including service to the profession, personal interest, and condition of employment. Many of the citations in this chapter represent HIM professionals in the role of researcher.

Second, HIM professionals in the health information services departments of healthcare enterprises assist researchers in several ways, including:

- Assisting members of IRBs in the review of proposed studies that relate to data in health databases or paper records
- Evaluating and summarizing for administration the content of proposed studies that relate to data in health databases or paper records
- Identifying the location of the desired health data in databases, records, logs, reports, registers, or indexes
- Directing researchers and other authorized users to the location of health data
- Discussing with researchers the format of the data, such as paper records, microfilm, microfiche, and database
- Noting caveats, such as time frames and residual codes, related to the data
- Running computer queries to find cases
- Arranging access to computer databases and paper records
- Managing the work area reserved for researchers
- Obtaining signed confidentiality statements

Third, HIM professionals are employees of research companies or agencies. These positions represent one of the roles from AHIMA's Vision 2006. This role is that of the research and decision support analyst. In this role, HIM professionals collaborate "with product and policy organizations on high-level analysis projects such as clinical trials and outcomes research" (AHIMA 1999, p. 131).

All HIM professionals can use the steps of research. Research provides a thorough, systematic approach. The problem-solving models of management and the decision-making models of decision sciences are based on the steps of research. Therefore, the logic of the approach allows HIM professionals to use research in their day-to-day activities. To find answers to common questions or solutions to everyday problems, research is a practical and effective tool. In the long term, the orderliness of the step-by-step approach saves time and results in the best decision.

Research results are made public in professional presentations, proceedings of meetings, and journals. The availability and accessibility of these results allow all HIM professionals to benefit. HIM professionals can put the results of the research into practice. For example, as a consequence of the medical sociologist's research on the chatter about patients in hospital elevators, orientation sessions specifically address the need to maintain confidentiality in all conversations and in all settings.

Relationship with the Professional Body of Knowledge

One of the defining characteristics of a profession is that it has a body of knowledge. By definition, a field of work without a body of knowledge becomes an occupation or a job. Therefore, as a means to build and expand knowledge, research is the foundation of a profession.

As an emerging profession, health information management is developing and articulating its body of knowledge. Leaders of AHIMA recognize the importance of knowledge in advancing practice and professional learning (Kloss 2000). HIM professionals are conducting research in issues and topics related to health information. These topics and issues involve health information technology and systems, health data security and quality, management, benchmarks in practice and education, and informatics. (See figure 16.20.) This research is defining, expanding, and refining the body of knowledge for the HIM profession.

Figure 16.20.   Research topics in health information management

Compliance	Best practices in health information services
Use of computer applications in HIM education	Unique HIM instructional techniques
Information security	Information technology
Distance learning	Adoption and implementation of electronic health record
Vocabularies and terminologies	Role of technology in healthcare
Clinical education	Quality and use of coded data
Management issues	Impact of data quality in health outcomes
Graduate education	Data mining
Workforce retention and satisfaction	
Impact of HIPAA	
Managed care	
HIM curricular changes and their effectiveness	

Use in HIM Practice: Data Quality

HIM practitioners can use research to improve their department's efficiency and effectivness. They also can use research to improve their own performance as managers and administers. But which results should they rely on? Recent contradictory reports about widely used drugs raise skepticism about the research enterprise. The following section gives HIM practitioners pointers and information on how to identify high-quality data in research.

Evaluating research begins with carefully, critically, and analytically reading the journal article. Cohen (1991) provides questions that analytical readers of research should ask themselves. As a demonstration, these questions will be applied to a journal article in *Perspectives in Health Information Management* (Watzlaf, Zeng, Jarymowycz, and Firouzan 2004).

Researchers Watzlaf, Zeng, Jarymowycz, and Firouzan conducted a research study to measure the awareness, use, and validity of the minimum content for electronic health records (EHRs) as recommended by the American Society for Testing and Materials (ASTM). (See figure 16.21.)

1. Is the problem clearly stated? Are terms defined as needed? Has the problem been appropriately delimited?

    Statements: "Therefore, it is important to assess if those who purchase and use these systems are aware that these standards exist, and to measure the extent of usage of these standards. It will also be helpful to see if the content of the standards are meeting users' needs, so future revisions can address any deficiencies or problem areas." "To our knowledge, no other survey-

based study has been performed that examines the awareness, use, and fulfillment of user's needs of the most recent ASTM E1384 standards and E1633 coded values for the EHR."

Based on these statements, it appears the conditions of the first set of questions are met.

2. Is the hypothesis stated? Does the hypothesis relate to the problem? Is the way the researcher intends to test the hypothesis clear?

    "The study is descriptive. Because there is no intent to make inferences, no hypothesis is needed."

    The conditions of the second set of questions are not applicable.

3. To the best of the student's knowledge, is the literature review thorough, complete, and pertinent? Is the literature review clear and organized? Is the student convinced this problem is important? Does the literature review synthesize rather than merely summarize?

    The authors explain the advantages of the EHR based on the Standard Guide. They cite Mary Brandt and Gretchen Murphy, AHIMA leaders. The authors also state, "To our knowledge, no other survey-based study has been performed that examines the awareness, use, and fulfillment of user's needs of the most recent ASTM E1384 standards and E1633 coded values for the EHR." "It is therefore important and timely to determine the awareness, use, and validity of the ASTM standards for the content and structure of EHRs and their corresonding coded values."

    The final statement is most convincing. Based on these statements and the citation of professional leaders, it appears the conditions of the third set of questions are met.

4. Does the study's design relate to the problem? Is the population clearly defined? Is the method of creating the sample clearly explained? Is bias reduced in sampling? Is the sample representative of the population?

    Yes, the design relates to the problem because there is little known on the topic. When little is known, the descriptive, cross-sectional design is appropriate. The population is stated in the article: U.S. healthcare facilities identified by the American Hospital Association; vendors of EHR/CPR systems as identified in Healthcare Informatics; vendors reviewed by the American Academy of Family Physicians; volunteers, organizations recognized by CPRI-HOST. Yes, sample creation is clearly explained.

    Stratified random sample (stratification by state and type) reduces bias.

5. Is the instrument specified? Is the instrument related to the problem? Does the researcher state the instrument's reliability and validity?

    The authors explain that they designed their own survey. The survey was piloted on a random sample of 5 to 10 facilities and organizations. To detect

Figure 16.21.   Key questions to evaluate research

1. Is the problem clearly stated? Are terms defined as needed? Has the problem been appropriately delimited?
2. Is the hypothesis stated? Does the hypothesis relate to the problem? Is the way the researcher intends to test the hypothesis clear?
3. To the best of the student's knowledge, is the literature review thorough, complete, and pertinent? Is the literature review clear and organized? Is the student convinced this problem is important? Does the literature review synthesize rather than merely summarize?
4. Does the study's design relate to the problem? Is the population clearly defined? Is the method of creating the sample clearly explained? Is bias reduced in sampling? Is the sample representative of the population?
5. Is the instrument specified? Is the instrument related to the problem? Does the researcher state the instrument's reliability and validity?
6. Does the researcher explain the method clearly enough and with sufficient detail that another person could replicate the study? Are confidential data protected?
7. Does the researcher use the best mode to present the results? Do tables, figures, and graphs have clear titles? Do the numbers "add up"?
8. Do the conclusions relate to the findings? Does the researcher provide alternative explanations? Does the researcher relate the findings back to the larger body of knowledge or theory?
9. Are all citations in the body of the article in the reference list? Is jargon kept to a minimum?

Source: Cohen 1991.

potential problems, two individuals were shadowed when completing the online survey. A draft of the survey was presented to the ASTM E1384 committee. Changes were made based on the comments. From the piloting it appears that the instrument relates to the problem. The instrument's reliability and validity were not stated. As a new instrument, reliability and validity would need to be established, particularly if the researchers wanted to use this instrument again. Based on this information, it appears the conditions of the fifth set of questions are partially met.

6. Does the researcher explain the method clearly enough and with sufficient detail that another person could replicate the study? Are confidential data protected?

Yes, because the method is very detailed, another researcher could replicate this study. It does not appear that confidential data were obtained; however, the researchers did go through their IRB.

Based on the clarity, I believe that the article met the conditions of the sixth set of questions.

7. Does the researcher use the best mode to present the results? Do tables, figures, and graphs have clear titles? Do the numbers "add up"?

Tables appear to be the best mode to present the results. Tables have clear titles. Authors explain when the numbers do not "add up." Tables contain lots of data and seem long. Perhaps selected findings relevant to the audience could have been extracted. Overall, the article appears to meet conditions of the seventh set of conditions.

8. Do the conclusions relate to the findings? Does the researcher provide alternative explanations? Does the researcher relate the findings back to the larger body of knowledge or theory?

The authors concluded, "This study was able to provide some beginning information on the type of EHR system healthcare facilities have in place, as well as their awareness of ASTM standards and the specific minimum data elements they believe should be included in an EHR."

Comparing these conclusions, the problem statement, and the findings, it appears that they all relate.

The authors did not provide alternative explanations as they were conducting a descriptive study. They linked to the larger body of knowledge by extrapolating how their study supported the development of the longitudinal record. Overall, the article appears to have met the conditions of the eighth set of questions.

9. Are all citations in the body of the article in the reference list? Is jargon kept to a minimum?

All citations in the body of the article are in the reference list. ASTM and healthcare jargon is employed; however, it may have been difficult to communicate with the study participants without employing jargon.

Also, the fields of healthcare and informatics seem particularly prone to jargon.

Overall, the article appears to have partially met the conditions of the eighth set of questions.

Reviewing a journal article requires that readers synthesize all they know about research with much of what they know about a topic. Practicing these skills keeps readers sharp and attuned to results that do not meet the characteristics of data quality.

Another skill to evaluate research is to sort out the meaning of statistics on the tables that report them. A sample statistical table from a research article is dissected below.

The researchers investigated the relationships between independent variables and dependent variables (Layman and Guyden 1999). The independent variables were the coping mechanisms of self-disclosure, self-directed[ness], confidence, acceptance, structuring, problem solving, and coping resources. The dependent variable was burnout with its three subscales of emotional exhaustion (EE), depersonalization (DP), and personal accomplishment (PA).

The word *relationship* clues the reader that correlational statistical techniques are likely. The table's title lists the statistical technique as Pearson product–moment correlation. This title confirms the initial impression that correlational statistical techniques would be used. (See table 16.15.)

In the footnote, the researchers provide a key to the symbols (*, **, and ***). The asterisks meant the ρ values were less than would be encountered through chance. The $\rho < .05$ means that the probability of obtaining this extreme of a test statistic is 5 percent. The $\rho < .01$ means that the probability of obtaining this extreme of a test statistic is 1 percent. The $\rho < .001$ means that the probability of obtaining this extreme of a test statistic is 0.1 percent. Therefore, the researchers' findings were unlikely to be due to chance. A relationship existed between the emotional exhaustion and coping resources (–.4536).

Some of the findings have minus (–) signs in front of them. The minus signs show that an inverse relationship exists between the emotional exhaustion and coping resources (–.4536). An inverse relationship means that the *more* emotionally exhausted the respondent was, the *fewer* coping resources the respondent had. Inverse relationships move in opposite directions. An alternative explanation of the relationship between emotional exhaustion and coping resources could be that the more coping resources the respondent had, the less emotionally exhausted the respondent was. Correlations cannot indicate which came first, the emotional exhaustion or the coping resources. We only know that the two variables are related.

The researchers state that the study was a cross-sectional, correlational design. As a quasi-experimental design, the study cannot show causation. Thus, the researchers cannot state what caused the lower levels of emotional exhaustion for some respondents. The researchers do not know whether

Table 16.15.   Pearson product–moment correlation of burnout subscales and selected coping mechanisms

	Self-Disclosure	Self-Directed	Confidence	Acceptance	Solving Structuring	Problem Resources	Coping
EE	2.2489 (287) $p = .000$***	2.3245 (287) $p = .000$***	2.3993 (287) $p = .000$***	2.2821 (287) $p = .000$***	2.2948 (287) $p = .000$***	2.3048 (287) $p = .000$***	2.4536 (287) $p = .000$***
DP	2.2952 (287) $p = .000$***	2.2172 (287) $p = .000$***	2.3004 (287) $p = .000$***	2.2895 (287) $p = .000$***	2.1808 (287) $p = .002$**	2.2712 (287) $p = .000$***	2.3653 (287) $p = .000$***
PA	.2984 (287) $p = .000$***	.3731 (287) $p = .000$***	.5332 (287) $p = .000$***	.3398 (287) $p = .000$***	.3904 (287) $p = .000$***	.4970 (287) $p = .000$***	.5576 (287) $p = .000$***

Note. (coefficient / (cases) / two-tailed test).
*$p < .05$. **$p < .01$. ***$p < .001$.

Source: Layman and Guyden 1999.

the high levels of coping resources caused the lower levels of emotional exhaustion. The most the researchers can say is that the more coping resources the respondent recorded, the less emotionally exhausted the respondent was.

Astute readers may note that the row of data labeled PA (personal accomplishment) does not have minus signs. The absence of the minus signs indicates that a positive relationship exists between the two variables. In positive relationships, the variables both move in the same direction. The *more* coping resources a respondent has, the *more* personally accomplished the respondent feels. To reiterate the correlational design of the study precludes statements about causation.

Being able to determine the meaning of tables with statistical data is a powerful tool. Articles report data in tables and other graphics because these formats efficiently deliver information. However, if one cannot decode the table, the benefit is lost. Acquiring skills in statistical reporting is valuable for HIM professionals because they are data driven.

Researchers provide much information in journal articles. As the field of HIM increasingly moves to data mining and evidence-based practice, skills in evaluating the quality of data reported in journal articles become ever more important. Honing skills in research and data quality is a key task for HIM professionals who are preparing to lead the practice in the future.

Check Your Understanding 16.9

Instructions: Answer the following questions on a separate piece of paper.

1. What should researchers who use large databases for secondary analysis know about them?

2. How do public databases and proprietary databases differ?

3. The researcher's informed consent form stated that the patients' information would be anonymous. Later, in the application form for IRB approval, the researcher described a coding system to track respondents and nonrespondents. The IRB returned the application to the researcher with the stipulation that the informed consent must be changed. What raised the red flag?

4. What is the Common Rule?

5. A researcher is at an institution that is a covered entity and received federal funding for research. Which set of regulations applies to the researcher?

6. Why is research particularly important to an emerging profession, such as health information management?

Real-World Case

Recent articles in the *Journal of the American Medical Association* (Lee et al. 2000) and the *Journal of Quality Improvement* (Schneider et al. 2001) have discussed the use of databases and patient records in the collection of data for the Health Plan Employer Data and Information Set (HEDIS).

These articles interested several physicians in a large, urban physician group practice. The physicians wanted to evaluate the quality of care and services that their practice provided. Because its performance measures were easily accessible, the physicians decided to use the HEDIS. In addition, because the evaluation was purely voluntary, the physicians decided that, initially, they would address one HEDIS performance domain per month.

Many of the physicians in the practice were familiar with the HEDIS from either their readings or past involvement with managed care organizations. They knew that data from claims (administrative data) and patient records (clinical data) were required to calculate performance rates. Therefore, the physicians gave the HEDIS project to the practice's health information manager because of her expertise in these areas.

Upon receiving the project, the health information manager decided to implement the step-by-step approach of a research study. She made this decision for three reasons. First, the clearly defined steps in research would divide the large project into tasks of a manageable size. Second, the systematic approach would reduce the likelihood of overlooking important aspects of the project. Third, the physicians, her supervisors, would understand the scientific approach of a research study. Therefore, the health information manager utilized her knowledge of research methods to approach a task in the workplace.

Summary

High-quality research depends on a carefully conceived plan and impeccable execution. Researchers' plans are similar to the blueprints that architects use to construct buildings. Researchers use their plans to conduct their studies and to build new knowledge. Research is systematic, and health information professionals can adapt its step-by-step approach to practical problems in the workplace.

Knowing the purpose of the research is a consistent theme in this chapter. Purpose drives decisions in each of the steps of research. These steps are defining the problem, reviewing the literature, determining the design and method, selecting the instrument, collecting and analyzing the data, presenting the results, and interpreting the findings.

The purpose of research determines the approach, whether qualitative or quantitative. Qualitative research is often exploratory and preliminary; quantitative research investigates numerically measurable observations or tests hypotheses.

Purpose also assists researchers in clarifying their research question. Considering their purposes helps researchers to concentrate or narrow the focus of the question to a researchable issue. Purpose also can ensure that researchers investigate meaningful problems that need solutions or significant questions that need answers.

The literature review is guided by purpose. In research, preference is given to articles in refereed journals. Purpose aids researchers in discriminating between relevant and irrelevant articles and between related and tangential articles. Finally, one purpose of the literature review is to identify gaps in the body of knowledge that researchers can fill with their studies.

There are six common designs of research: historical, descriptive, correlational, evaluation, experimental, and causal–comparative. The design a researcher chooses depends on the purpose of the research. Associated with each design are many methods of research, including survey, observation, case study, ethnography, experiments, secondary analysis, and meta-analysis. As with the choice of design, purpose is crucial in the choice of method.

Purpose also is crucial in selecting the research instrument. Instruments are standardized means to collect data. Although many factors should be considered in the selection of an instrument, the most important is the researchers' purpose.

The importance of purpose may be less obvious in the collection and analysis of data. However, the higher the stakes, the larger the sample. Moreover, research that involves many

variables also needs larger sample sizes. Therefore, purpose is a critical concern in the collection of data. Purpose also is involved in the analysis of data because statistical approaches vary by research design.

Moreover, purpose underlies the presentation of results and interpretation of findings. Researchers provide other HIM professionals with knowledge and techniques to answer questions and to solve problems in the workplace. Without presentation and interpretation, the knowledge and techniques would be unavailable to practitioners. Thereby, research in the field of health information management improves health information practices in the continuum of care.

HIM professionals are well suited to the role of researcher. Typically, persons in the field recognize their abilities to plan and organize. Their abilities with analytical expertise create a powerful toolbox of skills that HIM professionals can use to increase the field's body of knowledge.

References

Abdelhak, M. 1982. Hospital information systems applications and potential: A literature review. *Topics in Health Record Management* 3(1):8–18.

Abdelhak, M., P.A. Firouzan, and L. Ullman. 1993. Hospital information systems applications and potential: A literature review revisited, 1982–1992. *Topics in Health Information Management* 13(4):1–14.

AHIMA Data Quality Management Task Force. 1998. Practice brief: Data quality management model. *Journal of American Health Information Management Association* 69(6).

Aish, A.M., and D. Wasserman. 2001. Does Beck's Hopelessness Scale really measure several components? *Psychological Medicine* 31(2):367–72.

Alreck, P.L., and R.B. Settle. 2004. *The Survey Research Handbook,* 3rd ed. New York: McGraw-Hill/Irwin.

Amatayakul, M.K., and M.A. Shah. 1992. *Research Manual for the Health Information Profession.* Chicago: AHIMA.

American Health Information Management Association. 1999. *Evolving HIM Careers: Seven Roles for the Future.* Chicago: AHIMA.

Bailey, K.D. 1994. *Methods of Social Research,* 4th ed. New York: Free Press.

Barrows, R.C., Jr., and P.D. Clayton. 1996. Privacy, confidentiality, and electronic medical records. *Journal of the American Medical Informatics Association* 3(2):139–48.

Bedell, S.E., S. Jabbour, R. Goldberg, H. Glaser, S. Gobble, Y.X. Yinong, T.B. Graboys, and S. Ravid. 2000. Discrepancies in the use of medications: Their extent and predictors in an outpatient practice. *Archives of Internal Medicine* 160(14):2129–134.

Becker, H.S., B. Geer, E.C. Hughes, and A.S. Strauss. 1961. *Boys in White: Student Culture in Medical School.* Chicago: University of Chicago Press.

Bell, P.D. 1999. Evaluating the use of computer-assisted instruction in allied health professional education: A review of the literature. *Educational Perspectives in Health Information Management* 2(2):29–40.

Bell, P.D., and S. Hudson. 2001. Equity in the diagnosis of chest pain: Race and gender. *American Journal of Health Behavior* 25(1):60–71.

Bell, P.D., M.M. Micke, and R.M. Kasa. 1998. Equity in the diagnosis and treatment of chest pain: Gender, age, and comorbidity. *American Journal of Health Behavior* 22(6):443–50.

Berdie, D.R., and J.F. Anderson. 1974. *Questionnaires: Design and Use.* Metuchen, NJ: Scarecrow Press.

Bethell, C., J. Fiorillo, D. Lansky, M. Hendryx, and J. Knickman. 2004. Online consumer surveys as a methodology for assessing the quality of the United States health care system. *Journal of Medical Internet Research* 6(1):e2. Available online from jmir.org/2004/1/e2/.

Brodnik, M.S. 1993. Burnout and turnover potential among department leaders. *Journal of American Health Information Management Association* 64(8):64–67.

Brown, C., W.P. Moore, D. Hemman, and A. Yunek. 1996. The influence of instrumental activities of daily living assessment method on judgments of independence. *American Journal of Occupational Therapy* 50(3):202–06.

Buros Institute. 1938–1995. The Mental Measurements Yearbook: *The Yearbook 1938–1995.* Highland Park, NJ: Buros Institute.

Buros Institute of Mental Measurements. 2003. *The Fifteenth Mental Measurements Yearbook.* Available online from unl.edu/buros.

Burrington-Brown, J., and D.G. Wagg. 2003. Practice brief: Regulations governing research. *Journal of American Health Information Management Association* 74(3):56A–56D.

Byrne, M. 2001. Ethnography as a qualitative research method. *Journal of the Association of Operating Room Nurses* 74(1):82–84.

Campbell, D.T., and J.C. Stanley. 1963. *Experimental and Quasi-Experimental Designs for Research.* Chicago: Rand McNally.

Chadwick, B.A., H.M. Bahr, and S.L. Albrecht. 1984. *Social Science Research Methods.* Englewood Cliffs, NJ: Prentice-Hall.

Chun, K.T., S. Cobb, and J.R.P. French Jr., eds. 1975. *Measures for Psychological Assessment: A Guide to 3,000 Original Sources and Their Applications.* Ann Arbor, MI: Survey Research Center, Institute for Social Research.

Cohen, P.A. 1992. Meta-analysis: application to clinical dentistry and dental education. *Journal of Dental Education* 56(3):172–75.

Cohen, P.A. 1991. Criteria for evaluating research reports. Handout, Educational research course. Augusta, GA: Medical College of Georgia.

Colaianni, L.A. 1994. Peer review in journals indexed in Index Medicus. *Journal of the American Medical Association* 272(2):156–58.

Day, R.A. 1988. *How to Write and Publish a Scientific Paper,* 3rd ed. Phoenix: Oryx Press.

Department of Health and Human Services. 2002. Protection of human subjects. *Code of Federal Regulations* 45 CFR 46.

Dillman, D.A. 2000. *Mail and Internet Surveys: The Tailored Design Method,* 2nd ed. New York: John Wiley & Sons.

Edirisooriya, G. 1996. Research presentations in a democratic society: A voice from the audience. *Educational Researcher* 25(6):25–30.

Ericae.net. 2001. ERIC/AE test locator. ERIC Clearinghouse on Assessment and Evaluation. Available online from ericae.net.

Feldman, R.P., and J.T. Goodrich. 1999. The Edwin Smith surgical papyrus. *Child's Nervous System* 15(6–7):281–84.

Fenton, S., and M. Williams. 2005. Getting to know PubMed: An overview. *Journal of American Health Information Management Association* 76(3):60A–60D.

Flexner, A. 1910. *Medical Education in the United States and Canada: A Report to the Carnegie Foundation for the Advancement of Teaching.* 1960 Reissue. Washington, DC: Health and Science Publications.

Gall, M.D., W.R. Borg, and J.P. Gall. 2003. *Educational Research: An Introduction,* 7th ed. Boston: Allyn & Bacon.

Garrard, J. 2004. *Health Sciences Literature Review Made Easy: The Matrix Method.* Sudbury, MA: Jones and Bartlett Publishers.

Garvin, J.H. 2001. Building on the vision: Exploratory research in future skill areas of the clinical data specialist as described in evolving HIM careers. *Educational Perspectives in Health Information Management* 4(1):19–32.

Gay, L.R., and P. Airasian. 2003. *Educational Research: Competencies for Analysis and Application,* 7th ed. Upper Saddle River, NJ: Pearson Education.

Gibaldi, J. 2003. *MLA Handbook for Writers of Research Papers,* 6th ed. New York: Modern Language Association of America.

Gilles, K. 2004. Uncovering the relationship between IRBs and the HIPAA privacy rule. *Journal of American Health Information Management Association* 75(10):48, 49, 52, 55.

Giovannucci, E., M.J. Stampfer, G.A. Colditz, D.J. Hunter, C. Fuchs, B.A. Rosner, F.E. Speizer, and W.C. Willett. 1998. Multivitamin use, folate, and colon cancer in women in the Nurses' Health Study. *Annals of Internal Medicine* 129(7):517–24.

Glass, G.V. 1976. Primary, secondary, and meta-analysis of research. *Educational Researcher* 5(10):3–8.

Grove, C. 1980. Foundation for the future of quality assurance: A literature review of the past. *Topics in Health Record Management* 1(2):13–23.

Haas, L.F. 1999. Papyrus of Ebers and Smith. *Journal of Neurology, Neurosurgery & Psychiatry* 67(5):578.

Herndon, R.M., ed. 1997. *Handbook of Neurologic Rating Scales.* New York: Demos Vermande.

Hill, R.F., and E.P. Tyson. 1997. The culture of morning report: Ethnography of a clinical teaching conference. *Southern Medical Journal* 90(6):594–600.

Iverson, C., ed. 1998. *American Medical Association Manual of Style: A Guide for Authors and Editors,* 9th ed. Baltimore: Williams & Wilkins.

Jencks, C., and D. Riesman. 1977. *The Academic Revolution.* Chicago: University of Chicago Press.

Jha, A.K., G.J. Kuperman, J.M. Teich, L. Leape, B.Shea, E. Rittenberg, E. Burdick, D.L. Seger, M.V. Vliet, and D.W. Bates. 1998. Identifying adverse drug events: Development of a computer-based monitor and comparison with chart review and stimulated voluntary report. *Journal of the American Medical Informatics Association* 5(3):305–14.

Johnson, M. 1992. A silent conspiracy? Some ethical issues of participant observation in nursing research. *International Journal of Nursing Studies* 29(2):213–23.

Johnson, R.B., and A.J. Onwuegbuzie. 2004. Mixed methods research: A research paradigm whose time has come. *Educational Researcher* 33(7):14–26.

Kennedy, W.C., and E. Jacobs. 1981. Literature review of legal aspects of medical records. *Topics in Health Record Management* 1(4):19–32.

Kesh, S., and W. Raghupathi. 2004. Critical issues in bioinformatics and computing. *Perspectives in Health Information Management* 1(9):1–8.

Keyser, D.J., and R.C. Sweetland, eds. 1991. *Test Critiques.* Kansas City, MO: Test Corporation of America.

Khan, M. 1997. Basic components of a randomized clinical trial. *The Internet Journal of Anesthesiology* 1(1). Available online from ispub.com.

Kish, L. 1965. *Survey Sampling.* New York: John Wiley & Sons.

Kloss, L. 2000. Growing the HIM body of knowledge. *Journal of American Health Information Management Association* 71(10):27.

Koppel, R., J.P. Metlay, A. Cohen, B. Abaluck, A.R. Localio, S.E. Kimmel, and B.L. Strom. 2005. Role of computerized physician order entry systems in facilitating medication errors. *Journal of the American Medical Association* 293(10):1197–1203.

Lan, A.J., J.M. Colford, and J.M. Colford, Jr. 2000. The impact of dosing frequency on the efficacy of 10-day penicillin or amoxicillin therapy for streptococcal tonsillopharyngitis: A meta-analysis. *Pediatrics* 105(2):e19.

Layman, E.J., and J.A. Guyden. 1999. The relationships among psychological type, coping mechanisms, and burnout in directors of hospital health information management departments. *Educational Perspectives in Health Information Management* 1(2):29–41.

Layman, E., and V. Watzlaf. 2003. Manuscript characteristics affecting reviewers' decisions for journals in health information management. *Educational Perspectives in Health Information Management* 5(1):48–85.

Lee, F.W. 1996. Can computer-aided systems engineering tools enhance the development of health care information systems? *Topics in Health Information Management* 17(1):1–11.

Lee, T.H., J.I. Cleeman, S.M. Grundy, C. Gillett, R.C. Pasternak, J. Seidman, and C. Sennett. 2000. Clinical goals and performance measures for cholesterol management in secondary prevention of coronary heart disease. *Journal of the American Medical Association* 283(1):94–98.

Lewis, C.A. 1980. Cost containment in medical records: A literature review. *Topics in Health Record Management* 1(1):21–30.

Lippin, T.M., A. Eckman, K.R. Calkin, and T.H. McQuiston. 2000. Empowerment-based health and safety training: Evidence of workplace change from four industrial sectors. *American Journal of Industrial Medicine* 38(6):697–706.

Lloyd, S.C., and E. Layman. 1997. The effects of automated encoders on coding accuracy and coding speed. *Topics in Health Information Management* 17(3):72–79.

McDowell, I., and C. Newell. 1996. *Measuring Health: A Guide to Rating Scales and Questionnaires,* 2nd ed. New York: Oxford University Press.

Mechanic, D., and S. Meyer. 2000. Concepts of trust among patients with serious illness. *Social Science & Medicine* 51(5):657–68.

Mendonça, E.A., J.J. Cimino, S.B. Johnson, and Y.H. Seol. 2001. Accessing heterogeneous sources of evidence to answer clinical questions. *Journal of Biomedical Informatics* 34(2):85–98.

Metz, M.H. 2001. Intellectual border crossing in graduate education: A report from the field. *Educational Researcher* 30(5):12–18.

Meyer, G.S., and D. Blumenthal. 1996. TennCare and academic medical centers: The lessons from Tennessee. *Journal of the American Medical Association* 276(9):672–76.

Mikkelsen, G., and J. Aasly. 2001. Concordance of information in parallel electronic and paper-based patient records. *International Journal of Medical Informatics* 63:121–31.

Monsen, R.B. 1999. Mothers' experiences of living worried when parenting children with spina bifida. *Journal of Pediatric Nursing* 14(3):157–63.

Mulrow, C.D. 1994. Systematic reviews: rationale for systematic reviews. *British Medical Journal* 309(6954):597–99.

Nickels, J.C. 2005. Management of urinary tract infections: Historical perspective and current strategies, Part 1: Before antibiotics. *Journal of Urology* 173(1):21–26.

Oral, R., K.L. Blum, and C. Johnson. 2003. Fractures in young children: Are physicians in the emergency department and orthopedic clinics adequately screening for possible abuse? *Pediatric Emergency Care* 19(3):148–53.

Ornstein, S.M., L.L. MacFarlane, R.G. Jenkins, Q. Pan, and K.A. Wager. 1999. Medication cost information in a computer-based patient record system: Impact on prescribing in a family medicine clinical practice. *Archives of Family Medicine* 8(2):118–21.

Osborn, C.E. 2001. DRG analysis reveals potential problems, trends. *Journal of American Health Information Management Association* 72(7):78–84.

Osborn, C.E. 2000a. Practices and productivity in acute care facilities. *Journal of American Health Information Management Association* 71(2):61–66.

Osborn, C.E. 2000b. *Statistical Applications for Health Information Management.* Gaithersburg, MD: Aspen.

Osborn, C.E. 1999. Benchmarking with national ICD-9-CM coded data. *Journal of American Health Information Management Association* 70(3):59–69.

Osborn, C.E. 1998. A methodology for construction of a survey questionnaire. *Educational Perspectives in Health Information Management* 1(1):3–13.

Pamplona, M.C., A. Ysunza, M. Gonzalez, E. Ramirez, and C. Patino. 2000. Linguistic development in cleft palate patients with and without compensatory articulation disorder. *International Journal of Pediatric Otorhinolaryngology* 54(2–3):81–91.

Penslar, R.L. 2001. IRB Guidebook. Office for Human Research Protections. Available online from ohrp.osophs.dhhs.gov/irbguidebook.htm.

Ritter, P., K. Lorig, D. Laurent, and K. Matthews. 2004. Internet versus mailed questionnaires: A randomized comparison. *Journal of Medical Internet Research* 6(3):e29.

Roth, J. 2004a. Getting "hip" to other privacy laws, Part 1. *Journal of American Health Information Management Association* 75(2):50–52.

Roth, J.A. 2004b. Getting "hip" to other privacy laws, Part 2. *Journal of American Health Information Management Association* 75(3):48–50.

Roth, J.A. 2004c. Overdoes of privacy law creates headaches for student health clinics. *Journal of American Health Information Management Association* 75(8):64–65, 67.

Rudman, W.J., and D. Davey. 2000. Identifying domestic violence within inpatient hospital admissions using medical records. *Women & Health* 30(4):1–13.

Rudolph, F. 1990. *The American College and University: A History.* Athens: University of Georgia Press.

Salant, P., and D.A. Dillman. 1994. *How to Conduct Your Own Survey.* New York: John Wiley & Sons.

Schneider, K.M., R.T. Wiblin, K.S. Downs, and B.E. O'Donnell. 2001. Methods for evaluating the provision of well child care. *Journal of Quality Improvement* 27(12):673–82.

Shi, L. 1997. *Health Services Research Methods.* Albany, NY: Delmar.

Siemon, J.E. 1982. Case mix and data quality: A review of the literature. *Topics in Health Record Management* 2(4):13–22.

Singleton, R.A., Jr., and B.C. Straits. 1999. *Approaches to Social Research,* 3rd ed. New York: Oxford University Press.

Sollaci, L.B., and M.G. Pereira. 2004. The introduction, methods, results, and discussion (IMRAD) structure: A fifty-year survey. *Journal of the Medical Library Association* 92(3):364–71.

Spreen, O., and E. Strauss. 1997. *A Compendium of Neuropsychological Tests: Administration, Norms, and Commentary,* 2nd ed. New York: Oxford University Press.

Strunk, W., Jr., and E.B. White. 2000. *The Elements of Style,* 4th ed. New York: Longman.

Sudman, S. 1976. *Applied Sampling.* New York: Academic Press.

Sweetland, R.C., and D.J. Keyser, eds. 1991. *Tests: A Comprehensive Reference for Assessments in Psychology, Education, and Business,* 3rd ed. Austin, TX: Pro-Ed.

Thomas, E.J., and T.A. Brennan. 2000. Incidence and types of preventable adverse events in elderly patients: Population based review of medical records. *British Medical Journal* 320(7232):741–44.

University of Chicago Press. 2003. *The Chicago Manual of Style,* 15th ed. Chicago: University of Chicago Press.

Van de Mortel, T., and L. Heyman. 1995. Performance feedback increases the incidence of handwashing by staff following patient contact in intensive care. *Australian Critical Care* 8(2):8–13.

Van Vugt, M., P. Wilairatana, B. Gemperli, I. Gathmann, L. Phaipun, A. Brockman, C. Luxemburger, N.J. White, F. Nosten, and S. Looareesuwan. 1999. Efficacy of six doses of artemether-lumefantrine (benflumetol) in multidrug-resistant Plasmodium falciparum malaria. *American Journal of Tropical Medicine & Hygiene* 60(6):936–42.

Watzlaf, V., A. Katoh, and F. D'Amico. 1996. Obstacles encountered in the use of medical record and cancer registry abstract in breast cancer research. *Topics in Health Information Management* 17(1):25–33.

Watzlaf, V., X. Zeng, C. Jarymowycz, and P.A. Firouzan. 2004. Standards for the content of the electronic health record. *Perspectives in Health Information Management* 1(1):1–21.

Wilson, F.L., L.M. Baker, C. Brown-Syed, and C. Gollop. 2000. An analysis of the readability and cultural sensitivity of information on the National Cancer Institute's Web site, CancerNet. *Oncology Nursing Forum* 27(9):1403–409.

Wineberg, S. 2004. Must it be this way? Ten rules for keeping your audience awake during conferences. *Educational Researcher* 23(4):13–14.

Zhan, Chunliu, and Marlene R. Miller. 2003. Excess length of stay, charges, and mortality attributable to medical injuries during hospitalization. *Journal of the American Medical Association* 290(14):1868–874.

Chapter 17
Clinical Quality Management

Vicki L. Zeman, MA, RHIA

Learning Objectives

- To define quality within the context of clinical healthcare services
- To know who has ultimate responsibility for the quality of services provided by a healthcare organization
- To differentiate among the three types of performance measures used in clinical quality improvement (QI): structure, process, and outcome
- To understand the benefits of having a QI program and how each clinical department selects areas for review
- To describe the reason for an annual appraisal of a QI plan/program
- To understand and differentiate performance improvement initiatives of accrediting agencies, regulatory bodies, and payers
- To describe the significance of core performance measures in regard to data comparison, performance improvement, and data-driven accreditation
- To understand the rationale behind the patient safety initiatives and the role played by the private sector and the government
- To understand and explain Six Sigma as a quality measurement system and why its success in healthcare is dependent on physician and higher-level management buy-in
- To understand the similarities and differences of the various quality measurement systems used in the healthcare environment
- To explain the significance of outcomes management, case management, clinical practice guidelines, and benchmarking in quality management
- To understand the concept of sentinel event
- To recognize when root-cause analysis is required
- To understand the impact of the concepts of medical staff appointment/reappointment, credentialing, and clinical privileges on quality of care
- To recognize the functions of the executive committee and to discuss the relevance of medical staff bylaws/rules and regulations in quality improvement
- To describe the medical staff quality applications required by JCAHO standards and to summarize the medical staff's patient care review functions
- To understand the utilization review process and its impact on quality of care
- To understand the importance of integrating risk management into any QI program
- To recognize the role of severity indexing in a QI program
- To describe the impact of the Agency for Healthcare Research and Quality on performance improvement
- To appreciate the significance of the Medicare Prescription Drug, Improvement, and Modernization Act of 2003 incentive payment initiative
- To understand and value the importance of keeping QI data confidential and secure

Key Terms

Agency for Healthcare Research and Quality (AHRQ)
Agenda for Change
Benchmarking
Blood and blood component usage review
Bylaws/rules and regulations
Clinical privileges
Clinical Value Compass
Commission on Accreditation of Rehabilitation Facilities (CARF)
Core performance measures
Credentialing process
Emergency preparedness
Health Plan Employer Data and Information Set (HEDIS)
Health record review
Incident report review

Independent practitioners
Infection review
Institute for Clinical Systems Improvement (ICSI)
Leapfrog Group
Loss prevention
Loss reduction
Medical care evaluation studies (audits)
Medication usage review
Mortality review
National Association of Healthcare Quality (NAHQ)
National Quality Forum
Occurrence/generic screening
Orion project
ORYX initiative
Outcome measures
Peer review organization (PRO)

Performance improvement (PI)
Performance measure
Performance measurement system
Potentially compensable event (PCE)
Practice guidelines
Priority focus process (PFP)
Process measures
Quality
Quality assurance (QA)
Quality management
Quality gap
Quality improvement (QI)
Quality improvement organization (QIO)
Report cards
Risk prevention
Root-cause analysis

Safe practices
Scope of work
Sentinel event
Severity indexing
Surgical review
Six Sigma
Structure
Structure measures
Tax Equity and Fiscal Responsibility Act (TEFRA)
Temporary privileges
Ten-step monitoring and evaluation process
Universal Protocol
Utilization management
Utilization review (UR)
Verification service

Introduction

In healthcare, the term *quality* means one thing to the patient and another to the healthcare provider. But to both, the objective of quality is to arrive at a desired outcome. Providing the best care in the most effective manner and for the least cost is something every healthcare organization strives to do. Improving healthcare quality is a fundamental consideration of the U.S. healthcare system today.

The world is constantly evolving, and change is a sure thing. Whether making a change is chaotic or measured and controlled often speaks to the success of those involved in the change process. The more measured and controlled the change process, the greater the chance of success. People in healthcare are survivors of phenomenal change, both measured and chaotic, over the past two decades. Health information management (HIM) professionals have been a distinct part of the change process.

The gurus of managing the change process—Deming, Juran, and Crosby, for example—have developed methods to measure and monitor systems and processes in organizations. Their theories give managers methods to use in bringing about measured, focused change before crisis occurs. With encouragement from accrediting bodies and government agencies, healthcare organizations are trying to achieve continued, measured, and focused change with the purpose of improving healthcare.

Healthcare professionals are struggling to use the QI methods offered in the business sector. Healthcare is a highly complex environment involving many specially trained individuals with a strong commitment to their way of providing care. Finding ways to help such individuals work together effectively is a challenge.

This chapter discusses the history of **quality management** as well as how quality management is organized and evaluated in modern-day healthcare organizations. It then describes the clinical applications of QI efforts, focusing on the medical staff, nursing, and ancillary services. Finally, the chapter looks at using comparative data in the process of managing clinical quality.

Theory into Practice

Dr. Jeffreys, chief of orthopedics, has been collecting information on the outcomes of joint replacement surgery (hip and knee) for the past six months and is interested in following up on this information using **performance improvement** (PI) as the approach. She contacts Dorothy Davis, manager of the **quality improvement** (QI) department, to set up a meeting to get some action.

In their meeting, Dr. Jeffreys mentions that her review of the outcomes data has raised several concerns. Significant variations include the cost to the hospital of performing joint replacement procedures, length of stay, and the types of therapy following surgery. In addition, more and more

patients appear to be returning postoperatively because of problems. She believes that everyone in orthopedics needs to start thinking about "how we can do things to get better results."

Dorothy explains that the hospital uses a definite QI methodology. It is a basic problem-solving model developed by the Joint Commission on Accreditation of Healthcare Organizations (JCAHO) that looks like this:

Assess → Measure → Analyze →
Recommend Improvements/Changes → Measure → Analyze

She feels confident that she and Dr. Jeffreys can make general decisions, build a team of care providers to evaluate the current situation, and develop an action plan.

Dr. Jeffreys and Dorothy arrange a meeting with everyone who affects the care of patients undergoing joint replacement. They first will need to develop assessment information that is understandable to everyone involved. Dorothy asks the librarian to do a literature search of the orthopedic literature so they can benchmark their results. On her part, Dr. Jeffreys contacts the American Academy of Orthopaedic Surgeons to see whether it has any best practices available. Dorothy suggests that clinical **practice guidelines,** such as the ones adopted in the obstetrics department, be considered.

Dr. Jeffreys and Dorothy also decide to obtain information on the "change" process. Determined to "make a difference," Dr. Jeffreys is going to talk to all the orthopedic surgeons and the hospital's administration to ensure that everyone understands what she has found and how she plans to address the situation. Her goal is to improve the way the facility handles hip and knee joint replacement. However, improvement means change and change must be understood, encouraged, managed, and sustained if the healthcare environment is to improve.

QI is not an isolated event; it involves many people. Everyone from the physician to the housekeeping staff has an impact on the quality of care delivered. Understanding the QI process is a way to make a difference to the patients cared for at the hospital. QI is a problem-solving process used in a complex medical setting. Things will change only when everyone works together to achieve the common goal of improving patient care.

Overview of Clinical Quality Management

Clinical quality management involves the evaluation of direct patient care. Clinical performance is often measured around diagnosis, medical condition, or care processes along with outcomes. The relationship between the way care is provided and the outcomes or results of the medical intervention is the focus of clinical quality management. Clinical quality management includes the process of quality improvement as it is applied in healthcare organizations. Although both the administrative and clinical aspects of healthcare systems may be the subjects of QI processes, the focus is on the clinical applications of QI in healthcare systems today.

Quality Improvement and the Use of Aggregate Data

Quality is assumed to give an enhanced worth or value to a product or service. Each person brings his or her unique perspective to the quality of a product or service he or she receives. If a person sees a service as having quality, it follows that the service was perceived as being good. Further, cost affects the perceived quality of a product or service. Consumers believe that the greater the quality of a product or service and the lower the cost, the greater the value of that product or service. Americans demand high-quality products or services for the lowest possible cost. W. Edwards Deming stated that "Quality has meaning only in terms of the customer, his needs, what he is going to use it for" (Walton 1986, p. 28). The **Agency for Healthcare Research and Quality** (AHRQ) defines quality of healthcare as "The degree to which health services for individuals and populations increase the likelihood of desired health outcomes and are consistent with current professional knowledge" (Wachter and Owens 2004, p. 2).

Individuals involved in QI processes in healthcare organizations must determine who the customers are, what they want, and what must be done to meet their expectations. Expectations must translate into performance requirements so that healthcare professionals can evaluate whether customers' needs are being met. This leads to developing statements of expectation or performance called **performance measures.** Aggregate data are analyzed to determine whether expectations are being met. The data are frequently analyzed and compared against other internal and/or external data in a process called **benchmarking.** This allows the organization an opportunity to determine whether it is providing the highest-quality care possible.

History of Quality Management in Healthcare

The evaluation of healthcare quality has been evolving for many years. Hippocrates said, "Do no harm," thereby making the physician responsible for a patient's care. In 1854, Florence Nightingale introduced new protocols for her nurses during the Crimean War. Changes were made in the ventilation and sanitation systems and in how the nurses related to their patients. These changes dramatically reduced mortality rates. In 1917, the American College of Surgeons (ACS) established minimum standards of care. In following years, the ACS began an accreditation program.

These first steps led to the creation of JCAHO and standards for hospitals in 1952. JCAHO published its first set of standards for hospitals in 1953. In 1965, Congress passed the Social Security Amendments, which created Medicare and Medicaid, and initiated **utilization review** (UR) and **medical care evaluation studies (audits)** as a part of these programs. Evaluating clinical care was legislated in 1965 as part of Medicare/Medicaid. Medical care evaluation audits were mandated, and similar efforts were recommended by JCAHO by the late 1960s. JCAHO used the term *quality assurance* (QA) to identify its patient care improvement efforts with the introduction of accreditation standards in 1980. QA focused on hospitalwide problem solving focusing on the administrative or business operations of the organization. The QA standards allowed flexibility in the approach used by the organization. Problem lists were created, and many problems were solved. Mainly administrative in nature, the problems focused on the environment and personnel working in the organization. As problem lists became more legally challenging and the numbers of problems were reduced, JCAHO revised its standards in the mid-1980s.

The 1985 QA standards were revised as a process of monitoring and evaluating. The emphasis was still on an organization-wide effort, but the revised standards specified a **ten-step monitoring and evaluation process** to focus on the "important aspects of patient care and service" (JCAHO 1988, p. 12)." The new standards emphasized actions taken to improve care and the evaluation of those actions to ensure the effectiveness of the QA efforts.

In 1986, JCAHO launched a research and development project called the **Agenda for Change.** The Agenda for Change sought to develop better methods of evaluating healthcare effectiveness with regard to how the organization was governed and managed and how it provided clinical services. It included three initiatives that looked at the survey and accreditation process, education, and communication.

Developing valid and reliable quality performance measures that could be used as screens to identify potential problems became a major part of the survey and accreditation initiative. Another goal of this initiative was to have accreditation decisions more accurately reflect the quality of care rendered by the organization.

By 1990, the monitoring and evaluation process had been expanded to include medical staff review activities. In 1992, the accreditation manual began to transition from quality assurance to the QI processes used today. The monitoring and evaluation process was expanded to include a commitment to continuous improvement. In the mid-1990s, JCAHO introduced the chapter on improving organizational performance and reorganized the accreditation manual. The revised standards were organized around functions common to all hospitals and healthcare organizations.

The indicator measurement system (IMS) was introduced for hospital use beginning in the mid-1990s. An organization could use approved performance measures to screen their clinical performance to improve the quality of care. In addition, JCAHO's **Orion project** was launched in 1994. The Orion Project was an initiative to test accreditation models. JCAHO regional representatives worked with healthcare organizations; introduced measure-driven performance improvement systems; and attempted to coordinate JCAHO accreditation with other external review bodies, such as HCFA (renamed in 2001 as the Centers for Medicare and Medicaid Services [CMS]).

In 1997, the **ORYX initiative** began. Its purpose was to establish a continuous, data-driven accreditation process by using performance measurement data focused on core performance measures. With the help of advisory panels, JCAHO identified measures that give an overall picture of an organization's healthcare services. Data collection began in 2002. In an effort to coordinate accreditation with other external review bodies, data collected on several of the core measures are also required by **quality improvement organizations** (QIOs). At the heart of the ORYX project is the development of continuous improvement processes that focus on clinical areas. This is a work in progress, with data collection using five core measure sets continuing to be phased in over a period of years. Clinical QI efforts are more sophisticated and more clinically oriented today than at any other time in history.

Healthcare as an industry must strive to continually improve. It was slow to discover the link between improved processes and outcomes and increased effectiveness, efficiency, and cost savings. Some healthcare professionals still have a hard time recognizing the need to devote dollars to something that does not give an immediate payback.

The number of errors at any one hospital is likely to look insignificant, but the issue is compounded when data regarding errors are aggregated. In 2000, the Institute of Medicine (IOM) published information that brought attention to the issue of patient safety. *To Err is Human: Building a Safer Health System* asserted that 44,000 to 98,000 Americans die each year as a result of preventable errors. Shine (2002) states that, in actuality, these figures may be low because they do not include nursing home deaths or ambulatory care deaths. Moreover, many errors were never recorded in patient records. Shine further points out that all the evidence gathered needs to do more than point to individual doctors. Information must be used to develop safer systems and processes less likely to fail. The numbers of adverse events and costs to society go far beyond anyone's expectation. Error reports show a gap between average care and best care. The IOM identified six dimensions around which to frame the measurement of quality. These dimensions are (IOM 2001, p. 39–54):

- Safety
- Effectiveness
- Patient-centeredness
- Timeliness
- Efficiency
- Equity

Additionally, Wachter and Owens (2004) report in *The Genesis of Closing the Quality Gap* on the need for continued analysis of reasons for the **quality gap.** Finding ways to increase the rate effective practice as applied to actual patient care is being analyzed. Many reasons for the gaps between best, evidence-based practice and current treatment choices include:

- A gap in the dissemination of knowledge from research to practitioners
- Failure to implement best practice due to skepticism surrounding the cost effectiveness, environment, or organizational culture of practice setting
- Research setting effectiveness not equating to an individual's practice setting

There is much interest and ongoing research in developing ways to close the quality gap that involves research and a variety of organizations.

Check Your Understanding 17.1

Instructions: Answer the following questions on a separate piece of paper.

1. What is quality? Why is it important to meet customers' expectations?

2. What role have JCAHO initiatives played in the evolution of measuring healthcare quality?

3. What agencies have been important in the development of modern quality improvement processes?

4. What impact has the Institute of Medicine had on the measurement of healthcare quality? What has the development of performance measures contributed to the improvement of quality health care?

Organization of Quality Management in Healthcare Facilities

Quality management in healthcare facilities is organized to meet the needs of the organization. Today, most organizations have a program of continuous improvement in all functional areas. Data collection and analysis and resulting improvements have become an accepted way of doing business. An organization must address how it is going to achieve a successful QI program.

Organization, Accountability, and Ownership

The success of any QI program begins with a strong commitment from the executive level of the organization. This means that the governing body and the administration show, by example, their commitment to improving the quality of patient care. As an organization develops or revises a QI program, it must consider certain key elements. The elements of a QI program include:

- A clear statement of mission
- A supportive environment
- Available resources
- Leaders with adequate qualifications
- Adequate personnel
- An attitude of improvement
- Coordinated and integrated efforts
- Comprehensive and continuous care processes

Responsibility for QI activities must be clearly designated so that the program functions effectively. In addition, the methods of reporting should be made clear to all people involved in the QI program. (See figure 17.1.)

The governing body is ultimately responsible for the quality of care provided in any organization. Today, governing bodies are more involved in QI efforts than ever before. Board members are seeking training, asking questions, and insisting on seeing data confirming that care is improving within their organization. When a board expresses interest and concern about the quality of care being provided, it sets the bar for medical staff, administrative, and staff involvement.

The Role of HIM Professionals

Many different types of professionals work in quality improvement. From a historical perspective, HIM professionals have been involved in QI from the time of medical evaluation audits in the mid-1960s. HIM professionals are a natural fit for performance improvement activities because they know the health record (still the primary data source) and understand the documentation process. The HIM professional can be involved in several ways, including:

- Collecting data/information
- Organizing, interpreting, and reporting data in a meaningful way
- Knowing data sources
- Understanding clinical processes

Other professionals, such as registered nurses, are currently involved in QI in many facilities because of their understanding of clinical processes and clinical decision making.

Quality Improvement and Management Program

Every healthcare organization needs to find QI methods that work for it. Organization-wide QI may be completed as part of health information service responsibilities, part of

risk management, or a separate department in its own right. However they are designated, QI efforts must meet the needs of the facility.

JCAHO requires that the approach, processes, and **structures** be described in writing. (See figure 17.2.) The QI plan can be a separate document or incorporated into another planning document. CMS also requires a plan in writing. Items commonly found in a plan include, but are not limited to:

- Statement of mission/vision
- Objectives
- Values
- Leadership
- Organizational structure
- Methodologies
- Performance measures
- Communication
- Annual plan appraisal

The QI plan needs to be evaluated on a regular basis to determine its effectiveness. An annual appraisal should include a review of measurement and assessment activities and of documented improvements. The annual appraisal also should include a plan for the future direction of the program.

The most recent legislation to affect quality improvement at the federal level is the Medicare Prescription Drug, Improvement, and Modernization Act of 2003 (MMA) (PL 108-173). President George W. Bush signed this legislation into law on

Figure 17.1. Organizational communication and reporting

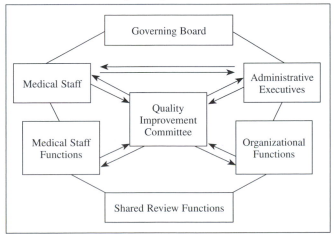

Figure 17.2. Organizational options for quality management programs

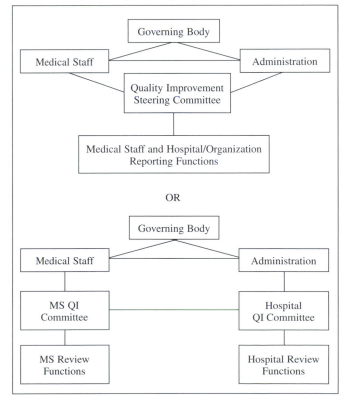

December 8, 2003. Section 646 is the portion of the legislation that directly affects healthcare quality. This section addresses the Medicare Health Care Quality Demonstration project. The goals are to:

- Improve patient safety
- Enhance quality of care
- Reduce scientific uncertainty and the unwarranted variation in medical practice that results in both lower quality and higher costs

The demonstration project is intended to identify, develop, test, and disseminate improvements to the U.S. healthcare system. It is hoped that CMS can encourage providers by giving them incentives to redesign systems that lead to safer, higher-quality, and lower-cost healthcare for everyone. (See figure 17.3.)

Definition of Quality Parameters

External regulators also are important factors in the quality puzzle. It is vital to understand who they are and what influence they have. The most influential external regulators in healthcare are voluntary accrediting agencies and the federal and state governments. A number of key judicial decisions also have had a profound impact on QI processes.

Judicial Decisions

Three landmark court decisions help explain the direction of quality improvement: *Darling v. Charleston Community Memorial Hospital* (1965), *Gonzales v. Nork and Mercy Hospital* (1973), and *Johnson v. Misericordia Community Hospital* (1981).

Figure 17.3.   Medicare healthcare quality demonstration system redesign incentives leading to improved quality of care

Incentives	Examples
Adopt and use decision support tools by physicians and patients	Evidence based medical guidelines Best-practice guidelines Shared decision-making programs
Reform of payment methodologies	Shared savings models Guaranteed-savings model Capitation model
Measurement of outcomes	Use IT effectively Redesign care processes Incorporate performance results
Enhanced cultural competence in healthcare delivery.	Care team delivery with patient interaction Patient centered care

Source: MMA 2003, section 646.

Darling is a landmark case that established a hospital's responsibility for patient care. Touching directly on quality are the issues of the facility's responsibility to have effective methods of credentialing in place and effective mechanisms for continuing medical evaluation. The facility is responsible for knowing whether the care it provides meets acceptable standards of care. The evaluation of medical care involves all professionals and must be done regularly so that both hospital and medical staff understand the results of patient care. The hospital must provide more than a place to practice and tools for physicians and other healthcare providers.

The *Gonzales* case supports a facility's responsibility for patient care. The hospital must establish a system to monitor the work and abilities of its physicians and other healthcare providers. In essence, the hospital owes its patients a duty to care.

The *Johnson* case further supports the duty of the healthcare facility to select its medical staff and grant privileges using carefully defined criteria. In addition, the **bylaws/rules and regulations** adopted by the medical staff must be followed. Further, the hospital has a legal duty to ensure that the guidelines are followed. It must appoint and supervise qualified medical staff and give the medical staff direct responsibility for the quality of care.

Federal Legislation

The federal government has had a profound impact on the development of quality improvement over the past 35 years. (See table 17.1.) The Social Security Amendments of 1965 and the Medicare Conditions of Participation that followed in 1967 laid the groundwork for medical evaluation audits and UR if a facility was going to accept Medicare/Medicaid patients. In 1972, professional standard review organizations (PSROs) were legislated. The PSROs began to monitor the quality and appropriateness of Medicare/Medicaid patient care.

The **Tax Equity and Fiscal Responsibility Act of 1982** (TEFRA) not only introduced diagnosis-related groups (DRGs) but also **peer review organizations** (PROs) to replace PSROs. In 1985, legislation was passed to deny Medicare payment for substandard care. In addition, the Conditions of Participation were revised to require a written QA plan in any facility accepting federal funds for Medicare/Medicaid patients. The term *quality assurance* later evolved into today's terminology, *quality improvement*.

In 1986, the Omnibus Budget Reconciliation Act (OBRA) required PROs to report adverse findings about healthcare providers to licensing and certifying agencies. That same year, the Health Care Quality Improvement Act (HCQIA) was passed to help protect peer review activities from liability and laid the foundation for the National Practitioner Data Bank.

The Agency for Health Care Policy and Research (AHCPR) was legislated in 1989. This agency began to develop outcome measures and was a resource in outcomes assessment. In the mid-90s, the agency name was changed to the Agency

Table 17.1. Major legislation relevant to clinical quality management

Date	Act	Description
1965	PL 89-97	Health coverage for citizens 65 years of age and older (effective July 1, 1966)
1972	PL 92-603	Professional standards review organizations created
1982	Tax Equity and Fiscal Responsibility Act	Peer review organizations and the prospective payment system (PPS) created
1983	PL 98-21	PPS for Medicare established
1985	Consolidated Omnibus Reconciliation Act	Denial of Medicare payments for substandard care authorized
1986	PL- 99-509	PROs required to report substandard care to licensing and certifying boards
1986	PL 99-660	Health Care Quality Improvement Act
1989	PL 101-239	Agency for Health Care Policy and Research created

Outcome measures research |
1990	PL 101-508	PROs required to inform licensing boards of physician sanctions
1996	PL 104-191	Health Insurance Portability and Accountability Act
2003	PL 108-173 Section 646	Medicare Modernization Act

for Healthcare Research and Quality (AHRQ). This agency has worked diligently to provide clinical evidence for best practice. In 2003, the AHRQ, together with Stanford-UCSF (University of California, San Francisco) Evidence-based Practice Center, developed a plan to analyze literature on QI strategies. These analyses focused on translating research into practice, concentrating on what would increase the rate of effective practices as applied to patient care in actual practice settings. The aim of this program is to close the quality gap (Wachter and Owens 2004, pp. 5–9).

In the 1990s, further federal efforts were undertaken to support QI in healthcare. In 1990, legislation was passed requiring PROs to report physician sanctions to licensing and medical boards. In addition, the National Practitioner Data Bank legislated in 1986 was activated.

In 2002, PROs were officially renamed quality improvement organizations (QIOs) to reflect changes in healthcare practice in recent years. The QIOs have developed their eighth **scope of work** to implement a performance incentive program that increases reimbursement when quality data are submitted and reported to CMS.

On January 24, 2003, CMS published the final rule in the *Federal Register* requiring hospitals to develop and maintain a quality assessment and performance improvement program (QAPI). Hospitals are required to show measurable improvement on designated performance measures that have

been linked to improved health outcomes and patient safety. Beginning in 2005, the MMA's incentive payment initiative is available to organizations that are willing to report quality data using 10 performance measures and to have their data publicly displayed. These data are available through the Department of Health and Human Services (HHS) Web page titled Hospital Compare (www.hospitalcompare.hhs.gov).

Legislative initiatives with the goal of improving the quality of care in the United States will most certainly continue. The federal government finances healthcare for a number of designated populations and has an interest in ensuring that the services provided are effective and appropriate within an increasingly integrated delivery system.

Accrediting Standards

As mentioned earlier, the idea of using standards to bring healthcare practice to a minimum level was initiated by the American College of Surgeons (ACS). Standards were used and refined over the years until the Joint Commission on Accreditation of Hospitals assumed responsibility for them. Today, the commission is known as the Joint Commission on Accreditation of Healthcare Organizations (JCAHO).

JCAHO's mission is to improve the quality of healthcare. Since 1953, it has worked to develop standards that help healthcare organizations measure and evaluate the care they provide. The use of clinical performance measures and continuous data-driven accreditation processes is currently being phased in.

However, JCAHO is not the only accrediting organization developing and using standards to encourage high-quality care. The **Commission on Accreditation of Rehabilitation Facilities** (CARF) has promoted high-quality healthcare in organizations serving patients who need rehabilitative treatment. The Accreditation Association for Ambulatory Health Care (AAAHC) is another private, nonprofit organization helping ambulatory healthcare organizations to improve the quality of their services. The Healthcare Facilities Accreditation Program (HFAP) of the American Osteopathic Association, one of two bodies authorized by CMS to accredit hospitals (the other being JCAHO), also has requirements for ongoing QI programs included in its accreditation standards.

In addition, QI efforts are being supported by organizations such as NCQA mentioned earlier. The **Health Plan Employer Data and Information Set** (HEDIS) is used to collect data on managed care plans. Other health plans have developed or are working to develop quality measures. For example, Blue Cross/Blue Shield is using healthcare performance measures from the **Institute for Clinical Systems Improvement** (ICSI). These efforts support the growing interest in the public reporting of healthcare performance data.

The **National Association of Healthcare Quality** (NAHQ) promotes continuous QI efforts in healthcare organizations by certifying qualified professionals. This organization offers QI professionals educational opportunities regardless of the healthcare setting they work in.

Quality Management Process

Each stage of the evolution of quality management has involved some aspect of data collection, data analysis, and a resulting change to improve areas that are problematic. The focus of data collection efforts has been driven by diagnosis/ procedure, problem, and, currently, clinical performance measures.

Performance Indicator Development

Performance measures are quantifiable indicators used over time to determine whether structure, process, or outcome supports quality performance. They usually represent important aspects of care provided by the organization, department, or unit of service. Performance measure development has been a linchpin for clinical quality improvement. After important aspects of care are identified, it is then possible to establish criteria or data elements that will determine care patterns.

The most common source of data is the health record. Data are collected, and the professionals involved in the QI process analyze them. A determination is made as to whether the data provide the information that is needed. A decision then is made about how best to improve the care provided. Key performance measures addressing best practice have been developed and addressed in various ways during the evolution of quality improvement.

JCAHO's Quality Monitoring and Evaluation Process

The evolution of quality management included the development of a ten-step monitoring and evaluation process by JCAHO. The idea behind monitoring and evaluation is to continuously collect and analyze data and to address findings. JCAHO's ten-step process was developed to help healthcare organizations have a more prescribed methodology for assessing quality. The basic premise is still applicable today. (See figure 17.4.)

Donabedian's Quality Assessment Model

Avidas Donabedian's QA model has been used and accepted for many years. The model's approach to the assessment of healthcare is based on the following three measures:

- **Structure measures** examine the organization's ability to provide services. Examples of measures of structure include policies and procedures, qualifications of staff, numbers of staff, physical space, and equipment.

- **Process measures** look at how care or service is provided to patients. The activities or protocols of care have some impact on the patient's outcome. Examples of process measures include protocols or methods of how treatment is delivered. For example, the patient's blood pressure is monitored hourly, patient education is completed before discharge, or the patient's discharge is determined to be appropriate. A healthcare provider (physician, nurse, or other allied health professional) usually carries out these functions.

- **Outcome measures** assess the end results of the care or services provided. Examples of outcome measures include mortality reviews, complications, or any adverse events. Any of these could indicate an undesirable outcome and indicate the need for further investigation.

JCAHO's Performance Measurement System

JCAHO's evolution to **core performance measures** is a story unto itself. In the late 1980s and early 1990s, JCAHO began to develop a **performance measurement system** they called an Indicator Monitoring System (IMS) that would focus on clinical applications. During this time, JCAHO determined that a program of continuous improvement was needed if a genuine impact on the quality of care was to be achieved. Additionally, JCAHO wanted to move from a process/structure orientation to one more focused on outcomes. The objective was to affect both administrative process and clinical patient care. One goal of the Agenda for Change initiative (discussed earlier) was to research and identify quality clinical performance measures. Identified performance measures represent sound clinical practice and reflect whether a healthcare organization is providing high-quality care to patients. The intention is to improve the quality of healthcare by improving performance in a given area of practice (for example, myocardial infarctions).

Figure 17.4.   JCAHO's ten-step monitoring and evaluation process

Step 1.	Assign Responsibility
Step 2.	Delineate Scope of Care
Step 3.	Identify Important Aspects of Care
Step 4.	Identify Quality Indicators
Step 5.	Establish Thresholds for Evaluation
Step 6.	Collect and Organize Data
Step 7.	Evaluate Data—Trends and Patterns
Step 8.	Take Actions to Solve Problems
Step 9.	Assess the Actions and Document Improvement
Step 10.	Communicate Relevant Information to the Organizationwide Quality Improvement Program

Source: JCAHO 1988.

The complexity of the IMS project led first to the Orion project and then to the current ORYX initiative. The ORYX initiative integrates outcomes with performance measures and makes them both a part of the accreditation process. The use of nationally standardized performance measures has been considered a part of this initiative from the beginning.

Core Performance Measures

Core performance measures are used to assess how well healthcare organizations provide care. They are currently being used by JCAHO and CMS, as well as healthcare plans such as Blue Cross. These organizations use data to understand what care is currently being provided and to determine where to focus QI activities. The use of statistically valid information becomes the basis for continuous performance improvement (PI). An organization can use the results of PI activities to determine its effectiveness in patient care over time. The organization can use the results to claim they provide high-quality care. The organization can literally "prove" its excellence. Measures are recommended by accrediting organizations (JCAHO) and the federal government (CMS/QIO) to allow comparability of like institutions.

Core performance measures are considered tools that provide an indication of an organization's performance. Core measures are defined as standardized sets of valid, reliable, and evidenced-based measures implemented by JCAHO for use within the ORYX initiative. In 1999, JCAHO gathered clinical professionals, healthcare provider organizations, state hospital associations, healthcare consumers, and performance measurement experts to determine where to focus attention. The following four initial core measurement areas were identified for hospitals:

- Acute myocardial infarction (AMI)
- Heart failure (HF)
- Pneumonia (PN)
- Pregnancy and pregnancy-related conditions

Discharge data collection on these measures began in July 2002. An additional hospital measure was added in the fall of 2003. Data collection for surgical infection prevention (SIP) began in July 2004. Other topics that have been identified for the development of performance measures include pregnancy and related conditions, children's asthma care, and pain management.

With the introduction of these core performance measures, healthcare facilities will be expected to select a performance measurement system that meets JCAHO's requirements and to send data to JCAHO on a routine basis. A performance measurement system must meet all parameters for data submission as determined by JCAHO. (See Table 17.2.) Data from similar organizations will be compared, and areas for improvement will be identified. If any undesirable patterns or trends are found, further monitoring and evaluation will follow.

Both JCAHO and CMS require the AMI, HF, PN, and SIP core performance measures. The intent is to reduce data collection requirements put on healthcare organizations. JCAHO and CMS have worked together to ensure that these measures are comparable. Data will be calculated in an identical fashion. (See table 17.3, p. 498.)

Hospitals are not the only healthcare organizations involved in JCAHO's ORYX initiative. Long-term care, home care, and behavioral health also are part of the initiative.

Data-Driven Accreditation

JCAHO is striving to make the accreditation process continuous and data driven. In January 2000, JCAHO surveyors used ORYX-specific presurvey reports to provide surveyors with information about performance measurement data. In the fall of 2002, JCAHO announced further changes to its accreditation process. The initiative was called Shared Visions-New Pathways. The intent of this initiative is to focus accreditation on operational systems critical to quality of care and safety issues. Sources to help target the accreditation survey include: ORYX core performance measure data, previous recommendations, demographic data related to clinical and diagnostic groups, complaints, **sentinel event** information, and MedPar Data.

Table 17.2.   Performance measurement system requirements for ORYX

Attribute 1	Performance Measure Characteristics	Refers to characteristics of the performance measures for use in the ORYX® initiative.
Attribute 2	Database (Measurement System Technical Capabilities)	Refers to the operational characteristics of measurement system.
Attribute 3	Performance Measure Accuracy	Refers to the extent to which performance measures correctly identify events they were designed to identify.
Attribute 4	Risk Adjustment/ Stratification	Refers to a process for reducing, removing, or clarifying the information confounding patient factors that differ among comparison groups.
Attribute 5	Performance Measure-Related Feedback	Refers to performance measure-related information that is available on a timely basis, to health care organization participating in the measurement system, for use in the organization's ongoing internal efforts to improve patient care and organization performance.
Attribute 6	Technical Reporting Requirements	Refers to requirement related to the transmission of accredited health care organization data to the Joint Commission by performance measurement systems.

Source: JCAHO 2004.

The core performance measure data will be instrumental in determining the focus of the clinical aspects of the survey. This approach to surveying uses the core performance measurement data, which is aggregated in an organization-specific manner. This is referred to as the **priority focus process** (PFP), which is an automated, rules-based tool. The intention is to make the accreditation process more relevant and valuable to healthcare organizations.

Patient Safety

Medical errors continue to make headlines in all parts of the U.S. We were shocked in 1999 when the Institute of Medicine reported that between 48,000 and 98,000 patients are killed by medical errors each year. In 2001, the IOM's report, *Crossing the Quality Chasm: A New Health System for the 21st Century,* laid the groundwork for the January 2004 IOM Crossing the Quality Chasm Summit. The purpose of the summit was to offer guidance at the community and national levels about how best to provide patient-centered, high-quality care. Reports made by reputable agencies, government and private, about safety concerns continue to express urgency about the need to address performance measures addressed in the "chasm in quality." (See figure 17.5.)

JCAHO and state and federal governments have been working to improve the safety of patients. JCAHO's Sentinel Event Advisory Group recommended National Patient Safety goals for 2005. Promoting patient safety is at the heart of the safety goals. Healthcare organizations are expected to comply with the safety goals in order to be accredited. The safety goals focus on known problematic areas. JCAHO recognizes that reliable system design, high-quality care, and evidence-based expert solutions all complement each other as organizations work to improve patient safety.

Universal Protocol for ambulatory care, critical access hospitals, hospitals, and office-based surgery is accepted by JCAHO, relevant clinical specialties, and professional medical associations and organizations. Universal Protocol incorporates the principles of eliminating wrong-site, wrong-

Table 17.3.   Comparison of JCAHO and CMS performance measures

Core Measures	JCAHO	CMS
Acute Myocardial Infarction (AMI)	• Aspirin on arrival • Aspirin prescribed at discharge • ACEI for LVSD • Adult smoking cessation counseling/advice • Beta blocker at discharge • Beta blocker at arrival • Time to thrombolysis • Time to PTCA • Inpatient mortality	• Aspirin at arrival • Aspirin at discharge • ACE inhibitor for LVSD • Beta blocker at arrival • Beta blocker at discharge • Thrombolytic agent received within 30 minutes of hospital arrival • PTCA received within 90 minutes of hospital arrival • Adult smoking cessation advice/counseling
Heart Failure	• Discharge instructions • LVF assessment • ACEI for LVSD • Adult smoking cessation advice/counseling	• LVF assessment • ACE inhibitor for LVSD • Discharge instructions • Adult smoking cessation advice/counseling
JCAHO: Community Acquired Pneumonia (CAP) CMS: Pneumonia	• Oxygenation assessment • Pneumococcal screening and/or vaccination • Blood cultures • Adult/pediatric smoking cessation advice/counseling • Antibiotic timing • Initial antibiotic selection consistent with current recommendation (ICU and Non-ICU)	• Initial antibiotic timing • Pneumococcal vaccination • Oxygenation assessment • Blood culture before first antibiotic received • Adult smoking cessation advice/counseling
Pregnancy & Related Conditions	Not comparable	Not comparable
Surgical Infection Prevention	Not comparable	Not comparable

Source: HHS 2005, JCAHO 2002.

Figure 17.5.   The chasm in quality select indicators from recent reports

- Between 44,000 and 98,000 Americans die from medical errors annually (IOM 2000; Thomas et al. 2000; Thomas et al. 1999)
- Only 55% of patients in a recent random sample of adults received recommended care, with little difference found between care recommended for prevention, to address acute episodes or to treat chronic conditions (McGlynn et al. 2003)
- Medication-related errors for hospitalized patients cost roughly $2 billion annually (IOM 2000; Bates et al. 1997)
- 41 million uninsured Americans exhibit consistently worse clinical outcomes than the insured, and are at increased risk for dying prematurely (IOM 2002; IOM 2003a)
- The lag between the discovery of more effective forms of treatment and their incorporation into routine patient care averages 17 years (Balas 2001; IOM 2003b)
- 18,000 Americans die each year from heart attacks because they did not receive preventive medications, although they were eligible for them (Chassin 1997; IOM 2003a)
- Medical errors kill more people per year than breast cancer, AIDS, or motor vehicle accidents (IOM 2000; CDC NCHS preliminary data for 1998, 1999)
- More than 50% of patients with diabetes, hypertension, tobacco addiction, hyperlipidemia, congestive heart failure, asthma, depression and chronic atrial fibrillation are currently managed inadequately (IOM 2003c; Clark et al. 2000; Joint National Committee on Prevention 1997; Legorreta et al. 2000; McBride et al. 1998; Ni et al. 1998; Perez-Stable and Fuentes-Afflick 1998; Samsa et al. 2000; Young et al. 2001)

Source: IOM 2001.

procedure, and wrong-person surgery. The steps involved in this protocol include

- Preoperative verification process
- Marking of the operative site
- "Time out" before starting any procedure

The private sector is actively involved in the patient safety initiative as well. The **Leapfrog Group,** a Washington-based coalition, is an example of a group that has effectively involved many healthcare organizations throughout the United States in its quality initiatives to make patients safe. Leapfrog has 30 **safe practices** endorsed by the National Quality Forum. (See figure 17.6.) A weighted system is used to prioritize findings to eliminate unsafe patient care practices. The Leapfrog Group

is working with CMS and the AHRQ to establish its initiatives. Leapfrog Group's approach and standards are similar to those established by JCAHO.

Government agencies also have been involved in the patient safety movement. The IOM led the way with its 1999 report on medical errors. CMS, AHRQ, and the Food and Drug Administration (FDA) have been involved in developing safe practice protocols. The HHS has awarded grants to help study safer healthcare delivery practices.

Individual states also have taken steps to provide safe environments for patients. In Minnesota, a new state law allows the public reporting of 27 serious adverse events. Included on the list are medication errors and surgery on the wrong patient or body part. Reports submitted by hospitals

Figure 17.6.   National Quality Forum endorsed set of safe practices

1. Create a healthcare culture of safety.
2. For designated high-risk, elective surgical procedures or other specified care, patients should be clearly informed of the likely reduced risk of an adverse outcome at treatment facilities that have demonstrated superior outcomes and should be referred to such facilities in accordance with the patient's stated preference.
3. Specify an explicit protocol to be used to ensure an adequate level of nursing based on the institution's usual patient mix and the experience and training of the nursing staff.
4. All patients in general intensive care units (both adult and pediatric) should be managed by physicians having specific training and certification in critical care medicine ("critical care certified").
5. Pharmacists should actively participate in the medication-use process, including, at a minimum, being available for consultation with prescribers on medication ordering, interpretation and review of medication orders, preparation of medication, dispensing of medication, and administration and monitoring of medications.
6. Verbal orders should be recorded whenever possible and immediately read back to the prescriber—for example, a healthcare provider receiving a verbal order should read or repeat back the information that the prescriber conveys in order to verity the accuracy of what was heard.
7. Use only standardized abbreviations and dose designations.
8. Patient care summaries or other similar records should not be prepared from memory.
9. Ensure that care information, especially changes in orders and new diagnostic information, is transmitted in a timely and clearly understandable form to all of the patient's current healthcare providers who need that information to provide care.
10. Ask each patient or legal surrogate to recount what he or she has been told during the informed consent discussion.
11. Ensure that written documentation of the patient's preference for life-sustaining treatments is prominently displayed in his or her chart.
12. Implement a computerized prescriber order entry system.
13. Implement a standardized protocol to prevent the mislabeling of radiographs.
14. Implement standardized protocols to prevent the occurrence of wrong-site procedures or wrong-patient procedures.
15. Evaluate each patient undergoing elective surgery for risk of an acute ischemic cardiac event during surgery and provide prophylactic treatment to high-risk patients with beta blockers.
16. Evaluate each patient upon admission, and regularly thereafter, for the risk of developing pressure ulcers. This evaluation should be repeated at regular intervals during care. Clinically appropriate preventive methods should be implemented consequent to the evaluation.
17. Evaluate each patient upon admission, and regularly thereafter, for the risk of developing deep vein thrombosis (DVT)/venous thromboembolism (VTE). Utilize clinically appropriate methods to prevent DVT/VTE.
18. Utilize dedicated antithrombotic (anticoagulation) services that facilitate coordinated care management.
19. Upon admission, and regularly thereafter, evaluate each patient for the risk of aspiration.
20. Adhere to effective methods of preventing central venous catheter-associated bloodstream infections.
21. Evaluate each pre-operative patient in light of his or her planned surgical procedure for the risk of surgical site infection and implement appropriate antibiotic prophylaxis and other preventive measures based on that evaluation.
22. Utilize validated protocols to evaluate patients who are at risk for contrast media-induced renal failure and utilize a clinically appropriate method for reducing risk of renal injury based on the patient's kidney function evaluation.
23. Evaluate each patient upon admission, and regularly thereafter, for risk of malnutrition. Employ clinically appropriate strategies to prevent malnutrition.
24. Whenever a pneumatic tourniquet is used, evaluate the patient for the risk of an ischemic and/or thrombotic complication and utilize appropriate prophylactic measures.
25. Decontaminate hands with either a hygienic hand rub or by washing with a disinfectant soap prior to and after direct contact with the patient or objects immediately around the patient.
26. Vaccinate healthcare workers against influenza to protect both them and patients from influenza.
27. Keep workspaces where medications are prepared clean, orderly, well lit, and free of clutter, distraction and noise.
28. Standardize the methods for labeling, packaging, and storing medications.
29. Identify all "high alert" drugs (for example, intravenous adrenergic agonists and antagonists, chemotherapy agents, anticoagulants and antithrombotics, concentrated parenteral electrolytes, general anesthetics, neuromuscular blockers, insulin and oral hypoglycemics, narcotics and opiates).
30. Dispense medications in unit-dose or, when appropriate, unit-of-use form, whenever possible.

Source: NQF 2003.

are analyzed by the Minnesota Department of Health and feedback is provided to the hospitals. Annual public reports describe adverse events, provide an aggregate analysis, and develop corrective action plans. Anyone can access information about safety in hospitals located in Minnesota. The numbers and variety of agencies and organizations looking at patient safety continues to grow (Minnesota Department of Health 2004).

Outcomes Management

Quality improvement during the late 1980s was strongly focused on outcomes as the best way to judge the quality of patient care. Many national organizations worked to develop databases that allowed the comparison of outcomes. JCAHO's IMS, the Maryland Quality Performance Measure Project, the Cleveland Health Quality Choice Program, and others were involved in developing performance measures, collecting data, and analyzing outcomes. The Agency for Health Care Policy and Research (AHCPR), now known as the Agency for Healthcare Research and Quality (AHRQ), was funded to research clinical outcomes. A physician, Dr. Paul Ellwood, introduced the concept of outcomes management as a method to improve the quality of care. Outcomes management is the systematic collection of healthcare results using outcomes measurement. A database of outcomes experience is used to compare treatment modalities.

As a method of improving the quality of care, outcomes management looks for the best treatment process. A treatment process is determined and used, and data are collected and entered into a database. The data are analyzed and the treatment process changed as necessary. The goal is to find the best practice possible to benefit patient care. These identified best practices then can be considered guidelines for the treatment of patients.

Historically, the diagnosis and treatment of patients by their physician or primary healthcare provider has been a very personal process. Practice guidelines are intended to use a best practice concept to detail the care and treatment of a patient for a specific diagnosis or procedure. Clinical practice guidelines are identified by the AHRQ as "systematically developed statements to assist practitioner and patient decisions about appropriate healthcare for specific clinical circumstances" (Schanz 1999, p. 3). Practice guidelines are taken from a combination of current literature and expert knowledge. Clinical practice guidelines (also known as practice parameters, Care Maps™, and clinical performance measures) are intended as tools to help make sound clinical decisions; they are not intended to replace sound clinical judgment.

Practice guidelines are intended to help standardize the care and treatment processes used by physicians. Deciding to use practice guidelines is an issue that every medical staff needs to address. The IOM has published criteria to evaluate practice guidelines. (See table 17.4.)

The decision to use practice guidelines must be made carefully, considering both the clinical and financial implica-

Table 17.4.   IOM criteria for practice guidelines

Criteria	Description
Validity	Leads to predictable health and cost outcome
Strength of evidence	Documented expert judgment and research
Estimated outcomes	Result of implementation projected with consideration given to patient preference and perceptions
Reliability and reproducibility	Same results if studied by another group
Clinical applicability	Populations defined for clarity of results
Clinical flexibility	Exceptions to clinical guidelines specified
Clarity	Written in clear direct manner
Multidisciplinary	Guidelines developed allowing collaboration with appropriately interested care providers
Scheduled review	Delineated time for assessment of accuracy and relevance
Documentation	Process of development well documented and includes personnel involved, data source, and procedures used

Source: Schanz 1999.

tions. If used appropriately, the best practices concept resulting from the use of practice guidelines can reduce cost and improve the quality of care.

Other Measurement Systems

A healthcare organization can measure the quality of the care provided in a variety of ways. Healthcare's complex nature has proved to be challenging, even difficult to evaluate. Evaluating the care provided to patients continues to evolve and change. Knowledge of current measurement systems being used in today's healthcare environment is necessary if one truly wants to provide the highest-quality healthcare.

Six Sigma

In the mid-1980s, William Smith, an engineer, developed the concept of **Six Sigma.** Motorola was the first company to adopt the concept and turn itself from a company on the edge of bankruptcy to a highly profitable firm. In 1996, General Electric, under the auspices of Jack Welch, adopted Six Sigma and the company is now famous for the quality of its products. It was not until 2001–2002, however, that healthcare organizations looked seriously at the Six Sigma concept. Healthcare has been slow to adopt this concept because the extensive training involved is expensive, and physician and administrative buy-in is hard to come by. In recent years, however, a number of healthcare organizations have implemented Six Sigma successfully.

Six Sigma uses a methodology not completely unique. It is reputed to use a "scientific methodology" that involves the following steps: define, measure, analyze, improve, and control (DMAIC). (See figure 17.7.) Each step has substeps that are referred to as "tollgates." The tollgates provide detailed directions on what must be done to complete each step before moving on to the next step (Eckes 2003, pp. 29–65).

Figure 17.7.   DMAIC improvement methodology

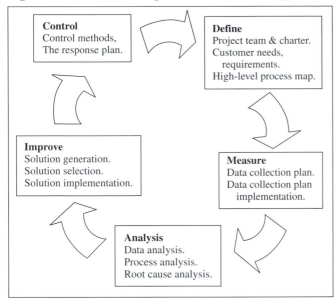

Source: Eckes 2003, p. 29.

Six Sigma uses many of the same tools used by other quality management systems. However, two tools unique to Six Sigma are (1) the critical quality tree (CQT) used in the define stage and (2) the process map used to identify the steps of a current process under review. In addition, Six Sigma uses "soft" tools that do not have a math basis; however, "soft" tools can be tricky to use because they have a subjective quality to them.

Six Sigma focuses on improving management and clinical processes. A unique attribute of the Six Sigma approach is that a company's strategic planning effort is a part of the Six Sigma process ensuring administrative buy-in. Statistical analysis is used to find the most defective part of a process, and rigorous control procedures are used to ensure sustained improvement. The goal of Six Sigma is to control for defects so that a .00034 percent defect rate is achieved (Lazarus 2003, p. 1).

Six Sigma can be used successfully in healthcare. It provides a systematic approach to validate data and focuses on the most meaningful improvements. As in other quality management concepts, the customer defines acceptable performance with the focus on delivery, quality, and cost. This definitely parallels the healthcare mainstay of cost, quality, and access (Lazarus 2003, p. 1). Successful implementation of Six Sigma in healthcare organizations has produced benefits such as the following:

- Higher productivity
- Fewer errors and adverse effects
- Improved organizational communication
- Improved patient satisfaction
- Better physician satisfaction
- Better nursing satisfaction
- Increased patient flow

- Short patient wait times
- Better use of advanced technologies

With 58 percent of all error-related deaths possibly preventable, healthcare must take the initiative to improve the quality of care. Six Sigma is another tool available to help close the quality chasm (Goedert 2004, p. 6).

National Quality Forum

The **National Quality Forum** (NQF) was created as a public–private partnership in late 1999 as a follow-up to the president's Advisory Commission on Consumer Protection and Quality in the Health Care Industry. Its mission is to improve healthcare quality by using a consensus-building approach to develop performance measures that are valid, reliable, and standardized. NQF has participation from a large number of groups from all parts of the U.S. healthcare system. National, regional, state, and local groups represent consumers, public/private purchasers, physicians, hospitals, other healthcare providers, accrediting bodies, supporting industries, and organizations involved in researching improvement in the quality of care. It uses its unique consensus-building process to develop common approaches to measure and report quality and patient safety standards with the goal of making improvements in the overall U.S. healthcare system.

The NQF is uniquely positioned to bring all interested parties together. However, challenges abound for this relatively new organization. Funding is unstable, some professional organizations are reluctant to give up or share their autonomy over quality and safety issues, and purchasers and payers continue to independently develop separate standards or fail to use national consensus standards. Few would argue the need to improve the quality of healthcare in the United States and the need for all interested parties to collaborate and move in a positive direction. The NQF is an organization positioned to provide a collaborative force to coordinate QI and safety improvement efforts.

Clinical Value Compass

The **Clinical Value Compass** is a PI approach developed to advance the association of quality and value. The "best care at the lowest cost" sums up this approach. A value equation may be represented as follows:

$$\text{Value} = f\,\frac{(\text{Quality} \times \text{Volume})}{\text{Costs}}$$

The name of this approach reflects its similarity to a directional compass. At the heart of the approach are four cardinal points:

- Functional status, risk status, and well-being (north)
- Costs (south)
- Satisfaction with healthcare and perceived benefit (east)
- Clinical outcomes (west)

The Clinical Value Compass gives providers a methodology to manage and improve healthcare services. (See figure 17.8, p. 502.)

Figure 17.8.   Clinical Value Compass example

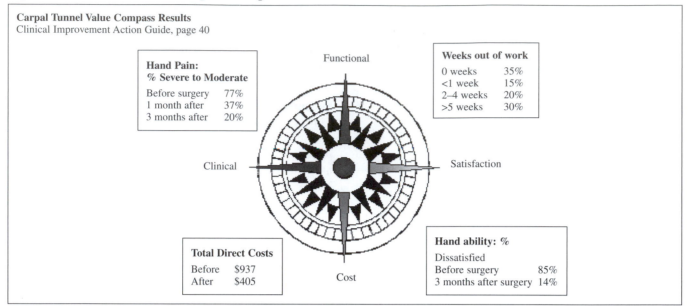

Source: Nelson et al. 1996.

Providers will measure the value of care for similar patient populations, analyze the delivery processes, change delivery processes, test the changes, and determine whether the changes lead to better clinical outcomes at lower cost (value). The process is straightforward and begins with a selection of a population set. Then value measures are selected and defined. There will be at least one value measure for each quadrant of the value compass. Performance measures can be structure, process, and/or outcome based. All key stakeholders can learn and see improvements that result in a healthcare experience that provides better value.

Managed Care Quality Criteria

The 1990s brought renewed interest in managed care and dramatic increases in the number of people who received healthcare services under its auspices. Health maintenance organizations, point-of-service plans, and preferred provider organizations have continued to evolve in the 21st century. Consumer pressure to be responsive to patient demands has changed the managed care scene in the early 2000s. Managed care organizations continue to develop methodologies that assess and compare healthcare plans. A number of organizations have jumped to the forefront in the development of methodologies that look at quality of access, service, and care provided. It is also worth noting that accreditation is becoming a more accepted norm among managed care organizations.

National Committee for Quality Assurance

The NCQA, a Washington-based nonprofit, private organization, is a leading source for information on quality of care provided by health plans. This organization accredits health plans and develops performance standards. Further, it sponsors, supports, and maintains HEDIS. HEDIS was developed through a combined effort of representatives from a variety of health plans and employers. This data set allows health plans to evaluate the quality of care provided by measuring their clinical practice using HEDIS performance standards (Millenson 1999, pp. 340–48).

Report cards can be developed using HEDIS information. The report card serves as a tool to inform employers about both the quality of care and the cost of the health plan and allows comparison of health plans. HEDIS measures include the following:

- Controlling high blood pressure
- Beta-blocker treatment after a heart attack
- Breast cancer screening
- Cervical cancer screening
- Childhood immunizations
- Cholesterol screening (after heart attack)
- Diabetic care (HbA1c testing)
- Timeliness of prenatal care

More than 60 different standards fall into the following five major categories:

- Access and service
- Qualified providers
- Staying healthy (wellness and preventative services)
- Getting better
- Living with illness

These data can help employers make decisions that are truly best for their organizations. The decisions can include both the cost and quality aspects of the health plan and can allow intelligent dialogue when making decisions about what health plan is best for an organization.

In 2004–2005, the NCQA continued to refine and evolve its commitment to quality. New initiatives begun by the NCQA included the Quality Plus program, which is a supplemental accreditation program. Its purpose is to highlight health plans that are innovative with regard to member communications, care management, physician compensation, and other activities in the healthcare industry. The desired result of Quality Plus is to acknowledge innovation and allow early acceptance.

In addition, the NCQA has introduced Quality Compass® 2004. This is a database with a wealth of information from the nation's health plans. Plus, the NCQA is presenting its interactive survey system (ISS), a Web-based survey that collects information more quickly than the paper-based system currently used. It is intended to promote a quicker improvement process for health plans. The NCQA Web site (www.ncqa.org) has a wealth of information about HEDIS and all NCQA initiatives.

Institute for Clinical Systems Improvement

The Institute for Clinical Systems Improvement (ICSI) is an independent, nonprofit organization dedicated to providing healthcare QI services to medical organizations in Minnesota. The medical organizations, located in North and South Dakota, as well as in Minnesota, range in size from 4 to 1,000 practitioners with a combined 7,000 physicians represented. Six Minnesota health plans sponsor ICSI. The primary financial sponsors are Blue Cross and Blue Shield of Minnesota, HealthPartners, and Medica. Associate sponsors are Metropolitan Health Plan, PreferredOne, and UCare Minnesota.

ICSI describes itself as an objective voice championing healthcare quality and helping to define and implement best practices for patients. It promotes the move to increased public reporting of healthcare performance, thereby enhancing the value of healthcare. The ICSI program includes the following three components:

- Scientific groundwork for healthcare
- Support for improvement
- The Minnesota health quality agenda

Carefully constructed clinical guidelines are made available to ICSI members. Each ICSI organization chooses at least four guidelines for intensive improvement and shares the results among all its members. ICSI tries to serve the healthcare community as an advocate for healthcare quality discussions. A unique approach ICSI has developed is that of providing best practice guidelines to patients and families in language they can understand. Visit www.icsi.org to learn more about this organization's commitment to quality.

Consumer Assessment Health Plan Survey

AHRQ has developed tools and information intended to help healthcare organizations document healthcare quality and help consumers make informed healthcare decisions about health plans. The focus of the Consumer Assessment Health Plan Survey (CAHPS) is to gather information that measures the consumer perspective. Questionnaires and reporting formats were developed, tested, and standardized to facilitate the collection and reporting of meaningful and reliable information about consumer experiences.

CAHPS products are intended to be flexible and of value to a variety of users. Currently, these tools are used by purchasers (employers, state and federal agencies), quality measurement organizations (accrediting organizations, state healthcare organizations), health plans, and survey vendors and consultants, among many others. (See figure 17.9.)

Moreover, new survey instruments are under development to address consumer assessment of inpatient care, provider groups, and individual providers. CMS, along with other regulatory agencies, will require hospitals, clinics, and nursing homes to collect data.

The National CAHPS Benchmarking Database (NCBD) contains five years' worth of data. The intent is to promote the comparison of results among users. For example, comparisons can be made between Medicaid agencies using the benchmarks from the database. The NCBD is the source of CAHPS information for all types of care. Another role of the NCBD is as a supplier of primary data for conducting research on survey design and health plan and enrollee characteristics. CAHPS is another tool that can be used to help improve the quality of healthcare in the United States.

Severity Indexing

Severity indexing is the process of identifying the level of resource consumption based on factors of clinical evidence. The more complications and comorbid conditions present, the sicker the patient and the higher the resource consumption. This method of trying to judge the level of illness is useful for reimbursement, utilization, and quality of care programs. Reimbursement should be higher when more resources are consumed, length of stay (LOS) should be longer or shorter based on resources needed and degree of illness, and quality could be compromised when a patient requires more care because of complications or comorbid conditions but does not receive it.

An organization using some form of severity indexing can use the information for a variety of purposes. Databases

Figure 17.9.   Consumer assessment health plan survey examples of current users

- U.S. Office of Personnel Management
- Centers for Medicare and Medicaid Services (CMS)
- National Committee for Quality Assurance
- Department of Defense
- Employers and business coalitions
- State Medicaid and State Child Health Insurance Program (SCHIP) agencies
- Health plans

Source: AHRQ 2003.

are available that allow the healthcare organization to make accurate determinations about the care rendered, the appropriateness of care, and the level of reimbursement. Adopting severity indexing also can affect reimbursement by providing a more complete picture of the patient care provided. Severity indexing can be especially effective when an organization wants to determine reasons for longer or shorter LOS or to provide information supporting or refuting statistics regarding the quality of care rendered. Examples of severity adjustment measures used today include:

- All-payer severity-adjusted (APS) DRGs, a product of HSS, Inc.
- All-patient refined (APR), a product of 3M Health Information Systems
- Disease staging, a product of Medstat
- AHRQ comorbidity measures

Both disease staging and AHRQ are clinically based measures. The all-payer severity-adjusted DRGs and all-patient refined DRGs are designed to help improve hospital payment systems, risk-adjusted medical outcome studies, and measurement of hospital case mix.

Check Your Understanding 17.3

Instructions: Answer the following questions on a separate piece of paper.

1. Define and describe how performance measures are used in performance improvement processes.

2. How are the assessment approaches of structure, process, and outcome and performance measure development tied together?

3. What are the similarities and differences of core measures, outcomes management, and clinical practice guidelines?

4. What core measures have JCAHO and CMS worked on together?

5. How do core measures contribute to making a data-driven accreditation process a reality?

6. What are five patient safety practices used by JCAHO, NFQ, Leapfrog, and CMS?

7. What federal agencies have been involved in developing safe practice protocols?

8. What contributions did managed care make to quality improvement?

9. Describe the role of the National Committee for Quality Assurance.

10. What other measurement systems are being used in the healthcare environment today?

11. How can severity indexing contribute to improved patient care?

Quality Management in Clinical Applications

The first QA efforts using JCAHO model from 1980 focused on problems. The problems were most often administrative in nature. For example, the mechanics of moving patients through admitting to their rooms and placing safety devices in patient rooms and hallways were addressed in the first wave of QA efforts. Making changes in the clinical practice of physicians was approached more slowly. Clinical applications are the current focus of QI efforts.

Medical Staff Applications

The medical staff is a key player in the evaluation of clinical services and any clinical process improvement efforts. The medical staff organization (MSO) works closely with the healthcare organization's administration but is directly responsible and accountable to its governing body. The bylaws/rules and regulations guide the medical staff regarding the organization's structure, functions, and responsibilities. In addition, the MSO must be responsive to internal requests from the administration or the governing body as well as external entities such as accrediting bodies and state and federal regulators.

Organization of the Medical Staff

Like any organization, the medical staff, as a self-governing entity, needs to have structure. JCAHO (2005) identifies key characteristics of the medical staff in its accreditation manual as:

- Being fully licensed independent practitioners as permitted by law and the facility
- Having delineated **clinical privileges** defining the scope of services
- Being subject to medical staff and departmental bylaws/rules and regulations and policies
- Being subject to review as part of the performance improvement activities

These characteristics help explain the role of the medical staff within the healthcare organization.

Committees are used to help most medical staffs to function. The executive committee is the only medical staff committee required by JCAHO. It is usually made up either elected or appointed medical staff officers, department directors, and an administrative representative. Actual membership (size, composition, functions) is defined in the medical staff's own bylaws/rules and regulations (discussed below). The majority of those serving on the executive committee must be fully licensed physicians. The members of the executive committee make decisions, determine policy, and act on behalf of the medical staff as a whole. In addition, this group provides leadership to the medical staff and works to support PI efforts.

The executive committee makes recommendations directly to the governing board on matters such as:

- Structure of the medical staff
- Mechanisms used to review credentials
- Medical staff membership
- Clinical privileges
- Participation in organizational PI activities
- Termination of medical staff membership
- Fair hearing procedures

Further, the executive committee receives and/or acts on reports from medical staff committees and/or departments/units and makes recommendations regarding those reports.

Many medical staffs today are departmentalized or divided into functioning units; only very small, uncomplicated medical staffs are not. JCAHO does not specify how a medical staff will organize. It is the responsibility of the medical staff to determine its method of self-governance with approval of the governing body. The bylaws/rules and regulations contain descriptions and definitions necessary to the operation of the medical staff.

A departmentalized medical staff must decide on the mechanism for acting and reporting. JCAHO recommends defining the leadership of each medical staff department. It further states that the department director must be qualified with appropriate education and training. The medical staff bylaws/rules and regulations specify the responsibilities of the department director. These responsibilities include:

- Determining clinical activities of the department
- Determining administrative responsibilities of the department
- Establishing mechanisms for the surveillance of the clinical activities performed by all individuals in the department
- Establishing criteria for clinical privileges for care provided within the department
- Recommending clinical privileges for each department member
- Determining the competence and qualifications of department personnel
- Integrating department functions into the organization
- Determining mechanisms for assessing and improving the quality of services and care provided within the department

The bylaws/rules and regulations of the medical staff provide the guidelines and framework or structure needed for the medical staff to function. In addition, the bylaws/rules and regulations define:

- Medical staff membership
- Credentialing procedures
- The process of awarding clinical privileges
- Committee structure (including the executive committee)
- Departmentalization
- Categories of the medical staff
- All the other areas determined appropriate for the medical staff to function effectively

The bylaws/rules and regulations must be approved by the medical staff and by the governing body of the organization. When approved, they are intended to provide an agreement between the medical staff and the organization's administration.

Credentialing of the Medical Staff

Since its inception, JCAHO has supported healthcare organizations by developing processes to ensure that only the most qualified professionals practice in healthcare organizations. JCAHO's standards guide healthcare organizations in the **credentialing process.** Each healthcare organization must have its own credentialing process; thus, each healthcare organization will have a different process. Using JCAHO standards results in a credentialing process with a certain commonality among healthcare organizations. A sound credentialing process is the foundation of high-quality care.

Credentialing is the process of reviewing and validating qualifications, granting professional or medical staff membership, and awarding delineated privileges. Specific policies and procedures are used by healthcare organizations to accomplish this process. The credentialing process verifies the education, training, experience, current competence, and ability to perform the privileges requested or any other background information pertinent to an individual requesting membership on the medical staff. The medical staff bylaws/rules and regulations delineate what needs to be collected and reviewed and the process of approval or denial of medical staff membership and clinical privileges.

The credentialing process begins with a potential medical staff member submitting an application to the medical staff for membership and a request for clinical privileges. After the information on the application has been verified, the department chair reviews the request for clinical privileges and makes a recommendation. The application, the results of the verification process, and the department chair's recommendations are reviewed by a selected group of medical staff members. The credentials committee commonly performs this function. The recommendation goes from the credentials committee to the executive committee. The executive committee then reviews the recommendations and makes its recommendation to the governing board. The governing board reviews the information and makes the final decision to accept or reject the application. (See figure 17.10, p. 506.)

The application to the medical staff contains categories of information as specified by the NCQA. Some of the suggested categories include:

- Licensure
- Hospital privileges
- Drug Enforcement Administration registration
- Medical education, including specialty board certification
- Malpractice insurance
- Liability claims history
- National Practice Data Bank (NPDB) queries (as required by law)
- Medical board sanctions
- Previous applications for medical staff membership/privileges

Items such as the above, plus additional items designated by the medical staff, are included on the application.

During the credentialing process, each applicant to the medical staff requests specific clinical privileges. According to JCAHO, granting clinical privileges refers to the authorizing of a practitioner to provide specific patient care services within well-defined limits. The criteria for awarding clinical privileges must be detailed in the medical staff bylaws/rules and regulations. Criteria include, but are not limited to, pre-established definitions of minimum levels of education, training, experience, and competence (JCAHO 2005, pp. MS13–15).

Figure 17.10.   Flowchart of the credentialing process

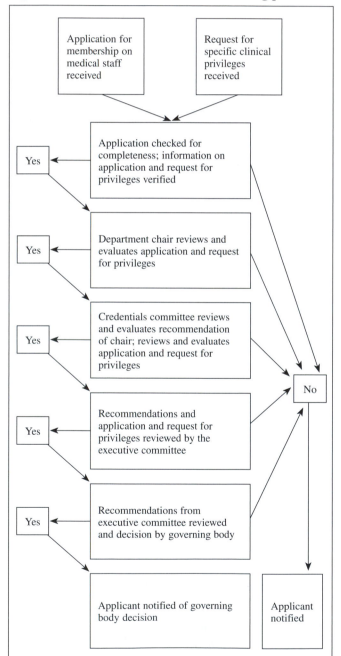

Most healthcare organizations maintain lists of the procedures, services, and/or treatments that are most likely to be requested based on the services they offer. After the request for clinical privileges is made, the verification process begins. If the medical staff is departmentalized, the department director uses the criteria to make recommendations regarding the appropriateness of the requested privileges. If the medical staff is not departmentalized, the chief (president) of the medical staff or designee performs this function.

Clinical privileges may be categorized in a variety of ways. JCAHO gives examples of ways to categorize clinical privileges, for example, by:

- Practitioner specialty
- Level of training or experience
- Patient risk categories
- Lists of procedures or treatments
- Any combination of the above

The delineation of privileges includes any limitations imposed on the individual provider, including the ability to admit, treat, or direct the course of treatment of patients admitted to the facility.

In today's healthcare environment, credentials are verified by either the healthcare organization (usually by a medical staff services professional) or a **verification service.** In either case, primary sources should be checked when possible. According to the Health Care Quality Improvement Act, the NPDB must be queried when verifying applicants to the medical staff. All queries must be completed before any appointments are made or privileges awarded. In all cases, the verification process needs to be done in a timely manner, which is usually specified in the bylaws.

Initial appointment and awarding of privileges is done for no more than a two-year period. Typically, appointment and designation of clinical privileges are done together. The credentialing process is ongoing. The reappointment and renewal or revision of clinical privileges is completed at least every two years. The reappointment/reappraisal process is continuous within the time line delineated in the medical staff bylaws.

The reappraisal process includes reviewing objective information collected on each individual who provides patient care services. Data are gathered and maintained on the practice patterns of all healthcare providers. Included in the data are the PI activities completed within the defined time line. A credentials file is maintained on each member of the medical staff. This information is considered confidential and must be handled in accordance with established policies and procedures contained in the medical staff bylaws/rules and regulations. State and federal peer review and confidentiality legislation should be reviewed.

The initial granting of medical staff membership and privileges, along with any revisions or revocations of clinical privileges, must follow the medical staff bylaws/rules and regulations. All applicants have the right to appeal decisions and to have a fair hearing before a panel of their peers.

Temporary privileges may be awarded when special circumstances arise. The medical staff bylaws/rules and regulations specify how temporary privileges are applied. JCAHO requires that the chief executive officer or designee base the granting of temporary privileges on the recommendation of the department chair, when possible, or the president of the medical staff. Temporary privileges must fall under state and federal regulations. Examples of when temporary privileges are appropriate include pending verification of credentialing information and the need for a highly specialized individual to provide care in an emergency situation.

Medical staff bylaws/rules and regulations must specify the criteria used to appoint/reappoint or award clinical privileges. The medical staff and governing board approve the criteria. The bylaws must be applied to all applicants equitably. All individuals providing patient care services in the healthcare organization must be included in the credentialing process. It is imperative that the information be provided as part of the application and that the request for privileges be reviewed and verified. Failure to verify information jeopardizes the healthcare organization from a liability standpoint. Courts consistently hold healthcare organizations liable for failure to verify application/request for privileges information. Cases where healthcare organizations were found liable include *Candler General Hospital, Inc. v. Persaud* (1994), *Purcell & Tucson General Hospital v. Zimbelman* (1972), and *Insinga v. LaBella* (1989). Case law in this area continues to evolve.

Independent Practitioners and Credentialing

Individuals who provide healthcare services without supervision or direction are considered to be **independent practitioners.** Independent practitioners may work as employees of the organization or may work privately or through a group of physicians. Physicians, dentists, podiatrists, and clinical psychologists most commonly practice as independent practitioners.

Licensed independent practitioners other than physicians also must go through a credentialing process as described in the section on medical staff credentialing. Medical staff bylaws will delineate the process for credentialing independent practitioners. Independent practitioners go through an appointment/reappointment process and have specific privileges delineated within the scope of their license and the rules and regulations of the organization and medical staff. Independent practitioners must seek appointment and request specific clinical privileges and practice within that framework. The objective of this process is to ensure patient safety by ensuring that only trained, competent, and qualified individuals provide healthcare services within the organization.

Other Medical Staff Quality Applications

Because the medical staff is responsible for ensuring the quality of care provided to patients treated in the healthcare facility, it is involved in collecting and analyzing data and improving both clinical and nonclinical functions in the organization. For the QI process to be successful, the medical staff must be engaged in QI activities. Data collection and analysis and recommendations are done on an ongoing basis, and changes are made to improve the patient care services offered in the organization. The medical staff and the healthcare organization can then judge whether the services provided are meeting standards of care.

Patient Care Review

Physician leadership is critical to the success of the continuous PI program of any organization. Medical practice has changed remarkably over the past century. The practice of medicine has moved into the 21st century with the medical paradigm shifting from individuality to one of teamwork and collaboration. Physicians still work in an atmosphere of infallibility and have great difficulty acknowledging mistakes or lack of knowledge (Shine 2002). Yet they persist in looking for ways to provide the best possible medical care for their patients. Physicians, the government, and accrediting agencies continue efforts to determine the best way to collect information about patient care that allows a consistent and objective patient care review process.

Currently, PI incorporates the evaluation of outcomes and processes. The medical staff must lead the way in improving clinical and nonclinical processes used in organizations. Involvement of the medical staff in patient care review is critical. This means the medical staff is involved in the measurement, assessment, and changes resulting from the review of patient care processes. JCAHO provides guidelines to the medical staff.

No matter how the medical staff implements performance improvement, the process of evaluating peers needs to be clearly defined, have identified participants, and have properly designed methods, time frames, and conditions for peer review functions. Characteristics of peer review are identified by JCAHO as:

- Consistent
- Timely
- Defensible
- Balanced
- Useful
- Ongoing

Using these guidelines, the medical staff can provide leadership in evaluating the clinical processes of peers.

Health Record Review

Health record review is necessary to ensure that the documentation captured is complete and accurate and reflects the care provided to the patient. At a minimum, the team involved in this improvement process consists of medical staff, nursing, HIM, and administrative services. The review includes health record documentation on both open and closed cases, with the total number of records being reviewed at approximately 5 percent of the overall discharges. Elements being evaluated are identified in JCAHO standards. Findings must be shared with the healthcare organization's healthcare providers. Problems identified should be corrected, and the healthcare organization must be able to demonstrate how this is done.

Surgical Review

Data collection systems must be developed and used by healthcare organizations to evaluate all operative procedures. Both invasive and noninvasive procedures should be included in this improvement process. All procedures are a potential risk to the patient, and so the appropriateness of the procedure must be determined. The procedures established to have the greatest risk are reviewed closely as part of a **surgical review.** Procedural processes and outcomes need to be addressed. Again, JCAHO helps guide the medical staff and healthcare organization in developing a system to measure the use of operative and other procedures. The procedural processes to be measured include:

- Selection of the appropriate procedure
- Patient preparation for the procedure
- Performance of the procedure and patient monitoring
- Postprocedure care
- Postprocedure patient education

Medication Usage Review

Medication use is an important method of treatment in healthcare. Because of the growing number of available medications and the potential for adverse effects, such as short-term side effects, interactions of medications, and toxicity, it is essential that the healthcare organization measure the administration and use of medications as part of a **medication usage review.** Moreover, the healthcare facility should evaluate medication use. Priority is based on:

- Number of patients receiving a medication
- Risk versus therapeutic value
- Known or suspected problem-prone drugs
- Therapeutic effectiveness

In addition, attention should be given to medication processes. Again, JCAHO provides guidelines for data collection regarding:

- Ordering or prescribing medications
- Preparing and dispensing medications
- Administrating medications
- Monitoring the effects on patients of medications

Blood and Blood Component Usage Review

Blood and blood components are used to treat patients. Treatment has the potential of offering patients risks as well as benefits. JCAHO provides standards to guide the healthcare organization and the medical staff in performing a **blood and blood component usage review.** PI processes should examine the ordering, distribution, handling and dispensing, administration, and monitoring of the effects of blood and blood components. Other considerations include when blood and blood components are ordered but not indicated, when they are indicated but not given, or when they are administered incorrectly.

Mortality Review

A **mortality review** is an important outcome performance measure. Establishing a meaningful evaluation of mortality (death) is essential in the analysis of ongoing outcome and process improvement.

Infection Review

The medical staff and the healthcare organization should work together to provide an environment that reduces the risk of infections in both patients and healthcare providers. The healthcare organization should support activities that look for, prevent, and control infections. An **infection review** is done with the involvement of the medical staff. Information is collected regularly on endemic and epidemic nosocomial infections. As appropriate, the healthcare organization must report significant information to both internal groups and public health agencies.

The organization also must take the necessary steps to prevent and reduce the risk of infection in visitors to the facility. Monitoring should be ongoing, and the healthcare organization should support a process focused on reducing risks and lowering infection trends. Moreover, in today's healthcare environment, processes must be in place to support the results of bioterrorism activities in preventing the transmission of disease.

Check Your Understanding 17.4

Instructions: Answer the following questions on a separate piece of paper.

1. Why is it essential to include the licensed, independent medical staff in the healthcare organization's quality improvement program?

2. How do the bylaws/rules and regulations support medical staff involvement in the organization's QI program?

3. How does the credentialing process help ensure the quality of care provided by the healthcare organization?

4. Why is it necessary to do regular reappointment/reappraisals of all members of the medical staff? Who is responsible for making sure this is done?

Nursing Staff Applications

Nursing leadership and nurses providing patient care services are part of the organization's overall quality improvement program. Nursing works with the governing body, medical staff, administration, and other healthcare providers to collect and analyze data, implement changes where necessary, and improve services. Focus is placed on areas where the largest numbers of patients are provided services, where there is highest risk, or where there are known problems.

Nurses provide the majority of hands-on care. They not only provide direct nursing care but also work closely with other professionals in carrying out treatment plans. Their impact on the patient is all-embracing. Nursing professionals must provide care that is consistent with current literature and meets nationally recognized standards.

Nursing executives and staff must provide the appropriate guidance for all nursing care. Policies and procedures, standards of nursing practice, nursing standards of patient care, and standards to measure, assess, and improve patient outcomes must be defined, documented, available, and used to improve patient care processes. Nurses must work in conjunction with management, the medical staff, and other healthcare providers as part of an organization-wide PI program.

Ancillary Services Applications

All patients should receive information about the care they are provided. Information about how data are collected, used, and evaluated can be incorporated into this message. A number of individuals are involved in the data collection and analysis and system/process redesign. Data may be collected from patients about their experiences by using patient satisfaction surveys. In addition, patients need to be informed of the healthcare organization's process improvement activities.

Utilization Management

Ensuring the appropriate and efficient use of a facility's or health plan's resources is the focus of **utilization management** (UM). Abdelhak et al. (2001) define UM as the systems and processes that ensure that the organization's resources, both human and nonhuman, are used most effectively to meet patient care needs. In addition to the appropriate use of the organization's resources, UM incorporates the process of utilization review (UR). A UM program helps ensure that patients receive appropriate care in an efficient and cost-effective manner. UM programs are required by CMS, the Medicare and Medicaid Conditions of Participation, many state regulations, and JCAHO. Data collected as part of this program offer insight into the quality of care provided.

UR is a formal review of patient resource use. Data collected during this formal review help determine the appropriateness of the services provided. UR ensures the medical necessity of treatment provided and the cost-effective use of resources and identifies over- or underuse of available services. Both the federal government and many state regulations require healthcare organizations to have a written UR plan. Although JCAHO does not require a written UR plan, it does require that UR incorporate a review of all patients, not just those who are federally funded.

History of Utilization Management

As healthcare organizations try to improve their efficiency, UM becomes a resource for collecting information to help determine how best to treat patients. To coordinate UM activities, a UR coordinator collects the required information, uses admission and continued-stay and discharge screening criteria, and works with physicians and the administration to ensure that patients are being treated appropriately for medically necessary reasons.

UR was legislated as part of the 1965 amendments to the Social Security Act. The focus of this legislation was on LOS

review using physician reviewers. It also initiated medical care evaluation studies or audits. UR affected only federally funded patients until JCAHO published standards in the early 1970s. It then was expanded to include at least a sampling of patients with private payment sources.

Utilization Management Staffing

UR coordinators have a variety of backgrounds. Registered nurses have moved into the field very successfully because of their clinical backgrounds and rapport with physicians. Health information managers also can be successful in the field because of their knowledge of documentation practices, their clinical backgrounds, and their understanding of reimbursement requirements. UR coordinators must be able to work with physicians and employees of insurance companies and managed care organizations. In addition, they must be able to work with various committee structures and must be active participants on the UM committee.

The UM committee consists of individuals who provide clinical services to patients and those involved in reimbursement. It should include representatives from administration, nursing, HIM, UM, physicians, and others who are thought to play a role in the care and treatment of patients. The composition of the committee should be detailed in the UR plan. The purpose of the committee is to review and evaluate the medical necessity of care provided to patients and the appropriateness of treatment. In addition, the committee may be involved with the QI studies initiated by the QIO.

Utilization Management Processes

In actuality, the UR process was implemented slowly. An organization must use screening criteria as a tool to make its determinations. Milliman and Robertson, a healthcare consulting organization, publishes the evidence-based guidelines used by many facilities today (Milliman and Robertson 2002). These screening guidelines are a collection of best practices drawn from a variety of sources. Time frames for review are determined by the facility and are a part of the UR plan. Several types of review are common in healthcare organizations today.

Preadmission Review
Preadmission review is done prior to the patient's admission. It is required by most managed care plans. Its purpose is to determine if the admission and/or procedure are medically necessary and appropriate in an acute care setting. The preadmission review identifies patients who are unsuitable for admission or for a particular procedure and then directs them to the appropriate care setting to obtain healthcare services.

Admission Review
Admission review is done at the time the patient is admitted to the facility. This review is done to determine/verify the medical necessity and appropriateness of admission.

Continued-Stay or Concurrent Review
Continued-stay/concurrent review ensures that the patient is remaining in the facility because of medical necessity

and is being treated appropriately. The review ensures that the patient is evaluated at preset intervals to determine the appropriateness of care rendered and that beds are utilized efficiently. The specific interval is commonly tied to the diagnosis and/or procedure.

Discharge Planning

Discharge planning ensures that a patient is ready for placement in a nonacute setting when he or she leaves the facility. This process often begins either at preadmission or upon admission to ensure that the patient is placed or receives services needed at the time of discharge. Client education is an important part of the discharge planning process. Readiness for discharge is determined by preestablished criteria.

Retrospective Review

Retrospective review is completed after patient discharge. Its purpose is to determine medical necessity and appropriateness of services rendered. When care is determined to have been inappropriate or medically unnecessary, reimbursement is denied. The QIO is responsible for performing retrospective review on federally funded patients. Insurance companies and managed care organizations also do retrospective reviews. Reimbursement can be withdrawn when documentation does not support the medical necessity or appropriateness of care rendered. In addition, retrospective review can help determine problems with overutilization, underutilization, inefficient scheduling of services, and patterns of nonacute days.

Observation care is appropriate for patients with a condition that requires some time to determine whether admission is medically necessary. Different managed care plans have different criteria to determine the appropriate use of observation beds. In any case, care must be taken because the time spent in an observation bed is billed as an outpatient service and may not be covered under the patient's insurance.

Ancillary Services Review

Ancillary services review is tied to ordering, scheduling, and preparation for and performance of various tests and services. Data should be collected to determine whether ancillary services are being used in an efficient and effective manner. QI programs frequently address the appropriate use of ancillary services.

Medicare Review

Medicare review began with introduction of professional standard review organizations (PSROs). PSROs were nonprofit agencies made up of physicians who examined the medical necessity of care. In addition, energy was put into ensuring that the most economical care was rendered to meet the needs of the patient. PSROs introduced the concept of denying payment for care determined to be unnecessary. In addition, quality objectives were introduced to healthcare through the PSROs. Their effectiveness was questioned until their demise in the early 1980s.

TEFRA replaced the PSROs with PROs. The PRO program was established to ensure that Medicare beneficiaries were provided services that are medically necessary, appropriate, and recognized as meeting professional standards of care. The name PRO was changed to QIO (quality improvement organization) in 2002.

QIOs review the appropriateness of admission, continued stays, and discharges. The QIO contracts with CMS to provide specific initiatives during a designated period of time (currently three years). Their current scope of work is focused on quality-related issues, payment error prevention, and other areas. The eighth scope of work involves a shift to a more national clinical QI focus with data being collected in collaboration with JCAHO. (See table 17.3, p. 498.)

Notices of noncoverage were required by both the PSROs and the PROs and are still a part of the UR process. A notice of noncoverage is required for various situations, including:

- *Preadmission notice of noncoverage:* In this situation, the client is made aware, prior to admission, that care or services may not be covered or may be obtained at a lesser level of care. The client then is informed that if admission takes place, he or she will be responsible for all charges that result from the stay.
- *Admission notice of noncoverage:* In this situation, the patient is informed that acute care is not required and that he or she will be responsible for charges resulting after a specific grace period (48 hours).
- *Continued-stay notice of noncoverage:* In this situation, the patient is notified that acute care services are no longer required and that he or she will be responsible for charges after a specific grace period (48 hours).

The content and wording of the notices is prescribed by CMS through the QIOs. A policy and procedure regarding these notices must follow the prescribed methodology. The QIO monitors each notice of noncoverage and closely reviews these cases.

External Agency Review

Third- and fourth-party reviewers complete external agency reviews. Reviewers include commercial health insurance companies, managed care plans, and auditors. The focus of the reviews includes resource utilization, quality of care, reimbursement issues, and cases meeting specific criteria, such as readmission within seven days after discharge.

Medicaid Review

The Medicaid program was established by Title XIX of the Social Security Amendments of 1965. Federal money is distributed to each state under a block grant methodology, and each state administers disbursement based on federal guidelines. Medicaid reviews differ from state to state. Range of services, qualifying factors, methods of payment, and LOS limitations are handled differently. UR plans also differ from state to state. However, most states do require a prior-approval process for inpatient care and selected outpatient procedures. Retrospective and prospective reviews may be a part of the process. Understanding each state's UR requirements is essential.

Managed Care Review

Managed care plans use UM to keep costs down and quality up. Each managed care plan will have a unique approach to doing UM. Managed care organizations frequently use preadmission certification. Continued-stay review is handled by the managed care organizations collecting information on the acuity and the timeliness of services. The managed care organization will request information both concurrently and retrospectively to determine medical necessity and appropriateness of care. UR coordinators work closely with a variety of managed care organizations to ensure that payment is made for services rendered.

Risk Management

Risk management is a program designed to reduce or prevent injuries and accidents and to minimize or prevent financial loss to the organization. The concept of reducing injuries and accidents has been around for thousands of years. The Code of Hammarabi (400 B.C.) actually addressed the issue of physician liability. When a physician inflicted certain injuries on a patient, punishment for the injuries was prescribed in the code. During the 1970s, the dramatic increase in malpractice claims supported the need for more aggressive management of risk in healthcare organizations. Risk management systems today are sophisticated programs that function to identify, reduce, or eliminate **potentially compensable events** (PCEs), thereby decreasing the financial liability of injuries or accidents to patients, staff, or visitors.

JCAHO and other accrediting bodies recommend risk management programs, state and federal laws and regulations give guidance with regard to risk management, and a variety of professional organizations offer professional guidelines that address the importance of risk management. Even third-party payers expect organizations to have systems in place to keep patients, staff, and visitors as safe as possible. Liability insurance carriers require and support an organization's efforts to develop and sustain risk management programs. Policies and procedures addressing risk must be developed and used to control injuries and accidents and to reduce the organization's financial liability.

Healthcare organizations today are faced with ever-increasing costs for liability insurance. Internally, an organization must collect information on injuries and accidents. Incident/event reporting is frequently organized with the help of the insurance carrier. Along with these data, occurrence/generic screening tools can be used to collect data on the risk management of patients. In addition, patient satisfaction surveys, mortality and morbidity reviews, infection control data, patient complaints, hazard reports, claims management, as well as the development of appropriate policies and procedures to collect and analyze the data, all contribute to the well-being of the organization.

The healthcare organization must provide personnel to support the efforts of risk management. This can be accomplished by hiring a risk manager who has adequate authority to make changes as necessary, or these duties can be part of the quality and safety areas of the organization. In either case, it is essential that the organization recognize the need to collect and analyze data, make changes, and improve current facility systems and to do so in conjunction with current efforts to improve the quality of care.

Risk Management Processes

For a risk management program to be successful, it must include certain processes. **Loss prevention** is a risk control strategy that includes developing and revising policies and procedures that are both facilitywide and department specific. It also involves educating staff, including medical personnel, healthcare executives, volunteers, and employees. Credentialing activities must be thorough. Compliance must be assured with federal, state, and accrediting bodies' standards, laws, and regulations. Complete and thorough patient education must be provided.

Another component of a successful risk management program is **loss reduction**. Loss reduction encompasses techniques used to manage events or claims that have already taken place. Ways to reduce losses incurred include:

- Investigating reported incidents or addressing occurrence reports promptly
- Reviewing claims made against the facility
- Managing workers' compensation programs
- Being knowledgeable about alternate dispute resolution processes
- Treating employee injuries on-site
- Implementing back-to-work programs
- Assisting with depositions or other pretrial activities
- Working closely with defense counsel

Another component of a successful risk management program is **risk prevention**. Some of the ways that risk prevention can be attained include:

- Educating all employees and medical staff to recognize and properly report all potentially adverse occurrences
- Ensuring that all employees and medical staff are doing their jobs to the best of their ability
- Developing early warning and reporting systems that identify areas of potential adverse effect
- Creating databases to track events and help point out areas where systems can be improved
- Making changes to systems requiring improvement and monitoring these areas to determine success
- Providing employees with appropriate safety training

Risk Management Reporting Tools

Several areas require special mention because they are basic tools in an effective risk management program.

Incident Report Review

Incident report review is a process in which incident reports are analyzed or descriptions of adverse events are evaluated. Common examples include needle sticks; patient, employee, or visitor falls; and medication errors. Reviewing incident reports and developing a database of incidents with report capability can help identify patterns or trends that signal potential adverse events.

Occurrence/Generic Screening

Occurrence/generic screening is a methodology where predefined criteria are used to review medical records to find cases that may indicate adverse patient outcomes. These criteria are not disease or procedure specific. Rather, they are generic in focus and include items such as whether an informed consent was signed, whether the patient was returned to the operating room, whether hospital-acquired infections were noted, and whether there was a failure to respond to significant x-ray or laboratory results.

Safety Programs

Every organization must have a safety program in place to focus on the environmental concerns of patient care. Fire, radioactive materials, and air quality are examples of areas addressed in a safety program. Federal and state laws require safety programs and accrediting bodies to have standards that address safety. Safety and risk are closely linked and data should be shared.

Internal/External Disaster Preparedness Programs

An **emergency preparedness** program addresses disasters and emergency situations both inside and outside the healthcare organization. The September 11, 2001, tragedy involving the World Trade Center and the Pentagon created new challenges for this program. Management plans the response to crisis situations. The organization must have protocols on how patients will be treated, admitted, and discharged. The plan must be developed in cooperation with agencies and organizations within the community. All entities responding to emergency situations must be ready to work together to handle any type of disaster. Additionally, everyone working within the organization must be trained to respond to emergency and disaster situations.

The emergency preparedness plan must address certain areas, for example, how the organization will address the need for backup utilities, communication systems, and radioactive and chemical decontamination and isolation. Personnel must know their roles and responsibilities in a crisis situation. Practice sessions, also called disaster drills, should be held to help personnel react appropriately. Whether the emergency is internal or external to the organization, the appropriate policies and procedures need to be in place and well understood by the organization's personnel to ensure that the response is timely and meaningful.

Informed Consent Review

Healthcare organizations deal with many liability issues, including ensuring that clients understand and agree to treatment through the informed consent processes. Consent can be given either orally or in writing (expressed consent). It also may be implied through the actions or circumstances of the client's behavior.

Appropriate informed consent is one in which the client or patient acknowledges his or her understanding of the nature of the treatment or procedure to be performed. In addition, he or she must understand the risks, benefits, and alternatives to the treatment or procedure. The informed consent process involves an exchange of information between the healthcare provider and the patient or client, along with permission or assent. Failure to obtain informed consent can result in liability issues for both the healthcare organization and the healthcare provider. See chapter 8 for additional discussion of informed consent.

Sentinel Event Review

JCAHO's Sentinel Event Policy went into effect on April 1, 1998. Its purpose was to improve the quality of care. A **sentinel event** is an unexpected occurrence involving death or serious physical or psychological injury, or the risk thereof. Serious injury is defined as the loss of a limb or function. Events are deemed sentinel because they signal the need for immediate investigation and response. Examples of clinical events needing this kind of response are significant medication errors, significant adverse drug reactions, and confirmed transfusion reactions.

The organization may need to perform an intense analysis when the following occur:

- Patterns, trends, or variations of performance are significant or unexpected.
- Performance differs significantly from performance in other, similar facilities.
- Performance varies significantly from accepted standards.
- A sentinel event occurs

Policies and procedures must be in place to respond to a sentinel event.

When a sentinel event occurs, organizational leadership must support the process of investigation, analysis, and improvement. The expectation is that the organization will respond to all sentinel events. **Root-cause analysis** is the process used to identify the cause of the event. The organization looks for ways to decrease the likelihood of such an event happening again. The focus should be on organizational and clinical systems and processes, not on the person or people involved in the sentinel event.

Root-cause analysis examines both the clinical and administrative reasons for the event. After data collection and analysis, the organization should develop an action plan and move to make improvements in order to make such future events as unlikely as possible. The focus of JCAHO's survey process will be on how the organization has handled the sentinel event.

An organization is encouraged (but not required) to report sentinel events to JCAHO. A root-cause analysis and an action plan must be completed regardless. Healthcare organizations reporting a sentinel event can benefit by having an outside, objective third party review their action plan and by obtaining consultation as needed. In addition, the organization should show the public a sincere effort to remedy problems and improve.

Check Your Understanding 17.5

Instructions: Answer the following questions on a separate piece of paper.

1. What do utilization review and utilization management contribute to quality of care?

2. How do the different types of review (for example, preadmission, admission, continued stay, and discharge planning) support medical necessity, appropriateness of services, and length of stay review?

3. How does the notice of noncoverage affect the denial of reimbursement?

4. How does risk management contribute to the overall quality improvement program?

5. How do sentinel event policy and root-cause analysis contribute to the quality of care provided to patients?

Integration of Comparative Data into Clinical Quality Management

JCAHO and the QIOs have developed performance measures requiring regular data collection. In addition, the healthcare organization needs to develop its own performance measures. Performance measures frequently are built around the categories of efficiency, effectiveness, safety, timeliness, and quality. Determining what data collection techniques will meet the needs of the QI process, which data displays and reporting methods are most effective, what to consider when analyzing and interpreting data, and how to affect systems and processes with meaningful changes all need to be considered.

Chapter 23 addresses the tools and techniques of PI. Those tools can be applied to clinical quality improvement.

Data Collection and Reporting Techniques

To collect the required data, performance measures must be developed or identified that focus on the correct data elements. Clinical measures need to be detailed, diagnosis/procedure specific (usually), focused on process or outcome (most commonly), and selected by high-volume, high-risk, or known problems. It is necessary to determine what you want to know and how you can say it in numbers. The data can be reported as either meeting the element (for example, 98 percent of patients were free of infection) or not meeting the element (for example, 2 percent of the patients experienced infection). Each data element collected must be clearly defined, clearly understood, and agreed on by everyone involved in the data collection process. This helps ensure that the data collected support what the organization wants to know.

The scope of performance measurement activities requires clarity. The important areas of service are usually based on volume, risk, or known problem. The population targeted must be clearly identified and defined, and the sample size must be representative and allow for valid and reliable statistical measurement. (See chapters 16 and 18.) Descriptions of the raw data and data sources must be identified precisely so that everyone understands what the data elements will tell them. The medical record remains as the main data source.

It also is important to identify who will be involved in collecting and assessing the data, determining improvements, and performing ongoing evaluation. Data gathering is frequently done using forms, check sheets, surveys, questionnaires, or computer screens using database or spreadsheet applications as the tool to maintain consistency and accuracy. Further, it is necessary to determine how often data will be collected (daily, weekly, or monthly) and whether they will be collected concurrently or retrospectively and for how long.

Data displays need to be functional and credible and must meet the needs of reviewers. It is important to remember that effective data displays are visual supports that allow reviewers to understand data at a glance. Likewise, it is important to keep the data display simple by emphasizing no more than one or two points. Avoid spreadsheets or data summaries that are complex and overwhelming. Data display tools include, but are not limited to, pie charts, histograms, scatter charts, line charts, and bar graphs. (See chapter 15).

Narrative data also can be used effectively. Narrative information can address performance goals, data sources, and data collection procedures.

Data Analysis and Interpretation

The analysis and interpretation of data demonstrates whether a performance measure is being met. Changes plotted over time can answer questions about whether systems are doing what they are intended to do or whether they require change. Analysis and interpretation can help point out what change will have the most impact. The HIM professional and others involved in the QI activity can work together to use the displayed information to improve patient care. The HIM professional can be instrumental in ensuring that the data collected and displayed are accurate and truthfully represent actual performance (Spath and Hale 2003, pp. 3–5).

The QI activities follow a problem-solving process of access, measure, analyze, and improve. Determining the best way to effect change can be challenging. Langley et al. (1996) recommend a combination of a thorough understanding of the current system or process, creative thinking, and use of improved technology, when possible. Some ideas for developing creative thinking include:

- Know current boundaries before making changes.
- Rearrange the steps of the process.
- Looks for ways to level the current flow of tasks or activities.

- Challenge why you are doing the QI activity.
- Describe what would be ideal.
- Do not allow the current process to continue.

Different techniques can be used to improve the patient care process. Traditional approaches include training or education of personnel and administrative changes such as decreasing wait times, more thorough credentialing, and working closely with risk management to decrease liability.

Results Reporting and Follow-up

Because QI is an organization-wide effort, reporting lines must be clear and direct. Reporting begins with a hospital and/or medical staff committee or some other organizational unit such as infection control, safety, or utilization management and follows a clear and defined route. It is essential that communication be thorough and complete. The QI plan must delineate how reporting will flow through the organization. All levels of the organization must know that results will be shared throughout the organization.

After changes are made to improve systems or processes, there must be a way to determine whether the change was meaningful. This involves determining what needs to be known and selecting a few data elements that will give that information. If the changes have been successful, it may be necessary to either reduce the frequency of review for this performance measure or make an alternative change if no significant improvement can be identified.

For a quality management program to be effective, the risk management, safety, and disaster programs must work in conjunction with the QI program. Data collected to meet the needs of the different programs designed to keep patients, staff, and visitors safe and to allow response to community needs must be shared to benefit the overall organization. Developing methods for reporting and evaluating the results of the different programs and systems is a complex, continuous challenge. Results from any of the above areas can give an indication of high-quality care or point out areas requiring improvement or change.

Data Security and Confidentiality

The confidentiality and security of QI data must be addressed through effective policies and procedures. QI information must move through the organization's communication systems and yet be protected. State statutes may be used to help develop policies that are supported by legislation. Peer review activities are addressed by legislation in every state. Data must be kept in a secure environment, and access to the data must be carefully delineated and supported by statute whenever possible. Release of QI information must be handled in accordance with statutes, policies and procedures, and medical staff bylaws/rules and regulations.

Use of Computer-Based Comparative Data

The computerization of healthcare data can offer healthcare providers, regulators, and payers a wealth of administrative and clinical information. Going back to Codman's pioneering work, it was recognized that good data can lead to the discovery of improved treatment practices (Newhauser 2002, Millenson 1999). Then, beginning with the IOM's *To Err Is Human* and continuing through its 2003 report, *Priority Areas for National Action: Transforming Health Care Quality,* it was recognized that the need to collect, analyze, and distribute large quantities of data will help transform healthcare to a standard of best practice/best evidence. Computerization of data will enhance the ability to bridge the gap between best-evidence-based practice and actual practice.

The use of computerized data allows comparison of actual practice to best practice (benchmarking) and is critical to both regulatory and accreditation processes in 2005. The enormous volume of data has not prevented continued efforts to try and use the data effectively. JCAHO's ORYX initiative relies on the review of data trends and patterns to determine where to focus survey efforts. JCAHO-accredited organizations are encouraged to review their own data against data from like organizations to determine their own PI opportunities. CMS is working with JCAHO to evaluate quality of care on designated diagnoses. Both JCAHO and CMS will utilize data submitted by organizations to analyze professional practice. This will give them information on whether an organization is exemplary, average, or substandard, which then gives focus for improvement opportunities/expectations. CMS is currently providing financial incentives to healthcare providers for submitting and publicly reporting their quality performance data to comply with the MMA.

Other computerized information systems are either available or under development. The true benefit of computers is their tireless ability to cross-check information and provide user feedback. Computerized physician order entry (CPOE) has received much attention in helping to reduce medication errors. More research is being done in this area to advance the safety of patients receiving healthcare services. Pharmacies also have gone to a variety of systems such as robotic medication distribution and bar-coding systems that help keep patients safe from receiving the wrong medication or wrong dosage. Alerts for drug interactions, smart systems that give clues to evidence-based practice, also will give necessary information to practitioners on the front lines. It is increasingly clear that insufficient access to, or management of, information plays a substantial role in the causes of medical errors. Further, physicians rarely recall *all* standards of care that can apply to a patient, especially in the time-limited, encounter-focused format based on patient complaint (Roland and Kannan 2003, p. 37).

The federal government is playing an instrumental role in accelerating the development and use of an electronic health record (EHR), and President Bush has stated on several occasions the need to develop one. The first annual National

Healthcare Quality Report (NHQR) stated that as a nation we are making progress. Key findings included:

- High-quality healthcare is not yet a universal reality.
- Opportunities for preventive care are frequently missed.
- There is more to learn.
- Greater improvement is possible.

President Bush named David Brailer, M.D., Ph.D., as the national coordinator for health information technology. Dr. Brailer is working to develop EHR systems that will enable physicians and other health professionals to electronically tap into a wealth of treatment information to better care for patients. Four major goals have been identified by federal leadership. They are (Rose 2004, pp. 15–17):

Goal 1: Inform Clinical Practice—Information tools at point of care;

Goal 2: Interconnect Clinicians—Interoperable health information infrastructure providing access to critical information;

Goal 3: Personalize Care—Give consumers more access to and involvement in making health decisions; and,

Goal 4: Improve Population Health—Expand public health monitoring, quality of care measurement and bring research advances into medical practice.

The federal legislative process continues to spawn bills related to technology and healthcare quality. In 2005, the following legislative efforts were introduced: the Information Technology for Health Care Quality Act, the Patient Safety and Quality Improvement Act, the National Health Information Incentive Act, the 21st Century Health Information Act, and the Health Technology to Enhance Quality Act. Many of these legislative efforts are directed at promoting the adoption of standards, interoperability, and government funding to help support the move to electronic health information. Watching developments in this direction should be of great interest to healthcare organizations.

It is unequivocally believed that health information technology can improve care quality, reduce medical errors, and lower administrative costs.

Healthcare is an information-intense process. It is unfortunate that patient records and methods used to move information along the continuum of care have remained virtually stagnant. Electronic health information has unknown potential, yet little of it has been realized in today's healthcare environment (Kizer 2004b, p. 1). As we plan for the future by developing standards at the national, regional, and local levels, we must remember that computerized data must be kept in a secure environment. Passwords, fingerprints, retinal scans, and limited access are basic security features used to protect QI data. (The handling of computerized information is addressed thoroughly in chapters 2 and 5.) Adapting security and confidentiality practices for general computerized information is essential.

Check Your Understanding 17.6

Instructions: Answer the following questions on a separate piece of paper.

1. Why is it necessary to clearly define performance measures, criteria, and/or data elements used in data collection?

2. What is the main source of data?

3. Explain how quality management, utilization management, risk management and patient safety are interrelated.

4. Why must quality improvement data be kept confidential?

5. What are three ways an electronic health record will improve the quality of patient care?

6. What impact could poor communication practices have on a quality improvement program?

Real-World Case

According to an Associated Press article published in the *News-Tribune,* March 25, 1995, an award-winning 39-year-old health columnist, who was being treated for breast cancer, died as a result of receiving the wrong dosage of cyclophosphamide (a cancer-fighting agent) and an overdose of another drug meant to keep her from suffering side effects. This happened at a reputable facility that specializes in the treatment of cancer.

At least a dozen doctors, nurses, and pharmacists missed the medication error for four days. Her husband reported that she suffered tremendously as the lining of her intestine was shed, resulting in her literally vomiting sheets of tissue. The doctors had reassured the patient and her husband that all was normal. Her heart failed after receiving four times the recommended amount of medication.

An autopsy revealed no visible signs of cancer in her body, which indicated that the treatment had worked. Another woman died of a similar mistake two days earlier. Human error was felt the only possible explanation, according to the treatment center. Incorrect doses of medication through either dispensing error, administration error, or prescription error can be deadly. Moreover, many adverse events go unreported. In November 1999, the Institute of Medicine reported that medical errors kill an estimated 44,000 to 98,000 Americans each year and affect every healthcare setting, and that medication errors are responsible for more than 7,000 deaths per year.

Summary

In the 20th century, the American College of Surgeons paved the quality improvement (QI) road by establishing standards of care. In the last half of the 20th century, the Joint Commission on Accreditation of Healthcare Organizations (JCAHO) and other accrediting bodies have clearly led the way in developing modern QI initiatives. The federal government, through the Medicare Conditions of Participation and quality improvement organizations (QIOs), also has contributed to the development of high-quality patient care. In addition, judicial decisions have made, and will continue to make, significant progress toward improving healthcare.

Every healthcare organization has its own version of quality. In general, however, the attributes of quality must be both administrative and clinical in nature and involve both the medical and facility staff. The organization's focus should be on customer satisfaction, professional standards of care, and process and system performance. The organization must collect and analyze data and use the results to make improvements in its processes and systems and in the healthcare it provides. Instituting a methodology of performance improvement will bring ordered change and improve the quality of healthcare.

Numerous QI methodologies have been used over the years, beginning with the medical care evaluation audit. JCAHO has introduced several methodologies and is currently moving toward a data-driven, continuous accreditation process. Other accrediting organizations have developed methodologies that require assessing, measuring, and improving the quality of healthcare. Outcomes management practice guidelines are examples of techniques frequently used in healthcare to help ensure that patients receive high-quality care.

The medical staff must be a part of the organization's QI efforts. The QI process begins with a well-functioning credentialing process to ensure that the medical staff is qualified to perform requested clinical privileges. The medical staff's bylaws/rules and regulations must support the QI processes. Medical staff leadership is critical when evaluating clinical processes as part of the performance improvement (PI) program. Moreover, the QI processes in any organization include a variety of programs.

The utilization management function contributes to high-quality healthcare by providing information on how effectively and efficiently the organization's resources are being used. Risk management contributes to patient safety by directly linking known risks to improving patient care. Use of generic criteria to monitor patient care helps to identify areas of risk, which enables the organization to be proactive in preventing or reducing injuries and accidents. The emergency preparedness program and safety programs also contribute to the quality of care.

Today, accrediting agencies, government agencies, and healthcare organizations use performance measures. Collecting information to evaluate an organization's processes is critical to improving the care the organization provides patients. Using effective data analysis and interpretation techniques helps determine whether the processes are effective.

Making meaningful changes is a constant challenge. Communicating performance measurement information to all parties who might benefit is difficult. Healthcare in the United States today is a highly technical, complex environment. All who practice in this environment must be aware of the need to continuously improve the processes and systems with which they work to achieve the quality and cost-effectiveness challenges facing the U.S. healthcare system.

References

Abdelhak, M., S. Grostick, M.A. Hanken, and E. Jacobs. 2001. *Health Information Management of a Strategic Resource,* 2nd ed. Philadelphia: W.B. Saunders.

Agency for Healthcare Research and Quality. 2005 (March). Fact sheet: Tools for hospitals and health care systems. AHRQ Publication No. 05-P016. Rockville, MD: AHRQ.

Agency for Healthcare Research and Quality. 2004 (August). *Closing the Quality Gap: A Critical Analysis of Quality Improvement Strategies.* Vol. 1 in *Series Overview and Methodology,* Technical Review. AHRQ Publication No. 04-0051-1. Rockville, MD: AHRQ.

Agency for Healthcare Research and Quality. 2003 (March). Fact sheet: CAHPS and the National CAHPS benchmarking database. Available online from ahrq.gov.

Agency for Healthcare Research and Quality. 2001 (March). Reducing and preventing adverse drug events to decrease hospital costs, in *Research in Action 1.* AHRQ Publication No. 010020. Rockville, MD: AHRQ.

Arrichiello, L. 2000. *HEDIS 101.* St. Paul, MN: Blue Cross/Blue Shield of Minnesota.

Brandt, M. 1994. Clinical practice guidelines and critical paths: Roles of HIM professionals. *Journal of American Health Information Management Association* 65(2):54–59.

Candler General Hospital, Inc. v. Persaud, 212 GA App. 762 (442 SE.2d 775) (1994).

Centers for Medicare and Medicaid Services. 2005a (January). Medicare begins performance-based payments for physician groups. Available online from cms.hhs.gov/researchers/demos/pgp.asp.

Centers for Medicare and Medicaid Services. 2005b. Medicare Program; Solicitation for Proposals for the Medicare Health Care Quality Demonstration Programs. Medicare Health Care Quality Demonstration System Redesign Incentives Leading to Improved Quality of Care. Available online from cms.hhs.gov/researchers/demos/mma646/SOLICITATION_09_07_2005.pdf.

Crosby, P.B. 1979. *Quality Is Free: The Art of Making Quality Certain.* New York: Penguin Books.

Darling v. Charleston Community Memorial Hospital, 33 IL 2d 326 (1965).

Department of Health and Human Services. 2005. Hospital Compare: Hospital Care Quality Measures. Available online from hospitalcompare. hhs.gov/Hospital/Static/About-HospQuality.asp?dest=NAV|Home|About| QualityMeasures#TabTop.

Donabedian, A. 1980. *Exploration in Quality Assessment and Monitoring,* Vol. 1: *The Definition of Quality and Approaches to Its Assessment.* Ann Arbor, MI: Health Administration Press.

Eckes, G. 2003. *Six Sigma for Everyone.* Hoboken, NJ: John Wiley and Sons.

Elliott, C., P. Shaw, P. Isaacson, and E. Murphy. 2000. *Performance Improvement in Healthcare: A Tool for Programmed Learning.* Chicago: American Health Information Management Association.

Goedert, J. 2004 (April). Crunching data: The key to Six Sigma success. *Health Data Management* 12(4):44–48.

Gonzales v. Nork and Mercy Hospital 20 CA 3d 500 (1978).

Governance Institute. 2000. *The Board's Role in Monitoring Quality.* Washington, DC: Governance Institute.

Graham, O.N., ed. 1995. *Quality in Health Care: Theory, Application, and Evaluation.* Gaithersburg, MD: Aspen.

Guidelines for reporting hospital quality data. 2004. *Clinician Review* 14(3):46.

Healthcare Cost and Utilization Project, Nationwide Inpatient Sample. 2004 (June 9). *Overview of disease severity measures.* Available online from hcup-us.ahrq.gov/db/nation/nis/OverviewofSeveritySystems.pdf.

Hospital Compare. 2005. United States Department of Health and Human Services. Available online from hospitalcompare.hhs.gov/Hospital/Static/Data-Professionals.asp?dest=NAV.

Institute of Medicine. 2000. *To Err Is Human: Building a Safer Health System.* Washington, DC: National Academy Press.

Institute of Medicine, Committee on Quality of Health Care in America. 2001. *Crossing the Quality Chasm: A New Health System for the 21st Century.* Washington, DC: National Academy Press.

Insinga v. LaBella FL (543 So.2d 209) (1989).

Johnson v. Misericordia Community Hospital, 99 WI 2d 708 (1981).

Joint Commission on Accreditation of Healthcare Organizations. 2005. *Comprehensive Accreditation Manual for Hospitals.* Oakbrook Terrace, IL: JCAHO.

Joint Commission on Accreditation of Healthcare Organizations. 2004. The Joint Commission announces the 2005 National Patient Safety goals and requirements. *Joint Commission: Perspectives* 24(8): 1–3.

Joint Commission on Accreditation of Healthcare Organizations. 2002 (March 18). A Comprehensive Review of Development and Testing for National Implementation of Hospital Core Measures. Available online from jcaho.org/pms/core+measures/cr_hos_cm.htm.

Joint Commission on Accreditation of Healthcare Organizations. 1996. *When Bad Things Happen to Good Health Care Organizations: Meeting the Joint Commission Sentinel Event Policy Requirements Leaders Guide, Part 1.* Oakbrook Terrace, IL: JCAHO.

Joint Commission on Accreditation of Healthcare Organizations. 1988. *The Joint Commission Guide to Quality Assurance.* Oakbrook Terrace, IL: JCAHO.

Kizer, K. 2004a (April 12). Conducting a dissonant symphony: NQF is working to bring more healthcare players into harmony on quality. *Modern Healthcare,* 34(14):20.

Kizer, K. 2004b (June 17). Submission for the record to U.S. House of Representatives, subcommittee on health, hearing on health care information technology. Available online from waysandmeans.house.gov/hearings.asp?formmode=view&id=2244.

Langley, G.J., K.M. Nolan, T.W. Nolan, C.L. Norman, and L.P. Provost. 1996. *The Improvement Guide: A Practical Approach to Enhancing Organizational Performance.* San Francisco: Jossey-Bass.

Lazarus, I. 2003 (Jan. 1). Six Sigma raising the bar. *Managed Healthcare Executive.* Available online from managedhealthcareexecutive.com/mhe/article/articleDetail.jsp?id=43331.

Leape, L. 1990. Practice guidelines and standards: An overview. *Quality Review Bulletin* 16:42–43.

Lee, K., and C. McGreevey. 2002. Using comparison charts to assess performance measurement data. *Journal on Quality Improvement* 28(3):129–38.

Lumsdum, K., and M. Haglund. 1993 (October 20). Mapping care. *Hospitals and Health Networks* 67(20):34–40.

Medicare Prescription Drug, Improvement, and Modernization Act of 2003 (Dec. 8). Public Law 108-173. Available online from cms.hhs.gov/medicarereform/MMAactFullText.pdf.

Mellott, Susan, ed. 1996. *NAHQ Guide to Quality Management,* 6th ed. Glenview, IL: NAHQ.

Millenson, M. 1999. *Demanding Medical Excellance.* Chicago: University of Chicago Press.

Milliman and Robertson. 2002. *Milliman Care Guidelines.* Seattle: Milliman.

Minnesota Department of Health. 2004. Adverse Health Events Reporting Law: Implementation Update. Available online from health.state.mn.us/patientsafety/aeupdatefs04.pdf

Morrissey, J. 2003. Leapfrog works on weighted evaluation system. *Modern Healthcare* 33(42):8.

Mosser, G., and S. Scheitel. 2004. *Public Reporting of Health Performance in Minnesota: A Position Paper of the Board of the Institute for Clinical Systems Improvement.* Bloomington, MN: ICSI.

National Quality Forum. 2003. *Safe Practices for Better Healthcare: A Consensus Report.* Washington, DC: NQF..

Nelson, E., J. Mohr, P. Batalden, and S. Plume. 1996. Improving health care, Part 1: The clinical value compass. *Journal on Quality Improvement* 22(4):243–55.

Neuhauser, D. 2002. Heroes and martyrs of quality and safety. *Quality and Safety in Health Care* 11:104–105.

Pozgar, G. 2004. *Legal Aspects of Health Care Administration,* 9th ed. Boston: Jones & Bartlett.

Prophet, S. 1997. Fraud and abuse implications for the HIM professional. *Journal of American Health Information Management Association* 68(4):52–56.

Purcell & Tucson General Hospital v. Zimbelman 18 AZ App. 75 (500 P.2d 335) (1972).

Roland, T., and P. Kannan. 2003. E-service: A new paradigm for business in the electronic environment. *Communications of the ACM* 46(6):37–42.

Rose, E. 2004. Life after go-live, Part 4: Preventing error with an EMR. *Journal of Healthcare Information Management* 17(4):15–17.

Rust, R. 2003. E-service: A new paradigm for business in the electronic environment. *Communications of the ACM* 46(6):37–42.

Schaffer, W.A. 1991. Introducing data to medical staffs. In *Quantitative Methods in Quality Management: A Guide for Practitioners,* edited by D.R. Longo and D. Bohr. Chicago: American Hospital Publishing.

Schanz, S.J. 1999. *Developing and Implementing Clinical Practice Guidelines.* Chicago: AMA.

Shine, K.I. 2002. Health care quality and how to achieve it. *Academic Medicine* 77(1):92.

Slee, V.N., and D.A. Slee. 1991. *Health Care Terms.* St. Paul, MN: Tringa Press.

Slovensky, D.J. 2001. Quality management and clinical outcomes. In *Health Information: Management of a Strategic Resource,* rev. ed., edited by M. Abdelhak et al. Philadelphia: W.B. Saunders.

Spath, P.L. 2000. *Fundamentals of Health Care Quality Management.* Forest Grove, OR: Brown-Spath & Associates.

Spath, P., and D. Hale. 2003 (January). Comparative performance data can be change agent. *Hospital Case Management* 11(1):3–5.

StratisHealth. 2000. *The Sixth Scope of Work: National Priorities and Performance Measures.* Bloomington, MN: StratisHealth.

Wachter, R., and D. Owens. 2004 (August). *The Genesis of Closing the Quality Gap.* AHRQ Publication No. 04-0051-1. Rockville, MD: AHRQ.

Walton, M. 1986. *The Deming Management Method.* New York: Putnam Publishing Group.

Youngberg, B. J. 1990. *Essentials of Hospital Risk Management.* Rockville, MD: Aspen.

Part V

Knowledge-Based Healthcare
Data and Information

Chapter 18
Biomedical and Research Support

Carol E. Osborn, PhD, RHIA

Learning Objectives

- To explain the role of biomedical research in evaluating the safety and efficacy of diagnostic and therapeutic procedures in order to solve human problems
- To relate the measures outlined by the Nuremberg Code, the Declaration of Helsinki, and the Belmont Report for the protection of human subjects
- To outline the contents of informed consent for the protection of human subjects as required by federal regulation
- To discuss the Health Insurance Portability and Accountability Act (HIPPA) and its privacy provisions for the protection of human subjects

- To outline the various research designs for conducting biomedical research
- To describe the purpose of outcomes and effectiveness research
- To describe the various types of outcomes and effectiveness measures
- To relate the purpose of the Health Plan Employer Data and Information Set (HEDIS®) sponsored by the National Commission for Quality Assurance (NCQA)
- To explain the purpose and requirements of the ORYX measurement process

Key Terms

Agency for Healthcare Research and Quality (AHRQ)
Attributable risk (AR)
Beneficence
Case-control study
Clinical trial
Cohort study
Controls
Core measures
Cross-sectional study
Double-blinded study
Epidemiological studies
Experimental study
Food and Drug Administration (FDA)
Health Plan Employer Data and Information Set (HEDIS)
Health Research Extension Act (1985)
Healthcare Cost and Utilization Project (HCUP)
Human subjects
Informed consent
Justice
Morality

National Committee for Quality Assurance (NCQA)
Observational study
Odds ratio
Office for Human Research Protections (OHRP)
Office of Research Integrity (ORI)
ORYX
Outcomes and effectiveness research (OER)
Principal investigator
Privacy Rule
Prospective studies
Protected health information (PHI)
Protocol
Quality indicators (QIs)
Randomized clinical trials (RCTs)
Relative risk (RR)
Respect for Persons
Retrospective study
Single-blinded study
Sponsor
Vulnerable subjects

Introduction

Biomedical research is a search for knowledge that often leads to advances in medicine. It uncovers what new drugs and other types of treatments, as well as new technology, are safe and effective for patients. When new treatments and/or technologies ultimately reach the consumers of healthcare, long-term studies of outcomes and effectiveness begin.

This chapter explores the various methods by which biomedical research is conducted. It also examines methods of assessing outcomes and effectiveness, including programs initiated by the **Agency for Healthcare Research and Quality,** the Joint Commission on Accreditation of Healthcare Organizations (JCAHO), and the **National Committee for Quality Assurance** (NCQA).

Theory into Practice

A physician in a healthcare facility is conducting a retrospective study of pathological fractures in women age 65 and over. He asks the HIM professional to provide medical records of these patients for the past five years.

The facility's information warehouse is queried for the number of cases that fall into DRG 239, Pathological Fractures and Musculoskeletal and Connective Tissue Malignancy, for the years 2001 through 2004. The cases selected have a principal diagnosis code of 733.xx.

The HIM professional is also asked to review the **informed consent** for a clinical trial that compares a new drug with the traditional drug for treating peripheral neuropathy. In the consent, the HIM professional notices the following paragraph (the consent is written in the first person):

> I understand that all or part of my medical record will be sent to the Gynecology Oncology Group (GOG) administrative office in Philadelphia, Pa., as well as to the GOG statistical data center in Buffalo, N.Y., to be reviewed and analyzed by physicians and other study personnel, along with the records of all other patients participating in this study from this and other institutions. I understand that hospital records, doctor's office records, and laboratory, operating room, and other records may be audited by representatives of the GOG and the National Cancer Institute.

The HIM professional has been asked to advise the principal investigator (PI) on whether this statement is in compliance with the privacy rule of the Health Insurance Portability and Accountability Act (HIPAA) (HHS 2004a). The HIM professional advises the PI that the statement adequately informs the subject on the parties that will have access to his or her protected health information (PHI). But the PI is also advised that there should be a separate HIPAA consent that informs the subject of the right to revoke the consent at any time, on procedures for revoking the consent, and whether treatment is contingent upon signing the consent.

Clinical and Biomedical Research

Biomedical research studies are conducted to evaluate disease processes and interventions and the safety, effective-ness, and usefulness of drugs, diagnostic procedures, and preventive measures such as vaccines and diets. The broad objective of these studies is to establish reproducible facts and theory that help solve human problems.

Ethical Treatment of Human Subjects

Human subjects are used in biomedical research studies. Because human subjects are involved, researchers are required to follow certain ethical principles that guide their behavior, **morality,** and character traits. Research ethics:

- Provide a structure for analysis and decision making
- Support and remind researchers to protect human subjects
- Provide workable definitions of benefits and risks

Risk versus benefit is critical in weighing the advantages of biomedical research. A benefit is a positive value of being part of the clinical research study. A benefit may be specific to the individual subject in that it provides a good therapeutic outcome, or it may be a direct advantage to society as a whole rather than to the individual subject.

Risks are concerned with the probability or magnitude of harm to the research subject. Stating that 1 in 100 patients may experience a certain risk suggests probability of harm. Stating that minor itchiness as a result of the treatment or liver failure as a major effect of the treatment caused death suggests magnitude of harm.

The challenge for the researcher is to weigh risks to the subject against potential benefits. This is difficult because not all potential benefits and risks are known in advance, and, as stated above, the benefit may be for society at large rather than for the individual subjects who assumed the risks.

The Nuremberg Code and the Declaration of Helsinki

International guidelines also govern the ethical conduct of human research. The Nuremberg Code outlines research ethics that were developed during the trials of Nazi war criminals following World War II. The code was widely adopted as a standard for protecting human subjects in the 1950s and 1960s. The basic tenet of the Nuremberg Code is that "voluntary consent of the human subject is absolutely essential" (Nuremburg Code 1949, p. 181). It is the duty and responsibility of the individual initiating, directing, or conducting the experiment to ensure the quality of the informed consent. Additionally, the Nuremburg code requires that research be based on animal work, the risks be justified by the anticipated benefits, only qualified scientists conduct the research, physical, and mental suffering be avoided., Research in which death is expected should not be conducted.

The Declaration of Helsinki is a code of ethics for clinical research approved by the World Medical Association in 1964. It was a reinterpretation of the Nuremberg Code directed toward medical research with a therapeutic intent. It is a statement of ethical principles that provides guidance to physicians and other participants in medical research involving human subjects, including research on identifiable human material or identifiable data. The document has been revised a number of times, most recently, at the Fifty-second World Medical Association Assembly held in Edinburgh, Scotland, in October 2000.

Despite the Nuremberg Code and the Declaration of Helsinki, controversial ethical practices in biomedical research continued to be a problem. In 1966, Dr. Henry K. Beecher, an anesthesiologist, described 22 examples of research studies with controversial ethics that had been published by prominent researchers in major journals. Beecher's article increased public awareness of the ethical problems related to biomedical research, including:

- Lack of informed consent
- Coercion of, or undue pressure on, volunteers
- Use of a vulnerable population
- Information being withheld
- Available treatment being withheld
- Information about risks being withheld
- Subjects put at risk
- Risks to subjects that outweigh the benefits
- Deception
- Violation of rights

The U.S. Public Health Services Syphilis Study

A study conducted in the United States that brought ethical issues in research to the forefront was the U.S. Public Health Services Syphilis Study. This study was designed to study the natural history of syphilis in African-American men. At the time the study began, there was no treatment for syphilis. However, by the 1940s penicillin had proved to be safe and effective. The men enrolled in the study were denied treatment. They continued to be followed until 1972 when the first public accounts began to appear in the national press. The study resulted in 28 deaths, 100 cases of disability, and 19 cases of congenital syphilis.

After the press blew the whistle, Congress formed an ad hoc panel that determined the study should be stopped immediately and that oversight of human research was inadequate. It was recommended that federal regulations be implemented to protect human research in the future. In 1974, Congress authorized formation of the National Commission for the Protection of Human Subjects in Biomedical and Behavioral Research. The commission was charged with identifying the basic ethical principles that underlie the conduct of human research.

In 1979, the commission published the *Belmont Report: Ethical Principles and Guidelines for the Protection of Human Subjects of Research*. The *Belmont Report* identifies the following three basic ethical principles that underlie all human subject research:

Respect for persons requires that individuals be treated as autonomous human beings and not used as a means to an end. Elements of autonomy include the ability to understand and process information

and the freedom to volunteer for research without coercion or undue influence from others. Respect for persons requires informed consent and respecting the privacy of research subjects.

Beneficence is minimizing harms and maximizing benefits. Beneficence requires the best possible research design to achieve its goals. It also requires that researchers be able to perform the research and handle the risks.

Justice requires that people be treated fairly and that benefits and risks be shared equitably among the population. Justice requires that subjects be selected equitably and that vulnerable populations or populations of convenience not be exploited.

The **Office for Human Research Protections** (OHRP) of the Department of Health and Human Services (HHS) monitors compliance with the federal regulations that govern the conduct of biomedical research (HHS 2005a). The federal regulations can be found in the *Federal Register* (1991, volume 56, number 117).

Check Your Understanding 18.1

Instructions: Answer the following questions on a separate piece of paper.

1. What is the origin of the Nuremberg Code? What are its basic tenets?

2. List the three principles outlined in the *Belmont Report*.

3. A researcher fails to inform a study participant of the reasonable risks in a study on the effectiveness of a new chemotherapy agent. What ethical principle was violated?

4. List five ethical issues in the conduct of biomedical research in the United States cited by Beecher.

5. What study led to establishment of the *Belmont Report* and ultimate federal regulations for human subject protection?

Informed Consent

In most cases, biomedical research requires that subjects be given informed consent. Informed consent is a person's voluntary agreement to participate in research or to undergo a diagnostic, therapeutic, or preventive procedure. It is based on adequate knowledge and an understanding of relevant information provided by the investigators. In giving informed consent, subjects do not waive any of their legal rights nor do they release the investigator, sponsor, or institution from liability for negligence. Federal regulations require that certain information be provided each human subject. This information includes the following:

- A statement that the study involves research, the purpose of the research, the expected duration of subject participation, a description of the procedures to be followed, and the identification of procedures that are experimental.
- A description of reasonably foreseeable risks or discomforts. The description must be accurate and reasonable, and subjects must be informed of previously reported adverse events.
- A description of the benefits to the subject or others who may reasonably benefit from the research.
- A disclosure of the appropriate alternative procedures or courses of treatment, if any, that might be advantageous to the subject. When appropriate, a statement

that supportive care with no additional disease-specific treatment is an alternative.

- A statement describing the extent to which confidentiality of records identifying the subject will be maintained. The statement should include full disclosure and description of approved agencies, such as the **Food and Drug Administration** (FDA), that may have access to the records.
- For research involving more than minimal risk, an explanation as to whether any compensation or medical treatments are available if injury occurs, and, if so, what they consist of or where further information may be obtained.
- An explanation of whom to contact for answers to pertinent questions about the research and research subjects' rights and whom to contact in the event of a research-related injury to the subject.
- A statement that participation is voluntary and that the subject may discontinue participation at any time without penalty or loss of benefits to which he or she is otherwise entitled

The regulations further require that additional consent information be provided when appropriate (Federal Policy 45 CFR 46.116), including:

- A statement that the treatment or procedure may involve risks to the subject (or embryo or fetus if the subject is pregnant) that are unforeseeable
- Anticipated circumstances under which the subject's participation may be terminated by the investigator without regard to the subject's consent
- Any additional costs that a subject may incur as a result of participating in the research
- The consequences of a subject's decision to withdraw from the research and procedures for orderly termination of participation by the subject
- A statement that significant new findings developed during the course of the research that may relate to the subject's willingness to continue participation will be provided to the subject
- The approximate number of subjects involved in the study

Federal regulations also require that informed consent be in a language that is understandable to the subject. If it is not, the consent form must be translated into the appropriate language. Subjects who are illiterate must have an interpreter present to explain the study and translate questions and answers between subject and investigator. A model consent form appears in figure 18.1.

In institutions where biomedical research is conducted, consent forms are usually maintained in storage facilities monitored by the **principal investigator.** Copies of the consent may or may not be kept in the medical record depending upon organizational policy. Consent forms often contain sensitive

Figure 18.1.   Template for informed consent for research involving human subjects

Consent to Investigational Treatment or Procedure

I, _____ , hereby authorize or direct _____ or associates of his/her choosing to perform the following treatment or procedure (describe in general terms), upon _____ (myself).

The experimental (research) portion of the treatment or procedure is:

This is part of an investigation entitled:

1. Purpose of the procedure or treatment:

2. Possible appropriate alternative procedure or treatment (not to participate in the study is always an option):

3. Discomforts and risks reasonably to be expected:

4. Possible benefits for subjects/society:

5. Anticipated duration of subject's participation (including number of visits):

I hereby acknowledge that _____ has provided information about the procedure described above, about my rights as a subject, and he/she answered all questions to my satisfaction. I understand that I may contact him/her at phone no. _____should I have additional questions. He/she has explained the risks described above, and I understand them; he/she has also offered to explain all possible risks or complications.

I understand that, where appropriate, the U.S. Food and Drug Administration may inspect records pertaining to this study. I understand further that records obtained during my participation in this study that may contain my name or other personal identifiers may be made available to the sponsor of this study. Beyond this, I understand that my participation will remain confidential.

I understand that I am free to withdraw my consent and participation in this project at any time after notifying the project director without prejudicing future care. No guarantee has been given to me concerning this treatment or procedure.

I understand that in signing this form that, beyond giving consent, I am not waiving any legal rights that I might have, and I am not releasing the investigator, the sponsor, the institution, or its agents from any legal liability for damages that they might otherwise have.

In the event of injury resulting from participation in this study, I also understand that immediate medical treatment is available at _____ _____ and that the costs of such treatment will be at my expense; financial compensation beyond that required by law is not available. Questions about this should be directed to the Office of Research Risks at _____.

I have read and fully understand the consent form. I sign it freely and voluntarily. A copy has been given to me.

information such as that related to genetic testing. Results of tests related to genetic testing are not to be provided to insurers or other parties, and sometimes not to the subject. To help ensure that this information is not released inadvertently in the regular course of business related to the release of information process, some organizations choose to maintain these important documents separately. Examples of documents that are kept in the study center files are listed in figure 18.2.

JCAHO also has specific requirements regarding the protection of human research subjects. These are identified in the patients' rights chapter of JCAHO accreditation manual (JCAHO 2005a). The specific requirements related to human subject research appear in figure 18.3.

Vulnerable Subjects

Federal regulations (DHHS regulation 45 CFR 46.111(b) and FDA regulation 21 CFR 56.111(b)) require that "when some or all of the subjects are likely to be vulnerable to coercion or undue influence, additional safeguards have been included in the study to protect the rights and welfare of these subjects." When a subject has limited mental capacity or is unable to freely volunteer, the subject is considered vulnerable. Examples of **vulnerable subjects** include:

- *Children* may be vulnerable depending on age, maturity, and psychological state. There is potential for control, coercion, undue influence, or manipulation by parents, guardians, or investigators. The risk is greater for particularly young children.

- *Mentally disabled individuals* have problems with capacity. They may not have freedom to volunteer because they may be institutionalized or hospitalized, are economically and educationally disadvantaged, and suffer from chronic diseases.

- *Educationally disadvantaged subjects* may have limitations on understanding the study they will be participating in; some may be illiterate. There is potential for undue influence and/or manipulation.

- *Economically disadvantaged subjects* may volunteer only because they will benefit economically. That is, because they will receive payment for participating in the research, they may "volunteer." They may enroll in research only to receive monetary compensation or medical care they cannot otherwise afford.

- Similarly, *individuals with incurable or fatal diseases* may "volunteer" to participate out of desperation. In many cases, these individuals have failed many treatments and view volunteering in biomedical research as their last chance at surviving their illness. Also, because of disease progression or effects of medications, they may not have the mental capacity necessary to make an informed decision. These individuals may accept high risk because they are desperate for a cure, even when there is little or no prospect of direct benefit.

- *Prisoners* have limited autonomy and may not be able to exercise free choice. They may believe that they will receive adverse treatment or be denied certain privileges if they refuse to participate in the research study. In addition, cash payments may be an inducement to participate

Figure 18.2.   Study center file contents

Investigator's brochure

Signed protocol

Revised protocols (if applicable)

Protocol amendments (if applicable)

Continuing review documents

Informed consent form (blank)

HIPAA consent form (blank)

Copies of signed consent forms

Curriculum vitae (resumes) of principal investigator and coinvestigators

Documentation of Institutional Review Board (IRB) or Ethical Review Board (ERB) compliance

All correspondence between the investigator, IRB, or ERB, and study sponsor or contract research organization, relating to study conduct

Copies of safety reports sent to FDA

Lab certifications

Normal laboratory value ranges for tests required by the protocol

FDA's Clinical Investigator Information Sheet

Clinical Research Associate monitoring log

Drug invoices

Study site signature log

Financial disclosure statement

Figure 18.3.   JCAHO standards for human subjects research

Standard: The hospital protects research subjects and respects their rights during research, investigation, and clinical trials involving human subjects.

Elements of Performance:
1. The hospital reviews all research protocols in relation to its mission, values, and other guidelines and weighs the relative risks and benefits to the research subjects.
2. The hospital provides patients who are potential subjects in research, investigation, and clinical trials with adequate information to participate or refuse to participate in research.
3. Patients are informed that refusing to participate or discontinuing participation at any time will not compromise their access to care, treatment, and services not related to the research.
4. Consent forms address the above elements of performance; indicate the name of the person who provided the information and the date the form was signed; and address the participants' right to privacy, confidentiality, and safety.
5. Subjects are told the extent to which their personally identifiable private information will be held in confidence.
6. All information given to subjects is in the medical record or research file along with the consent forms.
7. If a research-related inquiry (that is physical, psychological, social, financial, or otherwise) occurs, the principal investigator attempts to address any harmful consequences the subject may have experienced as a result of research procedures.

Source: JCAHO 2005a.

in research, thus it could be said that they are not truly volunteering but only participating for the cash benefit. Prisoners represent a population of convenience; that is, they are readily accessible and available. Studies on a contained population can be done more quickly and more cheaply. Lastly, prisoners may not realize benefits from their participation in research because of their incarceration and social and economic status.

Privacy Considerations in Clinical and Biomedical Research

In response to a congressional mandate in the Health Insurance Portability and Accountability Act (HIPAA) of 1996, HHS issued regulations entitled Standards for Privacy of Individually Identifiable Health Information. Known as the **Privacy Rule,** the regulations protect medical records and other individually identifiable health information from being used or disclosed in any form. The rule became effective on April 14, 2001, and organizations covered (covered entities) by the rule were expected to be in compliance by April 14, 2003.

The Privacy Rule establishes a category of **protected health information** (PHI), which may be used or disclosed only in certain circumstances or under certain conditions. PHI is a subset of what is called individually identifiable health information. It includes what healthcare professionals typically regard as a patient's protected health information, such as information in the patient's medial records as well as billing information for services rendered. PHI also includes identifiable health information about subjects of clinical research. Patient information considered "protected" is listed in figure 18.4.

The Privacy Rule defines the means by which human research subjects are informed of how their protected medical information will be used or disclosed. It also outlines their rights to access the information. The Privacy Rule protects the privacy of individually identifiable information while ensuring that researchers continue to have access to the medical information they need to conduct their research. Investigators are permitted to use and disclose PHI for research with individual authorization or without individual authorization under limited circumstances.

A valid Privacy Rule Authorization is an individual's signed permission that allows a covered entity to use or disclose the patient's PHI for the purpose(s) and to the recipient(s) stated in the authorization (HHS 2004b). When an authorization is obtained for biomedical research purposes, the Privacy Rule requires that it pertain only to a specific research study, not to future unspecified projects. Following are the core elements of the Privacy Rule Authorization:

- A description of the PHI to be used or disclosed, identifying the information in a specific and meaningful manner
- The names or other specific identification of the person or persons authorized to make the requested use or disclosure

Figure 18.4.   Deidentifying protected health information

The Privacy Rule allows covered entities to deidentify data by removing the following 18 elements that may be used to identify the individual or the individual's relatives, employers, or household members.

1. Names
2. All geographic subdivisions smaller than a state, including street address, city, county, precinct, ZIP code, except for the initial three digits of a ZIP code if, according to the current publicly available data from the Bureau of the Census:
   a. The geographic unit formed by combining all ZIP codes with the same three initial digits contains more than 20,000 people.
   b. The initial three digits of a ZIP code for all such geographic units containing 20,000 or fewer people are changed to 000.
3. All elements of dates (except year) for dates directly related to an individual, including birth date, admission date, discharge date, date of death; and all ages over 89 and all elements of dates (including year) indicative of such age, except that such ages and elements may be aggregated into a single category of age 90 or older.
4. Telephone numbers
5. Facsimile numbers
6. Electronic mail addresses
7. Social Security numbers
8. Medical record numbers
9. Health plan beneficiary numbers
10. Account numbers
11. Certificate/license numbers
12. Vehicle identifiers and serial numbers, including license plate numbers
13. Device identifiers and serial numbers
14. Web universal resource locators (URLs)
15. Internet protocol (IP) address numbers
16. Biometric identifiers, including fingerprints and voiceprints
17. Full face photographic images and any comparable images
18. Any other unique identifying number, characteristic, or code, unless permitted by the Privacy Rule for reidentification

Source: HHS 2004a.

- The names or other specific identification of the person or persons to whom the covered entity may make the requested use or disclosure
- A description of each purpose of the requested use or disclosure
- Authorization expiration date or expiration event that relates to the individual or to the purpose of the use or disclosure
- Signature of the individual and date (If the individual's legally authorized representative signs the authorization, a description of his or her authority to act for the individual also must be provided.)

In addition, the authorization must include statements indicating:

- that the individual has the right to revoke the authorization at any time and must be provided with the procedure for doing so
- whether treatment, payment, enrollment, or eligibility of benefits can be contingent upon authorization, including research-related treatment and consequences of refusing to sign the authorization, if applicable

- any potential risk that PHI will be redisclosed by the recipient and no longer protected by the Privacy Rule

In addition, the authorization must be written in plain language and a copy provided to the individual. Elements that are required in a HIPAA consent are shown in figure 18.5; optional elements are listed in figure 18.6 (p. 528).

It is believed that the Privacy Rule will promote participation in clinical trials. The reason cited most often is concern about health insurance discrimination and loss of privacy should the information be released.

Oversight of Biomedical Research

Because of past abuses of human subjects in the conduct of biomedical research in the United States, Congress began

hearings in 1981 to investigate scientific misconduct. Twelve cases of scientific misconduct were reported in the country between 1974 and 1981. Representative Albert Gore Jr., chairman of the Investigations and Oversight Subcommittee of the House Science and Technology Committee, held the first hearing. Continued abuses were reported throughout the 1980s, which resulted in the creation of several agencies that provide oversight of biomedical research.

Office of Research Integrity

In response to the public outcry over scientific misconduct in biomedical research, Congress passed the **Health Research Extension Act** in 1985 (PHS regulation 42 CFR 493). The act requires the secretary of HHS to issue a regulation requiring applicant or awardee institutions to establish "an administrative

Figure 18.5. Model HIPAA consent—required elements

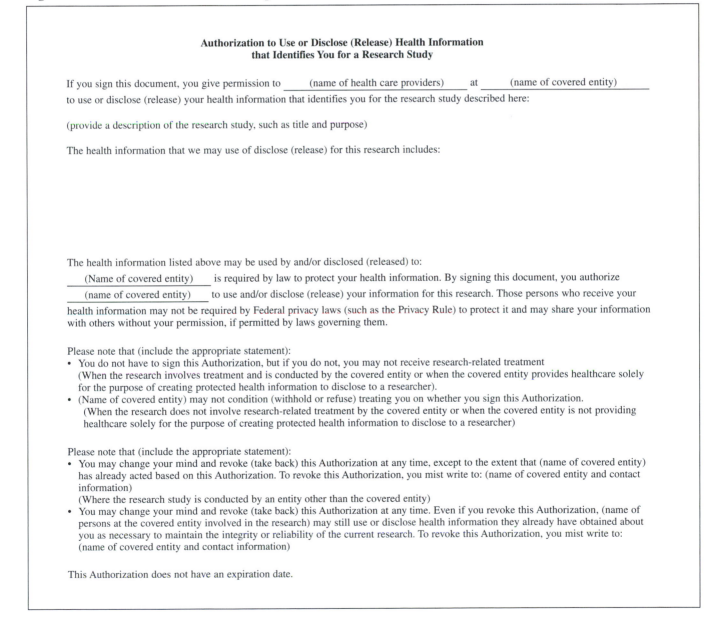

Authorization to Use or Disclose (Release) Health Information
that Identifies You for a Research Study

If you sign this document, you give permission to _____(name of health care providers)_____ at _____(name of covered entity)_____
to use or disclose (release) your health information that identifies you for the research study described here:

(provide a description of the research study, such as title and purpose)

The health information that we may use of disclose (release) for this research includes:

The health information listed above may be used by and/or disclosed (released) to:

_____(Name of covered entity)_____ is required by law to protect your health information. By signing this document, you authorize
_____(name of covered entity)_____ to use and/or disclose (release) your information for this research. Those persons who receive your
health information may not be required by Federal privacy laws (such as the Privacy Rule) to protect it and may share your information
with others without your permission, if permitted by laws governing them.

Please note that (include the appropriate statement):
- You do not have to sign this Authorization, but if you do not, you may not receive research-related treatment
  (When the research involves treatment and is conducted by the covered entity or when the covered entity provides healthcare solely
  for the purpose of creating protected health information to disclose to a researcher).
- (Name of covered entity) may not condition (withhold or refuse) treating you on whether you sign this Authorization.
  (When the research does not involve research-related treatment by the covered entity or when the covered entity is not providing
  healthcare solely for the purpose of creating protected health information to disclose to a researcher)

Please note that (include the appropriate statement):
- You may change your mind and revoke (take back) this Authorization at any time, except to the extent that (name of covered entity)
  has already acted based on this Authorization. To revoke this Authorization, you mist write to: (name of covered entity and contact
  information)
  (Where the research study is conducted by an entity other than the covered entity)
- You may change your mind and revoke (take back) this Authorization at any time. Even if you revoke this Authorization, (name of
  persons at the covered entity involved in the research) may still use or disclose health information they already have obtained about
  you as necessary to maintain the integrity or reliability of the current research. To revoke this Authorization, you mist write to:
  (name of covered entity and contact information)

This Authorization does not have an expiration date.

Figure 18.6.   Model HIPAA consent—optional elements

Authorization to Use or Disclose (Release) Health Information
that Identifies You for a Research Study

- Your health information will be used or disclosed when required by law.

- Your health information may be shared with a public health authority that is authorized by law to collect or receive such information for the purpose of preventing or controlling disease, injury, or disability, and conducting public health surveillance, investigations, or interventions.

- No publication or public presentation about the research described above will reveal your identity without another authorization from you.

- All information that does or can identify you is removed from your health information, the remaining information will no longer be subject to this authorization and may be used or disclosed for other purposes.

- **When the research for which the use or disclosure is made involves treatment and is conducted by a covered entity:** To maintain the integrity of this research study, you generally will not have access to your personal health information related to this research until the study is complete. At the conclusion of the research and at your request, you generally will have access to your health information that (name of covered entity) maintains in a designated record set that includes medical information or billing records used in whole or in part by your doctors or other healthcare providers at (name of covered entity) to make decisions about individuals. Access to your health information in a designated record set is described in the Notice of Privacy Practices provided to you by (name of covered entity). If it is necessary for your care, your health information will be provided to you or your physician.

- If you revoke this Authorization, you may no longer by allowed to participate in the research described in this Authorization.

process to review reports of scientific fraud" and "report to the Secretary any investigation of scientific fraud which appears substantial."

Before 1986, reports of scientific misconduct were received by funding institutes within the Public Health Service (PHS). In 1986, the National Institutes of Health (NIH) assigned responsibility for receiving and responding to complaints of scientific misconduct to its Institutional Liaison Office. This was the first step in creating a central locus of responsibility for scientific misconduct within the HHS. In March 1989, the PHS created the Office of Scientific Integrity (OSI) and the Office of Scientific Review (OSIR) in the Office of the Assistant Secretary for Health (OASH). In 1992, the OSI and the OSIR were consolidated to form the **Office of Research Integrity** (ORI) in the OASH (HHS 2005b). The creation of these groups removed responsibility for reviewing complaints of scientific misconduct from the funding agencies.

In 1993, the NIH Revitalization Act established the ORI as an independent agency within HHS. The role, mission, and structure of the ORI is focused on preventing misconduct and promoting research integrity principally through oversight, education, and review of institutional findings and recommendations. Responsibilities of the ORI include:

- Developing policies, procedures, and regulations related to the detection, investigation, and prevention or research misconduct and the responsible conduct of research
- Reviewing and monitoring research misconduct investigations conducted by applicant and awardee institutions
- Implementing activities and programs to teach the responsible conduct of research, promote research integrity, pre-

vent research misconduct, and improve the handling of allegations of research misconduct
- Providing technical assistance to institutions that respond to allegations of research misconduct
- Conducting policy analyses, evaluations, and research to build the knowledge base in research misconduct and research integrity

The Office for Human Research Protections

Protection of human subjects is required under the HHS Code of Federal Regulations (45 CFR 46). The Office for Human Research Protections (OHRP) is a federal agency that provides leadership and oversight on all matters related to the protection of human subjects participating in research conducted or supported by the HHS, as outlined in the regulations. It has formal agreements with more than 10,000 federally funded universities, hospitals, and other medical and behavioral research institutions in the United States and abroad. These organizations must agree to abide by the human subject protection regulations found in the Code of Federal Regulations. The OHRP's duties include:

- Establishing criteria for, and approving assurance of, compliance for the protection of human subjects with institutions engaged in HHS-conducted or HHS-supported human subject research
- Providing clarification and guidance on involving humans in research
- Developing and implementing educational programs and resource materials
- Promoting the development of approaches to enhance human subject protections

The OHRP also evaluates substantive allegations or indications of noncompliance with HHS regulations regarding the conduct of research involving human subjects (HHS 2005a). It also provides education and development on the complex regulatory ethical and regulatory issues relating to human subjects protection in medical and behavioral research. The OHRP helps institutions assess and improve their own procedures for protecting human subjects through a quality improvement program.

Check Your Understanding 18.2

Instructions: Answer the following questions on a separate piece of paper.

1. In signing an informed consent, a subject releases the research sponsor from any liability or negligence. True or false?

2. A patient agrees to be a subject in a clinical trial assessing the effectiveness of the combination of two cancer agents. Because the patient is part of this research, all medical expenses are covered by the sponsoring organization. True or false?

3. Medical records of subjects in a research study may be released without patient authorization. True or false?

4. A subject may withdraw from a research study at any time. True or false?

5. Individuals who may be subject to undue influence to enroll in biomedical research are considered vulnerable. True or false?

6. Individuals who participate in clinical trials and biomedical research must sign the HIPAA consent form. True or false?

7. A patient's medical record number is considered protected health information (PHI). True or false?

8. What basic elements should be contained in an informed consent for human subjects?

9. Describe the relationship of the HIPAA Privacy Rule to clinical research.

10. What federal agencies provide oversight to biomedical research?

Types of Biomedical Research Design

The more common types of designs for research involving human subjects include:

- **Epidemiological studies**
- **Case-control studies**
- **Cohort studies**
- **Cross-sectional study**
- **Clinical trials**

Epidemiological Studies

The purpose of an epidemiological study is to compare two groups of individuals, one group with the risk factor of interest and one without it. In such studies, the investigator attempts to identify risk factors for diseases, conditions, behaviors, or risks that result from particular causes, such as environmental factors and/or industrial agents.

Epidemiological studies are concerned with finding the causes and effects of diseases/conditions and/or the whys and the hows. The goal is to quantify the association between exposures and outcomes and to test hypotheses about causal relationships. Epidemiological research has several objectives, including:

- To identify the cause of disease and its associated risk factors
- To determine the extent of disease in a given community
- To study the natural history and prognosis of disease
- To evaluate new preventive and therapeutic measures and new modes of healthcare delivery
- To provide the foundation for public policy and regulatory decisions relating to environmental problems

Epidemiological studies may be observational or experimental. In an **observational study,** the exposure and outcome for each individual in the study is studied (observed). In an **experimental study,** the exposure status for each individual in the study is determined and the individuals are then followed to determine the effects of the exposure.

Observational studies are used to generate hypotheses for later experimental studies. They may consist of clinical observations at a patient's bedside. For example, Alton Ochsner observed that every patient he operated on for lung cancer had a history of cigarette smoking (Gordis 1996). If he had wanted to explore the relationship further, he would have compared the smoking histories of a group of his lung cancer patients with a group of his patients without lung cancer. This would be a case-control study. Research designs that are considered observational are prospective cohort studies, retrospective cohort studies, case-control studies, and cross-sectional studies.

In biomedical research, experimental studies consist primarily of randomized clinical trials. In randomized clinical trials, individuals are randomly assigned to experimental and control groups in order to study the effect of an intervention, such as an experimental drug.

A major purpose of epidemiological studies is to determine risk. In prospective studies, a 2×2 table is a tool that is used to evaluate the association between exposure and disease. (See table 18.1.) The table is a cross-classification of exposure status and disease status. The total number of individuals with the disease is $a + c$, and the total number without disease is $b + d$. The total number exposed is $a + b$, and the total number not exposed is $c + d$.

The number of individuals who had both exposure and the disease is recorded in cell a; the number who had exposure, but no disease, is recorded in cell b; the number who had the disease, but no exposure, is recorded in cell c; and the number who had neither the disease nor exposure is recorded in cell d.

Table 18.1. 2×2 table for classifying disease status and exposure status

		Disease Status		
		Yes	No	Total
Exposure Status	Yes	a	b	$a + b$
	No	c	d	$c + d$
		$a + c$	$b + d$	$a + b + c + d$

Case-Control Study

Case-control studies are the mainstay of epidemiological research. In them, persons with a certain condition (cases) and persons without the condition (**controls**) are studied by looking back in time. The objective is to determine the frequency of the risk factor among the cases and the frequency of the risk factor among the controls in order to determine possible causes of the disease. In a case-control study, if there is an association between exposure and disease, the prevalence of history of exposure will be higher in persons with the disease (cases) than in those without it (controls). For a case-control study, the 2×2 table in table 18.1 is modified in table 18.2. The proportion of cases exposed is a/a + c, and the proportion of controls exposed is b/b + d.

The advantages of case-control studies are that they are easy to conduct and cost-effective, with minimal risk to the subjects. Also, existing records are used to conduct the studies. Case-control studies also allow the researcher to study multiple causes of disease. Because they usually involve small groups, case-control studies are easily repeatable to determine whether the results are consistent.

Although the use of existing medical records is advantageous, there are problems associated with using them for retrospective research. One major problem is that the cases are based on hospital admissions. Admissions are based on patient characteristics, severity of illness and associated conditions, and admission policies. All of these vary from hospital to hospital, making standardization of the study difficult. In addition, there are problems related to poor documentation, illegibility, and missing records. Lack of consistency in diagnostic and clinical services between hospitals also makes comparability difficult. Further, validation of the information can be difficult. An important aspect of epidemiological studies is the identification of risk. In studies using medical records, the population at risk is generally not defined.

Cohort Study

A cohort study is a prospective study in which the investigator selects a group of exposed individuals and unexposed individuals who are followed for a period of time to compare the incidence of disease in the two groups. The length of time for follow-up varies from a few days for acute diseases to several decades for cancer and cardiac diseases. If there is an association between exposure and disease, the incidence of disease is greater in the exposed group (a/a + b) than in the unexposed group (c/c + d). New cases of the disease are identified as they occur so that it can be determined whether a time relationship exists between exposure to disease and development of disease. The time relationship must be established if the exposure is to be considered the cause of the disease. For a cohort study, the 2×2 table in table 18.1 is modified in table 18.3.

One of the most famous cohort studies is the Framingham Study, which began in the 1950s. The research project was designed to monitor the incidence of coronary artery disease in more than 5,000 residents who were examined every two years for a period of 20 years. This study has provided important data demonstrating the relationship between the development of heart disease and risk factors such as smoking, obesity, diet, and high blood pressure.

Cohort studies offer several advantages. First, the researcher can control the data collection process throughout the study. Also, outcome events can be checked as they occur; many outcomes can be studied, including those that were not anticipated at the start of the study. The disadvantages of cohort studies are that they are costly and there is a long wait for the study results. Also, subjects may be lost to death, withdrawal, or follow-up.

One difference between case-control and cohort studies is that the former is a **retrospective study** and the latter is a **prospective study.** A retrospective study is conducted by reviewing records from the past; a prospective study is designed to observe events that occur after the subjects have been identified. The advantages and disadvantages of retrospective and prospective studies are outlined in tables 18.4 and 18.5.

Another difference is that in a cohort study the subjects are individuals with or without the disease and the focus is disease status; in the case-control study, the subjects are individuals who have been exposed or not exposed to the disease and the focus is exposure status.

Cross-Sectional Study

In a cross-sectional study, both the exposure and the disease outcome are determined at the same time in each subject. A cross-sectional study also may be referred to as a prevalence study because it describes characteristics and health outcomes at a particular point in time. It provides quantitative estimates of the magnitude of a problem. After the population has been defined, the presence or absence of exposure and of disease can be established for each individual in the study. Each subject is then categorized into one of four subgroups that correspond to the 2×2 table that appears in table 18.6.

The prevalence of disease in persons with exposure (a/a + b) is compared with persons without exposure (c/c + d). Alternatively, the prevalence of exposure in persons with the disease (a/a + c) is compared to the prevalence of exposure to persons without the disease (b/b + d).

A major advantage of the cross-sectional study is that it is relatively easy to conduct and may produce results in a short period of time. The disadvantage is that, because exposure and disease are determined at the same time in each subject, the time relationship between exposure and onset of the disease cannot be established. It describes only what exists at the time of the study.

Clinical Trials

Clinical (medical) research is a specialized area of research that primarily investigates the efficacy of preventive, diagnostic, and therapeutic procedures. Efficacy involves both safety and effectiveness.

Table 18.2.   2 × 2 table for case-control studies

	Cases (with disease)	Controls (without disease)
Exposed	a	b
Not exposed	c	d
Total	$a + c$	$b + d$
Proportions exposed	$a/a + c$	$b/b + d$

Table 18.3.   2 × 2 table for cohort studies

	Disease Develops	Disease Does Not Develop	Totals	Incidence Rates of Disease
Exposed	a	b	$a + b$	$a/a + b$
Not Exposed	c	d	$c + d$	$c/c + d$

Table 18.4.   Advantages and disadvantages of retrospective studies

Advantages	Disadvantages
Short study time	Control group subject to bias in selection
Relatively inexpensive	
Suitable for rare diseases	Biased recall possible
Ethical problems minimal	Cannot determine incidence rate
Hospital medical record may be used	Relative risk is approximate
Small number of subjects	
No attrition problems	

Table 18.5.   Advantages and disadvantages of prospective studies

Advantages	Disadvantages
Control group less susceptible to bias	Requires more time
No recall necessary	Costly
Incidence rate can be determined	Relatively common diseases only
Relative risk is accurate	Ethical problems may be considerable and influence study design
	Volunteers needed
	Results may not be generalizable to a larger population
	Requires a large number of subjects
	Problems with attrition

Clinical trials are the specific, individual studies within the field of clinical research. They offer a systematic way to introduce, evaluate, and monitor new drugs, treatments, and devices prior to their dissemination throughout the healthcare system. As a result, they have proved to be effective means of advancing knowledge about medicine and health and, thus, improving the quality of healthcare in the United States. Because clinical trials involve patients, they can begin only after the researcher has shown promising results in the laboratory or the results have been well documented in the literature.

The NIH supports thousands of clinical trials (Clinicaltrials.gov). Private organizations such as drug companies and health maintenance organizations (HMOs) also support them. Trial sites are teaching and community hospitals, physician group practices, or health departments. Many clinical trials are multicentered; that is, a number of research institutions cooperate in conducting the study. In **randomized clinical trials** (RCTs), participants are assigned to a treatment or a control group. They may be **single-** or **double-blinded studies,** in which case the investigator, the participants, or both do not know who is in the treatment or control group until the end of the study.

Researchers conduct clinical trials using **protocols.** Protocols are sets of strict procedures that specify the language of informed consent, the types of subjects, the timing of treatments, the period of participation, and the evaluation of efficacy. For example, in RCTs, researchers must follow strict rules in assigning patients to groups. The rules ensure that both known and unknown risk factors will occur in approximately equal numbers between the group of patients receiving the treatment and the group of patients not receiving it.

Most clinical trials consist of three phases. In a phase 1 drug trial studies are performed on 20 to 80 healthy volunteers who are closely monitored. The objective of phase 1 drug trials is to determine the metabolic and pharmacological actions of the drug in humans, to determine the side effects associated with increasing dosages, and to gain early evidence of effectiveness. Historically, phase 1 trials are considered the safest and usually involve administering a single dose to healthy volunteers. But they also can pose a high level of unknown risk because this is the first administration of a drug to a human. When the drug is highly toxic, such as cancer chemotherapies, cancer patients are usually the subjects for phase 1 trials.

Table 18.6.   2 × 2 table for cross-sectional studies

	Disease	No Disease	Totals	Prevalence of Disease for Exposed/Not Exposed
Exposed	a	b	$a + b$	$a/a + b$
Not Exposed	c	d	$c + d$	$c/c + d$
Totals	$a + c$	$b + d$	$a + b + c + d$	$a + b + c + d$
Prevalence of Exposure for Disease/No Disease	$a/a + c$	$b/b + d$		

Group a: Persons exposed with the disease
Group b: Persons exposed without the disease
Group c: Persons with the disease, but not exposed
Group d: Persons without disease and without exposure

Table 18.7. Phases of clinical trials

Phase	I	II	III	IV
Number of Subjects	20–80	100–300	1000–3000	Multitudes postmarketing
Purpose	Evaluate safety Determine dosage Identify side effects	Evaluate safety Determine effectiveness	Collect more information about safe usage Confirm effectiveness Monitor side effects Compare to alternatives	Collect data on effect on specific groups (populations) Monitor long-term side effects

In the phase 2 drug trial, the number of participants is usually increased to between 100 and 200. The purpose of this trial is to evaluate the drug's effectiveness for a certain indication in patients with the condition under study and to determine the short-term side effects and risks associated with the drug. Subjects included in phase 2 studies are usually those with the condition the drug is intended to treat. Phase 2 studies are randomized, well controlled, and closely monitored. They may include randomization to treatment and control groups and be double-blinded. Treatment and control groups allow for comparison between subjects who received the drug and those who did not.

Phase 3 drug trials involve the administration of a new drug to a larger number of patients in different clinical settings to determine its safety, effectiveness, and appropriate dosage. The number of subjects involved may range from several hundred to several thousand. Phase 3 trials are conducted only after evidence of effectiveness has been obtained. Phase 3 studies are designed to collect more information on drug effectiveness and safety for evaluating the drug's overall risk benefit.

The FDA, in collaboration with the **sponsor,** may decide to conduct a phase 4 postmarketing study to obtain more information about the drug's risks, benefits, and optimal use. Phase 4 studies may include studying different doses or schedules of administration than what was used in phase 2 studies, the use of the drug in other patient populations or other stages of the disease, or the use of the drug over a longer period of time. See table 18.7.

Risk Assessment

As stated earlier, one objective of epidemiological studies is to assess risk. Risk is the probability that an individual will develop a disease over a specified period of time, provided that he or she did not die as a result of some other disease process during the same time period. It is usually expressed as **relative risk** (RR). RR is calculated from cohort studies and compares the risk of some disease in two groups differentiated by some demographic variable such as sex or race. The group of interest is referred to as the exposed group and the comparison group is the unexposed group. The risk ratio is calculated as:

$$\frac{\text{Risk for exposed group}}{\text{Risk for unexposed group}}$$

A relative risk of 1.0 indicates that there is identical risk in both groups. An RR that is greater than 1.0 indicates an increased risk for the exposed group; an RR of less than 1.0 indicates a decreased risk for the exposed group.

Odds Ratio

In a case-control study, the objective is to identify differences in exposure frequency associated with one group having the disease under study and the other group not having it. The incidence of disease in the exposed and unexposed populations is not known because persons with the disease (cases) and without the disease (controls) are identified at the onset of the study. Thus, RR cannot be calculated directly. So the question becomes, What are the odds that an exposed person will develop the disease? Put another way, What are the odds that a nonexposed person will develop the disease?

In a case-control study, the **odds ratio** compares the odds that the cases exposed to the disease with the odds that the controls were exposed. Using the 2 × 2 table in table 18.1 as a reference, the odds ratio is calculated as:

$$\frac{a/b}{c/d} = \frac{a \times c}{b \times c}$$

The odds ratio measures the odds of exposure of a given disease. For example, an odds ratio of 1.0 indicates that the incidence of disease is equal in each group; thus, the exposure may not be a risk factor for the disease of interest. An odds ratio of 2.0 indicates that the cases were twice as likely to be exposed as the controls. This implies that the exposure is associated with twice the risk of disease.

Attributable Risk

The **attributable risk** (AR) is a measure of the public health impact of a causative factor on a population. In this measure, the assumption is that the occurrence of a disease in an unexposed group is the baseline or expected risk for that disease. Any risk above that level in the exposed group is attributed to exposure to the risk factor. It is assumed that some individuals will acquire a disease, such as lung cancer, whether or not they were exposed to a risk factor such as smoking. The AR measures the additional risk of illness as a result of an individual's exposure to a risk factor. The AR is calculated as:

$$AR = \frac{(\text{Risk for exposed group}) - (\text{Risk for unexposed group})}{\text{Risk for exposed group}} \times 100$$

Outcomes and Effectiveness Research in Healthcare

The major objective of **outcomes and effectiveness research** (OER) is to understand the end results (outcomes) of particular healthcare practices and interventions. Examples of patient outcomes include ability to function, quality of life, satisfaction, and mortality. By linking the care that patients receive to the outcomes they experience, OER has become the key to developing better ways to monitor and improve the quality of care.

The history of outcomes research can be traced back to the 1860s when Florence Nightingale laid the foundation for collecting and evaluating hospital statistics. Hospital mortality rates were the basic measures used for evaluating patient outcomes. The major finding was that mortality rates varied significantly from hospital to hospital.

The Flexner Report (1910), the Codman studies (1914), the establishment of hospital standards by the American College of Surgeons (1913), and the founding of JCAHO (1952) are landmarks in the development of outcomes research. More recently, the passage of Medicare (1965) and subsequent legislation has accelerated interest in outcomes research.

Outcomes and Effectiveness Research Strategies

OER may be conducted at the community, system, institutional, or patient level. At the community level, outcomes research focuses on the population as a whole or on specific communities. For example, the Dartmouth Atlas of Musculoskeletal Health Care (Center for the Evaluative Clinical Sciences 2000) has found that the rate for leg amputations in the southern tip of Texas is more than two times higher than the national average. The amputation rate in the Corpus Christi region is 3.7 leg amputations per 1,000 Medicare patients, three times higher than in Amarillo.

OER at the system level refers to the healthcare system as a whole. It may include the entire country or a specific region. Examples of geographic variations in medical care at the national level cited by the Dartmouth Atlas of Health Care include:

- In Bend, Oregon, the rate for back surgeries is 7.3 for every 1,000 Medicare recipients, more than four times higher than in Syracuse, New York, where there are 1.5 surgeries for every 1,000 Medicare recipients.
- Heart patients in Elyria, Ohio, receive angioplasties at a rate more than seven times higher than in York, Pennsylvania, 360 miles away.
- Men in Baton Rouge, Louisiana, undergo prostate removal surgery at a rate more than eight times higher than do men in Tuscaloosa, Alabama.

OER at the institutional level refers to the sites in which healthcare is delivered: hospitals, clinics, or HMOs. At the patient level, interest is on the interaction between one provider and one patient. An example outcome study performed at the institutional level is a review of medical records and/or clinical data of patients with a principal diagnosis of acute myocardial infarction who expire during hospitalization. A second example is the ongoing assessment of patient satisfaction.

There is no standard method for conducting outcomes research at the institutional level or any level. Donabedian (1966) proposed the first model for evaluating patient outcomes. His model focused on measuring the structure, process, and outcomes of medical care. Structure is the setting in which the healthcare is provided and the resources available to provide it. Process is the extent to which professionals perform according to accepted standards. Process is a set of activities that take place between providers. Outcomes include changes in the patient's condition, quality of life, and level of satisfaction. Characteristics of structure, process, and outcome appear in table 18.8. Other models used for the study of outcomes include the disease model and the health and wellness model. Epidemiological approaches are often used to study outcomes. In the hospital setting, the medical record often serves as the data source for outcomes studies.

Table 18.8.   Characteristics of structure, process, and outcome

Structure	Process	Outcome
System characteristics: Organization Specialty mix Workload Access/convenience	Technical: Visits Medications Referrals Test ordering Hospitalizations	Clinical endpoints: Symptoms and signs Laboratory values Death
Provider characteristics: Specialty training Preferences Job satisfaction	Interpersonal: Interpersonal manner Counseling Communication level	Health-related quality of life: Physical Mental Social Role
Patient characteristics: Diagnosis/condition Severity Comorbidity Health habits		Satisfaction with care: Access Convenience Quality General

Outcomes and Effectiveness Measures

Several types of measures are used in OER. These include:

- *Clinical performance* measures are designed to evaluate the processes or outcomes of care associated with the delivery of clinical services. They allow for intraorganizational and interorganizational comparisons to be used to improve patient health outcomes. Clinical measures should be condition specific or procedure specific or should address important functions of patient care, such as medication use and infection control.
- *Patient perceptions of care* and/or services focus on the delivery of clinical services from a patient's perspective. Aspects of care that may be addressed are patient education, wait times, medication use, pain management, practitioner bedside manner, communication regarding current care and future plans for care, and improvement in health status.
- *Health status* measures address the functional well-being of specific populations, both in general and in relation to specific conditions. They indicate changes that have occurred in physical functioning, bodily pain, social functioning, and mental health over time.
- *Administrative/financial performance* measures address the organizational structure for coordinating and integrating service, functions, or activities across organizational components. Examples of administrative/financial measures are those related to financial stability, utilization, length of stay (LOS), and credentialing.

Defining expected clinical outcomes is a major section of the protocols for clinical trials. The principal investigator or organization sponsoring the study must specifically state the expected outcomes of the clinical trial before the investigation can begin. Investigators also must state at what point the research study will stop if adverse events occur. Examples of study objectives and outcome variables are listed in figure 18.7.

Current Outcomes Movement

The current outcomes movement gained momentum in the 1980s when the prospective payment system (PPS) for Medicare inpatient care was implemented. The public and policy makers were concerned that Medicare patients were being forced out of hospitals because "their DRG had run out." The fear was that patients were being discharged based on their LOS rather than when they were clinically ready for discharge. William Roper, who became HCFA (Health Care Financing Administration, now the Centers for Medicare and Medicaid Services [CMS]) administrator in 1986, promoted the use of Medicare databases to monitor the quality of care through measurement of mortality rates, readmission rates, and other adverse outcomes.

Simultaneously, others were advancing the outcomes movement, which contained elements of research, measurement, and management. John Wennberg, director of the Center for

Figure 18.7.   Sample objectives and outcome variables for clinical research

Objective: to determine whether the treatment drug is safe and effective in patients with advanced chronic heart failure and is effective in reducing the incidence of cardiovascular hospitalization and/or mortality due to all causes.

Primary Outcome Variable: The primary outcome variable is the time from entry into the study to mortality from all causes of cardiovascular hospitalization. A hospitalization is a nonelective admission for medical therapy that results in at least one overnight stay. A cardiovascular hospitalization is one that is due to heart failure, myocardial infarction, coronary insufficiency, stroke, atrial or ventricular dysrhythmias, or symptomatic heart block.

Secondary Outcome Variable:

Time from study entry to all-cause mortality or all-cause hospitalization

Time from study entry to all-cause mortality or worsening heart failure hospitalization

Patient global assessment at the six-month visit

Six-minute walk test at the six-month visit

Other Outcomes of Interest:

All hospitalizations, classified by cause (heart failure, cardiovascular, vascular, nonvascular) in regard to frequency, length of stay, and cost

Number of emergency department visits classified by cause (heart failure or nonheart failure)

Mortality classified by cause (heart failure, cardiovascular, vascular, nonvascular)

All-cause mortality, all-cause hospitalization, cardiac transplant, and left ventricular assist device insertion

Myocardial infarction and cardiac revascularization

The safety and tolerability of the drug as determined by the occurrence of adverse events, permanent treatment withdrawals, changes in laboratory tests, physical exam and ECG

the Evaluative Clinical Sciences at the Dartmouth Medical School, and others developed methods for exploring the impact of healthcare services on patient outcomes. Other research efforts on geographic variations in medical practice, appropriateness of care, and the poor quality of medical evidence to support various interventions and treatments resulted in establishment of the Agency for Health Care Policy and Research (AHCPR) in 1989. The Healthcare Research and Quality Act of 1999 changed the agency's name to the Agency for Healthcare Research and Quality (AHRQ). The mission of the AHRQ is to support research designed to improve the outcomes and quality of healthcare, reduce its costs, address patient safety and medical errors, and broaden access to effective services. The research sponsored by the AHRQ provides information that helps people make better decisions about healthcare. The goals and research priorities of the AHRQ include:

- Supporting improvement in health outcomes
- Strengthening quality measurement and improvement
- Identifying strategies to improve access, foster appropriate use, and reduce unnecessary expenditures

A component of the AHRQ is the AHRQ **quality indicators** (QIs). QIs are measures that address various aspects of quality. The various types of QIs include the following (AHRQ 2005a):

- *Prevention QIs* identify hospital admissions that could have been avoided, at least in part, through high-quality outpatient care.
- *Inpatient QIs* reflect quality of care inside hospitals, including inpatient mortality for medical conditions and surgical procedures. Four dimensions are used to assess inpatient quality: volume, mortality for inpatient procedures, mortality for inpatient conditions, and utilization indicators.
- *Patient safety indicators* also reflect quality of care inside hospitals but focus on potentially avoidable

complications and iatrogenic events. Patient safety indicators screen for problems that patients experience as a result of exposure to the healthcare system and that can be prevented by changes at the provider level or the area level. Provider-level indicators include only those cases where a secondary ICD-9-CM diagnosis code flags a potentially preventable complication. Area-level indicators capture all cases of potentially preventable complications in a given area either during a hospitalization or resulting in subsequent hospitalization. Area-level indicators are identified by both principal and secondary ICD-9-CM diagnoses codes.

Examples of AHRQ quality indicators appear in tables 18.9 through 18.11 (p. 536).

Table 18.9.   AHRQ inpatient quality indicators

Type of Indicator	Definition	Indicators
Volume	Indirect measure of quality based on evidence suggesting that hospitals performing more of certain intensive, high-technology, or highly complex procedures may have better outcomes for these procedures.	Esophageal resection volume Pancreatic resection volume Pediatric heart surgery volume Abdominal aortic aneurysm (AAA) repair volume Coronary artery bypass graft (CABG) volume Percutaneous transluminal coronary angioplasty (PTCA) volume Carotid endarterectomy (CEA) volume
Mortality Indicators for Inpatient Conditions	Conditions where mortality has been shown to vary substantially across institutions and where evidence suggests that high mortality may be associated with deficiencies in the quality of care.	Acute myocardial infarction (AMI) mortality rate Congestive heart failure mortality rate Acute stroke mortality rate Gastrointestinal hemorrhage mortality rate Hip fracture mortality rate Pneumonia mortality rate
Mortality Indicators for Inpatient Procedures	Procedures where mortality has been shown to vary substantially across institutions and where evidence suggests that high mortality may be associated with deficiencies in the quality of care.	Esophageal resection mortality rate Pancreatic resection mortality rate Pediatric heart surgery mortality rate AAA repair mortality rate CABG mortality rate PTCA mortality rate CEA mortality rate Craniotomy mortality rate Hip replacement mortality rate
Utilization	Procedures whose use varies significantly across hospitals and for which questions have been raised about overuse, underuse, or misuse. High or low rates are likely to represent inappropriate or inefficient delivery of care.	Cesarean delivery rate Primary Cesarean delivery rate Vaginal birth after Cesarean (VBAC) rate VBAC rate, uncomplicated Laparoscopic cholecystectomy rate Incidental appendectomy in the elderly rate Bilateral cardiac catheterization rate

Source: AHRQ 2002.

Table 18.10.   AHRQ patient safety indicators

Complications of anesthesia
Death in low-mortality DRGs
Decubitus ulcer
Failure to rescue
Foreign body left during procedure
Iatrogenic pneumothorax
Selected infections due to medical care
Postoperative hip fracture
Postoperative infection or hematoma
Postoperative physiologic and metabolic derangements
Postoperative respiratory failure
Postoperative pulmonary embolism or deep vein thrombosis
Postoperative sepsis
Postoperative wound dehiscence
Accidental puncture of laceration
Transfusion reaction
Birth trauma—injury to neonate
Obstetric trauma—vaginal with instrument
Obstetric trauma—vaginal without instrument
Obstetric trauma—Cesarean delivery
Obstetric trauma with 3rd degree lacerations—vaginal with instrument
Obstetric trauma with 3rd degree lacerations—vaginal without instrument
Obstetric trauma with 3rd degree lacerations—Cesarean delivery

Source: AHRQ 2002.

Table 18.11.   AHRQ prevention quality indicators

Indicator Name
Diabetes short-term complication admission rate
Perforated appendix admission rate
Diabetes long-term complications admission rate
Pediatric asthma admission rate
Chronic obstructive pulmonary disease (COPD) admission rate
Pediatric gastroenteritis admission rate
Hypertension admission rate
Congestive heart failure (CHF) admission rate
Low birth weight rate
Dehydration admission rate
Bacterial pneumonia admission rate
Urinary tract infection admission rate
Angina without procedure admission rate
Uncontrolled diabetes admission rate
Adult asthma admission rate
Rate of lower-extremity amputation among patients with diabetes

Source: AHRQ 2004.

One must use caution when evaluating the results of assessments using the inpatient quality indicators. The data collected for these indicators were collected using the ICD-9-CM codes that appear on the UB-92. This represents administrative data and not research data. Limitations associated with using administrative data include:

- *Coding differences across hospitals:* Some hospitals code more thoroughly than others, making "fair" comparisons across hospitals difficult.
- *Ambiguity about when a condition occurs:* Most administrative data cannot distinguish whether a specific condition was present at admission or whether it occurred during the inpatient stay.
- *Limitations in ICD-9-CM coding:* The codes are often not specific enough to adequately describe a patient's condition, which makes it impossible to perfectly risk-adjust any administrative data set. This makes fair comparisons across hospitals difficult.

However, despite these limitations, QIs can assist individual hospitals in comparing their organizations with averages at the national, regional, or state level. The information can be used to investigate potential quality problems. Investigation may reveal quality problems for which quality improvement programs may be initiated, uncover problems in data collect that can be remedied through coding education, or determine what additional clinical information is required to understand the quality issues, beyond that obtained through administrative data alone.

An analytical tool that the AHRP supports is the **Healthcare Cost and Utilization Project** (HCUP). The HCUP database, called HCUPnet, is an online query system that gives instant access to the largest set of all payer healthcare databases that are publicly available (AHRQ 2005b). It contains Web-based tools that can be used to identify, track, analyze, and compare trends in hospital care at the national, regional, and state levels. HCUP data are used for research on hospital utilization, access, charges, quality, and outcomes. This database can be queried for information when doing internal assessments related to the AHRQ QIs. Figure 18.8 provides a snapshot of the interactive databases available at HCUPnet.

As an example, an organization wants to evaluate its congestive heart failure (CHF) mortality rate. CHF is a progressive, chronic disease with substantial short-term mortality, which varies across organizations. To begin the process, the researcher must review the definition of CHF mortality rate, which appears in table 18.12, and the ICD-9-CM codes used to retrieve the CHF information (table 18.13). The organization's data then can be compared with AHRQ QIs available at the HCUPnet Web site. (National data for the CHF mortality rate is displayed in figure 18.9, p. 538.)

Figure 18.8.   Text from HCUPnet Web page (partial)

National Statistics	*Create your own statistics for national and regional estimates on hospital use for all patients from the HCUPNationwide Inpatient Sample (NIS).*
For Children Only	*Create your own statistics for national estimates on use of hospitals by children (age 0–17 years) from the HCUPKids' Inpatient Database (KID).*
State Statistics	*Create your own statistics on stays in hospitals for participating States from the HCUPState Inpatient Databases (SID).*
Quick Statistics	*Ready-to-use tables on commonly requested information from the HCUPNationwide Inpatient Sample (NIS), the HCUPKids' Inpatient Database (KID), or the HCUPState Inpatient Databases (SID).*
AHRQ Quality Indicators	*Ready-to-use national information on measures of healthcare quality based on the NIS, using theAHRQ Quality Indicators (QIs).*

Source: AHRQ 2005b.

Table 18.12.   Congestive heart failure mortality rate

Relationship to quality	Better processes of care may reduce short-term mortality, which represents better quality.
Benchmark	State, regional, or peer group average
Definition	Number of deaths per 100 discharges with principal diagnosis code of CHF
Numerator	Number of deaths with a principal diagnosis code of CHF
Denominator	All discharges with a principal diagnosis of CHF. Age 18 years and older. Exclude patients with missing discharge disposition, transferring to another short-term hospital, MDC 14 and MDC 15.
Type of indicator	Mortality indicator for inpatient conditions
Empirical performance	Population rate (2002): 4.61 per 100 discharges at risk

Table 18.13.   ICD-9-CM codes for congestive heart failure

398.31	Rheumatic heart failure	428.21	Acute systolic heart failure
402.01	Malignant hypertensive heart disease with CHF	428.22	Chronic systolic heart failure
402.11	Benign hypertensive heart disease w/ CHF	428.23	Acute or chronic systolic heart failure
402.91	Hypertensive heart disease w/ CHF	428.9	Heart failure NOS
404.01	Malignant hypertensive heart/renal disease w/ CHF	428.30	Diastolic heart failure NOS
404.03	Malignant hypertensive heart/real disease w/ CHF and renal failure	428.31	Acute diastolic heart failure
404.11	Benign hypertensive heart/renal disease w/ CHF	428.32	Chronic diastolic heart failure
404.13	Benign hypertensive heart/renal disease w/ CHF and renal failure	428.33	Acute or chronic diastolic heart failure
404.91	Hypertensive heart/renal disease NOS w/ CHF	428.40	Systolic/diastolic heart failure NOS
404.93	Hypertensive heart/renal disase w CHF and renal failure	428.41	Acute systolic/diastolic heart failure
428.0	Congestive heart failure	428.42	Chronic systolic/diastolic heart failure
428.1	Left heart failure	428.43	Acute/chronic systolic/diastolic heart failure
428.20	Systolic heart failure NOS		

Figure 18.9. National quality indicators—2001 national statistics
    Deaths per 1,000 adult admissions with congestive heart failure (CHF) (excluding obstetric and neonatal admissions and transfers to another hospital) (IQI 16), by patient and hospital characteristics, 2001

Patient/Hospital Characteristic	Adjusted Rate a/		
	Estimate	Standard Error	P-Value: Relative to Marked Group b/
Total U.S.	44.698	0.428	
Patient characteristic:			
Age Groups for Conditions Affecting Any Age			
18–44 b/	22.076	2.258	
45–64	25.679	0.967	0.142
65 and over	50.750	0.488	0.000
Age Groups for Conditions Affecting Primarily Elderly			
65–69 b/	35.905	1.379	
70–74	32.705	1.182	0.078
75–79	42.576	1.058	0.000
80–84	53.968	1.055	0.000
85 and over	72.328	0.927	0.000
Gender:			
Male b/	48.272	0.640	
Female	41.833	0.575	0.000
Median income of patient ZIP:			
Less than $25,000	42.678	1.475	0.232
$25,000–$34,999	45.843	0.818	0.258
$35,000–$44,999	44.267	0.827	0.739
$45,000 or more b/	44.627	0.699	
Location of patient residence:			
Metropolitan b/	43.573	0.479	
Micropolitan	47.994	1.251	0.001
Non-CBSA	50.439	1.470	0.000
Location of inpatient treatment:			
Northeast b/	49.514	0.939	
Midwest	43.447	0.920	0.000
South	44.069	0.649	0.000
West	41.512	1.129	0.000
Expected payment source:			
Private insurance b/	47.832	1.173	
Medicare	43.619	0.489	0.001
Medicaid	46.731	1.692	0.593
Other insurance	57.347	3.659	0.013
Uninsured/self pay/no charge	48.916	2.723	0.715
Hospital characteristic:			
Ownership/control:			
Private, not-for-profit b/	44.330	0.504	
Private, for-profit	43.841	1.101	0.686
Public	47.763	1.194	0.008

Figure 18.9.   (Continued)

Patient/Hospital Characteristic	Adjusted Rate a/		
	Estimate	Standard Error	P-Value: Relative to Marked Group b/
Teaching status:			
Teaching	44.817	0.823	0.863
Nonteaching b/	44.652	0.501	
Location of hospital:			
Metropolitan b/	43.344	0.470	
Micropolitan	49.545	1.312	0.000
Noncore	53.607	1.685	0.000
Bedsize:			
Less than 100	51.067	1.119	0.000
100–299 b/	44.933	0.658	
300–499	41.770	0.825	0.003
500+	43.189	1.061	0.163

Source: Agency for Healthcare Research and Quality's Healthcare Cost and Utilization Project, Nationwide Inpatient Sample. For relevant denominator sources, see Methods section.

a/ Rates are adjusted by age, gender, age-gender interactions, and APR-DRG risk of mortality score. When reporting is by age, the adjustment is by gender and APR-DRG risk of mortality score; when reporting is by gender, the adjustment is by age and APR-DRG risk of mortality score.

b/ Reference for p-value test statistics.

Weighted national estimate from HCUP Nationwide Inpatient Sample (NIS), 2001, Agency for Healthcare Research and Quality (AHRQ), based on data collected by individual statewide data organizations and provided to AHRQ through the HCUP partnership.

Total number of weighted discharges in the U.S. based on HCUP NIS = 37,187,641.

Source: AHRQ 2005b.

Use of Comparative Data in Outcomes Research

Healthcare organizations such as the NCQA and JCAHO have developed measures for evaluating the effectiveness of healthcare providers. The purpose of the measures developed by the NCQA is to provide purchasers of healthcare, primarily employers, with information about the cost and effectiveness of organizations with which they contract for services. JCAHO measures also are designed primarily to encourage organizations to improve their own performance and to provide a comprehensive picture of the care provided within the organization.

National Commission for Quality Assurance

The NCQA is an accountability system for managed care organizations. It was founded in 1990 as an independent organization with the support of the Robert Wood Johnson Foundation, the large employer community and the managed care industry's main trade association. The NCQA began accrediting managed care organizations in 1991. Its mission is to improve the quality of healthcare by generating useful, understandable information about healthcare quality to help inform consumer and employer choice, and working to generate information and feedback to help physicians, health plans, and others to identify opportunities for improvement and make changes that enhance the quality of patient care.

The Health Plan Employer Data and Information Set

As part of these efforts, the NCQA developed a set of performance measures known as the **Health Plan Employer Data and Information Set,** more commonly known as HEDIS. More than 60 different measures were designed to provide both purchasers and consumers of healthcare with information to compare the performance of managed care plans.

Three methods are used in collecting HEDIS data: examining claims data, reviewing health records, or a combination of both. The health record can provide the most complete information, but it is the more time-consuming, costly, and difficult method. Health record review is time-consuming because a statistically valid sample of records must be reviewed. The stated minimum is 411 charts. It is costly because the reviewers must have technical skills that require higher salaries. Moreover, health records must be reviewed from the offices of many physicians because there is usually more than one primary care provider in any health plan.

HEDIS performance measures cover a number of areas: effectiveness of care, access and availability of care, satisfaction with care, health plan stability, utilization of services, cost of care, healthcare choices, and health plan descriptive information. A list of specific HEDIS measures is provided in table 18.14 (p. 540).

Table 18.14.   Example HEDIS performance measures

Effectiveness of Care Measures	Customer Satisfaction Measures
Asthma medication use Controlling high blood pressure Antidepressant medication management Advising smokers to quit Beta blocker treatment after a heart attack Breast cancer screening Childhood and adolescent immunization status	Plan rating Claims processing Customer services Access to care

Source: NCQA 2004.

Providers and consumers of care are often interested in different performance measures. Providers are usually more interested in process and outcome measures, whereas consumers (patients) are more interested in measures that pertain directly to them. For patients, the most important reasons for choosing a healthcare plan are physician communication, respect toward patients, time spent with physicians, and location of the physician's office. (Detailed information about NCQA programs and HEDIS measures can be found online at www.ncqa.org.)

The ORYX Initiative

In 1987, JCAHO began developing a set of performance measures that became know as the as the **ORYX** initiative. ORYX is a performance measurement process that JCAHO has integrated into the accreditation process. It is a data-driven process that encourages healthcare organizations to examine their processes for providing care in order to improve the results of care. JCAHO-accredited hospitals, long-term care facilities, home care, and behavioral health organizations must participate in the program.

ORYX uses standardized performance measures, referred to as **core measures,** that are applied across accredited healthcare programs (JCAHO 2005b). The use of core measures allows for benchmarking based on processes and outcomes of patient care. Core measures are designed to provide a comprehensive picture of the care provided in a given area. A core measure must:

- Demonstrate that it will have a significant impact on the health of specified populations
- Be precisely defined and specify requirements for data collect and for calculation of the core measure value or score
- Consistently identify the events it was designed to identify across healthcare organizations (reliability)
- Measure or capture what it is intended to measure (validity)
- Be interpretable (that is, its results must be easily understood by the users of the data, including accrediting organizations, providers, and consumers)

- Have the ability to be risk-adjusted or stratified (that is, the extent to which differences among population groups can be controlled or taken into account)
- Be assessed for availability and accessibility of the required data elements and the effort and cost of abstracting and collecting data
- Be useful in the accreditation process and support the organization's quality improvement efforts
- Be under the provider's control to influence the processes and/or outcomes being measured
- Be publicly available

In ORYX's early stage of development, hospitals had considerable flexibility in that they could select among hundreds of performance measures that best served their strategic measurement goals. But this method did not allow for comparability of information across organizations. The ORYX initiative now requires use of standardized, evidenced-based measures permitting more rigorous data comparisons across organizations.

In 2004, to reduce duplication of effort, JCAHO and CMS announced that they were working to align current and future measures common to both organizations. These are referred to as hospital quality measures and considered integral to improving the quality of care provided to hospital patients (JCAHO 2005c, JCAHO 2005d, JCAHO 2005e). The hospital quality measure sets currently utilized by JCAHO and CMS are:

- Acute myocardial infarction
- Heart failure
- Pneumonia
- Surgical infection prevention

In addition, JCAHO has a core measure set for pregnancy and related conditions. Examples of core measures from each category appear in table 18.15. Note that they are similar to the AHRQ quality indicators.

Each facility selects its own core measures based on the services it provides. For example, a hospital that does not provide obstetrical services would not be required to select measures from the pregnancy and related conditions category. Hospitals that serve patient populations having conditions that match two or more of the core measure sets are required to choose two measure sets. Hospitals should select measures that correlate to the greatest degree of high-risk, high-volume, and problem-prone areas within the organization. Data are submitted quarterly to JCAHO.

The ORYX requirements have been simplified for small hospitals. A hospital is designated as small when it has an average daily census of less than 10 and outpatient visits of fewer than 150 per month. Small hospitals are required to collect data internally on all selected measures/measure sets; generate either run charts or control charts on each measure, at least quarterly, for use in internal quality improvement activities; make data reports available for review by surveyors during on-site surveys; and produce reports upon request of JCAHO for the purpose of data-monitoring activities.

Table 18.15.   Examples ORYX core measures

Core Measure	Type of Measure	Measure	Description	Rationale
Heart Failure	Process	Adult smoking cessation advice/counseling	Heart failure patients with a history of smoking cigarettes, who are given smoking cessation advice or counseling during hospital stay	Smoking cessation reduces mortality and morbidity in all populations. Patients who receive even brief smoking-cessation advice from their physicians are more likely to quit.
Pneumonia	Process	Antibiotic timing	Mean time from arrival at the hospital to the administration of the first dose of antibiotic at the hospital	There is growing clinical evidence of an association between timely inpatient administration of antibiotics and improved outcome among pneumonia patients.
Pregnancy and Related Conditions	Outcome	Inpatient neonatal mortality	Live-born neonates who expire before the neonate becomes age 28 days	Neonatal mortality continues to account for the largest proportion of infant deaths. Low birth weight is a very important risk factor of neonatal mortality.
Surgical Infection Prevention	Process	Prophylactic antibiotic received within one hour prior to surgical incision	Surgical patients who receive prophylactic antibiotics within one hour prior to surgical incision	Studies have found that the lowest incidents of postoperative infection was associated with antibiotic administration during the one hour prior to surgery.

Source: JCAHO 2005b.

How an organization uses its selected core measures is evaluated during a JCAHO accreditation on-site survey. The organization must demonstrate the reliability of the data, conduct credible analysis of the data, and initiate system and process improvements.

Check Your Understanding 18.4

Instructions: Answer the following questions on a separate piece of paper.

1. What is the purpose of outcomes and effectiveness research?
2. What types of outcomes are studied?
3. What is the mission of the Agency for Healthcare Research and Quality (AHRQ)?
4. Who sponsors the Health Care Utilization Project (HCUP)? What is the purpose of its database?
5. What is the focus of the AHRQ quality indicators? What are their limitations?
6. What types of performance measures are used in outcomes and effectiveness research?
7. What is the purpose of the HEDIS measures developed by the National Committee for Quality Assurance?
8. How are HEDIS data collected?
9. What is the purpose of the ORYX core measures developed by JCAHO?
10. What are the five ORYX core measurement areas?

Real-World Case

The director of quality contacts the HIM professional regarding a report posted at HealthGrades.com. Health Grades is an organization that helps consumers evaluate and compare hospital performance. To accomplish this objective, it purchases MedPAR data from CMS on all hospitals in the United States and provides hospital ratings on a variety of procedures and clinical conditions, free of charge, on its Web site.

The director of quality is concerned about the hospital's rating on treating heart attacks compared to its major competitor in the city (table 18.16) and asks the HIM professional to investigate the criteria used to establish the ratings.

Table 18.16.   Data for Real World Case

Hospital	Inhospital Mortality (Survival)	Inhospital +1 Month Mortality	Inhospital +6 Month Mortality	Cardiac Procedure Availability
Your Hospital	***	***	***	Full
Competitor	*****	***	***	Full
Legend: ***** — Best		*** — As Expected		* — Poor

Source: HealthGrades.com.

Summary

Biomedical research conducted on human subjects should follow guidelines set forth in the *Belmont Report*, the Nuremberg Code, and the Declaration of Helsinki. Further, biomedical research on human subjects requires informed consent. The Office of Research Integrity and the Office for Human Research Protections are federal agencies that provide oversight of biomedical research.

Many study designs are used to conduct biomedical research, including case-control studies, cohort studies, cross-sectional studies, and clinical trials. In a case-control study, the frequency of the exposure in the diseased cases is compared with the frequency of exposure in the controls. In a cohort study, a set of group characteristics by risk factor in a group of individuals is followed over time for outcome. In a cross-sectional study, the frequency of a risk factor and an outcome of interest in a geographically defined population is studied at one point in time. Clinical trials are controlled studies that involve human subjects. They are designed to evaluate prospectively the safety and effectiveness of new drugs, devices, or behavioral interventions.

A major objective of biomedical research is to quantify the risk of obtaining a particular disease resulting from exposure to a risk factor. Relative risk, odds ratio, and attributable risk are measures used to quantify or assess risk. Relative risk compares the incidence of disease in the exposed group to the incidence of disease in the control group. The odds ratio, the odds of exposure in a diseased group, is divided by the odds of exposure in the nondiseased group. Attributable risk is the proportion of total risk for a disease or outcome attributable to a particular exposure.

Various models for outcomes and effectiveness research are available. The Agency for Healthcare Research and Quality (AHRQ) serves as a resource for individuals engaged in outcomes research. The AHRQ sets a national agenda for the types of outcomes research that should be conducted. In addition, the Joint Commission on Accreditation of Healthcare Organizations conducts the ORYX program, which has a set of core measures for evaluation effectiveness of care in various types of healthcare organizations. Lastly, the NCQA administers HEDIS, a program for evaluating the quality of services provided by managed care organizations.

References

Agency for Healthcare Research and Quality. 2005a. *AHRQ Quality Indicators—Guide to Patient Safety Indicators.* Version 2.1, revision 3. AHRQ pub. no. 03-R203. Rockville, MD: AHRQ.

Agency for Healthcare Research and Quality. 2005b. *HCUPnet, Healthcare Cost and Utilization Project.* Rockville, MD: AHRQ.

Agency for Healthcare Research and Quality. 2004. *AHRQ Quality Indicators—Guide to Prevention Quality Indicators: Hospital Admission for Ambulatory Care Sensitive Conditions,* revision 4. AHRQ pub. no. 02-R0203. Rockville, MD: AHRQ.

Agency for Healthcare Research and Quality. 2002. *AHRQ Quality Indicators—Guide to Inpatient Quality Indicators: Quality of Care in Hospitals—Volume, Mortality, and Utilization,* revision 4. AHRQ pub. no. 02-R0204 (December 22, 2004). Rockville, MD: AHRQ..

Center for the Evaluative Clinical Sciences at Dartmouth Medical School. 2000. Dartmouth Atlas of Healthcare. Hanover, NH: CECS. Available online from dartmouthatlas.org.

Department of Health and Human Services. 2004a. *Clinical Research and the HIPAA Privacy Rule.* NIH pub. no. 04-5495. Available online from privacyruleandresearch.nih.gov/clin_research.asp.

Department of Health and Human Services. 2004b. *HIPAA Authorization for Research.* NIH Pub. no. 04-5529. Available online from privacyruleandresearch.nih.gov/authorization.asp.

Donabedian, A. 1966. Evaluating the quality of medical care. *Milbank Memorial Fund Quarterly: Health and Society* 44(3):166–203.

Gordis, L. 1996. *Epidemiology.* Philadelphia: W.B. Saunders.

Joint Commission on Accreditation of Healthcare Organizations. 2005a. *Comprehensive Accreditation Manual for Hospitals.* Oakbrook Terrace, IL: JCAHO.

Joint Commission on Accreditation of Healthcare Organizations. 2005b. Facts about ORYX for hospitals, core measures and hospital core measures. Available online from jcaho.org.

Joint Commission on Accreditation of Healthcare Organizations. 2005c. Specifications manual for national hospital quality measures. Available online from jcaho.org.

Joint Commission on Accreditation of Healthcare Organizations. 2005d. A comprehensive review of development and testing for national implementation of hospital core measures. Available online from jcaho.org.

Joint Commission on Accreditation of Healthcare Organizations. 2005e. Attributes of core performance measures and associated evaluation criteria. Available online from jcaho.org.

National Committee for Quality Assurance. 2004. *The State of Health Care Quality: 2004. Industry Trends and Analysis.* Washington, DC: NCQA.

The Nuremberg Code. 1949. Washington, DC: U.S. Government Printing Office. Reprinted in *Trials of War Criminals before the Nurembert Military Tribunals under Control Council Law* 2(10):188–82. Available online from nihtraining.com/ohsrsite/guidelines/nuremberg.

Chapter 19
Expert Systems and Decision Support

J. Michael Hardin, PhD

Learning Objectives

- To understand the concept of decision support and the process of decision making
- To recognize the valuable assets contained within the organization's current data systems and how to better use the data
- To understand the background and history of decision support systems in general
- To identify the different structures used to develop decision support systems
- To differentiate among decision support systems and other information systems
- To understand the general types of decision support systems and to recognize the key architectural differences
- To understand the concept of data warehousing and how it is applicable to decision support
- To understand the concept of data mining and types of data mining tools used in decision support systems
- To recognize the different classes of decision support systems found in healthcare
- To understand some of the basic models of artificial intelligence used in developing decision support systems
- To recognize some of the career opportunities related to decision support activities that are available to health information management professionals

Key Terms

Applied artificial intelligence
Artificial neural network (ANN)
Association rule analysis (rule induction)
Clinical decision support system (CDSS)
Clinical repository
Data miners
Data mining
Data warehouse
Data-based DDS
Decision support system (DSS)
Decision tree
Executive information system (EIS)
Expert system (ES)
Geographical information system (GIS)
Graphical user interface (GUI)
Graphics-based DSS
Health management information system (HMIS)
Hospital information system (HIS)
Hybrid online analytical processing (HOLAP)
Inference engine
Intellectual capital
Knowledge-based DDS
Linkage analysis
Machine learning

Model-based DDS
Multidimensional data structure
Multidimensional database management system (MDDBMS)
Multidimensional online analytical processing (MOLAP)
Natural language processing (NLP)
Normalization
Online analytical processing (OLAP)
Operations research (OR)
Relational database management system (RDMS)
Relational online analytical processing (ROLAP)
Return on investment (ROI)
Rule induction
Satisficing
Simon's decision-making model
Snowflake schema
SQL (structured query language)
Star schema
Structural decision
Supervised learning
Transactional systems
Unstructured decision
Unsupervised learning
Virtual reality (VR)

Introduction

In *Future Health: Computers and Medicine in the Twenty-First Century,* Kaufman and Paterson (1995) identified seven goals that must be addressed in order to meet the future computing needs of physicians. Of critical importance, they observed, was the continued development and research of **decision support systems** (Pickover 1995).

But what are expert and decision support systems? For many people in healthcare, the mention of these systems evokes notions of a computer application that assists the clinician in caring for patients. Based on symptoms and other data from the patient, the computer system formulates possible diagnoses for the patient's condition and presents these suggestions to the clinician. In difficult cases, possibly involving rare conditions, these suggestions may greatly assist the clinician in formulating a decision regarding the best course of treatment for the patient.

Computer systems that provide such aid and recommendations to clinicians in making clinical decisions for individual patients are an important group of expert and decision support systems used in healthcare. This group of systems typically is called **clinical decision support systems** (CDSS).

This chapter examines the many types of expert and decision support systems that are found in today's healthcare environment. It also describes the infrastructure requirements for decision support systems. Finally, the chapter looks at how artificial intelligence is applied in healthcare and discusses the roles of health information management (HIM) professionals in decision support.

Theory into Practice

Jewish Hospital HealthCare Services (JHHS) is a regional network providing healthcare services at 35 locations throughout Kentucky and southern Indiana. The JHHS network owns two acute care hospitals, one rehab hospital, a home health agency, and a hotel; manages six hospitals; and operates two primary care centers, nine outpatient rehabilitation centers, and three healthy lifestyle centers. In total, JHHS services more than 300,000 patients annually.

JHHS's corporate planning department is responsible for developing strategies and making recommendations on a variety of business issues with costs ranging from $5 to $50 million. Some of these business decisions include:

- Ambulatory care development
- Community needs assessments
- Optimal placement of physicians to maximize patient access and service
- Competitor analysis (physicians and facilities)
- Market analysis (customer location, market share by type of service)
- Employer analysis (where they are and how they use JHHS)
- Drive time and access studies
- Healthcare site selection

As an example, in planning a new healthcare facility, the group must advise corporate officers on the ranking of several sites using identified variables, determine which site is most optimal, and recommend what services each site should incorporate.

To accomplish its healthcare site selection model, the team uses a decision support system (DSS), in particular, a geographical information system, that incorporates healthcare statistics and business data in various planning and allocation models. The system is called ArcView Business Analyst from ESRI. (See www.esri.com/software/businessanalyst/index.html.) Using DSS, the corporate planning team has been very successful in helping the corporation to make good, strategic decisions and helping JHHS to remain competitive.

Decision Support Systems

As business in general and healthcare in particular have entered into the 21st century, a new economic reality has emerged. Known by many different names, this new reality often is called "a knowledge economy" (Hardin et al. 1999). Businesses in a knowledge economy are more reliant on information, and this information resides in their employees and in their corporate data systems. The sum of all this knowledge represents a new form of business asset: **intellectual capital** (Stewart 1997). To be competitive and provide high-quality products and services in a knowledge economy, a business must learn to make right decisions quicker than their competitors do (Senge 1990).

The key point here is decision making. Decision making is a critical task for managers and clinicians. There is no shortage of computers and information technologies. What is important is not simply having information technology to collect data (although in healthcare this is very important as has been seen in the earlier chapters), but how a healthcare organization uses its information to make decisions. Stewart notes that "a corporation becomes a true knowledge company when it becomes aware of and involved in the 'deeper level,' where information is pursued for its own intrinsic value and not simply to automate or report on other activities" (1997, p. 6).

Expert and decision support systems enable business (healthcare) to move beyond automation of activities and begin to use computers to gain knowledge about its customers and its operations. DSSs include the establishment of repositories and **data warehouses** to efficiently store the organization's data in such a way as to make them accessible to managers as they make decisions. It also includes activities associated with **data mining,** which is the process of sorting through the organization's data to identify unusual patterns or to apply analytical models that will assist in predicting future events. Current applications of data-mining activities in healthcare include models to support fraud detection, utilization review, and clinical pathways.

DSSs also assist hospital chief financial officers (CFOs) in allocating financial resources (Friend 1992) and assist health plan administrators in managing the medical care market and formulating appropriate payment plans (Forgionne 1991). Additionally, DSSs assist hospital administrators in evaluating resource utilization (Cunningham and McKenna 1993) and improving the distribution of pharmaceuticals for inpatient patients (Zaki 1989). DSSs are being used and evaluated as tools to prevent medical errors and adverse events (Berner et al. 1999) in response to the serious issues noted in *To Err Is Human: Building a Safer Health System* (Kohn, Corrigan, and Donaldson 2000). The study described in this book shocked many people when it reported that as many as 98,000 people die annually in the United States as a result of medical errors such as:

- *Adverse events,* which are injuries to patients caused by medical mismanagement instead of the patient's underlying disease or medical condition
- *Medication-related errors,* such as accidental drug poisoning
- *Medication adverse events,* which are injuries resulting when, for example, an antibiotic drug is prescribed for a patient with a history of allergic reactions to the antibiotic

The 2001 Institute of Medicine (IOM) report entitled *Crossing the Quality Chasm: A New Health System for the 21st Century* recommends that greater use of DSSs by healthcare providers and organizations will improve the quality of care for patients and help minimize the likelihood of the occurrence of these serious problems.

Definition and Types

Although computers are integral to the implementation of decision support and expert systems, these systems are really about people—how they solve problems, how they think, how they use information and decide which information to use. In essence, these systems indicate how people make decisions. Hence, a study of decision support and expert systems also must incorporate some discussion of people issues.

A DSS is a computer-based system that gathers data from a variety of sources and assists in providing structure to the data using various analytical models and visual tools in order to facilitate and improve the ultimate outcome in decision-making tasks associated with nonroutine and nonrepetitive problems. However, this is but one of many definitions of a DSS. Because the goals involved in these systems have such breadth, no universally agreed-upon definition exists (Turban 1995). Nevertheless, this is a good working definition and captures the important characteristics commonly identified for DSSs. Table 19.1 provides a list of some of these characteristics.

Table 19.1. Common characteristics of a decision support system

- Is used in semistructured or unstructured decision contexts
- Is intended to support decision makers rather to replace them
- Supports all phases of the decision-making process
- Focuses on the effectiveness of the decision-making process rather than its efficiency
- Is under the control of the DSS user
- Uses underlying data and models
- Facilitates learning on the part of the decision maker
- Is interactive and user-friendly
- Is generally developed using an evolutionary, iterative process
- Provides support for all levels of management from top executives to line managers
- Can provide support for multiple independent or interdependent decisions
- Provides support for individual, group-based, and team-based decision-making contexts

Source: Marakas 1999, p. 3.

Notice that the words *expert system* do not appear in the definition above. Was this an oversight? Well, yes and no. Most commonly, an **expert system** (ES) is a computer-based system that can perform problem-solving tasks equal to the performance of human experts and, in some cases, can actually exceed the abilities of human experts. ESs were developed as part of a branch of computer science known as **applied artificial intelligence,** and the vision of some of these efforts has been to replace human experts with computers.

Some people argue that although they have some unique features in their architecture, ESs also satisfy the concepts contained in the definition of DSS. Hence, an ES is simply one type of DSS. However, if the notion in the definition relating to the facilitation role of the DSS is seen as one in which the system suggests possible actions, but the final decision rests with the human decision maker, ESs may go beyond DSSs. Artificial intelligence and this view of ESs is discussed later in this chapter, but for now it suffices to include the ES as a type of DSS.

History and Background

The roots of DSS emanate from two articles that appeared in the early 1970s: "Models and Managers: The Concept of a Decision Calculus," by J.D. Little (1970), and "A Framework for Management Information Systems," by G.A. Gorry and M.S. Scott-Morton (1971). Using ideas from the research of Herbert Simon (1960, 1957) on how people, in particular, managers, make decisions, these two works proposed computer-based systems to assist in unstructured decision making.

Simon argued that decisions were arrayed on a spectrum from highly structured to unstructured. **Structured decisions** arise from very established, repetitive kinds of problems, ones for which standard solutions are available. Examples of areas that provide such decisions are accounts receivable, patient entry, and so on. **Unstructured decisions** depend on the context that produced the need for the decision to provide a framework for the solution.

During World War II, a new branch of applied mathematics, **operations research** (OR), was developed to analyze situations arising out of the war and to propose mathematical models for their solutions. OR proved very effective in providing solutions to structured problems arising in this context. After the war, this new discipline was applied to business problems and a new business discipline, management science, was launched. During the 1950s and 1960s, these new disciplines assumed that decision makers could follow logical and systematic processes for arriving at business decisions by applying the scientific method to business problems. Thus, business problems were analyzed and classified into various general groups (for example, inventory control and scheduling). The key features of each of these general problems were analyzed, and elegant mathematical models and solutions were developed for them. Computer programs then were developed to perform the computations in a quick and efficient manner. Thus, by the late 1960s, the use of computers to provide assistance and support in the solution of structured decisions had become an important tool for business decision makers.

However, more research was still needed for unstructured decisions. According to Simon, unstructured decisions arose from those contexts in which there were no clear-cut solutions and for which the particular problem or decision at hand may never have been encountered previously and may never be encountered again. The set of possible alternatives as well as the relevant data may not be available to the decision maker in these complex decisions.

Decision-Making Process

When faced with decisions, Simon (1960) observed that people use a three-phase approach. A schematic of **Simon's decision-making model** is shown in figure 19.1.

Figure 19.1. Simon's decision-making process

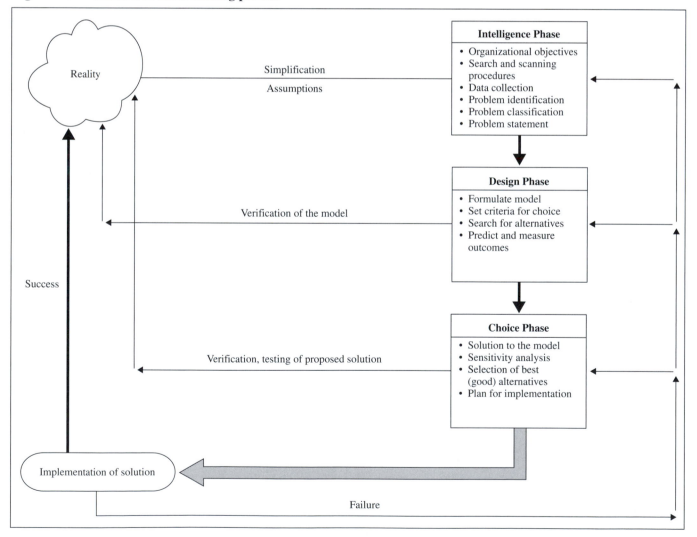

The Intelligence Phase

The first phase of Simon's decision-making model is the intelligence phase. In this phase, the decision maker is attentive to the organization's goals and is on alert for issues that run counter to those goals. The key activities of this phase are problem identification and organizational objective formulation, such as defining the objectives of the problem and what needs to be accomplished. Other activities during this phase may include breaking the problem down into smaller subproblems, problem classification, and data collection. However, the final outcome of this phase should be a careful statement of the problem to be solved or decision to be made.

The Design Phase

In the design phase of the decision-making process, the decision maker identifies possible courses of action and the varieties of decision alternatives, locates the various knowledge sources of relevance to the problem, formulates a basic model for the problem, and determines the criteria to be used to evaluate possible alternatives. Also in this phase, the decision maker may seek to gather various data pertinent to the problem. In developing a model, the decision maker identifies various sets of variables to be included.

The sets of variables used in the modeling aspect of this phase include:

- The outcome, or dependent or target variable(s)
- The variables that can be manipulated or controlled
- The variables that cannot be controlled but are simply part of the context of the problem

The relationships among these variables also must be specified.

Often the decision maker has available standard decision-making models. For example, models developed in management science (such as linear and nonlinear programming, goal programming, integer programming) are helpful in this process; the decision maker simply identifies and gathers the appropriate data and information from within the organization to apply these models accurately to a given situation. Illustrative of this phase, one main aim of a data warehouse is to provide a convenient location from which to obtain any data needed in formulating and then solving such models.

The Choice Phase

In the choice phase, the decision maker applies the criteria decided on in the second phase and searches for the appropriate decision alternative. When the decision has been chosen, it must be evaluated and then a recommendation made as to the final solution to the given problem. Certainly, there is overlap between phases two and three with respect to enumerating the possible alternatives and in evaluating and selecting a decision alternative. This concept of postulating various decision alternatives and then selecting from among them is the classic view of decision making and is illustrated in figure 19.2.

Figure 19.2. Classic view of decision making

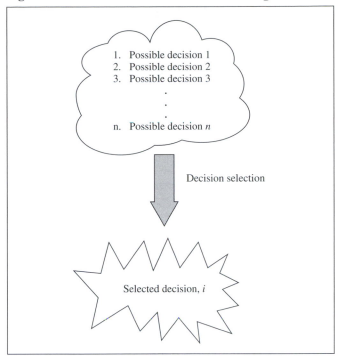

A number of interesting questions can be posed about this process, including:

- How are the alternative decisions postulated?
- How many alternatives should be identified?
- What if there are too many alternatives (as is possible in complex problems)?
- What are possible strategies for selecting among the alternative decisions?

The answer to how the alternatives are postulated lies to a large degree in the creativity of the decision maker; however, having as many sources of data and information available will enhance this activity. In choosing a possible criterion for selecting among alternatives, various options are available depending on the situation. For example, a problem involving the expenditure of capital may involve a large number of alternatives. Hence, the decision maker might select the criterion of maximizing the **return on investment** (ROI) and seek the alternative that gives the greatest ROI.

Because it can be difficult to determine exactly what the ROI will be for various investments, one might elect to use the criterion that the solution should make a "good" ROI possible. Because the definition of *good* in this case is fuzzy, some minimum ROI might be set and the first alternative accepted that exceeds this minimum. The general idea here is that the decision maker will accept any solution that meets the minimum requirements for a solution; it does not have to be the very best solution or even the optimal solution. Simply providing a solution to the problem that meets the requirements renders it a "good" solution. Such an approach is sometimes called a "good enough" solution or a **satisficing** solution (Simon 1977, 1976).

The examples above go through phase two of the decision-making process. The next question concerns how to go about searching through all the alternatives to identify one that fulfills the criterion. This search is part of phase three activities and has various options. One option is to use a "try-one-and-see" approach. The idea is simply to begin evaluating the criterion on a given alternative and see if it works. If it does, we are done; if not, we move on. Selection of alternatives is by chance, and so this option may be called a blind search.

Another option would be to use the mathematical optimization tools developed in operations research and management science and to attempt to select the analytically optimal alternative, one that either maximizes some objective such as ROI or minimizes something like loss. Both blind search and optimal searches, however, may take an exceedingly long time, even on a computer, so other options may need to be considered.

In some situations, other information might be incorporated into the search process. This additional information can be in the form of rules of thumb, hunches, or experience but is nevertheless felt to be accurate. When this type of information is used to help in the search, it is called a "heuristic" search. In cases where the criterion of satisficing is employed, search techniques such as genetic algorithms (a new area in artificial intelligence and machine learning) can be used.

Structure of Decision Support Systems versus Information Systems

Based on the account above of how people make decisions, it is easy to see various types of support that would be helpful to a decision maker. For example, having a data warehouse would facilitate the generation of solutions to ad hoc problems concerning patient case mix, patient payer mix, typical patient flow, length of stay, and so on. Another type of support is assistance in performing any of the searches mentioned. For any realistic problem, such searches would exceed the cognitive limits of most people. Computer-based DSSs were developed to meet these needs.

The functionality of a DSS will be much different from that of an information system (IS). ISs developed as managers began to recognize the need for periodic reports from the transactional or operational systems within the organization. **Transactional systems** perform electronic data processing and storage. They were among the first implementations of computer technology to business during the 1950s and 1960s and are still a primary application today. Such systems include payroll systems, patient billing systems, patient registration systems, accounting systems, and so on.

Tan (2001,1998) applies the term **hospital information system** (HIS) to the transactional systems found in healthcare and uses the term **health management information system** (HMIS) for those systems whose purpose is to pro-vide reports on routine operations and processing. Examples of HIMSs are pharmacy inventory systems, radiological systems, and patient tracking systems. Many of these systems have been discussed in earlier chapters of this book. Neither the HIS nor the HMIS has decision support as its explicit purpose.

As stated earlier, DSS is about people and making decisions, not about data processing. Thus, the structure or architecture of the DSS will reflect this emphasis. Figures 19.3, 19.4, and 19.5 may be used to compare the differences between an HIS, an HMIS, and a DSS. Figure 19.3 presents a conceptual model of a typical HIS (or data-processing system). The key elements of the system relate to data acquisition and entry, storage, retrieval, record keeping, and so on. Typical outputs would include a patient bill, a listing of patient charges, and a list of patients admitted on a given day.

The HMIS presented in figure 19.4 (p. 550) includes some of the same elements as the HIS, in particular, data entry and storage. The key difference is that a standard reports element is added to the system. Thus, the outputs from the system will assist managers in monitoring the operations of the organization. For example, the system may generate a standard report on the number of admissions per week for the past six months. In addition, it could generate a report on the average cost per patient over a given period of time.

Figure 19.5 (p. 551) focuses on the role of the system as a decision tool. First, there is the user interface element. This element provides a friendly and interactive environment for user interaction with system. Ideally, this will be through a **graphical user interface** (GUI), allowing the user to point, click, drag, and drop icon objects on the computer screen to accomplish desired tasks. Input devices include the standard keyboard and the computer mouse.

The second element of the model identifies the sources of data that populate the DSS. These sources are those that a decision maker would turn to in order to obtain more information and knowledge about the problem's background and setting. Such sources would include data from the organization's operational/transactional systems (HIS, HMIS) and could include other sources of external data such as state, regional, or national comparative data.

The DSS must contain some element or subsystem to manage all this information. This element may be divided into a database management subsystem and a model or knowledge-based management subsystem, depending on the sophistication of the DSS.

Perhaps the key element in the DSS is the one that assists in reasoning from the data and knowledge. This element enables the DSS to recognize and solve the problem. In expert systems, this element is often called the **inference engine.** Overall, it is where the DSS integrates the data and knowledge provided from the various sources, uses the structure of the problem as presented to it by the user, and applies its models/reasoning to suggest a feasible decision.

Finally, the DSS must communicate proposed decision options to the user/decision maker. Most often, this communication is accomplished through the same user interface that was used to specify the problem to the system, although it could use a separate system.

DSSs can be classified according to the exact nature of the various elements represented in its model. These elements are discussed in the following subsections.

Data-Based Decision Support Systems

A **data-based DSS** uses a database management approach for its overall organization. Its central focus is on providing access to the various data sources within the organization through one system. In essence, all the data and knowledge management is performed through the database subsystem. The input user interface generally allows the user to specify many forms of ad hoc queries through a graphical interface. The system uses its knowledge system to translate the user's requests into a query format acceptable to the database component. A typical implementation of this system allows the user to specify queries in a pick-and-click or drop-

down manner via the GUI. The system then translates those requests into the database language **SQL** (structured query language). The SQL is submitted to the database system containing the various data sources, and a report is sent back to the user. In healthcare, the STARS® system from ViPS, Inc., is an example of a databased DSS. Most data warehouse systems also fall into this category of DSS.

Model-Based Decision Support Systems

The famous statistician George Box once quipped, "All models are wrong, but some are useful" (1979, p. 202). A model is a generalized, abstract representation of the world in which the decision or problem is located. In fact, all individuals depend on models to help interpret and organize everyday experiences. Experiences and decisions are interpreted and formed in terms of these mental models. These models are constructed from our experiences and education and those of the society in which we live.

A good **model-based DSS** attempts to include as many different models as can be accommodated to provide the user the greatest flexibility in framing the decision situation. For

Figure 19.3. Conceptual model of a health information system

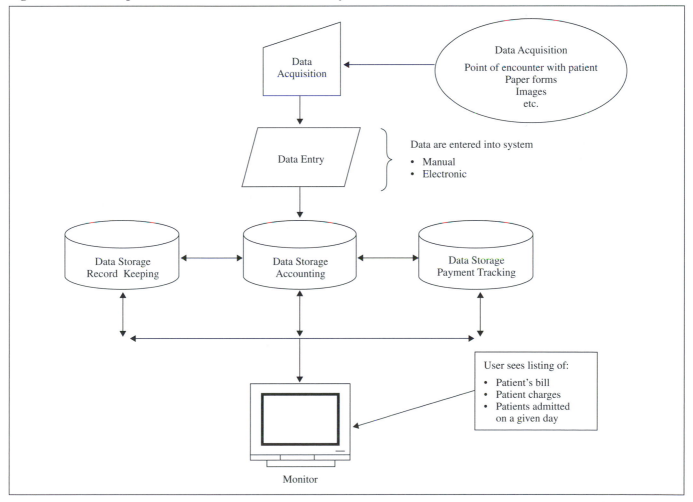

example, the SAS Enterprise Miner tool for data mining provides a large collection of models that the user can select and combine into an overall description of the problem. Other systems may provide specific models such as financial risk analysis or forecasting, depending on the area for which the DSS was developed.

In the model-based DSS, the key element is the subsystem that manages the system's models. The models make up the system's knowledge. The user describes the decision situation to the system in terms of the models available in the system or by using a modeling language. Internal and external data relevant to the needs of the model are accessed and supplied to it, The reasoning element in this system consists primarily of the modules needed to perform the computations or searches as required by the model. Results are provided via the user interface or output system.

Many examples of model-based DSS exist in healthcare. For example, the Episode Treatment Groups system from Symmetry Health Data Systems, Inc., can assist both buyers and providers of healthcare services with case-mix analysis of patients, provider profiling, and severity-of-illness adjustments when making quality of care and financial decisions.

Knowledge-Based Decision Support Systems

A **knowledge-based DSS** is one in which the key element is the knowledge base. Knowledge-based DSSs are often

Figure 19.4.   Conceptual model for a health information management system

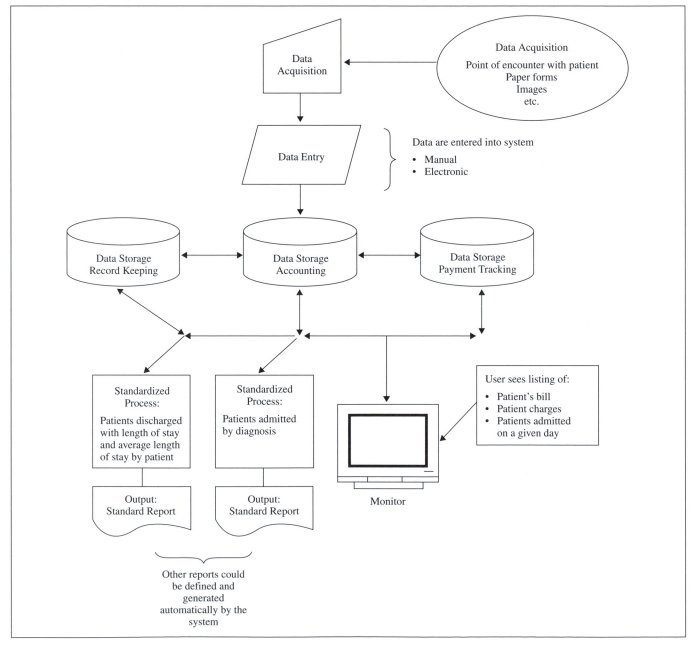

referred to as rule-based systems because the knowledge is stored in the form of rules. For example, a simple rule system is the familiar IF, THEN, ELSE format—if a certain condition is true, then this is an indication of a certain other condition, else the condition is not indicated. By applying general rules of this form to a given situation, a decision is suggested to the user. The form of the rules can be generalized to allow them to have a probabilistic nature. For example, a rule might state that if a given condition is present, there is some probability that another condition is present.

In a knowledge-based DSS, the reasoning element is usually referred to as the inference engine mentioned earlier. The inference engine is a module that can apply and link the appropriate rules together based on the inputs provided by the user. Often the user in a dialog format supplies the input in these systems. The user interface asks the user a question and the user responds. Through the inference engine, the DSS applies the appropriate rule or rules and determines whether more input is needed. This iterative process between user and DSS continues until the DSS either is able to make a suggestion or determines that its knowledge base is not sufficient to make a determination.

Because many of the ideas of the knowledge-based DSS arose from the early work in artificial intelligence in computer science, it is often considered under the framework of expert systems. Examples of knowledge-based systems in

Figure 19.5.   Conceptual model of a decision support system

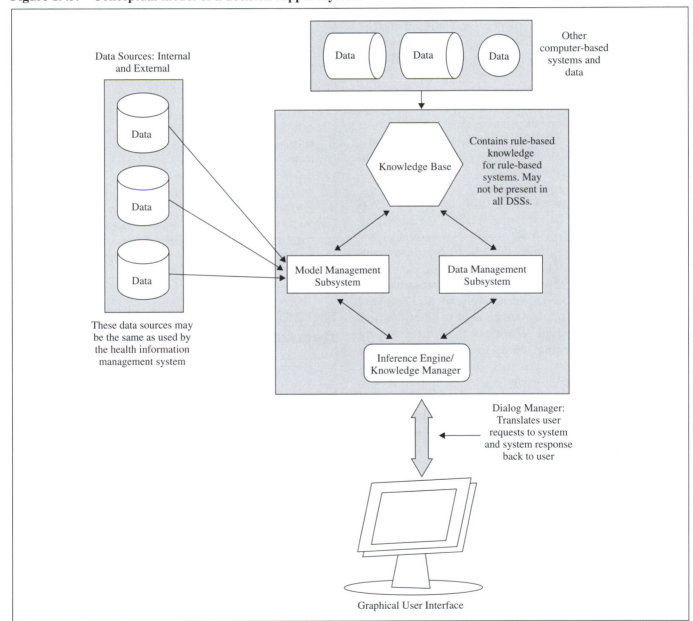

Adapted from Turban 1995, p. 88.

healthcare include the early work of Shortliffe (1976) on his MYCIN system. The MYCIN system provided assistance in diagnosis and therapy selection for patients with blood-borne bacterial infections. Other systems that developed later along these lines are QMR (Quick Medical Reference) by Miller, Masarie, and Myers (1986) and DXplain by Barnett et al. (1987). Artificial intelligence and these types of systems are discussed in later sections of this chapter.

Graphics-Based Decision Support Systems

Graphical tools are becoming more and more important in helping people make decisions. Perhaps the old adage that a picture is worth a thousand words is really true. **Graphics-based DSSs** exploit the human ability to glean patterns and insight from visual presentations of data. Thus, the key element in the architecture of a graphics-based DSS is the user interface. This interface must be carefully constructed and include both hardware and software. The hardware must be able to present detailed visualizations in a timely manner. Further, the type of graphic itself is of fundamental importance.

In a graphics-based DSS, the knowledge base is the collection of graphics that the system is capable of displaying. Common graphics include maps, histograms, and bar charts. However, many systems today involve a complex combination of various graphical displays for both output and input. Depending on the purpose of the DSS, various types of data also must be available to the system.

Many types of graphics-based DSSs have been developed for healthcare. In 1995, the Health Care Financing Administration (HFCA), now renamed the Centers for Medicare and Medicaid Services (CMS), contracted with Los Alamos National Laboratory to develop new techniques for reviewing Medicare claims to detect potentially fraudulent claims and/or providers (http://www.c3.lanl.gov/ccs3web/index2.html). Los Alamos used a variety of new mathematical models and algorithms from the emerging area of **machine learning** and data mining to accomplish their tasks. One result of this work was development of a visualization system that gave the user the ability to spot potential patterns of fraud and abuse. In this case, the data/knowledge element of the system is the claims data, the reasoning element consists of the models and algorithms, and the user interface is the graphical display.

Similar graphical techniques have been developed by other people to detect fraud. These methods use a data-mining technique called **linkage analysis.** Linkage analysis portrays relationships discovered within data sets by a linked network graph. The graph shows interactions among items in the data set and has been applied to fraud investigations in money laundering (for example, Davis 1981; Davidson 1993). Netmap from Alta Europe (www.altaeurope.com), Daisy (www.daisy2000.com), and SAS's Enterprise Miner are examples of general software programs that implement this approach. Today, many healthcare organizations as well as government agencies are investigating linkage analysis as

a DSS tool for containing the increasing cost of healthcare due to fraud and abuse.

Another important graphics-based DSS is the **geographical information system** (GIS). The example cited at the beginning of this chapter illustrates just one use of these types of graphics-based DSSs within healthcare. Other areas of application are also interesting. For example, Begur, Miller, and Weaver (1997) reported on their use of the package MAPINFO (www.mapinfo.com) for the development of a graphics-based GIS system to assist in the routing of home healthcare nurses during their daily visits to ensure the shortest commuting distances and thereby minimize travel expenses.

Check Your Understanding 19.1

Instructions: Answer the following questions on a separate piece of paper.

1. Why is decision support important for modern healthcare?

2. What are some of the challenges facing healthcare that decision support can assist in addressing?

3. What is a decision support system?

4. What is the key difference between a decision support system and an expert system?

5. Out of what discipline from World War II did the study and development of decision support systems come?

6. What are the three phases in Simon's model of the decision-making process?

7. Describe the classical view of decision making.

8. What is the key element in the architecture of a decision support system, and what does it do?

9. Name the four classes of decision support systems.

10. Name at least one important medical decision support system that can be classified as a knowledge-based DSS. Explain why it falls into this classification.

Infrastructure Requirements for Decision Support Systems

What types of organizational and technical infrastructure are required to enable the effective use of decision support systems? To implement effective DSSs, an organization first must have developed at least four key components: (1) a data warehouse or operational data store, (2) a set of data-mining or data-querying tools, (3) a trained group of data analysts or **data miners,** and (4) a trained group of data users. A definition and brief overview of these elements follows. Chapter 20 thoroughly explores data warehousing and data-mining concepts and tools.

Data Warehouses

Data warehouse is a popular concept in information technology (IT) circles today. Almost any conference on IT contains a presentation on some aspect of the corporate data warehouse. The term was coined primarily by William Inmon (1992). Basically, a data warehouse is a database that has the following functions:

- It serves as a neutral storage area for data extracted from an organization's transactional systems.
- It serves as a storage area organized around specific business functions or requirements.
- It provides easy access to business data for analysis or data mining (that is, decision support).

Although various people have proposed different definitions of the data warehouse, all agree that one of its critical aspects is that it is a database. Its content is organized in a subject-specific, integrated, time-invariant, nonvolatile manner using one of several possible data models.

Because its architecture is so important, some people simply define data warehouse as architecture and not as an application or thing. Its architecture refers to how the system is put together or constructed; it is the system's blueprint. Thus, a data warehouse could be thought of as a collection of software systems that includes:

- A database engine allowing access, manipulation, and storage of transactional data
- An application software that allows business analysts to conduct complex business tasks, such as decision support
- A connectivity system that allows the system to communicate with the data sources as well as the end users (that is, client and server[s])

A simplified model of a data warehouse is shown in figure 19.6.

A comparison of the database components of a data warehouse and a transactional system shows that their underlying goals are very different. In a transactional system, the database has been constructed according to well-established principles of relational database design, in particular, **normalization.** Normalization seeks to eliminate redundancy in data storage. The design goal of a transactional system is to eliminate potential errors arising from updating, deleting, or inserting new records into the system, as well as minimizing data redundancy. Thus, a data model for these systems includes many tables, each containing nonredundant data. A data warehouse, on the other hand, is designed to assist the user in querying corporate data. Thus, the underlying design sacrifices data redundancy for query speed and ease of access and use. The data warehouse is not highly normalized.

Two well-known data models are used in designing data warehouses:

- The **star schema** seeks to represent the data within the business context by key business dimensions (time, location, and so on) and by the quantities of interest that are characterized by these dimensions (units sold, dollars spent, length of stay, and so on). For example, suppose the data of interest pertain to patient costs and lengths of stay over time. The star schema organizes the data around a central fact table containing these key business data items and relates the other dimensions of these data items (for example, physician, patient information, procedures, hospital service, time, and so

Figure 19.6. Simplified model of a data warehouse

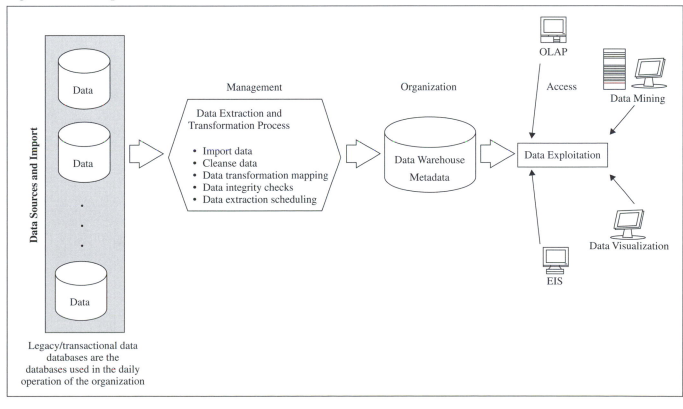

on) through tables linked to the central fact table. The links are accomplished through variables called keys (for example, patient_ID). Figure 19.7 illustrates the star schema.

- The **snowflake schema** allows the dimensions in the star schema to be normalized. Figure 19.8 illustrates the general notion of the snowflake schema.

In healthcare, a closely associated idea is the **clinical repository**. The clinical repository likewise is a database that has been developed using a consistent clinical data model and clinical vocabulary and provides accurate clinical data from the various patient care systems. The clinical repository requires that the other health information and patient care systems be integrated with it to allow data to flow between it and the other systems. Thus, the clinical repository is like the data warehouse in that it serves as a database for storing data from transactional systems.

However, the data warehouse and the clinical repository differ in architecture. Because the clinical repository is integrated into the overall information system, its architecture is best described by the systems with which it interacts. The star and snowflake schemas are typically not utilized in its design. Further, although nonclinical data warehouses are static in nature (their data do not change except as specified on a periodic basis), the clinical repository is constantly changing as new clinical data are available for patient care. And finally, the nonclinical data warehouse is focused on retrospective analyses of business data; the business analyst wishes to tap the corporate data to assist with future decisions. However, the clinical repository is focused on assisting with patient care in a near real-time environment. (Refer to chapter 20 for a detailed discussion of the steps involved in planning and implementing a data warehouse as a component of an organization's knowledge management program and decision support strategy.)

Figure 19.7.   Example star schema for a data warehouse

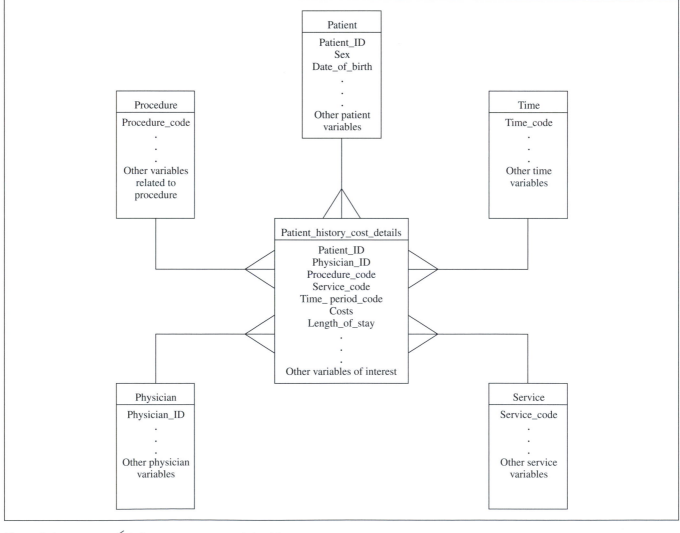

The symbol ————< indicates a one-to-many relationship.

Figure 19.8.   General snowflake schema

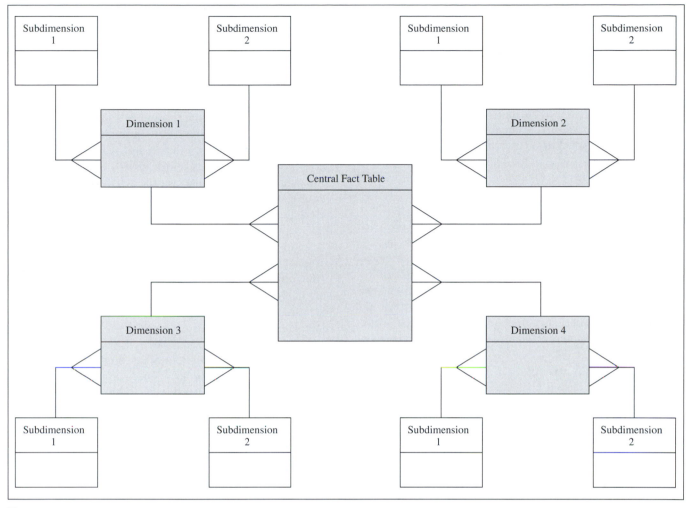

Notes:

1. All dimensions have been shown with exactly two subdimensions for illustrative purposes only. A dimension can have as many subdimensions as necessary.

2. Only generic table names are shown, for example, Dimension 1. In practice, the corresponding variables would appear in the table.

Introduction and Overview of Data-Mining Tools

Data-mining tools exploit the resources of the data warehouse. They enable the end user to query the warehouse, to drill down into the details of the information, to develop models for prediction, and to allow discovery algorithms to highlight new patterns of potential interest. (See chapter 20 for a discussion of the data-mining process and examples of OLAP analyses.)

Online Analytical Processing

One set of tools is **online analytical processing** (OLAP). In discussing the data warehouse, it was mentioned that a key design feature is to recognize that complex business problems are multidimensional in nature. Thus, the data warehouse attempts to identify the key business dimensions of the data and organize the data around those dimensions.

OLAP is an application architecture that was developed to explore the multidimensional aspects of such business data. OLAP stores the data in a **multidimensional data structure** (multidimensional database, or MDDB) and enables the user to examine and view the data along dimensions that may be specific to the context and will be defined by the business rules of the organization. For example, total cost of stay in a hospital has dimensions of time, type of charges involved, and so on. Often this data structure is conceptualized as a data cube, where its dimensions represent the dimensions of the data and the data item of focus, such as cost or length of stay, is viewed as being located in one of the cells of the cube. This process is often referred to as slicing and dicing or drilling down into the data.

The MDDB is often stored in memory, which results in a very fast response to the user. The data in the MDDB are usually aggregated, and many statistics are calculated prior to loading them into the system.

The OLAP database does not have to be part of the data warehouse, but it does extract data from it. The data warehouse database model, though, is often designed with OLAP in mind.

Although OLAP is based on the concepts of multidimensional databases, its implementation by different vendors has resulted in specialized data structures. Thus, OLAP tools have been categorized into several different groups, including:

- **Multidimensional online analytical processing (MOLAP):** MOLAP vendors developed specialized multidimensional data structures, that is, **multidimensional database management systems** (MDDBMSs). A typical business context in which this has worked well is decision support for business problems involving applications of trend or time series analyses.
- **Relational online analytical processing (ROLAP):** ROLAP vendors have sought to develop systems that can access the two-dimensional tables found in a typical **relational database management system** (RDBMS). Using these tables, the user can create a multidimensional view of the data without having to create the multidimensional data structure. ROLAP has been evolving rapidly among vendors, and various implementations are available.
- **Hybrid online analytical processing (HOLAP):** HOLAP is actually a catchall group. With the rapidly changing landscape of technologies, vendors are adopting system architectures that blur the lines of distinction among these various groups.

As mentioned, the data structure on which OLAP is based can provide a convenient platform from which to perform other data mining. However, one important distinction must be noted: Data mining and OLAP are different. As noted above, OLAP gives the user the ability to view and query the data in a multidimensional manner, but it is up to the user to determine which query to submit or what view is required to support a given decision problem. Data mining, on the other hand, seeks to learn from the data or to discover patterns not previously recognized by the user. Additionally, data mining seeks to search for new solutions to problems whereas OLAP must remain passive. Not all people agree with this distinction. Many vendors currently market systems as data-mining systems when, in essence, their true nature is OLAP. They simply provide the user an environment from which to provide drill downs into corporate data.

Machine Learning Techniques

Artificial neural networks (ANNs) and **decision trees** are examples of data-mining tools that use machine learning techniques called **supervised learning.** In supervised learning, the algorithm learns the inherent patterns hidden in the data that predict a specified outcome or target variable. This outcome or target variable must be present in the supplied data set in order for the supervised learning algorithm to proceed. (See chapter 20 for additional discussion of ANNs and decision trees.)

Another class of machine learning techniques is **unsupervised learning.** Unsupervised learning techniques seek to group cases or data records together that are similar or alike in certain respects. The goal of the analysis is to discover previously unknown groupings that exist in the data. A common unsupervised learning algorithm is k-nearest neighbor clustering, a technique applied when data attributes are numeric.

One last machine learning technique that has received a lot of attention for data mining is **rule induction,** or **association rule analysis.** Association rule analysis does not fit neatly into either of the previous categories of learning techniques. Rule induction seeks to uncover the co-occurrences of items within the database. For example, the classic illustration of association rule analysis is the "market basket" analysis. In this case, the analyst wished to determine customer-purchasing behaviors by examining associations among the various items customers place in their shopping baskets.

For instance, if the customer has placed milk in the basket, how likely is he or she to also place bread in the basket? If the customer has placed bread and cheese in the basket, how likely is he or she to also purchase soup? Thus, association rule analysis examines the co-occurrence of items in customers' baskets and produces sets of rules or associations that describe customer-buying behavior. A typical rule produced by an association rule analysis is as follows:

Milk & bread → cheese [support = 2%, confidence = 80%]

Support is the percentage of times that all three items occurred together in all the baskets examined; confidence is the percentage of time that cheese occurred given that both milk and bread were in the basket.

Although this type of analysis may seem of great use to retailers, how can it be used in healthcare? Suppose the "basket" was a person's tenure with a particular company. The various activities, projects, buildings, and jobs that the individual had or was involved in while with the company might be the items in the basket. Interesting questions that an association rule analysis could reveal include:

- Did people who worked in a specific building develop lung cancer?
- Did individuals in certain management positions also experience certain stress-related diseases?

Another example in healthcare is fraud detection. In this case, a "basket" would be a suspected provider or group of providers and the items in the basket would be the codes they billed. An association rule analysis then would suggest interesting co-occurrences of codes billed together. For example,

{short office visit and patient age >65} → {CBC ordered}
[support = 20%, confidence = 98%]

A payer integrity officer may find this association unusual and investigate whether the provider has some financial interest in the lab to which the patients are being referred.

Data Miners

Data miners are those individuals who use the data warehouse and the various analytical tools and software applications to support the decision-making activities of the organization. In this sense, they are decision support analysts. Moreover, data miners understand and can effectively use various data-mining algorithms such as those mentioned above.

In healthcare organizations, data miners may hold degrees in either a clinical or business area. Such an educational background is, in fact, very helpful because it enables the data miner to better understand the context of the decision support problem. However, data miners will need to have other skills as well, including the ability to use relational databases, advanced statistics, and computer programming.

Data Users

Data users include a range of individuals within the organization. At one end of the spectrum is senior management. A senior manager uses reports prepared from the data, often extracting data from the data warehouse, in managing and making decisions for the business. In some cases, a senior manager might use a DSS called an **executive information system** (EIS). An EIS can provide easy access to a variety of corporate data without the need for programming or making requests to other information technologists. Such systems provide predefined queries and reports specifically tailored to address issues of continuing concern to management. For example, the CEO of a health system would be interested in always knowing the past week's number of patients admitted, average length of stay, and total dollars billed and collected. Using available data, an EIS would allow the CEO to generate such reports in her or his office.

Other data users include clinical staff and business staff. Clinical staff use patient data in the routine care of their patients; business staff use data in determining bills, sending out invoices, and crediting accounts.

Thus, many individuals in an enterprise use data. Data miners use data to develop answers for specific issues currently facing the organization, and others use data in their day-to-day jobs.

Check Your Understanding 19.2

Instructions: Answer the following questions on a separate piece of paper.

1. What are the three functions of a data warehouse?

2. What does normalization seek to do in a database?

3. What two well-known data models are used in constructing a data warehouse?

4. How is a data warehouse different from a clinical repository?

5. What do the acronyms OLAP, MOLAP, ROLAP, and HOLAP stand for?

6. What is supervised learning? Unsupervised learning?

7. Name two important data-mining tools.

Uses of Decision Support Systems in Healthcare

Decision support systems are used in a variety of contexts in contemporary healthcare organizations.

Healthcare Decision Support

The term *healthcare decision support* is used here to cover a variety of DSSs used in healthcare, other than clinical decision support, executive decision support, or nursing decision support. In general, these systems all seek to provide the same assistance as a DSS in general, namely, to assist the user in the decision-making process within the domain of the system.

Examples of these systems include medication management and pharmacy order-entry DSSs. These systems assist in warning of possible drug interactions and prescribing errors (Poikonen and Leventhal 1999). Other examples of a healthcare DSS are alert and monitoring tools built into patient information systems.

During the last several years, healthcare has given a lot of attention to quality of care and has used the tools of total quality management (TQM) to measure progress in this arena. Various systems have been proposed and developed that assist in combining data from financial units within a hospital as well as from the clinical areas to allow both administrators and clinicians to examine quality improvement and cost efficiency of services provided to patients. Several recent articles discussing these systems can be found in Howe, Terpening, and Wadhwa (1999), Hohmann, Buff, and Wietecha (1998), and Dexter et al. (2001). These systems all fall within the definition of healthcare decision support.

Clinical/Medical Decision Support

CDSSs were mentioned at the beginning of this chapter. As noted earlier, for many people, the whole notion of the use of computers in medicine conjures up an image of the physician interacting with a computer system to reach a decision regarding a diagnosis for a patient. However, in the broadest sense, a CDSS is any computer system that assists a health professional in making clinical decisions. Some CDSSs include reminder and other alert systems as part of the integration with a general clinical information system.

The CDSS was one of the earliest applications of computers in healthcare. The research on CDSSs dates back to the late 1950s with papers by Ledley and Lusted (1959) and Warner, Garner, and Toronto (1964). Particularly illustrative of the early work in CDSSs is Shortliffe's (1976) seminal work on the MYCIN system. MYCIN was developed to assist physicians in the selection of appropriate antibiotic therapy and was evaluated for patients with blood-borne bacterial infections (Yu et al. 1979). The system was designed using ideas that emerged out of the computer science field of artificial intelligence. Research in artificial intelligence provided new models for developing computer systems that could process and reason from "rules" provided to the system. Most software systems process numbers as input. "Knowledge" of the context of the numbers resides within the program and is "hard-coded" into the system.

Work in artificial intelligence and the resulting area of expert systems provides a means for a computer system to be supplied with a collection of rules that the system can then reason with or chain together to draw new inferences or make new decisions. A typical rule from the MYCIN is given in figure 19.9. Basically, a rule is a conditional statement expressed in an if-then format. Given a condition such that the "if" part of the statement is true, the "then" part of the rule indicates what conclusions are indicated. These rules may be referred to as production rules, condition-action rules, situation-action rules, or if-then rules.

MYCIN used a collection of about 450 rules that were elicited from in-depth interviews with medical experts in the area of antibiotics. The rules then were stored in the system's knowledge base. A knowledge base is the collection of all rules from which an ES can draw in reaching a decision. The component of the system that chains the rules together or reasons from the rules is the inference engine. Two common methodologies for performing this chaining process are forward chaining and backward chaining (Russell and Norvig 1995).

During these early years of research in CDSSs, several other systems also were developed. Gorry and Barnett (1968) developed a model for diagnosis using a sequential Bayesian reasoning system. Using this work, F. T. de Dombal and his colleagues developed a CDSS for diagnosing abdominal pain (de Dombal, Hartley, and Sleeman 1969). In 1975, R. A. Miller and his associates presented the INTERNIST-I system (Pople, Myers, and Miller 1975; Miller et al. 1982). This system, initially called DIALOG, has undergone much development and research over the years and is now best known as QMR (Miller, Masarie, and Myers 1986). In the late 1980s, Otto Barnett and his colleagues proposed the DXplain system (Barnett et al. 1987).

Today, there are many CDSSs, each attempting to address various areas in clinical care. Currently, many researchers are examining how best to integrate these systems into overall medical work flow, in particular, linking these systems to a patient's computer-based health record (Berner et al. 1999). Several examples of recent work in this include Durieux et al. (2000), Gerbert et al. (2000), and Dayton et al. (2000). A recent commercial implementation of a CDSS is found at www.dynasty.com/goSolutions/triage. Two Web-based systems for patients are http://easydiagnosis.com and http://askred.dynasty.com/drd.

Executive Decision Support

Executive decision support systems, often called executive information systems (EISs), are special types of DSSs specifically designed to facilitate and support the decision-making needs of the organization's top executives. They provide easy access to both internal and external data sources relevant to monitoring critical success factors and making strategic decisions. EISs provide overall views of the organization's operations and offer a wide range of views of the data, including drill-down tools and various summarization tools. Table 19.2 lists some common characteristics of a typical EIS.

The term *EIS* was coined at the Massachusetts Institute of Technology (MIT) in the late 1970s and early 1980s (Marakas 1999). Originally, the EIS consisted of a mainframe computer program that pulled together various corporate data and packaged them in an easily readable and accessible format for decision makers. The intent was to assist corporate officers who were either unfamiliar or uncomfortable with working with computers.

Since the early days of EISs, however, the demand for such data and decision support has grown. Today, EISs support not only top-level executives, but also mid- and lower-level managers who require such support. With the advent of the PC and local area networks, such support can easily be offered to an organization's various levels of management.

Although EISs are types of decision support systems, it is important to note a few key differences. First, the EIS

Figure 19.9.   A typical rule from the MYCIN system

Rule 507	
IF:	(1) The infection which requires therapy is meningitis
	(2) Organisms were not seen on the stain of the culture
	(3) The type of infection is bacterial
	(4) The patient does not have a head injury defect, and
	(5) The age of the patient is between 15 years and 55 years
THEN:	The organisms that might be causing the infection are *Diplococcus pneumoniae* and *Neisseria meningitidis*

Source: Musen, Shahar, and Shortliffe 2001, chapter 16.

Table 19.2.   Characteristics of typical executive information systems

Characteristic	Description
Degree of use	High, consistent, without need of technical assistance
Computer skills required	Very low, must be easy to learn and use
Flexibility	High, must fit executive decision-making style
Principal use	Tracking, control
Decisions supported	Upper-level management, unstructured
Data supported	Company internal and external
Output capabilities	Text, tabular, graphical, trend toward audio/video in future
Graphic concentration	High, presentation style
Data access speed	Must be high, fast response

Source: Dobrzeniecki 1994.

generally will not provide the sophisticated modeling and database capabilities that a DSS does. The EIS targets the top-level view and is not intended for the more in-depth analyses provided by a DSS. Second, the EIS is intended to allow executives to gain a quick view or "snapshot" of the organization as a whole, whereas a DSS often provides more detailed support in a particular area of the organization's operation. Third, generally speaking, EISs incorporate external data into the information given to the user, whereas DSSs typically use internal data.

The use of EISs in healthcare has grown over the years. Dobrzeniecki (1994) listed four examples of EIS use in healthcare settings:

- Baylor University Medical Center uses an EIS system called Performance Advisor to assist in creating flexible budgets that allow for different levels of customer activity. The program is a mainframe, general-ledger system.
- Meriter Hospital, in Madison, Wisconsin, adopted a product called Alternative View from Gerber Alley. This product provides an EIS for the hospital's clinical applications and has been part of its TQM effort.
- Samaritan Health Services, in Phoenix, Arizona, adopted the IBM product, Destiny, as its EIS system. The system provides a "briefing book" feature, which organizes information into several folders on key areas of interest. Users can monitor the various areas by selecting the appropriate folder. The system provides summary and trend information in graphical formats.
- The Florida Acute-Care and Teaching Hospitals Healthcare Cost Containment Board adopted MAXPAR, which allows executives to monitor financial, productivity, and physician-related data in all 220 acute care and teaching hospitals in the state of Florida. MAXPAR is an EIS product specifically designed for healthcare. A variety of summary information is available (for example, comparisons of practice patterns and average length of hospital stays for particular procedures). (See chapter 20 for additional discussion of EISs and an example of an in-depth financial/clinical analysis done with an EIS.)

Nursing Decision Support

The role of nursing in the care and treatment of patients is best thought of as complementary to the role of the physician. Physicians diagnose diseases, obtain medical histories, identify disease risks, and prescribe treatments. Nurses, on the other hand, contribute to the cure of patients through their special role of patient care. Nurses assess how patients respond to treatment and therapy and are coping with their conditions and treatments. Nurses develop patient care plans and seek ways to assess patients and alleviate suffering.

Nursing DSSs assist nursing staff in their delivery of patient care. Clearly, the decisions faced by nurses are broad and complex, making the development of such systems difficult. For this reason, to date, there are few nursing DSSs, although some systems have been developed that are similar to the clinical diagnostic DSSs mentioned above. For example, Lagina (1971) developed a system for assessing the anxiety of patients awaiting surgery. A recent interesting study by Ruland (1999) examined the use of decision support to elicit patient preferences and include them in the nursing care plan.

In a broad sense, however, decision support is built into current nursing information systems, especially those that are a part of emerging comprehensive patient information systems. These systems provide nurses with important, timely data on the patient and include alerting and monitoring mechanisms.

Artificial Intelligence Applications in Healthcare

Throughout this chapter, applications in healthcare and decision support have been mentioned from a branch of computer science called artificial intelligence (AI). AI is actually a fairly new branch that originated formally in 1956 when the term was coined (Russell and Norvig 1995). Although AI is generally thought of as being the development of programs for playing games such as chess, making robots, or creating computer systems that talk and interact with people, it is concerned primarily with understanding and building intelligent entities or agents in addition to studying intelligence. Thus, all the things mentioned are part of AI, plus more.

Four areas of AI are discussed in the following subsections.

Natural Language Processing

In 1950, Turning proposed his now-famous test for defining computer or machine intelligence. He proposed a test in which a human integrator would ask questions and interact via teletype with a computer presumably in another location out of the integrator's sight. A computer passed the test when the integrator could tell whether he or she was interacting with a human or a computer at the other end.

For a computer system to pass this test, it must possess at least the capability of **natural language processing** (NLP). NLP is the ability of a computer to understand the full range of meaning contained in languages such as English. The system must be able to process the commands, instructions, or other input when provided by sentences as spoken in normal human discourse. Computer systems have excellent capabilities to process structured or constrained input where the user is limited to certain phrases or when a very specific manner in which to provide input to the system is prescribed. However, natural language has proved to be a very difficult capability for a computer system to acquire.

Recently, some systems have come to market with the ability to learn spoken language. Dictation programs that type as the user speaks have become widely available, and Microsoft Windows XP comes with speech recognition as a standard module. Nevertheless, the user must train these programs by providing as much as 30 minutes of spoken language to the system. Typically, these programs ask the user to read a predefined passage into the system. After the selection is read, training algorithms in the system process the recorded speech and train the system to recognize the user's unique speech patterns. Often such systems require additional training and adjustments. Once trained, however, the user can give verbal commands to the system and have them be performed.

In healthcare, NLP would be a tremendous tool for computer-assisted coding (AHIMA 2004). Such information could be entered directly into the patient's computer-based health record, thus enhancing other decision support tools. However, such systems are still some distance in the future. Although NLP is an active area of research within both the computer science and informatics communities, many challenges still must be overcome. Issues such as a consistent or standard medical vocabulary must be addressed in addition to other technical issues in the speech recognition process.

Expert Systems

Earlier in this chapter, a distinction was made between decision support systems (DSSs) and expert systems (ESs). Discussion of both the knowledge-based DSS and the CDSS, particularly the MYCIN system, has introduced many of the features that characterize an expert system.

An ES attempts to replicate a human expert's ability to solve complex problems in a particular domain. In solving a particular problem, the system employs a set of rules obtained through a knowledge-gathering or engineering process by the developers of the ES. Reasoning is accomplished via an inference algorithm (as mentioned previously) from AI. As mentioned previously, the reasoning component is the inference engine.

ES users are not experts in the particular problem domain. Rather, the ES is developed (ideally) as a surrogate for the expert. Thus, the user is typically inexperienced in the problem domain. In a sense, the goal of an ES is to capture an expert in the computer system.

One of the most difficult tasks in developing an ES is the capture of expert knowledge. This task is exceedingly difficult for several reasons. First, experts do not always know exactly how they arrive at their decisions. Often they have many years of experience and have developed an intuition about the problems and their solutions within the domain. Asking experts to state their knowledge in if-then rules becomes impossible. Second, even when if-then rules can be elicited from an expert(s), ensuring that the rules are consistent is a major challenge. Consistency of the rules means that when the rules are applied, the consequence will not contradict other rules in the collection or simply be circular.

Over the years, ESs have received mixed reactions from researchers and practitioners alike. The early work on MYCIN and other similar systems was groundbreaking. Many ES researchers and developers took as their goals the replacement of the expert with the computer. However, this goal was never fully accomplished. By the mid- to late 1980s, many clinicians questioned the idea of a system that treated the physician as a passive user, unable to solve a given diagnostic problem. Miller (1994) termed this early model of diagnostic support the "Greek oracle" model and noted its weaknesses. He observed that more recent systems have attempted to allow the user more control. The goal is no longer to allow the computer system to be the expert but, rather, to enhance the performance of the user.

In general, people are wary of giving a computer "expert status," especially in healthcare. In a few cases, ESs have been able to meet the goal of practically replacing the expert. An example is the XCON system developed in the 1980s by Digital Equipment Corporation (DEC) for use by sales and service people to configure DEC computer systems for customers. XCON was able to mimic the performance of computer engineers in configuring systems and was used by DEC for several years.

In healthcare, a variety of CDSSs have been developed using ES methodologies. Some of these systems have undergone rigorous evaluation (Berner et al. 1994). Yet, the reactions to these systems remain mixed. Carter observed the activity in this area as being one of "impressive creativity coupled with limited successes, small gains, [and] cynical resignation" (1999, p. 194). He concluded: "Do physicians really want help with the diagnostic process? This is a question of social and cognitive processes for which the answer to-date appears to be a very cool 'perhaps'" (1999, p. 194).

Artificial Neural Networks

ANNs are another important area in AI. They seek to provide mathematical models and computer algorithms that operate in a similar manner to the nervous system, in particular, the brain. The basis for ANNs consists of simple units called perceptrons (similar to the biological unit, neuron). These perceptrons are connected together and work in parallel. As data are presented to the ANNs, learning takes place through the adjustment and modification of weights embedded in the construction of the perceptron.

Research in ANNs began in the late 1940s and 1950s as an attempt to create programs that could reason similarly to human reasoning ability. Although the initial goal of the early researchers was never realized, over the years various ANN models have been developed that are very useful in pattern recognition, clustering, and predictive modeling. Many examples of ANN applications can be found in recent medical literature. Examples include applications involving the use of ANNs to assist radiologists in reading (classifying images), predicting patient outcomes, and developing clinical pathways.

Virtual Reality

Virtual reality (VR) is a recent area of AI. Jaron Lanier, founder of VPL research, coined the term in 1989 (Beier 2001). Since then, the term has been associated with a variety of closely related topics such as artificial reality, artificial life, virtual worlds, virtual environments, and cyberspace. VR is not purely an area of AI but, rather, combines elements from computer simulation and computer graphics and visualization to provide an interactive, computer-mediated experience for the user. In the typical application, the user actually perceives himself or herself as an active participant in the "virtual" world constructed by the computer. To achieve this highly interactive, "virtual" experience, VR applications often require the user to wear some type of sensory device to achieve the immersive experience. Such devices range from a sensory glove or a head-mounted vision display, or both, to recent devices in which the user wears a complete sensory suit. These devices register the user's reactions to various actions occurring in the virtual environment and provide visual feedback and, in some cases, even physical sensations.

The application of VR to medical and healthcare issues has been rapidly occurring. Many other examples are available on the Web as well as in numerous articles and reference materials (for example, Isdale 1993).

The application of VR to decision support, however, is still in its infancy. Some promising directions are in the application of VR to assist in simulating emergencies and training and in monitoring different healthcare workers' reactions. More business-oriented VR applications include examining the location of new facilities, studying traffic flow patterns, and modeling local residents' reactions to real estate development.

Check Your Understanding 19.3

Instructions: Answer the following questions on a separate piece of paper.

1. Name four types of decision support systems found in healthcare.
2. What are the main characteristics of a clinical decision support system?
3. What was the name of one of the earliest CDSSs?
4. What type of inference engine did the system given above use?
5. What are some of the difficulties in maintaining a CDSS?
6. What is a key characteristic of an EIS?
7. What makes the task of decision support for nursing so complex?

Future Roles for HIM Professionals

On March 10, 2003, a task force was convened by the American Health Information Management Association (AHIMA). The group met to discuss the strategic directions of AHIMA and the evolution of the e-HIM initiative. Through a number of dialogues among the participants, including industry and academic leaders, this group charted new roles for HIM professionals in response to identified needs within healthcare organizations today. A variety of new roles related to the area

of decision support were identified. Overall, the group found that HIM professionals will be increasingly required to provide, interpret, and use data as well as provide decision support over the continuum of healthcare. Several of the new roles identified by the group that are directly related to decision support are:

- Content expert (data sets, nomenclature, and classification standards)
- Data analyst
- Data facilitator/data information broker/data information presenter
- Data miner
- Data navigator
- Data quality and integrity monitor
- Data translator

Data analysts, navigators, and facilitators will perform many of the tasks often associated with a research specialist (RS). As outlined by Johns and Hardin (2006), the RS works to create and support decision- and knowledge-based activities within an organization by gathering and analyzing data. Typical job descriptions for RSs will include skills such as proficiency in Microsoft Access and/or SQL server, Visual Basic or Cold Fusion, and a statistical package such as SPSS or SAS.

In addition, these roles will require excellent communication skills and the ability to manage data (verification, examination, and collection).

The skills for a data miner and some data analysts are best described as a combination of the skills required above. In most cases, a data miner also should have at least a master's degree in an area such as health informatics, biostatistics (or applied statistics), epidemiology, or some quantitative health science field.

One difference between the data manager/navigator and some of the other roles listed is that the data miner will not necessarily be involved directly in the collection and management of data from the clinical or other setting. Instead, he or she will use the tools of data mining to better utilize the organization's data resources in making strategic and other business decisions.

Future Development of Decision Support Systems

Many directions are possible for future development of DSSs. The incorporation of NLP into patient information systems may enable quick capture (extraction of discrete data from free text) of physicians' clinical observations. Another avenue of development is to help consumers of healthcare services make more informed decisions. Examples of this direction of development include the APACHE system mentioned in the real-world case and systems such as one that assists low-literacy women in making decisions about options of care and treatment for breast cancer. Jimison and Sher (1999) have written a helpful review that summarizes much of the activity in this area. Future directions also may include the development of systems that can guide nonexpert individuals in providing care for critically injured individuals during catastrophic events such as natural disasters when trained medical personnel are taxed to their limits and unable to meet the needs of all the people who need care.

Real-World Case

According to an article published in the *Naples Daily News* on January 22, 2001 (www.naplesnews.com), Naples Community Hospital in Naples, Florida, recently completed the installation of a computerized decision support system for the hospital's intensive care unit (ICU). The software program assists both physicians and families in making decisions regarding treatment options for seriously ill or injured patients. Using the information available through the hospital's information systems, the new system is able to predict the mortality of the hospital's sickest patients. The system is called APACHE, which stands for Acute Physiology, Age, Chronic Health Evaluation, from APACHE Medical Systems, Inc. (www.apache-msi.com).

The physician, Dr. William Knaus, developed the APACHE manual (or paper-based) scoring system for critically ill patients in 1991. He wanted a way of tracking his patients to monitor their outcomes. According to Vi Shaffer, president of APACHE Medical Systems, Inc., in McLean, Virginia, since 1991, data collected by physicians using APACHE scoring has been obtained on more than 700,000 patients in critical care environments. These data have been used to develop the current APACHE-computerized DSS.

The predictive model that lies at the heart of the system is based on a set of 29 variables. These variables are a mix of various physiological and demographic information on a patient. A second set of data provides information on where the patient was before he or she was admitted to the ICU.

The APACHE system can assist hospital administrators in assessing and monitoring the quality of care within the intensive care area and in monitoring the care received by critically ill patients. Second, it assists physicians in planning the most appropriate course of treatment and care for the patient. Other hospitals that have implemented the system have realized millions of dollars in savings in variable costs because physicians were able to make improved decisions on treatment options for patients.

Naples Community Hospital has 34 ICU beds and is owned by the nonprofit NCH Healthcare System. Two other hospitals in Florida also have implemented the APACHE system: Sarasota Memorial Hospital in Sarasota and Baptist Memorial Hospital in Miami.

Summary

Decision support systems will play an important role in the future of healthcare. Clinical decision support systems, which have received much attention in the past, will continue to play a key role—and perhaps an even more important role than before. As computer-based patient record and patient information systems emerge and develop, the incorporation of clinical decision support in the form of clinical reminders, clinical alerts, medication alerts, and drug interaction monitoring offers great potential for improving the quality of patient care and for eliminating many of the medical errors cited in recent reports. With strong mandates from both consumers and the government, the opportunities for advances in clinical decision support are numerous.

Other areas of decision support also offer great promise for the future. The development of data warehouses, and the use of data-mining tools to exploit this vast mountain of data, will be an important competitive advantage for healthcare organizations. Many already are employing and studying the use of data-mining tools to identify medical errors and adverse events. In other examples, applications of this technology are proving beneficial in developing predictive models to assist in patient care and diagnosis, new facility location, clinical pathway development, identification of inappropriate utilization of healthcare resources, emergency vehicle scheduling in times of crisis, and improved quality of care for patients.

References

AHIMA e-HIM Work Group on Computer-Assisted Coding. 2004. Practice brief: Delving into computer-assisted coding. *Journal of American Health Information Management Association* 75(10):48A–H (with Web extras).

Barnett, G.O., J.J. Cimino, J.A. Hupp, and E.P. Hoffer. 1987. DXplain—An evolving diagnostic decision-support system. *Journal of the American Medical Association* 258(1):67–74

Begur, S.V., D.M. Miller, and J. Weaver. 1997. An integrated spatial DSS for scheduling and routing home-health-care nurses. *Interfaces* 27(4):35–48.

Beier, K.P. 2001. Virtual reality: A short introduction. University of Michigan Virtual Reality Laboratory (VRL). Available online from www-vrl.umich.edu/intro/.

Berner, E.S., et al. 1994. Performance of four computer-based diagnostic decision support systems. *New England Journal of Medicine* 330(25):1792–96.

Berner, E.S., R.S. Maisiak, C.G. Cobbs, and O.D. Taunton. 1999. A computer alert system to prevent injury from adverse drug events development and evaluation in a community teaching hospital. *Journal of the American Medical Informatics Association* 6(5):420–27.

Box, G.E.P. 1979. Robustness in the strategy of scientific model building. In *Robustness in Statistics,* edited by R.L. Launer and G.N. Wilkinson. New York: Academic Press.

Carter, J.H. 1999. Design and implementation issues. In *Clinical Decision Support Systems: Theory and Practice,* edited by Eta S. Berner. New York: Springer.

Cunningham, M., and O. McKenna. 1993. Market model addresses hospitals' need for decision support. *Journal of Medical Systems* 10:65–71.

Davidson, C. 1993. What your database hides away. *New Scientist* 137(1855):28–31.

Davis, R.H. 1981. Social network analysis: An aid in conspiracy investigations. *FBI Law Enforcement Bulletin* 50(12):11–19.

Dayton, C.S., J.S. Ferguson, D.B. Hornick, and M.W. Peterson. 2000. Evaluation of an Internet-based decision-support system for applying the ATS/CDC guidelines for tuberculosis preventive therapy. *Medical Decision Making* 20(1):1–6.

de Dombal, F.T., J.R. Hartley, and D.H. Sleeman. 1969. A computer-assisted system for learning clinical diagnosis. *Lancet* 1:145–48.

Dexter, P., S. Perkins, J.M. Overhage, K. Maharry, R. Kohler, and C.J. McDonald. 2001. A computerized reminder system to increase the use of preventive care for hospitalized patients. *New England Journal of Medicine* 345(13):965–70.

Dobrzeniecki, A. 1994. *Executive Information Systems.* Chicago: ITT Research Institute.

Durieux, P., R. Nizard, P. Ravaud, N. Mounier, and E. Lepage. 2000. A clinical decision support system for the prevention of venous thromboembolism effect on physician behavior. *Journal of the American Medical Association* 283(21):2816–21.

Forgionne, G. 1991. Effectively marketing prepaid medical care with decision support systems. *Health Marketing Quarterly* 8(3/4):107–18.

Friend, D. 1992. Building an EIS your CFO will really use. *Chief Information Officer Journal* 5(1):32–36.

Gerbert, B., A. Bronstone, T. Maurer, R. Hofmann, and T. Berger. 2000. Decision support software to help primary care physicians triage skin cancer: A pilot study. *Archives of Dermatology* 136(2):187–92.

Gorry, G.A., and G.O. Barnett. 1968. Experience with a model of sequential diagnosis. *Computers and Biomedical Research* 1:490–507.

Gorry, G.A., and M.S. Scott-Morton. 1971. A framework for management information systems. *Sloan Management Review* 13:55–70.

Hardin, J.M., P. Miller, A. Whelton, and S. Bellile. 1999. A new role for HIM in the knowledge economy. *Journal of American Health Information Management Association* 70(7):56–59.

Hohmann, S., E.L. Buff, and G. Wietecha. 1998. Monitoring performance improvement using decision support systems. *Journal of American Health Information Management Association* 69(10):36–39.

Howe, R. S., M.B. Terpening, and S. Wadhwa. 1999. Disease management and clinical decision support. *Journal of Healthcare Information Management* 13(2):53–66.

Inmon, W.H. 1992. *Building the Data Warehouse.* New York: John Wiley & Sons.

Institute of Medicine, Committee on Quality of Health Care in America. 2001. *Crossing the Quality Chasm: A New Health System for the 21st Century.* Washington, DC: National Academy Press.

Isdale, J. 1993. Jerry Isdale's VR Page. Available online from isdale.com/jerry/VR/index.html.

Jimison, H.B., and P.R. Sher. 1999. Decision support for patients. In *Clinical Decision Support Systems,* edited by E. Berner. New York: Springer.

Johns, M.L., and J.M. Hardin. 2006. Research and decision support. Ch. 7 in *Ethical Challenges in the Management of Health Information: Process and Strategies for Decision-Making,* edited by L.B. Harman. Sudbury, MA: Jones and Bartlett; Chicago: AHIMA.

Kaufman, D.M., and G.I. Paterson. 1995. Preparing future physicians: How will medical schools meet the challenge? In *Future Health: Computers and Medicine in the Twenty-first Century,* edited by C.A. Pickover. New York: St. Martin's Press.

Kohn, L.T., J.M. Corrigan, and M.S. Donaldson, eds. 2000. *To Err Is Human: Building a Safer Health System.* Washington, DC: National Academy Press.

Lagina, S. 1971. A computer program to diagnose anxiety levels. *Nursing Research* 20(6):484–92.

Ledley, R., and L. Lusted. 1959. Reasoning foundations of medical diagnosis. *Science* 130:9–21.

Little, J.D. 1970. Models and managers: The concept of a decision calculus. *Management Science* 16(8):B466–85.

Marakas, G.M. 1999. *Decision Support Systems in the 21st Century.* Upper Saddle River, NJ: Prentice-Hall.

Miller, R.A. 1994. Medical diagnostic decision support systems—Past, present, and future: A threaded bibliography and commentary. *Journal of the American Medical Informatics Association* 1(1):8–27.

Miller, R.A., F.E. Masarie, and J. Myers. 1986. Quick medical reference (QMR) for diagnostic assistance. *MD Computing* 3(5):34–48.

Miller, R.A., H.E. Pople, Jr., and J. Myers. 1982. Internist-I, an experimental computer-based diagnostic consultant for general internal medicine. *New England Journal of Medicine* 307(8):468–76.

Pickover, C.A., ed. 1995. *Future Health.* New York: St Martins.

Poikonen, J., and J.M. Leventhal. 1999. Medication-management issues at the point of care. *Journal of Healthcare Information Management* 13(2):43–52.

Pople, H.E., J.D. Myers, and R.A. Miller. 1975. DIALOG: A model of diagnostic logic for internal medicine. In *Proceedings of the Fourth International Joint Conference on Artificial Intelligence.* Cambridge, MA: MIT Artificial Intelligence Laboratory Publications.

Ruland, C.M. 1999. Decision support for patient preference-based care planning: Effects on nursing care and patient outcomes. *Journal of American Medical Informatics Association* 6(4):304–12.

Russell, S., and P. Norvig. 1995. *Artificial Intelligence: A Modern Approach.* Upper Saddle River, NJ: Prentice-Hall.

Senge, P. 1990. *The Fifth Discipline: The Art and Practice of the Learning Organization.* New York: Doubleday.

Shams, K., and M. Farishta. 2001. Data warehousing: Toward knowledge management. *Topics in Health Information Management* 21(3):24–32.

Shortliffe, E.H. 1976. *Computer-Based Medical Consultations: MYCIN.* New York: Elsevier.

Simon, H.A. 1976. *Administrative Behavior,* 3rd ed. New York: The Free Press.

Simon, H.A. 1960. *The New Science of Management Decision.* New York: Harper & Row.

Simon, H.A. 1977. *The New Science of Management Decision,* rev. ed. Englewood Cliffs, NJ: Prentice-Hall.

Simon, H.A. 1957. *Models of Man.* New York: John Wiley & Sons.

Stewart, T.A. 1997. *Intellectual Capital.* New York: Doubleday/Currency.

Tan, J.K. 2001. *Health Management Information Systems: Methods and Practical Applications,* 2nd ed. Gaithersburg, MD: Aspen Publishers.

Tan, J.K., and S.Sheps, eds. 1998. *Health Decision Support Systems.* Gaithersburg, MD: Aspen Publishers.

Turban, E. 1995. *Decision Support and Expert Systems: Management Support Systems,* 4th ed. Englewood Cliffs, NJ: Prentice-Hall.

Turning, A. 1950. Computing machinery and intelligence. *Mind* 59:433–60.

Warner, H.R., R.M. Garner, and A.F. Toronto. 1964. Experience with Bayes' theorem for computer diagnosis of congenital heart disease. *Annals of the New York Academy of Science* 115:2–16.

Yu, V.L., et al. 1979. Antimicrobial selection by a computer: A blinded evaluation by infectious disease experts. *Journal of the American Medical Association* 242(12):1279–82.

Zaki, A. 1989. Developing a DSS for a distribution facility: An application in the healthcare industry. *Journal of Medical Systems* 13:331–46.

Chapter 20
Knowledge Management

Kam Shams, MA,
and Mehnaz Farishta, MS

Learning Objectives

- To understand knowledge management as a business discipline
- To recognize the importance of knowledge assets
- To discern the components of a knowledge management initiative/program
- To further explore key knowledge management applications in healthcare, such as data warehousing, executive information systems, online analytical processing, data mining, and customer relationship management
- To apply knowledge management to decision making
- To describe the role of a chief knowledge officer in a healthcare organization

Key Terms

Analysis session
Branding communications
Business intelligence (BI)
Chief knowledge officer (CKO)
Core communications
Customer relationship management (CRM)
Data cube
Data mining
Data warehousing
Decision tree
Executive information system (EIS)
Explicit knowledge
Fuzzy logic
Genetic algorithms
Information assets
K-nearest neighbor (K-NN)
Knowledge
Knowledge assets
Knowledge management
Knowledge production
Knowledge refinement
Knowledge use
Knowledge workers
Learning organization
Multidimensional analysis
Neural networks
Online analytical processing (OLAP)
Online analytical processing (OLAP) engine
Operations support systems (OSS)
Predictive modeling
Relational database management system (RDMS)
Rule induction
Strategic communications
Structured analysis
Tacit knowledge
Unstructured analysis
Wisdom

Introduction

Hidden deep within the minds of individuals and embedded in business processes are nuggets of information and **knowledge** regarding the data, processes, and organizational components that can lead to effective strategic and tactical decisions. Leveraging this knowledge at the right time by the right people is necessary to add value to the healthcare organization's daily decision-making process.

All healthy organizations generate and use knowledge. As organizations interact with their environments, they absorb information, turn it into knowledge, and take action based on it in combination with their experiences, values, and internal rules. Without knowledge, an organization could not organize itself; it would be unable to maintain itself as a functioning enterprise (Davenport and Prusak 2000).

Hence, knowledge is increasingly recognized as a strategically significant resource of the firm and a critical source of competitive advantage (Grant 1996; Prusak 1996). Whereas individuals create knowledge, organizations play a critical role in stimulating knowledge creation, articulating and codifying such knowledge, and cultivating a culture of knowledge augmentation and sharing (Nonaka 1994). In this context, the National Electronic Library for Health defines **knowledge management** as "the creation and subsequent management of an environment which encourages knowledge to be created, shared, learned, enhanced, organized and utilized for the benefit of the organization and its customers" (Oxbrow and Abell 2002, p. 45).

The process of knowledge management, with its various components and applications, can enhance clinical and financial decision making and transform data into **business intelligence** (BI) and **wisdom.** By applying the knowledge management discipline, healthcare organizations can allow their knowledge base to be updated and maintained by **knowledge workers,** closing the gap between the knowledge worker and the organization. Reducing turnaround time for meeting business objectives results in a progressive organization that can maximize the use of its **knowledge assets** for tangible benefits.

This chapter discusses how healthcare organizations can transform data into information and then into wisdom through the process of knowledge management. In addition to defining knowledge management, the chapter presents a five-step framework for a knowledge management initiative and explains how the process can be applied in healthcare organizations using different performance improvement tools.

Theory into Practice

Hospital A began as a small community hospital in Texas. Over the past 10 years, it has become the largest medical center between Austin and Dallas. Founded in 1956 by a charity organization, the hospital has grown in response to growth in the area population. Today, hospital A has four campuses and is part of the ABC Regional Health Network. The health system provides a network of services, including a cancer center; home care health management; women's health centers; rural clinics; and family, emergency, cardiac, and psychiatric services. As part of the ABC Health Network, hospital A is operating as a private for-profit institution. For the past four years, it has been generating modest revenues for the network, whereas the other hospitals in the network have been operating at break-even levels.

Hospital A has undertaken an initiative to increase revenues for the entire network by improving current processes in the areas of data management and customer relationship management. The hospital has a valuable leader in its chief information officer (CIO), who is known for his leadership skills and innovation. The CIO has been promised that in the next fiscal year, he will be allocated a budget of $2 to $3 million to purchase information technology tools to help in the areas his initiative intends to address.

The CIO created a think tank composed of members from various hospital departments, including finance, scheduling/admissions, human resources, medical records, management information systems, accounting, nursing, and medical staff. The team identified the following areas that need data/information and reports:

- The insurance contracts that are currently making money for the hospital
- How to lower the cost for the largest employer in town and whether the hospital should consider direct contracting
- Accounts the collectors should go after when they come to work every morning
- Volume, cost, and profitability by service and location
- Trends in drug use and costs for pharmacy contract negotiations

The team decided to embark on a knowledge management initiative and identified the following tasks:

- Deciding which information technology (IT) tools or applications should be used to fulfill the hospital's data/reporting needs
- Cataloging the knowledge assets of the organization and sharing the findings, especially to determine what has already been achieved in those areas
- Identifying gaps that exist in the current system and explaining the underlying reasons
- Selecting the knowledge management application(s) to address the information needs identified
- Developing recommendations for creating a culture of knowledge management in the organization
- Deciding whether to recommend the creation of a chief knowledge officer role in the organization

From Knowledge to Wisdom

The U.S. healthcare system is complex and polarized with inexorable pressure on both payers and providers to achieve cost and quality improvements. To achieve shared cost and quality goals, payers, providers and healthcare management need rapid access to a broad range of reliable data, some of which traditionally reside with payers, others with providers (Cintron-Allen 2004). It also is a fact that the U.S. healthcare industry has been slow to adopt innovations in IT that can help streamline workflow to make sense of the wide range of healthcare data, citing the uniqueness of its business as the reason for the sluggishness. However, increased regulation and competitive market forces have required the industry to become more efficient, effective, and customer oriented similar to other leading industries. Thus, decision support systems and knowledge management applications have assumed an increasingly important role in enabling the industry to adjust to change. These applications are being applied in several healthcare areas in an effort to:

- Determine the cost-effectiveness of treatment protocols
- Understand the cost structures of services
- Find patterns in data that are of significance
- Forecast trends to make sense of the monumental amount of healthcare data
- Implement process redesign initiatives to enhance customer service

The creation, communication, and absorption of information within a system pose enormous challenges for healthcare management, especially when dealing with legacy healthcare information systems (HIS). Most legacy information applications still operate in a linear fashion, creating information in isolated stages in the same way that cars are manufactured (Loshin 2001).

Legacy systems focus primarily on providing operational applications to meet day-to-day hospital clerical and tactical needs. They are transaction based, with single platforms and hierarchical databases that provide fragmented decision support. Although this continues to be essential in running many aspects of today's healthcare environment, it poses an interesting challenge in the rapidly changing world of healthcare in which the acute care service component has shifted toward ambulatory care and there is renewed emphasis on chronic and long-term care management. Thus, in the new paradigm, the emphasis is on knowledge management applications rather than traditional HIS systems.

Knowledge management applications are end-user centric, with graphical user interface (GUI) and Web-based applications, and use the power of relational database technology to provide holistic decision support. (See figure 20.1 for a comparison of the paradigm shift in healthcare organizations.) Moreover, there is a tremendous need to integrate all components of the local healthcare delivery system, which

Figure 20.1.   Comparison of information management paradigms in healthcare organizations

Old Healthcare Paradigm	New Healthcare Paradigm
Health information system	Enterprisewide knowledge management system
Operation oriented	Analysis oriented
Hierarchical database	Relational database
Programmer centric	End-user centric
Silo based	Process based
Character based	GUI/WEB based
Fragmented decision support	Holistic decision support

is reflected in the new healthcare economy. Traditional HIS vendors have struggled to handle this evolving healthcare model. They also have struggled with the adaptation of emerging technology to meet the changing needs of the new marketplace.

Information growth is accelerating beyond the scope of most healthcare information systems. In 2000, for example, the International Data Corporation predicted that the information distributed through corporate intranets would undergo a phenomenal growth of more than 37 times by the year 2002. Regardless of the actual growth percent, this is a lot of information to deal with, and most healthcare IT systems and organizations will struggle with its effective management and utilization (Grammer 2000).

Thus, it is not surprising that most organizations are seeking new IT tools that are based on open systems and have the capabilities to perform knowledge management-related functions. In stride, the IT marketplace is exploding with options and software that allow organizations to add on to their current HIS systems in order to make them more useful, more productive, and less costly and, at the same time, to leverage their current investment. Hence, overall, IT spending is on the rise, albeit being plagued with periods of relatively low activity in the healthcare sector. According to Forrester Research, a Cambridge, Massachusetts–based technology research firm, technology spending by U.S. companies and governments has recovered from the downturn of 2001 to 2003 to grow by relatively modest annual growth rates of 6 percent from 2003 to 2008 (Bartels et al. 2004a).

In a postcapitalist society, Peter Drucker wrote: "The basic economic resource is no longer capital, nor natural resources, nor labor. It is and will be knowledge. Value is now created by 'productivity' and 'innovation,' both applications of knowledge to work" (Penny 2000). The organizations that can leverage technology to exploit their data through the use of data warehousing, **customer relationship management** (CRM), and **data mining** not only have BI as a corollary but also create a competitive advantage for themselves. By identifying trends, unusual patterns, and hidden relationships that a competitor may not realize, these organizations can create new opportunities for growth and will thrive in the changing healthcare marketplace. In this context, some can argue that the extent of use of IT in the organization is almost directly related to the adoption of knowledge management.

Knowledge Management Defined

Knowledge, or the awareness and understanding gained through experience, is not held within an organization itself but, rather, by the various individuals who make up the organization. An organization's viability directly depends on how the organization captures and harnesses knowledge to help it identify the best business practices and to refine and improve them during changing times.

As described in a white paper by Gallagher Financial Systems, Inc. (1999), knowledge management is a process that attempts to identify and capture knowledge to enable individuals to share it, to leverage existing knowledge in the creation of new knowledge, and to use it to define and improve business practices. Additionally, knowledge management may be defined as the practice of treating knowledge like any other business asset, in other words, as something to be used, maintained, and expanded to the benefit of the organization. From a practical standpoint, organizations need to know what, how, why, where, and when to use their knowledge in order to be successful. Hence, they need to view knowledge management as a strategic way of integrating organizational know-how, processes, and learning (Lau 2004).

It is only when healthcare leadership realizes the potential power of information in the creation of knowledge as a critical corporate asset that the foundation of a knowledge-centric organization can be laid. This signals the migration from an industrial-age view of data to a knowledge-age view, where many data sets are aggregated, fused, enhanced, and broadcast to share an enterprise-wide knowledge base (Loshin 2001). Thus, knowledge management accelerates learning and decision making and leverages expertise and technology to enable smart organizations to achieve peak performance. It is a process, not an end product.

Most corporate knowledge resides in the heads of employees digesting vast amounts of information. Although information is captured, knowledge usually is not. Bits of it leave at the end of every employee's tenure (Grammer 2000). Thus, knowledge management must be acknowledged as a business discipline that depends on various knowledge assets, or sources of knowledge, for an organization, and not merely as a software application. The Gartner Group captures this concept in its definition of knowledge management. According to its definition, knowledge management is a discipline that promotes an integrated and collaborative approach to the process of information asset creation, capture, organization, access, and use. **Information assets** include databases, documents and, most important, the tacit expertise and experience resident in the organization's employees. Simply put, "A simple definition for KM [knowledge management] is formalizing the management of an enterprise's intellectual assets" (Harris and Berg 2003). Another interesting perspective comes from Douglas Dotan in his paper presented at The Quality Colloquium, Harvard University: "Knowledge management is defined as the art and science of changing or transforming data and information into useful knowledge" (2003).

The key to the aforementioned perspectives is identifying knowledge management as a discipline rather than a technology. Healthcare management must recognize that, as a discipline, knowledge management requires cultural and process changes in order for the organization to have a return on investment (ROI). Technology is certainly the enabler to ascertain business/corporate intelligence, but without cultural change, organizations cannot reap the full benefits of adopting a knowledge management initiative. Knowledge management puts forth the goal of achieving competitive advantage by leveraging the vast knowledge of collective corporate memory.

Managing Knowledge

In this context, it is important to look at ways organizations can manage knowledge effectively. The following section lists some recommendations to successfully manage knowledge (Hughes 2001):

1. The organization must create a knowledge management vision supported by concrete principles and strategies to realize it
2. The organization must develop a knowledge management culture that celebrates diverse viewpoints and encourages collaboration and knowledge sharing.
3. The organization must provide materials that support knowledge management, for instance, databases, communication, and Web technology; groupware such as white boards, online conferencing software, or video-conferencing equipment; job aids such as knowledge maps and computer-based performance support; and physical structures such as learning centers, and so on.
4. The organization must establish and support staff in the acquisition of core competencies, including technical expertise and knowledge, the skills necessary to identify, categorize, save, and share knowledge, as well as the ability to locate or mine knowledge from human and computer sources.
5. The organization must develop and implement a mechanism to integrate knowledge residing in human minds with knowledge residing in documents.
6. The organization must establish systems to communicate, structure, categorize, analyze, and locate knowledge, as knowledge needs to be continually renewed, replenished, and expanded, as well as categorized and archived to avoid knowledge overload.
7. The organization must implement systems that will protect the organization's knowledge assets from unauthorized access and use.

Conceptual Framework of Knowledge Management in Healthcare

The concept of knowledge management in a healthcare setting can be understood further by breaking it down into the following key components as a conceptual framework:

- Knowledge production
- Knowledge use
- Knowledge refinement

These components are all within the social context of the underlying structures, values, and preferences of individuals and organizations. Briefly, **knowledge production** involves the creation of knowledge through collection, generation, synthesis, and identification. It also involves the organization of knowledge through codification, storage, packaging, and coordination. **Knowledge use** consists of distribution, sharing, application, and integration of knowledge. Finally, **knowledge refinement** consists of evaluation, reflection, adaptation, and sustainability (Lau 2004). (See figure 20.2.)

More details are necessary here to understand this framework as proposed by Dr. Francis Lau. It is important to remember that the author defines knowledge as information combined with experience, context, interpretation, and reflection. The knowledge source may be explicit or tacit depending on where it is located (for example, policy document versus individual expert). The author concludes that knowledge management, then, is the systematic approach to translating between the explicit and tacit forms of this knowledge in a given context. In this conceptual framework of knowledge management in healthcare, the three knowledge sources of particular interest to the author are policy synthesis, research findings, and local practices, referred to by the Canadian Health Services Research Foundation as policy, evidence, and experience, respectively.

Knowledge Production

Knowledge production refers to different means of creating and organizing policy, evidence, and experience. The creation of such knowledge in particular settings from policy syntheses, research findings, and local practices involves these subconcepts.

Figure 20.2.   A conceptual knowledge management framework in healthcare

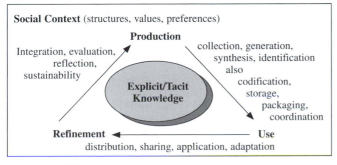

Source: Lau 2004, p. 8.

- The collection of local experience around specific clinical cases and health services/programs that reflect practice norms, organizational forms, and values/preferences in a particular health setting
- The generation of new understandings of relationships among specific factors, processes, and outcomes from primary research and policy development such as a randomized trial or case study in a particular health setting
- The synthesis of available research findings, policy advice, and local experiences in specific areas of health through a critical review process such as systematic review
- The identification of individuals, groups, and organizations as resources with expertise or experience in specific areas of health who are willing to share their tacit knowledge

As policy, evidence, and experience are being created, some formal means of organizing this knowledge is required. Depending on whether the knowledge is explicit or tacit, it may be stored in repositories as artifacts or acknowledged as intellectual resources for consultation. The subconcepts for organizing policy, evidence, and experience are:

- The codification of knowledge using appropriate nomenclature for its description, classification, and indexing (examples include the use of Systematized Nomenclature of Medicine, or SNOMED to codify practice experiences, structured abstracts for scientific literature, and policy synthesis briefs for options analysis)
- The storage of knowledge in computer-based repositories to allow its retrieval, updating, monitoring, and archiving
- The packaging of knowledge with different levels/types of content details and delivery modalities targeted at specific groups of policymakers, practitioners, and researchers
- The coordination of intellectual resources on such details as their expertise, experience, location, and availability

Knowledge Use

Knowledge use refers to the manner by which policymakers, practitioners, and researchers use policy, evidence, and experience as knowledge within the local setting. As such, this knowledge not only needs to be disseminated to the intended audience, but it also must be translated and even modified to suit local circumstances such as geographical, value, and cultural differences. The subconcepts for knowledge use are:

- The distribution of knowledge through different modalities such as newsletters, bulletins, policy briefs, and Web-based resources to targeted audiences
- The sharing of knowledge through interpersonal communications and dialogues via such forums as workshops

- The application of the knowledge within a local setting as new policies, guidelines, or practice routines
- The adaptation of the knowledge to suit local circumstances such as values, cultures, and norms for implementation in a specific health setting

Knowledge Refinement

Knowledge refinement refers to ways in which policy, evidence, and experience as knowledge sources are institutionalized with organizations over time as part of routine practices in a taken-for-granted fashion. The means of knowledge refinement are:

- The integration of knowledge with or without adaptations as part of existing work processes and practice norms in a taken-for-granted fashion within the local setting
- The evaluation of a specific knowledge source using different structure, process, and outcome/output measures such as quality of knowledge produced, extent of its use in a given setting, and effect on the organization and its staff
- The reflection on the knowledge source through subjective interpretations by policymakers, practitioners, and researchers (examples include personal experiences and lessons learned from those involved with producing and using the knowledge in a given setting)
- The sustainability of the knowledge management approach by ensuring that policymakers, practitioners, and researchers are committed to ongoing production, use, and refinement of the knowledge sources within the local setting

Social Context

The production, use, and refinement of policy, evidence, and experience as knowledge takes place in a complex and changing context, which renders these concepts unique and difficult to replicate. This evolving context is influenced by social structures, value systems, and personal choices as outlined below:

- *Structures* provide the organization, rules, and processes that make up the social environment where policymakers, practitioners, and researchers reside and operate.
- *Values* are personal viewpoints, morals, and standards used by policymakers, practitioners, and researchers as guiding principles for their beliefs and actions.
- *Preferences* are choices and priorities set by policymakers, practitioners, and researchers on a wide range of health issues based on their belief systems and needs.

Knowledge Management Process

Knowledge management also transforms data into information and then into knowledge, which eventually creates wisdom or BI for the organization. (See figure 20.3.) This section describes the constituents of BI or, rather, the end

Figure 20.3.   Transformation of data to information to knowledge to wisdom

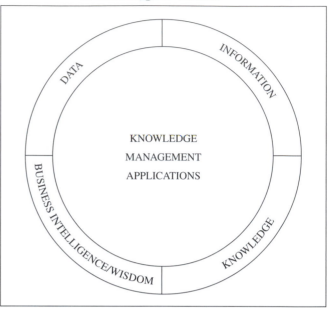

product of knowledge management, which improves an enterprise's ability to make good decisions and makes information available to everyone in the enterprise.

As explained in earlier chapters, data can be broadly defined as a collection of facts—facts about specific events and objects and about an industry in general—that can be analyzed. The facts originate from a variety of sources and include raw statistics such as demographic, billing, nursing, pharmacy, laboratory, and marketing information. Thus, data can form the basis of knowledge as they are gathered, analyzed, and synthesized by individuals within the organization. Healthcare relies heavily on transaction processing systems because they are capable of collecting and processing large amounts of data, which is crucial for knowledge management solutions.

Sometimes referred to as **explicit knowledge,** information results from the collection and communication of ideas and experiences. The process involves combining and/or summarizing data from different sources to create information that affects decisions because it influences the way people interpret their environment and the underlying trends in their day-to-day operations (Allison 2000).

Knowledge management or BI applications that have ad hoc query and reporting capabilities enable users to extract data from a database. By placing data in a context that produces meaning, these applications give users the ability to create information. The creation of information is an extensive process that involves constantly separating and regrouping data to extend their value. Applications that have **online analytical processing** (OLAP) **engines** allow users to analyze data and determine relationships, patterns, trends, and exceptions. An OLAP engine is an optimized query generator that can retrieve the right information from the warehouse to accommodate what-if business queries. This process further paves the way for the ultimate transition of information into knowledge and BI.

Knowledge involves much more than storing information and recalling it when the time is appropriate. Translating information into knowledge requires robust IT tools, experience, and reflection. Combining information with experience, knowledge helps provide a context in which new information can be created and interpreted when compared to previously acquired information. Because knowledge comprises ideas, experiences, and insights, true knowledge is often referred to as **tacit knowledge.** It is important to note that knowledge in itself means nothing if appropriate action does not follow. This leads to the end goal of the knowledge management process—creating BI for the organization. For this reason, intelligence, or wisdom, is defined as the empowerment and courage to act (English 1999).

Knowledge represents the intelligence that individuals apply to data and information in order to make decisions and draw conclusions. Without intelligence, information cannot become knowledge. Thus, the possession of knowledge, along with intelligence and the ability to create new knowledge, determines an organization's success in accelerating business processes and reducing and eliminating nonvalue-added activities, which is one of the major goals of a knowledge management initiative.

Return on Knowledge Assets

Implementation of knowledge assets in the organization's IT infrastructure maximizes its ROI. Data warehousing, data mining, CRM, and OLAP are all tools and applications that bring knowledge management to the forefront of the organization. Data stored in the organization's databases and other data sources are retrieved and used to perform various functions and to make important decisions. When data are inaccurate, missing, or used ineffectively, the processes performed and decisions made by the organization will be impaired. Therefore, it is important that the organization adopt the discipline of knowledge management to become a **learning organization.** A learning organization focuses on acquiring and sharing knowledge and making information available to all.

Knowledge management initiatives play a key role in the organization's overall health in numerous ways, including by:

- Reducing costs of information gathering and decision support that add no value to the business
- Improving customer support processes so that questions are answered faster and more accurately
- Identifying new market opportunities
- Reducing the knowledge gap that exists when key personnel leave an organization

When all identified knowledge assets are documented and communicated, it is possible to capture and retain informa-

tion as well as tacit knowledge. Finally, if a sound knowledge management mechanism is in place, the knowledge acquired can be shared among users, which raises the organization's strategic acumen in general. As workers share knowledge, they improve their performance, are able to make better decisions, and are transformed into knowledge workers. Thus, the organization is able to respond in a timely manner to changes in the marketplace. Moreover, as knowledge is documented and shared, it becomes easier to retain tacit knowledge for new employees and to reduce errors.

Knowledge management or BI applications that have data mining capabilities enable users to identify hidden trends and unusual patterns within the data. Without the use of a data mining application, this effort would be extremely time consuming. Similarly, data warehousing is a knowledge management application that aids knowledge acquisition and knowledge transfer. Using a variety of data sources, business processes, and organizational departments, data warehousing puts information into context. In addition, it extracts strategic knowledge from the raw data, enabling organizations to deliver the knowledge to the right people for timely and powerful responses to changing healthcare needs. This is how the adoption of knowledge management takes advantage of intellectual assets and increases business performance.

Knowledge Management Programs and Initiatives

Before embarking on a knowledge management initiative, it is important to identify the sources of knowledge, or knowledge assets, of an organization. (See figure 20.4.) These assets include printed documents, unwritten rules, work flows, customer knowledge, databases/spreadsheets, and human expertise and know-how. Knowledge as information in a context that supports proper decisions and actions exists as both explicit and tacit knowledge. Explicit knowledge refers to knowledge that is fully and clearly expressed and defined, and it includes documents, databases, and other types of recorded and documented information. On the other

Figure 20.4.   Knowledge assets in a healthcare organization

Explicit Knowledge
Documents
Spreadsheets
Databases
Recorded and documented information
Health information systems
Inventory of all applications and tools to leverage information
Tacit Knowledge
Human expertise and know-how
Actions, ideals, values, and emotions of individuals
Corporate culture
Work flow
Professional experience
Corporate memory
Intellectual assets

hand, tacit knowledge is implied by or inferred from actions or statements. Hence, the actions, experiences, ideals, values, and emotions of an individual constitute tacit knowledge. Tacit knowledge tends to be highly personal and difficult to communicate. Corporate culture, organizational politics, and professional experience are common examples of tacit knowledge.

It also is crucial to develop an organized framework to capture knowledge and transform it into BI. The basic framework of a knowledge management initiative consists of five steps. Underlying these steps are two general principles that help chart the course toward knowledge management. The first principle is to realize the challenges faced by the organization; the second is to develop principles for success. (See figure 20.5.) Principles for success include an emphasis on learning, integrating, and sharing data/information/knowledge across an enterprise, regardless of individual departments; on identifying the ROI; and finally, on selecting robust solutions, such as data warehousing, OLAP, data marts, executive information systems, data mining, and so on, that create BI.

The following five steps of a knowledge management initiative guarantee the transformation of an ordinary organization into a learning organization.

Step 1: Categorize the Organization's Knowledge Assets

As mentioned earlier, the organization's knowledge assets include both explicit physical assets (spreadsheets, documents, databases, and so on) and tacit intellectual assets (the collective knowledge, human expertise, and know-how of the organization's employees and staff). They also include an inventory of all applications and tools that are in place to leverage information, such as data warehousing applications, data marts, transaction processing systems, and so on. While categorizing explicit knowledge assets (even though this knowledge is documented), it is not always clear where to find the desired information because it exists in many locations and forms. Additionally, it can be difficult to determine correlations among different information components to form useful knowledge and to separate out-of-date information from current information. Similarly, grouping tacit

knowledge assets is a challenge. Tacit knowledge is shared via word of mouth and shared experiences, but at some point it becomes impractical to rely on word of mouth to convey appropriate tacit knowledge throughout an organization.

It is important to realize that data and information can exist in the absence of people. However, knowledge can exist only as a characteristic in people when they apply their experience and reason to recognize the significance of information. Wisdom requires actions that lead to the accomplishment of good results. It also requires empowered and motivated people to act on knowledge. Therefore, the first step in categorizing knowledge assets is to recognize that merely doing an audit is not sufficient. It is equally important to consider whether the knowledge assets can be shared with others in the organization. It is in this process of sharing lessons learned that knowledge can be leveraged, and it is this leveraging of knowledge and information that multiplies the value of the organization's knowledge assets (English 1999).

Steps 2 and 3: Analyze the Cost and Value of Current Knowledge Assets and Identify Problems That Current Assets Cannot Solve

Completion of the first step, creating an inventory of systems and information within an organization, makes it easier to determine the value of the information and its associated update and maintenance costs. Outdated information often makes it difficult to retrieve important information in a timely manner. Other times, new information is created that may or may not add to the overall picture. Thus, it is important to take stock of information that is of value to the organization.

In addition, a detailed analysis is prudent at this stage to ensure that the existing applications and systems (such as the HIS, online transaction systems, and others) are producing results that are in line with the organization's objectives. Key questions to consider include:

- Is the organization able to use the information effectively?
- Is the information readily available?
- Is the information accessible to all decision makers in a timely manner?
- Is the information creating a strategic advantage for the organization?

In addition, costs are associated with these systems and applications in terms of hardware, software, and manpower. When there is no ROI in terms of leveraging information and using these systems to their optimum potential, it is even more crucial to embark on a knowledge management initiative that can support these applications and add innovation where it is lacking to ensure an affirmative response to the preceding key questions.

Thus, analyzing the cost and value of current assets and identifying problems that current assets cannot solve are

Figure 20.5.   The course of knowledge management

Individual Challenge	Available
Admit that knowledge is inaccessible	Data warehousing
Identify business problems	OLAP tools
Identify target audience	Smart EMR
	DSS EIS
Principles for Success	Document warehousing
Analyze return on investment	
Integrate sharing of culture between HIS and HIM	
Learn! Learn! Learn!	
Keep WWW in mind	
Aim for robust solutions	

crucial steps in identifying gaps in the current system and seeking appropriate solutions that will bridge them and strategically maneuver the organization to survive in today's competitive healthcare environment.

Step 4: Build a Culture That Encourages the Capture of Knowledge Targeted to Achieve the Organization's Objectives and Goals

The emphasis on knowledge retrieval is a key component of this step to make explicit knowledge readily available to users and to have tacit knowledge documented. Additionally, this step requires organizations to use communication technologies and virtual teams to break down the cultural and geographic barriers to knowledge sharing (Penny 2000).

Another important part of this step is to create a process that will motivate employees to share knowledge. Employees sometimes hesitate to share their knowledge because of a perception that their job or role in the organization could become obsolete. Technology can enable the organization to overcome some of these cultural barriers (Penny 2000). Creating a culture of knowledge also requires that steps be taken to encourage the use of information by all users. For this purpose, information/knowledge must be easily available to knowledge workers across the organization.

Step 5: Deploy and Implement Knowledge Management and BI Applications

After a culture of knowledge management is adopted, the final step of a knowledge management initiative is to deploy and implement knowledge management and BI applications. The combination of data warehouses and analytical tool sets has given organizations the ability to drill down into integrated data to reveal cost savings and competitively differentiating findings. Organizations can rely on BI analysis to provide hard facts that will help them make better, more informed decisions and reap unforeseen rewards (Goldman 2001).

In this context, data warehousing is by far one of the most important knowledge management applications. It has the potential to eliminate the barriers between data and the business analysts who need them, improve data quality, and integrate internal and external data. All these promises make knowledge discovery more efficient, improve knowledge transfer, or provide information that, as a byproduct, points the organization to areas where it needs to gain more knowledge (Allison 2000).

Although data warehousing is vital to the data-intensive healthcare industry, it cannot be a panacea. A well-designed BI system also exploits technologies such as online analytical processing, an **executive information system** (EIS), client/server computing, the Internet and intranets, new **relational database management systems** (RDMSs), parallel processing, and advanced microprocessors. Success in adopting any of these BI applications lies in proper planning and implementation and in management support and leadership, which are necessary to remove barriers to change that may exist in the organization.

Check Your Understanding 20.1

Instructions: Answer the following questions on a separate piece of paper.

1. In what ways does knowledge management apply to healthcare services?
2. Where is knowledge found in healthcare organizations?
3. List and describe the five steps or components of a knowledge management program.
4. What is the difference between information and knowledge?
5. What is the difference between knowledge and wisdom?
6. What is the difference between explicit knowledge and tacit knowledge?

Knowledge Management Applications in Healthcare Organizations

Bill Gates, CEO of Microsoft, described the qualities of leadership in an interview in *Industry Week* as "vision, innovation, long-term thinking, and risk-taking" (*Industry Week* 1995). Maximizing the return on data warehousing requires these qualities. If healthcare leadership is ready to become a knowledge management organization, the sky is the limit.

As IBM chairman and CEO Louis V. Gerstner Jr. stated at the Securities Industry Association's annual convention in Boca Raton, Florida, in October 1997, "Today and in the future, companies that succeed will be those that know how to manage knowledge faster than competitors. It isn't a question of getting new information. It's the ability to extract information from your existing business, to see trends and insights faster than your competition" (Gerstner 1997). If knowledge is indeed power, the importance of knowledge management systems and applications for tapping into this power cannot be ignored. The healthcare industry is in a constant state of flux. It is only through the transition of data into knowledge that healthcare organizations can compete strategically in this evolving industry. Although most organizations have transitioned from data to analysis, only those that understand the value of data and technology have advanced to knowledge and wisdom, which has led to the competitive advantage these organizations currently enjoy. BI and/or knowledge management applications, such as data warehousing, EISs, OLAP, data mining, and customer relationship management, are the cornerstones of the healthcare landscape. These applications transform knowledge into wisdom, which gives organizations the ability to make decisions in a timely manner, improve their performance and operations, and respond to their most important customers—the patients.

In today's healthcare marketplace, fast and easy access to information about the key factors driving the business is paramount. To meet this need, most organizations are consolidating data from operational systems into BI and knowledge management applications (such as central data warehouses or data marts) that are structured to support decision making, enterprise/Web portals, data mining applications, and so on. In the past several years, industry research giants and independent vendor companies have presented interesting data and statistics on trends in IT spending in these sectors. For instance, in a survey conducted by a knowledge management company in the healthcare marketplace in December 2000, most of the healthcare clients surveyed had anticipated that the budgets for acquiring strategic knowledge management applications would grow at a healthy pace in 2001–2002. Specifically, 58 percent of the facilities surveyed believed that spending would increase, 29 percent stated that spending would remain the same, and 13 percent planned to spend less on new intelligence software. (See table 20.1.) Of those planning to increase software purchases in the next 12 months, the main reason given was their emphasis on improving decision making in a managed care environment. Similarly, according to the International Data Corporation, the worldwide BI tools market reached $3.9 billion in 2003 (Vesset 2004). IDC forecasts a continued steady growth in this market during the next five years with a compound annual growth rate of close to 5 percent. Although this growth rate does not match the spectacular performance of the market in the late 1990s, it does reflect an increased demand for software to analyze data, ranging from BI tools to packaged analytic applications (IDC 2004). (See figure 20.6.) Clearly, many IT organizations understand that although these robust and powerful BI tools and analytic applications are more expensive than the traditional character-based HIS applications, they succeed where traditional HIS applications struggle to meet the organization's needs, often increasing the cost in the long run because of inefficiency and difficulty of use. Evidently, the organization's eventual success with BI and analytic applications more than compensates for the initial IT investment.

These BI and analytic applications are designed to improve a healthcare organization's ability to make good business decisions by making necessary information available at all levels of the enterprise, from senior management to the knowledge worker. The healthcare industry is faced with making more complex decisions in shorter time frames and managing colossal amounts of data under tighter budgets and cost constraints in the delivery of high-quality services. It is more important than ever to empower more people within an organization to become knowledge workers. When knowledge workers use smart business intelligence or knowledge management applications, they can address these challenges in a consistent and effective manner and become the champions of a learning organization.

In a learning organization, the focus is on delivering information quickly, clearly, and visually to everyone within the organization, with a strong emphasis on data integrity and the ability to see every aspect of the business relationship in a true perspective. Therefore, data are given prime importance for developing trends, aggregates, and summarizations over time and for discerning valuable information.

The tools, often referred to as BI or knowledge management applications, that help accomplish this also share great importance and reverence in a learning organization. Howard Dresner of the Gartner Group coined the term *business intelligence* in the early 1990s to encapsulate the end-user query and reporting (EUQR) tools, decision support tools, and the OLAP tools market. Since the term was coined, BI has been driven by activities in data warehousing and data mart technology, including extraction, transformation, and loading (ETL); data cleansing; databases; information portals; data mining; and business modeling. Of these various knowledge management/BI applications, data warehousing, EIS, OLAP, data mining, and CRM applications play a key role in a healthcare setting.

Data Warehousing

Industry and market research indicates that knowledge management and strategic decision making powered by data warehouses have dominated IT industry attention since the 1990s (Boar 2000). Numerous companies in multiple industries, including healthcare, are achieving tremendous benefits from data warehousing, including faster and better decision making, employee empowerment, and leveraging of operational data and scenario analysis.

A data warehouse is a platform that contains all of an organization's data in a centralized and normalized form and in one place for deployment to users in order to fulfill simple reporting of data to complicated data analysis, decision support, and executive-level reporting/archiving needs. Typically, a data warehouse consists of a set of programs that extract data from the operational environment, a database that maintains data warehouse data, and systems that provide data to users (Lambert 1996). Physically, a data warehouse is a repository of information that businesses need to thrive

Table 20.1. Worldwide business intelligence revenue by segment, 2001–2008 ($M)

	2001	2002	2003	2004	2005	2006	2007	2008	2003–2008 CAGR (%)
BI tools	3,635.8	3,701.6	3,884.0	4,082.2	4,286.3	4,491.1	4,689.8	4,896.8	4.7
Growth (%)	N/A	1.8	4.9	5.1	5.0	4.8	4.4	4.4	

Source: IDC, June 2004.

**Figure 20.6.   Results of a healthcare industry survey
on future growth in the acquisition
of strategic information technology
applications**

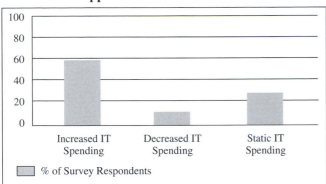

Figure 20.7.   Attributes of a data warehouse

DATA
INFORMATION
KNOWLEDGE
INTELLIGENCE

Periodic or real-time refreshment of the database from the source OLTP or OSS applications

Extended-time accumulation of data

Simple restore/recovery

Ability to "can" repetitive user requests

Flexible import/export facilities

Information sharing

Analyst workbench that may include graphics tools, report writers, statistical modeling tools, spreadsheets, simulators, query languages, word processors, desktop publishing, project management software, artificial intelligence tools, data-mining tools, information discovery/exchange tools, and development tools

Source: Boar 2000.

in the information age. Analytically, a data warehouse is a modern reporting environment that provides users direct access to data.

Data Warehousing Applications

Data warehousing applications include information retrieval, analysis, and reporting. The data sources for these types of applications are often triggered extracts from online transaction processing (OLTP) systems or **operations support systems.** Figure 20.7 lists the attributes of data warehouse applications.

Benefits of Data Warehousing

Data warehousing offers healthcare organizations a number of benefits, including:

- *Immediate information delivery:* Data warehouses shrink the length of time between the business event and the delivery of relevant event information for decision support.
- *Data integration from across and outside the organization:* Data warehouses combine data from multiple sources, such as billing systems and clinical management systems.
- *Ability to perform trend and outcome analysis:* Data warehouses contain multiple years of cross-departmental data for effective business analysis.
- *Unlimited query and reporting capability:* Data warehouses allow users to run any type of queries/reports to answer any strategic questions that arise during day-to-day operations.
- *Ability to analyze and present data to create business intelligence:* Data warehouses give users tools to look at data differently, for example, tables and graphs that make information available quickly and in easy-to-read formats.
- *Freedom from information systems department resource limitations:* With a data warehouse, users can create most of their reports themselves, thus saving considerable time.

Compared to the costs associated with implementing data warehouses (including hardware/software, development personnel/consultants, and operational costs), the benefits are infinite, including added revenue and reduced costs generated by process redesign. The success of data warehousing is most evident when data warehouses are conceptualized, implemented, and managed as a decision support tool for strategic decision making.

Data Warehousing as a Decision Support Tool

Data warehousing as a decision support tool is invaluable for an organization to incorporate BI. For healthcare organizations, using clinical, financial, and operational information in an integrated decision support database to provide immediate access to healthcare practitioners and management is becoming crucial. Many healthcare organizations struggle with the utilization of data collected throughout their legacy transaction processing HIS system, which is often not integrated for management, decision making, and clinical care processes.

Managed care pressures are on the rise, and the marketplace is observing government efforts to better manage Medicare/Medicaid. Expense control, cost avoidance, utilization management of resources, direct provider-to-employer contracting, utilization of data for competitive advantage, and adoption of information technology/automation for increased productivity are no longer mere buzzwords but, instead, are paramount strategic areas of the managed care marketplace. Hence, most healthcare facilities are giving precedence to case management, continuum management, and disease state management initiatives to manage cost, integrate care across the continuum, and align clinical pathways with clinical best practices for optimum patient care at lower costs. Unquestionably, a decision support strategy with data warehousing as its application is critical to meet these challenges.

Healthcare organizations that survive and thrive in today's information age are evolving toward a data warehouse–based decision support infrastructure to sustain transparent, knowledge-based, rapid decision making required by the healthcare revolution. This involves designing a data warehousing strategy that is robust enough to evolve with the growth and change in healthcare to lay a foundation for real-time, 360-degree views of an organization's key financial and clinical health/performance/outcome indicators. Hence, current technology demands for a sound data warehousing strategy include robust relational database architecture to leverage current and future data analysis across the continuum of care, executive information systems that help with physician best practice patterns analysis and provide evidence-based care, and online analytical processing.

With its powerful set of tools, data warehousing maximizes the user's ability to leverage and exploit the captured operational data and creates a strategic advantage for organizations. Time is the key factor. A data warehousing strategy allows organizations to compete across time by enabling employees to strategically learn from the past, adapt in the present, and position themselves for the future with the help of the powerful tools supported by this technology (Boar 2000). During the course of business, employees perform many tasks, control processes, share information, and make many decisions. When better information is made available in a timely manner and at the point of need, employees become more empowered, which creates leverage for the organization. Through data warehousing, potent information is made available to all employees so that they can solve problems and make good decisions. This is why data warehousing is considered a rising-tide strategy. When the tide comes in, it raises all the ships in the harbor; similarly, data warehousing raises the strategic acumen of all employees (Boar 2000). In the information age, data warehousing is a key strategic weapon for organizations.

Data Warehousing as a Performance Improvement Tool

As financial and marketplace pressures force healthcare organizations to better integrate all the components of the local healthcare delivery system, many forward-looking organizations have recognized the fact that they cannot improve what they cannot measure. More and more enlightened organizations are empowering their staff, including managers and key stakeholders, with data warehouse–based critical thinking and knowledge management tools to completely transform the way they do business. Instead of running the organization from stacks of paper reports received 30 to 40 days after the fact, managers can proactively identify opportunities for performance improvement, cost savings, and revenue enhancements by using point-and-click data mining tools. The backlog of reports that once existed in information systems is diminishing, and IS departments are shifting from being the total provider of reports to all

users to being a conduit and facilitator of knowledge management.

With the power of data warehousing, management can make more complex decisions and manage more data in a shorter time frame with tighter budgets and cost constraints. And, as mentioned earlier, employees are empowered with the right tools so that they can make better and timelier decisions for the benefit of the organization. Data warehousing and disease and case management are crucial for healthcare institutions if they are to integrate all critical service lines to create a healthcare delivery system that offers customers the best experience in a high-quality and cost-effective manner.

For healthcare organizations facing growing pressures to cut costs and maintain high-quality patient care, adopting a data warehouse strategy is a key decision to make. For this strategy to be successful, management must perform an analysis of current systems/processes to identify areas for improvement and target areas that can benefit from the powerful tool of data warehousing. By analyzing the organization's goals, objectives, and vision and comparing them to the decision support systems already in place, management can determine how best to implement a data warehousing strategy. For the healthcare facility without the ability to provide the right data to the right decision makers at the right time and in the right manner for the areas of patient care, budgeting, planning, research, process improvement initiatives, external reporting, benchmarking, trend analysis, and marketing, data warehousing is the right answer. Immediate access to accurate information is the driving force behind the adoption of a data warehouse strategy.

Planning and Implementation of a Data Warehouse

After management has decided to adopt a decision support strategy that involves establishment of a data warehouse, steps must be taken to properly plan and implement its application. These steps include:

1. The business objectives and goals of the healthcare organization must be identified, followed by gap analysis for data needs and finalization of hardware and software requirements.
2. The source systems used to collect data within the healthcare organization must be identified, along with the resources required to establish the data warehouse and data marts for each of the service lines. This includes selection of an implementation team. It is recommended that a decision support core team be designated as the primary repository for financial and clinical data. This core team must collaborate efforts with the IS team, including representation from clinical departments, health information management, information services, and administration. Additionally, it should work with the owners of the source systems to identify the core data elements to feed into the data warehouse.

3. The data to be fed into the data warehouse must be edited and cleansed. Also, time lines for downloading data from the source system to the data warehouse must be defined, along with audits within the warehouse to ensure data integrity.

4. Following the business objectives, data marts should be built and rolled out for identified service lines. The first data mart built should be the executive information system (EIS), with the data needed by administration to answer the questions that keep them up at night. Next, the identification, validation, and transfer of needed data from the data warehouse to the EIS follows. Other service line data marts can be built and customized as appropriate.

5. Finally, an education program should be implemented to enhance the transition of end users toward knowledge management.

To ensure successful implementation of a data warehouse decision support strategy, it is crucial to elicit organizational resources, including management support. Furthermore, measures of success should be delineated to evaluate the strategy's viability and durability. These measures could include the achievement of business goals and objectives such as increased revenue/market share, increased patient volume, improved patient outcomes, increased volume of activity on the data warehouse/data marts, increased number of requests for the development of new data marts, and the ability to respond quickly to changes in healthcare. In addition, implementation of a successful data warehouse decision support strategy can produce significant cost savings by eliminating the costly report-writing maintenance of legacy applications, reducing support costs by simplifying operations, and eliminating nonessential reports (Evans 1997).

Past studies have found that data warehousing generates significant return on investment for the organizations. In addition to cost savings and increased revenues, there are other benefits that magnify the ROI for this decision support strategy. These benefits include (Evans 1997):

- More timely information access for decision makers
- Customized information delivery for end users
- Ability of the system to handle large amounts of data while providing fast response time
- State-of-the-art analysis tools that require minimal training time
- Improved management ability to identify trends and change a course of action through increased access to data
- Integrated information from multiple systems in a process that organizes information to allow comparison of multiple time periods from multiple sources

Executive Information System

When it comes to making sense of the volumes of raw data collected in any industry, including healthcare, implementation of a data warehouse based on relational database technology, which extracts, transforms, aggregates, summarizes, organizes, and stores data in a format that is more conducive to reporting and analysis is surely the first step. As illustrated previously, the benefits of implementing a data warehouse are countless, notably, that data warehousing has the "potential" to turn raw data into valuable information that can be used in daily decision making as well as long-range strategic planning.

To realize this potential, raw data have to be enhanced via analyses and transformed into information and knowledge. In this analysis of data, ease-of-use is paramount so that users can easily make sense of the data analysis. The easier the process of getting to the relevant information, the faster the business decision can be made to adjust to the ever-changing business conditions (Makhani and Nanjee 2002). However, most organizations struggle with the ability to provide decision makers with the information they need in a timely manner. These organizations are confronted with this information struggle because they do not either understand what relevant information is needed and/or know how to obtain it efficiently (Wu 2000a). This is where EISs in conjunction with data warehousing lay the foundation for a powerful decision support strategy.

Overview of an Executive Information System

In his article subtitled "What Is Business Intelligence?" Jonathan Wu claims, "During the last 10 years, the names of information systems have changed from executive information systems (EIS) to decision support systems (DSS) and now to BI systems. But, more has happened than just a name change. The technology has significantly evolved from internally developed graphical user interfaces (GUI) to packaged applications that provide users with easy access to data for analysis" (Wu 2000b). Effective use of data warehouses and EISs leads to the development of knowledge, which provides the basis for efficient decision making. From a data analysis perspective, the EIS aids in the process of gathering high-quality and meaningful information about the subject matter being researched that will help the individual analyze information, draw conclusions, or make assumptions. From an IS perspective, the EIS provides users with analytical processing and data analysis to answer business questions and identify significant trends or patterns in the information being examined. In addition, EIS provides knowledge workers with the capability of multidimensional analysis as demonstrated in an example below.

EIS is a point-and-click analytical application that enables users to immediately retrieve existing information from many critical sources for better decision making. It aids in intuitive navigation through specific data sets. For a healthcare facility, an EIS can extend the analytical capabilities to a whole new level with financial and clinical data marts that allow for tailored analysis. The result is a constant source of information to fine-tune processes and policies that increase productivity. Work flows and processes can be tweaked via quantitative study of how work has been done. Combined with powerful data mining and drill-down tools, knowledge workers can retrieve information quickly and effectively, which results in superior decision making. Users can view the data from several aggregations, the most granular generally being the patient level. (See figure 20.8.) An EIS also provides extensive graphing capabilities and customized, user-driven analyses. By offering an array of breakdowns and filters on a subset of patient records selected by date range, an EIS can become a tool that is as easy to use as it is prolific with results, driven from the power of a data warehouse (Makhani and Nanjee 2002).

Benefits of an Executive Information System

An EIS offers several advantages, some of which are briefly summarized below:

- *Increased revenues, reduced costs, and the ability to compete effectively:* An EIS helps organizations achieve this by presenting holistic and timely information and knowledge for effective decision making.
- *Power to manage business complexity:* An EIS helps enterprises organize their data to facilitate data analysis and mining to unearth hidden patterns and trends.

- *Information democracy:* An EIS facilitates the sharing of information across all borders of the healthcare enterprise, offering all decision makers the tool to analyze data at their level and make better financial and clinical decisions.
- *Ability to make sound strategic decisions:* Perhaps the greatest benefit that an EIS offers is the ability to use all actionable information with the existing tacit knowledge within an organization and to create a synergy that empowers strategic decision makers to gain a competitive edge in the marketplace.

An EIS in Action: Example of Financial and Clinical Analysis in Healthcare

The following example illustrates how an EIS can aid in performing financial and clinical in-depth analyses with just a simple point-and-click. This example looks at physician comparison and profiling within a given time frame to discover how the physicians are performing with respect to parameters such as patient volume, length of stay (LOS), charges, costs, and financial bottom lines. In the beginning of the example, figure 20.8 shows an EIS dashboard for analysis, which is

Figure 20.8.   EIS dashboard: Example of financial and clinical analysis in healthcare using an EIS

Year	IN DIS	OUT	Total LOS	Average LOS	Charges	Average Charges	Reimb Actual	Total Cost	Profit Actual %	Profit Expected	Balance
Jan 99	307	0	1 Total LOS	5.6	$1,556,402	$5,070	$967,127	$178,917	81.50%	$1,122,910	$9,460
Jan 00	379	0	5599	14.8	$2,350,780	$6,203	$1,520,057	$1,604,684	-5.28%	$419,750	$20,508

Drg	IN DIS	OUT	Total LOS	Average LOS	Charges	Average Charges	Reimb Actual	Total Cost	Profit Actual %	Profit Expected	Balance
5	1	0	2	2.0	$6,486	$6,486	$5,519	$4,954	10.23%	$65	$00
12	2	0	2003	1001.5	$149,279	$74,639	$24,273	$83,478	-70.93%	-$58,936	$224
14	2	0	10	5.0	$15,139	$7,570	$9,122	$9,694	-5.90%	$5,445	$00
15	1	0	2	2.0	$3,194	$3,194	$2,833	$1,916	32.35%	$1,278	$00
20	2	0	13	6.5	$20,355	$10,177	$9,988	$11,721	-14.79%	$5,617	$00
24	1	0	6	6.0	$8,583	$8,583	$3,507	$6,507	-46.12%	$2,076	$00
25	2	0	5	2.5	$7,073	$3,536	$4,616	$6,009	-23.18%	$1,064	$00
53	1	0	3	3.0	$4,620	$4,620	$4,749	$4,167	12.25%	$453	$00
78	1	0	10	10.0	$13,060	$13,060	$5,305	$7,612	-30.31%	$5,448	$00
79	2	0	11	5.5	$15,742	$7,871	$12,594	$11,440	9.16%	$4,302	$00
87	4	0	40	10.0	$52,961	$13,240	$20,917	$26,710	-21.69%	$26,210	$00
88	21	0	80	3.8	$93,924	$4,473	$66,606	$68,860	-3.28%	$21,705	$773
89	37	0	131	3.5	$156,914	$4,241	$117,994	$103,907	11.93%	$33,825	$2,916
90	4	0	7	1.8	$8,414	$2,103	$8,849	$5,569	37.06%	$2,845	$00
91	2	0	7	3.5	$6,600	$3,300	$3,201	$5,902	-45.76%	$575	$00
96	4	0	13	3.3	$13,647	$3,412	$9,091	$10,255	-11.35%	$1,182	$00
97	2	0	4	2.0	$4,380	$2,190	$3,820	$2,351	38.45%	$2,024	$00
98	1	0	7	7.0	$6,307	$6,307	$1,226	$5,177	-76.32%	$1,129	$00
99	1	0	2	2.0	$1,668	$1,668	$2,611	$00	0.00%	$1,668	$00
116	1	0	3	3.0	$22,498	$22,498	$9,405	$5,812	38.20%	$15,882	$00
121	13	0	59	4.5	$80,804	$6,216	$61,200	$54,828	10.41%	$21,456	$04
122	2	0	5	2.5	$10,969	$5,484	$4,867	$7,463	-34.79%	$3,506	$00
127	19	0	152	8.0	$106,854	$5,624	$84,482	$74,232	12.13%	$32,622	$02

EXTRACRANIAL VASCULAR PROCEDURES   110 Drgs presented in the form of a numerical grid, enabling in-depth data investigation via traditional row and column tables. Data are broken down into valuable segments, providing rapid discovery of various win–loss situations. The grid can be ranked, customized, selected, and manipulated to best bring about results, while the application of breakdowns, filters, and drilldowns extract dynamic changes to the grid's size and content.

Continuing with the example, figure 20.9 shows how the grid has been changed to reflect a certain scenario. According to the row and column headers in the screenshot, for the time period dated January 2000, 10 attending physicians were treating inpatients with DRG 127 (heart failure and shock) and who had the insurance through Medicare, Blue Cross, and Medicaid. With this as the breakdown/filter combination, it is possible to look at how these physicians performed with respect to parameters such as patient volume, average length of stay, charges and costs, and profit/loss balances. An example of the potency of the visual/graphical representations made possible by an EIS, figure 20.10 (p. 580) presents another way to view data via the pattern analysis screen. This screen utilizes the "largest piece of the pie" analogy to graphically illustrate the analysis of data. Here, the 10 physicians

from the previous screen are now put together on one pie of results. The various categories on the left of the pie graph can be activated separately to quickly understand each physician's performance in each individual category. A quick reference of the actual numbers also is provided along with the graphical display. Yet another way to view the same information is via the LOS comparison, as shown in figure 20.11 (p. 581).

Because LOS tends to be a valuable form of performance evaluation, a bar graph is provided for immediate recognition of variations from the norm. As can be seen by the screenshot, physicians are analyzed together to evaluate how they compare to the LOS average. Details such as patient volume, costs, and charges can be seen below as a particular physician's bar is selected.

Profiling is another analysis that can be done when an item of interest has been obtained. This is shown in figure 20.12 (p. 582). Whether for a DRG, insurance, an employer, or a physician, any EIS breakdown can be profiled to obtain a closer look at the "who, what, and where" of that particular item. The physician profile in this screenshot takes one sample physician and illustrates summarized reports of details such as principal diagnoses, payer information, readmission reports, and patient

Figure 20.9.   EIS dashboard: Physician comparison across different financial and clinical data elements

Figure 20.10.   EIS dashboard: Physician comparison analysis—graphical representation via a pie chart

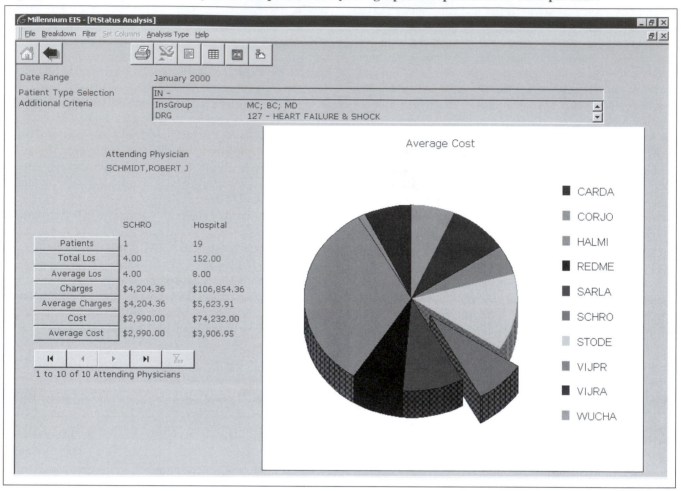

destination. Profiling provides an in-depth look at the history behind a given entity and insightful clues as to why a certain performance level has been attained (Makhani and Nanjee 2002).

Figure 20.13 (p. 583) shows the LOS comparison in the form of a bubble graph. Here, the axes represent two important measurements: LOS and charge comparisons. The size of the bubbles as well as their distance from the origin give an insight as to how near or far the physicians are from the average. Finally, figure 20.14 (p. 584) shows the EIS's ability to drill all the way down to the patient level. Here, several forms of analysis can be made of a variety of details related to the patient's medical experience. Charge transactions, charge categories, diagnoses, operations, and CPT codes all can be viewed in full detail with the click of a button. As an example, the charge transactions page can potentially illustrate anything and everything that occurred during the patient's experience on a day-by-day basis. Filters of these transactions, as well as intelligent ranking features, help to further enhance the data analysis endeavor.

As illustrated in the example above, it is clear that an EIS can prove extremely beneficial to healthcare manage-

ment in conducting key analyses that will ultimately help improve clinical outcomes and improve the financial bottom line. Relevant, timely, and customized information is the key ingredient that healthcare organizations and facilities need to stay competitive. Cutting costs, increasing revenue, and enhancing efficiency are needs for any healthcare facility today. An EIS, in conjunction with a data warehouse, can function as a powerful analysis tool that can provide fast response times and the ability to perform in-depth analyses with utmost ease. With this potent combination, management can identify key trends and change the course of strategic action more quickly due to increased access to knowledge-rich data (Makhani and Nanjee 2002).

Online Analytical Processing

Data stored in an organization's databases and other data sources are retrieved and used to perform various organizational functions and to make important decisions. Data that are inaccurate, missing or not used effectively will impair the processes performed and decisions made by the organization. "Garbage in, garbage out" is the reality to reckon with. In addition to needing good data, healthcare organizations need the right set of tools to harness and analyze the prolific data in the business environment (Makhani and Farishta 2002).

Therefore, successful data analysis is the golden key to successful results. As illustrated previously, organizations must implement knowledge management initiatives to make strides in leveraging data for better decision making. Data warehousing, EISs, data mining, and OLAP are tools and applications that bring knowledge management to the forefront in an organization (Makhani and Farishta 2002). The subsections below discuss OLAP and the data mining process.

Overview of Online Analytical Processing

OLAP is a computing technique for summarizing, consolidating, viewing, and applying formulae to and synthesizing data according to multiple dimensions. OLAP software enables users (analysts, managers, executives, and others) to gain insight into the enterprise's performance through rapid access to a wide variety of data views organized to reflect the multidimensional nature of the enterprise performance data (Kelkar 2001). By making use of intelligent and intuitive operations, OLAP applications based on a data warehouse provide an exceptional tool for conducting sophisticated analyses and examinations.

In other words, OLAP offers fast access to multidimensional information for exploitation in a wider BI context. OLAP is a function of software technology that enables analysts, administrators, and executives to gain key insight into crucial elements of data. This examination of information via rapid, consistent, and interactive access provides for a wide variety of possible views of information, transformed from raw data to reflect the various dimensions of reality. The information gained by an individual conducting this analysis can be said to represent the core data of an enterprise, but in a manner that is understood by the user. Because of its versatility in presenting data, OLAP provides its analysts with a profound level of comprehension for its multitude of medical information (Kelkar 2001).

In the area of leveraging an organization's operational data to create strategic acumen, OLAP also supports data warehousing as a decision support tool. Using OLAP, enterprises can drive decision support, do trend analysis, compare business units, and monitor strategic business decisions. OLAP data are a way that multiple business dimensions are reflected, for example, patients admitted per quarter by disease category, costs per service line by region, medical supplies shipped on

Figure 20.11.   EIS dashboard: Physician comparison analysis, LOS comparison

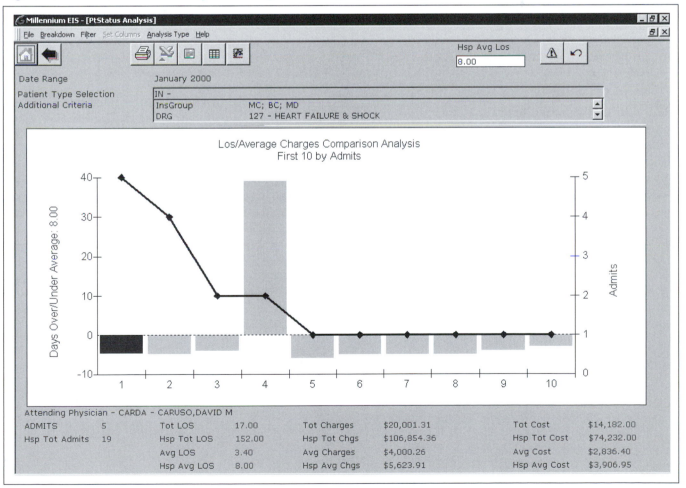

Figure 20.12.   EIS dashboard: Physician profiling, graphical representation via a pie chart

time per department per hospital, and so forth. This type of information allows managers to conduct comparison and trend analysis effectively (Makhani and Farishta 2002).

OLAP and Multidimensional Analysis

The multidimensional nature of a problem requires looking simultaneously at the data from more than one dimension. The key driver for OLAP technology is this aspect of multidimensional views. For example, a business analyst might want to get monthly (time dimension) reimbursement data for a set of services (service dimension) across all patient segments (patient dimension) and across all age groups (age dimension) to analyze payer patterns. This is a multidimensional expression of a real business problem. OLAP has the inherent ability to present data in many views and at different granularities by virtue of operations such as slicing, dicing, drill-down, pivoting, and filtering.

To elaborate, OLAP functionality is characterized by the dynamic, **multidimensional analysis** of consolidated enterprise data. This process makes it possible to analyze potentially large amounts of data with very fast response times, allowing users to drill down to the most granular levels of detail for optimal knowledge gain. OLAP helps the user to synthesize enterprise information through comparative, personalized viewing, and to analyze historical and projected data for various what-if data model scenarios. With such a wide variety of avenues by which a user can analyze data, OLAP is optimized for multidimensional query and report.

An increasingly popular data model for OLAP applications is the multidimensional database (MDDB), also known as the **data cube.** OLAP cubes store precomputed results of data at different levels and, hence, multidimensional query results are returned faster. Before examining the various components of OLAP, it is important to understand its foundation. Every application, or process, has an underlying core on which the entire function takes place. For OLAP, this underlying core is an element known as a data cube, an entity that holds the boundless amount of information on which analyses can be made. This cube is developed, manipulated, and transformed in different ways to produce the results that OLAP delivers (Makhani and Farishta 2002).

Data Cubes

A data cube is a collection of one or more tables of data assembled in a fashion that allows for dynamic analysis to be conducted on their joins, intersections, and overall integration. Because these tables are thoroughly populated with the information used for analysis, it is obvious to see how a data cube is a superlative structure. Creating an intelligent construction based on how information in these tables intersects and interrelates is the core property of a data cube, allowing for a powerful entity to be probed for analysis.

To understand a cube visually, it can be said that it is an accumulation of several two-dimensional tables or squares that can be attached together, strategically, to create a three-dimensional cube. A physical cube, after all, is simply a set of squares that have been put together; in a similar manner, a data cube is simply a set of tables that have been wisely compiled into one collective structure.

Using this cube structure, OLAP is able to properly present a wealth of insightful views and perspectives into various databanks of medical information. A cube is laid out in a manner that represents the row and column conventions of a common table but enhances this design with the addition of so-called pages. A page represents a filter of the current data being viewed. When a page is changed, it alters the view, purpose, or intent of that analysis to a completely different perspective. Where one page may filter the data for the highest expense by a particular department, another page may provide a breakdown of the patients and their particular treatments that contributed to the high cost. By passing an unlimited set of different magnifying glasses over the same set of data, different results and meanings emerge to provide a 360-degree analysis of how these data can provide the power of knowledge (Makhani and Farishta 2002).

OLAP and Data Analysis

Users can employ a variety of OLAP operations to gain the most out of their data analysis endeavors. Some common actions that can be conducted with OLAP are the ability to:

- Calculate and model across dimensions, through hierarchies, and across members
- Explore trend analyses over sequentially sectioned time periods

Figure 20.13. EIS dashboard: Physician profiling continued, LOS comparison via a bubble graph

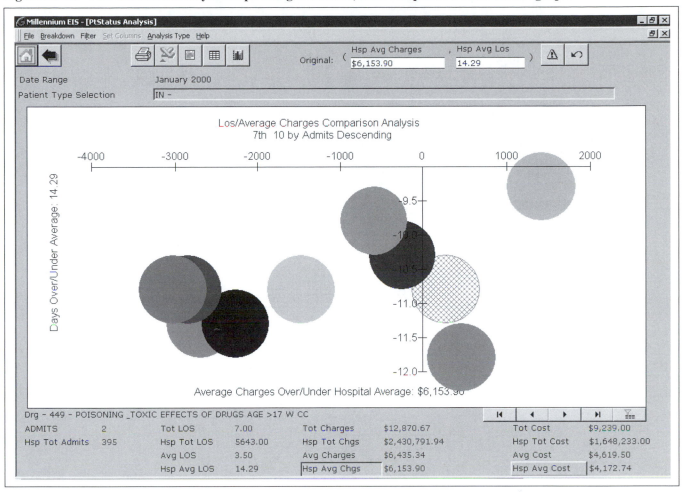

- Slice through various subsets for on-screen viewing
- Perform drill-down operations to deeper levels of consolidation
- Reach through to underlying detail data
- Rotate to new dimensional comparisons for investigation

Without proper data analysis, it is difficult to realize the full potential of data collected by healthcare organizations. Because of the incredible amount of data to be dissected and understood, it is very important that OLAP be used to successfully extract the greatest amount of value from seemingly disparate data.

Example of a Financial Analysis Using OLAP

To provide an actual illustration of how OLAP can be used, a simple and yet effective example of data analysis using OLAP in the area of final-billed analysis is provided. In this illustration, a knowledge worker/user uses a final-billed analysis cube created for a healthcare organization that represents the status of the organization's final-billed accounts. Opening up the data cube, screen one is depicted in figure 20.15 (p. 585).

To maximize cash flow, the goal is to ascertain how to collect the greatest amount of payment in the shortest amount of time possible. Looking at the first two columns of data in figure 20.15, the user can see that it represents the number of patients and how much they owe for the past 30 days. Users can immediately see that 961 people owe the hospital $25,439, 1,216 people owe $90,954, 56 people owe $476,902, and so on. Obviously, it is more efficient and advantageous to work with 56 accounts and gain $476,902 than it is to work with 961 accounts and collect $25,439. Already, the analysis has pointed the knowledge worker in the right direction for maximum monetary gain.

To expand further, perhaps this healthcare organization's policy is to aggressively pursue accounts that are 30 to 60 days past due. Using OLAP's drag-and-drop filtering, the user can focus on only those accounts. (See screen two in figure 20.16, p. 586.) The column in figure 20.16 clearly shows that the best and most rational approach for the knowledge worker to take is to pursue the four accounts that can produce $45,229. To learn more about these accounts and the details of the circumstances, the knowledge worker can utilize the various page filters to probe further. (See figure 20.17, p. 587.)

Figure 20.14.   EIS dashboard: Example of drilling down to the patient level

Millennium EIS - [PtStatus Analysis]

Patient Demographic Data

| Charge Txns | Chg Category | Diagnosis | Operations | CPT Codes |

Account: V82650847 Name:
Unit#: M000031682 Race:
Abs Status: FINAL Pt Status:
Birthdate: 9/15/1946 Drg:
Age/Sex: 53 M Prin Dx:

L47006911	1	0	88
V82650847	1	0	6
V82703968	1	0	5
V82680075	1	0	5
V82723495	1	0	4
V82712761	1	0	4
V82696576	1	0	4
V82690397	1	0	4
V82714726	1	0	3
V82698168	1	0	3
V82696626	1	0	3
V82692567	1	0	3
V82689019	1	0	3
V82670951	1	0	3
V82668260	1	0	3
V82667742	1	0	3
V82657479	1	0	3
V82653189	1	0	3
V82670365	1	0	2

Patient Charge Transactions

ACCOUNT: V82650847 NAME:
ADMIT DATE: 12/31/1999 DISCHARGE DATE: 1/6/2000

DAY	DATE	COUNT	PROCEDURE	DESCRIPTION	CHARGES	COST
Day 1	12/31/1999	3	2507690	LANOXIN 0.25MG TAB	$1.68	$0.00
Day 1	12/31/1999	1	3001480	BLOOD GASES, CAPILLARY	$66.65	$34.36
Day 1	12/31/1999	1	3001480	BLOOD GASES, CAPILLARY	$66.65	$0.00
Day 1	12/31/1999	3	4100011	ADDED AEROSOL TX DIAGNOSTIC	$135.00	$56.13
Day 1	12/31/1999	3	4100011	ADDED AEROSOL TX DIAGNOSTIC	$135.00	$0.00
Day 1	12/31/1999	1	3010170		$4.90	$2.53
Day 1	12/31/1999	1	3006110	METABOLIC PANEL, BASIC	$52.25	$26.94
Day 1	12/31/1999	1	3006110	METABOLIC PANEL, BASIC	$52.25	$0.00
Day 1	12/31/1999	1	2510310	HUMULIN 70/30 INSULIN	$45.88	$13.40
Day 1	12/31/1999	3	2507690	LANOXIN 0.25MG TAB	$1.68	$1.02
Day 1	12/31/1999	1	3011540	MYOGLOBIN, QUAN. SERUM	$58.10	$0.00
Day 1	12/31/1999	1	2000100	INTENSIVE CARE UNIT	$810.00	$728.43
Day 1	12/31/1999	1	3008350	TROPONIN	$90.20	$0.00
Day 1	12/31/1999	1	2718610	DRESSING OPSITE 10 X 14	$1.88	$0.00
Day 1	12/31/1999	1	7300020	ELECTROCARDIOGRAM	$78.00	$22.05
Day 1	12/31/1999	1	4100400	ARTERIAL PUNCTURE	$15.95	$0.00
Day 1	12/31/1999	1	4100400	ARTERIAL PUNCTURE	$15.95	$6.64
Day 1	12/31/1999	1	2600445	NONCOR PORT INFUSION SET	$18.00	$6.41
Day 1	12/31/1999	1	4500080	ER-INTERMEDIATE	$222.90	$134.09
Day 1	12/31/1999	1	2717190	URINAL DISP	$1.05	$0.55
TOTAL AMOUNT					$12,609.90	$6,894.19

By simply dragging down the account type and insurance page filters, the user can learn a great deal about the breakdown of various accounts. The bottom segment of figure 20.17 ($5,000–$25,000) illustrates the breakdown of the four accounts the user decided to monitor. From filtering, the user can see the various services these patients received (account type) and their insurance plans. If desired, the patient name and account number filters also can be dragged down for the patients involved in the analysis. This can be an incredibly beneficial tool for financial and/or clinical analysts who wish to know anything and everything about the accounts in question.

Certainly, data will grow at an exponential rate in all organizations, including healthcare. This growth rate and subsequent complexity underline the need for appropriate, fast, and more efficient data analysis solutions. Solving modern business problems with the help of clinical analysis, market analysis, and financial forecasting requires query-centric database schemas that are multidimensional. Hence, the incredible amount of time, money, and knowledge gained from successful data analysis using OLAP is definitely something that cannot be ignored. Healthcare organizations that place importance on data analysis and understanding

surely stand heads and shoulders above the crowd, reaping maximum benefits that lead to efficiencies in their overall operations. By implementing OLAP for their data-analyzing endeavors off a data warehouse, medical institutions can be sure they will always be up to speed with the trends, practices, and events of the ocean of data in which they perform (Makhani and Farishta 2002).

Data Mining

Successful healthcare organizations empower their management and staff with data warehousing–based critical thinking and knowledge management tools for strategic decision making. Many healthcare organizations struggle with the utilization of data collected through their OLTP system, which is not integrated for decision making and pattern analysis.

Healthcare data can be classified into four categories:

- *Patient-centric data,* which are directly related to patients
- *Aggregate data,* which are based on performance and utilization/resource management data
- *Transformed base data* for planning, clinical, and management decision support, which consist of data elements

from various sources that are combined, summarized, and made more relevant and meaningful to decision makers

- *Comparative data* for healthcare services research and outcomes measurement

The data source is usually the enterprise's OLTP system or operations support system. Thanks to years of accumulated disparate data, these systems are data rich but information poor (Shams and Farishta 2001). With the adoption of data warehousing and data analysis/OLAP tools, an organization can make strides toward leveraging data for better decision making.

Data mining, also known as database exploration and information discovery, brings the practice of information processing closer to providing the answers that organizations want from their data (Ferguson 1997). Healthcare involves massive amounts of data that have no organizational value until they are converted into information and knowledge. Data mining provides automated pattern recognition and attempts to uncover patterns in data that are difficult to detect with traditional statistical methods. Without data mining, it is difficult to realize the full potential of the data collected within an organization because the data under analysis are copious, highly dimensional, widely distributed, and uncertain (Ferguson 1997). For healthcare organizations to suc-

ceed, they must be able to capture, store, and analyze their data (Shams and Farishta 2001).

In the early days of data warehousing, data mining was viewed as a subset of the activities associated with the warehouse. Today, data mining is recognized as an independent activity that is paramount for success with data warehouse–based decision support systems (DSSs). It enables users to discover hidden patterns without a predetermined idea or hypothesis about what the patterns may be.

The Data Mining Process

The data mining process can be divided into two categories: (1) discovering patterns and associations and (2) using the patterns to predict future trends and behaviors (Ferguson 1997). As mentioned earlier, the power of data mining is that it can reveal patterns the user has not considered in his or her search, producing answers to questions that were never asked. This is especially helpful when dealing with a large database with an infinite number of patterns to identify. Interesting to note is the fact that "the more data in the warehouse, the more patterns there are, and the more data we analyze, the fewer patterns we find" (Parsaye 1996). What this means is that in a large database, it may be best to data-mine different data segments separately so that the influence of one pattern does not dilute the effect of another. At this junction, the user should not fear the loss of certain indicators or patterns

Figure 20.15.   Example of financial data analysis using OLAP, final-billed analysis cube (screen one)

Golap - [Galaxy On Line Analytical Processing]

File Edit Format Tools Export Admin Help

PatientName	InsuranceOrder	Insurance	FinClass	AccountType	AccountNumber1

	At AgeBucket							
	D000-030		D031-060		D061-090		D091-120	
BalanceBucket	PtVolume	Balance	PtVolume	Balance	PtVolume	Balance	PtVolume	Balance
$00000.01-00050	961	$25,439	155	$4,397	820	$20,506	435	$10,735
$00050.01-00100	1,216	$90,954	123	$8,678	541	$39,359	352	$25,242
$00100.01-00250	1,378	$227,992	151	$25,545	531	$88,384	341	$56,291
$00250.01-00500	645	$214,960	83	$28,483	280	$97,851	157	$54,584
$00500.01-01000	327	$224,313	45	$31,391	203	$147,188	134	$94,624
$01000.01-02000	342	$464,399	21	$29,137	87	$121,899	68	$99,212
$02000.01-03000	113	$276,930	9	$22,164	56	$139,203	26	$62,884
$03000.01-04000	82	$276,409	9	$29,495	23	$81,446	20	$70,515
$04000.01-05000	23	$105,469	2	$8,606	14	$62,387	7	$30,585
$05000.01-25000	56	$476,902	4	$45,229	31	$245,144	26	$207,175
$25000.01-50000	2	$75,072						
$50000+					1	$51,571		
Total BalanceBucket	5,145	$2,458,840	602	$233,125	2,587	$1,094,939	1,566	$711,846

Figure 20.16. Using OLAP's drag-and-drop filtering: A view of accounts that are 30 to 60 days past due (screen two)

in a smaller segment. When a trend or pattern is applicable in an entire database, it also is evident in a smaller segment. Thus, depending on the circumstances and the nature of data in a warehouse, data mining generally can be performed on a segment of data that fits a business objective rather than on the whole warehouse (Parsaye 1996).

Data mining technology and techniques are invaluable to healthcare management in analyzing clinical and financial data for strategic decision making. Such techniques can help organizations meet their business objectives for cost control and revenue generation, while maintaining high-quality care for the patients. Moreover, data mining tools and techniques can ease the burden for management and staff faced with the growing pressures of lower payer reimbursements, increased labor costs, and a highly competitive healthcare marketplace. These tools can work as strategic weapons to convert data into information, creating BI in the process.

In a data mine, analysis for pattern identification is done on a data segment and the process of mining this segment is called an **analysis session.** For example, management may want to predict the response to a flu vaccination initiative for the elderly in the community by analyzing previous initia-

tives or to know the patient sample over various geographic regions. When a user begins the analysis with a specific task, for instance, analyzing reimbursement by DRGs, the analysis is called a **structured analysis.** Structured analysis is generally done on a routine basis (for example, analysis of quarterly costs, revenues, expenses, and so on) to identify and forecast trends. When the user wanders through a database without a specific goal, he or she may discover interesting patterns or randomly hidden facts. In this case, the analysis is called an **unstructured analysis** (Parsaye 1996). For example, a supermarket may mine its customer data and find that 65 percent of the people who buy tuna fish in a can buy orange juice at the same time.

The following types of techniques are used in data mining:

- Decision trees
- Genetic algorithms
- Neural networks
- Predictive modeling
- Rule induction (associated rule analysis)
- Fuzzy logic
- K-nearest neighbor

Decision Trees

A **decision tree** is a tree-shaped structure that visually describes a set of rules that caused a decision to be made. For example, it can help determine the factors that affect kidney transplant survival rates.

Decision trees also are techniques that learn and discover patterns from data that have been presented to them. One nice feature of a decision tree is its ease of interpretation. Decision tree algorithms operate by searching through the data for the best possible variables on which to divide the data so that new groups resulting from the split will be more alike than the original overall group. The process continues again with each new group. That is, for each new group, the algorithm searches for the best variable on which to split so that the new groups that result from the split will be more alike. The process continues until the algorithm reaches a stopping point using criteria supplied by the user. A classic example of decision tree methodology is the DRG algorithm process used in Medicare reimbursement.

Genetic Algorithms

Genetic algorithms are optimization techniques that can be used to improve other data mining algorithms so that they derive the best model for a given set of data. For example, algorithms can help determine the optimal treatment plan for a particular diagnosis.

Neural Networks

Neural networks are nonlinear predictive models that learn how to detect a pattern to match a particular profile through a training process that involves interactive learning, using a set of data that describes what the organization wants to find. For example, neural networks can help determine what disease a susceptible patient is likely to contract. They are good for clustering, sequencing, and predicting patterns. Their

Figure 20.17.   Using OLAP's drag-and-drop filtering for account type and insurance filters: A detailed breakdown is available for individual accounts (screen three)

drawback is that they do not explain why they have reached a particular conclusion.

Predictive Modeling

Predictive modeling can be used to identify patterns. The patterns then can be used to predict the odds of a particular outcome based on the observed data.

Rule Induction

Rule induction, also referred to as association rule analysis, is the process of extracting useful if-then rules from data based on statistical significance.

(See chapter 19 to review examples of the use of the rule induction technique.)

Fuzzy Logic

Fuzzy logic handles imprecise concepts. It is more flexible than other techniques. For example, it can help identify patients who are likely to respond to hospital/community initiatives to raise awareness of the cause of AIDS prevention.

K-Nearest Neighbor

K-nearest neighbor (K-NN) is a classic technique for discovering associations and sequences when the data attributes are numeric (Ferguson 1997).

Forms of Data Mining

In the early days, organizations generally followed the "build a warehouse first, mine later" paradigm. Classified by Parsaye as the "sandwich paradigm," this "build first, think later" approach can be considered a "data dump paradigm" because in many cases it leads to the construction of a toxic data dump whose contents are not easily salvageable. A much better way is to "sandwich" the warehousing effort between two layers of mining. The first, preliminary round of mining is considered "premining." Thus, one understands the data before warehousing it. Then the warehouse is built based on information uncovered during premining. This approach ensures that data mining complements the data warehouse (Parsaye 1995, 1996).

Data mining can exist in the following basic forms:

- *Above the warehouse:* This form of data mining provides a minimal architecture for analysis and pattern identification and is prescribed only when data mining is not a key objective for the warehouse.
- *Beside the warehouse:* This form of data mining allows data mining to be done in specific data segments with specific business objectives, and the exploratory nature of the data mining exercise does not interfere with the warehouse's routine processes of query and reporting. Data are moved from the warehouse to the mine, restructured during the transformation, and then analyzed.
- *Within the warehouse:* This form of data mining works as a "republic within a republic" and is independent of the warehouse structures. However, it usually leads to loss of flexibility, most often because of the centralization within the warehouse. This form limits significant

benefits because problems with mining within the warehouse, once begun, multiply quite rapidly.

In most cases, the beside-the-warehouse approach is prescribed. Stand-alone data mines also can exist in situations where it takes too long for an organization to build its corporate warehouse. In fact, the stand-alone data mine can be used later as a guide to design the warehouse architecture following the sandwich paradigm mentioned above (Parsaye 1995, 1996).

Selection of Data Mining Tools

When selecting a data mining tool or product, it is important to consider how well it integrates with other components of the data warehouse. A two-way exchange interface with an OLAP tool should be done. This allows the OLAP tool to pass selected subsets of the data warehouse to the data mining tool to be mined for patterns that the OLAP tool has difficulty observing. The data mining tool then can forward its findings to the OLAP tool to verify them in a larger database.

Additionally, it is important that the data mining tool support rule conversion. Converting mined rules into queries using structured query language (SQL) allows OLAP and other analysis tools to use the mined rules immediately for data segmentation purposes and makes them available for reuse by other OLAP applications (Ferguson 1997). It is equally important that the data mining tool have visualization capabilities. The success of data mining relies on how well the user can view, evaluate, and act on discovered patterns through the user interface tool. He or she must have a natural way to view the results of a data mining activity, and the user interface must integrate seamlessly into the user's current environment for ease of use. The power of automatic pattern discovery is enhanced when patterns can be viewed via charts and tables using color, position, and size differentiators (Ferguson 1997).

Other requirements need to be considered to have success with a data mining product. The data mining product architecture must account for scalability and run-time performance in its design and must use multiprocessors to take full advantage of performance-enhancing technology. The product must support a full range of data mining activities and techniques to enable users to see the same problem from many different angles. In addition, it must support various possible data sources, both internal and external. Finally, the data mining tool should support data preparation activities, such as data cleansing, data description, data transformation, data sampling, and data pruning (Ferguson 1997).

Customer Relationship Management

Customer relationship management (CRM) is another key knowledge management/BI application. Today, the health-care industry has to react to empowered customers almost as much as any other industry. According to the Pew Internet & American Life Project May 2005 report, 8 in 10 Internet users have looked online for health information. Seventy-nine percent of Internet users have searched online for information on at least one major health topic, statistically the same portion (80 percent) the Pew Internet & American Life Project found in 2005. That translates to about 95 million American adults (18+) who use the Internet to find health information. Moreover, healthcare consumers are willing to spend their own money to get the kind of care they want. According to the National Health Expenditure–related data presented by the federal Health Care Financing Administration (now renamed the Centers for Medicare and Medicaid Services) from 1980 to 2003, private spending on healthcare was at a level of $631.1 billion in 1998, increasing to $913.2 billion in 2003, with the trend continuing in the projections from 2004 to 2014. Finally, consumers are dissatisfied with the current healthcare picture in which physicians spend less and less time with patients. Increasingly, patients want more personalized care and information. According to a study of patients and physicians conducted by Harris Interactive and AriA Marketing's research group, U.S. consumers want to manage their healthcare through a combination of online, phone, and nurse triage services. These findings are echoed by Price Waterhouse Coopers Healthcast 2010, which found that "speed and service will be the keys to consumer satisfaction" (Paddison 2001a, 2001b).

In this environment, healthcare must take the patient perspective and communicate with patients based on their needs, not solely on the healthcare organization's need to promote its strategic vision. This is not to discount the provider's responsibility to create and maintain organizational awareness and loyalty through more traditional marketing approaches, but it does call for a new model. This paradigm leads to event-driven, one-to-one marketing, which is enabled by CRM solutions (Paddison 2001a, 2001b).

CRM is all about providing products and services to meet customer need when and where the customer wants them. Therefore, CRM requires a focus on business strategy, organizational structure, and organizational culture, as well as technology. CRM aligns these elements with customer information and technology so that all customer interactions can be conducted to the long-term satisfaction of the customer and to the benefit and profit of the organization (Imhoff, Loftis, and Geiger 2001). Thus, the redefined CRM solution for healthcare is built on understanding customer needs and health histories and allowing practitioners to effectively implement and track health promotion and disease prevention programs targeted for specific patients and prospects. This is how CRM enables healthcare to build and maintain individual relationships to increase the lifetime value for each customer (Paddison 2001a, 2001b).

Core Communications Programs

In healthcare, the CRM philosophy is based on communications that include **core communications** at the center, supported and surrounded by branding and strategic com-

munications. (See figure 20.18). The term *core communications* refers to the basic communications that inform customers and others in the community about how they can maintain and improve their health. Core communications are a series of triggered, event-specific communications based on need and data, such as age, sex, and health profile, that give providers an appropriate time and personalized reason to communicate with the recipients. They include events such as recommended immunizations (for example, tetanus) and screenings (mammography and prostate cancer exams) as well as classes, newcomer programs, physician referral programs, satisfaction and outcome surveys, and customized newsletters.

Branding communications include messages sent to increase awareness and enhance image in the marketplace. A branding program should differentiate the organization from its competitors and persuade consumers that it is the best place to receive such care. Because most traditional tools used in branding (such as media advertising) are not necessarily launched from a CRM system, it is helpful to show how branding fits with, and benefits from, the CRM structure.

Finally, **strategic communications** are programs created to advance specific organizational goals such as promoting a new center or service, establishing a new program, or positioning the organization as a center of excellence in a specific discipline (for example, cardiology or oncology). Even though strategic goals differ from organization to organization, the CRM system can be used to identify the most attractive candidates for those strategies and to develop messages and offers that promote the organization to customers and track campaign results. These three layers form a complete CRM marketing approach, with core communications and strategic communications largely event driven (Paddison 2001a, 2001b).

Benefits of Core Communications Programs

The core communications program offers the organization several key benefits. Most healthcare organizations want to improve and maintain the health and wellness of their communities. The essence of a core communications program is to inform people of events designed to improve their health, thus making it an important and effective tool in achieving a wellness mission. Customer retention also will increase as

Figure 20.18.   Application of CRM philosophy in healthcare organizations

CORE COMMUNICATIONS
Triggered and event-driven communications based on need and data (for example, age, gender, and health profile)

BRANDING COMMUNICATIONS
Messages sent to increase awareness and enhance image in the marketplace

STRATEGIC COMMUNICATIONS
Programs created to advance specific organizational goals

organizations engage customers in activities that are of interest and importance to them. This, in turn, will increase loyalty and foster long-term relationships and greater customer lifetime value.

In addition, because these communications are targeted only to the individuals for whom they are most relevant, organizations can lower marketing costs significantly and either retain the savings or apply them to other marketing programs. Moreover, the core communications program is a great way to begin leveraging the several hundreds of thousands of dollars required to develop and implement the CRM solution. Finally, after an organization has identified the events to include in its core communications program and has created the messages for various channels, the program runs itself. An automated program sends out the event-triggered communications and notifies the appropriate individuals of the action (Paddison 2001a, 2001b).

Implementation of Core Communications Programs
Putting a core communications program into action involves the following steps:

1. Identify the need. Different individuals have different healthcare needs at different times in their lives. Identifying those needs and matching them to events the organization wants to promote is extremely crucial.
2. Identify the events to promote. Such events might include immunizations, screenings, wellness classes, and so on.
3. Define selection criteria. These criteria are used to determine who should receive each communication based on information in the CRM database. At a minimum, this information will include age and sex but also could include information such as payer type, health status, and so on.
4. Determine the timing for the campaign.
5. Determine the message to communicate. The message should go to the selected audiences with an offer that will prompt a response.
6. Determine how to communicate on a customer-by-customer basis, for instance, via the Internet, direct mail, or calls from the call center (Paddison 2001a, 2001b).

Adoption of a Customer Relationship Management Philosophy

Adoption of the true CRM philosophy will change the order of things within the organization. CRM implementation requires careful planning, an understanding of its critical success factors, and the ability to manage its success factors while continuing to facilitate change. A sustainable CRM-friendly culture must be established in an organization. Several factors can be monitored to ensure that the culture will enable a customer focus. Service staff must understand the positive impacts that can result from satisfied customers. They must be generally accepting and enthusiastic about the customer satisfaction aspects of their positions. Finally, their job skills must be assessed and be adequate for implementing a CRM strategy (Imhoff, Loftis, and Geiger 2001).

The presence of a knowledge management structure is very important in the adoption of a CRM philosophy. The information management infrastructure needs to be in place on both the IT and business sides. Building a CRM strategy without excellent customer information is similar to building a house without a foundation. Managing customers depends on being able to manage large amounts of information about them. And like every other asset, information should be controlled, maintained, and enhanced. However, unlike other assets, information is used by everyone in the organization. Controlling and maintaining information is a very complex task. As a supporting block of a CRM initiative, the information must be accurate and up-to-date. Therefore, customer information management is critical to CRM success (Meza 1998).

Many organizations today have legacy systems, and every line of business has its own customer database. The reality is that the information in these disparate databases is rarely shared effectively across business lines. This so-called silo approach creates an environment that breeds poor data quality and leads to a poor understanding of the organization's customers. Organizations must encourage enterprise-wide understanding of their customer relationships and ensure that all distribution channels and customer touch points share consistent information regarding customer relationships (Meza 1998).

In addition to the emphasis on a customer-based culture and the importance of a solid information management structure, technology plays a key role in the adoption of a CRM philosophy. The ability to develop the CRM program requires the creation of a marketing database powered by the Web. The unique blueprint or data model must be industry focused, market driven, and technology enabled (Paddison 2001a, 2001b). The components of a mature healthcare data repository that provides a near-complete view of individual patient and prospect activities are necessary. The correct tools must be applied to make the database fulfill the tasks for which it was designed, which include analyzing and mining the data for information opportunities. This software, based on algorithms and statistics, can be grouped into three categories: information delivery and data analysis, data mining, and campaign management. All information should be accessible to the user on the desktop through standard word-processing and spreadsheet software (Paddison 2001a, 2001b).

After the data warehouse is built, the organization must develop a strategic plan to take full advantage of the CRM program's capabilities. Key questions to consider include:

- What do I want to accomplish with my CRM program?
- Where are my opportunities?
- Who are my individual customers?

- What is the makeup of their household?
- What do they need? What is their health status?
- Are they insured?
- What message do I need to communicate to them?

A CRM market plan might include an overall evaluation of services and products for value and efficiency, an overall market evaluation for revenue opportunities and growth areas, identification of the size of the market by total number of customers and analysis of the current market share compared with the competitors' share, the development/marketing of programs that can improve wellness and quality of life, and the tracking and evaluation of communications efforts and annual refinement (Paddison 2001a, 2001b).

The CRM strategy must be flexible and remain relevant to changing times (Meza 1998). Understanding the customer base as an asset, with a strategy of differentiation through customer service, provides the foundation for a successful CRM solution (Byrne 2001). When implemented correctly, a CRM program can give organizations the ability to fully understand their customers' needs and expectations across the lines of business and at every point of interaction. Moreover, it can integrate sales, marketing, and customer service initiatives in a manner that optimizes the customer relationship and the customer experience (Meza 1998).

The degree to which an organization is able to change depends on its ability to strengthen customer relationships through improvements in the availability, access, and accuracy of customer information and to eliminate nonvalue-added activities to streamline business processes across the organization. It also is important to develop a learning organization that addresses the issues of training and change because information and processes alone are not sufficient when the right people to service the customer are unavailable.

A training program must include all levels of the organization and stress the importance of customer information management and data quality and how they relate to the successful implementation of a CRM strategy (Meza 1998). In conclusion, healthcare organizations must not forsake the ultimate goal of providing high-quality, consistent service to each customer during each interaction, regardless of the channel. CRM is the cornerstone for accomplishing this goal.

Check Your Understanding 20.2

Instructions: Answer the following questions on a separate piece of paper.

1. What is a learning organization?
2. What are the four categories of healthcare data?
3. What is a data warehouse? What purpose does it fulfill in knowledge management?
4. What function(s) does data mining play in knowledge management?
5. Name the three basic forms of data mining.
6. What is customer relationship management?
7. Explain the differences among core communications, branding communications, and strategic communications.

Application of Knowledge Management to Decision Making

The preceding sections of this chapter have focused on providing an overview of key knowledge management applications in healthcare—data warehousing, EISs, OLAP, data mining, and CRM. These applications play a key role in a learning or knowledge management organization in which data act as the primary source of manipulation to navigate through the decision-making process. Data can be used in several areas, including patient care, process reengineering, quality improvement, clinical and management decision making, basic and applied research, health services research, external reporting, strategic planning, market trend analysis, and more. Various sources of the healthcare data include operational information systems and OLTP systems, legacy systems, departmental databases, primary research data, and secondary research data sources.

As mentioned previously, there is immense data chaos in healthcare because of disparate data sources and extensive amounts of data. Hence, BI inquiry can rarely begin with a precisely framed question. Often knowledge workers need to navigate through the data and ask questions based on what they see at the time in order to discover valuable information in the form of trends and patterns. For this reason, data from different sources need to be analyzed and summarized to achieve meaningful insight, which needs to be presented to other users in the system for effective and timely decision making.

Thus, the decision-making process can be divided into the following three phases:

1. The *discovery phase* involves looking at comparisons and exceptions and examining data from many different dimensions to identify trends and patterns. Discovery tools include OLAP, data mining, and other query tools.
2. The *analysis phase* focuses on proving that the identified trends do exist, understanding them, forecasting them over time, and making solid predictions about their consequences. Analysis tools include modeling, market research, what-if analysis, and so on.
3. The *presentation phase* involves creation of the reports that are most appropriate for the organization's goals and objectives. Presentation tools include data visualization, geographical analysis, bubble charts, and multimedia viewers. These tools must be easy to use and data driven, with drag-and-drop functionality and summarization logic.

Online Analytical Processing as a Discovery Tool

It is important to note that OLAP serves as one of the discovery tools besides data mining. As previously outlined, OLAP is a software configuration that provides a fast way to view and analyze data from any perspective without having to specify the perspective and the exact level of detail required in advance. In other words, OLAP offers fast access to multidimensional information for exploitation in a wider BI context. To leverage an organization's operational data to create strategic acumen, OLAP supports data warehousing as a decision support tool. Using OLAP, enterprises can drive decision support, do trend analysis, compare business units, and monitor strategic business decisions.

In the context of a discovery tool, an OLAP engine is an optimized query generator that can retrieve the right information from the warehouse to accommodate what-if business queries. OLAP data are presented in a way that reflects multiple business dimensions: patients admitted per quarter by disease category, costs per service line by region, medical supplies shipped on time per department per hospital, and so on. This type of information enables managers to conduct effective comparison and trend analysis. OLAP makes it possible to analyze potentially large amounts of data with very fast response times. It also enables users to slice and dice through the data and drill down or roll up through various dimensions as defined by the data structure (Hettler 1997).

A knowledge worker may want to move progressively into more detail or drill down into summarized data. This capability is extremely valuable in investigating what exists at different levels of detail. By enabling multidimensional analysis, business performance reporting, and business modeling, OLAP data sources play a pivotal role in a data warehousing initiative. In addition, OLAP is ideal for meeting business users' requirements because with it, information is stored in an intuitive business structure, is easy to use, and can be delivered to many users within the enterprise. Users can ask questions of the data naturally—in the way they think—without worrying about how the database will interpret their queries. OLAP is also faster, which means users obtain answers more quickly and are likely to use it more often (Hettler 1997).

An organization's success depends on its ability to make timely and efficient decisions. Most healthcare organizations have the data but do not have the ability to turn the data into information and knowledge. This ability to provide complete and high-quality information and knowledge for better decision making will determine not only who survives, but also who thrives in today's constantly changing and competitive healthcare marketplace.

For healthcare organizations to survive under current market pressures, they must react quickly to seize growth- and quality-enhancing opportunities as they arise. Moreover, they must give their customers the ability to interact effortlessly with the organization. This requires that all departments and functions of the organization be integrated with coherent data and information flow among all users. Organizations must work collectively with all their departments to understand how to access the information to improve business and clinical decision making.

In addition, organizations must track progress toward goals and targets across the various departments to provide an integrated picture of where the hospital stands. Finally, they must provide a balanced view of the organization that transcends both financial and clinical data to create direct cause-and-effect relationships between operational and strategic directives.

Data warehousing, EISs, OLAP, data mining, CRM, and other knowledge management applications help organizations address these essential needs. They also help organizations meet their objectives for smart organizational planning and operations; process and outcomes improvement; disease, case, and care management; risk management; cash flow improvement; outcome measurement; cost and clinical effectiveness assessment; and so on. These applications help transform data into BI so that an organization can make strategic decisions and act on the knowledge it has acquired to improve overall performance.

Without question, an organizational culture that cultivates knowledge sharing is critical to the successful implementation of knowledge management applications. As economist Lester C. Thurow discusses in *Building Wealth: The New Rules for Individuals, Companies, and Nations in a Knowledge-Based Economy,* people tend to resist sharing their knowledge when they believe that doing so will undermine their value to the organization (Allison 2000). If the organization aims to successfully integrate knowledge management at its core, management must eliminate this barrier by creating an environment of trust. This is a distinguishing characteristic of a learning organization, which focuses on efficiently acquiring knowledge from different sources, both within and outside the organization. A learning organization uses technology such as data warehousing to ensure that information is available to all employees at the right time and in the right way in order to raise the organization's strategic acumen.

Chief Knowledge Officer

With the importance of a knowledge-sharing culture in mind, a healthcare organization can successfully implement knowledge management applications through creation of a **chief knowledge officer** (CKO) position. The individual in this position would oversee the entire knowledge acquisition, storage, and dissemination process and identify subject matter experts to help capture and organize the organization's knowledge assets. Management should give the CKO authority to research and obtain enabling technologies that would capture and leverage information from the various knowledge assets. To organize this process, the CKO creates a knowledge map to ensure that relevant information sources within the organization are identified and obsolete and/or incorrect information sources are discarded. The CKO also can ensure that an incentive system is in place to encourage knowledge workers to share their knowledge with others in the system. A useful technique might be to reward workers for reusing knowledge and contributing to the corporate knowledge base. This position also might create a "one-stop shop" where knowledge would be accessible to all. Finally, the CKO position can take the leadership in advocating constant change and innovation to capture and improve the use of knowledge.

Check Your Understanding 20.3

Instructions: Answer the following questions on a separate piece of paper.

1. What role(s) do knowledge workers play in organizational decision making?

2. Describe the roles of discovery, analysis, and presentation in the decision-making process.

3. What is OLAP, and what role does it play in decision support systems?

4. What role does the CKO play in a healthcare organization?

Real-World Case

Begun in 1935 as the 47-bed Gregg Memorial Hospital, Good Shepherd Medical Center (GSMC) has since grown to a 349-bed regional referral center for specialized care with the largest trauma center in Longview, Texas. A nonprofit medical center, GSMC is funded solely from patient revenue and community support and receives no public support from any taxing authority. In 1996, the center provided $28 million of uncompensated care to the residents of eastern Texas, largely through the ongoing support of the Good Shepherd Foundation, the Good Shepherd Guild, and the Good Shepherd Prospectors. In 1999, it was named one of the 100 top hospitals nationally for case management and its orthopedic departments and intensive care units.

Wiley Thomas, CIO at GSMC, was faced with the challenges of effective knowledge management that many hospitals face today. The hospital had embarked on a case management program, and data/administrative automation was critical to its success. As Thomas explained, "Appropriate clinical utilization is the name of the game. It is vital that we have technology that meets our very special needs of disease and case management, and also has the capability to empower our clinical decision makers, which includes physicians, to feel comfortable with the data to make clinically appropriate changes in practice patterns."

Thomas responded to these challenges by making data warehouse technology GSMC's computer-based patient record (CPR) foundation using a data warehousing/data repository solution. To date, the hospital has saved more than $3 million in case management and been recognized in *Modern Healthcare* for its success.

Before case management was implemented at Good Shepherd, the average length of stay (ALOS) for a coronary artery bypass patient also having a cardiac catheterization during his stay was 14.7 days. At that time, the HCFA ALOS for that patient type was 12.1 days. Two years after GSMC implemented its case management initiative, the ALOS for these patients plummeted to 10.3 days, less than the HCFA average of 10.8 days.

The case management software used by GSMC pinpoints areas where costs are excessive, allowing doctors and case managers to work together to find an equally effective and less costly treatment option. Quarterly reports consisting of charts and graphs show precisely which physicians are using effective, cost-efficient treatment options. The reports are seen by physicians and reviewed by administration and the executive board. One of the reports includes a top 10 DRG section that lists the physicians with the highest dollar charges. Another report shows the top five physicians with the highest expenditures.

Case managers are assigned to specific areas to determine the average cost of patient treatment and to compare it with Medicare. Case management software not only organizes and calculates the information but also allows each case manager to track individual patients and to tie them back to the physicians who treated them.

Financial outcome is another aspect affected by the case management software, which reduces the time required to track treatments and ALOS. Case management has grown tremendously since the software's implementation. Initially, one nurse was the liaison to cardiovascular patients, but because of the tremendous savings, 12 case managers now handle the steadily growing workload. The case management software helped give GSMC the means to cut costs without sacrificing patient care.

Summary

Knowledge management is the process of collecting and processing information, using it, sharing it, and enhancing it to improve the business practice of healthcare organizations. The maintenance of knowledge is crucial to an organization's viability and ability to reach its peak performance level. Knowledge management involves the transformation of data into information, then into knowledge. The process of knowledge management, with its various components and applications, can enhance clinical and financial decision making.

Before embarking on a knowledge management initiative, it is important to identify the sources of knowledge, or knowledge assets, of an organization. In addition, it is crucial to develop an organized framework to capture knowledge and transform it into business intelligence (BI). There are five steps in a knowledge management initiative that guarantee the transformation of an ordinary organization into a learning organization. The final step involves the deployment and implementation of knowledge management and BI applications. These applications play a key role in a learning or knowledge management organization in which data act as the primary source of manipulation to navigate through a decision-making process.

This chapter addressed five of these applications in detail, including data warehousing, executive information systems, online analytical processing, data mining, and customer relationship management, which are the cornerstones of the healthcare landscape. These applications help transform knowledge into wisdom, which gives organizations the ability to make decisions in a timely manner, improve their performance and operations, and respond to their most important customers—the patients.

Moreover, it important to understand the decision-making process and its phases and to have an organizational culture that cultivates knowledge sharing when the organization aims to successfully integrate knowledge management at its core.

References

Allison, B. 2000 (July 14). Catching the next wave. *DM Review.* Available online from dmreview.com/article_sub.cfm?articleId=2491.

Boar, B. 2000. *The Art of Strategic Planning for Information Technology,* 2nd ed. New York: John Wiley & Sons.

Byrne, R. 2001 (May 11). Unified customer interaction: Bridging the physical/virtual world gap. *DM Review.* Available online from dmreview.com/article_sub.cfm?articleId=3402.

Cintron-Allen, R. 2004 (December). Shared goals demand shared data. *Health Management Technology* 25(12):36–37. Available online from healthmgttech.com/.

Davenport, T., and L. Prusak. 2000. *Working Knowledge: How Organizations Manage What They Know.* Boston: Harvard Business School Publishing.

Dotan, D. 2003 (Aug. 24). Knowledge management for the 21st century hospital system. Paper presented at The Quality Colloquium, Harvard University. Available online from ehcca.com/presentations/qualitycolloquium1/dotanH1.doc.

English, L.P. 1999 (October). Information quality in the knowledge age. *DM Review.* Available online from dmreview.com/article_sub.cfm?articleId=1452.

Evans, J. 1997. Need for analysis drives data warehouse appeal. *Health Management Technology* 18(11):28–31.

Ferguson, M. 1997 (November). Evaluating and selecting data mining tools. *InfoDB* 11(2).

Fuscaldo, D. 2005 (Aug. 23). After years of stagnation, U.S. tech spending ticks upward. *TechnologyReview.com.* Available online from technologyreview.com/articles/05/08/ap/ap_082305.asp?p=1.

Gallagher Financial System, Inc. 1999. Knowledge management and knowledge automation systems. A white paper prepared by Gallagher Financial System Inc. from material provided by P. Haley and P.D. LeFebvre. Available online from gogallagher.com/Knowledge%20Management%20&%20Automation.pdf.

Gerstner, L.V. Jr. 1997. Presentation given at the Securities Industry Association's annual convention in Boca Raton, FL. Quoted in Grandy, C. Breakthrough performance for star schemas. Boulder, CO: Dynamic Information Systems Corp.

Goldman, L. 2001 (Nov. 5). Customer relationship management: Refine, not rebuild your data warehouse. *DM Review.* Available online from dmreview.com/article_sub.cfm?articleId=4253.

Grammer, J. 2000 (March). The enterprise knowledge portal. *DM Review.* Available online from dmreview.com/article_sub.cfm?articleId=1940.

Grant, M.R. 1996 (July/August). Prospering in dynamically-competitive environments: Organizational capability as knowledge integration. *Organization Science* 7(4):375–87.

Harris, K. and T. Berg. 2003 (June 23). *One More Time: What Is Knowledge Management?* Stamford, CT: Gartner Inc.

Hettler, M. 1997 (March). Data mining goes multidimensional. *Healthcare Informatics* pp. 43–50. Available online from healthcare-informatics.com/issues/1997/03_97/sys_rev.htm.

Hughes, G. 2001. Knowledge management: Another avenue for HIM professionals. *Journal of American Health Information Management Association* 72(1):70–71.

IDC.com. 2004 (June). Worldwide business intelligence by segment, 2001–2008. Available online from idc.com.

Imhoff, C., L. Loftis, and J. Geiger. 2001. *Building the Customer-Centric Enterprise.* New York: John Wiley & Sons.

Industry Week. 1995 (Nov. 20). "Gates wins respect." *Industry Week* 12(4).

Kelkar, B. 2001 (Dec. 21). Exploiting symbiosis between data mining and OLAP for business insights. *DM Review.* Available online from dmreview.com/article_sub.cfm?articleId=4446.

Lambert, B. 1996 (March 1). Data warehousing fundamentals: what you need to know to succeed. *DM Review.* Available online from dmreview.com/article_sub.cfm?articleId=1313

Lau, F. 2004 (Sept. 20). Toward a conceptual knowledge management framework in health. *Perspectives in Health Information Management* 1(8). Available online from library.ahima.org/xpedio/groups/public/documents/ahima/bok1_024634.html.

Loshin, D. 2001 (July). Intelligent information processing. *DM Review.* Available online from dmreview.com/article_sub.cfm?articleId=3693.

Makhani, T., and M. Farishta. 2002. The power of online analytical processing. *MUSE Matters* 13(2):23–25.

Makhani, T., and Nanjee, A. 2002. The new generation executive information system. *MUSE Matters* 13(3).

Meza, J. 1998 (Sept. 1). Customer information management: The critical foundation to a CRM strategy. *DM Review.* dmreview.com/article_sub.cfm?articleId=910.

Nonaka, I. 1994 (February). A dynamic theory of organizational knowledge creation. *Organization Science* 5(1).

Oxbrow, N., and A. Abell. 2002. CILIP in the knowledge economy: A leadership strategy. Chartered Institute of Library and Information Professionals. As quoted in Robertson, S. 2005 (March 14). Fact sheet: What is knowledge management? National Electronic Library for Health. Available online from http://libraries.nelh.nhs.uk/knowledgemanagement/.

Paddison, N. 2001a (Jan. 26). Benefits of event-driven CRM in healthcare, part 1. *DM Review.* Available online from dmreview.com/article_sub.cfm?articleId=2999.

Paddison, Nancy. 2001b (Feb. 2). Benefits of event-driven CRM in healthcare, part 2. *DM Review.* Available online from dmreview.com/article_sub.cfm?articleId=3052.

Parsaye, K. 1996 (September). Data mines for data warehouses. *Database Programming and Design.*

Parsaye, K. 1995 (April). The sandwich paradigm for data warehousing and mining. *Database Programming and Design* 9(9):s6–s11.

Penny, P. 2000 (Sept. 8). Knowledge management: Maximizing the return on your intellectual assets. *DM Review.* Available online from dmreview.com/article_sub.cfm?articleId=2678.

Pew Internet & American Life Project. 2005. Health information online. Available online from pewinternet.org/pdfs/PIP_Healthtopics_May05.pdf.

Prusak, L. 1996 (March–April). The knowledge advantage. *Strategy & Leadership* 24(2):6–8.

Shams, K., and M. Farishta. 2001. Data warehousing: Toward knowledge management. *Topics in Health Information Management* 21(3):24–32.

Vesset, D. 2004 (July). *Worldwide Business Intelligence Tools 2004–2008 Forecast Update and 2003 Vendor Shares.* Market analysis document #31472. Framingham, MA: IDC.

Wu, J. 2000a (Nov. 22). Business intelligence: The transition of data into wisdom. *DM Review.* Available online from dmreview.com/article_sub. cfm?articleId=2524.

Wu, J. 2000b (Feb. 10). Business intelligence: What is business intelligence? *DM Review.* Available online from dmreview.com/article_sub.cfm? articleId=1924.

Part VI

Management of Health Information Services

Chapter 21
Principles of Management

David X. Swenson, PhD

Learning Objectives

- To introduce the management discipline, the evolution of management thought, and the key functions and skills of management
- To identify significant trends in managerial models
- To understand that management approaches emerge in response to change drivers of a particular period
- To identify key theorists in the development of management practices

- To describe the four functions of management
- To describe the 10 roles of a manager
- To describe the relationship between management functions and skills and levels of management
- To identify different approaches to problem solving and decision making
- To describe key practices for effective communication

Key Terms

Acceptance theory of authority
Active listening
Administrative management
Balanced scorecard (BSC)
Baldridge Award
Bounded rationality
Break-even analysis
Bureaucracy
Business process reengineering (BPR)
Chain of command
Change drivers
Clinical communication space
Conceptual skills
Controlling
Critical path method
Decentralization
Discipline
Downsizing
Effectiveness
Efficiency
85/15 rule
Emotional intelligence (EI)
Esprit de corps
Evidence-based management
Executive dashboard
Forecasting
Fourteen principles of management
Gantt chart
Goals
Groupthink
Hawthorne effect
Hierarchy of needs
Human relations movement
Interpersonal skills

Intuition
ISO 9000
Leading
Line authority
Linear programming
Management by objectives (MBO)
Management functions
Maslow's Hierarchy of Needs
Nonprogrammed decision
Operational plan
Operations management
Organizing
Paradigm
Piece-rate incentive
Planning
Program evaluation and review technique (PERT)
Programmed decisions
Queuing theory
Revenge effects
Role theory
Satisficing
Scalar chain
Scientific management
Self-monitoring
Simulation and inventory modeling
Span of control
Staff authority
Strategic plan
Tactical plan
Technical skills
Theory X and Y
Time and motion studies
Total quality management (TQM)
Vertical structure

Introduction

Models for management originally were based on traditional ways of organizing people to accomplish tasks. For thousands of years, these typically involved small family cottage industries, military organizations, or church-directed structures. With the advent of the industrial revolution, migration to cities, and specialization of labor, the former methods of management no longer worked effectively. Workers did not necessarily carry on family traditions, could not be commanded to comply with orders, or did not serve out of dedication to some larger corporate value. New ways of thinking about management were needed.

Management theories are not just academic exercises; they are ways of describing how managers think about the way organizations work, which in turn influences their decisions and directs their efforts and behavior. The theories described in this chapter reflect the development of management theories over the decades, as well as newer approaches being developed. Many elements of even the early theories are still practiced widely. By being able to identify our working theories, we are better able to evaluate how appropriate they are for our settings and how we can revise them to work better.

In 1962, Thomas Kuhn published *The Structure of Scientific Revolutions.* Translated into 20 languages and cited by scholars in numerous fields, it has been a reference point for new management thinkers. Kuhn introduced the concept of a **paradigm,** a mental model or structure for perceiving, understanding, and responding to the world. Paradigms make thinking more efficient by drawing attention to certain things, but they also filter out exceptions to the rules where innovations may lie. He argued that scientific progress, rather than growing slowly and incrementally, more often occurs when complexity increases to a high degree and cannot be adequately dealt with by the current paradigm. A paradigm shift then occurs, and the old one is replaced with a new one.

A key idea in management is the recognition that management theories and practices grow out of the unique constellation of forces or **change drivers** that operate at the time. These large-scale forces consist of demographic, social, political, economic, technical, and, more recently, global and informational factors. In a competitive environment, each organization seeks to position itself to succeed against other organizations and does so by the effective and efficient allocation of its resources to respond to these demands.

In this chapter we will describe many of the historical and theoretical developments in management, most of which are still used today in organizations. The functions, skills, and roles of managers will be identified, along with trends in management theory related to problem solving. Finally, the importance of communication in organizations will be emphasized related to the increasing role of information in the healthcare workplace.

Theory into Practice

Three years ago, Northern General Hospital merged with St. Vincent Hospital. The merger was intended to take advantage of the complementary specialized services each hospital provided, and both had equally talented staff and strong reputations in the region. Although the organizations had blended rather well, unforeseen problems emerged.

After the merger, duplicate positions were eliminated, a single vision statement was formulated, and the organizational hierarchy was flattened. Yet, morale was low and turnover continued to be higher than expected, even among staff who were secure in their positions. Conflict among employees, and between managers and employees, became a constant concern.

As management began to examine the problem areas, it became clear that the two hospitals were financially, operationally, and organizationally compatible; however, much less attention and preparation had been given to the human aspects of organizational change. Although executed fairly, the **downsizing** disrupted long-standing relationships, job security, and management–employee trust. Knowing that merged organizations often experience two to three subsequent downsizings, employees were waiting for the next round of layoffs. The flatter structure and lower staff sizes required remaining staff to take on multiple roles and heavier workloads. High performers were encouraged to take on more leadership roles in addition to their regular work; many such ad hoc managers were talented in their fields but had little managerial or leadership experience.

Moreover, the cultures of the two facilities were markedly different, both a strength and a source of conflict. Before the merger, Northern General provided a wide range of health services including abortion and contraception; St. Vincent traditionally limited such services. Several groups of physicians left the merged facility to avoid ethical conflicts.

The health information management (HIM) department was at the heart of the organization in many ways. HIM staff were integrating two different information systems, taking on key roles in developing the new **balanced scorecard** (BSC), and trying to orient staff to the new forms of documentation, all the while dealing with their own uncertainties. They were discovering how essential it was to have a clear understanding of successful management styles and theories that could become the blueprint for the emerging organization.

Landmarks in Management as a Discipline

A **discipline** is a field of study characterized by a knowledge base and perspective that is distinctive from other fields of study. The knowledge base and perspective form a foundation for the discipline's practices, guide research for continuing refinement, and create its literature base. As the study of management found its way into academic settings, theories and practices of management began to emerge. Changing social conditions and growing technological innovations often contributed to the way that management theories were framed.

Scientific Management

The late 19th and early 20th centuries marked the emergence of many elements of modern management theory. The individuals profiled in the following subsections were key players in that development.

Max Weber

German sociologist, lawyer, and political economist Max Weber (1864–1920) was formulating his ideas of the ideal or prototypic organization. Recognizing the inefficiency that was occurring with high variability in standards, he proposed that organizations become bureaucracies. He believed that variability could be reduced by having a formally structured hierarchy of relationships, by formulating rules and regulations to standardize behavior, and by using trained specialists for jobs.

As a result, efficiency could be promoted, subjective judgment and favoritism could be eliminated, and planning could be based on the position rather than the person. At a time when organizational procedures were highly variable, bureaucratic theory offered the structure necessary to improve performance. In the modern marketplace where competitive advantage is maintained through innovation, **bureaucracy** has come more often to refer to slow decision making, unresponsiveness, ignoring the uniqueness of individuals, and rules without reasons.

Frederick Taylor

About the same time that Weber was forming his ideas about bureaucracy, Frederick W. Taylor (1856–1915) was a young engineer working at the Midvale Steel Company. He discovered that his company and most others had tremendous unused potential. Pay and working conditions were poor, waste and inefficiency were prevalent, and management decision making was unsystematic and not based on research of any sort. Taylor introduced new practices whose success led to his being recognized as the Father of Scientific Management. Although many of his ideas are commonly accepted today, they were revolutionary at the time.

Taylor defined the main objective of managers to be that of securing maximum prosperity for employer and employee. He viewed management and the workforce as interdependent and promoted the idea that people were inherently capable of hard work. The problem, he argued, was that the old management stifled workers and could be remedied by his four principles:

1. Management should develop a scientific approach to work, involving precise, measurable guidelines for output; pay could be linked to performance.

2. Management should select, train, and develop workers scientifically to be first class so that the right person has the right job.
3. Management and workers should collaborate to ensure that the job matches plans.
4. Management should provide equal division of work and responsibility between workers and management.

To implement his ideas, Taylor and his followers developed new techniques. **Time and motion studies,** for example, were conducted in which tasks were subdivided into their most basic movements. Detailed motions were timed to determine the most efficient way of carrying them out. After the one best way was found, the best worker match for the job was hired, tools and procedures were standardized, instruction cards were written to guide workers, and breaks were instituted to reduce fatigue. From implementing new practices, one mining company increased production from 12.5 to 47 tons of loaded pig iron per day and reduced the number of yard laborers from 600 to 140 with no reduction in output. A **piece-rate incentive** system also was developed in which workers received additional pay when they exceeded the standard output level for their task.

Taylor's principles were quickly embraced and later refined by Frank and Lillian Gilbreth, Henry Gantt, and others. The Gilbreths were a husband and wife team who developed many of the early ideas of ergonomics and work efficiency. Their original studies focused on bricklaying, part of Frank's background, in which they noticed that workers developed their own ways of working and that no two workers used the same method. The Gilbreths divided the process into detailed individual motions they called "therbligs" (Gilbreth nearly spelled backwards) to identify unnecessary or inefficient motions. Seeking the single best way to perform the tasks, they reduced the number of motions for bricklaying from 18 to 4.5, which resulted in much higher productivity, less fatigue, and better planning. Lillian (1878–1972) was known for her studies on finding innovative ways to design efficient kitchen and home living areas for patients with cardiac-limited conditions.

Frank Gilbreth

Frank Gilbreth (1868–1924) embraced time saving with a passion and gained notoriety with his experiments. For example, he would experiment to see whether it would be faster to button his vest from top to bottom or the reverse. He tried to shave with two razors, but the time saving was reduced by having to patch his several cuts. Two of his children wrote the popular book *Cheaper by the Dozen* in which they detailed the family's preoccupation with innovations.

Henry Gantt

Henry Gantt (1861–1919) worked for Taylor and was known for his promotion of favorable psychological work conditions. He may be best remembered for his development of the **Gantt chart,** which is still used for project management to show how the components of a task are scheduled over time. His chart contributed to development, in the late 1950s, of the **program evaluation and review technique** (PERT) developed by the U.S. Navy and the **critical path method** developed by Dupont. He also contributed his Task and Bonus Plan to management, which provided bonus payment for workers who exceeded their production standards for the day.

Many of these developments were rapidly applied to the growing market demand for popular products in the United States. Sears and Roebuck probably designed the first manufacturing assembly line for meeting mail-order delivery. In the automobile industry, Henry Ford (who employed Taylor) became intrigued by the moving conveyer belt of carcasses in a Chicago slaughterhouse. He quickly developed this idea into his assembly line for automobile manufacturing, streamlining production from a one-person assembly time of 12.5 hours to about 93 minutes per car. The idea was taken to its extreme in healthcare in the early 1970s when Russian ophthalmologists attempted to introduce assembly-line radial keratotomy, a surgery for correcting eye lens problems. The idea did not catch on widely, although there have been attempts in other countries to promote this idea to cut medical costs.

The legacy of scientific management is pervasive and persists in many areas of modern management. At a time when most businesses were growing in size and complexity, but lacked sound organization, Taylorism provided principles for increasing standardization and consistency. It emphasized the role of research in understanding how tasks were done, in selecting and training people, and in providing consistency in rules and procedures to promote efficiency. However, Taylorism was not without critics. Although scientific management helped managers routinize the internal workings of the business, it essentially ignored the external environment. In addition, critics complained that it was based on simplistic economic motivation, that workers were viewed as mechanistic parts of an organizational machine, and that senior management tasks were excluded from analysis.

Administrative Management

Attempting to compensate for scientific management's exclusion of senior management, **administrative management** argued that management was a profession and could be learned. The following subsections profile three individuals who played key roles in describing management functions.

Henry Fayol

Henry Fayol (1841–1925), a French engineer and director of mining, published a book summarizing his executive experiences in 1916. Fayol's major contribution includes a description of both five functions of management and fourteen principles for organizational design and administration.

Fayol's five **management functions** have persisted with some variation into modern organizations and identify key functions that define the manager's role. These managerial functions were:

- **Planning** consists of examining the future and preparing plans of action to attain goals.
- **Organizing** includes the ways in which the managed system is designed and operated to attain the desired goals. It involves the way that tasks are grouped into departments and resources are distributed to them.
- **Leading** (sometimes also called directing) is the process of influencing the behavior of others. It involves motivating, creating shared culture and values, and communicating with all levels of the organization.
- **Controlling** refers to the monitoring of performance and use of feedback to ensure that efforts are on target toward prescribed goals, making course corrections as necessary.

Fayol's fifth function, coordination or unifying and harmonizing activity and effort has been absorbed by the other functions (primarily controlling) in modern versions.

Fayol formulated **fourteen principles of management** to guide managerial activities within the total organization. (See figure 21.1.) Like his managerial functions, most have been incorporated into modern organizations and are widely accepted today. For example, authority was proposed as the right of an executive to give orders and expect obedience. Unity of command meant that each employee reports to only one boss. The **scalar chain,** or line of authority, ensured that everyone in the organization appears in the **chain of command** and reports to someone. **Esprit de corps** emphasized

Figure 21.1.   Fayol's fourteen principles

1. *Specialization of labor:* Work allocation and specialization allow concentrated activities, deeper understanding, and better efficiency.
2. *Authority:* The person to whom responsibilities are given has the right to give direction and expect obedience.
3. *Discipline:* The smooth operation of a business requires standards, rules, and values for consistency of action.
4. *Unity of command:* Every employee receives direction and instructions from only one boss
5. *Unity of direction:* All workers are aligned in their efforts toward a single outcome.
6. *Subordination of individual interests:* Accomplishing shared values and organizational goals take priority over individual agendas.
7. *Remuneration:* Employees should receive fair pay for work.
8. *Centralization:* Decisions are made at the top.
9. *Scalar chain:* Everyone is clearly included in the chain of command and line of authority from top to bottom of the organization.
10. *Order:* People should clearly understand where they fit in the organization, and all people and material have a place.
11. *Equity:* People are treated fairly and a sense of justice should pervade the organization.
12. *Tenure:* Turnover is undesirable and loyalty to the organization is sought.
13. *Initiative:* Personal initiative should be encouraged.
14. *Esprit de corps:* Harmony, cohesion, teamwork, and good interpersonal relationships should be encouraged.

the work climate in which harmony and cohesion promoted good work.

Chester Barnard

Chester Barnard (1886–1961), a former president of the New Jersey Telephone Company and the Rockefeller Foundation, published *The Functions of the Executive* in 1938. In this book, he elaborated the role of top executives. He proposed that the leader needed information from those below, that the communication system is designed and implemented by the executive, and that the role of middle management is to implement plans and solve problems.

Barnard developed the **acceptance theory of authority,** which proposes that people have free will to choose whether they follow work orders. In addition, he emphasized that the measure of organizational cooperation is effectiveness and efficiency. **Effectiveness** refers to the degree to which the organization achieves its intended outcomes; **efficiency** refers to how well a minimum of resources is allocated to achieve the outcomes.

Mary Parker Follett

Another major contributor to the administrative approach was Mary Parker Follett (1868–1933). In contrast to what was often considered a mechanistic view by Taylor, she was interested in broader social ideas and championed the role of relationships in organizations. Although she drew mixed attention in the late 1920s, she foresaw the development of a systems view of business, the role of empowered employees in organizational development, and the use of workgroups to implement solutions. Her ideas have enjoyed a revival in recent years, acknowledged by such management gurus as Peter Drucker and Henry Mintzberg. Follett promoted using teamwork and creative group effort, involving people in organizational development, and integrating the organization, which contained many elements of systems theory.

Humanistic Management

Although the United States has always touted itself as the home of democracy, the equity of power in the workplace has not always existed between workers and management. By the early 1900s, there were growing social pressures to treat workers in a more enlightened manner. Building on Barnard's and Follett's ideas that people should be treated fairly and that effective controls come from individual workers, the stage was set for a shift in management thought stimulated by an experiment at an electric power plant.

Hawthorne Studies

At the turn of the century, gas and electricity companies were intensely competitive about their respective products, and it appeared that electricity had edged out gas. To firm up its advantage, Thomas Edison and the Committee on Industrial Lighting proposed a study that would confirm the advantage of electric lighting. The Hawthorne plant of the Western Electric Company was elected to serve as the laboratory for examining the effects of illumination. From 1924 to 1932, Harvard professors Elton Mayo and Fritz Roethlisberger conducted the series of experiments. In some cases, the lighting in the plant was changed to see how it affected productivity. Although performance initially increased when illumination was improved, it paradoxically also improved when lighting was lowered to about the level of moonlight. The study concluded that although light was not the motivator they intended, positive attention and human relations improved performance—the so-called **Hawthorne effect.**

The Human Relations Movement

The human relations movement revolutionized thinking about how to treat workers to improve productivity and initiated the **human relations movement.** Sometimes referred to as the contented cow approach (contented cows give more milk), the belief was that satisfied workers are more productive. Interestingly, reexamination of the original research design and data suggests that financial incentives had a good deal to do with motivating people, and yet the impact of the human relations emphasis continues (Parson 1974). This movement reached its peak during the 1960s and 1970s.

Human Resources Management

In the 1950s, the field of psychology in the United States was just coming into its own prominence, as were theories of motivation. Observing that many problems derived from an inability to meet needs, Abraham Maslow (1908–1970) suggested that a hierarchy of needs might help to explain behavior and provide guidance for managers on how to better motivate workers.

His now-famous hierarchy, **Maslow's Hierarchy of Needs,** began with physiological existence needs and progressed through safety, social belongingness, self-esteem, and finally self-actualization or creativity needs. This developmental view of needs meant that to motivate people, lower-order needs should be satisfied before higher-order needs could serve as motivators. Although these were useful generalizations, in the emerging global economy with diverse populations, motivators can vary considerably by culture. What works as a management approach in American organizations may not work as well in other countries or cultures. (See chapter 24 for a full discussion of current human resources management principles, issues, and practices.)

Douglas McGregor

Douglas McGregor (1906–1964) recognized the shift in conceptual models from assumptions that workers were incapable of independent action to beliefs in their potential and high performance. He formulated the contrasting views as **theory X and Y** (1960). Theory X presumed that workers inherently disliked work and would avoid it, had little ambition, and mostly wanted security; therefore, managerial direction and control was necessary. Theory Y took a more enlightened view and assumed that work was as natural as play, that motivation could be both internally and externally driven, and that under the right conditions people would seek responsibility and be creative. Although theory Y is most favored at present, theory X may still be appropriate in some military, corrections, and immature workforce settings. In contrast, the innovative Saturn Corporation has based nearly all its auto manufacturing practices on theory Y.

Despite its simplicity, the human relations view brought management to focus on the human side of enterprise (to use McGregor's term). Managers and researchers began to consider the possible role of social and psychological factors on performance. This gave balance to a view of workers that was too heavily laden with mechanistic and economic explanations.

Operations Management

The innovations resulting from wars, the space race, and other international crises have often been the impetus for innovation. With World War II came the problems of planning, organizing, distributing, and monitoring huge collections of troops and materiel on a global basis. Advances in the fields of statistics, mathematics, and quantitative methods were brought to bear on decision making and strategy in an approach called operations research. **Operations management** later emerged as an application of these techniques in the business setting to better understand how products and services could be manufactured and delivered.

Techniques

A variety of techniques is now commonly found in many organizations, including:

- **Forecasting** is regularly used for planning in which previous conditions (such as sales and inventory) are projected into the future. Increasingly sophisticated software can provide projections of changes in technology, demographics, and human resources needs. However, in a rapidly changing environment, predictions based on past performance can be uncertain.
- **Linear programming** is used to identify an optimal decision given a set of planned constraints or limited resources.
- **Break-even analysis** helps planners determine when a project "breaks even," that is, the level of sales at which total revenues equal total costs. Revenues beyond that are profits.
- **Queuing theory** is a mathematical technique for determining the flow of customers or for designing optimal wait times for services.
- **Simulation and inventory modeling** is a recent development in management science based on computerization and systems concepts. The key components and processes of a system are represented in a computer model so that planners can experiment with different operating strategies and designs to get the best results before committing to their actual implementation.
- **PERT** was originally developed by the Navy in 1958 to coordinate the building of submarines. Now facilitated by powerful computer packages, PERT allows large, long-term, and complex projects to be shown graphically in order to clarify critical task sequences, potential bottlenecks, and the time required for them. For complex situations such as healthcare systems, computer decision support can help explore and optimize decisions.

Although many of these programs and techniques are challenging to learn, their ability to deal with vast amounts of data provides considerable advantage to the managers who can fully use them.

Contemporary Management

Although many aspects of older theories of management are still widely practiced in most organizations, research and practical experience have led to many new developments in the field. More contemporary approaches to management include **management by objectives** (MBO), **total quality management** (TQM), and an emphasis on excellence. Each of these has made a contribution to better understanding how effective management works, but none of them alone has yet succeeded in producing a comprehensive solution for managing organizations.

Peter Drucker and Management by Objectives

Often referred to as the guru of management gurus, Peter Drucker (1909–) more clearly formulated the practice of strategy by integrating formulation, tactical planning, and budgeting into a single system of management (Kerker 2001). He revolutionized the role of strategy by wresting it from the hands of top management and making it everyone's job, helping workers understand how mission, strategy, goals, and performance were related. Because strategy was action oriented, starting in the 1950s, Drucker elaborated on the technique of management by objectives (MBO), in which clear target objectives could be stated and measured and could direct behavior. The four elements of an MBO system include (Drucker 1986):

- Top management's planning and setting of goals
- Managers with subordinates setting individual objectives related to organizational goals
- Autonomy in the means of achieving objectives
- Regular review of performance in obtaining objectives

W. Edwards Deming and Quality

From the late 1970s to the mid-1980s, the United States was beset with a series of economic setbacks. Serious recessions, a growing trade deficit, government deregulation, and huge operating losses led to the downsizing of hundreds of thousands of workers. Quality became the focus as a means of increasing competitive position, and much of the idea was derived from W. Edwards Deming (1900–1993), an American statistician. Deming had initially developed his ideas in the 1940s (Walton 1986), but the American economy was booming at the time and seemed to believe it had found the "one best way" to do things. Consequently, American industry was inattentive to Deming's ideas about improvement and his statistical control procedures for monitoring quality. However, the Japanese were suffering from an all-but-destroyed economy and were eager to hear new ideas about production. They quickly adopted the concept of total quality management (TQM).

Total Quality Management

TQM purported to overcome the limitations of MBO, criticizing the use of quotas because workers too often spent too much time trying to look good or protect themselves by seeking short-term objectives and ignoring long-term and critical outcomes. TQM offered a way to build in high performance by maximizing employee potential and continuous improvement of process. The **85/15 rule** of TQM proposes that 85 percent of problems encountered are the result of faulty systems rather than unproductive employees. The manager's job, then, becomes one of anticipating and removing barriers to high employee performance. Deming proposed his fourteen principles for TQM implementation. (See figure 21.2.)

Variations of TQM also were promoted by Juran and Crosby, and many of the ideas now find expression in a variation called **business process reengineering** (BPR). In the 1990s, when recognition of the high level of business competition was reaching a peak, Hammer and Champy (1993) published *Reengineering the Corporation.* They proposed that a radical redesign of the organization might be necessary to reduce costs, streamline operations, and improve quality of service. By the mid-1990s, the idea was often used to justify downsizing, or the reduction of labor costs by laying off portions of the workforce, often without achieving the improvements desired.

The popularity of these approaches has demonstrated the growing importance of customer satisfaction, benchmarking, employee involvement, and teamwork. Quality has become a national goal. In 1987, Congress established a national award to recognize excellence in the manufacturing and service industries, small business, and, in 1999, healthcare and education. The **Baldridge Award,** named after the Secretary of Commerce, is based on meeting several criteria: leadership, strategic planning, customer focus, information and analysis, human resources and process focus, and business results.

ISO 9000 is another example of the drive toward quality improvement. ISO 9000 is an internationally agreed-upon set of standards for quality management established in 1987. Adopted by more than ninety countries, the generic standards can be applied to organizations of any size. It involves defining, executing, and auditing best practices in production or service delivery (ISO Online 2002).

Peter and Waterman's *Search for Excellence*

Although elements of most major theories can be found within the practices of successful managers, new developments and refinements in thinking continue to thrive. In 1982, Peters and Waterman published *In Search of Excellence.* Based on a sample of highly successful business firms, they described the management practices that led to their success. Eight characteristics were described that became the rage in management circles for a time, with managers hoping to reproduce in their own organizations what top firms had done. (See figure 21.3.) Although the eight practices are very

Figure 21.2.   Deming's fourteen principles

1. Create a constancy of purpose toward continual improvement of products and services, with the objectives to stay in business, be competitive, and provide jobs.
2. Adopt the new philosophy for a new economic age by correcting superstitious learning, calling for a major change, and looking at the customer rather than competition.
3. Cease dependence on inspection to achieve quality by eliminating emphasis on mass inspection and building quality in from the beginning.
4. Don't award business based on price tag alone, and minimize total costs by developing trusting and loyal long-term relationships with single suppliers.
5. Constantly and continually improve production and service systems and thereby improve quality and decrease costs.
6. Institute training on the job, where barriers to good work are removed and managers provide a setting that promotes worker success.
7. Institute leadership with the aim of revising supervision to better help people, machines, and processes do a better job.
8. Drive out fear so everyone can work effectively toward company goals.
9. Break down barriers between departments so that various departments can work as a team and anticipate problems of production or use of a product or service.
10. Avoid asking for new levels of productivity and zero defects through slogans and targets because most problems of low productivity lie with the system rather than the worker.
11. Replace work standards such as quotas, numerical goals, and MBO with good leadership.
12. Remove barriers that rob people at all levels of their pride of workmanship; shift from numbers to quality.
13. Institute a program of education and self-improvement by emphasizing lifelong learning and employment.
14. Transformation of the workplace occurs through everyone's action.

Figure 21.3.   Characteristics of highly successful firms

1. *A bias for action:* They establish a value for action and implementation rather than overanalyzing and delaying with endless committees.
2. *Close to the customer:* They listen and respond to customers to satisfy their needs.
3. *Autonomy and entrepreneurship:* They empower people and encourage innovation and risk taking.
4. *Productivity through people:* They increase employees' awareness that everyone's contributions lead to shared success.
5. *Hands on, value driven:* Their managers should be visible, involved, and know what is going on.
6. *Stick to the knitting:* They stay with the core business, what they do well, and avoid wide diversification.
7. *Simple form, lean staff:* They have fewer administrative layers and keep the structure simple.
8. *Simultaneous loose–tight properties:* They maintain dedication to core principles but encourage flexibility and experimentation in reaching goals.

important, a follow-up of the same organizations four years later showed disappointing results. In that short time, 66 percent had fallen from a top position and 19 percent were in a troubled position (Pascale 1990).

Although researchers continue to search for the essential ingredients that will make firms most successful, the lesson from the excellence studies highlights some important principles, including:

- Whether you succeed or fail, try to understand what brought that about.
- When you succeed, recognize that the success factors are not static but, rather, are continually changing.
- Do not let past success strategies keep you from discovering new ones for the future.
- What may contribute to the success of one type of organization or competitive setting may not be as useful to other types and settings or at other stages of organizational development.

Check Your Understanding 21.1

Instructions: Answer the following questions on a separate piece of paper.

1. What are some of the important management concepts that have persisted over the decades? Why have they persisted?

2. Why have some management ideas been rapidly accepted, and others have required years to become popular?

3. Using the example of the Gilbreth time-motion study, identify some complex activity you engage in (such as packing for a trip, dressing in the morning, and so on) and see how you can streamline the sequence to become more efficient.

4. Explore reasons why the top companies identified in Peters and Waterman's *In Search of Excellence* dropped from their top position within a few short years. How might that have been prevented?

Functions and Principles of Management

As mentioned earlier, Fayol identified four functions of management. Related to these functions are certain categories of skills that are needed to carry them out.

Managerial Functions

As theories of management began to be refined, so too did the formal nature of the manager's role. As organizations increased in diversity, complexity, and size, managers often shifted their expertise from expert knowledge in doing a task to expert knowledge in managing other people. As Mary Parker Follett is reputed to have said, "Management is the art of getting things done through people" (Stoner and Freeman 1989). Specific functions of management came to be defined, as did a range of skills and subroles that contribute to successful problem solving.

Fayol's management functions of planning, organizing, leading, and controlling continue to be useful categories for examining the work of the manager. After the enterprise is begun, these four stages become a cycle for continuous improvement in which the last function of control is fed back into planning for plan revision.

Planning

Planning is the first step in management and involves determining what should be accomplished and how. Although planning occurs at all levels, top-level or strategic planning is most critical in formulating the mission and providing direction for change. When these strategies are defined, they can be implemented at the lower levels of the organization. Planning provides competitive advantage over those who minimize the importance of planning, as reflected in higher levels of performance such as profits (Shrader, Taylor, and Dalton 1984).

Plans are usually organized hierarchically, with a mission statement driving the enterprise by defining exactly what business the organization is in and what is valued. The **strategic plan** follows from the mission. It is formulated by top management, sets the priorities and positioning of the organization for a time period, and is based on the constellation of internal strengths and weaknesses and external opportunities and threats. These are translated through the lower levels of the organization by middle management, which formulates **tactical plans** for the organization's major divisions. At the lower departmental levels, these finally become **operational plans** that are implemented as daily activities.

Plans are usually expressed in terms of **goals.** Goals are statements of intended outcomes that provide a source of direction and motivation as well as a guideline for performance, decision making, and evaluation. Good goals cover key result areas of the strategy; have the characteristics of being specific, measurable, and challenging, but achievable; and are set for a given period of time.

Organizing

After the goals have been specified, the task changes to deciding how resources can be allocated to achieve them. Traditionally, division of labor has been used to divide work into separate jobs. This specialization allows for development of greater expertise and standardization of tasks and for clear selection and training criteria. However, too narrow or specialized a task, as in assembly-line work, may produce more boredom than productivity. As Bridges notes (1994), the emerging economy with downsized and flatter organizations may require workers to take on multiple roles and, consequently, to have portfolios of skills rather than highly defined job descriptions.

Jobs are most often organized by positions, and the positions are arranged hierarchically in the business by an organizational chart. (An example of a typical hospital organizational chart is shown in figure 21.4.) The organizational chart often includes departmental subdivisions and follows the scalar principle and unity of command discussed earlier. The **vertical structure** of the organization refers to the formal design of positions within departments and divisions,

Figure 21.4.   Sample hospital organizational chart

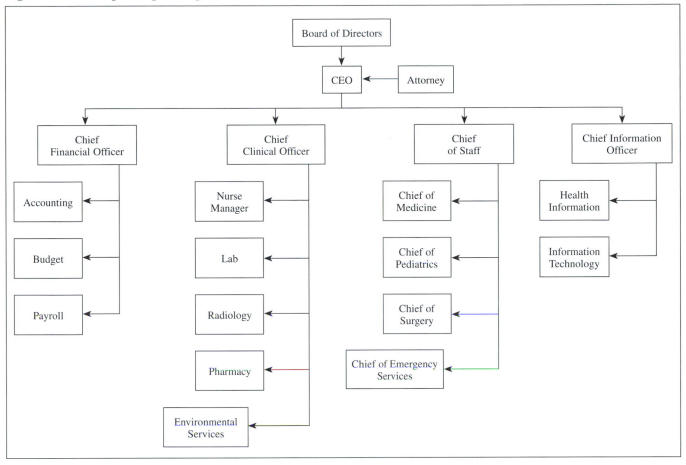

the lines of authority and responsibility, and the allocation of resources to them. Two kinds of authority are found in organizations. **Line authority** is the right of managers to direct the activities of subordinates under their immediate control; **staff authority** is related to the expert knowledge of specialists and involves their advising and recommending courses of action.

Each supervisor has a certain number of people who report to him or her, which is referred to as the span of management or the **span of control.** Although the span of control is determined more often by tradition or accident, there are several factors to consider in optimally balancing it. In general, the span is larger when work is routine and homogeneous, workers have similar tasks, rules and guidelines are available, people are well trained and motivated, workers are located together, and task times are short (Jacques 1996). Deciding how a combination of factors leads to a particular span has been facilitated by technology. For example, the Healthcare Management Council (HMC) provides a comprehensive measurement of organizational factors leading to a span of management recommendation. The HMC Span of Control Analysis considers organizational flatness, departmental fragmentation, and layers of management using organizational charts. The HMC report can be used by managers to

optimize organizational structure, set staffing and financial targets, and determine needs (HMC 2001).

Related to span is delegation, in which managers transfer authority to subordinates to carry out a responsibility. With an increasing focus on customers and rapid response, frontline workers are now trained to make decisions that once were made levels above them. When authority and responsibility move from the organization's top levels to its lower levels where they can be competently exercised, centralized decision making becomes decentralized. Although **decentralization** enables top managers to take on new responsibilities or spend time with other priorities, it places an additional burden on workers. (See chapter 23 for further discussion of organizational structures and charts.)

Leading

The third managerial function accomplishes goals by influencing behavior and by motivating and inspiring people to high performance. At the turn of the century, an autocratic view of leadership was considered to be appropriate, but as humanistic views have prevailed over the decades, leadership has become decentralized and distributed throughout the organization.

Leading is most often accomplished by communicating, directing, and motivating, all intended to influence behavior to perform well. Power, the ability to influence, is central to leadership and derives from several sources, including:

- *Authority* or legitimate power comes from the right of the position in the organization to direct the activities of subordinates.
- *Reward power* is based on the leader's ability to withhold or provide rewards for performance.
- *Coercive power* maintains control over punishments.
- *Referent power* exists when the leader possesses personal characteristics that are appealing to the constituency, and the constituency follows out of admiration, charismatic impact, or the desire to be like the leader.
- *Expert power* occurs when the leader has knowledge or expertise that is of value (French and Raven 1959).
- *Information power* is based on the persuasive content of the person's message, apart from personal characteristics (Raven 1983).

Leadership behaviors and most models of leadership fall into two categories: task-oriented behaviors, and social or group-oriented behaviors. Task-oriented behaviors are directed toward defining tasks, creating structure and rules, ensuring production, and placing emphasis on quality and speed of output. Social orientation focuses on interpersonal behaviors that develop and maintain harmonious work relationships, encourage morale, reduce stress and conflict, and build worker satisfaction. Several models of leadership, such as the Blake-Mouton Managerial Grid, use these two dimensions and are discussed in a later section of this chapter.

Controlling

The final managerial function refers to the monitoring of performance, determining whether it is on or off course in achieving the goals and making course corrections as needed. Managers are obligated to ensure that progress is made toward achieving goals, although recent trends indicate that employees are empowered to monitor themselves and each other, rather than being monitored from the top. This obviously requires selecting employees who have the maturity and integrity to accept this responsibility, but it corrects for the distortion and delay that can occur in a very hierarchical organization.

Significant breakthroughs have occurred in control with the development of the **executive dashboard** and balanced scorecard (BSC) introduced in 1992 (Kaplan and Norton 1996). The executive dashboard is often characterized as a manager's version of a pilot's cockpit dashboard; it contains all the critical information for leading the organization. The dashboard typically contains regularly updated information on key strategic measures such as forecasts, customer satisfaction, billings, profit, and so on.

The BSC is an extension of strategic planning in which key performance indicators are measured at all levels of the organization and progress with workers and management receiving ongoing feedback. Categories of feedback

usually include financial, customer satisfaction, internal processes (for example, quality, response time), and learning and growth. For example, the Health Information Department at New Hampshire Hospital worked to develop greater efficiency by asking staff to suggest best practices. Their suggestions resulted in reorganizing the clinical signature requirements for the discharge summary, rewriting and clarifying the release of information form, adding a "Transcription Corner" to the hospital's newsletter to better inform staff of the transcription process, and creating a customer satisfaction survey (Damour 2000).

The four functions of management vary in emphasis according to the level of management involved. (See figure 21.5.) In general, as one moves from first-line to middle management to top managers, planning increases, organizing increases, leading decreases, and controlling stays about the same (Mahoney, Jerdee, and Carroll 1965).

Managerial Skills

The categories of skills required to perform the four management functions are conceptual, interpersonal, and technical skills (Katz 1974). As management has become increasingly complex, the requisite skills for carrying out the four managerial functions also vary by level in the organization. (See figure 21.6.)

Conceptual Skills

The need for **conceptual skills** has increased significantly over the decades. Where it once was important only to have good technical skills, now a successful manager must be able to understand diverse fields and deal with complex situations.

Figure 21.5.   Management functions by level in the organization

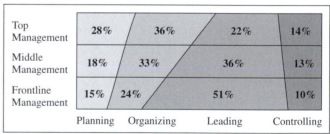

	Planning	Organizing	Leading	Controlling
Top Management	28%	36%	22%	14%
Middle Management	18%	33%	36%	13%
Frontline Management	15%	24%	51%	10%

Figure 21.6.   Functional skills by level in the organization

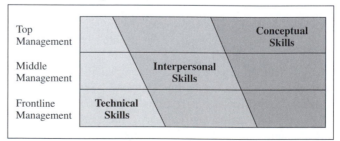

Top Management		Conceptual Skills
Middle Management	Interpersonal Skills	
Frontline Management	Technical Skills	

According to Tenner (1996), the lack of sufficient conceptual and planning skills has led to revenge effects. **Revenge effects** are unexpected and usually undesired outcomes that emerge from good intentions but failure to understand the long-term or ripple effects of an action in an interconnected organization or system (Swenson 2001).

For example, the HIPPA privacy rule was intended to provide greater patient privacy protection and quality of care, while also enabling better information access to providers. The strong emphasis on privacy and apprehension about the consequences of inappropriate information release has led some facilities to be overly cautious in releasing information. The *Seattle Times* reported an incident in which a man was unable to obtain information on his injured mother when she was transferred from an assisted living facility to an emergency department with a broken ankle. In another instance, Leo Greenawalt, 20-year president of the Washington State Hospital Association, could only obtain information that his elderly father was in intensive care, despite the fact that Greenawalt thoroughly explained to the facility that HIPPA allowed him access to such information. As a result of overzealous restriction, patients, relatives, and other care providers have experienced frustrating delays in obtaining information (Burrington-Brown 2004).

Interpersonal Skills

Interpersonal skills involve the ability to work with and through others to accomplish goals. Depending on the nature of the work and the level of interaction needed among individuals, interpersonal skills may or may not be a critical skill for employee success. However, managers, in their interactions with employees and with each other, need to cultivate impeccable interpersonal skills.

That the interpersonal domain is important is shown in a review of top management texts in which this was the only category that they all shared in common (Bigelow 1993). However, as the Institute for Employment Studies reports, managers too often have a skill gap between what is required and the actual level of interpersonal effectiveness (Kettley and Strebler 1997).

Interpersonal competency is based on self-awareness and understanding, and the best managers are those who can articulate both their strengths and weaknesses (Goleman 1998). Yet, self-awareness is not enough and consistently high performers also demonstrate **self-monitoring** (Church 1997). Self-monitoring refers to the ability to observe the reactions that one's behavior elicits in others and then adjusting one's behavior to improve the relationship. Other important interpersonal skills include communicating, motivating and influencing, managing conflict, credibility, and learning how to complement different ways of interacting (Page, Wilson, and Meyer 1999).

Emotional Intelligence

Effective managers are different from successful managers (Luthans, Hodgetts, and Rosenkrantz 1988). Effective managers are identified as those who have satisfied and committed subordinates and produce results; in contrast, successful managers are those who have been promoted rapidly. Such promotions are often related to their interpersonal effectiveness.

Some people believe that emotions do not have a role in the workplace, but others, such as Mathew Jeuchter, president of the American Society for Training and Development, assert that "leadership is almost all emotional intelligence" (Goleman 1998). Although it has been around for a long time, Daniel Goleman popularized the idea in his 1995 book, *Emotional Intelligence,* and it is currently one of the most widely discussed topics in psychology. Advocates of **emotional intelligence** (EI) believe that awareness and use of feelings complements rational intelligence and experience, and it is the combination of these that is the key to success. (See table 21.1.)

EI has caught the interest of many prominent organizations: Nearly 10 percent of Fortune 500 firms have used IE concepts in employee development efforts, and Johnson & Johnson initiated EI aptitude measuring for employees being considered for managerial potential in its consumer products division (Carey 2004). There is some supportive evidence for such use. Air Force recruiters who were selected based on their high scores on an EI measure were found to be more successful in attracting new recruits. They scored higher on assertiveness, empathy, happiness, and emotional self-awareness. The scores enabled the Air Force to predict successful recruiters by threefold and realize an annual savings of $3 million. In a multinational consulting firm, partners were assessed on EI and those who scored high on 9 or more of the 20 scales generated $1.2 million more from their accounts than lower scorers—a 139 percent gain (Boyatzis 2001).

Critics of the EI concept argue that it is not a distinct ability but, rather, a conglomerate of personality traits such as emotional stability, conscientiousness, and agreeableness. They believe that EI does not meet conventional standards of psychological measurement and that the criteria for measurement change over time. Additionally, they are concerned

Table 21.1.   Attributes of Emotional Intelligence

- Self-awareness: The ability to monitor, notice, and label one's feelings as they occur. This allows one to be more certain about feelings and to identify early vague feelings.
- Self-regulation: The ability to manage one's emotions and impulses. A person with this skill is often viewed as being reflective, comfortable with change and ambiguity, and able to control impulsiveness.
- Motivation: Being highly motivated is essential for focusing attention, mastering situations, showing creativity, and being productive and successful.
- Empathy: The ability to recognize emotions in others. This is important for teamwork as well as for helping adjust one's behavior to the emerging reactions of others.
- Social skills: The ability to handle relationships with others is central to being perceived as popular, effective with others, and having the qualities of a leader.

Source: Adapted from Goleman 1995.

that claims of its predicting success are exaggerated and that self-reports used are subject to bias (Matthews, Zeidner, and Roberts 2002).

Regardless of the criticism, organizations are eager to find something that will give their employees, managers, and leaders a competitive edge. Training programs, self-help books, and self-assessment instruments proliferate on EI. However, professionals should be cautious in expecting that a brief workshop will produce significant increases in these skills or personality features.

Technical Skills

Finally, understanding and mastering the technical information, methods, and equipment involved in a discipline constitute the **technical skills.** Although most important at the employee level of the organization, technical skills are still required for upper management so that there is a comprehensive understanding of the workings of the organization. However, conceptual and interpersonal skills are probably more useful in obtaining promotion in most organizations. This is true because, at higher levels in organizations, these types of skills are used more often and are more important than technical skills. For example, conceptual skills are more useful in the leading and planning function because they involve understanding the systems view of the total organization.

Managerial Roles

The activities of managers and leaders are typically organized around several roles. A role refers to a set of expectations about how a person is to behave from the perspective of oneself, peers, superiors, subordinates, consumers (patients), and others (such as legislators). **Role theory** has been a prominent framework for examining behavior in the field of sociology for decades, and it has been applied in management to clarify the wide range of responsibilities held.

Mintzberg's Role Studies

Henry Mintzberg (1939–), Cleghorn Professor of Management at McGill University, completed his dissertation at MIT on the roles of managers. Suspecting that what managers did might be difficult to classify in the categories covered in this chapter, he shadowed managers and recorded their actual activities. His findings defied many common assumptions about the work that managers do. It is widely believed that managers are systematic, reflective thinkers who carefully analyze situations before making decisions and acting. In practice, Mintzberg (1992) found that most chief executives spent less than 10 minutes on any activity and that supervising foremen in industry averaged one activity every 48 seconds. Managers opened 36 pieces of mail, attended eight meetings, and toured a building. Whatever was planned, something unexpected usually emerged. Another study of British middle and top-level managers showed that they were able to secure a half hour for concentrated work without interruption only once every two days. Mintzberg summarized his findings by saying that manag-

ers completed a great deal of work at an unrelenting pace, but the activities were characterized by variety, fragmentation, and brevity.

Mintzberg's subsequent research with managers showed that their activities could usually be described by 10 roles organized into three categories (table 21.2):

- *Interpersonal activity* arises from the manager's formal authority in the organization and is supportive of the informational and decisional activities. It includes the roles of figurehead for ceremonial and formal occasions, leadership for motivating and using power, and liaison to link and network for information and support.
- The *informational activity* includes the roles of monitor of performance information, disseminator of values and information, and spokesperson for the organization with outside groups.
- The *decisional activity* includes the roles of entrepreneur to promote improvement and change, disturbance handler to deal with disruptions, resource allocator for overseeing resources and setting priorities, and negotiator for arrangements with other organizations.

These roles are intricately intertwined and not easily separated by a particular problem when it comes to team management, where responsibilities are often distributed among team members. However, they provide a realistic portrayal of the wide range of skilled behaviors required of effective managers.

Comparing the workings of organizations during the 20th century with those emerging in the 21st century, there is a clear

Table 21.2.   Mintzberg's managerial roles

Managerial Activities	Related Roles
Interpersonal	• *Figurehead:* The manager represents the organization and is a symbol for ceremonial, social, legal, and inspirational duties. • *Liaison:* The manager maintains networks of relationships outside his or her organizational unit to gather information and favors. • *Leader:* The manager directs, guides, motivates, and develops subordinates.
Informational	• *Monitor:* The manager oversees internal and external information sources. • *Disseminator:* The manager communicates facts and values to others in the organization. • *Spokesperson:* The manager communicates with others outside the organization.
Decisional	• *Entrepreneur:* The manager promotes development and planned change in the organization. • *Disturbance handler:* The manager resolves crises and unexpected problems. • *Resource allocator:* The manager uses authority to allocate budget, personnel, equipment, services, and facilities. • *Negotiator:* The manager resolves dilemmas and disputes and determines the use of resources.

need for a new way of thinking on the part of managers. Although the managerial skills used in conceptualization, relationships, and technology will persist, they will have to be applied in a different manner. The change drivers of globalization, demographic and marketplace diversity, information and technological changes, and others will mean that managers will seldom be able to focus on the status quo as they have in the past. The new status quo is one of change and how people can be helped through transitions.

Again coming full circle, Taylor and other proponents of scientific management emphasized an important criterion for managerial success: It should be based on research whenever possible. As Pascale (1990) demonstrated in his diagram of the managerial fads from the 1960s to 1990s, many ideas were without empirical foundation, were short-lived, had limited application, and in some cases caused more problems than they solved.

In healthcare, as well as other fields of management, decisions are based more on political and value considerations than on empirical sources. With the increased interest in alternative approaches to healthcare (for example, acupuncture, nutrition), determining which methods are legitimate and produce the best outcomes can reduce liability and enhance sound program promotion. An emphasis on **evidence-based management,** or information-based management, is emerging in which more informed decisions are made based on the best clinical and research evidence that proposed practices will work. For example, Australia-based CSIRO works with healthcare organizations to determine factors that influence the use of health information by at-risk segments of a population and also develops performance measures for staff. Their procedures have increased the use of data and information by senior managers in strategic and daily planning. Increasingly, all levels of managers are having information available on performance evaluation and the outcomes of the decisions they make.

Check Your Understanding 21.2

Instructions: Answer the following questions on a separate piece of paper.

1. Discuss reasons for the four management functions changing in emphasis over the three levels of management. For example, why would there be less emphasis on the leadership function for top-level managers compared with the strong emphasis for first-line managers?

2. Examine a job description for a position in your field. What is the distribution of conceptual, interpersonal, and technical skills required?

3. Make a list of daily activities engaged in by observing or asking a manager what he or she does. Then, categorize the activities into Mintzberg's 10 managerial roles.

4. Draw an organizational chart of your college, a hospital, or some other organization with which you are familiar. Be sure to designate both line and staff positions.

5. What does quality mean in your work? Identify several tasks you perform, define quality for each task, and consider how you would measure it.

Trends in Management Theory

What we have seen in the several management theories presented in this chapter is that as change drivers have an impact on the marketplace and organizations, organizations must adapt in order to survive and thrive. Management theories become a template for thinking about the structure and processes by which business is conducted. As the marketplace changes, old theories may lose their explanatory power and be replaced with more accurate theories and principles for managing the organization. (See table 21.3.) At the same time, as managers become accustomed to, and develop expertise with, a certain viewpoint, they may become biased in its use and fail to see exceptions to it. A requisite skill for managers is to know when to use a particular framework and when to change it.

Although Taylor and others at the turn of the 20th century faced a host of changes, the unrelenting pace of change is an even more constant companion to managers today. The successful manager must be able to see patterns of change and prepare others to respond to them.

Problem Solving and Decision Making

Problems are defined as impediments to the attainment of goals. While some managers view problems as negative and something to be avoided, problem solving can also be viewed as an opportunity for managers and organizations to build experience and resilience. Solving problems requires that they be framed or defined in useful and understandable ways, that creative approaches are applied to them, and that efficient methods are applied to recurrent problems. Problem

Table 21.3.   Paradigm shift in management

Traditional Management Paradigm	The New Management Paradigm
Multilevel hierarchical organizations	Flatter organizations
Centralized decision making	Decentralized decision making
Status measured by the amount of turf controlled	Status reflected in success in achieving outcomes
Quantity	Quality
Individual leadership	Teamwork
Think local	Think global and systems
Maintain stability	Change and adapt
Job security	Job flexibility
Focus on profit	Focus on customers
Short-term view	Long-term view
Homogeneous workforce and market	Diverse workforce and market
Competition	Collaboration
Work at office	Telecommuting and home office
Capital	Information
Physical labor	Knowledge workers
Terminal education	Continuous learning

solving involves understanding and resolving the barriers to goal attainment, while decision making refers to making the best choices from among available alternatives.

Steps in Problem Solving

Two primary responsibilities of managers are solving problems and making decisions. In the early years of management practice, these activities were often based on personal preferences and limited experience, with little regard for long-term consequences. Since then, however, formal models of dealing with issues have been developed and managers are encouraged to proceed systematically through several stages, including:

1. Defining the problem and the desired outcome
2. Analyzing and understanding the nature of the problem
3. Generating alternatives
4. Selecting desired alternatives (decision making)
5. Planning and implementing the alternative
6. Evaluating and gathering feedback about the attained outcome

At each step in the problem-solving model, decisions need to be made that lead to the final choice of how to implement a means for solving the problem. Given the changing circumstances of the modern healthcare marketplace, it is unlikely that all the information managers desire will be available. They will need to decide using less than perfect or less than complete information, and under ambiguous or risky circumstances.

Rational versus Administrative Decision Making

In recent years, the importance of rational decision making has become essential in management, and a variety of models have been developed. The Vroom-Yetton (1971) normative decision tree, which is discussed in detail in a later section of this chapter, is an example of a system for responding to key questions, branching to alternatives, and arriving at a conclusion. For more complex decision making where there are several choices and criteria for selection, but the criteria cannot be ordered sequentially as in the Vroom-Yetton model, a decision matrix can be constructed for evaluating and comparing alternatives. (See figure 21.7.)

Using this method, the decision maker lists the criteria for a good outcome and then rates each possible alternative for the solution to the problem. Each alternative is identified, and each is rated on the extent to which it fulfills the desired outcome criteria. Finally, the criteria weightings are multiplied by the choice ratings and totaled. The alternative with the highest total is considered to provide the best combination of characteristics that meet the most important criteria. This can be a tedious process with very complex problems, and various computer programs and expert systems have been developed to systematically walk the user through the decision process and perform the calculations. An example is StatCon or "statistical consultant," a simple expert system that prompts the user to answer questions about research data, and then recommends which statistical procedure to use to analyze it (Andrews et al. 1981).

Although this classical model of problem solving illustrates what managers should do, the most accurate assessment of a manager's effectiveness is determined by what he or she actually does.

Bounded Rationality

Most, if not all, problem solvers and decision makers operate within the limits of **bounded rationality.** Bounded rationality recognizes that problem situations can be overwhelmingly complex and in states of constant change, that not every fact about a situation can be known, and that people are not always rational. As a result, bounded rationality accounts for the limits of time and information, and encourages action despite uncertainty.

Figure 21.7.   Decision matrix

Example—Choosing the Job Offer That Best Meets Your Career Criteria				
Key decision criteria for a good job	Rating of the Importance (1 = high)	Rating of extent to which this job meets each criterion (1 = high, 5 = low)		
		Job Choice 1 Rating : Product	Job Choice 2 Rating : Product	Job Choice 3 Rating : Product
Criterion 1: Good pay	5	3 : 15	4 : 20	2 : 10
Criterion 2: Preferred region of country	2	2 : 4	3 : 6	4 : 8
Criterion 3: Interesting work	4	3 : 12	5 : 20	4 : 16
Additional criteria Total ratings for each choice		↓ 31	↓ 46	↓ 34

Step 1: Identify and rate (1–5, 5 high) the importance of the criteria for your desired job.

Step 2: Rate the extent to which each of the job choices meet your criteria (1–5, 5 high).

Step 3: Multiply each rating by the criteria rating.

Step 4: Total the products for all ratings and compare across the choices.

Decision: The higher product total of job choice 2 (for example, 46) offers greater fit with the applicants preferred criteria than do choices 1 and 3.

Intuition and Satisficing

Because of bounded rationality, managers often tend to rely on intuition and satisficing. **Intuition,** unconscious decision making based on similar conditions, can be useful as a quick way for highly experienced persons to make decisions when the current problem is similar to prior experiences. This kind of decision making is neither impulsive nor arbitrary but, rather, is based on decision pathways that have become so automatic as to become unconscious.

Satisficing is a less precise method than intuition and refers to a manager adopting the first alternative that is sufficient to meet the minimum requirement for a solution to the problem. Although this method is efficient and saves time and effort, it may have unexpected long-term effects. For example, the first apparent solution is not necessarily the most efficient in terms of time and money or the most appropriate. Without further analysis, the first solution is simply the first idea that appeared.

Programmed and Nonprogrammed Decisions

Decisions can be programmed or nonprogrammed. **Programmed decisions** are those in which a problem is so predictable, uniform, and recurring that rules have been developed to standardize or automate the procedure. Such rules enable managers to delegate authority to others to make decisions using predetermined criteria or to develop expert systems in which computers can make decisions. An example of such automation is an inventory system that automatically requests an order for restocking by a supplier when stock reaches a certain level.

Nonprogrammed decisions involve situations that are unpredictable, extremely complex, or ill defined. These situations defy simple decision criteria and usually require careful deliberation, often in consultation with others. Examples of nonprogrammed decisions include those found in market development, strategic management, and new product or service development.

Groupthink: The Hazards of Team Decision Making

The disasters of the Bay of Pigs invasion of Cuba, Nixon's Watergate break-in debacle, the *Exxon Valdez* oil spill, the Union Carbide gas leak tragedy in Bhopal, India, Reagan's contra-arms deal, and the *Challenger* space shuttle accident all shared the common feature of **groupthink.** Coined in 1972 by psychologist, Irving Janis, the term refers to the tendency of a highly cohesive team to seek consensus. Subsequent research has shown this tendency to be relatively widespread and occurs when a team is very cohesive, there is high external pressure to perform, and few mechanisms are in place to correct for poor decision making.

The role of cohesion is an interesting one because most work teams desire to have high cohesion: close familiarity and homogeneity of styles, strong pride in and commitment to the team, and a shared mission and vision (Michalisin, Karau, and Tangpong 2004). The problem arises when cohesion is so high and pressure to succeed so great that pressure is exerted on members to conform to team processes that can result in poor decisions.

Conditions for the Emergence of Groupthink

Janis originally proposed eight symptoms of groupthink grouped around three risky tendencies (table 21.4).

- *Overconfidence* in the team's prowess can manifest as an illusion of invulnerability that leads team members to be overconfident and take excessive risks. They develop a collective rationalization that is used to discount warnings that would lead them to reconsider their underlying assumptions.
- *Tunnel vision* restricts the range of factors considered and can lead to a belief in the inherent morality of their cause, thereby ignoring the ethical consequences of their decisions. Outsiders are often viewed in stereotypical ways in which their threats are minimized.
- *Team pressures* further contribute to groupthink. Loyal members will disapprove of a member who questions the team and bring sanctions until he or she again conforms. Members also may self-censor when it appears that there is silent consensus, tunnel vision for viewing the problem, and group pressure to conform.

Consequences of Groupthink

The pressures to conform in groupthink often result in the restriction of information and the risk of poor decision making.

Table 21.4.   Symptoms of groupthink

Team's overestimation of its own power and morality
- *Illusion of invulnerability.* The illusion that they cannot go wrong leads to excessive optimism and risk taking.
- *Unquestioned belief in team's inherent morality.* Members believe their actions are correct leading them to ignore moral and ethnical implications.

Close-mindedness
- *Team rationalization to discount warnings.* They collectively minimize indications that would lead them to reconsider their assumptions and commitments.
- *Stereotypes of the opposition.* Outsiders are viewed as negative, evil, stupid to justify negotiations or to consider they could counter the team's efforts.

Pressure toward uniformity
- *Self-censorship.* Members tend to minimize and withhold expression of their dissenting views and counterarguments.
- *Illusion of shared unanimity.* Self-censorship and the false belief that silence means consent leads to the shared illusion that everyone agrees with the decision.
- *Pressure to conform.* Members who deviate from team norms by expressing doubts or arguing against its position are implicitly and explicitly pressured to conform.
- *Self-appointed "mind-guards."* Some members appoint themselves to protect the team from adverse information that might challenge their illusions.

Source: Janis 1982.

Such restrictions can limit considerations of objectives, information search, alternative courses of action, examination of the risks of the preferred choice, and reassessment of the preferred choice. Moreover, they can bias the discussion and processing of the problem-solving process, and lead to a level of confidence that results in contingency plans being are ignored or minimized.

In spite of, and in contrast to, these limitations, groupthink can have a beneficial effect on a group by contributing to morale following a devastating defeat and can provide encouragement when an otherwise positive outcome appears doubtful (Janis 1982).

Countermeasures for Groupthink

The conditions that contribute to groupthink are ubiquitous, and it requires deliberate action by the team to minimize their adverse affects. By being aware of the risk of groupthink, alert to the symptoms, and intentionally implementing countermeasures, the team can maintain adequate cohesion without sacrificing decision quality. Instruments such as The Groupthink Profile (Swenson 2003) enable the team to better assess and discuss the implications of team cohesion, organizational self-correcting processes, pressure on the team, symptoms of groupthink, and countermeasures.

The use of countermeasures is especially important, and they can be internal or external. *Internal procedures* to reduce risk include using brainstorming, revisiting important decisions, monitoring the degree of consensus and disagreement, rotating the devil advocate's role among members, actively seeking contradictory information, and developing norms to challenge and question each other. In addition, the leader can refrain from stating an opinion that might affect opinions too early and the team might be divided into subgroups to encourage different conclusions. *External procedures* include discussing decisions with outside experts and nonteam members and inviting external observers to provide feedback on meetings, decisions, and team processes. Such procedures increase awareness of group processes and enhance skills at arriving at better decisions.

Check your understanding 21.3

Instructions: Answer the following questions on a separate sheet of paper.

1. In what ways could you increase the feelings of cohesion for a team? What would be some indications of that cohesion?

2. What are some indications that cohesion has become excessive (for example, signs of groupthink)?

3. What actions might be taken to reduce the risks of groupthink?

Managerial Communication

The exchange of information is central to health information management and one of the most frequently used definitions of *communication*. Although we often take communication for granted, miscommunication poses problems and risks in the healthcare field. It is important for professionals to understand important aspects of communication, including channels and barriers, the challenge of diversity, and ways communication can be improved.

Importance of Communication

As noted earlier in this chapter, Follett observed that managers get things done through people, and this in turn is accomplished by communicating with them. Communication is the interpersonal process by which information is transferred from one person to another. Nearly everything we do can potentially communicate something to someone, or more economically stated, "You cannot not communicate" (Watzlawick, Beavin, and Jackson 1968). About 75 percent of the working time people spend in organizations is used for interpersonal interactions. Still, ineffective communication remains a significant problem in most organizations. For example, a survey of workers who voluntarily quit their organizations found that about 25 percent of their reasons were because they perceived their managers to be poor communicators (Supplee Group 2002). Executives tend to agree, citing that as much as 14 percent of a 40-hour work week is wasted due to poor staff–manager communication (Mills 1998).

Formal and Informal Channels

Communication can take place through formal or informal channels. *Formal communication* consists of those intentional messages that are directed to people through their role relationships in the organization and usually through established channels such as e-mail, phone, face-to-face interaction, memo, letter, or other forms of announcement. This kind of communication usually focuses on task accomplishment and related matters. In contrast, *informal communication* may occur across role or department boundaries or organizational levels. It tends to employ face-to-face interactions and focuses on the interpersonal aspects of work, such as rumors and topics outside the immediate scope of the workplace. It is through informal communication that most relationships develop between employees and that influence is exercised.

Barriers to Communication

Complex organizations also have a variety of barriers to the richness or completeness of communication, both structural and interpersonal. *Structural barriers* include the distortion that can occur when a message is passed through several people, each adding or deleting information based on their own perceptions and needs. The increasing use of e-mail in organizations also eliminates the nonverbal cues of voice tone, volume, and inflection, as well as facial cues and gestures that add so much to face-to-face communication. *Interpersonal barriers* include distraction and partial listening, tendency to judge, assumption that we know what others mean, and fear of asking questions. In general, low-richness channels are one-way communication tools such as reports, bulletins, memos, and e-mail and high-richness channels include telephone and face-to-face interactions.

Diversity

As the workforce continues to become more diverse, there will be greater challenges to managerial communication. A Los Angeles multinational firm, for example, provides new employee orientation in 17 different languages. In many Asian countries where courtesy and "saving face" is very important, a person might say maybe when he really means no in order to avoid hurting feelings. Whereas most task-oriented Americans prefer to get right down to business, many South Americans prefer to spend time getting to know whom they are doing business with, and Arabs may have conversations where they shift from business to personal and other interests and then loop back several times.

Nonverbal communication also differs culturally: What may be a benign gesture in one place may be very offensive in another (Axtell 1991). For example, many Americans feel quite comfortable crossing their legs and leaning back in a chair, but showing the sole of the foot in such a manner is very offensive to most Arabs, and most Japanese would consider a slouched posture a sign of poor character. Beckoning by curling the index finger back is a common way for Americans to say "come here," but in Indonesia and Australia, such a gesture is used only for calling animals. Appreciating communication differences and customs is an important part of being an effective communicator, cosmopolitan traveler, and respected manager.

Suggestions for Increasing the Accuracy of Communications

To communicate effectively, managers must pay just as much attention to how their message is received and interpreted as they do to its content. The following practices can enhance the accuracy and acceptance of communication (Okum 1987; Morgan and Baker 1985):

- Minimize "noise" that can distort the message. Make sure all parties are minimally distracted, can give their undivided attention, and have sufficient time to get their message across.
- Know what outcome you want to communicate through your message and then check to see if you get it.
- Monitor others' nonverbal behaviors for cues that they are following or are confused.
- Consider the effect that different interpersonal styles, cultural backgrounds, and experiences may have on interpretation of the message or how it is delivered.
- Use **active listening** in which you (or the other person) restate in your own words what you have heard the other person say.
- Respond to the feelings, attitudes, and values in the message as well as the content. Show empathy, concern, and compassion, as appropriate.
- Use examples or visual aids to make the message clearer.
- Ask for feedback and listen to it without being judgmental.
- Write clearly and concisely.

Remember that how well you model communication skills sets the norm for others.

Clinical Communication Space

As discussed throughout this chapter, communication is central to understanding error rates, providing performance feedback, and facilitating transition during change. **Clinical communication space** is the context and range of electronic and interpersonal information exchanged among staff and patients in the healthcare facility. Although electronic information is readily available, electronic medical records account for only about 10 percent of information exchange, with voice and e-mail accounting for another 25 percent. Fifty to 60 percent of the preferred communication among staff involves informal, synchronous, or face-to-face encounters (Coiera 2000; Safran, Sands, and Rind 1999; Tang et al. 1996). However, the pace of work sometimes leaves staff passing comments in the hall, calling on cell phones, and leaving Post-it notes where they hope they will be seen.

The work environment is characterized by many interactions and multiple interruptions, both electronic (pagers, telephones, e-mail) and interpersonal. These distractions, as well as information overload and memory limitations, create the risk of information errors and deficits (Patel, Arocha, and Kaufman 2001). Most communication errors are usually between healthcare professionals in different disciplines (Gardner 2003). In addition, the hierarchical nature of most healthcare organizations is a source of miscommunication. As messages travel through several layers and channels, information is added or dropped out or modified.

Miscommunication rather than incompetence is at the root of twice as many errors that plague healthcare facilities (Wilson, et al., 1998). One error often begets another error, thereby producing a cascade of miscommunication. In a study of 75 error reports involving 15 physicians across five states, it was discovered that such a cascade was involved in 77 percent of the errors. Eighty percent of the cascades involved some form of miscommunication between physicians and medical records, including mishandling of patient requests and messages, inaccessible records, and inadequate reminder systems (Robeznieks 2004). In another study of 30 medical malpractice case files and 30 medical incident investigations, communication problems accounted for 76 percent of the cases (Stone 2002). Medical errors have been estimated to cost the U.S. economy between $17 and $29 billion annually (IOM 1999).

Although medical errors and injury to patients has been heavily documented and the analyses continue to grow, other outcomes from staff miscommunication have been less examined. Executives believe that as much as 14 percent of each 40-hour week is wasted due to poor communication between managers and their staff—an equivalent of seven weeks a year that lowers employee morale and performance (Krell and Sammer 1998). Moreover, it has been estimated that improved telecommunications could save the healthcare industry $30 billion annually (Little 1992).

Guidelines for Giving Feedback

Feedback enables people to monitor their own behavior and the reactions of others and to adjust their behavior and communication to be more effective. Feedback enables correction before (or soon after) errors occur and prevents their accumulation. Yet, effective feedback is not just "speaking your mind" to express yourself. If the purpose is to influence behavior, feedback must be used respectfully and strategically. The following characteristics of useful feedback should be kept in mind:

- *Relationship:* Become acquainted and develop a positive working relationship with people before giving feedback.
- *Requested:* People are most receptive when feedback is solicited rather than imposed on them.
- *Confidentiality:* Give feedback in private, especially when it is sensitive.
- *Needs of the recipient:* Effective feedback takes into consideration what the person needs rather than just serving your needs; it should be given to help, not hurt.
- *Practical:* Feedback focuses on the what is said or done rather than why; the latter takes us away from a solution focus and toward speculation about motives.
- *Descriptive:* Feedback describes specific behavior and the recipient's reaction rather than judgments. Basing it on direct observation and providing examples can help reduce defensiveness and focus efforts.
- *Manageable amount:* Feedback should be given in a manageable amount; don't give too much feedback or too fast.
- *Balanced:* Provide both positive and negative constructive feedback; start with the positive, then present areas needing improvement, and end with positive.
- *Timing:* Give the feedback soon after the behavior has occurred.
- *Realistic:* The behavior to be changed should be something the receiver can do something about.
- *Listen and check:* The recipient may be asked to paraphrase what he or she has heard in the feedback to ensure accuracy of perception. Be attentive to the recipient's response to the feedback, and clarify and explain where needed.
- *Climate:* Create an environment in the organization in which the seeking and sharing of feedback is an expectation and a common occurrence.

Real-World Case

Western Memorial Hospital recognizes the need for regular and timely feedback for staff development, the same way it had come to value rapid information reflecting the nature of key operating variables such as patient load, length of stay, medical errors, and so on. The staff reasoned, correctly, that if people had more information about their performance,

they would be able to refine their efforts and become more efficient. Perhaps they would even reduce their stress by reducing performance problems; fewer hassles would be passed on to others in the chain of service delivery. All that remained was to provide people with the information and to look forward to improvements.

The feedback would include patient ratings of care, data regarding patient turnover in the department, timeliness of performance, and perceptions of performance by other staff. On a weekly basis, staff would receive a three-page sheet of more than 40 performance-related behaviors rated as poor, fair, adequate, good, and excellent. The sheets were printed in each office and distributed to staff mailboxes that were secure. It seemed like a good thing to do.

Soon after implementation of the performance feedback system, however, difficulties began to arise. The clerical staff distributing the rating forms began to notice and report that the reports were beginning to pile up in the mailboxes. Furthermore, tracking of the performance problems failed to show the expected improvement. Admonitions by supervisors to staff to "be sure to read your feedback reports" apparently went unheeded. As a result of the lack of use, supervisors were directed to mandate weekly removal of the reports and any left in boxes would be a source of reprimand. Although most of the reports disappeared on schedule from the boxes, there remained only marginal indications of performance change. It was time to find out what was going on.

The human resources (HR) department, which had received enthusiastic support from department heads, initiated "informal conversations" with random staff members in each department. They asked what people thought about the new feedback forms, how the forms were used, and why they thought the forms were not being used as expected. Results were mixed: Some staff reported that they thought it was a fine idea, but that they just had little time to implement it. Others said that they had looked over the reports and tried to do something with them, but their efforts at change were sporadic. A few asked, "What reports?"

In consultation with department heads, HR considered that although the effort was a good idea, they had underestimated what was necessary to effectively implement the feedback. They finally asked the department heads to return to their staffs and hold a meeting specifically on the performance feedback reports. The results were enlightening and led to a revision of the entire process. Employees indicated a variety of concerns: They had not been asked initially what was important for them to know, and they were given feedback on some variables that were of unknown utility to them. The frequency of reports did not show sufficient lag between data points for them to see meaningful differences on variables. The reports were delivered by clerical staff who could read the reports, and there were some instances where staff performance had become lunch conversation among the clerks. The reports were usually distributed on Fridays when large volumes of paper were already in the mailboxes and people were ready to leave for weekends. As a result, many of the reports simply got lost on desks or tossed in wastebaskets. Finally, these efforts were mostly problem focused for reducing errors and there was little discussion with supervisors tying performance to the discussions and reinforcement of developing new behaviors. As a result, many staff did not find the information attractive and grew passive-avoidant in reading them.

This information confirmed that HR had misjudged the feedback plan. By revising the system, the utility rate of information went from 32 to 78 percent in six months. The HR department modeled effective receptiveness to feedback, and the change was finally implemented successfully, although with significant modifications.

Summary

As the marketplace has expanded to a global perspective and workplace settings have become more diverse and complex, the discipline of management has likewise evolved. Classical management theories focused on formal authority, hierarchical avenues of communication and accountability, and operational efficiency. Weber's concept of bureaucracy, Taylor's scientific management, and Gilbreth's and Gantt's operational innovations provided such structure.

As management became professionalized, effective practices and responsibilities became more formal and were incorporated into the administrative model of management. In addition to describing the functions of planning, organizing, leading, and controlling, Fayol formulated 14 principles for management. Prior to emergence of the humanistic approach to management, Bernard proposed the acceptance view of authority and emphasized the balance of effectiveness and efficiency. The Hawthorne effect marked the shift from operations and authority to the human relations movement and attention to worker motivation. Maslow described a hierarchy of needs that provided managers with a model for targeting efforts to motivate workers, and McGregor recognized the shift from authoritarian to humanistic orientation in his Theory X and Y.

As technology and strategy were emphasized in response to international conflicts and competition, management science developed a variety of new tools. Operations management, statistical forecasting, break-even analysis, queuing, modeling, and PERT were used to reemphasize production to balance the renewed emphasis on people.

More contemporary approaches to management have emphasized improved quality of products and services through greater efficiency and increased focus on people. TQM, the Baldridge Award, and the search for best practices have fine-tuned many management and business processes.

Effective management involves not only understanding Fayol's four functions, but also understanding and developing conceptual skills for strategy, emotional intelligence or interpersonal skills for working effectively with people, and technical skills for dealing with the specific business field.

Moreover, managers must learn to perform multiple roles while working at an unrelenting pace.

More recent theories have emphasized the complexity of modern organizations. Senge's (1990) emphasis on systems theory, for example, helps managers understand how the organization's components are connected much as a living system, and that change in one component can affect other components.

Change management requires strong leadership. Managers traditionally maintain a highly efficient workplace and establish procedures; leaders look to the future and promote change. Both solve problems and make decisions. Recurrent problems lend themselves to clear rules for programmed decisions that can be used routinely; unique, complex, or changing situations require careful thought when nonprogrammed decisions are made. Formal decision making progresses through several stages, including problem definition, problem analysis, generation of alternatives, selection of alternatives, plan implementation, and evaluation and feedback. In practice, managers more often use intuition or satisficing. Groupthink can produce riskier decisions and requires review of team norms periodically as well as implementation of countermeasures. Clear communication with consideration of all stakeholders can further reduce distortion and error.

References

Andrews, F., et al. 1981. *A Guide for Selecting Statistical Techniques for Analyzing Social Science Data*. Ann Arbor, MI: University of Michigan Institute for Social Research.

Axtell, R.E. 1991. *Gestures: The Do's and Taboos of Body Language around the World*. New York: John Wiley & Sons.

Bernard, Chester. 1938. *The Functions of the Executive*. Cambridge, MA: Harvard University Press.

Bigelow, J. 1993. Managerial skills texts: How do they stack up? *Journal of Management Education* 17(3):399–415.

Boyatzis, R.E. 2001. Developing emotional intelligence. In *The Emotionally Intelligent Workplace*, edited by C. Cherniss and D. Goleman. San Francisco: Jossey-Bass.

Bridges, W. 1994. *Jobshift: How to Prosper in a Workplace without Jobs*. Reading, MA: Addison-Wesley.

Burrington-Brown, J. 2004. Does the Privacy Rule hinder patient care? *Journal of American Health Information Management Association* 75(9):72–73, 76.

Carey, B. 2004 (July 14). A different kind of smart. *Los Angeles Times*.

Church, A.H. 1997. Managerial self-awareness in high performing individuals in organizations. *Journal of Applied Psychology* 82(2):281–92.

Coiera, E. 2000. When conversation is better than computation. *Journal of the American Medical Information Association* 7:277–86.

Damour, C. I. 2000. Striving to be the best: Practice solutions for today. *Journal of the American Health Information Management Association* 71(7):51.

Drucker, P. 1986. The appraisal of managerial performance. *Management Decision* 24(4):67–78.

French, J.R.P., and B. Raven. 1959. The bases of social power. In *Studies in Social Power*, edited by D. Cartwright. Ann Arbor, MI: Institute for Social Research.

Gardner, A. 2003 (Nov. 18). Tracking of medication errors rising: Report finds elderly most at risk in hospitals. Originally published by healthday.com. Available online from hon.ch/News/HSN/516102.html.

Gilbreth, F.B., Jr., and E.G. Carey. 1945. *Cheaper by the Dozen.* New York: Thomas Y. Crowell Company.

Goleman, D. 1998 (Nov.–Dec.). What makes a leader? *Harvard Business Review* 74(6):92–102.

Goleman, D. 1995. *Emotional Intelligence.* New York: Bantam.

Hammer, M., and J. Champy. 1993. *Reengineering the Corporation.* New York: Harper.

Healthcare Management Council. 2001. hmc-benchmarks.com.

Institute of Medicine. 1999 (November). *To Err Is Human: Building a Safer Health System.* Washington, DC: National Academy Press. Available online from iom.edu/Object.File/Master/4/117/0.pdf.

ISO Online. 2002. iso.ch.

Jacques, E. 1996. *Requisite Organization.* Arlington, VA: Cason Hall.

Janis, I.L. 1982. *Groupthink: Psychological Studies of Policy Decisions and Fiascos.* Boston: Houghton Mifflin.

Kaplan, R.S., and D.P. Norton. 1996. *The Balanced Scorecard.* Boston: Harvard Business School Press.

Katz, R.L. 1974. Skills of an effective administrator. *Harvard Business Review* 52:90–102.

Kerker, S. 2001. Kerker reflects: Drucker's development of the strategy-focused organization. *New Corporate University Review* 9(1).

Kettley, P., and M. Strebler. 1997. Changing Roles for Senior Managers. Institute for Employment Studies, IES Report 327. Available online from employment-studies.co.uk/summary/summary.php?id=327.

Krell, E., and J. Sammer. 1998 (December). A costly game of telephone. *Business Finance.* Available online from businessfinancemag.com/magazine/archives/article.html?articleID=4750&Print=Y

Kuhn, T.S. 1962. *The Structure of Scientific Revolutions.* Chicago: University of Chicago Press.

Little, A.D. 1992. *Telecommunications: Can It Help Solve America's Health Care Problems?* Cambridge, MA: Arthur D. Little.

Luthans, F., R. Hodgetts, and S. Rosenkrantz. 1988. *Real Managers.* Cambridge, MA: Ballinger.

Mahoney, T.A., T.H. Jerdee, and S.J. Carroll. 1965. The job(s) of management. *Industrial Relations* 4(2):97–110.

Matthews, G., M. Zeidner, and R.D. Roberts. 2002. *Emotional Intelligence: Science and Myth.* Cambridge, MA: The MIT Press.

McGregor, D. 1960. *The Human Side of Enterprise.* New York: McGraw-Hill.

Michalisin, M.D., S.J. Karau, and C. Tangpong. 2004. Top management team cohesion and superior industry returns: An empirical study of the resource-based view. *Group and Organization Management* 29(1):125–40.

Mills, K. 1998. Failure to communicate costly for companies. *NARTE News* 16(3).

Mintzberg, H. 1992. The manager's job: Folklore and fact. In *Managing People and Organizations,* edited by J.J. Gabarro. Boston: Harvard Business School Publications.

Morgan, P., and K. Baker. 1985 (November). Building a professional image: Improving listening behavior. *Supervisory Management.* 34–38.

Okum, B.F. 1987. *Effective Helping: Interviewing and Counseling Techniques,* 3rd ed. Pacific Grove, CA: Brooks/Cole.

Page, C., M. Wilson, and D. Meyer. 1999. A three domain, two dimensional model of managerial effectiveness. Paper presented at the Academy of Business and Administrative Sciences Conference, Barcelona, Spain.

Parson, H.M. 1974. What happened at Hawthorne? *Science* 183:922–32.

Pascale, R.T. 1990. Managing on the Edge. New York: Simon & Schuster.

Patel, V.L., J.F. Arocha, and D. R. Kaufman. 2001 (July/August). A primer on aspects of cognition for medical informatics. *Journal of the American Medical Information Association* 8(4):324–43.

Peters, T.J., and R.H. Waterman. 1982. *In Search of Excellence: Lessons from America's Best-Run Companies.* New York: Harper & Row.

Raven, B.H. 1983. Interpersonal influence and social power. In *Social Psychology,* edited by B.H. Raven and J.Z. Rubin, pp. 399–444. New York: John Wiley & Sons.

Robeznieks, A. 2004 (August). Communication problems often initiate "cascades" of errors. *American Medical News,* American Medical Association.

Safran, C., D.Z. Sands, and D.M. Rind.1999. Online medical records: A decade of experience. *Methods of Information in Medicine* 38(4–5):308–12.

Senge, P. 1990. *The Fifth Discipline: The Art and Practice of the Learning Organization.* New York: Currency/Doubleday.

Shrader, C.B., L. Taylor, and D.R. Dalton. 1984. Strategic planning and organizational performance: A critical appraisal. *Journal of Management* 10(2):149–71.

Stone, F. 2002 (April). An examination of the role of communication problems in preventable medical adverse events. Report no. AU/ACSC/110/2002-04 submitted in partial fulfillment of graduation requirements. Maxwell Air Force Base, AL. Available online from research.airuniv.edu/papers/ay2002/acsc/02-110.pdf.

Stoner, J.A.F., and R.E. Freeman. 1989. *Management.* Englewood Cliffs, NJ: Prentice-Hall.

Supplee Group. 2002 (Jan. 28). Employees cite poor managers as primary reason for quitting. Press release.

Swenson, D.X. 2003. The Groupthink Profile. Behaviortrends.com

Swenson, D.X. 2001. The Ouroboros Effect: The revenge effects of unintended consequences. Available online from faculty.css.edu/dswenson/web/Revenge.htm.

Tang, P., M.A. Jaworski, C.A. Fellencer, N. Kreider, M.P. LaRosa, and R.C. Marquardt. 1996. Clinical information activities in diverse ambulatory care practices. In *Proceedings of the American Medical Informatics Association, Annual Fall Symposium,* 12–16. Bethesda, MD: AMIA.

Tenner, E. 1996. *Why Things Bite Back: Technology and the Revenge of Unintended Consequences.* New York: Alfred A. Knopf.

Vroom, V., and P. Yetton. 1971. *Leadership and Decision Making.* Pittsburgh: University of Pittsburgh Press.

Walton, M. 1986. *The Deming Management Method.* New York: Perigee Books.

Watzlawick, P., J.H. Beavin, and D.D. Jackson. 1968. *The Pragmatics of Human Communication.* New York: Norton.

Wilson, R.M., W.B. Runciman, R.W. Gibberd, B.T. Harrison, L. Newby, and J.D. Hamilton. 1998. The quality in Australian health care study. *Medical Journal of Australia* 169:458–71.

Chapter 22
Leadership Theory and Change Management

David X. Swenson, PhD

Learning Objectives

- To describe the functions of leadership
- To explain the differences between managers and leaders
- To discuss the key ideas of prominent leadership theories
- To recognize that a leadership approach needs to adjust to various situations
- To explain how leaders can fail in performance
- To identify the traits related to leadership effectiveness
- To appreciate how leadership theories have evolved from simple and two-dimensional models to complex, multi-dimensional and situational models
- To recognize the stages and impact of organizational change
- To understand how to facilitate a transition in order to minimize stress to people and production

Key Terms

Adopter groups
Androgynous leadership
Appreciative inquiry
Autocratic leadership
Champion
Change agent
Change drivers
Charisma
Consideration
Contingency model of leadership
Critic
Delegation
Democratic leadership
Diffusion S curve
Early adopters
Early majority
Ending

Exchange relationship
Expectancy theory of motivation
Great person theory
Icarus Paradox
In-group
Initiating structure
Innovators
Inventor
Laggards
Late majority
Leader–member exchange
Leader–member relations
Leadership grid
Learning history
Least Preferred CoWorker (LPC) scale
Lewin's stages of change

Neutral zone
New beginnings
Normative Decision Model
Organization development (OD)
Organizational lifeline
Out-group
Path–goal theory
Peter Principle
Position power
Reductionism
Reflective learning cycle
Refreezing
Self-efficacy
Servant Leadership Model
Situational model of leadership
Sponsor

Stages of grief
Survey feedback
Synergy
System
Systems theory
Task structure
Team building
360-degree evaluation
Trait approach
Transactional leadership
Transformational leadership
Unfreezing
Values-based leadership
Vertical dyad linkage
Worker immaturity– maturity

Introduction

Permanent whitewater is the phrase often used to describe the turbulent nature of the emerging business environment that managers must understand and operate in daily (Vaill 1996). It is difficult enough to bring knowledgeable people together to plan for specific problems within a given time period, but change is now continuous and ubiquitous. Compounding the complexity of such planning is the growing uncertainty about the future and the need for an ongoing revision of plans to match the turbulent environment. Such a situation requires excellent leadership and an understanding of, and participation in, innovation throughout the organization.

This chapter examines the importance and role of leadership, several theories of leadership, and how organizations need to be prepared to manage continuous transitions.

Theory Into Practice

Northwestern Clinic was a small healthcare facility. For several years it had operated in a cost-effective manner under the leadership of a physician executive. Following his retirement, the board of directors proposed that a change in leadership style was needed to remain competitive and responsive to the community. The directors recognized that such a shift, while desirable, would not be easy for the groups of stakeholders who were accustomed to their traditional way of operating.

The board invited an organization development consultant to assist in their restructuring efforts. They expected the consultant to spend some time diagnosing their facility and prescribe management solutions, much as the staff would deal with a patient. No such luck! The consultant explained that even a patient's response to treatment was more effective when they were fully engaged in their own health—so, too, was organization change. The consultant encouraged them to survey all staff, (providing them confidentiality) regarding what did and did not work, what their image of a more effective organization might look like, and ideas to make their own departments work better.

The information was presented to the board and administrative team, and rather than telling the collected group what it mean, instead the consultant asked them to consider what it reflected about the organization. Overcoming initial reluctance to tell the "expert" what they expected him to tell them, they began a lively exploration of perceptions, problems, and hopes.

In the weeks and months that followed, the consultant encouraged the board, administrative team, and all levels of management to continue to involve staff in the shaping of the new organization. He suggested that it was the people who made the organization, and they should be involved in decisions that affected them. He also emphasized that they now had the skills to continue the change process without relying on him. Although the transition from recipient of advice to creator of their own organizational future was not an easy one, subsequent years were marked by high morale, lower turnover, improved communication, and better patient service.

Functions and Principles of Leadership

Leadership is the art of setting a direction and influencing people to move in that direction. Given the changing nature of the workplace and marketplace, leaders are in a unique position to influence the shaping of vision and mission in order to inspire people to put forth their best effort. Leaders also are the ones who others rely on to help make organizational change meaningful and to facilitate the transition to a new direction. Yet, clarifying exactly who leaders are and what they do is not an easy task. Several specialists in the field have lamented that despite so much research on the subject of leadership, there is little to show for it in the way of real insight and practical results (Bennis 1959; Burns 1978; Yukl 1998). Even in an inspiring study by the Gallup Organization in which 80,000 managers from 400 companies were examined, the managers were found not to share a great deal in common other than "breaking rules" (Buckingham and Coffman 1999).

Functions of Leadership

Leadership is a central strategic concern for most organizations because it makes a difference. Each year, Fortune magazine and the Hay Group conduct a survey of the world's most-admired companies (Hay Group 1999). Hay interviewed the top companies in 21 industrial groupings and found that they were differentiated from the other companies by their exceptionally strong focus on several leadership areas. They put a great deal of effort into identifying and selecting people with leadership potential. In addition, they matched people whose needs fit the company's culture and strategic goals. Moreover, their organizational cultures emphasized the importance and value of people. Finally, they intentionally developed leadership competencies, such as orientation to achievement, self-confidence, self-management, empathy, and teamwork. Asked about their level of satisfaction with leadership, 91 percent expressed satisfaction with the quality and breadth of their leadership, compared to a group of global 500 companies that showed only a 72 percent satisfaction.

In addition, the top companies reported that leadership success was related to emotional intelligence and social skills; technical skills were considered only half as important. Supporting this was another Hay study in which CEO failure was most related not to flawed strategy or vision but, rather, to poor execution and problems in interpersonal relations (Charan and Colvin 1999). There is still some controversy about the extent to which leadership affects an organization. However, a growing body of evidence suggests it can make a strategic difference. Effective leadership has been found to improve the financial performance of an organization, with fiscal improvements ranging from 7 to 15 percent (Salancik and Pfeffer 1977) to a high of 44 percent (Weiner and Mahoney 1981). The essential role of the leader during organizational change also has been explored (Burke, Richley, and DeAngelis 1985).

In modern organizations, leadership does not just reside at the top but, instead, permeates the organization. In a CIO survey of 300 information management executives, 78 percent identified "inculcating leadership in their staff" as their most important job (Blodgett 1999). Every few years, a Human Resource Development National Executive Survey is conducted to assess organizational trends in training. The findings from a 1998 survey show that the importance of leadership development is increasing. About 84 percent of organizations reported that they promote some form of leadership training and employee development. Although it is still reserved primarily for managerial positions, leadership development is gradually finding its way throughout all levels of organizations (ASTD 1998). The most commonly mentioned skills of effective leaders included communication (57 percent), vision (53 percent), interpersonal skills (50 percent), strategic planning (40 percent), and change management (37 percent). Regardless of what the desired characteristics include, they appear deficient, as reflected in the topics the organizations preferred to see in training: change management (74 percent), leadership styles (73 percent), and performance management (65 percent).

The trend in modern organizations is to develop each employee's leadership potential to its full capacity. This allows the employees to exercise the empowerment they are given, demonstrate their value to the organization, and perhaps participate in leadership succession in the organization.

Leadership versus Management

As seen in several chapters of this text, the workplace and the marketplace are beset with continuous adaptations to large-scale **change drivers** over which there is little control. Management must provide stability and consistency for workers and at the same time prepare them for the transition to new structures and processes. Managers and leaders must collaborate closely to ensure clear understanding and smooth transitions in ways that minimize disruption to people and production. Although the activities of leaders and managers can be distinguished, there is considerable overlap between the roles and effective leaders and managers usually carry out both functions to some degree.

The terms *leader* and *manager* are often used interchangeably. Although they overlap, the two terms are technically—and in some aspects, practically—different. In general, the responsibility of managers is to ensure that current operations run smoothly whereas leaders strive to help the organization adapt to changing conditions. Managers tend to focus more on structured and analytical modes of thinking whereas leaders tend to use more flexible and creative modes. Managers are often more attentive to danger and uncertainty whereas leaders seek opportunities in undefined and unknown risk areas. Managers are said to determine the scope of problems whereas leaders search for alternative solutions. Managers seek methods and ask how something can be done whereas leaders seek motives and wonder why things are as they are and how they can be different. In general, then, managers work to create efficiency with the status quo whereas leaders move the organization into its unfolding future. (See table 22.1.)

These differences have been attributed to the influence of different developmental experiences in these individuals' lives. When asked about their early family and personal experiences, managers often describe uneventful early childhoods and see life as a steady normative progression of positive events and security. Being involved in social and organized activities from an early age, they tend to gain a strong sense of belonging, identity, and self-esteem from others. In contrast, leaders more often describe disruptive experiences in early family and childhood in which they were confronted by conflicts and stresses. These crises required reflection and mastery through which **self-efficacy** was developed. Because confidence grows out of problem solving rather than relationships, leaders may be more attached to a vision that drives their achievement and inspires others than to an immediate situation (Hickman 1990; Kotter 1990; Zaleznik 1977).

Attesting to the relevance of developmental experiences, biographical data have been found to be predictive of good leadership. At a time when human resources directors use caution about the types of questions they can ask in employment interviews, inquiring about the kinds of experiences that have led managers and leaders to be the kind of people they are can be insightful. It is important to remember that both roles are required in organizations, and it is in collaboration

Table 22.1.   Differences between managers and leaders

Managers	Leaders
Administer, replicate, and maintain	Innovate, originate, and develop
Emphasis on structure	Emphasis on people
Short-range view	Long-range view
Focus on bottom line	Focus on the horizon
Relies on control and rules	Relies on trust and inspiration
Avoids risks as problems	Takes risks as opportunities
Does things right	Does the right thing
Uneventful early childhood	Developmental conflicts requiring reflection and mastery
Life seen as steady progression of positive events and security	Life punctuated with series of disruptions and challenges
Feel strong sense of belonging	Feel separateness; create rather than inherit identity
Transactional	Transformational

that leaders and managers provide balance for organizations in transition.

Flawed and Failed Leadership

A browse through most bookstores will show a series of unusual titles in the business section: *Crazy Bosses, When Smart People Work for Dumb Bosses, How to Work for an Idiot, Dinosaur Brains,* and so on. Such books reflect a serious problem in many organizations. The base rate for failed leadership has been estimated between 60 and 75 percent based on employees reporting that the worst aspect of their job is their immediate supervisor (Hogan, Raskin, and Fazzini 1990). In other studies, the failure rate of corporate executives in the United States from the 1980s to1990s was about 50 percent (DeVries 1992) and 45 percent for new executives by mid-2000 (Ballard 2005). Incompetent management has been cited as 60 percent in one large hospital (Shipper and Wilson 1991) and 50 percent in one large aerospace organization (Milliken-Davies 1992). Even Fortune 500 companies report an average turnover of 2.3 CEOs over the past decade (Andersson 1999).

The consequences of these failures also are tragic. For example, it was found that about 25 percent of bosses abuse their employees to the extent that the employees call in sick, slow production, or leave the job (Lesly 1992). Such malfeasance costs industries and the economy up to $5 billion annually, and it is estimated that half of the company's reputation is tied to the CEO's reputation. The risk and consequences also extend to the executives, and upwards of 75 percent have even considered quitting at some time (CEOGO 2003).

How is it that prominent organizational leaders such as Kenneth Lay of Enron, Dennis Koslowski of Tyco, John Rigas of Adelphia, Martha Stewart of Omnimedia, and others in nearly daily news can fail their organizations? How is it that such talented people fall from success? It appears that there are three reasons: abuse of power, limited capacity, and personal impairments (Hale 2002).

Leaders throughout the organization and executives in particular have the right to exercise power to influence others and produce change. Power can become abused when a crisis requires a directive decision, but leadership continues the directive approach long after the crisis has passed. When there are insufficient checks and balances in the organization, such power can become excessive and often self-serving. This can even produce blind spots or compartmentalized thinking in which the person can entertain completely inconsistent values. For example, in the year before the accounting scandal brought down Enron, CEO Kenneth Lay toured the country presenting a training series on leadership ethics.

In other cases, the successes and skills that led a person to promotion may be based on performance in a previous position but be unrelated to the new position. A successful manager who arose in a large or small company may not fare as well in the opposite-sized organization (Jahna 2002). Once referred to as the **Peter Principle** in which some people were promoted to their level of incompetency (Peter and Hull 1969), leaders also may find themselves in a changing organization where their previous skills are outdated. For example, some managers may have an excellent understanding of such components as the financial process, but be unable to see the broader systemic view necessary for sound strategic planning.

Finally, leaders may have personal flaws or problems that interfere with a once successful style. Stress, alcohol abuse, anxiety, depression, and personality disorders can adversely affect a leader's judgment. Even unbridled success can exaggerate personality qualities and impair judgment as reflected in the *Icarus Paradox* (Miller 1990). In Greek mythology, Icarus was the son of Daedalus, who used wax to cover their arms with feathers so that they could fly like birds. Overcome with the thrill of flying, Icarus flew too near the sun. The heat from the sun melted the wax, causing Icarus to fall.

The **Icarus Paradox** proposes that successful styles, unrestrained, can become their extreme: Builders become imperialists, pioneers become escapists, salespersons become drifters, and craftspersons become tinkerers. For example, Harold Geneen, the financial wizard and CEO of the diversified conglomerate ITT, led his company to a series of highly successful acquisitions in the 1970s. In less than 10 years, Geneen had acquired 100 companies, with 375,000 employees in 80 countries. The corporate culture became infused with growth values, yet at the same time such growth could not be coordinated. People and divisions engaged in cutthroat political competition, divisional strategy suffered, product lines were outdated or ignored, and serious operations problems emerged. By the late 1970s, a new CEO had to downsize by 60 percent and sell more than 100 business units to keep the corporation afloat.

Although there are no completely successful prevention strategies, there are several practices that can reduce flawed leadership. When leaders are chosen or succession plans are in place, the "fit" between the leader's experience, style, and ability and the organization's culture and needs should be considered. Control mechanisms should be in place in the organization, usually a well-trained board of directors that monitors executive performance and development. Although charismatic leaders are inspiring and needed, especially during downturns and crises, they should be cautious in taking the organization in their personal direction rather than a strategic direction. Other warning signs include believing that they "own" the organization, having a short-term strategic focus, not wanting to hear adverse feedback, not modeling valued behavior, and contributing to intra-organizational competition.

Trends in Leadership Theory

The purpose of a theory is to serve as a template for examining some phenomenon, such as leadership. The theory labels important features, then uses them to describe, explain, and help predict what might happen if certain actions were pursued. Yet, unlike other areas of management, leadership theories have not coalesced into a clear picture; indeed, there are as many views on leadership currently as there were before the millennium. For example, Ralph Stogdill, one of the foremost researchers on the topic opined, "four decades of research on leadership have produced a bewildering mass of findings. . . . The endless accumulations of empirical data have not produced an integrated understanding of leadership" (1974, p. vii).

That leadership makes a difference is undisputed, but exactly how and why it makes a difference is still not well understood and research reflects an inconsistent picture. For example, leadership is been found to be related to job satisfaction, productivity, and organizational commitment (Dunn 1999; McNeese-Smith 1997). Supportive studies have shown that leadership accounts for between 32 and 40 percent of the variance in organizational productivity and profits (Lieberson and O'Connor 1972; Weiner and Mahoney 1981). In contrast, other studies suggest that although leaders shape organizational members' beliefs and behaviors, many external factors that affect the performance of organizations are beyond the influence of leaders (Bass 1993). It also may be the case that when organizations are successful, such performance is attributed to leaders whereas the opposite attribution is made following failure. It is likely that such inconsistencies are due to methodological and measurement differences, as well as different styles of leadership being more or less effective in different situations (Smith, Carson, and Alexander 1984). Nonetheless, some generalizations can be made.

Recently, several leadership theories have emerged to focus more attention on the interpersonal role of managers. In addition, as opposed to focusing on roles at the top leadership levels, recent theories encourage and explore a flatter distribution of leadership roles and responsibilities within an organization.

Early theories were more basic views of leadership, consisting primarily of traits that leaders were expected to possess. As the limitations of these simple conceptualizations became evident, and the workplace and the marketplace became increasingly complex, the definitions and characteristics of effective leadership necessarily broadened to account for different circumstances. These situational or contingency views emphasize a leader's skills in assessing a situation and adjusting behavior accordingly. Although leadership theories have attempted to account for more complex behavior over time, nearly all of them continue to include task-oriented and people-oriented aspects.

Classical Approaches to Leadership Theory

The classical approaches to leadership refer to those early theories that formed the foundation for thinking about leadership and provided a basis for advancing research and new practices. Based on hierarchically structured organizations of the time, classical leadership theories tended to focus on the principled and effective use of authority. This emphasis began to change with the many social changes emerging in the early to mid-1900s. Inventions and innovations in manufacturing increased competition, which made managers more open to new ideas. Workers became increasingly better educated and skilled, thereby requiring managers with authoritative styles to adopt more democratic approaches. The workforce also became increasingly diverse, much like today, and this required a broader understanding of different cultures and motivational approaches.

Great Person Theory

The course of human history is marked with the contributions of great people. Such outstanding individuals originally led to the conception of leadership as an inborn ability, sometimes passed down through family, position, or social tradition, as in the cases of royal families in many parts of the world. The problem with the **great person theory** is that some of those who took positions of such greatness were terribly lacking, as in the case of such notables as Caligula in Rome, Idi Amin in Uganda, and Pol Pot in Cambodia. In the United States, there have been people who were leaders in one sphere, but who failed in others. General Ulysses S. Grant excelled as a general, which largely got him elected president, a role he performed miserably. Braniff Airlines struggled with the leadership of Harding Lawrence who, despite his strategic brilliance, demotivated employees. On flights, his tantrums were notorious and he resorted to screaming and throwing food—violent behaviors that would be considered arrestable offenses today (Harris 1982).

Trait Approach

The **trait approach** gradually replaced the great person model and proposed that leaders possessed a collection of traits or personal qualities that distinguished them from nonleaders; in other words, they had "the right stuff." During the 1930s and 1940s, hundreds of studies on the trait approach to leadership were conducted, and as many as 18,000 traits were identified (Allport and Odbert 1936). Traits were often grouped into categories related to physical needs, values, intellect, personality, and skill characteristics. Some researchers have organized traits on the three leadership requirements of conceptual, interpersonal, and technical skills. Others add a fourth category, administrative skills, which includes the four managerial functions of planning, organizing, directing, and controlling (Yukl 1998).

Unfortunately, in much of the early research, only a weak relationship was discovered between traits and individuals who would emerge as leaders and many leaders did not share all the traits in common. During later studies in which traits and skills were correlated with leader effectiveness rather than leader emergence, stronger connections appeared. Some of the more important traits included adaptability, social alertness, ambition, assertiveness, cooperativeness, decisiveness, dominance, energy, stress tolerance, and confidence. Skills included intelligence and conceptual abilities, creativity, tact, verbal fluency, work knowledge, organization, and persuasion (Stogdill 1974). Despite this extensive work, it appears that no single traits are absolutely required for leadership. Having certain traits and skills leads to a greater likelihood that such attributes may be more helpful in a situation and to leader effectiveness.

Autocratic versus Democratic Leadership

As Douglas McGregor noted in his formulation of Theory X and Y, two types of environments and leaders corresponded to autocratic and democratic behaviors. In the late 1950s, stimulated by the cold war between political democracies and communism, researchers at Iowa State University conducted studies on democratic and autocratic leaders (White and Lippitt 1960). They found that groups under **autocratic leadership** performed well as long as they were closely supervised, although levels of member satisfaction were low. In contrast, **democratic leadership** led members to perform well whether the leader was present or absent and members were more satisfied. This kind of research led to the emphasis on participative management in many organizations, although the studies have been strongly criticized for studying groups of young boys at a summer camp and then generalizing the findings to corporate behavior (Lee 1982).

However, the autocratic—democratic dimension was useful for understanding a range of managerial behavior. Tannenbaum and Schmidt (1973) designed a continuum that described seven degrees of managerial involvement in a decision. (See figure 22.1.) At one end of the continuum, the manager makes a decision alone and announces it; at the other, the manager encourages his or her subordinates to make their own decisions within prescribed limits. This model reflected a shift away from looking at the leader in isolation or in terms of a rigid or permanent style and suggested that a person had available a range of behaviors depending on the situation. But what behaviors made leaders successful?

Behavioral Theories of Leadership

Earlier theories focused on what leaders should do and what was expected of them. In contrast, the emerging behavioral theories described what managers actually do. The emerging theories clearly emphasized a leader's orientation toward both tasks and people and enabled leaders to describe a variety of styles rather than just the "right" style.

Normative Decision Tree

Victor Vroom and Philip Yetton (1971) developed the **Normative Decision Model** in the early 1970s. Using a continuum similar to Tannenbaum and Schmidt's, they identified a series of intermediate questions and decisions, which could be answered yes or no, that would lead to each outcome. (See figure 22.2.) Crucial aspects of the situation related to the quality of the decision required, the degree of subordinate support for the decision, the amount of information available

Figure 22.1.   Tannenbaum and Schmidt's leadership continuum

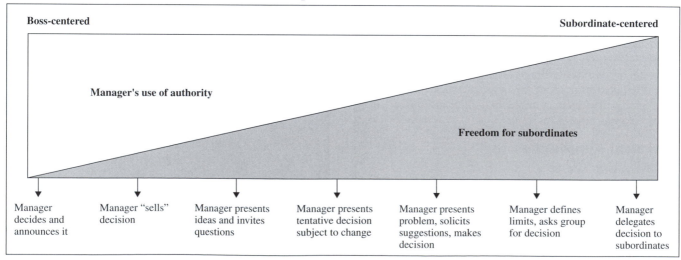

Figure 22.2.   Normative decision tree

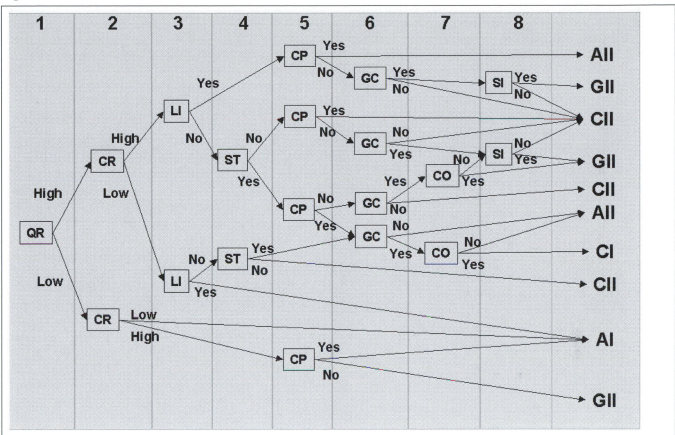

At each step in the process, a question is asked and the response determines the next branch and question. Each node of the tree has a critical criterion for determining the outcome, including:

- *Quality requirement (QR):* How important is the technical quality of the decision?
- *Commitment requirement (CR):* How important is subordinate commitment to the decision?
- *Leader's information (LI):* Do you (the leader) have sufficient information to make a high-quality decision on your own?
- *Problem structure (ST):* Is the problem well structured (e.g., defined, clear, organized, lends itself to solution, time limited, etc.)?
- *Commitment probability (CP):* If you were to make the decision by yourself, is it reasonably certain that your subordinates would be committed to it?
- *Goal congruence (GC):* Do subordinates share the organizational goals to be attained in solving the problem?
- *Subordinate conflict (CO):* Is conflict among subordinates over preferred solutions likely?
- *Subordinate information (SI):* Do subordinates have sufficient information to make a high-quality decision?

Decision Outcome	Description
Autocratic I (AI)	Leader solves the problem alone using information that is readily available.
Autocratic II (AII)	Leader obtains additional information from group members, then makes decision alone. Group members may or may not be informed.
Consultative I (CI)	Leader shares problem with group members individually and asks for information and evaluation. Group members do not meet collectively, and leader makes decision alone.
Consultative II (CII)	Leader shares problem with group members collectively but makes decision alone.
Group II (GII)	Leader meets with group to discuss situation. Leader focuses and directs discussion but does not impose will. Group makes final decision.

to leaders and followers, and how well structured or defined the problem was. A decision made exclusively by the leader without member input could create problems in acceptance, just as delegating a decision to a group could be costly in time and effort, if unnecessary. The Vroom-Yetton model enables a manager to decide on the level of decision-making involvement: autonomous, consultative, or delegative. A more recent revision of the model by Vroom and Jago (1988) replaced the limiting features of the yes-no response options with five choices. It also incorporated consideration for subordinate development, decision time, and the manager's rating of the criteria as new decision rules. The resulting formula is complex and most easily applied with a software program.

Another way to view both autocratic and democratic leadership continuum models is by describing them along a task-social dimension. For example, both the linear models of Tannenbaum and Schmidt and of Vroom and Jago allowed behavior to be described from a task to a social orientation. However, these linear models only allowed leaders to be placed along a single point on the continuum and did not allow them to favor both aspects at the same time. By "bending" the linear continuum into orthogonal axes (figure 22.3), it is possible to create a grid or a two-by-two table that has a greater area for describing more varieties of leadership behavior. Using this matrix format, a person could be described as having both task and social orientations, not just one or the other.

Ohio and Michigan Studies

During the 1950s and 1960s, researchers at The Ohio State University examined the behavior of leaders in several hundred studies and reduced them to two categories: **consideration** and **initiating structure** (Shartle 1979). Consideration referred to attention to the interpersonal aspects of work, including respect for subordinates' ideas and feelings, maintaining harmonious work relationships, collaborating in teamwork, and showing concern with the subordinates' welfare. Initiating structure was more task focused and centered

on giving direction, setting goals and limits, and planning and scheduling activities. During the same period, researchers at the University of Michigan developed a similar model. Comparing effective and ineffective managers, they found that a key difference was that the former employee-centered managers focused more on the human needs of their subordinates whereas their less effective job-centered managers emphasized only goal attainment (Likert 1979).

Leadership Grid

Building on the Ohio State and Michigan studies, Blake and Mouton (1976) at the University of Texas identified the same two dimensions: concern for people and concern for production. Their **leadership grid** marked off degrees of emphasis toward orientation using a nine-point scale and finally separated the grid into five styles of management based on the combined people and production emphasis. For example, a score of 9,9 (emphasizing both people and production) was called "Team Management." Blake and Mouton considered it the best orientation because it emphasized harmonious cooperation in production to achieve goals. A score of 9,1, an "Authority-Compliance" orientation with an emphasis on production and operational efficiency, afforded little attention to human needs. The 1,9 "Country Club" orientation emphasized group harmony, esprit de corps, and cooperation over production. The 1,1 "Impoverished" orientation reflected inattention toward both relationships and work production. A mix of both dimensions, but less than a team orientation, is the 5,5 "Middle-of-the-Road" approach, which tries to balance the two. (See figure 22.4.)

Later Models of Leadership

To this point, most theories have emphasized identifying a cluster of traits or a single style or orientation for leadership. As research in leadership has continued, it has become apparent that successful leadership does not depend on style or skills alone but, rather, on matching a leader's style with the demands of a specific situation.

Figure 22.3.   The shift from leadership continuum to matrix leadership model

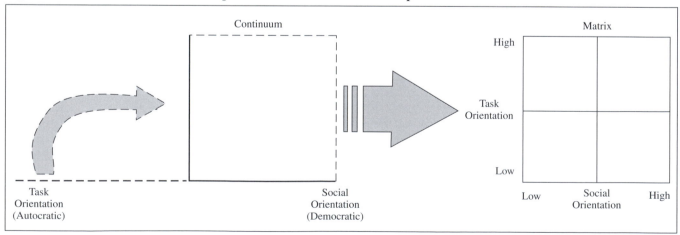

Figure 22.4. Leadership matrix models

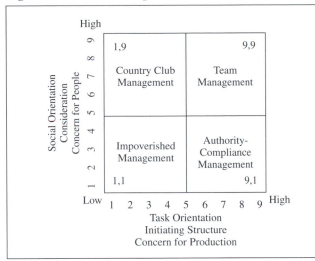

Fiedler's Contingency Model

Fred Fiedler at the University of Illinois designed his **contingency model of leadership** to compensate for the limitations of the classical and behavioral theories of leadership (Fiedler 1967). Fiedler kept the social-task orientation as the cornerstone of his theory and designed an innovative test to determine the leader's preferred style. The **Least Preferred CoWorker (LPC) scale** presented a series of 16 to 22 bipolar adjectives along an eight-point rating scale. Sample items included unfriendly to friendly, uncooperative to cooperative, and hostile to supportive. When the leader described a least-preferred coworker with positive terms, he or she was considered to have a relationship orientation. That is, although the leader might not want to work with the coworker, the leader's interpersonal orientation allows him or her to still perceive the coworker in a positive light. In contrast, a task-oriented leader would be one who described the LPC in negative terms; if he or she cannot work with the coworker, this biases the leader's view of the person on other behaviors.

The second aspect of Fiedler's model was the favorability of the situation in which the leader would operate. Because contingency means "depends on," the favorability or fit of a leader depends on the following three situational factors:

- *Leader–member relations,* or "group atmosphere," is much like social orientation and includes the subordinates' acceptance of, and confidence in, the leader and the loyalty and commitment they show toward the leader.
- *Task structure* is obviously related to task dimension described by other theories above and refers to how clearly and how well defined the task goal, procedures, and possible solutions are.
- *Position power* refers to the authority the leader has to direct others and to use reward and coercive power.

In general, the greater the favorability to the leader, the more the subordinates can be relied on to carry out the task

and the fewer challenges to leadership. Situations more favorable to leadership are those in which leader–member relations are positive, task structure is high, and position power is high. Situations in which these factors are reversed are considered unfavorable to leaders because they have less leverage to influence their followers. Task-oriented leaders tend to perform better in situations that are either high or low in favorability; relationship-oriented leaders do better under moderately favorable conditions.

Although the idea of a contingency or leadership style varying in effectiveness depending on circumstances has gained in popularity, research has not shown extensive support for certain aspects of Fiedler's model and its utility remains in dispute. The LPC, for example, does not appear to be exclusively related to task and relationship styles and may measure other, unrelated features. Fiedler originally believed that personality was "fixed" and that one should engineer or change a situation to be more compatible with a leader's style. Although Fiedler introduced a variety of useful strategies for changing the three contingencies, it is now clear that leaders have much more flexibility in applying their style than was once thought. Finally, several studies have shown that leaders in high- or low-favorability situations are about equally effective in goal attainment. Nonetheless, Fiedler's important contribution was his promotion of the idea of contingency.

Hersey and Blanchard's Situational Model

One of the more popular leadership models used for training, and one that has attempted to integrate other ideas from management, is Hersey and Blanchard's **situational model of leadership** (Hersey, Blanchard, and Johnson 1996). As Dubrin (2001) points out, this is more a model than a theory because it does not explain why things happen but, rather, offers recommendations for behaving differently under various conditions.

To the already widely used task and social dimensions, Hersey and Blanchard added a third: the maturity of the followers. **Worker immaturity–maturity** is a concept borrowed from Chris Argyris, who suggested that job and psychological maturity also influences leadership style. Job maturity refers to how much work-related ability, knowledge, experience, and skill a person has; psychological maturity refers to willingness, confidence, commitment, and motivation related to work. Behaviors associated with maturity include initiative, dependability, perseverance, receptiveness to feedback, goal orientation, and minimal need for supervision. Argyris (1957) suggested that to apply a directive approach with mature workers can result in stifling their maturity and even in forcing them back to lower levels of maturity. Hence, adjusting leadership style to worker maturity is an important consideration. (See figure 22.5, p. 628.)

Hersey and Blanchard also adapted the grid format of their predecessors and structured it in a developmental sequence. Borrowing the idea that teams and organizations progress through developmental stages of a life cycle

**Figure 22.5.   Argyris's worker immaturity–
                 maturity continuum**

Assertiveness & initiative	Passivity
Independence	Dependence
Wide behavioral choices	Limited behavioral range
Deep and strong interests	Shallow & casual interests
Past–future perspective	Present-centered perspective
Self-awareness & control	Low self-awareness

Figure 22.6.   Situational leadership model

(Miller and Friesen 1984; Tuckman 1965), they suggested that leadership style should be adjusted to the stage of team development. For example, their Situation-1 (S1) involves high-task, but low-social, emphasis, thereby indicating that the leader should focus on task duties such as setting goals, identifying resources and constraints, and so on. As the team moves to Situation-2 (S2), task and social functions of the leader are both involved as members attempt to influence each other and to explore how their styles may conflict with or complement each other. In Situation-3 (S3), members clearly know the task and need little direction, but social interaction around team norms may require intervention and guidance. Finally, Situation-4 (S4) is the stage of high team performance in which both task and relationships require little intervention by the leader. Worker maturity is high, and the leader may be active only in encouraging higher performance and removing barriers to performance. Hersey and Blanchard also incorporated Tannenbaum and Schmidt's autocratic–democratic continuum, which they distributed across the developed stages and labeled telling, selling, participating, and delegating. (See figure 22.6.)

Path–Goal Theory

A more recent model of leadership, initially introduced by House (1971), is **path–goal theory.** This theory was based on the **expectancy theory of motivation** that proposes that one's effort will result in the attainment of desired performance goals. Path-goal theory states that a person's ability to perform certain tasks is related to the direction and clarity available that lead to organizational goals. For example, if a worker is unclear about what a task involves and what should be done, performance will be improved when clear instructions are given. The role of leaders, then, is to facilitate the path toward the goal by removing barriers to performance.

Path-goal theory identifies four different situations, each requiring a different facilitative response from leadership. (See figure 22.7.) When workers lack self-confidence, leaders provide support by being friendly, approachable, concerned about needs, and equitable. This increases the worker's confidence to achieve the work outcome. When the worker has an ambiguous job, the leader is more directive in providing the worker with direction, schedules, rules, and regulations that clarify the path. When workers do not have sufficient job challenge, the leader uses an achievement approach by setting challenging goals, continually seeking improvement, and expecting high performance. Finally, when the reward is mismatched with worker needs, the leader takes a more consultative or participative role in which workers share work problems, make suggestions, and are included in decision making to ensure more appropriate rewards. All four strategies result in improved task performance and satisfaction—again, the task and social dimensions.

Dyadic Relationship Theory

Some leadership theories are macro theories and attempt to explain leadership across large domains; but there also are micro theories that focus on a specific context for leadership. **Leader–member exchange** (LMX) (Graen and Skandura 1987) and closely related **vertical dyad linkage** (VDL) represent micro theories that focus on dyadic relationships, or those between two people, or between a leader and a small group. More specifically, they explain how **in-group** and **out-group** relationships form with a leader or mentor, and how **delegation** may occur.

VDL was first formulated in 1975 (Dansereau, Graen, and Haga 1975) to describe the single-person mentoring relationships that occur in organizations and was later supplemented by leader–member relations theory that applied the same idea to the leader's relations with groups. In these situations, leaders look for subordinates with high-performance and leadership potential that distinguishes them from subordinates with less potential. The best predictors of being selected for in-group, in addition to competence, include compatibility of the subordinate with the leader, interpersonal liking for each other, and being extraverted. Once identified, the leader and subordinates form an **exchange relationship,** in which a leader offers greater opportunities and privileges to a subordinate in exchange for loyalty, commitment, and assistance. The leader may delegate special responsibilities, offer interesting and desirable tasks, give opportunities for highly visible or skill-building projects, and provide mentoring.

Figure 22.7. Path–goal theory

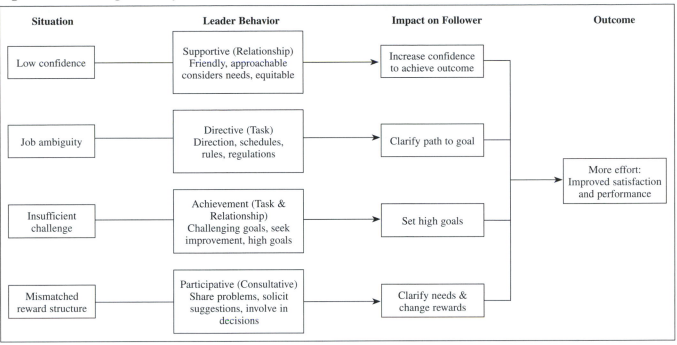

Those subordinates who form a group around the leader are referred to as the in-group; those subordinates not included form the out-group. Being in the in-group may sound attractive, but it involves performance "beyond the call of duty." In-group members may spend longer hours, take work home or work during off-hours, and take on more difficult tasks compared to members in the out-group. The out-group expects to be treated fairly by the leader, and as long as the exchanges are viewed as fair, there is little or no conflict between the in- and out-groups; they can remain fairly stable over time. However, when the out-group perceives that the in-group is receiving greater privileges for doing the same work as the out-group, the latter can feel resentment, alienation, and hostility, and show lower performance. There is evidence that once in the in-group, the halo effect can take over and ratings of the subordinate may be inflated (Duarte, Goodson, and Klitch 1993). The leader must ensure fair treatment and clear expectations for both groups. In addition, leaders can promote high-quality relationships with all employees by speaking with people personally, using active listening, not imposing the leader's view on issues discussed, and sharing expectations about the job and working relationship.

Theories of Transactional and Transformational Leadership

This discussion goes back to the difference between managers and leaders discussed earlier. In 1978, when James MacGregor Burns published his Pulitzer prize-winning *Leadership,* he emphasized this distinction among political leaders, calling them transactional and transformational styles. **Transactional leadership** refers to the role of the manager who strives to create an efficient workplace by balancing task accomplishment with interpersonal satisfaction. In contrast, **transformational leadership** is considered more complex and powerful. In this leadership style, leaders promote innovation and organizational change. In the mid-1980s, Bernard Bass extended the model into the business world (1985).

An important aspect of transformational leadership is **charisma,** or the ability to inspire and motivate people beyond what is expected with exceptionally high levels of commitment (Bass and Avolio 1993; Klein and House 1995). Charisma refers to influence by force of personality in which the leader inspires commitment, loyalty, and faith in a vision. Examples of people who have wielded such power include Martin Luther King, Normal Schwarzkopf, Winston Churchill, Adolph Hitler, and David Koresh. Although the rhetoric and imagery can be stimulating to followers, there is a risk that with the leader's passing, leadership succession may fail and progress may falter.

In a five-year study, Bennis and Nanus (1985) conducted extensive interviews with 90 top leaders. Their study reinforced differences between transformational (leaders) and transactional (managers) roles, finding that transformational leaders were distinguished by their "four Is": idealized influence (leader as role model), inspirational motivation (team spirit and meaningfulness), intellectual stimulation (innovation and creativity), and individual consideration (mentoring).

Attempting to define the leadership practices of transformational leaders, Kouzes and Posner (1989) surveyed 550 middle and senior managers in private and public sectors. They used a series of questions that identified how leaders performed during their personal best leadership achieve-ments. They reduced the results into five leadership practices and 10 behavioral commitments:

- Challenging the process included the search for oppor-tunities and taking risks.
- Inspiring a shared vision involved envisioning the future and enlisting others.
- Enabling others to act was based on fostering collabora-tion and strengthening others.
- Modeling the way included setting an example and planning small wins.
- Encouraging the heart referred to recognizing and cel-ebrating accomplishments.

Kouzes and Posner stressed that the relationship between leaders and followers has a **synergy,** in which the combina-tion of their efforts produces more than either acting alone. This enthusiasm for change is essential in dealing more effectively with the innovations and changes that face mod-ern organizations.

Values-Based Leadership

The demoralizing impact of corporate scandals, layoffs due to downsizing, and stress, especially in the healthcare indus-try, has led to the resurgence of a focus on values and ethics in the workplace. Values are core beliefs that guide and moti-vate attitudes and actions and both form and express an orga-nization's culture. Values make a difference to most people. The 2000 Global Employee Relationship study showed that (WalkerInformation 2001a) employees who believed that they worked for an organization and leader who were ethical were 55 percent more loyal than the average employee.

Role of Values

One of the significant consequences of the organization and its leaders not being perceived as highly ethical is that employ-ees feel less loyalty and commitment and tend to leave the organization. In 2002, the national healthcare annual turnover rate averaged 19 percent (Gering and Connor 2002), and the cost of staff turnover ranged from 25 to 200 percent of annual compensation and benefits (Berk 2003; Burkholder 2003). By 2004, the turnover of allied health staff had become as high as 49 percent (Waldman et al. 2004).

Many organizations find that there are widespread conditions that mitigate employee retention. In our global marketplace, an international study of 10,000 employees in 32 nations reflected that only 34 percent are really loyal to their organizations, two-thirds do not believe their organization operates ethically, and 40 percent question their leader's personal integrity (Kidder 2000). Within the United States, "true loyalty," or the combina-tion of high loyalty and commitment, is only 24 percent. Although two-thirds to three-quarters of employees are often proud of their work, would work above and beyond their requirements, and are highly motivated, they still consider leav-ing current positions. This discontent is related to questioning

the fairness of pay and policy execution, as well as low recogni-tion of achievement and insufficient job performance measures. Less than half of employees feel a sense of caring and concern for them in the organization, perceive that their judgment is trusted, or feel encouraged to be innovative (WalkerInforma-tion 2001a). Clearly, to retain talented people as well as to maintain a competitive position, organizational leadership must reestablish and promote ethical behavior and a culture of strong, consistent, and compatible values.

Many organizations believe that merely sending managers off to training will provide sufficient skill in ethical manage-ment. However, for the 75 percent of organizations that pro-vide such training and consulting to their leadership teams at a cost of $15 billion, only about 10 percent actually translate it into behavior change (Hunter 2004). To fully effect change, managers and leaders must implement the values to be devel-oped in an organization into their own behavior.

Servant Leadership

The **values-based leadership** theories are similar to Burns's transformational leadership (1978), as well as other contin-gency theories such as path-goal leadership in which the lead-er's role is to empower and facilitate employee satisfaction and productivity. Prominent among values-based approaches is Robert Greenleaf's concept of servant leadership (Greenleaf 1991). Greenleaf was director of management research at AT&T for 38 years, as well as a Quaker with a strong contem-plative orientation. To Greenleaf, servant leaders are those who put the needs, interests, and aspirations of others above their own. Larry Spears, CEO of the Greenleaf Center for Servant Leadership, describes it as seeking to "involve others in decision making, is strongly based in ethical and caring behavior, and it enhances the personal growth of workers while improving the caring and quality of organizational life" (1995, p. 142).

The values-based organization, represented by the **Ser-vant Leadership Model,** promotes 10 essential values (Greenleaf 1991):

- *Listening* intently to clarify the will of the group as well as to hear one's own "inner voice" and seeking to discover what one's body, mind, and spirit are commu-nicating
- *Empathize* with and understand others, assuming their good intentions, even when behaviors must be rejected
- *Healing* as a force for transformation and integration using the subtle communication of valuing the whole
- *Awareness* with courage to persist in recognizing and discussing what may be sensitive issues
- *Persuasion* rather than positional authority to build consensus and make decisions
- *Conceptualization* or vision must be balanced with daily realities
- *Foresight* requires learning lessons from the past, reali-ties of the present, and consequences in the future using intuition

- *Stewardship* in which all stakeholders hold as their goal the greatest good for the larger society
- *Commitment* to the personal, professional, and spiritual growth of people
- *Community building* within the organization to replace what has been lost socially

Although servant leadership does not have strong evidence to support its effectiveness, its popularity has spread worldwide as well as to many of the best companies in the United States. A 2001 *Fortune* survey showed that 35 of the top 100 organizations were using a servant leadership approach; among them, Southwest Airlines, TDIndustries, and Synovus Financial were ranked second, fourth, and fifth, respectively (Levering, Moskowitz, and Katz 2000).

The strengths of the servant leadership concept include the following:

- It is compatible with the current surge of values and faith-based orientation in the lives of many people.
- There is anecdotal evidence of its success in prominent organizations.
- It has an intuitively desirable focus on values given a scandalous and postmodern environment.
- It contrasts serving others with the more traditional directive and hierarchical approach.

The weaknesses of the theory include the following:

- Some secular and nonfaith-based settings may not be receptive to its religious overtones.
- The concepts are vaguely defined and difficult to measure.
- Its popularity exceeds its evidence.
- It may not account for all the facets of leadership.
- It is unclear how the concept works in a highly competitive or crisis environment.

Gender and Leadership

The idea of the "glass barrier" or "glass ceiling" was originally coined by Carol Hymowitz and Timothy Schellhardt in a 1986 *Wall Street Journal* article. The term refers to an unofficial barrier imposed to prevent certain groups, especially women, from progressing to higher levels of management in organizations. Since its introduction, the concept has raised awareness of the role and contribution of women and the importance of diversifying the workforce. There have been substantial increases in women's ascension into management and leadership in all fields and questions whether there are really differences between women and men's styles of management.

Women in Organizations

The role of women in organizations has changed dramatically over the decades. In 1972, women occupied only 17 percent of the supervisory and management positions in U.S. firms. However, by 2003, about 40 percent of all such positions were held by women. A gender-centered perspective on leadership would propose that, through socialization, women develop a feminine leadership style that can be characterized by an emphasis on relationships through caring and nurturing, such as in collaborative projects and participatory decision making. In contrast, men develop a masculine style characterized by a focus on competition, domination, and task orientation. Early research on gender tended to support this dichotomy and that males were more often viewed as having desired leadership qualities (Megargee 1969). More recently, with the women's movement, challenges to the "glass ceiling," and the increase in numbers of women entering managerial and leadership positions, there is a societal shift in gender perceptions.

Yet, even this view of men and women is changing. An extensive study of 900 male and 900 female managers from 143 companies was conducted in which they received a **360-degree evaluation** of their leadership abilities (totaling 17,491 assessments). The results were unexpected: male managers were more likely to delegate tasks; female managers were perceived as more assertive and competitive while maintaining control of their assigned projects. Furthermore, the stereotype of women managers being more participatory was not reflected in the study. Overall, ratings by supervisors of the managers showed no significant difference in their effectiveness (Kabacoff 1998).

Gender Differences

In general, there is more evidence that there are actually few differences between men and women leaders in behavior, but that there are differences in perceptions of those behaviors (Bass and Avolio 1994; Kolb 1999). Leadership does not exist in a person but, rather, is a perceived relationship between people. The same behavior exhibited by men and women may be interpreted and labeled differently by the perceiver. This is due to gender-based stereotypes that include expectations about how gender roles should be performed.

In what has become a classic, the 1987 *Price-Waterhouse v. Hopkins* case reflected the prominent role of gender stereotype. Ann Hopkins was a high-performing and rapidly rising employee who during five years had brought in more clients than other candidates for company partnership. When she was denied partnership status, she sued. Allegedly, partners at Price Waterhouse perceived her direct and assertive behavior as inappropriate for what they believed should be a feminine role. They told her she was "too macho, abrasive and overbearing" and would be more promotable if she wore jewelry and makeup and walked and talked more femininely (Price-Waterhouse 1987). Price-Waterhouse was cited for sex discrimination, and the impact of gender stereotypes on people and organizations was brought to prominence. Although there may be advantages to women's leadership styles in some organizations, in organizations with a masculine culture women may experience prejudicial evaluations (Eagly and Carly 2003).

Androgynous Leadership

When the combination of leader effectiveness and gender is questioned, the answer becomes clearer, and middle managers who were described as successful more often possessed a combination of stereotypic masculine and feminine qualities or were **androgynous leaders** (Korabik 1990). As organizations continue to be diverse in the workforce and markets and complex in applying organizational strategy, androgynous managers and leaders may have greater flexibility in style to deal with such situations. The also may be perceived by others as more balanced.

Studies of gender leadership, particularly those examining the glass ceiling, have focused on external barriers to women's emerging as leaders. Although there is evidence for this, recent studies on self-efficacy show that the expectations by the women themselves may have a functional influence on their role seeking. Self-efficacy, or confidence in one's personal capabilities to do a job, affects the level of aspiration of potential leaders; those with low self-efficacy do not see themselves as capable and are less likely to seek a leadership role (McCormick, Tanguma, and Lopez-Forment 2003).

Self-efficacy also is related to how long a person will persist at a difficult task, use self-encouraging thoughts, and be resilient against setbacks. High-efficacy women faced with a high-stress situation tend to perceive it as a challenge whereas low-efficacy women tend to view it as threatening (Hoyt 2002).

Check Your Understanding 22.2

Instructions: Complete the following activities on a separate piece of paper.

1. Think of a decision you might be confronted with as a supervisor at work. Use the Vroom-Yetton decision tree to trace how you might choose whether to make the decision yourself, consult with others, or delegate the decision making to someone else.

2. Describe how your approach to leading people should change as they move through the stages of worker maturity. Explain what might happen if your style mismatches what they need at these stages.

3. Make two columns of leadership behaviors related to stereotypes of male and female roles. Make a third column in which you blend the two into an androgynous role. What are the advantages of this intermediate role over the other two?

The Learning Organization: Understanding and Participating in Change

When Peter Senge published *The Fifth Discipline: The Art and Practice of the Learning Organization* (1990), it was likely that not many people expected his ideas to influence management thinking as much as they have. As with Taylor's theory, the marketplace was ready for, and receptive to, new ways of thinking about increasingly complex organizations and how they could adapt to equally complex competitive environments.

Systems Theory

When introduced in the 1940s by von Bertalanffy and others, **systems theory** was a reaction against **reductionism** in which complex processes were reduced to their constituent elements and analyzed by their parts. Proponents of systems theory believe that important information is lost by too specific a focus and thus emphasize the interconnections, organization, and wholeness of these constituents rather than their inspection in isolation. In management, systems decisions implemented in good faith and with planning may have an adverse ripple effect in other parts of the organization or in relationship to the external environment.

The learning organization was an idea with a good fit for the questions that managers were asking: How do we adjust to all the changes in the marketplace (Argyris and Schon 1996; Senge 1990)? Systems theory's answer was learning. All **systems** (individual, team, organizational) adapt to a changing environment by learning. The more rapidly they learn, the faster they can take a stronger competitive position. This has led Robert Weiler, CEO of GIGA Information Group, to paraphrase the Darwinian principle: "It's not the strongest that survive, it's those most responsive and adaptive to change" (Pratt 2000). Arie de Geus (1997), a retired Royal Dutch/Shell Group executive who wrote *The Living Company,* takes an even stronger stance comparing organizations to living organisms that must adapt and evolve in competitive environments.

Proponents of systems theory suggest that organizational learning best takes place when a culture is formed that supports it. Such a culture is often described as emphasizing openness and communication, inquiry and feedback, adequate time for tasks, and mutual respect and support. This kind of organization also employs reflective learning in which people are alert to their experiences, consider what they reflect about the organization, and explore ways of improving performance. The Japanese push for quality has derived an interesting term, *Kaizen,* or "continuous improvement," to describe the importance of people in the learning organization. Like a *tsunami,* if each person learns from experience and applies something new each day of work, by the end of a year the organization has a "tidal wave" of small innovations that make a great difference.

Systems Thinking Skills

Contributing to the development of the learning organization are the disciplines or systems thinking skills identified by Senge (1990):

- *Personal mastery* refers to the lifelong discipline of continually clarifying personal values and vision, creativity, commitment, and intuition.
- *Mental models* are the conceptual maps we make of how things operate. They are representations based on our assumptions and beliefs that can limit our understanding of possibilities.

- *Building shared vision* emphasizes the consensual formulation of a compelling image of what the future or other goal might be.
- *Team learning* refers to the process of the team learning from its own experience that contributes to improving its performance.
- *Systems thinking* involves a way of thinking that considers the relationships among events, cycles and patterns of behavior, and awareness that everything is connected to everything else to some degree.

Consequences of Decisions

When managers do not consider the ripple effect of decisions throughout the organization, they can eventually face unexpected consequences that have adverse effects. For example, a mental health center had been losing staff due to stress, low morale, and overwork as well as having fewer billable contact hours. The center decided to involve staff in more administrative planning to increase their sense of involvement and buy-in. As a result of the mandatory involvement, staff members had even less time for clients, more conflict with administration, and fewer billable hours. As a result,

even more staff left because of the unexpected pressures of seeing the larger administrative problem. In another example, lawmakers recognized the growing problem of an aging population and eagerly approved the concept of home health care. The intention was to make visits to ill persons in their homes and thereby save large costs to insurance companies, Medicare, and the patients themselves. Instead of saving money, however, many healthcare facilities came to rely on the services as a strong source of revenue and therefore encouraged more service. In 1998, the average home healthcare patient received about 80 visits a year, nearly four times as many as 10 years earlier (Daft 2000).

As organizations grow, expand their involvement with other organizations, and develop more complicated information systems in a continually changing and competitive environment, they will need to find better ways to respond. Efforts have been made to model some of these complex environments using systems theory. Simulation software such as PowerSim and Vensim can help managers create representations of various processes such as patient flows in order to identify bottlenecks, critical points, and intervention points. Figure 22.8 is a stock-and-flow diagram showing the

Figure 22.8.   A stock-and-flow diagram showing the management of psychiatric patients

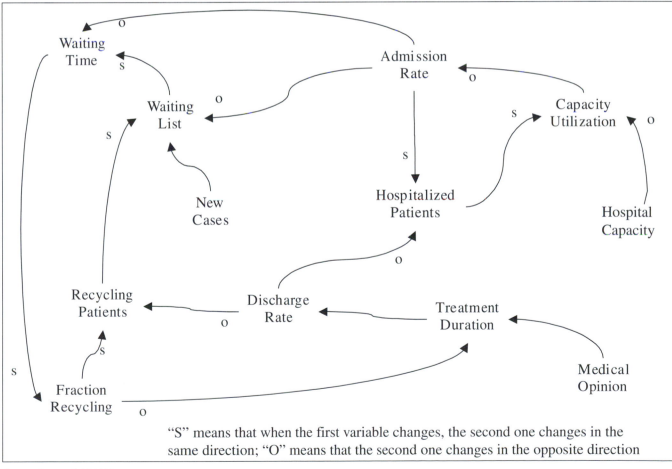

"S" means that when the first variable changes, the second one changes in the same direction; "O" means that the second one changes in the opposite direction

Source: Dangerfield 1999.

management of psychiatric patients. Although these programs require much training, they exemplify the direction that systems thinking is going with regard to management. Such modeling will eventually enable managers to explore how various innovations may affect their organizations.

Diffusion of Innovations

Innovations have occurred throughout history, but little attention was given to exactly how they were adopted until Rogers and Shoemaker (1971) clarified the process in their book, *Communication of Innovations.* Although Rogers and Shoemaker were not the first to develop ideas about diffusion, their presentation of the adopter categories or stakeholders and the **diffusion S-curve** came at a time when businesses were eager to understand consumers.

Categories of Adopter Groups

Viewing the organization in much the same way that marketers view market segments, Rogers and Shoemaker identified five categories of adopters of an innovation that generally fits the normal curve (figure 22.9):

- *Innovators:* This venturesome group comprises about 2.5 percent of the organization and individuals who are eager to try new ideas. These individuals tend to be more cosmopolitan, to seek out new information in broad networks, and to be willing to take risks.
- *Early adopters:* This respectable group accounts for about 13.5 percent of the organization. The individuals in this group have a high degree of opinion leadership. They are more localized than cosmopolitan and often look to the innovators for advice and information. These are the leaders and respected role models in the organization, and their adoption of an idea or practice does much to initiate change.
- *Early majority:* This group comprises about 34 percent of the organization. Although usually not leaders, the individuals in this group represent the backbone of the organization, are deliberate in thinking and acceptance

of an idea, and serve as a natural bridge between early and late adopters.
- *Late majority:* This skeptical group comprises another 34 percent of the organization. The individuals in this group usually adopt innovations only after social or financial pressure to do so.
- *Laggards:* The traditional members of this group are usually the last ones to respond to innovation and make up as much as 16 percent of the organization. The laggards are often characterized as isolated, uninformed, and mistrustful of change and **change agents,** but they may serve a function by keeping the organization from changing too quickly.

When planning a change, each of these groups should be considered as a market segment whose needs must be responded to by leaders. In general, people who are more receptive to innovation are better educated and more literate and have stronger aspirations. In addition, they have higher socioeconomic status, occupational prestige, more income, and social mobility. Moreover, they are better socially networked, cosmopolitan, diverse in interests, and well integrated into the organization and the community (Rogers 1995).

Diffusion Curve

Each of the adopter categories engages innovation at a different time and a different acceptance rate, as shown by the diffusion S curve. (See figure 22.10.) Note that during the early stages of diffusion, there is a shorter period between becoming aware of an innovation and adopting it. Over time, each adopter category becomes aware of the innovation but increasingly takes longer periods to adopt it, which can affect how well an innovation is introduced into the marketplace or how fully it is practiced in the organization. In addition, how quickly an innovation is accepted is based on a number of factors, including whether it offers an advantage relative to its alternative, its compatibility with the potential adopters' values and lifestyles, how easy it is to understand and use, the degree to which it can be experimented with, and the degree to which the results are visible to others (Rogers 1995).

Figure 22.9.   Characteristics of innovation stakeholders

Figure 22.10.   The diffusion S-curve

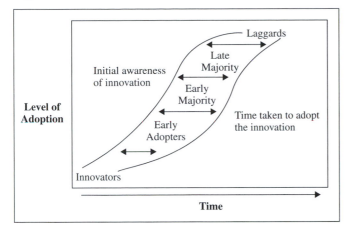

Innovator Roles

In the late 1960s and early 1970s, the literature reflected a new interest in the roles of innovators within organizations who become gatekeepers or nodes for the flow of information (Allen and Cohen 1969). Four roles have been identified for the successful implementation of an innovation (Daft and Marcic 1998):

- The **inventor** (innovator) is the individual who develops a new idea or practice in the organization. However, it is not sufficient to merely originate and understand the new idea. Rather, the idea must be facilitated by several other roles in the organization before it is adopted or brought to market (Daft 2000).
- The **champion** is someone in the organization who believes in the idea, acknowledges the practical problems of financing and political support, and assists in overcoming barriers.
- The **sponsor** is usually a high-level manager who approves and protects the idea, expedites testing and approval, and removes barriers within the organization.
- The **critic** is a crucial, but sometimes overlooked, role. This role is essential in challenging the innovation for shortcomings, presenting strong criteria, and, in essence, providing a reality test for the new idea.

In an innovative environment, all these roles are important and good examples of how role responsibilities are distributed in an organization.

Management, Fads, Fashions, and Trends

Innovations are not limited to products and services; they also extend to management theories and practices themselves. The competitive nature of most industries, including healthcare, as well as the need to use resources wisely, has led to a rich development of management techniques and practices. Although many of these are based on successful limited applications, they are too often quickly promoted beyond their evidentiary base and followed enthusiastically by a group. They become fads when they rise and fall quickly, fashionable when they rise quickly and fall slowly, and trends when they persist over a longer time (Aldaq 1997). (See figure 22.11.)

Fads tend to proliferate during periods of uncertainty, when organizations search for innovative ways to fill what is perceived as a performance gap and to gain competitive advantage. Additional influence to adopt fads is often from popular management consultants and the popular media (who in turn are competing to sell their ideas) who speak to people's naive fascination with novelty. Many common practices have been considered as fads at some time in their emergence, such as total quality management, managing by objectives, zero-based budgeting, managing by walking around, decentralizing, downsizing, and so on. Figure 22.12 shows the rise and fall of management practices based on their frequency of citation in Business Source Premier (a database of 4,600 journals) from 1950 to 2004.

Figure 22.11.   Fad, fashion, and trend curves

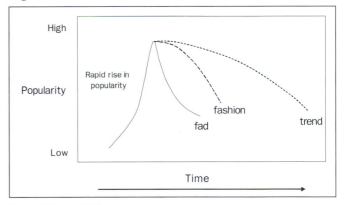

Source: Wasson 1978.

Figure 22.12.   Patterns of management practices

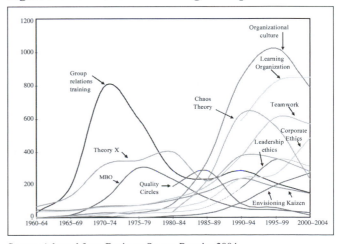

Source: Adapted from Business Source Premier 2004.

In 1993, a study of 4,000 organizations in 15 countries found that fads are popular across all countries and industries. The average executive in the United States, Britain, France, and Japan reported using from 11 to 14 of the top 25 fads (Rigby 1998). Despite the sparse initial evidence to support them, it appears that fads will continue to be a part of organizational strategies for improvement efforts.

The Problem with Fads

The major problem with fads is that they present the illusion of easy implementation, singular changes, and a quick fix to organizational problems. In practice, most significant changes require years. For example, shifting from traditional structures to team-based organizations has been estimated to take three to five years (Armstrong n.d.), and implementation of the balanced scorecard typically requires the same duration (Kaplan 2002). It took Motorola, the originator of the Six Sigma approach, 10 years to fully implement the concept. Such changes are clearly not a quick fix.

The overuse of fads can adversely affect employees who tend to become discouraged by unrealistic expectations, revised work procedures, and wasted resources (Birnbaum 2000; Byrne 1997). The initial enthusiasm fails to produce the expected results; in other cases, management support is lacking. As a result, even when good practices are initiated, many employees consider them just the next fad and fail to commit to them.

Though fads have often been implemented with high enthusiasm, they have just as frequently failed to perform. Between 1992 and 1996, 450 large and medium-sized European companies were studied regarding their adopting innovative management practices (Pettigrew 1999). In these organizations, partial or piecemeal implementation tended to fair poorly, although they did better when used across several fronts. The most successful changes occur when they are implemented across several fronts in an organization, with the recognition that they will take time and effort to be effective.

The enthusiasm with which fads are received appears to wax and wane over time, comprising what is typified as a fad life cycle. The steps of the fad life cycle are:

1. Some deficiency is perceived that requires a solution.
2. A management technique or theory is discovered that appears to solve the problem.
3. The euphoria of the fad's supporters leads to promotion within the organization.
4. Extension of the fad beyond its sound application ensures its eventual failure.
5. Derision and lowering of regard for the innovation begins to pervade the organization.
6. The fad is abandoned and may be replaced by a search for another solution (Right cited in Chaulk and Sexty 2002).

The Failure of "Excellence"

Despite the wide popularity of Peters and Waterman's *In Search of Excellence,* the fad nature of the promotion became obvious after only a few years. As noted previously, of the 43 companies they profiled, only a third remained in the top position. (See figure 22.13.) In a 2001 interview with *Fast Company* magazine, Peters admitted that he had no idea what he was doing when he wrote the book, he identified the eight principles only under pressure of a pending presentation (not after thoughtful consideration and data analysis), and he selected many companies on a much-less-than-rigorous basis (Peters 2001). Nonetheless, the book was a useful turning

Figure 22.13.   The 43 "excellent" companies five years later

Excellent	Still Performing but Weakened Leadership	Weakened Position	Troubled Position
Rockwell	Bristol-Myers	Amdahl	Atari
Disney	Delta	Bechtel	Chesebrough-Ponds
Boeing	Dow	Caterpillar	Avon
DEC	Dupont	Dana	Data General
Emerson	Hughes	Hewlett-Packard	Fluor
Frito-Lay	(GM)	Kodak	Kmart
IBM	Levi Straus	Raychem	National Semiconductor
Intel	Marriott	Schlumburger	Revlon
Johnson & Johnson	Proctor & Gamble	Texas Instruments	
Mars	Standard Oil	Tupperware	
Maytag	Amoco	(Dart)	
McDonalds	3M	Wang	
Merck			
Wal-Mart			

Source: Adapted from Peters 2001.

point for many managers who started paying more attention to the human element in their organizations.

Fad management probably fails for four reasons. First, executive leadership for, and commitment to, the initiative lags and mid-level managers carry the burden for implementation. Second, there is a failure to deploy the innovation. There are no mechanisms to maintain the innovation, spread it beyond the pilot group trying it, or training beyond the introduction. Third, management seeks shortcuts and easy, superficial applications rather than try to understand in-depth how the organization must customize the process. Fourth, proper metrics or measurements are not used as feedback to gauge progress and success, and thereby help revisions (Marash, Berman, and Flynn 2003).

Not everyone agrees that management fads are a bad thing. Robert Cole of the University of California Haas School of Business has argued that adaptable companies learn how to use fads to improve quality and productivity (Cole 1999). Fads can motivate employees and bring attention to important organizational processes for revision. Exemplifying this is the American response to the Japanese Aquality challenge of the early 1980s. America was unprepared for the high market demand for high-quality goods, and the competition spurred U.S. businesses to focus more on quality.

From the end of World War II to the mid-1980s, management often held the belief that bigger is better and growth is good. By the end of the 1980s, productivity was declining, managerial overhead was increasing, and organizations were more seriously considering smaller size and efficiency (Tomasco 1987). Downsizing was popularly embraced as a way of reducing labor costs and improving performance, and nearly all the Fortune 1000 firms have utilized it. Reaching such faddish proportions, unfortunately downsizing has rarely delivered on its promise. (See table 22.2.) A survey of senior managers reported that 74 percent believed that downsizing adversely affected morale, trust, and productivity (Henkoff 1990). Another survey of nearly 1,500 firms found that their performance deteriorated following downsizing. Healthcare facilities fared no better, with a study of 281 acute care hospitals reporting increases in mortality and morbidity rates of 200 to 400 percent after downsizing (Cameron, Freeman, and Mishra 1993). It has been estimated that 68 percent of downsizing, restructuring, and reengineering is unsuccessful (Clark and Koonce 1995), yet many organizations continue the practice without carefully considering its implications.

Thinking Critically about New Approaches

New approaches should not be dismissed out of hand but, rather, should be thoughtfully examined for their utility in an organization or incorporation into a manager or leader's style. Several questions should considered:

- What is the source of the new idea or practice? Does it come from a source that can be generalized to other settings?

Table 22.2.   Failed achievements of downsizing

Expected Downsizing Outcome	Actual Results (%)
Expense reduction	46
Profit increase	32
Cash flow improvement	24
Productivity increase	22
ROI increase	21
Competitive advantage increase	19
Bureaucracy reduction	17
Decision-making improvement	14
Customer satisfaction increase	14
Sales increase	13
Market share increase	12
Product quality improvement	9
Technological advances	9
Innovation increase	7
Avoid takeover	6

Source: Bennet 1991.

- What is the evidence that it works?
- Can clear linkages between the practice and specific outcomes be measured?
- What does the level of enthusiasm or desperation about the fad suggest about the organization and what it really needs?
- What is needed to really implement the practice? It is rarely as simple or singular as the fad implies.

Change Management

A more global role for practitioners of organizational change is often referred to as the change agent. The change agent is a specialist in organizational development and facilitates the change brought about by the innovation. He or she may be internal or external to the organization, as in the case of a consultant specifically hired to assist with the change. **Organization development** (OD) is the process in which an organization reflects on its own processes and consequently revises them for improved performance. Beckhard has provided a widely accepted definition of OD: "Organization Development is an effort planned, organization-wide, and managed from the top, to increase organization effectiveness and health through planned interventions in the organization's processes, using behavioral-science knowledge" (1969, p. 9).

OD Consultant Functions

Blake and Mouton (1976) suggested that OD consultants might perform a range of five functions with management:

- The *acceptant function* uses counseling skills to help the manager sort out emotions to gain a more objective perspective of the organization.
- The *catalytic function* helps collect and interpret data about the organization.
- In the *confrontation function,* the change agent challenges the manager's thinking processes and assumptions.
- In the *prescriptive function,* the consultant may tell the manager what to do to correct a given situation.
- The *theory and principle function* involves helping the client system internalize alternate explanations of what is occurring in the organization.

Internal and External Change Agents

Change happens on its own but is usually most desirable when intentionally directed toward the benefit of the organization and its members. The role of the change agent is to facilitate this change process by utilizing reflective learning: drawing attention to important processes, helping people understand what the processes mean, and considering and implementing plans of action. Exactly who performs this role can be critical (Weick and Quinn 1995). There are advantages and disadvantages to using change agents from within the organization as well as from outside the organization. (See table 22.3.)

Advantages and Disadvantages of Using Internal Change Agents

Internal change agents have the clear advantage of being familiar with the organization, its history, subtle dynamics, secrets, and resources. Such people are often well respected, securely positioned, and have the strong interpersonal relationships to foster change. Moreover, there is an advantage

to recognizing the internal expertise of employees, maintaining confidentiality of the process, and using people who are invested in the success of the outcome.

Yet, the strengths of internal change agents can be weaknesses. Coming from the inside, however reputable they are, their previous relationships with others in the organization could lead to accusations of bias. As a product of the organizational culture, internal change agents may be as blind to certain problems as those they seek to facilitate. Another disadvantage is that they are taken away from their regular duties to conduct the facilitation or perhaps become overextended in trying to handle both responsibilities. Finally, internal change agents may be subject to pressures and sanctions regarding the outcome whereas an external change agent would have no such obligations.

Advantages and Disadvantages of Using External Change Agents

The external change agent has the advantage of providing a fresh, outside view as well as having the knowledge base to compare performance across organizations. Not having direct connections to the organization, he or she usually feels more comfortable challenging norms and culture, questioning unusual or unfair practices, and generally noting events that others may be reluctant to comment on. Being from the outside, he or she may be seen as having new skills and being more objective, or at least less biased than an internal agent.

The weaknesses of the external agents include not having a history with their client organization that could enhance their awareness of important dynamics. Becoming familiar with the organization takes time, and during a crisis they may move too quickly to conclusions based on limited information. Additionally, external change agents may be strongly influenced by the viewpoint of the administrators who contracted with them. External change agents must thoroughly evaluate the relevant people and processes of the organization. Moreover,

Table 22.3. Advantages and disadvantages of internal and external change agents

	Internal Change Agent	External Change Agent
Advantages	1. Knows the environment, culture, people, issues and hidden agendas 2. Develops and keeps expertise and resources internal 3. Creates and maintains norms of organization renewal from within 4. Provides higher security and confidentiality 5. May have trust and respect of others 6. Has strong personal investment in success	1. Provides fresh, outside, objective perspective 2. Willing to assert, challenge, and question norms 3. May have more legitimacy to insiders by not taking sides 4. Brings skills and techniques not available from within organization 5. Brings diverse organizational experiences to bear; benchmark comparisons
Disadvantages	1. May be biased; has already taken sides, or may be disliked or mistrusted by some stakeholders 2. Previous relationships may contribute to subgrouping or fragmentation 3. Takes CA away from other duties 4. May be enculturated and is "part of the problem" or does not see it 5. Is subject to organizational sanctions and pressures as an employee	1. May or may not be available when needed by the organization; may split time and commitments with other clients. 2. High expense 3. Takes time to become familiar with the system 4. May create codependency or may abandon the system.

Source: Weick and Quinn 1995.

external agents can be expensive, charging tens to hundreds of thousands of dollars for their consultation. For example, in one hospital system, a consulting group contracted over four years to implement a balanced scorecard system for the fee of about $2.3 million. Finally, a highly charismatic, directive, and successful agent could foster dependency with a client organization, leaving the organization reluctant to learn to manage its own change processes.

Internal versus External Change Agents

When an organization plans to use internal or external change agents, it should consider several questions, including:

- How confidential and proprietary is the information involved? Would either type of agent present a disclosure risk?
- Are there conflicts of interest? Is the external agent working with any competitor or internal agent loyal to conflicting parties?
- What level of commitment and availability is required? What is the potential effect of an external agent with many other clients or an internal agent with other work obligations?
- What skills are required for a successful change effort? What constellation of experience and skills do the external and internal agents offer?
- How important is it that stakeholders view the agent as being objective, fair, and neutral? Which type of agent would best be viewed this way? Explain your answer.
- To what extent does the culture of the organization require changing? Which type of agent is better positioned to influence the change?

Stages of OD

The work of change agents is captured in the seven stages of OD (Kolb and Frohman 1970):

1. *Scouting stage:* The change agent inquires and observes to determine how receptive the organization is, where the leverage points for change are located, and what the fit is between his or her skills and the system's requirements.
2. *Entry and contracting stage:* The working relationship between the change agent and key organizational members is built, expectations are set, roles are clarified, credibility is established, and resources and constraints are identified.
3. *Diagnosis, or data-gathering and feedback, stage:* This stage is one of the central features of OD. Rather than using the so-called medical model in which an expert makes the diagnosis and delivers it to the patient, the OD practitioner obtains data from the organization and involves the organization in interpreting the data and considering their implications.

4. *Planning stage:* The system moves toward a conclusion about the information. Responsibility is shifted from the change agent to the organization, which commits to the change and often formulates policy regarding it.
5. *Implementation stage:* The plan is carried out as designed and agreed to, with the change agent available for further consultation as needed.
6. *Evaluation stage:* This stage involves selecting appropriate measurements, monitoring the change process and its outcomes, and keeping people informed.
7. *Termination stage:* The change agent meets with key organizational members to review the change process, to determine what and how they have learned from the experience, and to end the consulting relationship.

Methods of OD

OD methods are quite varied and have grown out of extensive research and innovation in the behavioral sciences. Cummings and Huse (1989) identified more than 20 different techniques that practitioners use to promote change, and new ones are emerging regularly. Popular examples are discussed in the subsections below.

Survey Feedback
Survey feedback is widely used, especially during the diagnostic stage when questionnaires are used to identify attitudes and values about aspects of the change process. The results of the survey are presented to decision makers as feedback, with the intention that any discrepancies between what they believe and what is actually occurring in the organization will prompt corrective action.

Team Building
Team building involves identifying performance goals and then building cohesion by involving members in activities that enhance acquaintance, resolve conflicts, build healthy group norms, and build skills in reflecting on team processes to continue performance improvement.

Appreciative Inquiry
Appreciative inquiry is based on the belief that whatever is needed in organizational renewal already exists somewhere in the organization. It seeks to identify where the change already works and how it can be amplified and transferred elsewhere in the organization.

Learning History
Learning history is the extensive and relatively long-term process of eliciting stories, experiences, and critical events in the life of the organization and its employees. These are collated into themes that reflect the values and processes of the organization that can be discussed by organization members. (See figure 22.14, p. 640.)

Figure 22.14. Learning history

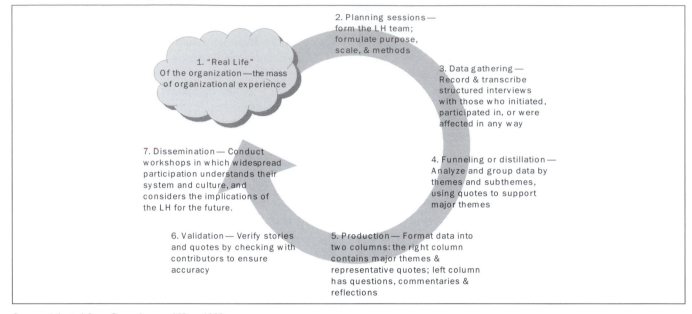

1. "Real Life"
Of the organization—the mass of organizational experience

2. Planning sessions—form the LH team; formulate purpose, scale, & methods

3. Data gathering—Record & transcribe structured interviews with those who initiated, participated in, or were affected in any way

4. Funneling or distillation—Analyze and group data by themes and subthemes, using quotes to support major themes

5. Production—Format data into two columns: the right column contains major themes & representative quotes; left column has questions, commentaries & reflections

6. Validation—Verify stories and quotes by checking with contributors to ensure accuracy

7. Dissemination—Conduct workshops in which widespread participation understands their system and culture, and considers the implications of the LH for the future.

Source: Adapted from Cummings and Huse 1989.

Organizational Lifeline

Organizational lifeline is a graphic time line with annual demarcations that show important events in the life of the organization over the years. It can be used to assist new employees in understanding how the organization has arrived where it is and to identify issues and change themes that are recurrent.

Stages of Change

People and organizations move through stages of change, and as they do, they have different needs and require different skills from the leader.

Lewin's Stages of Change

One of the first models of change was proposed by Kurt Lewin (1951), one of the early behavioral scientists who contributed to the knowledge base of information on group work, leadership, and organization development.

Lewin's model, or **Lewin's stages of change,** identified the initial stage of change as **unfreezing** the status quo, often by presenting the discrepancies between the status quo and the desired goals. Unfreezing often creates a state of cognitive dissonance, which is an uncomfortable awareness of two incompatible perceptions or beliefs, in this case, the discrepancy.

This motivates the person to resolve the dissonance, usually by changing the situation to make the perceptions congruent. This step marks the second stage of change or moving to the new desired state for the organization.

In the final stage of **refreezing,** the new behaviors are reinforced to become as stable and institutionalized as the

previous status quo was. Lewin originally conceptualized this three-stage process as one in which the organization would plateau and stabilize for a time before the next change was required. More recent beliefs about organizational change characterize the change process as continuous with little respite for workers, managers, or leaders. The status quo has become one of dealing with continual change, which can be stressful.

Stages of Grieving

Elizabeth Kubler-Ross (1969) examined the stress of change in her classic study of the **stages of grief** experienced by terminally ill patients and their families. Change in the healthcare system often involves mergers, acquisitions, downsizing, and other transitions that usually involve losses and grief. Her five-stage model has become useful in anticipating and working with people in a dramatic transition (Rogers 2000). The five stages of her model are (figure 22.15):

Figure 22.15. Kubler-Ross's stages of grief

Normal Level of Performance

1. Shock & denial
2. Anger & resentment
3. Bargaining & negotiation
4. Depression & despair
5. Acceptance & reorientation

Source: Adapted from Kubler-Ross 1969.

1. In the *shock and denial stage,* workers have difficulty believing the proposed transition. They may deny that change is imminent and go about business as usual rather than prepare for the adjustment. News of the change also may stun workers to the extent that they cannot concentrate or work efficiently, and they may isolate themselves.

2. In the *anger stage,* workers begin to understand the inevitability of the change. They may direct their resentment at the organization or the managers for allowing it to happen. In addition, they may engage in unproductive complaining, organize resistance, or even sabotage operations in attempts to reduce the threat.

3. In the *bargaining stage,* workers make a final attempt to avoid the change. They may actually try to bargain with managers to delay the change or work intensively to prove their value and reduce the risk of loss.

4. In the *depression stage,* workers may lose their self-esteem and be unresponsive to encouragement.

5. In the *acceptance stage,* workers begin to redirect their energy toward the new organization.

Resistance to Change

Kurt Lewin is credited with saying, "If you wish to understand something, try changing it." What he was referring to was the observation that when one attempts to change a system, the mechanisms that maintain it spring to its defense. Change does not come easily to most people, and in organizations, "resistance to change is experienced at almost every step" (DeWine 1994, p. 281). The first step for leaders who are trying to reduce resistance to change is to understand its source.

Resistance to change occurs for a number of reasons, including self-interest and anxiety about the unknown, different perceptions, suspiciousness, and conservatism. When confronted with change, the first thing most workers want to know is how it will affect them and their jobs. Because the turbulence of the marketplace makes many changes uncertain, workers may not receive satisfactory answers to their questions. Those who have attained expertise and status from their positions now may face new job descriptions or expanded or new duties. For example, many managers in downsized organizations have been reassigned as coaches to newly formed teams. This new role raises questions about their authority, status, and responsibility.

Other workers may resist change simply because they perceive the situation differently and believe the proposed change is unjustified. The result of ongoing change is to make many people uneasy about, and even mistrustful of, any innovation. Some people view all change as just another fad based on the whim of management rather than a survival strategy for the organization. And finally, some people are very conservative in their beliefs, are isolated in their social networks and information, and dislike the inconvenience of change.

Resistance can distract workers from their tasks, preoccupy them with gossiping, and contribute to stress and workplace violence. To confident change leaders, indications of resistance can be viewed as useful information about what stakeholders need before the transition can continue.

Facilitation of Change

The purpose of transition management is to make the potential upheaval and chaos posed by planned changed less disruptive to the people and processes of healthcare. It might be helpful to think of a transition as a series of stages through which people move as they adjust to changes. Each stage has its own set of challenges and tasks to master, the successful completion of which forms the foundation for moving on to the next stage. The role of managers and leaders is to facilitate the movement from stage to stage.

Bridges's Stages of Facilitation

In recognition of the stresses that change imposes on the organization's employees, Bridges (1980) extended Lewin's three-stage model with recommendations for transition management to ease the struggle. The stages of his model are as follows:

1. The transition process begins with the recognition that the old way of doing things is **ending.** Workers begin to anticipate and experience losses with resulting grief, blame, shock, and fear. They need help in letting go of the way things were. The organization can facilitate the transition by providing reasons for the ending and by indicating what will not change. It is usually best to overcommunicate to ensure that everyone has sufficient information about ongoing developments. Acknowledging losses and accepting grieving also can assist people in the ending stage.

2. The second stage, the **neutral zone,** begins when the old system has been left behind, but the new one has not yet been fully accepted. This stage fosters anxiety, uncertainty, and confusion. The organization can facilitate the transition by providing support, encouragement, protection, reassurance, and protection. The employees need to know where they are and where they are going. One creative approach to gaining acceptance of the transition is to have employees generate innovative ideas about how they can move toward the new organization.

3. In the third stage, **new beginnings,** people accept, orient themselves, and engage in the new organization. New goals are created to provide direction, and the workers' relationships with the organization and their jobs are reinvented and integrated. Attitudes and behaviors that support the new beginning are

supported by workers and role-modeled by leaders. Retraining, performance feedback and recognition of new behavior serve to reinforce the transition.

Importance of Reflection

Reflection is the process of examining one's experience. It is an essential skill for developing leadership skills and an important component of team and organization development. However, reflection alone is not sufficient for changing behavior. Reflection involves awareness. Reflective learning, on the other hand, uses awareness to formulate an interpretation of what has been observed, considers what difference can be made by applying what has been learned, and executes the efforts toward change through deliberate action.

Several remarkably similar models of the **reflective learning cycle** have been developed over the years, including those by John Dewey (1938), David Kolb (1970), W. Edwards Deming (1986), and Donald Schon (1983). These models share the following four stages in common (figure 22.16):

1. *Doing:* At this stage, people are concentrating and working directly on a task. Although most people reflect on a task after it is accomplished, this is often too late to make midcourse or more frequent changes. The reflective process should be used often, although too much reflection sometimes is used to avoid task completion.
2. *Reflection:* At this stage, the task is paused and the individual or team members reflect on how they have been working. What do they notice? The raw data become information as reflection progresses to the interpretation stage.
3. *Interpretation:* At this stage, one considers what the information means, what it reflects about the work process, and how various observations might be related.
4. *Application:* The application stage follows as information becomes knowledge and is applied to the work by doing something differently. Finally, the new knowledge is used to return to the action stage.

Figure 22.16.   Reflective learning process

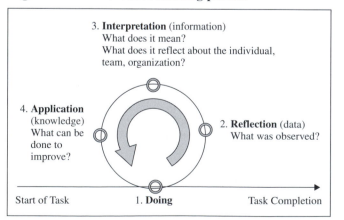

As the marketplace continues to change, organizations will have to adapt in order to maintain their competitive advantage. Organizational leaders play a key role in helping employees to reduce their resistance to change and to inspire and motivate them to accept it. By understanding leadership theories and the stages and techniques of planned change, and by using the reflective learning cycle, managers will be better prepared to meet the challenge.

Check Your Understanding 22.3

Instructions: Answer the following questions on a separate piece of paper.

1. If you were an OD consultant, what would you tell an executive team about a pending reorganization? What should the executive team expect?

2. If you were informed that your job was being eliminated due to reorganization, but that you could reapply for a new position, how would you react? What would you need to cope with the stress?

3. Make a list of reasons that people resist change. For each reason, suggest a way to reduce resistance.

4. Use the reflecting learning process to examine a group meeting. What did you notice? What do you think your observations reflected about the group processes? What might you do differently to improve the next meeting?

Real-World Case

Several reports in recent years from the Institute of Medicine have highlighted the need for new initiatives to improve patient safety, quality of care, and enhanced efficiency of the process of caring for patients. Specifically, the IOM recommended that new strategies be developed for educating health professionals. Supporting this, a survey of health care organizations in Minnesota revealed that three-quarters of respondents believed that having competence in using health information technologies would be "very to extremely important" for healthcare professionals by 2007–2012, and 70 percent had plans to implement computer-based documentation by 2007. Driven by these needs, the College of St. Scholastica in Duluth, Minnesota, proposed the Advancing Technology and Healthcare Education Now at St. Scholastica (ATHENS) initiative. The challenge is to provide students in health information management, nursing, physical therapy, occupational therapy, exercise physiology, and social work with the education necessary to competently use computer-based health information software applications and apply these tools to enhance their respective professions.

There is growing evidence that poor communication among professionals in different disciplines is a common source of medical errors. The new health professions' curriculum evolving from the ATHENS initiative will enable students to collaborate across disciplines using the electronic health record as a real-time, shared communication medium. Students will use software applications that are embedded with decision rules and alerts and evidence-based practice references, enabling more efficient and accurate clinical documentation, care planning, and results reporting, and creating a clinical data repository that integrates patient/client data from all sources for shared problem solving and decision making. This kind of professional development effort will reduce the communication barriers and challenges to transition management currently faced by most healthcare facilities (Athens Project 2005).

Summary

More recent theories have emphasized the complexity of modern organizations. Senge's emphasis on systems theory, for example, helps managers understand how the organization's components are connected much as a living system and that change in one component can affect other components.

Change management requires strong leadership. Managers traditionally maintain a highly efficient workplace and establish procedures; leaders look to the future and promote change. Both solve problems and make decisions. Recurrent problems lend themselves to clear rules for programmed decisions that can be used routinely; unique, complex, or changing situations require careful thought when nonprogrammed decisions are made. Formal decision making progresses through several stages, including problem definition, problem analysis, generation of alternatives, selection of alternatives, plan implementation, and evaluation and feedback. In practice, managers more often use intuition or satisficing. Groupthink can produce riskier decisions and requires review of team norms periodically as well as implementation of countermeasures. Clear communication with consideration of all stakeholders can further reduce distortion and error.

Leadership theories provide a way to examine what is required in a situation to facilitate change through people. Classical approaches to leadership emphasized collections of traits that became unwieldy in practice. However, as society embraced democratic ideals, management began to reflect greater worker participation and involvement in decision making. Vroom and Yetton's normative model of decision making enables managers to decide when to make a decision alone and when to delegate. Studies from Ohio State University, The University of Michigan, and Blake and Mouton have enabled leadership styles to be described along a continuum of task and social dimensions. Building on the need for leaders to adjust their styles to meet the unique characteristics of each situation, more recent models have emerged, including Fiedler's leadership contingency model, work done by Hersey and Blanchard, path–goal theory, leader–member exchange, and servant leadership. Some theories appear first as fads, although even fads can increase organizational awareness of important processes.

Change goes through different stages in an organization, and each stage has its own group of stakeholders. Plotting actual change results in an S-shaped curve with a slow start, rapid development, and a plateau of saturation and adoption. Within the organization, innovations require the key roles of inventor, champion, sponsor, and critic. The change agent spearheads the organization's change efforts, though there are advantages and disadvantages to internal and external change agent roles.

A variety of tools and techniques for helping organizations change has been developed. Surveys, team-building activities, appreciative inquiry, and learning history are examples of structured approaches to helping organizations examine how they deal with change. Understanding the stages of change also can relieve resistance to change. The stages of change often parallel the stages of grief identified by Kubler-Ross in her classic study. Similarly, the stages of organizational change can be thought of as an end to the old ways, a neutral time of transition, and new beginnings.

References

Aldag, R. 1997 (March). Moving sofas and exhuming woodchuck. On relevance, impact and the following of fads. *Journal of Management Inquiry* 6(1):8–16.

Allen, T. J., and S. I. Cohen. 1969. Information flow in two R&D laboratories. *Administrative Science Quarterly* 14(1):12–19.

Allport, G. W., and H. S. Odbert. 1936. Trait-names: A psycho-lexical study. *Psychological Monographs* (47):171–220.

American Society for Training and Development. 1998. National HRD executive survey: leadership development, first quarter survey report. Available online from astd.org.

Andersson, D. 1999. Avoiding the new executive failure trap. *Channel* 12(4). Available online from dom.semi.org/web/wchannel.nsf/0/6c527687b377f64b88256792007dd5ca?OpenDocument.

Argyris, C. 1957. *Personality and Organization.* New York: Harper & Row.

Argyris, C., and D. Schon, 1996. *Organizational Learning II: Theory, Method & Practice.* Reading, MA: Addison Wesley.

Armstrong, R.V. (n.d.). FAQs about team-based organizations. Available online from rvarmstrong.com/TBOFAQs.htm.

Athens Project. 2005. Advancing Technology and Healthcare Education Now at St. Scholastica. Available online from css.edu/programs/athens.

Ballard, A. 2005 (February 1). CEO boot camp to focus on early landmines to survive and thrive in new positions. Korn/Ferry International press release. Available online from kornferry.com/Library/Process.asp?P=PR_Detail&CID=914&LID=1.

Bass, B.M. 1985. *Leadership and Performance beyond Expectations.* New York: Free Press.

Bass, B., and B.J. Avolio. 1994. Shatter the glass ceiling: Women may make better managers. *Human Resource Management* 33:549–60.

Bass, B.M., and B.J. Avolio. 1993. Transformational leadership: A response to critics. In *Leadership Theory and Research: Perspectives and Directions,* edited by M.M. Chemers and R. Ayman. San Diego: Academic Press.

Beckhard, R. 1969. *Organization Development: Strategies and Models.* Reading, MA: Addison Wesley.

Bennet 1991 (June 6). Management: Downsizing does not necessarily bring an upswing in corporate profitability. *The Wall Street Journal.*

Bennis, W. 1959. Leadership theory and administrative behavior: The problem of authority. *Administrative Science Quarterly* 4:259–301.

Bennis, W., and B. Nanus. 1985. *Leaders: The Strategy for Taking Charge.* New York: Harper & Row.

Berk, B. 2003 (September). Bringing up the middle. *Healthleaders Magazine.* Available online from healthleaders.com/magazine/feature1.php?contentid'42127.

Birnbaum, R. 2000. The life cycle of academic management fads. *Journal of Higher Education* 71(1):1–16.

Blake, R.R., and J.S. Mouton. 1976. *Consultation.* Reading, MA: Addison Wesley.

Blodgett, M. 1999. Teaching Johnny to lead. *CIO Magazine.* Available online from cio.com.

Bridges, W. 1980. *Transitions: Making Sense of Life's Changes.* Reading, MA: Addison Wesley.

Buckingham, M., and C. Coffman. 1999. *First, Break All the Rules: What the World's Greatest Managers Do Differently.* New York: Simon & Schuster.

Burke, W.W., E.A. Richley, and L. DeAngelis. 1985. Changing leadership and planning processes at the Lewis Research Center, National Aeronautics and Space Administration. *Human Resources Management* 24(1):81–90.

Burkholder, N. 2003 (November). The real cost of turnover. Available online from staffing.org/updates/archive11062003.asp.

Burns, J.M. 1978. *Leadership.* New York: Free Press.

Business Source Premier. 1950–2004. Proprietary database available to scholarly libraries containing articles from scholarly and trade business journals on companies, industries, products, management, marketing, accounting, real estate, finance, insurance, business law, and technology.

Byrne, J. 1997 (June 23). Management theory: Of fashion of the month? *Business Week* 47.

Cameron, K.S., S.J. Freeman, and A.K. Mishra. 1993. Downsizing and redesigning organizations. In *Organizational Change and Redesign,* edited by G.P. Huber and W.H. Glick, pp. 19–63. New York: Oxford University Press.

CEOGO. 2003. CEO reputation study 2003. Burson-Marsteller. Available online from ceogo.com/.

Charan, R., and G. Colvin. 1999 (Jule 21). Why CEOs fail. *Fortune,* 69.

Chaulk, D., and R. W. Sexty. 2002. The management fad lifecycle phenomenon. Canadian evidence. Administrative Sciences Association of Canada/IFSAM Conference, Winnipeg, Manitoba.

Clark, J., and R. Koonce. 1995. Engaging organizational survivors. *Training and Development* 49(8):232–30.

Cole, R.E. 1999. *Managing Quality Fads: How American Business Learned to Play the Quality Game.* New York: Oxford Press.

Cummings, T.G., and E.F. Huse. 1989. *Organization Development and Change.* New York: West.

Daft, R.L. 2000. *Management.* Fort Worth, TX: Dryden.

Daft, R.L., and D. Marcic. 1998. *Understanding Management.* Fort Worth, TX: Dryden.

Dangerfield, B.C. 1999. Health systems model: UK cases. *Journal of the Operational Research Society* 50(4):345–53.

Dansereau, F., G. Graen, and W. Haga. 1975. A vertical dyad linkage approach to leadership within formal organizations: A longitudinal investigation of the role-making process. *Organizational Behavior and Human Performance* 13:46–78.

de Geus, A. 1997. *The Living Company.* London: Nicholas Brealey Publishing.

Deming, W.E. 1986. *Out of the Crisis.* Cambridge: Massachusetts Institute of Technology, Center for Advanced Engineering Study.

DeVries, D.L. 1992. Executive selection: advances but no progress. *Issues and Observations* 12:1–5.

Dewey, J. 1938. *Experience and Education.* New York: Collier.

DeWine, S. 1994. *The Consultant's Craft: Improving Organizational Communication.* New York: St. Martin's Press.

Duarte, N.T., J.R. Goodson, and N.R. Klitch. 1993. How do I like thee? Let me appraise the ways. *Journal of Organizational Behavior* 14:239–49.

Dunn, M.W. 1999 (November). The impact of leadership on employees' commitment to the organization: An international perspective. PhD dissertation, Nova Southeastern University.

Eagly, A.H., and L.L. Carly. 2003. The female leadership advantage: An evaluation of the evidence. *Leadership Quarterly* 14(6):807–35.

Fiedler, F.E. 1967. *A Theory of Leadership Effectiveness.* New York: McGraw-Hill.

Gering, J., and J. Connor. 2002 (November). A strategic approach to employee retention. *Healthcare Financial Management,* 40–44.

Graen, G., and T.A. Skandura. 1987. Toward a psychology of dyadic organizing. *Research in Organizational Behavior* 9:175–209.

Greenleaf, R.J. 1991. *Servant Leadership.* Mahwah, NJ: Paulist Press.

Hale, B. 2002. Kenneth Lay: A fallen hero. BBC News. Available online from news.bbc.co.uk.

Harris, B. 1982 (July). The man who killed Braniff. *Texas Monthly,* 116–20, 183–89.

Hay Group. 1999. New Fortune/Hay Group ranking of The world's most admired companies. Press release.

Henkoff, R. 1990. Cost cutting: How to do it right. *Fortune* 121(8):26–33.

Hersey, P., K.H. Blanchard, and D.E. Johnson. 1996. *Management of Organizational Behavior: Utilizing Human Resources,* 7th ed. Upper Saddle River, NJ: Prentice-Hall.

Hickman, C.R. 1990. *Mind of a Manager, Soul of a Leader.* New York: John Wiley & Sons.

Hogan, R., R. Raskin, and D. Fazzini. 1990. The dark side of charisma. In *Measures of Leadership,* edited by K.E. Clark and M.E. Clark, pp. 343–54. West Orange, NJ: Leadership Library of America.

House, R.J. 1971. A path-goal theory of leader effectiveness. *Administrative Science Leadership Review Quarterly* 16:321–39.

Hoyt, C. 2002 (fall). Women leaders: The role of stereotype activation and leadership self-efficacy. Kravis Institute *Leadership Review.* Available online from leadershipreview.org/2002fall/article2_fall_2002.asp

Hunter, J.C. 2004. *The World's Most Powerful Leadership Principle: How to Become a Servant Leader.* New York: Random House.

Hymowitz, C., and T. Schellhardt. 1986 (March 24). The glass ceiling: Why women can't seem to break the invisible barrier that blocks them from the top jobs. Special report: The corporate woman, cover article. *The Wall Street Journal.*

Jahna, S. R. 2002. Failure: The dreaded word in the CEOs' lexicon. *The CEO Refresher.* Available online from refresher.com/!jahnasr.html.

Kabacoff, R. 1998. Gender differences in organizational leadership: A large sample study. Paper presented at the 106th annual convention of the American Psychological Association, San Francisco.

Kaplan, R.S. 2002. Building strategy focused organizations with the balanced scorecard. Available online from www-ddc.moph.go.th/module/webadmin/download_module/pdf/Kaplan_BSC.pdf.

Kidder, R. M. 2000 (October). Want a loyal workforce? Build an ethical corporation. *Ethics Newsline*. Available online from globalethics.org/newsline/members/issue.tmpl?articleid=10090003003140.

Klein, K.J., and R.J. House. 1995. On fire: Charismatic leadership and levels of analysis. *Leadership Quarterly* 6(2):183–98.

Kolb, J.A. 1999. The effect of gender role, attitude toward leadership, and self-confidence on leader emergence: Implications for leadership development. *Human Resource Development Quarterly* 10(4):305–11.

Kolb, D.A., and A.L. Frohman. 1970. An organization development approach to consulting. *Sloan Management Review* 12(1):51–65.

Korabik, K. 1990. Androgyny and leadership style. *Journal of Business Ethics* 9:283–92.

Kotter, J.P. 1990. *A Force for Change: How Leadership Differs from Management*. New York: Free Press.

Kouzes, J., and B. Posner. 1989. *The Leadership Challenge: How to Get Extraordinary Things Done in Organizations*. San Francisco: Jossey-Bass.

Kubler-Ross, E. 1969. *On Death and Dying*. New York: Simon & Schuster/Touchstone.

Lee, James. 1982. *The Gold and Garbage in Management Theories and Prescriptions*. Athens: Ohio University Press.

Lesly, E. 1992 (September). Goodbye Mr. Dithers (Abusive bosses). *Business Week* 52.

Levering, R., M. Moskowitz, and M. Katz. 2000. *100 Best Companies to Work for in America*. Reading, MA: Addison Wesley.

Lewin, K. (1951). Field theory in social science. New York: Harper and Brothers.

Lieberson, S., and J.F. O'Connor. 1972. Leadership and organizational performance: A study of large corporations. *American Sociological Review* 37:117–30.

Likert, R. 1979. From production- and employee-centeredness to systems 1–4. *Journal of Management* (5):628–41.

Marash, S.A., P. Berman, and M. Flynn. 2003. *Fusion Management: Harnessing the Power of Six Sigma, Lean, ISO9001: 2000, Malcolm Baldrige, TQM and Other Quality Breakthroughs of the Past Century*. Fairfax, VA: QSU Publishing.

McCormick, M. J., J. Tanguma, and A. S. Lopez-Forment. 2003 (spring). Gender differences in beliefs about leadership capabilities: Exploring the glass ceiling phenomenon with self-efficacy theory. Kravis Institute *Leadership Review*. Available online from leadershipreview.org/2003spring/article2_spring_2003.asp.

McNeese-Smith, D.K. 1997. The influence of manager behavior on nurses' job satisfaction, productivity, and commitment. *Journal of Nursing Administration* 27(9):47–55.

Megargee, E.I. 1969. Influence of sex roles on the manifestation of leadership. *Journal of Applied Psychology* 53:377–82.

Miller, D. 1990. *The Icarus Paradox: How Exceptional Companies Bring about Their Own Downfall: New Lessons in the Dynamics of Corporate Success, Decline, and Renewal*. New York: Harper Business.

Miller, D., and P.H. Friesen. 1984. A longitudinal study of the corporate life cycle. *Management Science,* 1161–83.

Milliken-Davies, M. 1992. An exploration of flawed first-line supervision. PhD dissertation, University of Tulsa.

Peter, L.J., and R. Hull. 1969. *The Peter Principle: Why Things Always Go Wrong*. New York: William Morrow & Company.

Peters, T. 2001 (December). Tom Peters's true confessions. *Fast Company* 53:78.

Peters, T.J., and R.H. Waterman. 1982. *In Search of Excellence: Lessons from America's Best-Run Companies*. New York City: Harper & Row.

Pettigrew, A. 1999. Report warns companies to avoid quick fixes and management fads. University of Warwick press release. Available online from warwick.ac.uk/news/pr/business/126.

Pratt, D. 2000 (Sept. 14). Adaptation is key in the digital economy. *Barnstable Patriot*. Available online from barnstable-patriot.com/news_september_adaptation_is_key_in_the_digital_economy_archives_48_514.html.

Price-Waterhouse v. Ann B. Hopkins. 1987. Supreme Court of the United States. No. 87-1167. Available online from usdoj.gov/osg/briefs/1987/sg870104.txt.

Rigby, D. 1998 (September). What's today's special at the consultant's café? *Fortune* 138(5):76–77.

Rogers, K.A. 2000. Transition management as an intervention for survivor syndrome. *Canadian Journal of Leadership Nursing* 13(4).

Rogers, E. 1995. *Diffusion of Innovations,* 4th ed. New York: Free Press.

Rogers, E., and F.F. Shoemaker. 1971. *Communication of Innovations: A Cross-Cultural Approach*. New York: Free Press.

Salancik, G.R., and J. Pfeffer. 1977. Constraints on administrator discretion: The limited influence of mayors in city budgets. *Organizational Dynamics* 12(4):475–96.

Schon, D.A. 1983. *The Reflective Practitioner*. New York: Basic Books.

Senge, P. 1990. *The Fifth Discipline: The Art and Practice of the Learning Organization*. New York: Currency/Doubleday.

Shartle, C.L. 1979. Early years of the Ohio State University leadership studies. *Journal of Management* 5:126–34.

Shipper, F., and C.L. Wilson. 1991. The impact of managerial behaviors on group performance, stress, and commitment. Paper presented at the Research Conference on Leadership, Center for Creative Leadership, Colorado Springs.

Smith, J.L., K.P. Carson, and R. A. Alexander. 1984. Leadership: It can make a difference. *Academy of Management Journal* 27:765–76.

Spears, L. 1995. *Reflections on Leadership: How Robert K. Greenleaf's Theory of Servant Leadership Influenced Today's Top Management Thinkers*. New York: John Wiley & Sons.

Stogdill, R.M. 1974. *Handbook of Leadership: A Guide to Understanding Managerial Work*. Englewood Cliffs, NJ: Prentice-Hall.

Tannenbaum, T., and W. Schmidt. 1973 (May–June). How to choose a leadership pattern. *Harvard Business Review,* No. 73311. First published in 1958 (March–April) Harvard Business Review 36:95–101

Tomasco, R. 1987. *Downsizing: Reshaping the Corporation for the Future*. New York: AMACOM.

Tuckman, B.W. 1965. Developmental sequence in small groups. *Psychological Bulletin* 63:384–99.

Vaill, P.B. 1996. *Learning as a Way of Being*. San Francisco: Jossey-Bass.

Vroom, V., and P. Jago. 1988. *The New Leadership? Managing Participation in Organizations*. Englewood Cliffs, NJ: Prentice-Hall.

Vroom, V., and P. Yetton. 1971. *Leadership and Decision Making*. Pittsburgh: University of Pittsburgh Press.

Waldman, J.D., F. Kelly, S. Arora, and H.L. Smith. 2004 (January–March). The shocking cost of turnover in healthcare. *Health Care Management Review* 29:2–7.

WalkerInformation. (2001a). Commitment in the workplace: The 2000 global employee relationship benchmark report. Walker Information

Global Network and Hudson Institute. Available online from askemployees.com/why/docs/global.pdf.

Wasson, C. 1978. *Dynamic Competitive Strategy and Product Life Cycles.* Austin, TX: Austin Press.

Weick, K.E., and R.E. Quinn. 1995. Organizational change and development. *Annual Review of Psychology* 50:361–86.

Weiner, N., and T.A. Mahoney. 1981. A model of corporate performance as a function of environment, organization, and leadership influences. *Academy of Management Journal* 24:453–70.

White, R.K., and R. Lippitt. 1960. *Autocracy and Democracy: An Experimental Inquiry.* New York: Harper.

Yukl, G. 1998. *Leadership in Organizations.* Upper Saddle River, NJ: Prentice-Hall.

Zaleznik, A. 1977 (May–June). Managers and leaders: Are they different? *Harvard Business Review* 55:68–78.

Chapter 23
Work Design and Performance Improvement

Madonna LeBlanc, MA, RHIA

Learning Objectives

- To explain how standards can be applied to each of the resources of management and to identify alternative ways in which they can be communicated
- To identify the criteria for effective standard setting
- To explain the purpose and function of work measurement and work measurement techniques and to assess the strengths and weaknesses of each as a management tool
- To express production (quantitative) standards in terms of time/unit and units/time and to calculate quantitative standards using data obtained via various methodologies
- To identify the steps involved in a work-sampling effort and the tools that can be used with certain steps
- To determine sample size for a work-sampling effort by using the precision interval method and by a formula involving various scenarios of desired certainty factor and acceptable error in the study results
- To identify potential areas for improvement in the health information services (HIS) functions given data obtained through work measurement activities and appropriate benchmarks
- To develop production standards for HIS functions
- To forecast staffing requirements for HIS functions on the basis of predicted work volume increases/decreases

- To distinguish between quantitative and qualitative standards and to identify examples of each for HIS functions
- To write effective quantitative and qualitative performance standards
- To identify common symptoms of process problems, generally and specific to HIS
- To differentiate among the terms *effectiveness, efficiency,* and *adaptability* as goals of process improvement
- To describe the components of a system and how they are related
- To summarize the steps of the systems analysis and design process
- To describe the tools that can be used to assist managers in determining the efficiency of work flow and the distribution of work responsibilities in a work unit
- To discuss the principles incorporated in the philosophy of continuous quality improvement (CQI)
- To explain the purposes of the various CQI tools and techniques
- To discuss the similarities and differences among systems analysis and design, CQI, and reengineering

Key Terms

Affinity grouping
Benchmarking
Brainstorming
Check sheet
Common cause variation
Certainty factor
Closed systems
Compressed workweek
Continuous data
Continuous quality improvement (CQI)
Cybernetic systems
Cyclical staffing
Ergonomics
Fishbone diagram
Flextime
Float employee

Flow process chart
Flowchart
Force-field analysis
Full-time equivalent (FTE)
Goal
Histogram
Job procedure
Job sharing
Key indicator
Movement diagram
Multivoting technique
Nominal group technique
Objective
Open systems
Parallel work division
Pareto chart
Part-time employee

PDSA Cycle
Performance measurement
Precision factor
Productivity
Qualitative standards
Quantitative standards
Reengineering
Run chart
Scatter diagram
Serial work division
Service
Shift differential
Shift rotation
Six Sigma
Special cause variation
Standard

Statistical process control chart
System
Systems analysis and design
Systems thinking
Telecommuting
Time ladder
Unit work division
Volume logs
Work distribution analysis
Work distribution chart
Work division
Work flow
Work measurement
Work sampling

Introduction

Management has been defined as getting work done through and with people. It may be thought of as both a science and an art. Management is a science because it is based on theory and principles that have been—and continue to be—tested and explored. It is an art because effective management depends on the use of sound judgment, intuition, and communication and interpersonal skills. Managers engage in specific functions, including planning, organizing, directing, and controlling. These functions enable work processes to flow smoothly. It is the manager's responsibility to create and facilitate effective work processes so that the desired outcome can be achieved in a cost-efficient manner.

Management of human resources is one of the most challenging and critical functions in healthcare organizations. Whether as a lead staffperson, a supervisor, an assistant director, or a health information management (HIM) department director, the key to success lies in the practitioner's people and performance management skills. Performance management does not occur by accident or by osmosis. Careful consideration of the resources available and their organization is key to the effectiveness and efficiency of HIM departmental services, as is a well-designed set of tools and strategies to facilitate staff management.

Budgets need to be met, and variances in those budgets need to be addressed intelligently and swiftly. In order to respond to both service and fiscal demands, it is essential to have a plan of action, which includes staffing, **work division,** job procedures, ergonomic considerations, and performance or work measurement.

This chapter introduces key concepts, tools, and techniques associated with designing/redesigning and implementing effective and efficient work processes within an organization. It also discusses components of work processes and the development as well as the use of performance standards and various methodologies to achieve and sustain performance improvement.

Theory into Practice

Health information services in any healthcare setting is a complex array of task-oriented functions. It is a strongly customer **service**-driven department and needs to be in constant communication with its different customers.

Following is a pointed example of one department's ready response to customer concerns taken from "Using Benchmarking for Performance Improvement" by Gwen Hughes in the February 2003 issue of *Journal of the American Health Information Management Association:*

An HIM director at a large physician clinic has 21 transcriptionists who average about 140 lines per hour using conventional word processing software and cassette tapes. The transcription unit supports 80 physicians at a cost of 15 cents per line.

The HIM director contacts the Medical Group Management Association and, with its data, is able to determine that in similar settings

one transcriptionist generally supports four physicians. She knows transcription processes are not state of the art in her organization and wonders to what extent departmental performance might be improved by applying best practices.

First, she conducts a literature search of transcription best practices on the AHIMA and American Association for Medical Transcription Web sites. Then she searches AHIMA's Communities of Practice for best practice and transcription threads. She also talks to her peers on the local HIM association board and posts a discussion thread on the Ambulatory Care Community of Practice. She attends a national convention, visiting vendors and attending lectures on best practices and transcription technology.

She identifies 10 transcription departments of similar size and scope and interviews the HIM director or transcription manager at each, using an interview form she developed. She finds one department that is producing an average of 275 lines per transcriptionist per hour at a cost of 12 cents per line. During the interview, she finds out that this organization:
- has an incentive program
- uses software in which abbreviations typed onto the keyboard produce phrases and entire paragraphs
- uses templates that can be personalized for particular patients for routine procedures
- uses digital dictation from which to transcribe
- does not require transcriptionists to perform any clerical duties or cover for other HIM functions after hours
- has several telecommuting transcriptionists

On the basis of this information, the HIM director talks to her staff and decides to pursue abbreviation software, templates, and a digital dictation system. Once those technologies and processes are implemented, she intends to develop an incentive program and explore allowing transcriptionists to work from home. She presents the idea to administration, they accept the idea, and she obtains the necessary funding. As she implements each of these processes, the productivity of the transcription unit continues to increase. She provides administration with monthly progress reports and an annual cost-benefit analysis.

Health information managers can successfully address customer issues and performance variances by fully understanding the components of work processes and the application of performance/work measurements.

Methods of Work Division

Staffing involves the determination of which types of employees are needed, how many of each type are needed, and what kind of work schedule is needed. Employee selection depends on the skills, experience, and education required by the work. The number of employees needed depends on the volume of work and the pattern of work division that has been selected. Work scheduling is based on when employees are needed and/or what services are required.

Work Division Patterns

Any of a number of basic work division patterns can be followed in process-oriented departments. The type of pattern depends in large part on the type of work to be performed and the number of employees available to perform it. Three types of work division patterns are:

- *Serial work division:* The consecutive handling of tasks or products by individuals who perform a specific function in sequence. Often referred to as a production line-type of work division, serial work division tends to create task specialists. For example, three transcriptionists might be used to transcribe medical reports. A transcription clerk would support their work by performing functions such as sorting copies, answering telephones, and duplicating and disseminating the completed transcriptions. In this staffing model, the transcription clerk cannot perform his or her duties until the transcriptionists have completed their work.

- *Parallel work division:* The concurrent handling of tasks. Multiple employees do identical types of tasks and basically see the process through from beginning to end. In parallel work division, the transcription function might include four transcriptionists, each responsible for transcribing medical reports, sorting copies, answering telephones, and duplicating and disseminating the transcribed reports. Thus, all four transcriptionists would be expected to perform the same duties independent of the others.

- *Unit work division:* Simultaneous assembly in which everyone performs a different specialized task at the same time. The tasks are all related to the same end product but are not dependent on each other. The work is specialized, but the sequence of tasks is not fixed. Unit assembly is rarely referred to in HIS departments but is typical of manufacturing. Examples of unit assembly in an HIS department might include discharge record analysis and registry data abstracting. Both functions are vital to the completed medical record and may be performed by several individuals simultaneously, but independently.

Work Distribution Analysis

Work distribution analysis is a function of effective work process management and is one element of organizational analysis. It is used to determine whether a department's current work assignments and job content are appropriate. Making time to perform this analysis can lead to one or more of the following observations:

- Large amounts of time are being dedicated to functions of minor importance.
- Small amounts of time are being dedicated to functions of key importance.
- There is too much or too little job function specialization.
- There is duplication of efforts or functions.
- Some employees are overloaded with work assignments.
- Some employees do not have enough work to keep busy.
- Staff are performing tasks inappropriate to their positions.

Basic distribution data can be collected via a **work distribution chart,** which is filled out by each employee and includes all responsible task content. (See table 23.1.) Task content should come directly from the employee's current job description. In addition to task content, each employee tracks each task's start time, end time, and volume or **productivity** within a typical unit of a workweek.

Work Scheduling

After management has determined the equity of work distribution within a department and made adjustments accordingly, a work-scheduling system can be developed. Determining the work schedule for departmental staff involves more than simply assigning hours. Effective scheduling results in the following:

- A core of employees on duty at all times when services must be provided
- A pattern of hours (shifts) to be worked and days off that employees can be reasonably sure will not be changed except in extreme emergencies

Table 23.1. Work distribution chart

Position/ Employee	Supervisor/J. Johnson		Admissions Clerk/A. Jones		Discharge Clerk/B. Olson		File Clerk/R. Smith	
Activity	*Task*	*# of Hours*	*Task*	*# of Hours*	*Task*	*# of Hours*	*Task*	*# of Hours*
Release of information	Post requests; give depositions	2 10	Photocopy	8	Certify content	15	Retrieve records	10
Analysis	Chart IRS	2	File in MD box	3	Tag for incomplete	15	Collect charts	9
Filing	Audit file room	2	—	—	Pull for MDs	4	File and pull records	20
Administrative overhead	Attend meetings; supervise employees	12 10	Receive visitors; typing	14 14	Generate MD letters	5	—	—
Training	Read literature, etc.	2	Attend software training	1	Attend computer training	1	Attend computer training	1
Totals	40 hours/40 hours		40 hours/40 hours		40 hours/40 hours		40 hours/40 hours	

- Fair and just treatment of all employees with regard to hours assigned

Several staffing issues should be considered when devising an effective staff schedule. Answers to the following questions will help determine the department's course of action:

- How is the workweek defined by policy? The workweek is generally established to begin on Sunday, but organizational policy may dictate otherwise.
- What days of the week is the department open? How many and what hours/days are covered? When the coverage policy has been set, the number of personnel can be set.
- What functions must be performed each day and within what time frame?
- How many **full-time equivalents** (FTEs) are needed on the basis of the organization's definition of full-time? The Fair Labor Standard Act Wage and Hour Law defines the full-time standard as 40 hours per week, 80 hours per two-week period, or 8 hours per day. The act also defines the difference between exempt (management) and nonexempt (nonmanagement or hourly) employees.

HIS departments often are on a standard Monday through Friday, eight-hour-day pattern but also may need evening/weekend coverage to handle specific functions that must be provided 24 hours per day, seven days a week. Uninterrupted work stretches should be no less than two days and no more than seven days. In other words, avoid scheduling staff either every other day or for more than seven days in a row.

Shift Rotation and Shift Differential

Employee schedules may involve **shift rotations** and **shift differentials** when the department has more than the standard Monday through Friday, eight-to-five staffing needs. Rotation among morning, afternoon, and evening shifts is not the ideal scheduling situation but is often necessary when coverage is needed and personnel have not been specifically hired to work afternoons or evenings on a regular basis. Specific start and end times should be determined for every shift, and at least 12 hours should elapse between the time an individual ends one shift and begins another. Time spent on the more undesirable shifts should not exceed time spent on the preferred shift. For example, a schedule of two weeks of days, one week of afternoons, and one week of evenings is acceptable, but a schedule of one week of days, one week of afternoons, and two weeks of evenings can create problems. In this case, it would be prudent to adopt **cyclical staffing,** which is the rotation of work schedule for a group of employees to allow for a fair distribution of evening and/or weekend shifts for each person within the group. **Float employees,** staff that are cross-trained in a number of departmental functions, can often be utilized to enable this particular type of scheduling flow.

In situations where weekend coverage is an issue, employees should have at least alternate weekends off. Many employers pay a slightly higher hourly wage to employees who work less desirable shifts (evening, night, weekend). This is referred to as a shift differential.

Mandatory activities and the minimal staff needed to cover them should be defined when determining weekend or holiday coverage. All employees should participate in holiday/weekend rotation. Holiday rotations should be posted one year in advance and weekend rotations at least three months in advance. Employees should be required to provide their own holiday or weekend replacements but should not be responsible for providing replacements when their absence is due to illness.

Vacation and Absentee Coverage

To keep productivity optimal, the HIS department manager must plan appropriately for vacation staffing and absentee coverage. Temporary FTEs hired to cover for vacationing employees are most desirable, but not always feasible financially. Moreover, some positions are too complex to be filled with FTEs. For example, it is unlikely that a temporary assistant director could be hired to fill in for an assistant director on a two-week vacation.

When additional employees are unavailable, the department must determine which of the absent employees' tasks must be done and distribute the work among the available employees. A week or more of absent staff can add undue stress on the remaining employees and adversely affect department service levels; thus, it would be advisable to hire temporary help when more than one week of absence is expected.

Alternate Work Schedules

Another aspect of determining work schedules is that of considering alternatives to the regular workweek. Following are some examples:

- *Compressed workweek:* A compressed workweek is a week in which more hours are combined within fewer days (for example, four 10-hour days, three 12-hour days, seven 10-hour days with seven days off [seven on/seven off], and so on). This type of scheduling has advantages but may present child care issues and psychological/physical fatigue that could reduce efficiency and productivity.
- *Flextime (also called gliding time or bandwidth flextime):* On flextime, employees choose their arrival and departure times around a fixed core. For example, if management feels full coverage is essential between 10 a.m. and 2 p.m., employees could start as early as 5:30 a.m. or end as late as 6:30 p.m. and still provide the department with core coverage.
- *Job sharing:* Job sharing divides one job between two **part-time employees,** each with partial benefits (as they apply). In some organizations, the two employees

split full-time benefits (for example, one takes insurance coverage and one takes vacation time). Job sharing may work very well in some cases, but it also can be problematic depending on the compatibility of the two individuals involved. And should one person terminate employment, finding a compatible new job-sharing partner could present a challenge.

- *Telecommuting:* In this scenario, employees work full- or part-time in their own homes. The first employees in HIS departments to take advantage of telecommuting were transcriptionists; they were soon followed by at-home coders. These telecommuters use computers (often provided by the facility) at home to transcribe or code information and then transmit it electronically back to the HIS department. The advantages to this type of work scheduling are that it saves space in the department, reduces long commutes to the workplace, retains parents who prefer to be home in the workforce, and offers work opportunities to the physically challenged. On the other hand, employers may feel a loss of control when employees telecommute. And some employees in alternative work situations, such as telecommuters, need contact hours with other employees to avoid feeling disconnected from the department. (See chapter 23 for further discussion on managing telecommuters.)

In general, the benefits to employers of alternative work schedules include easier staff recruitment and better retention, increased morale, decreased absence and tardiness, and some productivity improvements. For employees, the benefits can include less home stress, reduced commuting time, and a perception of greater autonomy in the workplace.

Outsourcing
Competitive and regulatory forces are causing healthcare organizations to "right-size" with a focus on core functions and analyzing if they actually do what they exist to do. In addition, there is a move toward emphasizing performance improvement (PI) to ensure the quality of work being done and that the organization is getting the "biggest bang for its buck."

Right-sizing tactics include outsourcing, contracted services, and home-based services because they provide access to staff as needed, even in a tight labor market; free up internal resources for other things; get rid of some process and/or service "headaches"; provide access to newest technologies quickly; and accelerate change.

When healthcare organizations decide to use outsourcing or contracted services, a manager is challenged to select the most appropriate vendor to provide the services desired. Specific key factors to consider when selecting a vendor or partner include:

- Commitment to quality
- Price
- References/reputation
- Cultural match

- Flexible contract terms
- Value-added capability
- Existing relationship

What leads to success when adopting an outsourcing vendor or contracted service? Senior executive support is a requisite for achieving success in outsourcing. The administration's confidence in the process is essential to creating the seamlessness necessary for continued, smooth functional operation. Administrative support can best be engaged when the manager understands the organization's goals for each outsourcing or contracted service effort being planned. Selecting the right vendor also will be a defining variable for the relative success of the outsourcing plan. Good management of the relationship between the healthcare organization and the vendor includes properly constructed contracts, open communications among partners, and careful attention to personnel issues.

Contracting for Services
Knowing what you need and knowing what you want are imperative to the success of contracting services. Defining the scope of work and description of services as well as the deliverables or performance of services will clarify each party's expectations and responsibilities. Service-level agreements detail the actual functions and labors proposed to meet expectations. Price and payment terms must be very carefully considered and understood to avoid future misunderstandings. The relationship of the parties must be determined and specified in the contract to ensure that everyone involved understands the reporting chain of command.

In addition, terms for termination of the relationship must be specified in the contract. Confidentiality expectations of the vendor and its employees also are a critical consideration to ensure privacy and security of patient information viewed or created during the work process. Finally, the specifics of notifications of all kinds, such as notifications 60 days prior to termination, should be spelled out in the body of the contract.

When a manager is planning to contract for staffing in a transitional situation in order to meet organizational goals, various types of arrangements must be considered, including:

- *Full-service:* When a backlog is evidenced because of a newly assumed level of production, it may be necessary to engage a full complement of services to maintain productivity.
- *Project based:* When the scenario is simply above and beyond the ability or scope of current staffing, a project-based staff may serve the process until the particular project is completed.
- *Temporary:* When a backlog is a transient event, temporary staff can be the solution to bringing productivity back into line with the department's goals.
- *Permanent:* When a newly assumed level of productivity is needed due to, for example, the assumption of a new specialty group, a permanent level of staffing may be essential.

Management of Work Procedures

Staff must know the detailed specifics of a job or function in order to understand its full scope. Management's responsibility is to create a directive for employees that will fully aid them in carrying out the functions for which they were hired. One of the first steps is to determine the competencies necessary for each function and to address them in an instructional **job procedure.**

A job procedure is a structured, action-oriented list of sequential steps involved in carrying out a specific job or solving a problem.

Rules of Procedure Writing

To be effective, the writing of procedures requires considerable attention to detail. The following criteria facilitate the development of well-written procedures:

- Display the title accurately and clearly.
- Number each step of the procedure for ready reference.
- Begin each activity with an action verb.
- Keep sentences short and concise.
- Include only procedures, not policies. Policy manuals should be maintained as separate documents.
- Identify logical beginning and end points to simplify directions.
- Consider the audience and construct the procedure to be of most help. For example, new staff, temporary staff, or cross-trained staff who perform these procedures only occasionally need a basic, simplified version to ensure completion of a new or seldom-performed task.

In addition, the written procedure should provide completed ("filled in") samples of forms used during the procedure being documented.

It is considered best practice to have the individual who does the job write (or at least draft) the procedure because he or she knows it best. Supervisory personnel should collect all the written procedures and determine whether they are complete and follow a consistent format.

Procedure Formats

When determining the appropriate format for a procedure, the HIS manager needs to consider the audience as well as the complexity of the task. Several formats can be followed in documenting procedural documentation, including:

- *Narratives:* Narrative formats are the most common for procedure writing. The author details the processes of the procedure in a step-by-step description method.
- *Playscript:* This format describes each player, the action, and the player's responsibility regarding the process from start to completion of a specific task, function, or procedure.
- *Flowcharts:* Flowcharts use standard flowcharting symbols provided in software programs such as Power-Point™ and VISIO¨ to depict the steps associated with a procedure. Figure 23.1 shows an example of flowcharting applied in the HIS setting.

Sometimes a combination of narrative and flowchart formats is used. However, whatever format is chosen, all procedures should be available to employees at any time.

Procedure Manuals

A procedure manual is a compilation of all of the procedures used in a specific unit, department, or organization. Procedure manuals may be kept as hard copies that have been printed out and bound together in a book or binder, or they may be maintained on an organization's secure Web site or intranet. The functions of procedure manuals include:

- Promoting teamwork
- Promoting conformity
- Reducing training time
- Establishing guidance on standards
- Explaining what is expected of employees
- Answering employee questions

The manual's content and format are relatively straightforward. Procedure manuals should include the following elements:

- *Title page:* Name of the facility, name of the manual, name of the department, and date
- *Foreword:* Paragraph form, purpose of manual, suggestion for use by employees
- *Table of contents:* List of all procedures in the manual referenced to page number
- *Job instruction and execution:* Step-by-step procedures to be followed, including forms used in each procedure, preferably completed ones together with explanations
- *General rules and regulations:* Information that includes department- or unit-specific details often influenced by state or federal law and/or regulatory agencies
- Index: Alphabetical list of topics covered in the manual (optional)

Work Environment

Considering the fact that the average FTE spends more waking hours in the work environment than in the home, it would be prudent for management to create a workplace ambiance that evokes comfort and productivity. Whether creating new space or evaluating current space, development of the work environment involves certain fundamental principles that address space and equipment, aesthetics, and **ergonomics.**

Work Flow

The **work flow** in a departmental setting is the established path along which tasks are sequentially completed by any number of staff to accomplish a function. According to Keister (2001), "Workflow has been defined as the automation of a business process, in whole or in part, during which documents, information, or tasks are passed from one participant to another for action in a way that is governed by a set of procedural rules."

Figure 23.1.   Loose chart filing flowchart

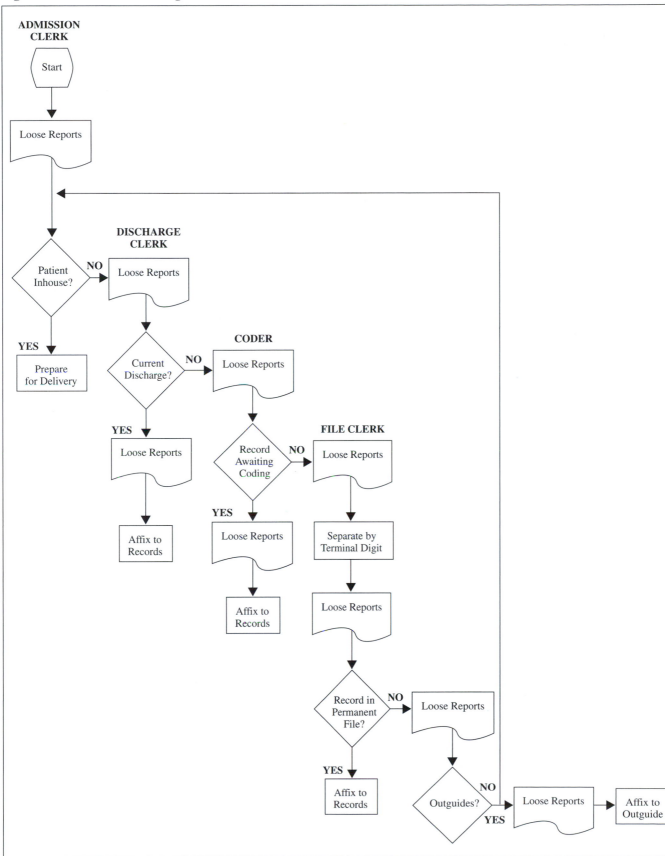

Well-designed work flow is critical to achieving optimal efficiency and productivity when a function requires the coordinated activity of a group of employees. In a manual process environment, spatial relationships among people who perform tasks and the equipment required to perform them are critical factors in planning efficient work flow.

In such situations, creating a layout diagram, sometimes called a **movement diagram** or layout flowchart, helps the manager to visualize the functions and related tasks performed in a defined work area and how they are related. (See figure 23.2.)

Space and Equipment

Workspace design can influence morale, productivity, and job satisfaction. The design of efficient office space involves a number of considerations, the first of which is typically location. If the department is located on any floor other than ground level, it is important to determine how much weight the suspended floor can support. This is especially critical when planning for additional shelving to store paper medical records. The combined weight of the records and shelving can be extreme, and the floor must be designed to support weights of potential proportion.

The amount of space designated for the department is the determining factor in considering office design and equipment specifications. Space is considered a precious and costly commodity in healthcare facilities and must be used efficiently. Designing efficient office space is a highly specialized and intricate process.

Department managers should understand basic facility planning techniques. They also must consider the facility's master plan in developing a plan for the department. This ensures maximum efficiency, consistency, and flexibility. The department plan also should address:

- The department's physical environment
- Office space utilization
- Space planning techniques, guidelines, and standards
- Office furniture and equipment

In an ideal situation, a move into a new space is the reason for engaging in space planning. Reorganization of a department because of changes in workforce numbers resulting from downsizing or from taking on new functions constitutes a space planning process. Departmental reorganization in response to changes in methods or functions, such as a move to home-based transcription or implementation of an electronic health record (EHR), can trigger a call for revised space planning. Sometimes the basic need to improve work flow and/or the appearance of a department can be a pivotal reason for space planning.

Remodeling existing space, as opposed to designing new space, presents special challenges. There may be space problems that cannot be changed, such as walls and pillars that cannot be moved and inadequate wiring. In addition, employees may resist changes and find it difficult to think creatively. In such instances, managers need to be inventive and creative in their space utilization.

Hard space and soft space are other considerations in designing efficient and effective space utilization. Hard space is space that cannot be converted easily to service another function. For example, a file area could have certain structural needs or radiology may require lead walls. Soft space is space that is readily expandable or contractible to adjust to changing needs.

Determining how soft and hard space will be utilized is a major component of office space planning. Effective space planning has the following characteristics:

- Keeping costs to a minimum
- Contributing to the quality of the work
- Contributing to employee satisfaction
- Contributing to services provided by the department

Space needs change in the course of time and should be reevaluated periodically to determine whether principles of good space planning are being followed.

Four separate, self-explanatory types of office space are needed:

- Private office space
- General office space
- Service area
- Storage area

Another space consideration is personal space or the area of privacy surrounding an employee. Territoriality is a natural development because employees instinctively control the physical areas where they work.

Aesthetics

The physical environment factors, or aesthetics, of the workplace have the most physiological as well as psychological effects on employees. Aesthetic elements include the lighting of both the office and the workspace, the colors of the walls and furniture, auditory impacts, and atmospheric condition and temperature.

Light should be of sufficient brightness and diffusion for the work situation. Exposures (north, south, east, and west in order of preference) to natural light must be considered when creating new space because natural light is best and easiest on the eyes. Luminance is the quality of light, and lux is a unit of measure. (Candlelight equals 10 lux. A well-lit office equals 500 to 700 lux whereas the noonday sun produces 160,000 lux.) Desk or task lighting is more physically supportive than overhead florescent lighting alone. Many HIS functions include PC monitors, and the contrast between the print and the background can influence the employee's comfort level. Typically, a light background with dark print is least taxing on the eyes. Glare from light sources or PC screens can cause discomfort. Display screen fixtures can be used to help reduce glare. In addition, it is important to factor in the age of the staff; people over 40 have an increased

Figure 23.2.   Movement diagram: Inefficient (top) and efficient (bottom)

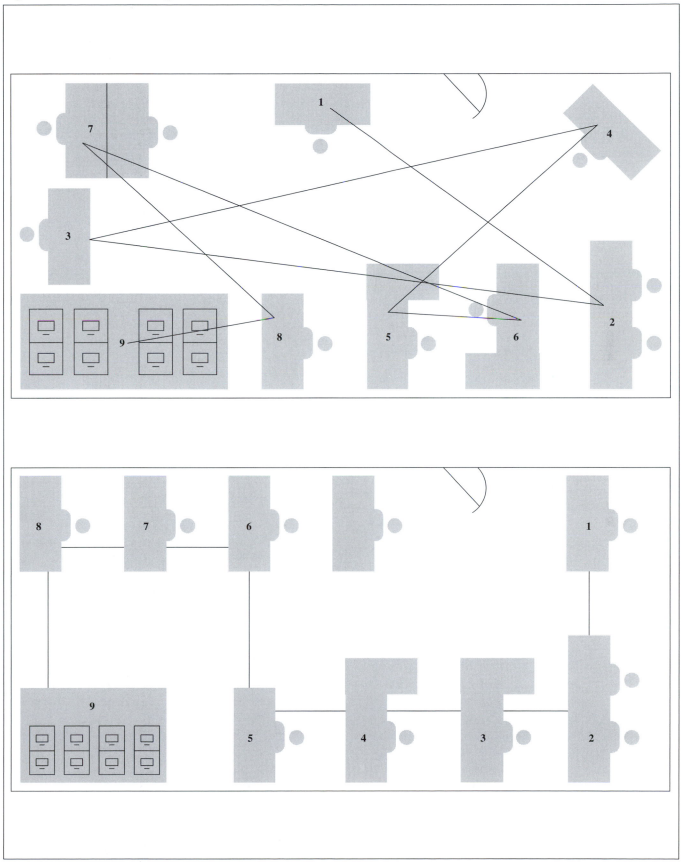

level of discomfort from glare. (For additional information on office light, visit IBM at www.pc.ibm.com/ww/healthy computing/vdt19c.html.)

Color influences how people feel. For example, dark areas feel brighter and/or lighter when painted with light colors. Moreover, certain colors evoke a variety of sensations and feelings. Blues are cool, reds are warm, greens evoke luxury, and so on. When choosing color schemes, it is important to consider the area and who will occupy it. Neutral colors can have a calming effect and help avoid the subliminal friction that some primary colors trigger. Also, the finish of the paint should be considered. Matte surfaces absorb more light and reduce glare but are typically not cleanable. On the other hand, gloss surfaces are cleanable, but reflective, and can exacerbate glare.

Music and sound can be incorporated to improve working conditions and relieve both mental and visual fatigue. Certain kinds of music can reduce tension and make employees generally feel better. Sound conditioning and soundproofing are important considerations because a noisy office is seldom efficient. A certain level of routine office background noise is expected and usually is not irritating. However, loud or abrupt sounds can be alarming, distracting, and disruptive. Planning separate space for noisy work processes, such as copying and printing, is effective because it addresses the source of the noise. Carpeting, drapes, and partitioning can offer noise control because they absorb significant amounts of sound.

Air-conditioning regulates temperature, circulation, and moisture content and determines cleanliness. When considering normal ventilation for the space, at least 2,000 cubic feet per person per hour should be configured to maintain a healthy respiratory atmosphere. Air that is too warm or too cold is equally distracting, and a balance can be difficult to maintain. A range of 68 to 72 degrees Fahrenheit is generally acceptable to most people.

Ergonomics

The word *ergonomics* is derived from the Greek word *ergon,* which means "work," and *nomos,* which means "natural laws of." Developed in the 1950s by a group of scientists and engineers, the discipline of ergonomics has helped redefine the employee workspace with consideration for comfort and safety.

Questions to consider in office layout and design include:

- Do staff members assume fixed working postures that remain static for the majority of the workday? For example, do they sit at a keyboard all day?
- Do staff members perform repetitive motions such as filing, stamping, hole punching, and so on?
- Has the psychological stress caused by uncomfortable workstations been taken into consideration?

In effective ergonomic planning, the designer must know the work requirements of the job and the tasks involved. The physical traits of the worker assigned to each workstation also influence ergonomic considerations. For example, height or leg length or back waist length will determine specific needs. Another consideration is whether a single person or multiple persons share one workstation throughout the workweek. Finally, one must consider what equipment is currently available at the workstation and what equipment must be purchased to create an ergonomically correct work environment?

When the work environment is not ergonomically sound, common cumulative trauma disorders and repetitive strain injuries associated with office personnel can occur, including:

- Carpal tunnel syndrome is considered an occupational illness rather than an injury because it takes a long time to develop to the point of debilitation. The syndrome causes flexion, with ulnar deviation. Symptoms include tingling, numbness, and pain in the wrist and lower arm.
- Upper back and neck strain is caused by poor posture. Symptoms include tension headaches and muscle pain.
- Eyestrain is caused by incorrect viewing distances and poor illumination. Symptoms include burning, watery eyes, and headaches.

Good preventative, proactive ergonomic management includes educating staff on how to care for themselves to reduce potential ergonomic injuries or discomfort. A few simple principles help raise employees' awareness of their physical relationship with the work environment. Managers should encourage, if not insist, that staff working at a PC for the majority (more than two-thirds) of a shift take hourly neck, shoulder, and wrist roll breaks, along with stretch routines. In addition, employees should be aware of, and assessed on their use of, the ten basic principles of good sitting posture. (See figure 23.3.)

Figure 23.3.   Ten basic principles of good sitting posture

- Feet should rest flat on the floor or footrest.
- A fist-width space should be measurable between the back of the knees and the edge of the seat pan of the chair.
- The hips should be at a 90-degree angle (or slightly greater) in relation to the body. To help ensure this angle, the knees should be at or below hip height.
- The lower back (lumbar region) should be supported.
- Shoulders should be relaxed, not shrugged, slouched, or rolled forward.
- Elbows should rest comfortably at the side or on armrests. When typing, elbows should be at 90-degree angles and preferably supported by an adjustable armrest at an appropriate height.
- Wrists should be maintained in a neutral (straight) position while typing or using any variety of keyboard.
- Head and neck should be in an upright position. To confirm this, the ears should be directly over the shoulders, which are directly over the hips.
- Computer monitors should be positioned directly in front of the worker. The top line of print should be horizontal with the eyes when looking directly forward.
- Ergonomic aids should be used to help maintain comfortable posture. Examples include footrests, wrist rests for keyboard and mouse, antiglare screens for computer monitors, copy stands, and adjustable chair height for those working at a multitask station.

These basic activities can help employees to stop the tension cycle and can reduce potential long-term discomfort.

Careful consideration and professional assessment of individual needs will help reduce or eliminate physical barriers to employee comfort and productivity. Preemptive, ergonomically correct practices markedly reduce employee absence and worker's compensation usage due to workplace injury.

Check Your Understanding 23.1

Instructions: Answer the following questions on a separate piece of paper.

1. Looking at the sample vacation schedule in table 23.2, for which weeks would the department be well advised to secure temporary help?

2. List the potential problem areas a work distribution analysis can reveal.

3. Who should write a job description? Who should collect the necessary information?

4. What is the best way to plan an efficient work flow?

5. Name the elements of good work environment planning.

Performance and Work Measurement Standards

Work is the task to be performed; performance is the execution of the task. Effective management involves discerning what work is to be done, what performance standards are achievable and appropriate, how performance can be measured in terms of efficiency and efficacy, and how performance can be monitored for variances from the standards set. Most employees simply want to know what tasks they are responsible for, what is expected of them, and how they are performing with regard to that expectation. Through performance standard-setting and measurement processes, managers can determine success or opportunities for improvement.

A **standard** may be defined as a performance criterion established by custom or authority with the purpose of assessing factors such as quality, productivity, and performance. Managers are responsible for controlling the resources available to them, including men (staff), materials, machines, methods, and money. Thus, managers are expected to set standards for each of these resources and then use them as ways to judge (assess, evaluate) the quality, productivity, and/or performance of those resources.

Criteria for Setting Effective Standards

To create viable, significant standards, it is important to identify the criteria for effective standard setting. Effective standards are:

- *Understandable:* The persons affected by the standard know what it means, and it makes sense to them.
- *Attainable:* It is reasonable to expect that the person(s) affected by the standard can actually achieve it.
- *Equitable:* If more than one person is affected by the standard, all are held accountable for it.
- *Significant:* Meeting the standard is important to the goals of the work unit or organization; the effort it takes to meet the standard is worth it.
- *Legitimate:* The standard has been formally accepted within the organization and is documented in appropriate places and ways.
- *Economical:* The standard can be met and monitored without incurring costs that are beyond the value of that which is gained by having it. In other words, is the standard worth the expense?

Keeping the definition of effective standards in mind, it is possible to set about writing new standards for the staff or reviewing and revising current standards. Several examples of effective resource management standards include:

- Standards related to human resources (staff)
  —*Quality:* Coders code inpatient services with 98 percent accuracy.
  —*Productivity:* Coders code 25 to 30 inpatient discharges per eight-hour workday.
  —*Performance:* Employees maintain an acceptable or better rating on peer evaluations of effectiveness as team members.
- Standards related to supplies (materials)
  —*Quality:* Paper-based health record forms must be printed on 20-pound paper stock, or pens used for

---

Table 23.2. Sample vacation schedule

Employee	Title	Hire Date	Week #	7/1	7/8	7/15	7/22	7/29	8/5	8/12	8/19
Brown	Transcriptionist	2001	1					x			
Dorsey	Transcriptionist	2000	2	x							x
Grunch	Transcriptionist	1999	3		x				x	x	
Glass	Clerk	2000	2			x	x				
Diewell Community Hospital Vacation Policy											
General Employees			**Department Managers/Administrators**								
3 years or less = 1 week 4 to 7 years = 2 weeks 8 to 10 years = 3 weeks 11 years and over = 4 weeks			3 years or less = 2 weeks 4 to 7 years = 3 weeks 8 years and over = 4 weeks								

health record documentation must contain water-proof ink.

—*Performance:* Paper-based health record forms must be two-hole punched on the top margin and three-hole punched on the left-hand margin to accommodate both the chart binder used on the care unit and the permanent file folder.

- Standards related to budgetary resources (money)

—*Performance:* Major budget expense categories (salaries, supplies, postage, telephone, travel, and maintenance) must remain within plus or minus three percent of the budgeted amount monthly.

—*Performance:* Paid dollars per key statistic (P$PKS) must be less than $2 plus or minus the target P$PKS indicator established for the department.

- Standards related to methods

—*Quality:* Health record forms must be assembled (organized) in accordance with the organization's standard chart order guidelines, or the health record of a discharged patient must be logged into health information services for processing by 7:00 a.m. the day following discharge.

—*Performance:* The health record of a discharged patient must follow this work flow pattern in the department's assembly, analysis, coding, chart completion (when appropriate), and permanent file.

- Standards related to equipment (machines)

—*Quality:* Each file shelf unit must support up to 100 pounds of file weight.

—*Productivity:* The copier must be able to collate and staple up to ten 50-page packets at a time.

—*Performance:* The printer must be able to produce prints (hard-copy paper and transparencies) from PowerPoint™ software using at least four different types of design templates.

Methods of Communicating Standards

After the standards have been created, they must be communicated to staff. All the above types of standards can be provided to staff in a number of ways, including through:

- *Written specifications,* as used in job descriptions, equipment specification sheets, and forms design guidelines
- *Documented rules, regulations, or policies,* as used in policy manuals, procedure manuals, regulations manuals, and employee handbooks
- *Demonstration models,* as in sample health records
- *Verbal confirmations,* as in the reinforcement of a standard whenever possible and appropriate

Standards are worded differently at various levels within the organization depending on whether they reflect a **goal** or an **objective.** A goal is a generalized statement of a unit, departmental, or organizational standard, typically without measurable content. An objective is a statement of end result

in measurable terms with time and cost limits, as applicable. For example, the HIS department might have a general standard (most commonly called a goal) for its transcription function, such as "to support patient care through accurate and timely transcription of medical reports." The transcription function then might state an objective-level standard in more specific language to make it more understandable and more measurable, for example, "to report routine history and physical, operative, and consultation dictation within twelve hours of dictation." This objective is related directly to the timeliness aspect of the preceding goal.

Qualitative and Quantitative Standards

Standards are also characterized in two other ways: as **quantitative standards** and as **qualitative standards.**

Qualitative standards specify the level of service quality expected from a function, such as:

- Accuracy rate (For example, assignment of diagnostic and procedure codes for inpatient records is at least 98 percent accurate.)
- Error rate (For example, mistakes in the assignment of diagnostic and procedure codes occur in no more than two percent of inpatient records coded.)

Quantitative standards specify the level of measurable work, or productivity, expected for a specific function, such as:

- Number of units of work per specified period of time or amount of time allotted per unit of work (For example, 70 records per FTE per day or no more than 15 minutes are allotted to coding an inpatient record.)
- Turnaround time (For example, dictation must be transcribed within 24 hours.)
- Response time (For example, requests are responded to within seven working days of receipt.)

Quantity standards (also called productivity standards) and quality standards (also known as service standards) are generally used by managers to monitor individual employee performance and/or the performance of a functional unit or the department as a whole. To properly communicate performance standards, managers need to make the distinction between quantitative and qualitative standards and identify examples of each for the HIS functions.

Key Indicators

Key indicators are live (versus retrospective) measurement thresholds that alert a department or work unit to its level of competent customer service. After the department's standards have been determined, the focus is on compliance. Managers must watch the key indicators to determine whether the department is on course. Two red flags that indicate that targets are being missed are:

- The number and severity of complaints increase. When the number or severity of complaints increases, the circumstances surrounding the complaints need to be assessed immediately so that corrections to the process or personnel involved can be made.

- Surveys to assess performance on accreditation, legal, or regulatory standards indicate that the organization has failed to comply in one or more areas. When the organization fails to comply with one or more external standards during a survey, the organization needs to correct the variance(s) and return to compliance.

Methods of Developing Standards

Any of a number of methods can be used to develop standards for productivity (the creation of products using an organization's financial and human resources) in a work unit. Two approaches are commonly used: **benchmarking** comparable performance and measuring actual performance.

Benchmarking Comparable Performance

Benchmarking is based on research into the performance of similar organizations and programs or on standards established by national or local sources, such as professional associations and standard-setting organizations. It has become a more prevalent approach in HIS management in the past few years because this type of information is now being published more regularly.

To engage in a benchmarking effort, the manager should first select key functions of the department that will be benchmarked (coding service, transcription service, release of information [ROI] service, and so on). Relating benchmarks to the specific process is critical. Thought must be given to the types of performance measure(s) desired as indicators (for coding, for example, payments remaining in accounts receivable due to uncoded records and payments remaining in accounts receivable due to coding disputes; for transcription, for example, turnaround time [dictation to charting] for consultations, operative reports, history, and physicals).

When the key functional areas have been selected and the types of indicators identified, the research of benchmarks through published sources (preferably) may begin. Investigation of benchmark standards involves assessment of their relevance to the department's specific situation; then the idea can be sold to the rest of the organization. Benchmarking involves the following steps:

1. Identifying peer organizations/departments that have achieved outstanding performance based on some key indicator (for example, 98 percent of health records coded within two days postdischarge)
2. Studying the best practices within the organization that make it possible to achieve that performance level
3. Acting to implement those best practices in one's own organization to achieve a similar performance

Routinely gathering performance data enables a manager to monitor actual performance against the benchmark and then evaluate factors in department processes that must be changed to move actual performance into the benchmark range.

Measurement of Actual Performance

Work measurement is the process of studying the amount of work accomplished and the amount of time it takes to accomplish it. It involves the collection of data relevant to the work, such as the amount of work accomplished per unit of time. Its purpose is to define and monitor productivity.

Work measurement can support a manager in many activities, including:

- Setting production standards
- Determining staffing requirements
- Establishing incentive pay systems
- Determining direct costs by function
- Comparing performance to standards
- Identifying activities for process/methods improvement

Gathering the information available through work measurement efforts will be invaluable to the manager in making administrative decisions. But how do managers know which work measurement will serve them best?

When selecting the work measurement technique that best suits his or her department, the manager should consider the following factors:

- The amount of financial resources available
- The availability of qualified personnel to take part in the study
- The amount of time available to devote to study
- The attitudes of employees toward participation in a study

Work measurement can be accomplished through a variety of techniques, including:

- *Analysis of historical (past performance) data:* The analysis of historical data generally uses work volume (direct or estimated) and hours paid from past records to establish the standard. When using historical data, managers are cautioned to keep in mind that volume figures are not adjusted for the level of quality and the number of hours paid is different from the number of hours actually worked.
- *Employee self-logging:* Employee self-logging is a form of self-reporting in which the employees simply track their tasks, volume, and hours worked. Employee logging incorporates a **time ladder,** which is a form used by the employee to document the amount of time spent (worked) on various tasks. It can be modified to include the number of units produced per task throughout the day. **Volume logs** are sometimes used in conjunction with a time ladder to obtain information about the volume of work units received and processed in a day by simply keeping track of the number of products produced or activities done. (See table 23.3, p. 660.)

• *Scientific methods:* The scientific methods of work measurement include time studies and the use of preestablished time/unit standards. For example, time studies use a stopwatch to record and document the time required to accomplish a specified task.
• ***Work sampling:*** Work sampling is a technique of work measurement that involves using statistical probability (determined through random sample observations) to characterize the performance of the department and its work (functional) units.

Each one of the varieties of work measurement techniques offers calculations of employee productivity in either unit/time or time/unit. For example, with the completion of a daily time ladder summary (table 23.4), a manager can determine simple unit/time productivity statistics by dividing the number of units produced by the number of hours worked. Table 23.4 also contains the type of data needed to calculate the weekly activities of coders and a clerks weekly activities.

Work sampling is an especially valuable technique in the development of performance standards. Work-sampling data can help the manager to:

• Catalog the activities being performed
• Determine the time devoted to each activity
• Identify inefficiencies
• Set employee performance standards

Table 23.3. Sample volume log

Task	Number of Worked Hours	Number of Units
Coding	40 worked hours	120 records
Loose filing	36 worked hours	48 inches

The coding standard calculates at three records per worked hour for this employee (120 records/40 hours) and a filing standard of 1.3 inches per worked hour (48 inches/36 hours). It does not capture any interruptions or unworked time in the eight-hour day but is a simple way to arrive at a ballpark figure.

Work-sampling projects follow an established sequence of steps and use specific tools:

1. Decide which work activities to monitor during the study.
2. Design the form that will be used to record the observations collected during the study. The sample observation record form shown in table 23.5 captures activities by individuals and by units of function (supervisory, transcription, clerical, and coder).
3. Determine the best size of the study sample by using the precision interval method, a standard formula used to determine sample size. The formula allows for various scenarios of desired **certainty factor** (confidence factor) and **precision factor** (acceptable error) in the study results. The certainty factor is a numerical representation of the confidence the manager has that the results will show the level of acceptable error. The precision factor is the level of tolerable error in the sampling process.

$$\text{Sample size} = 0.25 \times \left[\frac{\text{certainty factor } \%^2}{\text{precision factor } \%} \right]$$

*Note that the 0.25 is a fixed (not variable) part of the formula.

If the precision factor is 5 percent, the confidence factor needed is 95 percent. (Note that the precision factor plus the confidence factor equal 100 percent.) For example:

$$25 \times (0.95 \div 0.025)^2 = 0.25 \times (38 \times 38) = 361$$

4. Determine the length of the study and establish appropriate observation times. When the sample size (total number of observations required) has been determined, the number of observations per day can be determined on the basis of the number of days, weeks, or months available to complete the study. The actual time of each observation each day must be determined by using a random observation generator (figure 23.4)

Table 23.4. Sample daily time ladder summary

Unit: <u>Reception</u>   Date: <u>07-04-02</u>

Note: 7.5 worked hours (two 15-minute breaks)

Employee	Code/Task	Total Time (%)	Work Units
Jane	A. Answer phones	3hr/40%	64
	B. Write requisitions	1.75 hr/23%	92
	C. Personal/set up, etc.	.5 hr/7%	NA
	D. Mail handling	2.25 hr/30%	Incoming 80 **Outgoing 100**
Betty	A. Answer phones	5 hr/66%	100
	B. Write requisitions	.5 hr/7%	15
	C. Personal/set up, etc.	.5/7%	NA
	D. Mail handling	0	NA
	E. Stat chart delivery	1.5/20%	10

Table 23.5.   Sample observation record form

Activity	Mason	Davis	Perry	Kent	Martin	Carter	Roth	Evans	Larson	Owens .5 FTE	Total
	Supervisor	Transcriptionists			Clerical				Coders		
Supervision											
Coding											
Transcription											
Record A & A											
Record retrieval/filing/transport											
Release of Information											
Assisting physicians											
Other clerical											
Idle: Gone, rest											
Total observations											

Observation Times:

1.   6.
2.   7.
3.   8.   Recorded by: _____
4.   9.
5.   10.   Date: _____

Figure 23.4.   Observation generator

Time Block Number	Clock Time	Time Block Number	Clock Time
0	8:00 a.m.	25	12:10 p.m.
1	10	26	20
2	20	27	30
3	30	28	40
4	40	29	50
5	50	30	1:00 p.m.
6	9:00 a.m.	31	10
7	10	32	20
8	20	33	30
9	30	34	40
10	40	35	50
11	50	36	2:00 p.m.
12	10.00 a.m.	37	10
13	10	38	20
14	20	39	30
15	30	40	40
16	40	41	50
17	50	42	3:00 p.m.
18	11:00 a.m.	43	10
19	10	44	20
20	20	45	30
21	30	46	40
22	40	47	50
23	50	48	4:00 p.m.
24	12:00 p.m.	etc.	

and a random numbers table (figure 23.5). To create the observation generator, list the period of time the study will take place in a workday (in figure 23.4, from 8 a.m. until 4 p.m., with 10-minute increments) and number each predetermined time increment. Then using a random numbers table (figure 23.5 is a partial table of tables found in any statistics book), randomly select the first number and then a direction to read the numbers (horizontally, vertically, or diagonally). Looking at the first number, refer to the observation generator to find the time of day assigned that corresponding number. If it does not exist, proceed to the next number until the optimal number to complete the study has been selected. For example, if 500 observations were needed and 50 workdays were allotted to complete the study, 10 observations would need to be made each day of the 50-day study. (See figure 23.6, p. 662.)

Figure 23.5.   Random numbers table (partial)

69	18	82	00	97	32	82	53	05	27
90	04	58	54	97	51	98	15	06	54
73	18	95	02	07	47	67	72	62	59
54	01	64	90	04	66	28	13	10	03
75	75	87	64	90	20	97	18	17	49
08	35	86	99	10	78	53	24	27	85
28	30	30	32	64	81	33	31	05	91
53	84	08	62	33	31	59	41	36	28
etc.									

Note: Entry may be made at any point, proceeding horizontally or vertically.

Figure 23.6.   Example of a first day's observation times

Observation Times		
1. 8:50 a.m.	6. 1:00 p.m.	
2. 9:40 a.m.	7. 1:10 p.m.	
3. 10:20 a.m.	8. 1:20 p.m.	Recorded by: _____
4. 12:00 noon	9. 2:20 p.m.	Department: _____
5. 12:40 p.m.	10. 2:30 p.m.	Date: _____

5. Explain the purpose of the study and how it is conducted to observers and staff. Orientation of observers and personnel is very important because it encourages consistency in data collection among observers and ensures that unbiased and reliable observations are collected on the basis of the observation schedule. At this point in the study, those who will be observed also must be informed of its purpose. It is important that workers perform normally throughout the process. They also should understand that the outcome of the study will be shared with them at the conclusion of the study period.

6. Collect and record observation data at random points. (See table 23.6.)

7. Report the results of the study. (See tables 23.7 and 23.8 and table 23.9.)

Performance Measurement

Performance measurement is the process of comparing the outcomes of an organization, work unit, or employee to preestablished performance plans and standards. The results of the performance measurement process are expressed as percentages, rates, ratios, averages, and other quantitative assessments. Performance measurement is used both in assessments of quality of clinical care and for management applications. Examples of performance measures maintained by acute care hospitals include the rate of nosocomial infection, the percentage of surgical complications, the average length of stay, and the ratio of live births to stillbirths. Examples of performance measures maintained by an HIS department include transcription lines transcribed and turnaround times per report type, turnaround times for ROI and chart retrieval, and loose filing inches filed and existing.

Performance measurement is a fundamental managerial activity that supports two of the basic functions of management: controlling and planning. The control function is concerned with ensuring that the work unit or organization is doing what it should be doing in the right way. The function of planning is to define the expectations of performance (or standards), the processes required for achieving those expectations (or objectives), and the desired outcomes of performance (or goals). The goals, objectives, and standards established during the planning process become the criteria used in the control process to evaluate actual performance.

Performance Controls

In the control process, specific monitors (controls) are established and outcomes data are collected. The outcomes data are then analyzed to determine the extent to which actual performance corresponds to the performance expectations established during the planning process.

The characteristics of effective controls include:

- *Flexibility* refers to the fact that controls must be adaptable to real changes in the requirements of a process. For example, a budget is a control on the use of money. Money budgeted in one category (equipment) may need to be spent in another category (travel) because of a change in a program, a new law/regulation, and so on.
- *Simplicity* refers to the fact that those involved in the process must find the controls understandable and reasonable.
- *Economy* implies that controls should not cost more than they are worth. The time and money spent to implement a control should be in line with the level of risk (loss) involved if the process fails to meet performance expectations. For example, loss of a life calls for a significant investment in controls; criminal liability

Table 23.6.   First day's observations, Cure-All Hospital's HIM department

	Mason	Davis	Perry	Kent	Martin	Carter	Roth	Evans	Larson	Owens .5 FTE	
Activity	Supervisor	Transcriptionists			Clerical				Coders		Total
Supervision											2
Coding											0
Transcription											24
Record A & A											10
Record retrieval/filing/transport											16
Release of information											8
Assisting physicians											8
Other clerical											15
Idle: Gone, rest											10
Total observations	10	10	10	10	10	10	10	10	10	3	93

Table 23.7. Observation summary, Cure-All Hospital's HIM department

Activity	Previous Observation Days	3/10/00	Study Total	% Total
Supervision	—	2	90	2.2
Coding	—	0	18	0.4
Transcription	—	24	1,053	25.9
Record A & A	—	10	540	13.3
Filing/retrieval/transport	—	16	618	15.2
Release of information	—	8	381	9.4
Assisting physicians	—	8	273	6.7
Other clerical	—	15	711	17.5
Idle: Gone, rest	—	10	378	9.4
Total observations	—	93	4,062	100.0

Note: This particular work sampling effort involved a total work sampling of 500 planned observations (10 observations per workday for 50 days). This number of observations gives a ±2.75% precision interval for = >10% activities, a 5.5% accuracy rate, and 94.5% confidence level.

calls for significant investment in controls; a day of overtime to correct clerical errors calls for a minimal investment in controls.

- *Timeliness* suggests that controls should be implemented so as to detect potential variances within a time frame that allows for corrective action before any adverse effect has occurred. For example, the accuracy of a record number assignment should be confirmed at the time of registration or the coding checked before a bill is mailed or transmitted to avoid the adverse effects associated with errors that are transmitted to other areas of the organization or to the insurance carrier.

- A *focus on exceptions* demands that controls be targeted at those aspects of a process that are most likely to vary significantly from expectation. For example, a new transcriptionist who is likely to make more errors that could do damage to customer service ratings is generally monitored more closely and more often than one who is experienced and has performed well for the past year.

Table 23.8. Work sampling results, Cure-All Hospital's HIM department: Actual activity vs. expectations

Activity	Normal Range of Expectations	Department Expectations	Department Actual	Estimated Variation
Supervision	NA	15%	2.2%	−13%
Coding	2–4.5%	3%	0.4%	−2%
Transcription	30–40%	30%	25.9%	−4%
Record A & A	10–13%	12%	13.3%	+1%
Record retrieval/filing	2–5%	3%	15.2%	+12%
Release of information	6–9%	7%	9.4%	+2%
Assisting physicians	6–10%	8%	6.7%	−1%
Other clerical	8–13%	10%	17.5%	+7%
Idle: Gone, rest	7–14%	12%	9.4%	−3%
Total	NA	100%	100%	NA

Table 23.9. Work sampling results, Cure-All Hospital's HIM department

Activity Area/Expected %	% of Time	Minutes*	Hours*	Work Volume for Period	Work Units
Supervision/15%	2%	4,560	76	NA	NA
Coding/3%	1%	0.01 × 228,000 or 2,280	0.01 × 3,800 or 38 hours	775	Dx coded
Transcription/30%	26%	0.26 × 228,000 or 59,280	0.26 × 3,800 or 988	150,000	Lines transcribed
Record assembly and analysis/12%	13%	29,640	494	2,964	Records analyzed
Record filing, retrieval, etc./3%	15%	34,200	570	11,400	Records pulled/filed
Release of information/7%	9%	20,520	342	1,050	Requests handled
Assisting physician/8%	7%	15,960	266	NA	NA
Other clerical/10%	18%	41,040	684	NA	NA
Idle: Gone, rest/12%	9%	20,520	342	NA	NA
Total	100%	—	—	—	—

Notes: Working days in the period: 50 days
Current workforce: 9.5 FTE, including the supervisor
Work minutes/day per FTE: 480 minutes (8 hr × 60)

Total study work hours: 3,800 hours (9.5 FTE × 8 × 50)
Total study work minutes: 228,000 minutes (9.5 FTE × 480 × 50) or (3,800 × 60)

*Minutes and hours are calculated based on the percentage of total time represented by each activity area. For example, 2% of 228,000 minutes = 4,560 minutes; 2% of 3,800 hours = 76 hours.

There are two general types of controls: preventive (self-correcting) and feedback (nonself-correcting). Preventive controls are front-end processes that guide work in such a way that input and/or process variations are minimized. Simple things such as standard operating procedures, edits on data entered into computer-based systems, and training processes are ways to reduce the potential for error by using preventive controls.

Feedback controls are back-end processes that monitor and measure output, and then compare it to expectations and identify variations that then must be analyzed so correction action plans can be developed and implemented. Processes with feedback controls in place are also called cybernetic processes or systems. Some may be self-regulating (such as thermostatic systems), but most are nonself-regulating, meaning that they require intervention by an oversight agent (a supervisor, manager, or auditor) to identify the variance and take action to correct it.

Variance Analysis

When variations are identified (when actual performance does not meet or significantly exceeds expectations), further analysis is called for. Analysis of the performance factors involved in the work (people, supplies, equipment, and money) is conducted to help determine what, if any, changes should be made. Changes may involve activities such as additional staff training; modifications in procedures, work flow, or policies; purchases of updated equipment; or improvements in maintenance procedures. The analysis may lead to changes in performance criteria and expectations.

Assessment of Employee Performance

When establishing an employee performance assessment program, the steps in the control (evaluation) process include:

1. Monitoring and measuring outcomes performance
2. Comparing performance to established goals and standards
3. Evaluating variance and developing action plans
4. Taking appropriate action

Monitoring and Measuring Outcomes Performance

Monitoring and measuring performance involves taking an aggregate look at performance over a period of time. Options include operating on a self-reporting method such as self-logging, using computerized monitoring to audit productivity, manually auditing work samples, or relying on customer feedback to measure departmental performance.

Outcomes performance monitoring depends on employee productivity and management execution. Focus is on indicators such as turnaround time, cost/revenue reports, and customer feedback. The indicators highlight collective performance as a department and at the same time present discrepancies in goals and standards.

Consider this practical application of performance monitoring. Assume that one established expectation of the transcription function in a department is that the routine ROI in

response to a consent for use or a disclosure of health information request occurs within five working days of receipt in the department.

The first step in controlling a function would be to set up a data collection and reporting activity to obtain information that can be used to monitor the time it takes the department to respond to a routine ROI. (See table 23.10.)

Next, the department should determine the kinds of controls it wants to establish. The department wants to monitor routine requests, but how are "routine requests" defined? They may be any requests that are not stat or emergency or do not have to be handled within minutes, hours, or some stipulated amount of time under five working days. For example, a subpoena for a record that must be handled within three days or a request for a record needed for an appointment in a clinic the next morning would not be considered routine requests.

The line related to ROI requests in the middle of the performance report shown in table 23.11 indicates the average number of days it took the HIS department to respond to all the routine ROI requests in January (3), February (3), March (6), and April (5). However, the numbers tell nothing about the routine ROI requests the department has received, but not yet responded to.

The average turnaround time number is calculated by dividing the total response days attributed to the volume of routine requests responded to within the reporting period by the volume of routine requests responded to. For example, if the department responded to 300 routine requests in the month of May and 100 were responded to in six days, 100 in two days, and 100 in four days, the average turnaround time in May would be four days:

$$\frac{(600 \text{ days} + 200 \text{ days} + 400 \text{ days})}{300 \text{ requests}} = 4 \text{ days (average)}$$

The data used to arrive at the average turnaround time for the report also are quite useful because they allow the department to see what really makes up the four-day average and to focus on aspects of a process that might need some attention in order to prevent a crisis later on. Having the information

Table 23.10.   ROI requests

On June 6, 2000, Total Routine ROI Requests in Processing: 130					
Days Since Receipt	**6–10 Days**	**11–15 Days**	**16–20 Days**	**>20 Days**	**Summary**
Number of total	12 9%	15 12%	2 2%	1 1%	30 24%
Unable to locate record	0	2	0	1	3 10%
Incomplete record	12	12	2	0	26 87%
Issue with authorization	0	0	0	0	0
Unavailable record	0	1	0	0	1 3%
Other	0	0	0	0	0

Table 23.11.   Sample health information services performance report

Indicator	January 2006	February 2006	March 2006	April 2006
DCEs	5,000	5,400	5,360	5,500
Labor cost per DCE: <$10.00	$10.00	9.25	9.33	9.90
FTE budgeted at 50	50	50	50	48
Days in assembly/analysis at end of month <2days	1	2	2	3
Delinquency rate <50%	35%	40%	43%	45%
Coding: Days in AR due to uncoded records <5 days	3	5	4	5
Lines transcribed	120,000	130,000	128,000	132,000
Transcription: TAT for H&Ps <24 hours	12	16	18	26
ROI requests received	200	245	300	260
Release of Info: TAT <5 days	3	3	6	5
File pull requests	2,000	2,200	2,300	2,500
Retrieval rate: >95%	%94	%96	%93	%91%
Loose filing inches received	100 average 25/week	120 average 30/week	80 average 20/week	130 average 32/week
Loose filing inches at end of month: <16	15	20	12	15
Filing: Misfiles <1%	.05%	.08%	.06%	.08%
Resignations: <1%	0	0	0	2/50 = 4%
Education hours	4	16	2	8
Unproductive hours (sick, vacation): <15%	10%	12%	20%	10%

on a monthly basis to include as part of the regular performance reporting within the organization allows the manager to review monthly trends and identify potential focus areas for future process improvement activities.

In addition, the underlying data indicate that a considerable number of requests are not responded to within the five-working-days expectation (for example, 33 percent were responded to in six working days). A direct supervisor of the ROI activity would likely want access to information of this nature more often than once a month. For example, a weekly report showing the number of routine requests in the system for five days or more that have not yet been answered would allow the supervisor or ROI clerk to identify problem requests and take corrective actions over the course of the following week.

Comparing Performance to Established Goals and Standards

The next step in monitoring and measuring outcome performance is to compare current performance against established goals (standards). Continuing with the example in the preceding section, when comparing performance against the standard performance indicator of responding to routine ROIs within five days, the data in table 23.11 show an upward trend in March and April. The trend was appropriately reversed in May, which indicates that the function appears to be under control but obviously needs to be monitored.

Evaluating Variance and Developing Action Plans

When comparisons are done, the manager should evaluate any variances and develop an action plan specific to

each. The routine response to consent for use or disclosure of health information performance information does not indicate the need for significant action. Other variances in department functions may take priority, such as transcription turnaround time for H & Ps; days in assembly/analysis, coding; days in accounts receivable; and so on.

In an evaluation of variances, it is important to routinely collect data that provide the following types of information to disclose the triggers of the variances:

- Are any open ROI requests in the department with a date of receipt of more than five working days? (This is the focus on exceptions rule in action.)
- If so, what is the total number and what is the percentage of the total open ROI requests? How many are 6 to 10 working days, 10 to 15 working days, 16 to 20 working days, or more than 20 days?
- If so, what are the reasons the requests are still open?
- If so, on what date(s) has the requesting party been notified of the reason for the delay?

After the variances have been evaluated, action plans can be formulated to address them as follows:

- Establish a procedure to ensure weekly contact with the requestor to determine continuing need for the information and update on the status of the request.
- Flag the incomplete record with a ROI REQUEST PENDING to ensure that it is routed to ROI immediately when required documentation is complete.
- Track the missing record.

- Check the status of the unavailable record and contact user to obtain it so that ROI can occur and then (if necessary) the record can be returned to the user.

Taking Appropriate Action

Continuing with the consent for disclosure requests, appropriate actions are taken to put the plan in place and to monitor its effectiveness. Action plans should be revisited often to ensure that they are the appropriate approach to the problems originally identified by the data collecting and analysis.

Identification of Improvement Opportunities

When defining processes and identifying common symptoms of process problems generally and specific to HIS services, how do we know whether we have process problems? We need only be observant to:

- Inaccuracies and errors in work
- Complaints from customers
- Delays in getting things done or lots of interruptions
- Low employee morale or high rates of absenteeism/turnover
- Poor safety records and on-the-job injuries

Efforts to measure employee performance will alert management to the inaccuracies and errors in the work processes. The accuracy rate can be realized in a performance measurement plan. Any and all variances of quality must be addressed with expedient performance data collection and analysis.

Customer complaints indicate that a system or performance is not meeting expectations. Managers need to consider each complaint and determine whether it is circumstantial or a signal of something bigger. When chart delivery is delayed, customer expectations and patient needs should be examined and adjusted accordingly.

Delays in getting things done or continuous interruptions to a process can warn of roadblocks to success. Delays give time to revisit the current work flow and analyze what might be improved. If transcribed operative reports are not on the patients' charts within the prescribed time, how can the reason for the delay be identified and how can the improvement activity be planned to eliminate the delay?

Low employee morale and a high rate of absenteeism or turnover are serious indicators that procedures need to be improved. A lack of job satisfaction is typically caused by a lack of or incomplete training. High turnover and absenteeism are budget draining and call for a defined plan of action to avert a continued pattern. High turnover in positions that are especially difficult to fill can be exceptionally taxing to the budget and department alike because of the retraining and redistribution of workloads caused by reduced FTE levels.

Poor safety records or injuries are indicative of urgent process improvement opportunities. Work-related injuries and accidents are management markers regarding a poorly designed process, failing equipment, or poor training. Again, work injuries are a costly burden for the department and the goals and standards it has labored to establish. Are the charts too tightly packed on the shelves, creating extraordinary resistance to storing and retrieving records? Are personnel consistent in checking that aisles are clear before operating an automated movable filing system?

Being alert, collecting meaningful data, and observing and listening to customers and key staff are all ways to identify improvement opportunities. It is a continuous process that has no tolerance for complacency. Excellence is not an accident;it is a carefully planned outcome.

Principles of Performance Improvement

The general principles of work improvement, process improvement, and methods improvement are essentially synonymous. They all relate to a management philosophy that is systems oriented; that is, a management philosophy that views the work processes in an organization as being systematic in nature and seeks to constantly improve them by adjusting various components of the system.

A **system** is set of related elements (components) that are linked together according to a plan in order to meet a specific objective. Systems come in both manual and automated forms. The basic systems model demonstrates that a system is made up of the following components (figure 23.7):

- *Input* refers to human resources (attitudes, abilities), money, procedures (documents that describe how the department does things), equipment, supplies, and data.
- *Process* refers to the transformation of the inputs. What is done to or with the inputs results in something being accomplished. For example, assembling a medical record and coding the medical record are processes.

Figure 23.7.   Basic systems model

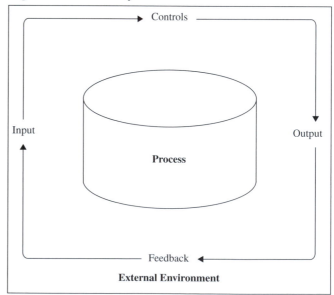

- *Output* is the finished product or the result of the process, such as an educated student, a transcribed report, a coded record, and so on.
- *Controls/standards* are the expectations of what the output should be and the mechanisms in place to monitor, track, and observe how well actual performance measures up to expectations. Examples of controls/standards are quality and production standards, such as 24-hour turnaround time, ROI requests responded to within five working days from receipt, and records coded within three days postdischarge. Also, laws, policies, and established procedures are standards that must be incorporated into the systems the facility manages.
- *Feedback* refers to the fact that when monitoring efforts indicate that expectations have been exceeded, it is time to compliment the folks involved and celebrate. Conversely, when expectations have not been met, it is time to sit down to discuss what can or should be done differently the next time. Feedback includes receiving complaints as well as indicators that something is not meeting customer expectations.
- *External environment* refers to anything outside the system that affects how it functions (for example, laws or regulations set by the local, state, or federal government). External factors that affect how the system functions include:
  —The HIPAA regulations related to patient information security
  —Medicare's Conditions of Participation requirements for what must be kept in a patient's medical record
  —The ICD-9 (soon to be ICD-10) coding systems, which drive the reimbursement systems in hospitals
  —A tight labor market, which makes it difficult to find well-educated employees

Systems such as those described here also are called **open systems** because they are affected by what is going on around them and must adjust as the environment changes and **cybernetic systems** because they have standards, controls, and feedback mechanisms built into them. On the other hand, a **closed system** operates in a self-contained environment; that is, it is not affected by outside factors. A mechanical system (engines, motors, and so on) is the best example of a closed system.

Thus, work improvement, process improvement, and methods improvement are simply three different phrases that are very closely related as concepts. They all relate to systematic approaches that managers take to determine what needs to be changed in the systems they manage in order to get the systems to meet expectations.

The aim, then, of all performance/method/process improvement efforts is to determine why actual output varies from expected output and then to take actions to increase the effect.

- *Effectiveness* indicates how closely the output from a process matches what is expected of the process. If a department is effective, it is getting done what it is supposed to get done.
- *Efficiency,* on the other hand, indicates how well the department is using its resources. Is it getting the most bang for its buck, or is it wasting time, money, energy, and other resources?
- *Adaptability* refers to the ease with which the system can adjust when circumstances require it to change to meet new demands or expectations. Adaptable systems respond appropriately to changing needs.

Customer Service

Customers are the people, external and internal, who receive and are affected by the work the healthcare facility does. They have names and needs, and are the reason(s) for the collective work of the organization.

Internal customers are located within the organization. They may be anyone within the work unit who is affected by the HIS function. Physicians and clinical staff need high-quality, expedient patient health information in order to deliver high-quality patient care. Administrative staff members are customers of the information harvested from collective databases for use in planning facilities and services. And not the least of internal customers are the HIM associates who rely on HIS to provide access to timely, reliable data to assist in clinical decision making.

External customers reside outside the organization. Physicians seen by patients who originated at the facility for care are considered external customers, as are purchasers and payers who need information so they can reimburse their enrollees in a timely manner. Regulatory agencies look to HIS for data on conditions of accreditation or participation. Vendors assist HIS, with the department's direct input, in making optimal selections of products. Communities look to HIS for information and data on their state of collective health and to earmark services the population needs to maintain a healthy existence.

All process improvement environments today focus on the customer and work to create a true customer orientation within the work environment by listening and responding to customers, thinking about their needs, and using that information to modify and improve the way our systems work for them.

In the process of customer orientation, management and staff must:

- Identify who the customers are
- Define quality from a customer perspective
- Determine how to judge service
- Obtain regular feedback

The Joint Commission on Accreditation of Healthcare Organizations (JCAHO) has standards that specifically require accredited organizations to have PI efforts as an integral aspect of their day-to-day operations, as follows:

PI.1. The leaders establish a planned, systematic, organization-wide approach to process design, performance measurement, analysis, and improvement.

PI.2. New or modified processes are well designed.

PI.3. Data are collected to monitor the stability of existing processes, identify opportunities for improvement, identify changes that will lead to improvement, and sustain improvement.

PI.4. Data are systematically aggregated and analyzed on an ongoing basis.

PI.5. Improved performance is achieved and sustained.

Performance Improvement Methodologies

Three principal methodologies are available to healthcare facilities interested in PI: **systems analysis and design, continuous quality improvement,** and **reengineering.** All three approaches have the same goal and use many of the same tools. However, they differ in focus and breadth of improvement effort.

Systems Analysis and Design

Systems analysis and design can be applied to any type of system. For example, it can be applied to the selection of a new information system or it can be applied to the redesign of a work process. Included in this section are discussions of the concept of **systems thinking,** steps of the systems analysis and design process, and tools frequently used in systems analysis and design.

Systems Thinking

When considering PI< a fundamental concept to understand is systems thinking. Systems thinking has been defined as "a conceptual framework, a body of knowledge and tools that have been developed over the past fifty years, to make patterns clearer and to help us see how to make changes effectively in the system" (Senge 1990, p. 7). It enables us to recognize and better view a process in its entirety, rather than just focusing on its individual parts.

It is impossible to appropriately examine systems, detect potential problems, and offer constructive suggestions without understanding what systems are and how they work. All organizations, departments, and work units can be viewed as systems. Johns defines a system as "a group of components that have the ability to self-adapt and that interact through defined relationships working to accomplish a goal or objective" (1997, p. 310). (From this definition, it is clear that a variety of entities that have complex, interrelated elements working together toward a common purpose are systems.)

Systems may be classified as:

- *Mechanical:* A heating and air-conditioning system is an example of a mechanical system.

- *Human:* A human system would be a family unit or employees working in a particular department.

- *Man–machine:* A man–machine system relies on either human–human interactions or human–technology interactions, for example, a monitoring system for patient care or a unit in HIM that uses the organization's health information system.

Most complex systems have numerous subsystems, and these subsystems frequently have still smaller subsystems.

All systems and subsystems are affected by resource constraints and are subject to certain controls. Controls may originate from within the entity or from outside. Internal controls include organizational policies and procedures or the prevailing organizational culture that helps shape and influence the organizational norms and values of the employees operating in the system. External controls include laws, regulations, or societal values. Both internal and external controls shape and constrain the system to function in a particular manner.

As mentioned earlier, all systems and subsystems have four components: inputs, conversion processes, outputs, and a feedback loop. Inputs may include the knowledge, abilities, skills, and attitudes of employees, as well as supplies and equipment. They are processed in some manner and transformed into an output. The actual output is then compared to the anticipated output to determine whether it complies with what was expected. This information is the feedback. In most cases, good inputs and good processes produce desirable outputs. The feedback loop is critical for determining whether changes should be made with either the input component or the process component to produce an actual output that is in line with the expected output.

Outputs of subsystems frequently become inputs of other subsystems. Consider a new patient being seen in a physician office. This encounter initiates a number of systems. Looking at the system from a macro level, the inputs would be the patient, the physician, the physician's staff, and the computer and instruments the physician used. The conversion processes could include registration, examination, assessment, treatment, and reimbursement. The outputs for the patient might be prescriptions and a bill or receipt.

However, a closer examination of the patient–physician encounter reveals activation of multiple subsystems, each with its own inputs, conversion processes, outputs, and feedback. For example, the registration process is a subsystem consisting of several smaller subsystems. The patient first completes the information form. The pencil, the patient's knowledge, and the patient's insurance card are all inputs into this subsystem. As the patient completes the form, he is engaging in the process. The completed form is the output.

The output of the registration subsystem becomes the input for the next subsystem initiated. The receptionist takes the completed form and, using the computer and her knowledge of the process (inputs), enters the patient's data into the practice information system (process). At this point, the output is the start of the encounter form. The physician uses the registration information as input, along with interview information, and then begins to examine the patient (process). After completing the examination, the physician may make notes in the patient's chart, write some prescriptions, and complete a form noting what was done so that the clerk can generate a form for billing.

The Systems Analysis and Design Process

The systems analysis and design process includes six distinct steps:

1. *Determine the need for the system and the system requirements.* The need for the system is often expressed as objectives established by management. Information must be obtained on the purpose of the system. Interviewing the people who participate and interact with the system is one way to determine the system requirements.

2. *Analyze the system requirements.* System analysis involves gathering, organizing, and evaluating facts about the current system. Data may be gathered by interviewing employees who participate in or interact with the system, conducting a focus group, administering a survey, reading organizational documents, and so on. The facts then must be organized in some systematic, meaningful way (for example, according to problems or steps in the process). The information then can be evaluated to determine whether the system's goal or purpose is being achieved currently in the most efficient and effective manner or whether it could be better achieved through a redesign.

3. *Propose a system design or redesign.* Actually designing the new system requires input from many personnel. Both managers and employees must buy in to the potential benefits of the new or redesigned system and be committed to working out the "bugs" that always accompany the implementation of something new. A number of systems or redesigns should be considered. From these alternatives, the design that seems to have the best potential for producing the desired outcome should be selected.

4. *Evaluate the proposed system.* Evaluation of the proposed system must take into consideration its impact on all the system components. Does the proposed system appear capable of meeting organizational goals and satisfying employee needs? Critical success factors should be developed that permit comparison of what is wanted with what is actually produced. At this point, it may be helpful to pilot-test the proposed system on a small scale to see how well it meets its objectives. Data should be collected and compared to the critical success factors identified earlier. Conducting a small test of change can provide valuable information and perhaps spare the organization the expense of implementing a system that may have unanticipated and negative consequences. If the proposed system appears to meet the criteria for success, it is ready to be implemented.

5. *Implement the system.* The implementation phase takes a great deal of time and planning. For example, the people involved in the system change must be given adequate training. Documentation of the changes, accompanied by **flowcharts** and revised policies and procedures, also can contribute to a smooth transition. Information obtained during the pilot test mentioned above may be used to facilitate the implementation organization-wide.

6. *Conduct ongoing evaluation and maintenance of the system.* Systems, particularly new and newly revised systems, will always need monitoring and maintenance to ensure that they are providing the desired results. Again, it may be helpful to think about the feedback loop. A method should be included in the design that would indicate whether the system is performing as expected.

Basic Tools of Systems Analysis

Tools are frequently used to gather the facts used in systems analysis. Three tools that provide valuable information on work flow and employee work activities are the work distribution chart, the movement diagram, and the **flow process chart.**

Work Distribution Chart

A work distribution chart can be very helpful in determining the nature of the work being performed in the unit, which employees are performing the activities, and the amount of time spent on each activity. As mentioned earlier, a work distribution chart shows job activities, time spent on them, and the names or titles of the employees who perform them. It can be very helpful in determining whether adequate time is available and appropriate for each task and whether employees are overburdened or have time for additional responsibilities. In addition, it can help the manager assess whether the work is organized and distributed appropriately.

Work distribution charts can be formulated in a variety of ways but frequently are tables with work tasks forming the row headings and a double column of employee names and hours spent on tasks forming the column headings. (See table 23.1, p. 649.) Data for the work distribution chart come from self-reported activities and hours or parts of hours spent on tasks gathered by employees over a designated period of time. Actual data collection time varies depending on what is needed to get a representative sample of activities and times. When adequate data have been collected, the manager compiles them, clusters similar job tasks together, and completes the chart.

Movement Diagram

A movement diagram is a visual depiction of the layout of the workspace with all the furniture, equipment, doorways, and so on sketched in. Superimposed on the layout are the movements of either individuals or things (for example, documents, files, etc). (See figure 23.2, p. 655.) The movement diagram can be used to evaluate the workflow and to redesign one that is more efficient. An inefficient workflow is depicted in figure 23.2 (top), that is, long distances between connected points in the workflow, crisscrossing paths and paths that backtrack in the work space. A redesigned movement diagram in figure 23.2 (bottom) depicts a smoother workflow resulting in improved efficiency.

Flow Process Chart

A flow process chart is useful in operations analysis. (See figure 23.8.) It charts the flow of work of a material or a task but is limited to the flow of only one unit at a time. Each step of a particular process is shown in chronological order and in great detail (for example, the distance a material moves in each step, the time needed, the quantity moved, and specific notes about the process). Standard symbols are used on the chart to indicate specific processes. An operation is symbolized with a circle, transportation with an arrow, storage with a triangle, inspection with a rectangle, and a delay with a figure resembling an uppercase *D*. When the symbols are connected with a line, the manager can see the actual flow of work.

The flow process chart is an excellent method for indicating time problems with work flow. It can show duplication and inefficiency and also can be very useful in verifying procedures or planning a workstation redesign (Liebler, Levine,

and Rothman 1992). Some flow process charts include two charts in one, a chart showing the current flow of work and a second chart proposing a redesigned work flow.

Check Your Understanding 23.2

Instructions: On a separate sheet of paper, indicate whether the following sentences are true or false and correct any false statement to make it true or to explain why it is false on a separate sheet of paper.

1. The output of one system is frequently the conversion process of another system.

2. A change that may result in an improvement in one subsystem may also cause a problem in a related subsystem or in the larger system.

3. One purpose for conducting a systems analysis is to determine if a redesign of the current system is necessary.

4. Pilot tests are sometimes helpful but often require more effort to implement than is warranted.

Continuous Quality Improvement

Continuous quality improvement (CQI), frequently referred to as total quality management (TQM) or service excellence, is a management philosophy that seeks to "involve healthcare personnel in planning and executing a continuous flow of improvements to provide quality health care that meets or exceeds expectations" (McLaughlin and Kaluzny 1999, p. 3). Its focus is on improving the quality of services provided to customers, whether internal (employees) or external (patients, physicians, payers). The approach is to make efforts to meet or exceed customer expectations by conducting small tests of

Figure 23.8.   Flow process chart

	PRESENT		PROPOSED		DIFFERENCE		
	NO.	TIME	NO.	TIME	NO.	TIME	
◯ OPERATIONS							Job_____
TRANSPORTATIONS							Date_____
☐ INSPECTIONS							Man Material
D DELAYS							
▽ STORAGES							Chartered by _____
DISTANCE TRAVELED		FT.		FT.		FT.	

DETAILS OF (PRESENT/PROPOSED) METHOD	OPERATION	TRANSPORT.	INSPECTION	DELAY	STORAGE	DISTANCE IN FEET	QUANTITY	TIME	ANALYSIS — WHY	NOTES	ACTION — CHANGE
1	◯		☐	D	▽						
2	◯		☐	D	▽						
3	◯		☐	D	▽						
4	◯		☐	D	▽						
5	◯		☐	D	▽						
6	◯		☐	D	▽						

change aimed at improving the quality of services. Of course, not all customer expectations can be met at the same time. In fact, some customers have expectations that conflict with the expectations of other customers. However, the goal is worth pursuing, even when only partly achievable.

CQI casts off the notion of ignoring problems until they become too big to ignore. Rather, it subscribes to the theory of seeking ways to improve the system through the testing of small, incremental changes with the expectation that, over time, the changes will continually improve the quality of care that health facilities provide to their patients (Berwick 1989). To achieve this, CQI relies on the gathering and analysis of data that can be used to make informed decisions.

More than the latest buzzword in healthcare, CQI is a way of thinking, a way of being, a way of managing, a way of conducting business. It can be applied to individuals as well as organizations. The expression "If it ain't broke, don't fix it" is alien to the CQI philosophy. Moreover, CQI does not seek to blame problems on individuals but, instead, suggests that systems or processes may have inherent flaws that contribute to problems.

CQI attempts to involve people in the examination and improvement of existing systems. Several principles are incorporated into the CQI philosophy, including:

- *Constancy of variation:* Systems will always produce some normal variation in their output; the manager's job is to reduce the amount of variation as much as possible so that the process can become more stable and produce a more reliable output. Managers should not assume that any variation is a defect but, rather, should monitor and measure data over time to ensure that any variation is, in fact, caused inherently by the system. This type of variation is **common cause variation.** A greater-than-expected variation is a **special cause variation.** Sometimes a change is initiated with the express purpose of producing an improvement effort, in which case it should be encouraged. Other times, changes result in negative outputs and these must be eliminated.

  An example of variation in HIS departments might be found in the coding and processing of records. A coder may complete 20 records one day, but only 18 the next. The variation is not due to the clerk's lack of productivity, but perhaps to the size of the records that day. In other words, the change is attributed to common cause variation. A significant drop in coding might indicate that a special cause is in effect. Perhaps the coder was assigned duties that day in addition to coding.

- *Importance of data:* Far too often, decisions for improvement are based on faulty assumptions. CQI recognizes the importance of collecting sufficient data so that informed decisions can be made. Omachonu states "that the ability to collect, analyze, and use data is a vital component of a successful performance improvement process. Health-

care organizations that do not devote sufficient attention to data collection may be able to speak of only marginal success in their process improvement journey" (1999, p. 71). Individuals planning a CQI effort must take time to develop appropriate data collection methods and instruments (written surveys, direct observation, focus group interviews, reviews of medical records with criteria forms). Appropriate analysis must follow data collection to provide the knowledge on which improvement efforts can be built (White 2002).

- *Vision and support of executive leadership:* CQI gurus such as W. Edwards Deming and Brian Joiner stress that acceptance of the CQI philosophy must funnel down from the top to truly permeate the organization's culture. Executive leadership must communicate a clear vision and mission statement that every employee can understand and share.

- *Focus on customers:* To be successful, the organization must know and understand what its customers need and want. One way to obtain customer feedback is to administer satisfaction surveys on a regular basis. Any needs that are identified should be addressed.

- *Investment in people:* The CQI philosophy assumes that people want to do their jobs well. However, because this philosophy is relatively new, some employees may need training on how they can more adequately serve their customers. Management can empower employees by giving them opportunities to learn and grow and feel more competent in performing their jobs.

- *Importance of teams:* Because CQI seeks to improve processes that may extend beyond the boundaries of individual departments, the people directly involved with the processes must work together. Teams should include individuals with different expertise and from different levels of the organization. Team members should be knowledgeable about portions of the process and able to contribute to the improvement effort. Having members from different areas on the team brings fresh perspectives and opens communication. A good team also is able to communicate its purpose and activities to other parts of the organization.

Improvement Models

Several models exist for structuring PI. One that is frequently used in hospitals is Hospital Corporation of America's FOCUS-PDCA model. This model includes five steps before initiating its PDCA (Plan, Do, Check, Act) cycle (described below in the Foundation for Improvement Model as the **PDSA Cycle**). The five initial steps of the FOCUS-PDCA include:

1. Find a process to improve.
2. Organize a team that knows the process.
3. Clarify the current knowledge of the process.
4. Understand causes of special variation.
5. Select the process improvement.

A different, but highly effective, model that can be used for any process targeted for improvement is the Langley, Nolan, and Nolan Foundation for Improvement Model (1994). It is presented here because of its simplicity. The model has two parts. The first part requires an individual or team to answer three fundamental questions; the second part requires initiation of the PDSA cycle.

The three fundamental questions that must be answered for any improvement project are:

- *What is my aim?* This question forces the responder to determine his or her overall goal.
- *How will I know a change is an improvement?* This question requires the responder to define measures (preferably quantitative, but also some qualitative) that will indicate progress made toward his or her goal. These measures will enable the individual or team to collect data.
- *What changes have the potential to result in improvement?* This question requires the responder to brainstorm a number of changes that might lead to improvement. He or she must recognize that not all changes do result in improvement.

After changes have been brainstormed, one change deemed to have significant potential for effecting improvement should be tried. This is a small test of change made with one change strategy. If it is successful, other changes may be added. The change strategy is tested using the PDSA cycle.

PDSA stands for Plan, Do, Study, and Act. It is actually a trial and learning cycle. (See figure 23.9.) The phases of the cycle break down as follows:

1. During the plan phase, preparations are made for implementing the selected change. This is the time to consider who, what, where, when, and how. In addition, this is the time to plan how to collect data that will be used in determining the progress of the implementation. It may be necessary to develop a data collection instrument. Having already determined what the measurements will be, it also may be necessary to collect baseline data before

implementing the change. Finally, this phase is the time to decide how often and how long to collect data before the results are analyzed.

2. During the do phase, the change strategy is implemented and data are collected. Perhaps the change strategy and the data collection will go on for two weeks before the analysis. The length of time depends on how frequently data were collected and how long the PDSA cycle is intended to last.

3. During the study phase, the data are analyzed. Is progress being made toward the defined aim? Are there any unanticipated problems? This phase indicates whether a change is an improvement. If it appears to be, the decision will likely be to continue the change strategy. If it is not showing as much improvement as expected, it may be necessary to adjust the change strategy. If it shows no improvement, it may be time to abandon the change strategy and test another one.

4. During the act phase, the knowledge obtained from the PDSA trial and learning cycle is applied, which leads to three possible actions: continue with the current change strategy, adjust it, or try a new one. At this point, a second PDSA cycle is implemented to continue the quest for knowledge about what affects the process and what permits progress. The more knowledge, the greater the likelihood of a successful improvement effort.

Basic CQI Techniques and Tools

A number of tools and techniques are frequently used with PI initiatives (Brassard and Ritter 1993; Johnson and McLaughlin 1999; Cofer and Greeley 1993). Some of them are used to facilitate communication among employees; others are used to assist people in determining the root causes of problems. Some tools show areas of agreement or consensus among team members; others permit the display of data for easier analysis. The following section presents a brief description and discussion of the purpose of tools and techniques commonly used by improvement teams (White 2002).

Brainstorming

Brainstorming is a technique used to generate a large number of creative ideas. It encourages team members to think "out of the box" and offer ideas. There are some variations in using the technique—one can use an unstructured method for brainstorming or a structured method. The unstructured method involves having a free flow of ideas about a situation. The team leader writes down each idea as it is offered so all can see. There should be no evaluative discussion about the worthiness of the idea because we want to do nothing that will inhibit the flow of ideas. Each idea is captured and written for the team to consider at a later point.

Structured brainstorming uses a more formal approach. The team leader asks each person to generate a list of ideas for themselves and then, one by one, the team leader proceeds around the room eliciting a new idea from each mem-

Figure 23.9.   PDSA cycles expedite improvement

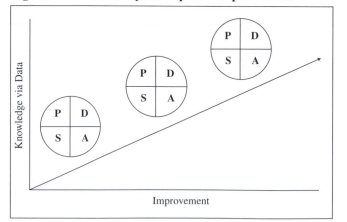

ber. The process may take several rounds. As team members run out of new ideas, they pass and the next person offers an idea until no one can produce any fresh ideas.

Brainstorming is highly effective for identifying a number of potential processes that may benefit from improvement efforts and for generating solutions to particular problems. It helps people to begin thinking in new ways and gets them involved in the process. It is an excellent method for facilitating open communication.

Affinity Grouping

Affinity grouping allows the team to organize and group similar ideas together. Ideas that are generated in a brainstorming session may be written on Post-it notes and arranged on a table or posted on a board. Without talking to each other, each team member is asked to walk around the table or board, look at the ideas, and place them in groupings that seem related or connected to each other. Each member is empowered to move the ideas in a way that makes the most sense. As a team member moves the ideas back or places them in other groupings, the other team members consider the merits of the placement and decide if further action is needed. The goal is to have the team eventually feel comfortable with the arrangement. The natural groupings that emerge are then labeled with a category. This tool brings focus to the many ideas generated. (See figure 23.10.)

Nominal Group Technique

Nominal group technique (NGT) is a process designed to bring agreement about an issue or an idea that the team considers most important. It produces and permits visualization of team consensus. In NGT, each team member ranks each idea according to its importance. For example, if there were six ideas, the idea that is most important would be given the number 6. The second most important idea would be given the number 5. The least important idea would have the number 1. After each team member has individually ranked the list of ideas, the numbers are totaled. The ideas that are deemed most important are clearly visible to all. Those ideas that people did not think were as important are also made known with their low scores. NGT demonstrates where the team's priorities lie.

Figure 23.10.   Affinity grouping

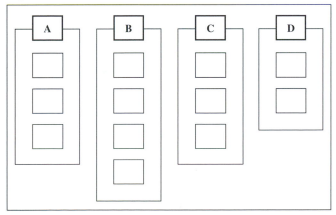

Multivoting Technique

The **multivoting technique** is a variation of NGT and has the same purpose. Rather than ranking each issue or idea, team members are asked to rate the issue using a distribution of points or colorful dots. Weighted multivoting is a variation of this process. For example, a team member may be asked to distribute 25 points among ten total issues. Thus, one issue of particular importance to him may receive 12 points, four others may receive some variation of the remaining 12 points, and five others may receive no points. After the voting, the numbers are added and the team is able to see which issue has emerged as particularly important to the team.

This process also can be done with colored dots. For example, if there are eight items on a chart, each team member may be given four dots to distribute on the four items that are most important to him or her. This method particularly enables team members to see where consensus lies and what issue has been deemed most important by the team as a whole.

Flowchart

Whenever a team examines a process with the intention of making improvement, it must first thoroughly understand the process. Each team member comes to the team with a unique perspective and significant insight about how a portion of the process works. To help all members understand the process, a team will undertake development of a flowchart. (See figure 23.1, p. 653.) This work allows the team to thoroughly understand every step in the process and the sequence of steps. It provides a picture of each decision point and each event that must be completed. It readily points out places where there is redundancy and complex and problematic areas.

Root-Cause Analysis (Fishbone Diagram)

When a team first identifies a problem, it may use a **fishbone diagram,** also known as a cause-and-effect diagram, to help it determine the root causes of the problem. (See figure 23.11, p. 674.) The problem is placed in a box on the right side of the paper. A horizontal line is drawn, somewhat like a backbone, with diagonal bones, like ribs, pointing to the boxes above and below the backbone. Each box contains a category. The categories may be names that represent broad classifications of problem areas (for example, people, methods, equipment, materials, policies/procedures, environment, measurement, and so on). The team determines how many categories it needs to classify all the sources of problems. Usually, there are about four. After constructing the diagram, the team brainstorms possible sources of the problem. These are then placed on horizontal lines extending from the diagonal category line. The brainstorming of root causes continues among team members until all ideas are exhausted. The purpose of this tool is to permit a team to explore, identify, and graphically display all the root causes of a problem.

After identifying a number of causes of a problem, a team may decide to begin working to remove one of them. CQI involves continually making efforts to improve processes;

Figure 23.11.   Fishbone diagram

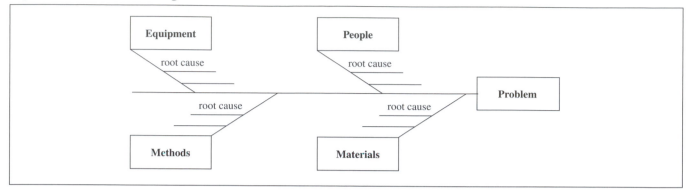

certainly removing one cause and then working to remove another cause will eventually improve the process. The question may arise, however, about which cause to remove first. Techniques such as multivoting or NGT, discussed above, can help bring consensus among the team about what to work on first.

Pareto Chart

When a team decides to use multivoting or NGT to determine consensus among the members about the most important problem to tackle first, each team member places a number or mark next to an item indicating his or her opinion about the item's importance. When the numbers are tallied, the items can be ranked according to importance. This ranking can then be visually displayed in a **Pareto chart.** (See figure 23.12.) A Pareto chart looks very much like a bar chart except that the highest-ranking item is listed first, followed by the second highest, down to the lowest-ranked item. Thus, the Pareto chart is a descending bar chart. This visualization of how the problems were ranked allows team members to focus on those few that have the greatest potential for improving the process. The Pareto chart is based on the Pareto principle, which states that 20 percent of the sources of the problem are responsible for 80 percent of the actual problems. By concentrating on the vital few sources, a large number of actual problems can be eliminated.

Force-Field Analysis

A **force-field analysis** also visually displays data generated through brainstorming. The team leader draws a large T formation on a board. (See figure 23.13.) Above the crossbar and on the left side of the *T* is written the word *drivers,* and above the bar and written on the right side of the *T* is written the word *barriers.* Team members are then asked to brainstorm and list on the chart under the crossbar the reasons or factors that would contribute to a change for improvement and those reasons or factors that can create barriers. Thus, the force field enables team members to identify factors that support or work against a proposed solution. Often the next step in this activity is to work on ways that either eliminate barriers or reinforce drivers.

Figure 23.12.   Pareto chart

Figure 23.13.   Force-field analysis

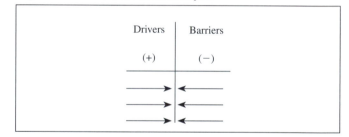

Check Sheet

A **check sheet** is a data collection tool permitting the recording and compiling of observations or occurrences. It consists of a simple listing of categories, issues, or observations on the left side of the chart and a place on the right for individuals to record checkmarks next to the item when it is observed or counted. (See figure 23.14.) After a period of time, the checkmarks are counted and the patterns or trends can be revealed.

A check sheet is a simple tool that allows a clear picture of the facts to emerge. It enables data to be collected. After data are collected, several tools can be used to display the data and help the team more easily analyze them.

Scatter Diagram

A **scatter diagram** is data analysis tool used to plot points of two variables suspected of being related to each other in some way. For example, to see whether age and blood pressure are related, one variable, age, would be plotted on one line of the graph, and the other variable, blood pressure, would be plotted on the other line. After several people's blood pressures are plotted along with their ages, a pattern might emerge. If the diagram indicates that blood pressure increases with age, the data could be interpreted as revealing a positive relationship between age and blood pressure. (See figure 23.15.)

In some cases, a negative relationship might exist, such as with the variables "age" and "flexibility" or with the number of hours of training and number of mistakes made. Whenever a scatter diagram indicates that the points are moving together in one direction or another, conclusions can be drawn about the variables' relationship, either positive or negative. In other cases, however, the scatter diagram may indicate no linear relationship between the variables because the points are scattered haphazardly and no pattern emerges. In this case, the conclusion would have to be that the two variables have no apparent relationship.

Histogram

A **histogram** (figure 23.16) is a data analysis tool used to display frequencies of response. (See also chapter 15.) It offers a much easier way to summarize and analyze data than having them displayed in a table of numbers. A histogram displays **continuous data** values that have been grouped into categories. The bars on the histogram reveal how the data are distributed. For example, an HIM administrator may want to show the number of minutes it takes to respond to patient requests for information. Minutes may be categorized into four groupings, for example, 1–30 minutes, 31–60 minutes, 61–90 minutes, and more than 90 minutes. Checkmarks may be recorded indicating the category of minutes taken to respond to the request. After a period of time, the checkmarks are added and the histogram is plotted with the frequencies shown on the vertical, or *y* axis, and the minute intervals shown on the horizontal, or *x* axis.

This graph indicates the different intervals patients had to wait for their requests to be filled. A histogram can give an excellent idea of how well a process is performing. Thus, it can show how frequently data values occur among the various intervals, how centered or skewed the distribution of data is, and what the likelihood of future occurrences is.

Run Chart

A **run chart** displays data points over a period of time to provide information about performance. (See figure 23.17.) Measured points of a process are plotted on a graph at regular time intervals to help team members see whether there are substantial changes in the numbers over time. For example, suppose an HIS manager wanted to reduce the number of incomplete records in the HIS department. The manager might first plot on a graph the number of incomplete records each month for the past six months and then enact a change in the processing of records designed to improve the process.

Figure 23.14.   Check sheet

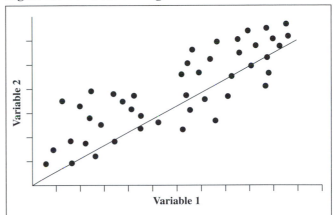

	1	2	Total
A	⊬⊬⊬	/ / /	8
B	/ / / /	/ / / /	8
C	/ /	/	3

Figure 23.15.   Scatter diagram

Figure 23.16.   Histogram

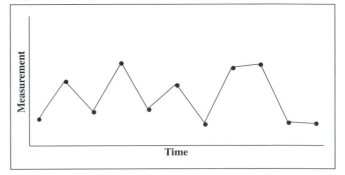

Figure 23.17.   Run chart

Following the improvement effort, data would continue to be collected on the number of incomplete records and would continue to be plotted on the graph. If the run chart shows that the number of incomplete charts has actually decreased, the HIS manager could attribute the decrease to the improvement effort.

A run chart is an excellent tool for providing visual verification of how a process is performing and whether an improvement effort appears to have worked.

Statistical Process Control Chart

A **statistical process control** (SPC) chart looks very much like a run chart except that it has a line displayed at the top, called an upper control limit (UCL), and a line displayed at the bottom, called a lower control limit (LCL). (See figure 23.18.) These lines have been statistically calculated from the data generated in the process and represent three units of dispersion above and below the midline (three standard deviations) (Omachonu 1999).

Like the run chart, the SPC chart plots points over time to demonstrate how a process is performing. However, the two control limit lines enable the interpreter to determine whether the process is stable, or predictable, or whether it is out of control. CQI statisticians Walter Shewhart and W. Edwards Deming first presented the idea of variation that routinely occurs in systems. Remembering the constancy of variation principle, it is easy to see the purpose of the SPC chart. The SPC chart indicates whether the variation occurring within the process is a common cause variation or a special cause variation. It indicates whether it is necessary to try and reduce the ordinary variation occurring through common cause or to seek out a special cause of the variation and try to eliminate it.

Six Sigma

Healthcare historically has been a follower with regard to CQI methods. Industry icon, Motorola, was one of the first high-profile companies to realize the benefits of the **Six Sigma** quality path in the 1980s under new leadership. When Motorola won the coveted Malcolm Baldridge National Quality Award in 1988, the "best-kept secret" was suddenly on the lips of all the nations' CEOs. That best-kept secret, in actuality, is not innovative in the sense that it is new knowledge; actually, it embraces tenets similar to Deming's PDCA. More emphatically, it is a culmination of "old notions" with a technology twist: data informatics. The evidence that gave the old innovation a new visibility is the evidence that success of the Six Sigma initiative is modeled and measured by data that are collected, cleaned, and considered strategically both in the lines of service and as an outcome. They are data that are, in most cases, already being captured, but not leveraged.

Some doubted that the likes of Six Sigma could be applied to the healthcare industry, in part or at large, because of the human variability of patients. However, the 1991 Institute of Medicine report highlighting the alarming statistic of 98,000 deaths linked to medical errors soon resulted in a movement to review statistical data in the healthcare industry with industry eyes. Industry is customer driven and so is healthcare. Industry relies on feedback regarding success and failure in relevant data and so does healthcare. Healthcare leaders became invested in enlisting this philosophy of excellence, reducing costs, lowering lengths of stay, and raising the bar for high-quality healthcare. The healthcare industry leaders that have embraced Six Sigma are quick to share their successes as the industry continues to come to understand the richness of the data that are captured and how to understand their inherent value. (For more information on Six Sigma, visit http://www.isixsigma.com.}

Business Process Reengineering

Unlike CQI, which focuses on conducting small tests of change to achieve continuous, but incremental, improvement over time, business process reengineering focuses on the potential revamping of the entire process from head to toe to achieve improvement. (See table 23.12 for a comparison of reengineering and quality management.) Reengineering implies making massive changes to the way a facility delivers healthcare services. In *Reengineering the Corporation: A Manifesto for Business Revolution,* Hammer and Champy (1993) defined reengineering as "the fundamental rethinking and radical redesign of business processes to achieve

Figure 23.18.   Statistical process control chart

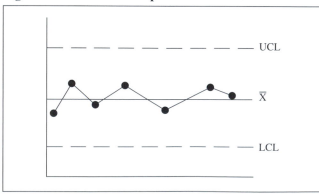

Table 23.12.   Reengineering compared to quality management

Reengineering		Quality Management	
Rethinking and Radical Redesign	Focus	Incremental Improvements	Focus
Rethink	Think out of the box	Quality planning	Focus on the customer
Redesign	Think both process and outcome	Quality control	Measure and monitor performance
Retool	Use technology to control and define work processes	Quality improvement	Use data, eliminate boundaries, and empower work

dramatic improvements in critical contemporary measures of performance such as cost, quality, service, and speed" (McBrierty 1995, p. 46).

Philosophy of Reengineering

Business process reengineering has entered the healthcare sector after first being successfully applied in the wider business community. In reengineering, the entire manner and purpose of a work process is questioned. The goal is to achieve the desired process outcome in the most effective and efficient manner possible. Thus, the results expected from reengineering efforts include:

- Increased productivity
- Decreased costs
- Improved quality
- Maximized revenue
- More satisfied customers

However, it should be clearly understood that the main focus is on reducing costs (Palmer 1995).

Used extensively in the mid-1980s and early 1990s, reengineering has met with significant criticism in the healthcare sector because of the fear it has invoked among healthcare workers. As would be expected, reengineering frequently results in the loss of jobs. Because salaries and benefits comprise 50 to 60 percent of a healthcare facility's total expenses, a drop in personnel can have a significant impact on reducing expenditures and is often used as an effective strategy in reengineering.

Process of Reengineering

When an organization decides to use reengineering as an improvement strategy, it commits itself to looking at selected processes within the organization in fine detail. Processes are selected for reengineering based on a number of criteria, including:

- Frequency and severity of problems created by the process, such as slow turnaround time or excessive waiting time
- Impact on customer satisfaction
- Complex processes involving multiple departments, procedures, and employees
- The feasibility of actually creating improvement (Umiker 1998)

Selecting a process for reengineering raises several questions, including:

- What is the intended purpose of the process? Is that purpose being accomplished efficiently?
- Is the process absolutely necessary? Could any redundancies or non-value-added activities be eliminated?
- Which employees are involved in the process, and which ones are actually needed? In other words, what are the minimum qualifications and minimum number of employees needed to do the job?

- Is the process as efficient as it could be, or are there more efficient means for accomplishing the goal?
- Is the process contributing to the efficiency of other processes that may be affected by its results?
- Is there an opportunity to combine processes and to train or use employees to perform more functions than they currently perform?
- Can any steps of the process be eliminated?
- Is outsourcing a feasible and more cost-effective alternative?
- Would new equipment or new technologies improve the process?

Many of the tools and techniques used in systems analysis and CQI also are used in reengineering. In reengineering, it is essential to thoroughly understand how the process contributes to how the organization functions and to determine whether a better method exists. Therefore, observation of processes, customer input, interviews with employees, and the use of cross-functional teams to discuss the current steps of the process are frequently used methods for obtaining data. Data must be collected for a sufficient period of time to actually reflect the effectiveness of the process.

In addition, the data must be analyzed appropriately and the analysis should include the input of individuals qualified to interpret the findings. Thus, a team composed of individuals involved in various aspects of the process should be permitted access to the data and should give input about alternative strategies. Moreover, the team can investigate the acceptability of new technologies that might allow for greater efficiency. Before new technologies are adopted, however, the team should thoroughly analyze the potential benefits, costs, and feasibility of using them in the organization.

After a reengineered process has emerged, new policies and procedures must be written and distributed to the people involved in the process. In addition, employees should be thoroughly trained in the redesigned process. However, it is very important that they be given adequate time to master the process. Managers play an important role in reengineering through their support, encouragement, and commitment to the process.

Factors for Success in Reengineering Efforts

One critical factor for the success of the reengineering effort is the visible and persistent commitment of senior administration. A second critical factor is management's commitment to excellence. Managers must demonstrate a can-do attitude in working through the change. In addition, the fact that change is needed to address an unacceptable problem must be effectively communicated throughout the organization. Having everyone, or almost everyone, acknowledge that a problem exists creates a great deal of buy-in. Employees, including physicians, should be encouraged to overcome any reluctance to participate in the change process due to fears about restructuring. Many healthcare organizations make the mistake of not including their physicians in critical decision making. The likelihood of a successful reengineering effort increases when every stakeholder is involved in the process.

Reengineering takes anywhere from one to three years to achieve. The organization should realize that change cannot be achieved overnight and should avoid trying to change too many processes at one time. Instead, it should focus its efforts on a few processes at a time. A great deal of planning, information gathering, and analysis must occur before an actual redesign can be implemented. When the planning phase has been completed, the organization should revise or develop policies and procedures accordingly and distribute them throughout the organization.

Finally, implementation of the redesigned processes requires patience. Glitches may occur with any new system, but with careful monitoring and persistent adjusting, reengineering can produce significant PI.

Check Your Understanding 23.3

Instructions: On a separate piece of paper, indicate whether the following statements are true or false. Then correct any false statement to make it true or explain why it is false.

1. ___ The goal of CQI—to meet and/or exceed the expectations of all the organization's customers—is generally attainable and achievable.

2. ___ A manager's job with regard to performance improvement is to seek ways to reduce the amount of normal variation that occurs within systems and processes.

3. ___ Obtaining and using actual data to inform managers who need to make decisions is a critically important element of the CQI philosophy.

4. ___ Six Sigma came to the attention of healthcare CEOs in the late 1990s as a completely new and innovative approach to managing quality and cost in healthcare.

5. ___ Reengineering is particularly focused on efficiency.

Real-World Case

On January 4, 2001, the *New York Times* published an article about an innovative redesign of the appointment system at the Kaiser Permanente Medical Center in Roseville, California. The physician office practice appeared very successful: the waiting rooms were usually filled with patients, and the appointment books showed several weeks of nonemergency patient appointments. Of course, problems would routinely occur when patients needed to be seen immediately and worked into the schedule. This situation usually backed up everything and created long waits. Patients, who already were feeling ill and irritated, became more irritated and physicians and staff had to apologize and find something or someone else to blame. In addition to creating an uncomfortable situation for everyone, the physicians often had to work longer hours than expected to see all their patients.

Dr. Mark Murray, a family practice physician, questioned whether there might not be a better way to manage the situation. However, his colleagues assured him that the situation was typical of successful physician office practices. "After

all," they said, "economically, it was better to have too many patients than too few patients, and as long as everyone eventually got seen, what really is the harm?" Nevertheless, Dr. Murray wondered if there might not be another way.

Dr. Murray was aware of the work being done by the Institute of Healthcare Improvement, a Boston-based, nonprofit organization committed to CQI principles. The proponents of this organization were physicians who had used many CQI methods, appreciated their benefits, and reported the improvements they had noted in the management of their own practices. Dr. Murray was eager to see if he could improve services for his patients, cut down on their wait time, and perhaps even create more consistency in working hours for his colleagues. He began to use several of the methods discussed in this chapter.

Realizing that neither he nor the staff really understood how the current system was working, he determined that it was essential to begin collecting data to learn what the process was like for their patients. The results were both surprising and validating. One surprising finding was that patients had to wait an average of 55 days to get nonemergency appointments. Not surprising was that there were more calls for appointments in the fall and winter than in the spring and summer. Generally, there were from 16 to 25 calls for appointments each day for each physician, with each physician generally seeing about 21 patients per day. Data also revealed and supported the supposition that more patients came to the office on Mondays than on any other day. As a result, Monday appointments were generally backed up, which contributed to patient irritation and physician and staff exhaustion. This information equipped Dr. Murray to make appropriate recommendations about supply and demand.

He presented his findings to his colleagues and proposed several changes to improve patient service. His goal was to significantly reduce wait time for both patients trying to make appointments and those in the waiting room. He suggested that practice physicians plan to work longer hours on Mondays, particularly during the winter. They were working longer hours anyway, so why not just set their expectations at that level? He further suggested that physicians work longer hours temporarily to reduce the practice's current backlog of patients. Dr. Murray's ultimate goal was very ambitious: He wanted patients to be able to make appointments with their own physicians on the very day they called.

His colleagues agreed that his goal would be very satisfying to patients, but it were achieved, they were very concerned about not having the comfort of seeing several weeks of appointments listed in the appointment book. Could this new system actually work? When the goal was communicated to patients, they seemed pleased, but skeptical. No one had ever heard of such a thing. They were used to long wait times and could not imagine quick response times. Enlisting the support of his colleagues was quite a challenge, but eventually they agreed to implement the changes. Success was not immediate; it took about a year for the goal to be realized. Now, however, patients can get an appointment with their own physician generally on the same day they call. Everyone is much happier.

Summary

Competencies pivotal to excellence in management include being knowledgeable about the components of work processes and how to define, execute, and monitor performance/work measurements. The elements that are part and parcel to strategically managing staff productivity include employing appropriate numbers of FTEs to operate the functions of an HIS department and creating an effective environment in which to do just that.

Performance improvement involves three major approaches: systems analysis and design, continuous quality improvement, and reengineering. These approaches share many similarities: all are focused on bettering the system to provide high-quality service in a cost-effective manner. They also use similar data-gathering and analysis tools. The differences in the approaches may reflect the breadth of change, the duration of the change effort, and the specific area of interest. Systems analysis and design often occurs with the design of a new system. CQI is a test of small changes with the intention of improving services to customers over time. Six Sigma involves leveraging routinely collected data to strategically measure, monitor, and improve services and outcomes. Reengineering is a massive reexamination and redesign of processes with the main purpose of reducing costs. All these approaches have their place in improving healthcare service delivery.

References

Berwick, D.M. 1989. Continuous improvement as an ideal in health care. *New England Journal of Medicine* 320(1):53–56.

Brassard, M., and D. Ritter. 1993. *The Memory Jogger II.* Methuen, MA: GOAL/QPC.

Cofer, J.I., and H.P. Greele. 1993. *Quality Improvement Techniques for Medical Records.* Marblehead, MA: Opus Communications.

Hammer, M., and J. Champy. 1993. *Reengineering the Corporation: A Manifesto for Business Revolution.* New York: HarperBusiness.

Hughes, G. 2003. Practice brief: Using benchmarking for performance improvement. *Journal of American Health Information Management Association* 74(2):64A–D.

Johns, M.L. 1997. *Information Management for Health Professionals.* Albany, NY: Delmar.

Johnson, S.P., and C.P. McLaughlin. 1999. Measurement and statistical approaches in CQI. In *Continuous Quality Improvement in Health Care,* edited by C.P. McLaughlin and A.D. Kaluzny, pp. 70–101. Gaithersburg, MD: Aspen Publishers.

Keister, J. 2001. Workflow automation: Streamlining the way things get done. *For the Record* 13(16):16–20.

Langley, G.J., K.M. Nolan, and T.W. Nolan. 1994 (June). The foundation of improvement. *Quality Progress,* pp. 81–86.

Liebler, J.G., R.E. Levine, and J. Rothman. 1992. *Management Principles for Health Professionals,* 2nd ed. Gaithersburg, MD: Aspen Publishers.

McBrierty, L. 1995. Reengineering: a step beyond CPR. *Journal of American Health Information Management Association* 66(2):46–48.

McLaughlin, C.P., and A.D. Kaluzny. 1999. *Continuous Quality Improvement in Health Care: Theory, Implementation and Applications,* 2nd ed. Gaithersburg: MD: Aspen Publishers.

Omachonu, V.K. 1999. *Healthcare Performance Improvement.* Norcross, GA: Engineering and Management Press.

Palmer, L. 1995. Reengineering healthcare: The future awaits us all. *Journal of American Health Information Management Association* 66(2):32–35.

Senge, P.M. 1990. *The Fifth Discipline: The Art and Practice of the Learning Organization.* New York: Currency/Doubleday.

Umiker, W. 1998. *Management Skills for the New Health Care Supervisor,* 3rd ed. Gaithersburg, MD: Aspen Publishers.

White, A. 2002. Performance improvement. In *Health Information Management Technology: An Applied Approach,* edited by M.L. Johns. Chicago: AHIMA.

Chapter 24
Human Resources Management

Shirley Eichenwald Maki, MBA, RHIA, FAHIMA

Learning Objectives

- To differentiate among the concepts of chain of command, scope of command, and unity of command
- To differentiate among the hierarchical, bureaucratic, and team-based approaches to organization and management
- To develop organizational charts that accurately represent an organization's formal structure
- To construct mission, vision, and values statements
- To differentiate the unique responsibilities associated with each level of management in the organization: supervisor, middle manager, executive manager, and board director
- To identify the activities associated with the human resources management function in an organization
- To associate key federal legislation with each of the human resources management activities
- To develop position descriptions, performance standards, staffing structures, and work schedules for use as tools in human resources management
- To explain how job descriptions are used in employee recruitment and selection.
- To identify effective steps in conducting an interview

- To discuss the roles that employee orientation and communication plans play in the development and retention of staff
- To articulate the benefits of teamwork in an organization and identify the steps in creating an effective team (team building)
- To identify and differentiate among the four methods of job evaluation
- To describe the relationship among performance standards, performance review, and performance counseling
- To identify the key steps a manager should take in performance counseling and/or disciplinary action
- To select the appropriate conflict management technique to use in each specific conflict situation
- To explain the process for handling employee complaints and grievances
- To identify the obligations an organization has to maintain the security of employee information and records
- To anticipate the impact of current workforce trends on the organization's human resources management activities

Key Terms

Ability (achievement) tests

Age Discrimination in Employment Act (1967)

Americans with Disabilities Act (ADA) (1990)

Aptitude tests

Authority

Behavioral description interview

Benefits

Board of governors (board of trustees, board of directors)

Bureaucracy

Chain of command

Civil Rights Act, Title VII (1964)

Civil Rights Act (1991)

Communication plan

Compensable factors

Compensation and benefits

Compromise

Conflict management

Constructive confrontation

Control

Delegation of authority

Disciplinary action

Discrimination

Effort

Employee record

Employment-at-will

Equal Employment Opportunity Act (1972)

Equal Pay Act of 1963 (EPA)

Executive managers

Exempt employees

Exit interview

Factor comparison method

Fair Labor Standards Act of 1938 (FLSA)

Family and Medical Leave Act of 1993 (FMLA)

Flexible work schedules

Grievance

Grievance procedures

Harassment

Hay method of job evaluation

Hierarchy

Hiring

Honesty (Integrity) tests

Interviews

Job description

Job classification method

Job evaluation

Job ranking

Job specification

Labor-Management Reporting and Disclosure Act (Landrum-Griffin Act)

Labor-Management Relations Act (Taft-Hartley Act)

Labor relations

Layoffs

Mental ability (cognitive) tests

Middle managers

Mission statement

National Labor Relations Act (Wagner Act)

Nonexempt employees

Occupational Safety and Health Act of 1970 (OSHA)

Organization

Organizational chart

Orientation

Panel interview

Performance counseling

Performance review

Performance standards

Point method

Policy

Position (job) description

Pregnancy Discrimination Act (1978)

Procedure

Progressive discipline

Recruitment

Reference check

Reliability

Responsibility

Resume

Retention

Scope of command

Selection

Skill

Staffing structure

Structured interview

Supervisory managers

Team building

Termination

Testing

360-degree evaluation

Uniformed Services Employment and Reemployment Rights Act (1994)

Union

Unity of command

Validity

Values statement

Vision statement

Workers' Adjustment Retraining and Notification (WARN) Act

Working conditions

Introduction

The process of management cannot be practiced or examined meaningfully outside the social, cultural, and ethical contexts in which human organizations of all kinds operate. In modern industrial societies, human resources represent every organization's most valuable asset.

Healthcare organizations are extremely complex. They must operate as effective and efficient businesses in a very tight financial environment. They also must employ a variety of well-educated technical specialists and professional employees to provide or support increasingly sophisticated healthcare services. Contemporary healthcare managers work in a unique environment that is characterized by the need to control costs and at the same time meet the needs of healthcare consumers and healthcare workers.

Managers work at many levels within healthcare organizations: as supervisors of functional units, as **middle managers** of departmental units or service lines, and as **executive managers** of multiple departmental units or service lines. At each level of management, the practice of managing the human resources within the prescribed scope of authority and **responsibility** is critical to the manager's success and the success of the entire organization.

Managing human resources (HR) is both an art and a science. Managers can learn much in this arena by partnering with HR management specialists, observing experienced colleagues, reflecting regularly on their own experiences, and continuing to develop their competencies throughout their careers.

This chapter is not meant to provide a comprehensive background in human resources management. The purpose of this chapter is to present a general introduction to the subject of managing human resources within the context of health information management (HIM) operations. The chapter begins with a brief overview of the principles and nature of organizations and a discussion of the roles of the various levels of management. Its primary focus is the interrelationship of HIM managers and HR professionals and the roles of the supervisor and middle manager as frontline implementers of the human resources policies and practices of healthcare organizations.

Theory into Practice

In 2000, healthcare organizations were challenged by the introduction of the ambulatory payment classification (APC) system and the outpatient prospective payment system (OPPS) for Medicare beneficiaries. The leadership of one hospital's HIM department needed to develop a plan to ensure compliance with the new reimbursement system. First, the department collected information about the regulations and APCs. Then, the department manager and the coding supervisor met to discuss the staffing changes and workload issues involved in implementing the new system.

It was decided that all emergency room visits, nuclear medicine and invasive radiology procedures, and cardiac diagnostic tests would be coded individually. That is, coders would no longer rely on a chargemaster. However, all of the outpatient chargemasters would need to be updated and a regular review schedule established.

The number of cases was projected on the basis of estimated Medicare patient volumes for the next budget cycle and current patient volumes. Time studies were then undertaken to identify how much time it would take to code each case. It was determined that this new coding function would require 0.75 full-time equivalent (FTE) positions. In addition, a 0.25 FTE would be needed to accommodate the increased **effort** associated with the updating and continuous review of the hospital's chargemasters as well as the quality control of all outpatient coding and documentation. As a result of the workload analysis, a new 1.00 FTE position was added to the next year's budget. In addition, the organization decided to contract with an appropriately experienced HIM professional to update all existing chargemaster documents on a preimplementation time line. This plan gave the HIM department and the HR department several months before implementation to finalize the **position description**, recruit and select a qualified candidate, and establish policies and procedures for the new system.

Principles of Organization

Organization is the planned coordination of the activities of more than one person for the achievement of a common purpose or goal. It is accomplished through the division of labor, and it is based on a hierarchy of authority and responsibility (Schein 1980). Jobs and the people who perform them are arranged in a way that accomplishes the goals of the organization. Various organizational tools are used to communicate the structure, the purpose, and the methods for accomplishing the shared work of the organization's members.

Organizations are somewhat like sports teams in that they have specific positions, a predefined set of rules, and a shared goal (in the case of sports teams, the goal is winning). Organizations also use communications tools that are similar to a player's roster (position descriptions), a rule or playbook (policies and procedures), and a record of wins and losses (a budget and financial records).

Like other types of businesses, healthcare institutions are a type of formal organization. That is, they have established goals and a specific purpose for existing. Although purpose, structure, and methods vary widely, all healthcare organizations use common systems and tools to achieve their goals.

Nature of Organizations

By nature, humans are social creatures. They are biologically designed to live within groups of their own kind. Moreover, they continuously form and reform informal and formal groups of various sizes (two members to billions of members) and longevity (a few seconds to a few centuries). No two groups have identical purposes, membership, or rules. Therefore, every human group is unique.

There is an endless variety of groups. Groups range from relatively informal friendships, families, and social clubs to extremely formal businesses, educational institutions, and national governments. They can be loose, unstructured, and temporary. An example of an extremely loose, short-term group might be that of a dozen people who ride on a bus together on a given morning. But even the most informal groups have a purpose and a set of more or less well-communicated rules. In this example, the group's purpose is to get from point A to point B. The rules required that the bus driver follow a pre-established route and that the riders pay a preestablished fare.

Although every group of humans is unique, interactions among humans follow predictable patterns. Human behavior has been studied for centuries. Theories on organizational behavior have been offered ever since humans learned how to communicate with each other. Although few principles of organizational behavior go unchallenged, centuries of observation have produced some basic rules. For example, one unchanging principle of organizational behavior seems to be that the group's structure affects the way its members interact with each other. And these structural effects can have both positive and negative consequences for the group as a whole as well as for its individual members.

Organizational Structures

At least until recent decades, formal organizations such as healthcare and manufacturing institutions have tended to be structured as relatively inflexible hierarchies. In a **hierarchy,** every member of the organization is assigned a specific rank. Each rank, in turn, carries a specific level of decision-making authority as well as specific responsibilities within the institution. Hierarchies are authoritarian in nature. In other words, they are strictly controlled by a powerful elite group working "at the top" of the organization. These few individuals make almost every significant decision on behalf of the entire organization.

Historically, large governmental institutions have tended to be organized as rigid bureaucratic structures. In a **bureaucracy,** as in a hierarchy, positions within the formal organization are assigned specific ranks. Hierarchical ranks are based on levels of decision-making **authority.** In contrast, bureaucratic ranks are based on levels of technical expertise.

The purpose of bureaucratic organizations is to conduct highly complex and regulated processes. The structure of the bureaucratic organization reflects the processes it was designed to carry out. Therefore, bureaucracies operate according to well-established and often-inflexible rules. Each individual within the bureaucracy is responsible for carrying out only a small, well-defined element of the larger process.

The Social Security Administration is a good example of a government bureaucracy. It was created in 1935 with the sole purpose of implementing the Social Security Act.

Both hierarchies and bureaucracies depend on authoritarian **chains of command. Scope of command** (that is, one manager oversees the work of many employees) and **unity of command** (that is, each employee is accountable to only one boss) are principles that are inherent in a traditional chain-of-command structure. The structures of military organizations, for example, are organized around extremely rigid chains of command.

In modern times, organizational structure has been studied systematically since the early 20th century. In the subsequent decades, a number of new management theories were suggested, and each theory seems to have required innovations in organizational structure. The period of economic rebuilding after World War II ushered in the current era of business thinking. Business and management theorists W. Edwards Deming and Joseph M. Juran began developing modern management systems during the early 1950s.

Today's management systems are modern in that they are moving away from the traditional authoritarian models that have prevailed since the Industrial Revolution. Most of all, they are modern in that they recognize the potential value of change and treat change as an opportunity rather than as a threat.

Modern management systems are based on the objective statistical analysis of data and information. They emphasize the **benefits** of sharing authority among employees and managers. They also favor interdisciplinary and cross-functional cooperation and teamwork over bureaucratic regulation and authoritarian control. Modern management systems value continual learning and demand systems thinking (Senge 1990, pp. 6–8). Systems thinking is simply an objective way of looking at work-related ideas and processes with the goal of allowing people to uncover ineffective patterns of behavior and thinking and then find ways to make lasting improvements.

In large part, modern management systems represent a rejection of the traditional authoritarian, hierarchical, and bureaucratic approaches to organization and management. However, because traditional management systems have been the accepted norm since the Industrial Revolution began in the early 18th century, they have proved difficult to displace. They continue to be the core organizational structures in place in most businesses today. Management theorists continue to lead the movement to establish information-based management systems and team-based organizational structures in all types of business endeavors, including the business of healthcare delivery. (See chapter 21 for a fuller discussion of the evolution of management theory.)

Organizational Charts

An **organizational chart** is a graphic representation of an organization's formal structure. It shows the organization's various activities and the specific members or categories of members assigned to carry out its activities. The chart for a very small organization might list the actual names of employees or individual position titles. The chart for a very large organization might list the various functional groups or departments responsible for each area of operations.

Traditionally, the reporting relationships among individuals and groups also are indicated according to accepted labeling conventions. For example, a solid line between two elements on a chart indicates a direct reporting relationship and a broken line indicates an indirect reporting relationship. (See figures 24.1, 24.2, and 24.3 for examples of organizational charts developed for different types of healthcare organizations.)

Today's healthcare organizations are somewhat less concerned with official lines of authority. Instead, they are concerned with the interrelationships of work groups and functions. Individual departments and interdepartmental work groups sometimes develop detailed organizational charts as a first step in redesigning work processes. The charts then can be used as the basis for creating work flow diagrams and flowcharts. The purpose of these graphic tools is to help work teams visualize current and proposed processes and then suggest and implement improvements.

Some organizations also include organizational charts in their official position (job) descriptions. In this context, the charts put the work of a specific position or employee into the larger context of how the whole organization works as a system of interdependent processes.

Figure 24.1.   Sample organizational chart for an acute care hospital

Figure 24.2.   Sample organizational chart for an ambulatory care clinic

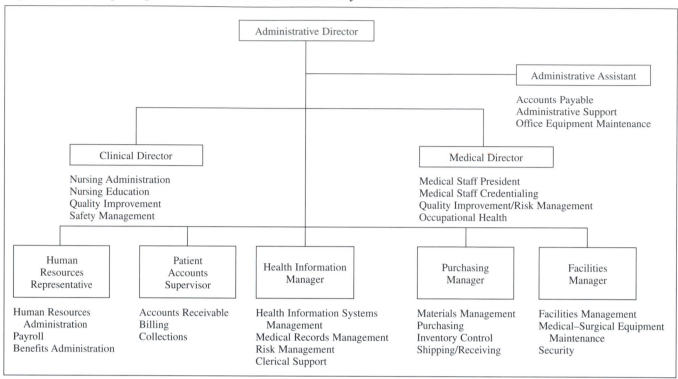

Figure 24.3.   Sample organizational chart for a managed care organization

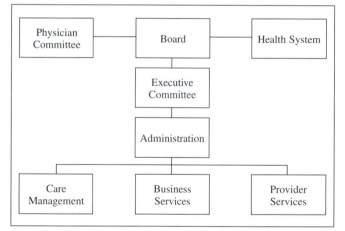

Mission, Vision, and Values Statements

Modern organizations use a variety of communication devices to convey their purpose and goals to their members and the communities they serve. A **mission statement** is a short description of the general purpose of an organization or group. For healthcare organizations, the mission statement usually includes a broad definition of the services the organization provides and the communities/customers it serves. Similarly, a **vision statement** is a short description of the organization's ideal future state. One way to make the distinction between an organization's mission and its vision is to think of the concepts in the following way:

- The mission is a *realistic* expression of what the organization actually does at the current time.
- The vision is an *idealistic* portrayal of what the organization would like to become sometime in the future.

Most healthcare organizations update their mission and vision statements regularly as part of the strategic planning process. The organization shares its mission and vision statements internally with its employees and medical staff and externally with its customers and the community it serves. The statements are meant to inform, guide, and inspire.

Healthcare organizations use mission and vision statements at many different levels. An individual organization usually develops statements for the enterprise as a whole. A multi-facility healthcare system usually develops statements for the system as a whole as well as for each individual facility within it. Departments, work teams, and even temporary task forces often develop vision and mission statements. These groups use the statements to express and communicate their specific purpose and goals. Figure 24.4 provides examples of vision and mission statements from healthcare organizations. (See chapter 28 for a broader discussion of strategic planning.)

Many healthcare organizations also develop **values statements** that communicate their social and cultural belief system. The organization's values statement provides a way to support the type of behavior the organization wishes to encourage among its members. For example, the Benedictine Health System based in Duluth, Minnesota, clearly identifies "hospitality, stewardship, respect and justice" as its organizational core values (Benedictine Health System 2002, p. 1).

Figure 24.4. Sample mission and vision statements

General Hospital Affiliated with a Larger Healthcare System

Lutheran Hospital's **mission** is to improve the health of the communities we serve by providing high-quality services in a responsible and caring way.

Our **vision** is to become the leader in promoting healthy life-styles in an atmosphere of spiritual support, dignity, compassion, and mutual respect for all.

Community General Hospital

Anytown General Hospital's **mission** is to provide quality health services and technology to meet the changing healthcare needs of the people of southwestern Minnesota.

Anytown General Hospital's **vision** is to become the hospital of choice for residents of Polk, Sunny Isle, and Spring counties, a position we strive to strengthen by our long-term commitment to:

- Teamwork
- Service excellence
- Compassionate care
- Cost consciousness
- Continuous improvement

Academic Medical Center

Prairie University Hospital's **mission** is to provide the most up-to-date medical and surgical services available in the three-state area and to train medical students and graduate physicians to meet current and future challenges in healthcare.

Our **vision** is the achievement of healthy communities and progress toward the future of healthcare for Montana, western North Dakota, and northwestern South Dakota.

Specialty Hospital

The **mission** of Women's Hospital of Somewhereville is to meet the healthcare needs of our patients and to exceed their service expectations.

Our **vision** is of a hospital:

- Providing services with compassion and kindness
- Striving for performance improvement
- Fostering pride and integrity
- Aiming for increased cost-effectiveness and productivity

Specialty Clinic within an Academic Medical Center

The **mission** of the Midwest Asthma Center is to:

- Provide optimal medical care for persons with asthma and related illnesses
- Develop new knowledge about asthma and its management through medical research
- Promote improved understanding about asthma and related illnesses through providing educational programs and materials for our patients, for other healthcare providers, and for the community

The **vision** of the Midwest Asthma Center is to provide the highest quality of integrated comprehensive care for persons with asthma and related illnesses and to be one of the centers of excellence in the world for asthma treatment, research, and education.

Primary Care Physicians' Practice

The **mission** of Coastal Shores Primary Care Associates is to serve the unique needs of individuals and families by providing high-quality, coordinated, primary care medical services through an efficient, accessible, and responsive network of caring providers.

Our **vision** is to be the primary care medical group of choice in the Atlantic County area by delivering high-quality, individualized, and efficient patient care.

Check Your Understanding 24.1

Instructions: On a separate piece of paper, indicate whether the following statements are true or false (T or F).

1. Systems thinking is a subjective way to look at work-related ideas and processes.
2. Bureaucratic ranks are based on levels of technical expertise.
3. Today's healthcare organizations are increasingly concerned with official lines of authority.
4. Healthcare organizations develop mission statements to communicate their social and cultural belief systems.

Levels of Management

As noted earlier in this chapter, the various levels of management in organizations have different levels of responsibility and decision-making authority.

Supervisory Management

Supervisory managers (supervisors) oversee the organization's efforts at the staff level and monitor the effectiveness of everyday operations and individual performance against preestablished standards. Further, supervisory managers are responsible for ensuring that the organization's human assets are used effectively and that its policies and procedures are carried out consistently.

Supervisory managers work in small (2- to 10-person) functional work groups or teams. They often perform hands-on functions in addition to supervisory functions. They play an important role in staff training and **recruitment/retention** efforts. Supervisory managers direct daily work, create work schedules, and monitor the quality of the work and the productivity of the staff. They are important resources in revising procedures and conducting performance reviews because they are familiar with the work of the unit and the performance of individual staff members.

Supervisory managers usually have advanced technical **skills** that allow them to perform the most complex functions of the work team. However, most supervisors have limited financial authority and must seek the approval of higher-level managers before spending money or **hiring** staff. Depending on the size and structure of the organization, HIM supervisors report to another supervisory-level manager or to a department-level manager or assistant manager.

Effective supervisory managers are extremely important in healthcare organizations because the greatest part of the healthcare organization's resources is expended at the operational level. Labor costs represent the greatest investment the organization makes. Staff and supervisory healthcare workers include nurses, clinical therapists, diagnostic technicians, dietary workers, laboratory workers, environmental support staff, and administrative support staff.

In healthcare organizations, health information technicians (HITs) or health information administrators (HIAs) often fill roles as supervisory managers. They provide vital administrative services and support patient care by protecting the accuracy and confidentiality of clinical databases and health records. They also ensure the financial health and future of their organizations by providing high-quality clinical coding services.

Middle Management

Middle management is concerned primarily with facilitating the work performed by supervisory- and staff-level personnel as well as by executive leaders. The responsibilities of middle managers include the following:

- Developing, implementing, and revising the organization's policies and procedures under the direction of executive managers
- Executing the organizational plans developed at the board and executive levels
- Providing the operational information that executives need to develop meaningful plans for the organization's future

Middle managers oversee operations of a broader scope in their work as managers or assistant managers of departments or disciplinary functions. For example, they may be responsible for overseeing all the functions in a health information services (HIS) department or for directing the functions in two or more related departments, such as (HIS), admission/registration services, and quality improvement services.

Middle managers can change department-level policies and procedures when necessary. For example, when a department manager finds that an employee is not following a specific procedure, he or she investigates and analyzes the department's systems and processes to determine whether the problem is with the employee's performance or with shortcomings in the processes themselves. In contrast, supervisory managers enforce the policies and procedures that relate directly to the activities of their own work group or team. For example, when a supervisor finds that an employee is not following a specific procedure, he or she takes action to correct that individual's performance.

Typically, middle managers are responsible for performing a limited number of hands-on analytical and/or decision-making functions related directly to the departments they manage. In an HIS department, for example, an HIM professional in an assistant director position might be responsible for tracking the quality of clinical databases and overseeing coding compliance programs. HIS department managers participate on a number of permanent and temporary interdisciplinary committees within the organization and serve as resources to the committees on subjects that relate to the organization's information resources. They also initiate interdepartmental efforts to address issues that go beyond department-level operations. In small healthcare organizations, the HIM director may play additional managerial roles in risk management, quality management, and/or utilization management.

Depending on the size and structure of the organization, HIS middle managers report to a department-level director or an executive-level manager (vice-president) on the organization's senior management team. In a multifacility healthcare delivery network, the HIS director might report to the vice-president of operations (sometimes referred to as the chief operating officer, or COO) or the vice-president of information services (sometimes called the chief information officer, or CIO). In a small community hospital, the HIS director might report to the CEO (chief executive officer), the CFO (chief financial officer), or the COO.

Executive Management and Governance

The third managerial level in healthcare organizations can be divided into executive management and governance. The governance body is often called the **board of directors** or the **board of trustees.**

Role of Executive Management

Executive managers are directly employed by the organization. They are hired by either the board or the organization's CEO with the board's approval. In publicly owned organizations, the stockholders elect board members. In privately owned organizations, the board members are appointed.

Executive managers are primarily responsible for working with the board to set the organization's future direction and establish its strategic plan. To that end, executive managers work to ensure that the organization uses its assets wisely, fulfills its current mission, and works toward achieving a meaningful vision for the future. Executive managers oversee broad functions, departments, or groups of departments. Executive managers are also responsible for establishing the policies of healthcare organizations and leading their quality improvement and compliance initiatives. In addition, executive managers work with community leaders to make sure that the healthcare organization contributes to the well-being of the community it serves.

Depending on the complexity of the organization, the titles of executive managers vary. The different titles include chief executive officer, president, executive vice-president, senior vice-president, vice-president, and director. Executive managers may report to other executive managers, to higher-level vice-presidents, or to the CEO.

In most organizations, the CEO is the highest-ranking executive manager. CEOs sometimes hold more than one title. For example, the head of an organization might have the title president and CEO. The CEO and/or president reports directly to the organization's board of directors.

Role of the Governing Board

Healthcare organizations such as hospitals, healthcare businesses, and multifacility healthcare delivery networks are organized as legal entities, or corporations. Every state has laws that dictate how corporations are to be structured and run within its jurisdiction. However, all state incorporation laws are consistent in one area: Responsibility for the operation of each healthcare organization ultimately lies with its board of governors. Thus, the board is the final authority in setting the organization's strategic direction, mission and vision, and general philosophy and ethical base. The name and structure of the board depend on the profit-making status of the organization, among other factors.

Typically, the board consists of a chairperson and 10 to 20 board members. It represents the interests of the organization's owners. Any number of different entities may own large healthcare organizations, including federal, state, and local governments; investment groups; educational institutions; and religious organizations. Moreover, healthcare organizations may be owned privately or publicly. In publicly owned for-profit entities, investors purchase stock on national and international stock exchanges and receive a share of the profits in the form of dividends. Many private healthcare organizations operate as not-for-profit charitable organizations. In not-for-profit organizations, any excess income is reinvested in the organization rather than being paid out in profits or dividends.

Check Your Understanding 24.2

Instructions: On a separate piece of paper, indicate whether the following statements are true or false (T or F).

1. Supervisory managers set the organization's future direction and establish its goals.

2. In general, middle managers perform the daily work of the organization.

3. Vice-presidents are representatives of the executive level of management.

4. The ultimate responsibility for the organization's operation lies with its chief executive officer.

5. In publicly owned healthcare entities, investors buy stock and receive dividends.

Role of the Human Resources Department

Payroll and benefits consume the majority of most healthcare organizations' financial resources. Therefore, adequate time and attention must be paid to the management of human resources. Effective HR management is also important for reasons beyond financial impact. HR management factors affect the attitudes and morale of healthcare workers and other employees and, therefore, affect their ability to perform their work effectively, as well. Obviously, employee morale becomes extremely important when the work involves car-

ing for patients directly or indirectly supporting those who provide hands-on care.

Entities such as hospitals, large physician groups, and managed care organizations commonly have a dedicated HR department that acts as a reference and support for managers at all levels. However, every manager must have an understanding of the principles of HR management in order to implement them effectively within the scope of the manager's authority and responsibility. Every manager must also know how to appropriately and effectively work with the organization's HR department.

The HR department is responsible for several types of interrelated activities. Mathis and Jackson (2002) describe HR management as a set of closely related activities focused on contributing to an organization's success by enhancing its productivity, quality, and service. Each of these interrelated activities is shown in figure 24.5. Mathis and Jackson also emphasize the importance of performing HR activities with the organization's unique mission, culture, size, and structure in mind as well as the greater social, political, legal, economic, technological, and cultural environment in which it operates.

Human Resources Planning and Analysis

HR planning and analysis ensure the long-term health of the organization's human assets. Internal trends such as the aging of the workforce or the changing nature of the skill mix required to handle the organization's evolving product lines must be addressed. The impact of external trends such as workforce shortages and evolving workforce expectations also must be assessed.

Figure 24.5. Human resources management activities

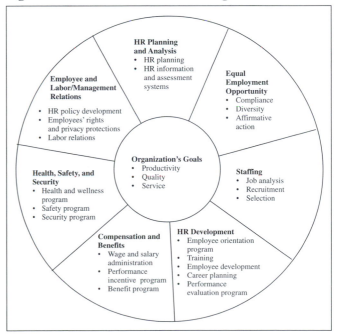

Adapted from Mathis and Johnson 2002, p. 4.

Equal Employment Opportunity Practices

The HR department takes the lead in ensuring that the various laws and regulations associated with equal employment opportunity (EEO) laws are scrupulously applied in the organization's hiring and promotion practices. Federally enacted EEO legislation includes the **Age Discrimination in Employment Act** (ADEA) of 1967, the **Americans with Disabilities Act** (ADA) of 1990, the **Civil Rights Acts** of 1964 and 1991, the **Equal Employment Opportunity Act** of 1972, the **Pregnancy Discrimination Act,** and the **Uniformed Services Employment and Reemployment Rights Act** of 1994 (Anthony, Perrewe, and Kacmar 1996; Buhler 2002). The Equal Employment Opportunity Commission (EEOC) was created as the agency responsible for investigating discrimination claims emanating from the Civil Rights Act of 1996.

Discrimination and **harassment** are two important concepts related to fair employment practices. Discrimination refers to practices that result in people being treated differently based solely on their differences. Harassment refers to practices that create a hostile work environment. Both are clearly illegal under the EEO laws.

Rights of Employees and Employers

Although many of the basic rights of employees are defined in law, others are expectations that may be debated within organizations. For example, **employment-at-will** is a well-established concept: Either an employer or an employee can terminate an employment relationship without providing either notice or reason. On the other hand, what are the privacy rights of employees? Can an employer monitor employees' e-mail and voicemail? Organizations are well advised to address the rights of employees and the rights of the employer in an employee handbook to clarify expectations for employees and supervisors. A well-developed employee handbook also improves the organization's legal position should the organization be called on to defend its actions in a court proceeding.

Staffing

The HR department also helps managers to define staffing needs; develop job descriptions; and recruit, screen, and select staff. After an employee is brought into the organization, the HR department plays a significant role, in partnership with the employee's direct supervisor, by spearheading the employee's immediate **orientation** to the organization's policies, practices, and procedures. The HR department is also active in addressing the employee's ongoing training and development requirements.

Compensation and Benefits Program

The organization's **compensation and benefits** program is probably the most prominent activity associated with HR management because it is so directly connected to the employee's pocketbook. This activity involves the establishment of basic definitions of employment and compensation status for the organization (for example, full-time versus part-time, temporary versus permanent, independent contractor versus employee, wage versus salary). The **Fair Labor Standards Act of 1938** (FLSA) and the **Equal Pay Act of 1963** (EPA) serve as fundamental legislative mandates in this area.

The HR department also leads the development and administration of the organization's benefits program, **job evaluation** and classification systems, wage and salary systems, and incentive pay systems.

Social Security, unemployment compensation, and workers' compensation are three benefits organizations are required to offer. Other common benefits offered to employees voluntarily by the organization are health insurance, retirement plans, wellness programs, holidays (time off with pay), vacation time, and employee assistance programs.

The **Family and Medical Leave Act of 1993** (FMLA) is an example of one legislative initiative that has had a major impact on the benefit programs, as well as on staffing activities (Anthony, Perrewe, and Kacmar 1996). Leaves of absence can be granted for a variety of reasons, including personal or family illness, pregnancy, or military service.

Health and Safety Program

The HR department is also involved in activities designed to protect the health, safety, and security of the workforce. Healthcare organizations have given substantial attention to safety management since the enactment of the **Occupational Safety and Health Act of 1970** (OSHA). The act's intended purpose is "to assure, so far as possible, every working man or woman in the Nation safe and healthful **working conditions** and to preserve our human resources." This act established a national reporting system for accidents and injuries on the job and led to the development of specific safety management programs in most businesses. More recently, health-related hazards associated with the use of technology or chemical substances in the workplace, injuries due to workplace violence, and employee security concerns have begun to receive special attention by HR professionals (Anthony, Perrewe, and Kacmar 1996).

Labor Relations

Employee and labor/management relations are established through the day-to-day interactions between employees and their managers. However, the organization's managers and employees often seek leadership and support from the HR department. The HR department sets the stage for developing and sustaining the quality of these critical relationships by establishing and communicating to both managers and employees the contracts, policies, practices, and rules that constitute the organization's expectations of its employees.

HR management activities associated with **unions** and collective bargaining are referred to as **labor relations.**

Labor organizations (unions) enter into negotiations with employers on behalf of groups of employees who have elected to join a union. The negotiations relate to compensation and safety and health concerns. In a unionized environment, three laws that came into existence over a period of 25 years (1935–1960) constitute a code of practice for unions and management. HR departments pay strict attention to these three acts (Mathis and Jackson 2002; Anthony, Perrewe, and Kacmar 1996):

- **Wagner Act (National Labor Relations Act)**
- **Taft-Hartley Act (Labor-Management Relations Act)**
- **Landrum-Griffin Act (Labor-Management Reporting and Disclosure Act)**

For the manager who oversees a group of employees covered by a union contract, these laws represent the basic rules for their interactions with employees in the areas of pay, benefits, safety, health, and performance evaluation.

Check Your Understanding 24.3

Instructions: On a separate piece of paper, indicate whether the following statements are true or false (T or F).

1. Internal and external environmental trends are significant factors in HR planning and analysis.
2. The Fair Labor Standards Act is one piece of the EEO legislation package passed in the early 1960s.
3. A national system for reporting workplace accidents and injuries was mandated by the Americans with Disabilities Act.
4. Orientation for new employees and the ongoing training of employees are solely the responsibility of the HR department.
5. The Fair Labor Standards Act, the Wagner Act, and the Equal Pay Act provide key guidelines for managing union relationships.

Role of the HIM Manager in Human Resources

Because the day-to-day management of the organization's human resources is the responsibility of supervisory, middle, and executive managers, every manager is responsible for the same HR activities as the HR professionals. In an HIS department, for example, the supervisor of coding services would be responsible for the day-to-day management of clinical coding specialists. Managers at all levels can use any of a variety of HR tools and processes to handle these responsibilities efficiently and effectively.

Tools for Human Resources Planning

Several tools may be used to plan and manage staff resources. Position descriptions, for example, outline the work and qualifications needed to perform a job. Performance standards establish the organization's expectations of how well a job must be done and how much work must be accomplished. Routine staff meetings and regular written communications

(via departmental Web sites, bulletin boards, and newsletters, for example) establish a routine process for up-to-date information flow for employees.

Staffing Structures and Work Scheduling

In addition to these basic tools, managers establish **staffing structures** and use work schedules to ensure that there is adequate coverage and staff to complete the required work. Schedules are developed first to provide adequate coverage during the hours the organization or department is open for business.

In hospitals, it is not uncommon to find some part of the HIM department open 24 hours a day, seven days a week. This schedule ensures that HIM staff will be available to provide information for admissions to the hospital and emergency department, support patient discharges and transfers, and handle other HIM functions. In some healthcare organizations, the demand for HIM services outside regular business hours is limited. In such cases, HIM functions can be provided by business office staff, nursing staff, and/or emergency department staff who have been cross-trained to perform basic HIM tasks.

Another scheduling consideration is space. Space limitations on the number of workstations in the department or the number of employees who can work in the file room may require that employees work in shifts or on weekends.

In addition, staff preferences need to be considered in creating the work schedule. Balancing the demands of the organization with individual requests for flexible start times makes scheduling an important part of the manager's responsibility. Organizations are commonly establishing **flexible work schedules** to accommodate employee needs to adjust work schedules to lifestyles. (These flexible scheduling options—compressed workweek, flextime, job sharing, and telecommuting—are discussed in detail in chapter 25.)

Written policies and procedures that explain the department's staffing requirements and scheduling procedures help the manager to remain fair and objective and help the staff to understand the rules. The amount of personal time off, such as sick leave or vacation, also factors into the development of a staff schedule and the overall assessment of the number of staff positions required.

In addition, most healthcare organizations establish some type of job classification system that combines jobs with similar levels of responsibility and qualifications into job grades that determine salary ranges and benefit packages. For instance, all supervisory-level managers might be classified into one salary and benefit category, but each would have a unique job description. Job classifications also may determine whether an employee belongs to a union or is a candidate for unionization at the time a union attempts to organize the workforce.

Position Descriptions

A **position (job) description** outlines the work to be performed by a specific employee or group of employees with the same responsibilities. Position descriptions generally consist of three parts: a summary of the position's requirements and purpose, its functions, and the qualifications needed to perform the job. Position descriptions also include the official title of the job.

A **job specification** is a document (or a section of the position description document) that is focused on the knowledge, skills, abilities, and characteristics required of an individual in order to perform the job. These specifications may include the following (Buhler 2002):

- Educational level and/or professional certifications
- Experience
- General characteristics (team player, good writing skills)
- Specific knowledge (foreign language proficiency, software program proficiency)

Position descriptions, including the job specification, are used during the recruitment process to explain the work to prospective candidates. They also enable managers and human resources staff to set appropriate salaries and wages for the various positions. Moreover, they may be used to resolve performance problems. The manager can use the position description to clarify the tasks the employee is expected to perform.

Generally, job descriptions are needed in the following circumstances:

- When an entirely new kind of work is required
- When a job changes and the old description no longer reflects the work
- When a change in technology or processes dramatically affects the work to be accomplished

Sometimes top performers outgrow their job descriptions. They may find more efficient ways of doing part of their assigned tasks and/or want more interesting or meaningful work. Some employees request updated job descriptions to support an increase in salary and benefits or a change in title.

When writing new position descriptions, managers may use existing descriptions of other, related jobs or interview staff who are currently performing some of the tasks intended for the new job. They also might ask staff members to keep a record of how they spend their time for a period that reflects a comprehensive cycle of their work. Staff with more repetitive daily activities may only need to record their activities for a week. In contrast, staff with more diverse tasks may need a month to document the scope of their duties.

Performance Standards

In addition to a position description, **performance standards** are often developed for the key functions of the job. These standards indicate the level of acceptable execution for each function. Performance standards are usually set for both quantity and quality and should be as objective and measurable as possible.

Some organizations establish measures that reflect various levels of performance. For example, one measure of a

coder's performance might be coding a specified number of charts per day, perhaps no fewer than 20 charts per day. Other organizations might establish several levels of expected performance, for example:

30–35 charts per day	Outstanding
25–29 charts per day	Exceeds expectations
20–24 charts per day	Meets expectations
15–19 charts per day	Needs improvement
Fewer than 14 charts per day	Unsatisfactory

The following example shows how a quality standard might be used as a performance indicator of coding accuracy. For example:

96%–100% accuracy	Outstanding
92%–95% accuracy	Exceeds expectations
89%–94% accuracy	Meets expectations
84%–88% accuracy	Needs improvement
Less than 84%	Unsatisfactory

In the preceding example, a definition for coding accuracy might be helpful. For example, accurate coding includes capturing accurate codes and sequencing them appropriately for all diagnoses and procedures that affect reimbursement.

Standards that are measurable and relevant to an employee's overall performance are helpful in setting clear expectations. They also are useful in providing constructive feedback. (See chapter 23 for a full discussion of performance standards and measurement.)

Policies and Procedures

Policies and procedures are critical tools that may be used to ensure consistent quality performance. A **policy** is a statement about what an organization or department does. For example, a policy might state that patients are allowed to review their health records under certain conditions such as when a clinical professional is present or in the HIM department. Policies should be clearly stated and comprehensive. They must be developed in accordance with applicable laws, and they must reflect actual practice. And because they may be used as documentation of intended practice in a lawsuit, policies should be developed very carefully.

A **procedure** describes how work is to be done and how policies are to be carried out. Procedures are instructions that ensure high-quality, consistent outcomes for tasks done, especially when more than one person is involved.

One of the benefits of developing a procedure is that time is taken to analyze the best possible method for completing a process. This analysis may begin by developing a flowchart to document work flow, decision points, and the flow required to complete a procedure. (Flowcharting is discussed in detail in chapter 23.)

After a flowchart is completed, the steps in the process are written down in the order in which they are to be performed. When more than one person is involved in completing a procedure, each person who performs a task is documented. Anyone generally competent to perform a task should be able to complete it after reading a well-written procedure.

This usually takes several drafts that have been reviewed by people who actually perform the work. Moreover, it might be useful to ask someone unfamiliar with the job to try to complete the task according to the written procedure.

Writing a procedure also offers a great opportunity to identify ways to streamline the process. Are supplies available and organized in a way that makes work efficient? Would it be faster to complete one type of task for all of the work, or should each job be completed before the next task is begun?

For example, a procedure for the process of logging in information requests might include the following steps:

1. The receptionist opens all incoming mail daily before 10 a.m. He or she then confirms that the date on the date stamp is accurate and stamps all mail in the upper right-hand corner.
2. The receptionist sorts requests for medical information into three categories: legal, medical, or insurance. He or she then counts the requests in each category, clips or binds the requests for each category together, writes the count on a Post-it® note, and places the note on the top request of each bundle. The bundles are then delivered to the release of information (ROI) inbox. (The inbox is located on the ROI coordinator's desk.)
3. The ROI coordinator picks up the external medical requests for information from the ROI inbox each morning after 10 a.m. He or she enters the request details into the ROI module of the department's computerized information system.

This example, although only the first three steps in a procedure, shows how a detailed procedure would be useful in training a new receptionist or ROI coordinator or in providing instructions to anyone needed to perform this task in the regular employee's absence. It also highlights the fact that the receptionist would need to be trained to identify different types of information requests and the ROI coordinator trained on the ROI module of the department's computerized information system.

Several tools may be used to effectively communicate the purpose, scope, and details of the work done by employees in the organization. The manager is responsible for developing and maintaining these tools. However, the manager's role does not end here. Given the tools described so far, he or she is ready to hire, train, and interact with employees.

Tools for Recruitment and Retention

Recruitment is the process of finding, soliciting, and attracting new employees. Retention is the ability to keep valuable employees from seeking employment elsewhere.

Staff Recruitment, Selection, and Hiring

Armed with a position description, the manager is ready to begin recruiting candidates for a new or open position. However, the manager should be sure to understand the organization's recruitment and hiring policies and to seek the assistance of the HR department before the vacancy is publicized. This preparation ensures that the organization's legal obligations and policies and procedures are followed throughout the recruitment, **selection,** and hiring process.

Recruitment

The first thing to consider in recruiting candidates to fill a staff opening is whether to promote someone from inside the organization or to look for candidates outside the organization. The advantage of promoting from within is that the practice often motivates employees to perform well, learn new skills, and work toward advancement. To advertise a vacancy internally, the organization might post it on facility bulletin boards or list it in the organization's newsletter or Web site. The department manager may announce an opening at a routine staff meeting or use any other communication channels available. Management must communicate an opportunity for promotion to all staff rather than to just the employee who is the most likely candidate. Because employees see widespread posting as a fair practice, it communicates the underlying message that internal candidates are considered first whenever possible.

When the position cannot be filled from within, however, there are several ways to advertise it externally. For example, the organization might run an ad in a newspaper, post the job on Internet recruitment sites, announce the opportunity at professional meetings, contact people who have previously applied or expressed interest in working at the organization, or work through a professional recruiter.

In most cases, the approach used depends on the nature of the open position. For example, the facility might run an ad for a file room position in a local newspaper, but not in a professional journal. On the other hand, the facility might turn to a professional recruiter when trying to fill a department director or experienced coding position.

As in every industry, job seekers looking for professional-level healthcare positions submit detailed resumes. A **resume** describes the candidate's educational background and work experience and usually includes information on personal and professional achievements. Candidates often submit a cover letter describing the type of position in which they are interested along with the resume. Today, it is common for candidates to submit, and organizations to accept, application letters and resumes through electronic systems.

Most organizations ask every candidate to complete a formal job application. People seeking entry-level positions may be asked to complete an application rather than to submit a resume. In many cases today, completion of applications can be done online.

Selection

When a sufficient pool of applicants has been recruited, the selection process can begin. The goal of the selection process is to identify the candidate most qualified to fill the position.

Testing applicants with reliable and valid instruments designed to objectively assess the applicants' fit for the position and **interviews** are the two basic tools employed in the selection process. **Testing** is commonly conducted during the applicant's first visit to the facility. **Reliability** of a test refers to the consistency with which a test measures an attribute. **Validity** refers to a test's ability to accurately and consistently measure what it purports to measure. Testing practices are under increasing legal scrutiny, which places a special burden on organizations to ensure that tests used are clearly job related. HR professionals are generally familiar with a variety of **ability (achievement) tests, aptitude tests, mental ability (cognitive) tests,** personality tests, and **honesty/integrity tests** that are suitable for use in the organization (Anthony, Perrewe, and Kacmar 1996; Buhler 2002). Many healthcare organizations also perform routine drug testing on candidates for employment in order to create a drug-free work environment.

Mathis and Jackson (2002) agree that the selection interview is generally considered the most important phase of the selection process. They also describe three effective interview formats:

- The **structured interview** uses a set of standardized questions that are asked of all applicants.
- The **behavioral description interview** requires applicants to give specific examples of how they have performed a specific procedure or handled a specific problem in the past.
- The **panel interview** includes a team of people who interview applicants at one time.

Interviewing is one of the most important skills that managers need for selecting new staff. Unfortunately, many managers receive little formal training in interviewing techniques and/or have little practical experience. Even supervisors and managers with many years of experience sometimes dread the interviewing process. This shortcoming can be overcome through self-education, mentoring by more experienced managers, or instructional sessions with HR professionals in the organization.

Failure to adequately prepare for conducting the interview has consequences that are very serious for the organization and the applicant. Reviewing the position description, reading the applicant's resume and/or application form, and preparing appropriate and relevant questions are important steps to take before beginning an interview.

The interview itself has four basic purposes:

- To obtain information from the applicant about his or her past work history and future goals
- To give information to the applicant about the organization's mission and goals and the nature of the employment opportunity
- To evaluate the applicant's work experience, attitudes, and personality as a potential fit for the organization
- To give the applicant an opportunity to evaluate the organization as a potential fit for his or her current and future employment goals

EEO regulations dictate the types of questions that may be asked during interviews and on job applications. For example, questions pertaining to age, religious affiliation, and marital status should be avoided in most cases. These regulations apply during all activities associated with the interview, including during formal interview sessions and during less formal lunches or dinners or hallway/elevator small talk when it is very easy to inadvertently lapse into discussions on these topics. Managers should always seek the advice of HR professionals when they are uncertain about which questions to ask.

Healthcare organizations, like other employers, must be certain to conduct careful background checks of potential employees. Managers or HR professionals also check the references of candidates and communicate with the past employers of candidates via telephone or correspondence. Checking references involves confirming the information provided by applicants on resumes and applications. **Reference checks** and/or a background investigation should also be conducted specifically to assess the applicants' fit with the position and to validate the accuracy of information the applicants provide on their applications and during their interviews. According to Mathis and Jackson (2002, p. 73), a recent survey of employers revealed that the false information furnished most commonly by candidates for employment dealt with past lengths of employment, salary history, criminal record, and job titles.

Hiring

After all the internal and external interviews, tests, and reference/background checks are complete, the hiring manager usually has enough information to make a hiring decision. In some organizations, the manager shares the hiring decision with key department staff, HR staff, and/or executive staff, depending on the level of the position.

When the details of the job offer have been approved by the HR department, a formal job offer should be made. The HR department should prepare a letter that describes the duties and responsibilities of the position, states the employment start date, and explains the salary and benefits package. In addition, the hiring manager may choose to communicate the offer to the candidate through a personal telephone contact, which is subsequently confirmed by an official letter (Anthony, Perrewe, and Kacmar 1996).

Staff Retention

It is normal to have a certain level of staff turnover. Employees move, retire, or seek other careers. A manager can do little to prevent turnover resulting from changes in the personal lives of employees. However, the actions of managers and the policies of the organization can have an impact, either positive or negative, on staff retention. The following questions should be considered:

- Does the organization support continued education either financially or through flexible work schedules?
- Do employees have opportunities to advance their careers within the organization?

- Are salaries and benefits competitive with similar organizations?
- Do working conditions provide a comfortable and safe environment?

Although individual managers may have limited influence on some of these factors, they must always be aware of the impact that broader organizational HR policies and practices have on employees. Gone unnoticed or left unaddressed, concerns in these areas are often what make employees look for other jobs. For example, employees can become dissatisfied when they feel that they are being treated unfairly or that HR practices are needlessly rigid. In some cases, employees become dissatisfied simply because they do not know the rationale for a particular HR policy or because a concern they have voiced about an unsafe condition in their work area is not acted on by the manager. The challenge to the manager is to anticipate or, at the very least, to find ways to be informed as soon as possible when employees express an HR-related concern.

Staff turnover is expensive in terms of both lost productivity and recruitment and training costs. To ensure effective management, turnover should be monitored across time and benchmarked with the rest of the organization and/or other organizations in the community or geographic area. Routine employee satisfaction surveys can help provide information about how employees feel about their jobs and insights into how the facility might improve working conditions. Conducting routine **exit interviews** with employees who leave the organization is another way to obtain information on how employees feel about their jobs and what issues cause them to leave.

New Employee Orientation and Training

One of the key ingredients in employee satisfaction is the feeling of being knowledgeable and competent. This feeling begins with an effective orientation and training program for new employees. Just as the manager prepared for the interview and selection of the new employee, he or she must plan how the new employee will learn about the organization, the department, and the job.

Most large organizations have a formal new employee orientation process. This process may involve a one-on-one session with human resources, group training with new employees from all over the organization, and/or some form of computer-based training.

In general, orientation programs in healthcare organizations address the organization's mission and vision, goals, and structure; general employment policies; employee conduct standards; communication processes; and confidentiality policies. Orientation also may include a tour of the facility and cover computer access and responsibilities. When the organization provides this type of orientation, the manager must understand the material covered and feel comfortable answering any questions or directing the new employee to the appropriate resource for follow-up.

The manager must be very patient during the employee's first days and schedule adequate time to spend with the new hire. Everyone learns in different ways and at a different pace. The first days not only establish how the employee will do the job but also contribute to the employee's ongoing relationships with the manager and other staff. (A full discussion of the development of new employee orientation programs is presented in chapter 25.)

Tools for Effective Communication

Maintaining regular and effective communication with staff is one of the ongoing challenges in managing human resources. Communication is very important because it contributes significantly to the morale of the staff and their ability to contribute to the department's operations as a whole. To address this challenge, a manager should establish a **communication plan** that includes routine and timely opportunities for both verbal and written information sharing within the department or work group. The plan should include, at minimum, the following types of communication:

- Daily personal contact with every employee to maintain a sense of connectedness and, as necessary, to create opportunities for casual discussions of emerging work-related changes or issues
- Web-based or traditional bulletin boards located in an area convenient to staff to publicize official announcements, permissible personal news, written status updates, and written highlights from departmental meetings
- Weekly status update meetings with the staff for each functional unit in the department in larger organizations or the entire department in smaller organizations
- Monthly departmental meetings with highlights recorded for posting
- Quarterly performance discussions with individual employees
- Ad hoc verbal or electronic (e-mail) status updates, as appropriate, to alert staff to information of interest from organizational meetings

On a day-to-day basis, when problems emerge that require resolution within the department or when decisions are made that affect the employees in the department, the management team is responsible for establishing a unique communication plan that conforms to the situation. Such a plan identifies the full range of employees affected by the problem or the decision and defines the specific approach that managers will take to engage or inform each person appropriately.

In general, keeping staff well informed is a key factor in developing and sustaining a healthy level of trust in the relationship between employees and managers. Communication plans are simple tools that managers can use to ensure that this very critical aspect of their responsibilities is handled with the level of routine and regular attentiveness it requires.

Tools for the Empowerment of Staff

Creating an environment that encourages and allows employees to use and develop their problem-solving and decision-making competencies is an established HR management practice that has many benefits. For example, it increases the manager's capacity and productivity, improves the quality and timeliness of decision making, enhances employee morale, and contributes to improved employee retention.

Team Building

Most people today want to work in a team. The team may consist of people who perform the same function within the same department, for example, a coding team. The team may bring together people who perform different functions within the same department to solve a shared problem or people from across the organization with different expertise to implement a new computer system or to study an issue that would affect the overall organization (for example, improvements in the employee evaluation system).

At their best, teams increase the creativity and improve the quality of problem solving. Often team-based decisions are more widely accepted than managerial decisions because team members enlist support for the decisions from their peers and coworkers. In addition, teams can use their collective energy to produce more work than individuals can. Moreover, teamwork establishes strong relationships among employees. Teamwork also can enrich jobs and provide variety in work assignments. Finally, teams can develop new leaders and expose employees to issues that would not be within the usual scope of their jobs.

One thing that binds team members together is having a common purpose. The purpose for an ongoing work team, for example, might be to ensure cross-training, improve procedures, and monitor quality and/or productivity. In other cases, teams are created for a specific purpose. Some teams exist for long periods of time because they have an ongoing reason to exist. Other teams function for limited periods of time and disband after their purpose has been fulfilled.

However, having a common purpose is only one element of an effective team. The team also must have an effective leader. This individual must be able to create agendas and organize meetings, lead discussions, and ensure that the work moves forward. The team may either appoint or elect its leader, depending on its purpose and the experience and expertise of its members.

In addition, effective teams set ground rules. For instance, team members might decide that all meetings will start on time, minutes will be recorded, decisions will be reached by consensus, and everyone will participate in discussions. The early establishment of rules can reduce conflict as the team moves forward. Teams work through the same type of decision-making process described earlier in this chapter. However, their strength lies in engaging the collective brainpower of all of their members, and so the team leader should use techniques that effectively engage every member of the team.

Not all teams are effective, and the causes for problems vary. For example, a team without a clear purpose could create a product that does not accomplish the work it was designed to accomplish. A leader who dominates the team could reduce its effectiveness and frustrate its members. Members who do not participate, have insufficient expertise, or are unconcerned with the team's success could cause the team to fail. And members who work outside the team or do not support its decisions can create dissension and reduce support for the outcome.

Managing staff teams is an important aspect of every manager's responsibilities. Careful consideration should be given to developing the team's purpose and composition. Team members need to feel that their work is important and that their contributions make a difference. A well-run team can be an effective and productive force. A poorly run team can waste time and frustrate and demoralize its members.

Delegation of Authority

Managers have specific responsibilities and the authority to act within the scope of those responsibilities. A manager's responsibilities can never be delegated to another person; that is, the manager always remains the one accountable for outcomes in areas within his or her designated scope. However, with appropriate preparation and decision-making guidelines in place, managers can and should delegate the authority to make and act on decisions to employees as individuals or teams. **Delegation of authority** expands the manager's capacity, improves the timeliness of decisions, and develops the competencies of other staff members.

When delegating authority, managers make it possible for staff to succeed by preparing them in advance as follows:

- By explaining exactly what needs to be done
- By describing clear expectations
- By setting clear deadlines
- By granting authority to make relevant decisions
- By ensuring appropriate communication and outcomes reporting
- By providing the resources needed to complete the assigned task

(See chapter 25 for an expanded discussion of empowerment and delegation as work force retention strategies.)

Check Your Understanding 24.4

Instructions: On a separate piece of paper, indicate whether the following statements are true or false (T or F).

1. To lead effectively, every manager should have an understanding of human resources management principles.

2. Position descriptions outline the work that employees are expected to perform.

3. Performance standards are developed to indicate the time frame in which each function of a job must be executed.

4. Procedures are written explanations of how to perform tasks.

5. In healthcare organizations, individuals applying for entry-level positions must submit a resume and a cover letter.

6. Staff turnover is expensive in terms of lost productivity and recruitment and training costs.

7. A manager's responsibilities include new employee orientation and training.

8. One thing that teams have in common is that their members are usually from the same department.

9. Managers can delegate responsibilities, but not authority.

10. The interview process is intended to give the applicant an opportunity to evaluate the organization as a potential fit for his or her current and future employment goals.

11. To be effective, communications with employees should be expressed in written form.

12. Trust between managers and employees is enhanced by keeping employees well informed.

Compensation Systems

Employee compensation systems basically serve to reward employees equitably for their service to the organization. Organizations also use compensation systems to enhance employee loyalty and encourage greater productivity.

The FLSA, the EPA, and several of the EEO laws (for example, Title VII of the Civil Rights Act, Age Discrimination in Employment Act, and the ADA) all have provisions that affect compensation systems. Provisions of the FLSA, for example, cover minimum wage, overtime pay, child labor restrictions, and equal pay for equal work regardless of sex. Federal regulations specify exemptions from some or all of the FLSA provisions for a number of groups of employees (Myers 1998). These groups are referred to as **exempt employees.** Covered groups are referred to as **nonexempt employees.**

Managers who control employee work schedules and process employee timecards at the close of each pay period become quite familiar with the provisions of the FLSA that relate to overtime pay. In general, the FLSA requires that employers pay time and a half for all hours that covered (non-exempt) employees work in excess of forty per week. Some organizations institute overtime pay for all worked hours in excess of eight hours per day. In calculations of worked hours, the FLSA specifies that rest periods of up to 20 minutes each be counted as worked time, but meal periods of thirty minutes or more are not counted as worked time. Time spent in mandated job-related training is considered worked time, and significant travel time (beyond the usual time required to commute to and from work) associated with a work-related event is counted as worked time. Compensatory time, taken in lieu of overtime pay, may be used when it is part of the organization's compensation plan (Myers 1998).

Because of the complexities and sensitivities associated with compensation issues, HR professionals are a manager's best advisor when questions related to compensation regulations and practices arise.

Compensation Surveys

The HR department routinely consults compensation surveys published by government agencies and professional and trade associations. In some cases, an HR department may choose to conduct an independent survey to obtain data more specific to the organization's needs. Often consultants experienced with survey design and data analysis are employed by the organization to either assist in or do the survey project to ensure a successful outcome from this costly activity. Compensation surveys provide benchmark data that the organization can use to evaluate or establish its compensation system for unique jobs within the organization or for jobs throughout the organization (Myers 1998).

Job Evaluations

Job evaluation projects are undertaken by an organization to determine the relative worth of jobs as a first step toward establishing an equitable internal compensation system. Job evaluation is the process of applying predefined **compensable factors** to jobs to determine their relative worth (Myers 1998, p. 630). Myers defines a compensable factor as "a characteristic used to compare the worth of jobs" and adds that "the EPA requires employers to consider [several] compensable factors in setting pay for similar work performed by both females and males." These factors include skill, effort, responsibility, and working conditions.

Four job evaluation methods are commonly used:

- **Job ranking** is the simplest and the most subjective method of job evaluation. It involves placing jobs in order from highest to lowest in value to the organization.

- The **job classification method** involves matching a job's written position description with a description of a classification grade. Jobs in the federal government are graded on the basis of this method of job evaluation.

- The **point method** is a commonly used system that places weight (points) on each of the compensable factors in a job. The total points associated with a job establish its relative worth. Jobs that fall within a specific range of points fall into a grade associated with a specific wage or salary.

- The **factor comparison method** is a complex quantitative method that combines elements of both the ranking and point methods. Factor comparison results indicate the degree to which different compensable factors vary by job, making it possible to translate each factor value more easily into a monetary wage (Mathis and Jackson 2002).

In recent years, the **Hay method of job evaluation,** officially known as the Hay Guide Chart-Profile Method of Job Evaluation, has been used extensively. It is adaptable to many types of jobs and organizations and easy for individuals within organizations to learn to use. The method is essentially a modification of the point method that numerically measures the levels of three major compensable factors: the know-how, problem-solving, and accountability requirements of each job (Myers 1998; Mathis and Jackson 2002).

Performance Management

Most organizations use some form of **performance review** system to evaluate the performance of individual employees. Although performance reviews should be a part of regular communications between managers and employees, formal performance review discussions are routinely held on an annual or biannual basis. The functions of performance reviews include the following:

- Assessment of the employee's performance compared to performance standards or previously set performance goals
- Development of performance goals for the future year
- Development of a plan for professional development

Reviews also may include employee self-assessments. In some organizations, other employees may contribute information to the reviews of colleagues and coworkers. In the case of a supervisory manager, his or her staff may participate in the evaluation. This form of evaluation to which managers, peers, and staff contribute is called a **360-degree evaluation.**

Many organizations base pay increases on the results of annual performance reviews. Whether or not the evaluation affects salary, the annual review is an opportunity to formally discuss past accomplishments, career development, and expectations for future performance.

Periodic Performance Reviews

Performance management is an ongoing challenge. Information about performance should be collected regularly and shared with employees, whether their jobs involve coding clinical records or directing a department. Good performance results should be shared to encourage and reward ongoing success.

Performance issues are rarely resolved by ignoring them. Understanding the causes of problems and working with employees to resolve them are important management tasks. Actions that can be taken to improve performance include retraining, streamlining responsibilities, reestablishing expectations, and monitoring progress.

Performance Counseling and Disciplinary Action

When actions taken to improve performance are unsuccessful, more formal counseling and even **disciplinary action** may be required. Most organizations have formal processes in place to ensure that all staff is treated fairly and that employment laws are followed. Managers should consult with the HR department to ensure that any disciplinary actions comply with approved procedures.

The steps described in establishing performance standards, hiring and training employees, and conducting routine performance reviews are all necessary before doing **performance counseling** or taking disciplinary action. Moreover, steps to improve performance should be taken in all cases.

Performance counseling usually begins with informal counseling or a verbal warning. No record of these actions is maintained in the employee's file.

The **progressive discipline** process begins with a verbal warning. When a second offense occurs, the process progresses to a written reprimand with formal documentation of the problem and delineation of the steps needed to correct it. Employees may be required to submit a step-by-step action plan to resolve issues and improve their performance. A third offense results in suspension, and a fourth offense generally results in dismissal.

In some environments, disciplinary actions include suspension from employment without pay or demotion to a job with lower expectations and less pay. In some cases, more than one of these actions may be taken. Generally, however, suspension and demotion are less popular than the use of binding performance improvement plans because suspension and demotion create a punitive atmosphere. Such punitive actions also affect the morale of other employees and staff. Empowering employees to create a plan of action places the responsibility for performance improvement in their own hands.

Regardless of the counseling and disciplinary actions mandated by the organization, managers should take some key steps of their own, including:

- Discussing performance problems and consequences for poor performance with the employee in a clear and direct manner
- Supporting the employee's efforts to improve performance or resolve performance issues
- Documenting the steps taken to improve performance
- Carefully following the organization's HR policies
- Consulting HR professionals before taking action
- Keeping performance issues confidential
- Following the same process for all employees

Termination and Layoff

One of the most difficult duties of a line manager is delivering the actual notification of **termination** to an employee. The HR department is a vital resource for advising and supporting the manager through this process to ensure that accepted HR practices as established by the organization are adhered to. Buhler (2002) presents these simple, general guidelines:

- State your position and end the discussion
- Be sensitive to appropriate timing for the discussion
- Be prepared with all of the appropriate severance information
- Treat the employee with dignity and respect

Layoffs are essentially unpaid leaves of absence initiated by the employer as a strategy for downsizing staff in response to a change in the organization's status (for example, an unexpected or a seasonal downturn in business volume). In many cases, employees may be called back to work at some future date.

The **Workers' Adjustment Retraining and Notification (WARN) Act** requires that organizations employing more than 100 people give the employees and the community a 60-day notice of its intent to close the business or to lay off 50 or more members of its work force.

Conflict Management

Sometimes problems arise because of conflicts among employees. It is not unusual for people to disagree. Indeed, sometimes a difference of opinion can increase creativity. However, conflict can also waste time, reduce productivity, and decrease morale. When taken to the extreme, it can threaten the safety of employees and cause damage to property.

Conflict management focuses on working with the individuals involved to find a mutually acceptable solution. There are three ways to address conflict:

- **Compromise:** In this method, both parties must be willing to lose or give up a piece of their position.
- **Control:** In this method, interaction may be prohibited until the employees' emotions are under control. The manager also may structure their interactions. For example, the manager can set ground rules for communicating or dealing with specific issues. Another form of control is personal counseling. Personal counseling focuses on how people deal with conflict rather than on the cause of specific disagreements.
- **Constructive confrontation:** In this method, both parties meet with an objective third party to explore their perceptions and feelings. The desired outcome is to produce a mutual understanding of the issues and to create a win-win situation.

Grievance Management

Employees have the right to disagree with management and can express their opinions or complaints in a variety of ways. They should be encouraged to bring problems and concerns directly to their manager. When they do not achieve satisfaction at that level, the manager should explain other options to the employee. For example, dissatisfied employees should understand that they can either take their issues to the next management level or discuss them with HR staff.

Organizations establish **grievance procedures** that define the steps an employee can follow to seek resolution of a disagreement they have with management on a job-related issue. A complaint becomes a **grievance** when it has been documented in writing. At that point, the formal grievance procedure is set in motion.

Employees who belong to a union should follow the grievance procedures set by their union. Union contracts usually specify the types of actions employees can take and the time frames for filing grievances. The contracts usually specify time frames for responses and define the formal process for elevating the consideration or resolution of a grievance. Grievances taken to the highest levels will likely have to be resolved through mediation or arbitration.

Each of these steps takes time and can cost money. Therefore, managers should try to avoid grievances by maintaining open and effective communication with their staff.

Maintenance of Employee Records

Official **employee records** must be maintained under the control of the HR department. Any personnel records maintained under the control of the manager must be kept secure at all times.

Federal legislation such as Title VII of the Civil Rights Act of 1964, the Age Discrimination in Employment Act, the Immigration Reform and Control Act, and the FLSA place numerous record-keeping and reporting requirements on the HR department. The Environmental Protection Agency (EPA) and the Occupational Safety and Health Administration (OSHA) also have record-keeping requirements. Myers (1998, pp. 125–26) outlines several additional record-keeping obligations, as follows:

- Employers must protect the confidentiality of personnel records and files.
- Employers must protect the health records of employees.
- Employers must avoid intruding into the personal lives of employees, such as their other associations, alcohol use, spending habits, and financial obligations unless there are valid job-related reasons for making such intrusions.
- Employers must prevent the public disclosure of personal information that may be embarrassing to an employee.
- Employers must protect the results of employment-related tests, including written tests used in making selection decisions, and the results of both preemployment and random drug testing.

Current Human Resources Trends

According to the U.S. Department of Labor (2004), the following workforce trends in employment are likely to affect the labor market in the United States during the first decade of the 21st century:

- Total workforce growth was slower between 2000 and 2006 than in previous decades.
- Only one-third of the entrants to the workforce between 2000 and 2006 were white males.
- Women will constitute a greater proportion of the labor force than in the past, with 59 percent of all U.S. women in the workforce in 2004. In the healthcare

industry, over 75 percent of the workforce are women. Slightly over 70 percent of the women in the workforce have children under the age of 18, and 3 out of every 10 women in the workforce hold college degrees.

- Minority racial and ethnic groups will account for a growing percentage of the overall labor force. Immigrants will expand this growth.
- The average age of the U.S. population will increase, and more workers who retire from full-time jobs will work part-time.
- As a result of these and other shifts, employers in a variety of industries will face shortages of qualified workers.

From this information, it is obvious that employers must be prepared to function with an increasingly diverse workforce in terms of gender, age, health status, race, and ethnicity. In general, the management of an increasingly diverse workforce is receiving considerable attention in the HR literature, and some organizations are initiating diversity-training programs. Mathis and Jackson (2002, p. 39) identify three content areas that are often included in diversity training programs:

- *Legal awareness:* Federal and state laws and regulations on equal employment opportunity and the consequences of violating these laws and regulations
- *Cultural awareness:* Attempts to deal with stereotypes, typically through discussions and exercises
- *Sensitivity training:* Attempts to sensitize people to the differences among them and how their words and behaviors are perceived by others

According to Gillian Flynn (1998), mixed reviews regarding the effectiveness of the diversity training received from both public- and private-sector organizations suggest that either the programs or their implementation is ineffective. There seems to be considerable work still to be done within healthcare organizations and HIM departments to prepare for the anticipated growth in the multicultural profile of HR assets over the coming decade.

The Department of Labor data also indicate that employees will increasingly seek ways to gain more control over their time. The time pressure associated with trying to balance work and personal lives (especially when both parents are working outside the family home) coupled with the time pressure associated with increasingly long commutes appear to be driving this concern to the surface in HR management. Flextime, job sharing, and home-based (telecommuting) staffing options are emerging as viable solutions to the workforce retention issue. Within transcription and coding work units in HIM services, flextime and home-based staffing options are being implemented to address the labor shortages already affecting departmental operations. (See chapter 25 for a full discussion of these staffing alternatives.)

Check Your Understanding 24.5

Instructions: On a separate piece of paper, indicate whether the following statements are true or false (T or F).

1. Employee compensation systems are used to enhance employee loyalty.
2. Minimum wage and overtime policies are impacted by the Taft-Hartley Act.
3. All employees are subject to the provisions of the Fair Labor Standards Act.
4. Trade associations and government agencies are routine sources for compensation benchmark data.
5. The Equal Pay Act requires employers to consider compensable factors when setting pay for similar work performed by both females and males.
6. Job ranking is the most commonly used method for conducting job evaluations.
7. The Hays method is a popular, specialized point method for conducting job evaluations.
8. Formal performance review sessions are routinely done on an annual basis.
9. A 180-degree evaluation involves evaluation feedback from supervisors, peers, and self-assessment.
10. The first step in a progressive disciplinary process is a verbal, undocumented warning.
11. Compromise is a method of conflict resolution with the goal of arriving at a win-win outcome.
12. Grievances taken to the highest levels for resolution will likely be resolved through mediation or arbitration.
13. Organizations are obliged to avoid intrusions into an employee's personal life unless there is a valid job-related reason for doing so.
14. U.S. Department of Labor statistics indicate that a surplus of qualified labor will be available in most industries over the next decade (2000–2006).
15. Flextime and home-based staffing alternatives are being employed in health information services to address labor shortage issues.

Real-World Case

A coding specialist position is being added to the health information services department of a large metropolitan medical center. The purpose of the new position is to help the current staff to handle its increased workload since the implementation of the outpatient prospective payment system for Medicare patients earlier in the year. Figure 24.6 shows the resume of one of the numerous candidates applying for the coding specialist position. The director of the department has already developed a detailed job description for the new position. (See figure 24.7, p. 702.) A registered health information administrator (RHIA) was hired six months ago to supervise the department's five-person outpatient services team, and this new supervisor is a bit nervous about taking on this part of her new job. The director of the department has delegated responsibility for leading the process of selecting the person to fill the new coding specialist position to the new supervisor.

Figure 24.6.   Sample resume

RESUME

Stephen Jeremy Johnsen
222 Brickpath Way   Born 1/23/1971
Chicago, ILL 60622   Height 5 ft 9 in
773/222-2222   Weight 180 lbs

Goal: Looking for a job that lets me use my education and my knowledge of hospital coding and billing

Salary: $30,000+, opportunitie for advancement

2001	Code Lincoln Valley Community Hospital	
	I left to move to Chicago to be with my girlfried	

2001   Billing specialist University Medical Center, Chapaigne,Illinois
          Was here for almost a year; disliked manager; needed more money

1999   School Oakwood Community College

          Worked as a orderly to earn money for classes, majored in health information technology and computer programming

1995   Army Stationed in South Carolina, Germany, trained as medical corpsman

1989   School, majored in business but dropped out to join Army and earn money for school

1989   Graduated Glenview high school, Computer club, Music Camp, Varsity football, worked in father's landscape business during summers

*References available

Summary

Management is key in setting the healthcare organization's direction, establishing its policies, and maximizing its assets. Included among its assets are the people who carry out the organization's mission: the human resources staff. Managers are diffused throughout the organization with different responsibilities assigned at different levels and yet all have important roles to play in creating and maintaining an environment that is prudent in handling its financial resources, focused on providing high-quality services to its customers, and attentive to the basic human needs its workforce.

Effective management of human resources begins with attention given to the adoption of appropriate policies, procedures, and practices in each of the seven HR activity areas: HR planning and analysis; equal employment opportunity; staffing; HR development; compensation and benefits; health, safety, and security; and employee and labor/management relations. HR professionals working in close partnership with the organization's managers hire and retain qualified employees by following these guidelines and fostering good working relationships between employees and management.

Effective recruitment, selection, and hiring practices involve the consistent use of the tools designed to identify the best-qualified candidates for each position. Once hired, ensuring that employees are well oriented and trained is the critical first step toward a successful long-term outcome. Subsequently, maintaining open and meaningful communications with employees, setting realistic performance expectations for employees, engaging employees in ways that give them appropriate control of their work schedule and environment, delegating appropriate levels of decision-making

Figure 24.7. Sample job description for the Real-World Case

Position Description

Position Title:	APC Coordinator
Immediate Supervisor:	Director of Health Information Management
General Purpose:	The purpose of this position is to create consistency and efficiency in outpatient claims processing and data collection to optimize APC reimbursement and facilitate data quality in outpatient services.

Responsibilities:

- Performs data quality reviews on outpatient encounters to validate the ICD-9-CM, CPT, and HCPCS Level II code and modifier assignments, APC group appropriateness, missed secondary diagnoses and/or procedures, and compliance with all APC mandates and outpatient reporting requirements.

- Monitors medical visit code selection by departments against facility-specific criteria for appropriateness. Assists in the development of such criteria as needed.

- Monitors outpatient service mix reports and the leading medical visit, surgical service, significant procedure, and ancillary APCs assigned in the facility to identify patterns, trends, and variations in the facility's frequently assigned APC groups. Once identified, evaluates the causes of the change, and takes appropriate steps in collaboration with the right department to effect resolution or explanation of the variance.

- Continuously evaluates the quality of clinical documentation to spot incomplete or inconsistent documentation for outpatient encounters that impact the code selection and resulting APC groups and payment. Brings identified concerns to medical staff committee or department managers for resolution.

- Provides and/or arranges for training to facility healthcare professionals on the use of coding guidelines and practices, proper documentation techniques, medical terminology, and disease processes appropriate to the job description and function as it relates to the APC and other outpatient data quality management factors.

- Maintains knowledge of current professional coding certification requirements and promotes recruitment and retention of certified staff in coding positions when possible.

- Reports to the facility Compliance Committee each quarter.

- Abides by the Standards of Ethical Coding as set forth by the American Health Information Management Association and monitors coding staff for violations and reports to the HIM Director when areas of concern are identified. Concerns involving compliance issues are forwarded to the Compliance Committee for action.

- Develops reports and collects and prepares data for studies involving outpatient encounter data for clinical evaluation purposes and/or financial impact and profitability.

- Serves as the facility representative for APCs by attending outpatient coding and reimbursement workshops and bringing back information to the appropriate departments. Communicates any APC updates published in third-party payer newsletters/bulletins and provider manuals to all facility staff that need this information.

- Keeps abreast of new technology in coding and abstracting software and other forms of automation and stays informed about transaction code sets, HIPAA requirements, and other future issues impacting the coding function.

- Demonstrates competency in the use of computer applications and APC Grouper Software, OCE edits and all coding, software and hardware currently in use in the HIM department.

- Performs periodic claim form reviews to check code transfer accuracy from the abstracting system and the chargemaster.

- Evaluates, records, and responds to the Peer Review Organization APC change and/or denial notices. Provides appropriate documentation from required source to the PRO when appealing a PRO decision.

- Monitors outpatient unbilled accounts report for outstanding and/or uncoded outpatient encounters to reduce Accounts Receivable days for outpatients.

- Serves on the Chargemaster maintenance committee.

Qualifications:

- Minimum of associate's degree in a health services discipline. Formal HIM education with national certification, RHIA or RHIT preferred.

- Coding certification required from the American Health Information Management Association or the American Academy of Professional Coders.

- Minimum of five years progressive coding or coding review experience in ICD-9-CM, CPT, and HCPCS with claims processing and/or data management responsibilities a plus.

- Good oral and written communication skills and comprehensive knowledge of the APC structure and regulatory requirements.

- Prefer someone with past auditing experience or strong training background in coding and reimbursement.

authority, and providing them with opportunities for ongoing staff development all serve to enhance employee morale and increase job satisfaction.

Managing human resources is both a science and an art. As such, it is learned through a combination of study and observation. Published HR management resources are readily available to provide the knowledge foundation associated with this field. In the workplace, HR professionals are available to serve as advisors to managers who want to handle this complex aspect of their management responsibilities knowledgably and artfully.

References

Anthony, W.P., P.L. Perrewe, and K.M. Kacmar. 1996. *Strategic Human Resource Management.* Orlando, FL: Harcourt Brace & Company.

Benedictine Health System. 2002. Advancing the BHS ministry through a renewed commitment to mission, values. *BHS System Spirit & Life* 6(3):1.

Buhler, P. 2002. *Human Resources Management.* Avon, MA: F+W Publications.

Department of Labor, Bureau of Labor Statistics. 2004. Women in the labor force: A databook. bls.gov/cps/wlf-intro-2005.pdf.

Flynn, G. 1998. The harsh reality of diversity programs. *Workforce* 12:26–35.

Mathis, R.L., and J.H. Jackson. 2002. *Human Resource Management: Essential Perspectives,* 2nd ed. Cincinnati: South-Western Publishers.

Myers, D.W. 1998. *1999 U.S. Master Human Resources Guide.* Chicago: CCH.

Senge, P.M. 1990. *The Fifth Discipline.* New York: Doubleday/Currency.

Schein, E.H. 1980. *Organizational Psychology,* 3rd ed. Englewood Cliffs, NJ: Prentice-Hall.

Chapter 25
Training and Development

Karen R. Patena, MBA, RHIA

Learning Objectives

- To understand the continuum of employee training and development
- To appreciate the role of staff development in retaining a competent workforce
- To understand how to respond to various learning styles and to the needs of adult learners
- To understand how to respond to the needs of a culturally diverse workforce or the needs of employees with disabilities
- To understand how to apply appropriate delivery methods to various training needs
- To learn how to develop an orientation program for new employees

- To learn how to prepare and conduct appropriate in-service education programs for various healthcare employees
- To prepare employees for e-HIM™ roles
- To identify alternative staffing trends and discuss their role in workforce retention
- To understand how to apply appropriate methods for developing employee potential
- To learn how to assess the needs of current employees for continuing education
- To be able to prepare a training and development plan for a health information management department
- To be able to comply with the requirements of laws and regulations affecting workforce training

Key Terms

Accountability
Adult learning
Asynchronous
Audioconferencing
Authority
Blended learning
Career development
Coaching
Competency
Compressed workweek
Computer-based training
Continuing education
Cross-training
Cultural competence
Customer service training
Delegation
Development
Distance learning
Diversity training

e-HIM™
e-learning
Electronic performance support system
Employment contract
Empowerment
Ethics training
Flex years
Flextime
Habit
Incentive
In-service education
Intranet
Job description
Job rotation
Job sharing
Job specification
Just-in-time training
Learning curve

Learning content management system
Learning management system
Lecture
M-learning
Massed training
Mentor
Motivation
Needs assessment
Offshoring
On-the-job training
Orientation
Outsourcing
Pay for performance
Productivity
Promotion
Reinforcement
Reverse mentoring

Role playing
Self-directed learning
Simulation
Socialization
Spaced training
Strategic management
Synchronous
Task analysis
Team building
Telecommuting
Trainee
Train the trainer
Trainer
Training
Training and development model
Web-based training

Introduction

As a service industry, healthcare relies on the availability of competent workers. The growth of new technologies, the application of new vocabulary and processes, and the decreasing numbers of employees with adequate skills to respond to the new environment mean that healthcare organizations must frequently assume responsibility for preparing and developing their own labor pool, unless they choose to outsource or use employees overseas. Providing the necessary training to workers is costly in terms of both money and time. Using overseas workers creates its own training needs in areas such as ethics or the English language. Moreover, after the organization has made the investment, it must do what it can to protect its investment by retaining its workforce.

Human resources are the healthcare institution's most valuable asset. Managing employees requires recognizing and meeting the needs of the employees as well as those of the organization. Healthcare organizations must provide employees with the tools for career success and personal achievement if they are to win their long-term commitment.

This chapter focuses on training and retaining employees in the healthcare organization. It describes the orientation process and different methods for training new employees as well as current employees taking on new job responsibilities. It discusses **adult learning** strategies, techniques for delivering employee training, including the increasing use of e-learning methods, and ways to enhance job satisfaction. Special training issues, such as diversity, offshoring of employees, and preparing for e-HIM™ roles are addressed. Finally, the chapter describes how to implement a departmental employee training and development plan.

Theory into Practice

Nancy New has just started her position as director of health information management (HIM) for a large academic medical center on the West Coast. The department includes employees who have been hired in the past few months as well as employees who have been there as long as 10 years. Her most recent employee, Susan, is a newly credentialed RHIT with excellent coding skills. She is very enthusiastic about her job but sometimes fails to follow procedures that she feels are unnecessary. Some of the long-time coders are resentful of Susan's skills and new ideas and have called in sick on several occasions. Hospital management has been reluctant to send employees to **continuing education** (CE) programs because of the cost and time that employees lose away from work.

One of the best coders in the department, Julie, has recently returned from maternity leave. Although she enjoys her job, she has informed Nancy that she is thinking of resigning. Paying someone to care for her baby is expensive, and Julie often has difficulty concentrating on her work because she feels guilty about not being at home.

As part of a cost-reduction effort, transcription services have recently been outsourced to a company using employees who live in other countries, and there have been concerns about the quality of their work.

A new physician on staff has asked Nancy's help to train his office staff to interface with the hospital's electronic health record system.

Nancy has discovered that a formal **training** program has never been implemented for HIM department employees. Although the medical center provides a basic **orientation** for new employees that includes a review of basic policies and procedures, benefits, and fire safety protocols, it has no plan or budget in place for CE. Nancy felt that her own orientation was not comprehensive enough, and she has had to learn a great deal about her department on her own.

Concerned about all these issues, Nancy has determined three major areas of focus. First, her coders are in need of updated skills. Second, she wants to upgrade the morale and interpersonal skills of both her new and long-term employees. Finally, she does not want a good employee to resign.

With her supervisor's approval, Nancy prepares an employee development plan for the department. She begins with a **needs assessment** on the individual as well as departmental level. She sets learning objectives for new and existing employees and prepares a departmental orientation plan to supplement the one provided by the medical center. The orientation plan includes an introduction to policies and procedures, a review of privacy regulations, and **on-the-job training** in the employee's specific work area. To improve cooperation within the department and to build morale, Nancy plans to involve long-term employees in revising policies and procedures and in assisting in the training efforts for the electronic health record. Before long-term employees are permitted to train, however, they must attend a **train-the-trainer** session.

Nancy next requests additional funding to provide CE for her employees. She plans to use programs such as AHIMA's Web-based coding programs to provide high-quality material that can be delivered to the work site, thus reducing both the cost of travel and time away from the job. All employees will be required to demonstrate competencies through annual assessments. Those with outstanding scores will be considered for promotional opportunities and merit-based salary increases.

Nancy has reviewed the contract with the transcription company and will express her concerns about quality to her administrator as well as suggest training topics. She also has proposed development of a Web-based program on using the electronic health record that physicians can access from their offices.

Finally, Nancy proposes that employees be given the option to use **flextime** or even to work at home, provided they continue to demonstrate the ability to work independently, meet quantity and quality standards, and successfully complete periodic competency assessments.

Six months after implementing her plan, Nancy sees a marked improvement in her employees' skill levels and the elimination of unnecessary steps following a review of policies and procedures. There is a cooperative attitude among the staff, and Julie continues to work for the department as a home-based coder. The transcription company has implemented an English skills improvement training program. A Web-based training program has been developed and is accessible through the hospital's **intranet** for physician office staff regarding the use of electronic records. Susan supported and adhered to the new processes, as did the other coders in the department.

Training Program Development

Traditional management theory differentiated between training for lower-level, technical employees and **development** for management staff who needed to improve skills such as decision making and interpersonal communication. However, this distinction has become outdated in the 21st century as organizations take a more comprehensive approach to improving employee performance. Today, the terms *training* and *development* are often used interchangeably, with the primary goal being to improve knowledge, skills, abilities, attitudes, and social behavior of workers at all levels. As employees who make up the organization grow, so does the organization.

Training programs should accommodate employees with special needs, such as providing equipment and locations that are accessible to those with disabilities or instructions in another language for employees for whom English is a second language. In addition, the organization should develop diversity-training programs. **Diversity training** facilitates an environment that fosters tolerance and appreciation of individual differences within the organization's workforce.

Training and development programs should be viewed as a vital part of the **strategic management** of healthcare institutions. The standards of accreditation organizations as well as healthcare plans require the demonstration of high-quality, efficient healthcare delivery. To remain financially viable, healthcare organizations must emphasize **productivity,** performance, and profitability. Managers should identify first goals and objectives for their departments and then individual employees, and then define the skills and knowledge necessary to achieve the objectives. This goal-oriented approach should challenge and encourage the workforce to achieve organizational goals while helping individual employees reach their highest potential.

Investment in training programs helps the organization to accomplish goals on an individual, group, and organizational level. Other important reasons for providing employee training and development include:

- To introduce new employees to the organization
- To provide a path for employee **promotion** and retention
- To improve employee performance and productivity
- To update skills for employees in new or restructured positions resulting from organizational or technological change
- To reduce organizational problems caused by absenteeism, turnover, poor morale, or substandard quality
- To deliver high-quality healthcare within budgetary constraints

One way to view training and development needs is as a continuum of five conceptual areas, beginning with orientation and extending into **career development.** Healthcare organizations are unique and so should their development programs be. A 50-bed long-term care facility has very different staffing and training needs than a large acute care academic medical center does. Table 25.1 presents an employee

Table 25.1.   Employee development continuum

Concept	Objectives	Scope of Skill Diversity	Emphasis on Personal/Career Growth	Training Site	Frequency
Orientation training	To introduce staff to the mores, behaviors, and expectations of the organization	Narrow	Narrow	Internal	Single instance
Training	To teach staff specific skills, concepts, or attitudes			Internal	Sporadic
In-service education	To teach staff about skills, facts, attitudes, and behaviors largely through internal programs			Internal	Continuous
Continuing education	To facilitate the efforts of staff members to remain current in the knowledge base of their trade or profession through external programs designed to achieve external standards			External	Continuous
Career development	To expand the capabilities of staff beyond a narrow range of skills toward a more holistically prepared person	Broad	Broad	Internal and external	Continuous

Source: Fottler et al. 1998, p. 201.

development continuum (Fottler, Hernandez, and Joiner 1998, p. 201). Each concept differs in objectives, diversity of skills, degree of emphasis on career development, training location, and frequency of delivery. There is no best way to deliver training; it must fit the context of the institution.

However, investment in employee development does not end with training. Organizations need to find ways to gain the commitment of employees so that they will remain productive. Retaining good employees and developing their potential is an area of great importance, particularly in an industry that has a shortage of qualified workers.

Elements of Workforce Training

The goal of any institution's training program is to provide employees the skills they need to perform their jobs. Because employees are at different stages in their career development, the training program must be flexible and able to adapt to meet many needs. At any given time, some new employees will need to know basic information about the organization and long-term employees will want to improve their ability to contribute at higher levels within the organizational structure. Today's workforce needs both technical skills and so-called soft skills, such as **team building** and critical thinking. For example, electronic health records are increasingly becoming an integral part of the healthcare work setting. Thus, whatever the primary task, most employees need to develop skills in using personal computers and related devices.

New Employee Orientation

After employees have been recruited and selected, the first step is to introduce them to the organization and their immediate work setting and functions.

Definition
New employee orientation includes a group of activities that introduce the employee to the organization's mission, policies, rules, and culture; the department or work group; and the specific job he or she will be performing. In addition to the basic skills needed to do the job, the employee needs to experience a period of **socialization** in which he or she learns the values, behavior patterns, and expectations of the organization.

Needs Assessment
As with all training programs, the orientation must be customized to the particular employee. New employees will require a more in-depth orientation than current employees who are starting a different position within the same institution. In a large facility, new employee orientation is usually coordinated by human resources (HR); in a small facility, it may be performed entirely by the employee's supervisor. The orientation may consist of a brief and informal presentation, or it may be a formal program that takes place over several days on a regularly scheduled basis. Formal programs typically begin with presentations by HR and other department heads before the new employee is introduced to his or her immediate supervisor. The supervisor then continues the orientation process within the employee's assigned department.

To develop an orientation program, it is helpful to begin with a **task analysis** to determine the specific skills required for the job. The **job description** and the **job specification** are excellent sources for this part of the process. Beyond specific tasks, all new employees need to understand matters common to the institution, such as personnel policies, benefits, and safety regulations. Federal and state governments and accreditation organizations also may require certain subjects to be included in the orientation program.

Requirements
Although the orientation program is typically done at a single point in time, a new employee may not feel completely competent for as long as a year from the date he or she was hired. The program should attempt to make employees feel that they made the right choice in accepting the position. For this to happen, they should feel welcome, comfortable in their new environment, positive about their supervisor, and confident that they are learning the skills they need to do the job. An orientation program should not just be for completing paperwork.

An effective tool used in orienting new workers is the orientation checklist. (See figure 25.1.) The orientation checklist helps the employer know that the employee is receiving the information he or she needs to begin the job and serves as an agenda for presenting the information in a logical manner. Rather than presenting everything the new employee needs to know all at once, it is helpful to spread the orientation over several days.

In addition, it is helpful to present policies and requirements that all employees must know, such as insurance programs, payroll requirements, and personnel policies, in an employee handbook given to new employees during the orientation. The handbook provides a handy reference after the immediate orientation period has ended. However, the facility must be careful not to include content that expresses or could imply conditions of an **employment contract.** If the employee views the handbook as a contract, it becomes a legally binding agreement. Employer or employee could be held liable if any conditions set out in the handbook are not strictly followed. Thus, the employee handbook must be viewed as advisory in nature and not as a legal document.

The requirements of an orientation program may be expressed on three levels: organizational, departmental, and individual.

At the *organizational level,* the orientation program provides the information that every employee who works for the company needs to know. This information typically includes:

- Background and mission of the organization
- Policies and procedures that apply to all employees, such as confidentiality agreements or infection control procedures

- Employee benefits (paid time off, insurance coverage)
- Safety regulations
- Employee/orientation handbook
- Tour of the facility

At the *departmental level,* orientation information typically includes:

- Departmental policies and procedures
- Introduction to other employees
- Tour of department
- Work hours
- Time sheet requirements
- Training in operation of equipment (for example, photocopying machines or computers)
- Safety regulations specific to the department

At the *individual level,* the new employee learns specific job tasks that, at a minimum, should include:

- Specific, measurable objectives for productivity and performance
- An explanation of each job task by the supervisor, followed by a demonstration and an opportunity for the employee to demonstrate the task

The new employee's individual orientation is usually the longest portion of the orientation program.

Components of an Orientation Program

An orientation program should be developed with input from HR, other department heads, and the employee's supervisor. For a typical new employee in the HIM department of an acute care hospital, the orientation program might follow the schedule shown in figure 25.1. The first portion of the program introduces the employee to the institution and is typically led by the director of education or the director of HR. The employee is given a handbook and any required forms to complete for payroll and insurance.

Figure 25.1.   Sample orientation checklist

Orientation Checklist

Supervisor _____   Date _____

Employee _____   Department _____

Before Worker Arrives

(Check off tasks when completed.)

____ 1. Prepare other employees.
____ 2. Have desk and supplies ready.
____ 3. Arrange for luncheon escort.

First Day

____ 1. Attend hospital orientation program.
____ 2. Receive employee handbook and (if applicable) union contract information.
____ 3. Receive benefit information.
____ 4. Review safety and security regulations, including infection control procedures.
____ 5. Introduce to immediate associates.
____ 6. Introduce to the workplace.
____ 7. Give overview of the job.
____ 8. Ask whether new employee has any questions.

Second Day

____ 1. Discuss confidentiality policy.
____ 2. Give job instructions.
____ 3. Review compensation.
____ 4. Explain hours of work.
____ 5. Discuss attendance requirements.
____ 6. Explain performance review.
____ 7. Explain quality and quantity standards.
____ 8. Encourage employee to ask questions.
____ 9. Explain where to store work overnight.

Orientation Completed _____ (Date)

Signature of Employee _____

Third Day

____ 1. Explain telephone system, computer system, and fax and copier machines.
____ 2. Explain reasons for rules and policies.
____ 3. Explain insurance plans.
____ 4. Ask whether the new employee has any questions.

Fourth Day

____ 1. Give employee opportunity to describe how he or she is getting along.
____ 2. Discuss departmental policies in addition to hospital policies.
____ 3. Explain hospital continuing education program.

Fifth Day

____ 1. Describe vacation system.
____ 2. Explain bulletin board policy.

Sixth Day

____ 1. Encourage employee to talk to supervisor when necessary.
____ 2. Administer postorientation assessment.
____ 3. Give orientation evaluation form to employee to complete.

Signature of Supervisor _____

Source: Adapted from Keeling and Kallaus 1996, p. 148.

The director of safety and security then introduces safety regulations.

To introduce the employee to the individual job setting as quickly as possible, the general portion of the orientation could be completed within the first half-day. The employee then could meet the immediate supervisor and be matched with a "buddy" to escort him or her to lunch and back to the department. Ideally, the buddy should have the same job as the new employee. On the afternoon of day one, the new worker should be introduced to coworkers, given a tour of the department, and shown his or her workstation. The first day could end with a basic overview explanation of the job's duties, including an opportunity for questions.

The individual portion of the orientation should continue as described in the suggested schedule, with some portion of each day devoted to job training and work rules so that the new employee can gradually understand the requirements of the job and become socialized to the work environment. As the new employee is trained and tested in each important aspect of the job, the supervisor should document his or her demonstrated competency. This documentation will help the organization to comply with the standards of the Joint Commission on Accreditation of Healthcare Organizations (JCAHO).

Assessment

After the orientation process, all the participants should be asked for feedback. A form should be developed and completed by the new employee. Figure 25.2 presents an example of a form for evaluating the general portion of the orientation program. Typical questions include:

- Was the program relevant to your job and needs?
- What part of the program was most useful to you?
- What part of the program was least useful to you?

In addition, supervisors should be asked to evaluate the effectiveness of the orientation process. For example, they should be asked for feedback on the employee's ability to apply his or her newly acquired job skills and for an assessment of the employee's comfort level with the department.

On-the-Job Training

Preparing staff to carry out the tasks and functions of their particular jobs should be an ongoing effort for both new and experienced employees. A variety of methods are available to employers. Effective training programs begin with a needs assessment and blend an appropriate combination of methods, media, content, and activities into a curriculum that is matched to the specific education, experience, and skill level of the audience.

Definition

On-the-job training is a method of teaching an employee to perform a task by actually performing it. Along with teaching basic skills, on-the-job training gives employees and supervisors opportunities to discuss specific problem areas and initiates socialization among the new employees and their coworkers. On-the-job training offers a number of advantages, including its relatively low cost compared to outside training programs and the fact that work is still in progress while the employee is being trained. However, employees may feel burdened if they are held responsible for work they do not accomplish during the training period and the learning process may be less than optimal if the work setting is disrupted by ongoing distractions and pressures.

Training may be performed by either a supervisor or a coworker with particular expertise. The selection of an appropriate trainer is critical to the success of this method. Even though they are very capable at performing the job being taught, some employees may not be effective teachers and may omit vital steps if not motivated to do the teaching.

Requirements of the Job

The training program should begin by reviewing the job description and the job specification. Job descriptions and job specifications should include a list of tasks performed for a job; the skills, ability, and knowledge required; and the expected quality and quantity standards of performance. Next, a performance analysis should be completed to assess the gap between expected performance and the employee's current performance level. In the case of a new employee, this may be verified through a written **competency** assessment. What the employee does not know or cannot do becomes the basis for on-the-job training. The requirements may include any of the following:

- Physical skills (for example, operation of equipment)
- Academic knowledge (for example, medical terminology or English spelling and grammar)
- Knowledge of institutional policies (for example, safety regulations)
- Technical skills, which may include both physical and mental skills (for example, use of computer programs)

Components of on-the-Job Training

On-the-job training offers a variety of delivery options, including:

- One-on-one training by a supervisor or an experienced peer
- Job rotation
- Computer-based training
- Coaching or mentoring
- Informal learning during meetings or discussions with supervisors and peers

One-on-one training is the technique used most often. In this type of training, the employee learns by first observing a demonstration and then performing the task. For this type of training to be effective, organizations may offer train-the-trainer workshops in which the **trainer** learns skills in communication and instruction. It is important to select a person to serve as a trainer who is not only competent in the job content, but also able to teach and interact effectively with the **trainee.** One-on-one training by the supervisor gives the supervisor an opportunity to observe how the trainee is doing and to make adjustments to meet the employee's skill level. A trainee who learns quickly can move through the steps at a faster pace; a trainee who learns slowly may need an opportunity for additional practice or a second demonstration.

In **job rotation,** the employee moves from job to job at planned intervals. This method is most useful for supervisory jobs, where the employee needs to learn a variety of tasks performed by several different employees, as well as their interrelationships. In **cross-training,** the employee learns to perform the jobs of many team members. This method is most useful when work teams are involved.

Computer-based training, including **Web-based training,** provides an opportunity to supplement job task performance with additional knowledge and/or simulation. It is effective in situations where repetition aids learning, for example, with medical terminology and tasks that cannot be duplicated entirely in the practice session, such as role-playing with different release of information (ROI) scenarios.

Figure 25.2. Sample orientation evaluation form

Employee Orientation Program Evaluation Form

Date: _____

Job Title: _____

1. Please rate each of the following items to indicate your reaction to the session. If ranking is less than average, please comment on the back of this form.

Item	Poor	Adequate	Average	Good	Excellent
Objective 1: Applicability to your job, responsibilities, and needs					
Objective 2: Enough examples and chances to practice so you can apply your new skills at work					
Objective 3: Opportunity for discussion with other participants					
Objective 4: Length of the program relative to its objectives					

2. Which part of the program was of most value to you? Why?

3. Which part of the program was of least value to you? Why?

4a. Please use the following scale to comment on each instructor's ability to lead the program where:

   1 = Needs improvement   2 = Adequate   3 = Good   4 = Excellent

Item	Instructor 1	Instructor 2
Organization/preparation of subject matter	1 2 3 4	1 2 3 4
Presentation of subject matter	1 2 3 4	1 2 3 4
Clarity of instructions	1 2 3 4	1 2 3 4
Ability to control time	1 2 3 4	1 2 3 4
Ability to link content to your job functions	1 2 3 4	1 2 3 4
Ability to stimulate productive discussions	1 2 3 4	1 2 3 4
Ability to create a productive learning environment	1 2 3 4	1 2 3 4

4b. Please comment on the instructors' abilities to lead the program:

5. How would you rate your overall reaction to the program?   1 2 3 4

6. How would you rate your level of skill/knowledge:
   a. Before the program?   1 2 3 4
   b. After the program?   1 2 3 4

7. Other comments:

Source: O'Connor et al. 2002.

After the trainee has demonstrated the ability to do the job, **coaching** should continue by the supervisor or an expert peer on an ongoing basis. The experienced worker observes or reviews the work of the employee in a nonthreatening manner, offering advice and suggestions for revising techniques to improve productivity and efficient work performance. In a formalized arrangement in which a specific person is assigned to follow up on a regular basis, the coach is referred to as a **mentor.** In this scenario, the mentor meets with the trainee on a regular basis and often gives advice on career growth and development within the organization.

It is estimated that approximately two-thirds of training actually results from informal interactions between the employee and his or her coworkers. Learning occurs even though it is not formally designed or monitored by the organization, for example, during hallway conversations or on lunch breaks when a work topic is discussed and other employees or supervisors offer suggestions or corrections.

On-the-job training methods can be used individually or in combination and should be adapted to each learner. Whatever technique is used, on-the-job training should follow the steps presented in figure 25.3.

Assessment

By its nature, on-the-job training provides an opportunity for immediate assessment of its effectiveness. The trainer can observe the employee's skills as part of the performance tryout and can question the employee on his or her knowledge of policies, procedures, and other academic knowledge that may be required. If the assessment reveals areas of weakness, the training can be adjusted to reinforce knowledge or repeat steps performed incorrectly.

When the employee is working on his or her own, the supervisor should check the quantity and quality of the employee's work against performance standards from time to time. If the employee's performance is below standard, the training can be repeated before bad performance becomes a **habit.**

Finally, the employee should be encouraged to ask questions both during and after the training and should receive positive and negative feedback as appropriate.

Staff Development through In-Service Education

The healthcare industry grows and changes constantly. Whether it is a new law passed by the state or the federal government, new reimbursement regulations, updates to ICD-9-CM or CPT codes, new or revised accreditation standards, or new **e-HIM**™ roles, change is a permanent factor. Preparing workers for such changes requires continuous training and retraining.

Definition

In-service education is the third step in the employee development continuum. (See table 25.1, p. 707.) It is a continuous process that builds on the basic skills learned through new employee orientation and on-the-job training. In-service education is concerned with teaching employees specific skills and behaviors required to maintain job performance or to retrain workers whose jobs have changed. Although in-service education may include external programs, it is primarily developed and delivered at the work site or through computer-based training.

Needs Assessment

The need for in-service education may be triggered by many events, including:

- A restructuring of the department and/or organization
- Annual updates to coding or reimbursement requirements
- Implementation of electronic health records
- A decline in productivity or morale or an increase in absenteeism
- A new organizational policy or procedure

Figure 25.3.   Steps in on-the-job training

Step 1: Preparation of the learner
   a. Put the learner at ease; relieve the tension.
   b. Explain why he or she is being taught.
   c. Create interest, encourage questions, find out what the learner already knows about his or her job or other jobs.
   d. Explain the whole job and relate it to some job the worker already knows.
   e. Place the learner as close to the normal working position as possible.
   f. Familiarize the worker with the equipment, materials, tools, and trade terms.

Step 2: Presentation of the operation
   a. Explain quantity and quality requirements.
   b. Go through the job at the normal work pace.
   c. Go through the job at a slow pace several times, explaining each step. Between operations, explain the difficult parts or those in which errors are likely to be made.
   d. Again, go through the job at a slow pace several times; explain the key points.
   e. Have the learner explain the steps as you go though the job at a slow pace.

Step 3: Do a tryout
   a. Have the learner go through the job several times, slowly, explaining each step to you. Correct mistakes and, if necessary, do some of the complicated steps the first few times.
   b. Run the job at the normal pace.
   c. Have the learner do the job, gradually building up skill and speed.
   d. As soon as the learner demonstrates ability to do the job, let the work begin, but don't abandon him or her.

Step 4: Follow-up
   a. Designate to whom the learner should go for help if he or she needs it.
   b. Gradually decrease supervision, checking work from time to time against quality and quantity standards.
   c. Correct faulty work patterns that begin to creep into the work, and do it before they become a habit. Show why the learned method is superior.
   d. Compliment good work; encourage the worker until he or she is able to meet the quality/quantity standards.

Source: Dessler, 2005, p. 276.

- An external requirement imposed by accreditation or licensing organizations, such as an annual renewal of CPR certification or retraining in infectious disease precautions or safety procedures

The amount of in-service education needed varies with the event and the education and experience of the employee. Downsizing or reorganizing organizational structure often causes changes in an individual employee's job responsibilities. Employees may need to learn other job functions within the work group or may even be placed in a new department. This can require a series of formal training sessions, including on-the-job training.

Renewal of training, required by external organizations, may be subject to defined content and duration, often including a test and/or demonstration of the employee's competence. On the other hand, implementation of a new policy or procedure may simply include distributing the information accompanied by a short meeting.

Decisions need to be made regarding the appropriate format of the in-service education. The following types of questions should be asked:

- Should the instruction be given as **massed training** in a highly concentrated session or as **spaced training** in several shorter sessions?
- Should the task be broken down into parts or be taught as a single unit?
- How will competence be assessed? Is the topic a skill that needs to be demonstrated by the learner, or is it a level of knowledge that should be tested with a written assessment?

As with other training categories, periodic analysis of actual-versus-desired job performance will create a list of topics that should be addressed with in-service education.

Requirements

Unlike orientation programs, which are delivered primarily at one point in time, in-service education programs need to be available on an ongoing basis. Depending on the size of the organization, some programs, such as a refresher on the response to the institution's disaster plan, may be offered on a monthly basis. The HR department may coordinate programs on topics that affect the organization as a whole. Programs specific to health information management, such as a coding update, are more likely to be developed by a supervisor or manager in the HIM department.

Finally, some topics serve the needs of more than one department. For example, a program on coding updates may be given by the coding supervisor to employees from the HIM, patient accounting, and physician billing departments. This type of program probably would take place in a more formal setting and require coordination with other department managers.

Examples of in-service education topics and the individuals within the organization who are likely to have responsibility for them are shown in figure 25.4.

Figure 25.4.   Examples of responsibility for in-service education

Organizationwide: The human resources department typically assumes responsibility for the following topics and may include staff from other departments in the planning and presentation:
- Fire and safety awareness
- Disaster plan implementation
- Infectious disease/universal precautions
- Diversity training
- Team building
- HIPAA training

Multiple Departments: The health information manager may work with managers of several departments to coordinate presentation of the following topics:
- ICD-9-CM or CPT annual updates
- Medical terminology training
- Use of office productivity software for employee productivity measurement
- Health record documentation

Health Information Management Department: The health information manager may develop in-service training within the department for the following topics:
- Release of information
- Fire, safety, and disaster preparedness
- Electronic health record (EHR) implementation
- Use of new photocopier

Steps in Conducting In-Service Education

Presenting an effective in-service program requires planning. The time frame depends on the complexity of the material and the number of participants but should include enough time to prepare materials and publicize the event. Generally, a formal in-service program should follow these steps:

- *Step 1: Set objectives.* Is the purpose of the program to teach a new job task to an individual or to improve morale within the department?
- *Step 2: Determine the audience.* Is the training intended for one employee or 50 employees? Are the participants from the same department or from several departments?
- *Step 3: Determine whether the content should be delivered as a unit or in parts (massed or spaced).* This may be determined by the availability of the employee as well as the topic.
- *Step 4: Determine the best method of instruction.* The education and experience of the audience, the time available, and the cost of preparing and delivering the instruction should all be taken into consideration. Is there a qualified expert in-house? Are videotapes or computer-based materials available for rent or purchase? Is space available to train a large group at one time? (See the discussions of adult learning strategies and delivery methods later in this chapter.)
- *Step 5: Prepare a budget.* If a specific amount has been allocated, the plan should be compared to the predetermined budget and revised, if necessary. Approval should

be obtained if the proposal is a new one. In addition, the proposal should include the costs of photocopying materials, speaker fees, and training resources.

- *Step 6: Publicize the program.* Flyers and/or electronic notices should be posted to announce the program and should include the date, time, location, topic, and a summary of the content. When it is important to know the number of attendees in advance, the notice should include a method for RSVP.
- *Step 7: If appropriate, prepare handout materials.* Handouts would include materials to be used for instruction as well as documents to reference following the program. At a minimum, an agenda of the topics and a schedule should be developed.
- *Step 8: Practice, practice, practice!* The person presenting the program should be adequately prepared and comfortable with the content. Also, a training room should be scheduled ahead of time, and any needed equipment should be checked to ensure that it is available and in good working order. Anyone planning to use a computer or a projector should know how to operate it.
- *Step 9: Use a variety of methods, and be alert to your audience.* In addition to the lecture, the presenter should engage the audience through interactive questioning and activities. People learn by doing. Opportunities should be provided from time to time for questions and periodic breaks when the program lasts more than two hours.

- *Step 10: Obtain feedback from the audience.* It is important to give the participants an opportunity to document their reactions to the training. To that end, an evaluation form should be created and distributed. A sample in-service education evaluation form is shown in figure 25.5.

Assessment

Because some amount of cost, in terms of both time and resources, is usually involved with in-service training, it is important to determine whether its objectives have been met. Three methods for assessing the impact of in-service education are:

- *Completion of an evaluation form at the conclusion of the program:* Immediate feedback provides an assessment of the effectiveness of the delivery methods. Is the employee energized and ready to put the material to use, or was the material overwhelming?
- *Formal or informal feedback from the employee's supervisor:* Within a few days of the program, the supervisor should be contacted to determine whether the learner has applied the new skills and knowledge on the job.
- *Follow-up with the employee at a later time:* Thirty days after the in-service program, the attendees should be asked to validate the value of the program. Are they able to perform their job better? Is there something they feel they did not learn that should have been included? This may be accomplished easily via an e-mail message.

Figure 25.5.   Sample in-service education evaluation form

In-Service Education Evaluation Form

To help us improve the quality of future programs, please complete the following evaluation of today's session.

Please use the following scale to answer questions 1–5:

1 = Needs Improvement   2 = Satisfactory   3 = Excellent

1. How satisfied were you with the content of the presentation?		1	2	3
2. How would you rate the organization of the presentation?		1	2	3
3. How would you rate the effectiveness of visual media used in the presentation?		1	2	3
4. How would you rate the delivery of the presentation?		1	2	3

5. How satisfied were you with the following aspects of the program?

a. Meeting location	1	2	3
b. Parking	1	2	3
c. Accessibility	1	2	3
d. Registration process	1	2	3
e. Meeting room setup/seating	1	2	3
f. Handout materials	1	2	3

6. What is one thing you learned that you did not know prior to attending?

7. What would you like to have learned more about?

8. Please provide any additional comments that could improve future programs.

Preparing the HIM Staff for e-HIM®

In 2003, AHIMA convened a task force of industry professionals with extensive experience in healthcare, HIM, academics, information systems, technology, and government to articulate a vision for the future state of HIM. The e-HIM initiative seeks to promote the migration from paper to an electronic health information infrastructure, reinvent how institutional and personal health information and records are managed, and deliver measurable cost and quality results from improved information management. The report of the task force described future roles for HIM professionals and an action plan to achieve the vision.

Future roles include:

- Business process engineer
- Clinical research protocol designer and manager
- Clinical trials manager
- Clinical vocabulary manager
- Consumer advocate
- Data analyst
- Data facilitator
- Data/information broker
- Data/information presenter
- Data sets, nomenclature, and classification standards developer
- Data miner
- Data navigator
- Data quality and integrity monitor
- Data resource manager
- Data security, privacy, and confidentiality manager
- Data translator
- Information system designer
- Work and data flow analyst

The task force recommended that HIM professionals continuously transform their knowledge, skills, and abilities to keep pace with the competencies needed for the new roles. Competencies are needed in areas such as data analysis, data integration, privacy and security, methods of encryption and deidentification, clinical vocabulary development and maintenance, and public health surveillance. Providing training for these topics should become a focus of the HIM department's training and development plan for all employees.

Other examples of career roles in information technology include:

- Applications analyst
- Project manager
- Team leader
- Marketing or sales associate

Special Issues for Training

Several issues must be considered in training programs that apply to all levels, from orientation programs to staff development.

Diversity Training

The September 11, 2001, terrorist attacks had a profound effect on training in the United States. Awareness of the impact of culture on the workforce became an important issue, yet people were afraid to discuss differences for fear of offending others. Organizations found it was important to learn about issues such as the effect of culture on communication and learning styles.

Diversity training attempts to develop sensitivity among employees about the unique challenges facing diverse religious, ethnic, and sexual orientation groups, as well as those with disabilities, and strives to create a more harmonious working environment. It is important to help all employees from diverse backgrounds feel part of the team, committed, and productive. Training should be provided for the entire organization, with additional specific training for management staff.

A training course about ethnic minorities might begin with a review of various cultures from a social studies perspective (that is, location of the country, climate, customs, or food preferences). Other topics that might be included later would be cultural norms, such as communication styles (strong eye contact or standing close when conversing), use of first versus formal names, or tolerance of jokes. Of particular importance to the HIM employee is the perspective of some cultures on the issue of privacy, which may require that permissions be obtained to comply with the Health Insurance Portability and Accountability Act (HIPAA) of 1996.

A booklet might be prepared about each group that provides knowledge of the culture, communication helps, and tips for nonjudgmental respect. Employees might be advised to read the material and then follow up with a discussion. When the training course has been completed, an employee advisory group might be formed to advise management staff regarding barriers and issues of concern to diverse employees. A calendar with various cultural and religious celebrations might be posted on the company intranet.

For those employees needing training in the English language and American culture, topics might include English reading and writing skills, focusing on general as well as medical terms. Interpersonal skills, customer service, and the U.S. corporate culture also might be helpful.

Suggested stages for diversity training include:

- Antiharassment and sensitivity training
- Cultural awareness and competence
- Development of multicultural teams
- Full inclusion of minority groups into every level of the organization

Many companies produce materials to help with diversity training, including videotapes, facilitator materials, printed materials, and cases for **role playing.**

Training for Offshoring

A shortage of skilled workers in the United States in specialties such as coding and transcription has resulted in companies and organizations using employees who live overseas,
a practice known as **offshoring.** This has resulted in some
unique requirements for training. To ensure quality control,
training should be included as a requirement within the service contract.

Areas of training for overseas workers may include English proficiency, privacy and security requirements (including HIPAA), American etiquette, and cultural differences.
For those desiring career advancement, topics such as leadership development and supervision should be added.

For those in the United States supervising the workers,
issues of **cultural competence** are essential. For example,
many Asian countries are much more respectful of the
impact of personal lives of employees, which requires breaks
for religious practice and other personal obligations.

Ethics Training

Ethics training helps employees focus on "right" versus
"wrong" behavior in the workplace. The focus of this training is to help employees recognize ethical dilemmas, using
codes of conduct to resolve problems. Training might be Web
based, using what-if scenarios. It is suggested that initial
training be part of the employee's orientation program, with
annual refresher training.

Team Training

Team-building training helps employees learn to work in
groups that have the authority to make decisions. Emphasis
is on the group rather than individual achievement. Skills
are taught that help members diagnose and devise solutions to problems. Exercises such as constructing items
within a group encourage creativity. Conflict-resolution
training focuses on communication skills needed to resolve
gridlock. Facilitators may work with a group, asking group
members and leaders to identify problem issues at the
beginning of the session. The group then ranks the themes
identified, and that becomes the agenda for problem solving. A byproduct of team training is improved employee
attitudes and satisfaction.

Customer Service Training

Customer service training identifies skills needed to meet
and exceed customer expectations. These include communication and listening skills. Often sensitivity training may
be taught as a part of customer service training, which helps
individuals learn how others perceive their behavior. Sensitivity training is based on the assumption that individuals
working in an unstructured situation will develop working
relations with each other. Typically, 10 to 15 people meet in
an off-site location. A skilled trainer serves as the facilitator.
The purpose is to develop an awareness of processes that
facilitate or inhibit group functioning.

Adult Learning Strategies

Training has been defined as the process of providing individuals with the materials and activities they need to develop the
knowledge, skills, abilities, attitudes, and behaviors desired in
the workplace. Learning is what occurs in the individual, the
changes in behavior, knowledge, attitudes, abilities, and skills
that are desired. In the healthcare work environment, learning
translates into achieving the goals of the institution, including
improved job performance. The objective is for employees to
develop effective work habits. To accomplish this objective, it
is important to understand how employees learn and the factors that affect the learning environment.

Learning Styles

Just as there are many personalities, there are many ways people
learn. It would seem appropriate, then, that the greatest amount
of learning will take place if the teaching method matches the
learning style of the learner. If relevancy, meaning, and emo-
tion are attached to the material taught, the learner will learn.
Learners tend to progress only as far as they need to in order to
achieve their goal. Therefore, the best time to learn is when it is
seen as useful, which has made **just-in-time training** popular.

Although there may be a preferred learning style, other approaches may be used, but not as often. Learning styles are influenced by factors such as age, maturity, and experience, and they may change over time. In general, active learning is more effective than passive learning. Younger workers prefer concrete, sequential learning, whereas older adults prefer more ambiguity, which permits them to draw on their own experience. Following are various models for categorizing learning styles:

- *Sensory:* Is the learner auditory (prefers to listen), visual (prefers to read), or kinesthetic (prefers to practice)?
- *Personality:* Various personality traits shape our orientation to the world.
- *Information processing:* People differ in how they receive and process information.
- *Social interaction:* Gender and social context determine learning style.
- *Instructional and environmental preference:* Sound, light, structure, and learning relationships affect perceptions.

Various teaching techniques may be used to address different learning styles. These include:

- Individual tasks (reading, answering questions)
- Working with a partner (exchanging ideas, problem solving)
- Lecture to a group
- Working in groups (role playing, simulations)

When addressing a group with various ages and learning styles, the trainer might offer a project with broad guidelines for group completion. Some students might contribute text, some might create graphics, and some might build a database, for example.

Computer technology and the advent of **e-learning** have offered the ability to deliver content to match a variety of learning styles. Some students may prefer to read text; others may prefer to interact with graphics or solve problems. The material can be delivered in a variety of modes in a cost-efficient manner and at a pace consistent with an individual's learning style.

Characteristics of Adult Learners

One of the most difficult tasks faced by employees is achieving balance. Ideally, people shift their time between the demands of work, the demands of home, and their own needs. Everyone wants to accomplish more with fewer and fewer hours. Although a low level of stress is positive, too much can lead to burnout. Therefore, training must be viewed as an integral part of the work environment and not as an add-on requirement. The individuals responsible for training need to understand that time is a very valuable resource.

Because time is scarce, employees need to see relevance in the activities that consume their time. They will be more willing to accept tasks that can be accomplished quickly, pro-vide satisfaction or tangible benefits, and can be completed within short time frames.

Three fundamental concepts in helping adults learn are motivation, reinforcement, and knowledge of results.

Motivation

Motivation is the inner drive to accomplish a task. At different stages in life, adults are motivated by specific needs. Understanding that employees differ in the relative importance of these needs at any given time is important in designing a training program. For example, a newly credentialed health information technician in his early 20s with no dependents may be interested in working long hours. He may demonstrate an eagerness to devote extra hours to training that will advance his career. On the other hand, a young parent may value time to attend his or her children's school activities and want to limit time spent away from home.

Employees will be more motivated when they perceive a need for the training. The trainer should call attention to the important aspects of the job and help employees understand how to perform these tasks efficiently and effectively.

Moreover, employees should see a direct connection between the knowledge learned and the work goal. It is helpful when the trainer explains the reason for performing a task in a certain order and relates policies to objectives. For example, coders may be instructed to review a record in a specific order, beginning with a discharge summary and then lab reports. It is helpful when the trainer explains that the purpose of this process is to ensure appropriate evidence of diagnoses to comply with reimbursement requirements.

Reinforcement

Reinforcement is a condition following a response that results in an increase in the strength of that response. It is associated with motivation in that the strength of the response is a factor of the perceived value of the reinforcer. For example, the young parent mentioned above who values time with his or her children may be negatively reinforced by a pay increase given after a training course when the increase requires additional work hours. However, money would serve as a reinforcer for the new health information technician discussed above. Reinforcement is most effective when it occurs immediately after a correct response.

Incentive pay systems are a form of positive reinforcement. For example, transcriptionists might be compensated based on the number of lines correctly transcribed rather than on an hourly rate.

Knowledge of Results

Adults like feedback on their performance. It is important to understand the concept of the **learning curve.** When a new task is learned, productivity may decrease while a great deal of material is actually being learned. Later, there is little new learning, but productivity may increase greatly. Either situation can be frustrating, so guidance and feedback are important to help employees understand what they have accomplished. In addition, it is important to explain that the employee may reach a plateau where improvement slows or levels off and that this is normal.

Education of Adult Learners

When an organization wants its workers to improve their work habits, it must demonstrate that it values the effort behind the improvements. The organizational climate must support the continued learning and growth of its employees. Some actions the administration might take to indicate this commitment include:

- Providing training during work hours rather than outside the employees' regular work schedules
- Conducting the training off-site to avoid interruptions from day-to-day activities
- Compensating voluntary education with incentives such as bonuses and/or promotions

Adults will remember and understand material that is relevant and has value to them. Therefore, it is important to present an overall picture along with the objectives they are expected to accomplish. Performance standards should be realistic and attainable. Setting artificially high standards reduces motivation and results in feelings of frustration, anxiety, and stress. Thus, employees should feel challenged, but not overwhelmed.

Consideration should be given to the importance of motivation, reinforcement, and knowledge of results. Setting individual goals that challenge employees and satisfy their particular motivators is the ideal. Training methods that allow for the design of individualized programs, such as computer-based training or print-based programmed learning modules, should be considered. Programmed learning modules lead learners through subject material that is presented in short sections, followed immediately by a series of questions that require a written response based on the section just presented. Answers are provided in the module for immediate feedback.

Learning is accomplished best by doing; therefore, it is important to provide as many hands-on activities as possible. Correct responses should be reinforced immediately. Recognition by the trainer or feedback about achievement may be just as effective as monetary rewards in providing reinforcement.

Adults learn better in small units because their attention span is usually not long. In addition, they want to be in control of the situation and learn at their own pace. Where possible, training should be delivered in a modular fashion over a longer period of time. The employee who learns quickly can move forward whereas the slower learner can devote more time to a specific activity.

Additional resources for information about adult learning are the American Society for Training and Development, the association for workplace learning and performance pro-

fessionals (www.astd.org) and Workforce, an organization that provides a variety of human resources tools, including a magazine and an electronic newsletter (www.workforce.com/section/11/).

Education of Learners with Special Needs

Trainers should be aware of the necessity of addressing issues of diversity and disability when preparing training programs.

Diversity

Content of training programs should be developed in a culturally sensitive manner. For example, speaking in an informal, or offhanded manner, may be offensive to some. It also is inappropriate in some cultures to question or challenge an instructor, or communal learning may be more valued than success of the individual. Males may be more used to dominating a discussion; females may need to be encouraged to contribute.

Disabilities

When designing training programs for use on computer, keep in mind that users need to be able to read and write with the help of a keyboard and monitor. Some programs may be developed using voice recognition software or screen readers. Web design should be compliant with requirements of the Americans with Disabilities Act (ADA). If graphics, audio, or video are to be used, a text alternative should accompany them to be accessible with a screen reader.

Check Your Understanding 25.2

Instructions: Answer the following questions on a separate piece of paper.

1. Describe the five models for categorizing learning styles.
2. What role does motivation play in developing a training program?
3. Give an example of a reinforcer other than a monetary reward.
4. Performance standards should be set higher than may reasonably be accomplished. Explain why you agree or disagree with this statement.
5. What two characteristics of adult learners should be considered when developing training programs?
6. What adaptations should be made to accommodate diversity and disability issues in training?

Delivery Methods

There are many techniques for delivering training, just as there are many purposes of training. Factors that influence selection of a training method include:

- Purpose of the training
- Level of education and experience of the trainees
- Amount of space, equipment, and media available for training
- Number of trainees and their location
- Cost of the method in comparison to desired results
- Need for special accommodation due to disability or cultural differences among the trainees

When the purpose of training is to increase the level of knowledge or to introduce new policies, a different method is appropriate than when the goal is to teach a hands-on skill. Training that requires a lot of room and equipment located near the employees' work area will require a different method than training that needs to be delivered across a distance. Instruction in essential skills or license requirements may justify a higher expenditure than instruction that is helpful, but not mandatory.

Table 25.2 presents the time and location requirements for various training delivery methods. Some subjects, such as demonstration of a new fire safety procedure, are best taught to a group of learners at the same time and place, for example, in a traditional classroom setting. Other subjects, such as use of computers, may be taught at a time and place convenient for employees to learn. **Audioconferencing** is a method used to train people located in different offices, but at one time. Each office can be equipped with a speaker and a transmitter, which enables learners to listen and respond to the same material presented by an instructor located at another site.

A recent trend is toward **blended learning,** using several delivery methods, therefore gaining the advantages and reducing the disadvantages of each method alone.

Traditional Training Methods

Teaching students in a face-to-face environment is still the preferred method for many teachers and students. It enables immediate feedback and can improve communication skills. Traditional methods of training groups include classroom learning, seminars and workshops, and role playing. In addition, many subjects lend themselves to individual learning using programmed texts.

Table 25.2. Location and time factors of various training methods

	Same Time	Different Time
Same Space	Traditional: Face-to-face meetings Classes	Work station: VCR Computer Interactive video disk
Different Space	Real-time distance learning: Audioconferencing Interactive television (two-way video and two-way audio) Satellite courses (one-way video and two-way audio) Synchronous computer communications	Asynchronous distance learning: Correspondence courses Video-based telecourses Online computer courses (computers and modems) Multimedia on demand (just-in-time)

©2002 Michigan Virtual University.
Source: Levenburg, N., and H. Major. 1998. Distance learning: implications for higher education in the 21st century. Originally published in *The Technology Source.*
This information is reprinted here with permission of the publisher.

Classroom Learning

Classroom learning is still the most popular method of instruction. When the goal is to train a large number of employees on largely factual knowledge within a short period of time, classroom learning may be the best choice. When the intention is to convey information, this method is effective and economical. However, it is not as appropriate for developing problem-solving skills or improving interpersonal competence.

Teaching a class used to mean using the **lecture** method in which the instructor delivers content and the student listens and observes, primarily one-way communication. This technique usually involves little active participation by the learner. However, because students learn more by doing, today's classroom instruction usually combines lecture with small group discussion, role playing, student presentations, videotapes, or other means where dialogue is facilitated. Using a combination of methods has proved to be highly effective. Videotape is useful for presenting events or demonstrations not easily accomplished in lectures, such as scenarios on interpersonal communication or conflict resolution or viewing surgical procedures. The class itself may be videotaped and the videotape used to deliver the same material to other shifts or workers unable to attend the class.

Seminars and Workshops

The purpose of in-service and CE is to develop new skills or to retrain employees whose jobs have been affected by changes in the organization, external requirements, or new policies or procedures. This type of training is best suited for a more formal setting. Seminars or workshops are typically conducted by experts on a subject and may be held in-house or offered by professional organizations, public or private colleges, or vocational schools.

A workshop or seminar may be offered over the course of one or more days and usually consists of several sessions on specific topics related to an overall theme. Some sessions are large, general classes and others are small, "break-out" classes on topics of limited interest. The cost of workshops and seminars, especially when they are held outside the workplace, is usually high because of the costs of materials, room rental, refreshments, and speaker fees. However, the opportunity to learn from experts in the field is very worthwhile.

Role playing

Role playing is an activity where learners are presented with a hypothetical situation they may encounter on the job, and they respond by acting out the response. It is useful for tasks such as interviewing, grievance handling, team problem solving, or communication difficulties.

Self-Directed (Programmed) Learning

Self-directed learning allows students to progress at their own pace. It presents material, questions the learner, and provides immediate responses with either positive or negative reinforcement. Providing an employee with the opportunity to control the learning situation is a clear advantage. It is suitable for delivery to one or many employees and is a solution for employees who cannot attend sessions outside work hours because of home or family responsibilities.

Self-directed learning (sometimes called programmed learning) was originally delivered via textbooks. Although computers have replaced them in some cases, textbooks still work very well at a relatively low cost. Learners are presented with text and diagrams and then respond to questions. Answers to the questions are provided on another page in the same book for easy checking and feedback. Other advantages to using texts are that they are easily portable and may be supported by other media, such as audiotapes. One disadvantage is that learners may not learn much more than the information in the traditional textbook, and the cost of development may not be paid back unless the book is used several times.

An example of a subject using a programmed text is medical terminology. Text and diagrams of a body system are presented, for example, and the learner is asked to label anatomical structures and to answer multiple-choice or fill-in-the-blank questions. An audiotape may be provided to give the pronunciation of the terms introduced in the text.

E-learning

E-learning refers to training courses delivered electronically. Although most often used to designate Web-based training, the term also may be used to refer to self-directed computer-based training, video or audioconferencing, or **electronic performance support systems** (EPSS). The use of e-learning increased dramatically following the events of September 11, 2001, as fear of travel increased. There is increased demand for online training because traditional methods lack the flexibility and broad-based delivery necessary to meet the rising demand for updated skills in many areas of healthcare.

Electronic training is most successful when:

- There is a large audience to train.
- Employees are geographically dispersed at several sites and/or work varied schedules.
- Just-in-time training is required.
- The purpose is to gain knowledge or learn applications.

Advantages of e-learning include flexibility of class time and place, consistency of delivery, reduced time and cost of training, and the ability to reuse and easily maintain content. Drawbacks include technical problems, such as connectivity or availability for large blocks of time, and student issues with motivation or distraction. Trainers may not be available for some time, and therefore a lag may occur between the time a problem arises and the time it can be solved. Figure 25.6 shows a breakdown of frequency of common e-learning delivery methods, and table 25.3 shows classroom versus e-learning advantages and disadvantages.

Success depends on an appropriate blend of solid instructional design, creativity, and proven technology.

Computer-Based Training

Computer-based training (CBT) is a method designed to provide individual learners with flexible training at their own pace. The students must have access to a computer on which the program is installed. Similar to text-based programmed learning, the explanatory material is presented and followed by a series of questions. The text is accompanied by sounds or drawings to maintain interest and to present the material in a creative way. After each question is answered, there is an immediate response or reinforcement by the computer. In most systems, students can repeat sections of the material until they have mastered it. Students can work on different topics, at varying speeds, and in several languages. The cost of developing CBT courses is higher than classroom instruction or texts, but once developed, the cost of delivery is less because the course can be used multiple times. It is especially useful for content that does not change frequently, such as basic medical terminology or general ROI policies.

CBT is usually delivered via CD-ROM or DVD-ROM. Both provide an excellent way to deliver text, audio, video clips, and animation, and both are particularly useful for providing simulations of work situations. The advantage of DVD-ROM is a large storage capacity and high quality, with up to two hours of full-screen digital video.

The advantages of CBT include lower training costs, reduction in travel or time away from work for workshops, and better learning retention than with traditional classroom teaching. In addition, interactive technology has been demonstrated to reduce learning time by an average of 50 percent.

Simulations

Simulations are training approaches that utilize devices or programs replicating tasks away from the job site; they are

Figure 25.6.   E-learning delivery methods

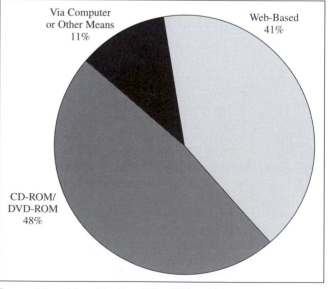

Source: Adapted from Mondy and Noe 2005, p. 214.

Table 25.3. Classroom versus E-learning advantages and disadvantages

	Classroom	Asynchronous Web-based	Synchronous Web-based
Advantages	• High-quality delivery • Immediate Q and A	• Just-in-time training • Self-paced learning • Consistency • Training materials easy to update • Flexible time and place • Cost-effective	• High-quality delivery • Immediate Q & A • Rapid, low-cost content
Disadvantages	• Expensive • Training too soon or too late	• Motivation can be difficult • Lack of classroom collaboration • Delay in trainer response	• Higher cost per student than asynchronous • Instructor and students need to be available at same time
Best for:	• Multiple students with similar skills • Training in single location • Interpersonal skills	• Basic training • Students in multiple locations	• Basic training • Students in multiple locations • Highly interactive knowledge sharing
Worst for:	• Students of varying skill levels • Consistency across learner groups	• Observing interpersonal skills/feedback • Real-time knowledge sharing	• Students of varying skill levels • Observing interpersonal skills/feedback

Source: Adapted from *Workforce Management Magazine* 2001.

often computer based. A typical simulation provides the learner with a scenario of a problem, and the learner must decide what action to take next. Learning occurs in two parts. First, the learner is immersed in a true representation of an actual situation, and second, the learner is required to manage several rules and relationships involved in the process. Learning is acquired through understanding the relationships among the complex processes. Simulation is helpful for training managers or supervisors.

Electronic Performance Support Systems

EPSSs are sets of computerized tools and displays that automate training, as well as documentation, and integrate this automation with the computer application. It is true just-in-time training, providing information at the time it is needed. These systems are especially useful for complex jobs with multiple steps. An EPSS prompts the user through a series of questions, similar to a checklist. Training time can be reduced significantly through the use of an EPSS, and quality of work is enhanced. An EPSS is relatively easy to update as policies or requirements change, ensuring that the user has the most up-to-date information available.

Distance Learning

Distance learning offers a delivery mode in which the physical classroom, the instructor, and the students are not all present at the same time and in the same location. Distance-learning systems remove barriers associated with location and timing, both individually and simultaneously. This is a particularly important issue for adult learners. In addition, distance learning supports self-directed and individual learning styles.

Methods that support different locations, but same-time delivery, include live audio- or videoconferencing or **synchronous** computer conferencing via Internet or intranet

delivery. Delivery of courses at both different locations and times is accomplished via **asynchronous** Internet or intranet Web-based courses or independent study courses offered through a combination of print-based, video, and computer-based training materials.

Live Audio/Video-Based Courses

With audio- or videoconferencing, employees in several locations can learn together via telephone lines or satellite transmission. Audioconferencing enables students to listen to material delivered by a presenter while looking at handout material or books. At selected points in the presentation, the instructor pauses and students interact and share comments or ask questions about the material. The advantage of audioconferencing is its relatively low cost compared to video or computer delivery. Moreover, it eliminates the time and expense of travel to the instruction site. It is useful for the same kind of purpose as the lecture method, which is to deliver specific content to a large group of people.

Interactive videoconferencing is delivered via satellite, television, or, most recently, computer and offers one- or two-way video together with two-way audio. With one-way video, students receive the image of the instructor and demonstrations and can both see and hear the presenter, but the instructor cannot see the students. Two-way video permits both parties to see each other and to interact. Improved technology is enhancing the quality as well as reducing the cost of this delivery method.

A teleconferencing network usually consists of video and audio recording equipment and a satellite service to broadcast the signal to televisions in a remote location. Videoconferencing permits additional flexibility in delivering courses that may be enhanced through visual as well as audio presentation, such as those that include demonstrations or simulation exercises. It is useful for training employees in organizations with multiple sites, such as integrated delivery networks with inpatient and outpatient facilities. The expense is justified for large organizations that do extensive training.

Web-Based Courses

The Internet has become a familiar entity in the lives of most people. Internet-based training permits on-demand training, removing both time and space barriers. The medium is familiar to most individuals and requires a minimum of instruction in the specific courseware used to deliver the course. This method provides instruction when, where, and at a pace suited to each learner. The instruction can be delivered in several forms.

Web-based courses can be delivered synchronously, with employees and trainers interacting via chat rooms at a predetermined time following review of materials. This closely mimics a traditional classroom setting. Another option is asynchronous delivery, where students and instructors interact through e-mail or discussion forums. It is not necessary to be online at the same time and is therefore more convenient than synchronous delivery. The discussion board format is the most frequently used, where students post comments and then review and respond at different times. Materials also can be posted for review at the student's convenience.

Software can be distributed simultaneously to students via e-mail. Students can interact with other students and the instructor via a listserv. The most common form of delivery today is to access courses developed by training organizations or universities via a Web site. Employees are issued a log-on name and password to access the course. Material can be presented using a variety of methods, including text, audio, or video. Relevant material can be accessed through hypertext links embedded in the Web site, which students can access with the click of a mouse.

Software for delivering Web-based courses is developed as **learning management systems** (LMSs) and **learning content management systems** (LCMSs). LMSs manage the learning process, tracking grades and access, presenting the content, and collating statistics on use. LCMSs provide a technical framework to develop the content and permit sharing and reusing content. Most courseware used by colleges and universities has both components.

Intranets are private computer networks that use Internet technologies but are protected with security features and can only be accessed by employees of the organization. Many hospitals use intranets to distribute policies, procedures, and education courses on a variety of topics. Material on CD-ROM can be installed and delivered via intranets for employee self-study, as well as other customized courses for specific employee needs.

The advantages of Web-based courses include the availability of the delivery medium (the Internet or intranet), which brings the course to the employee's computer at home or work, and the ability to easily update materials.

Multimedia materials, including audio, video, graphics, and animation, provide an interesting way to deliver material and have been shown to result in faster learning and greater retention. They also are well suited to adult learners, meeting their needs for education on their terms of time and location. Although sometimes expensive to develop, the cost of using multimedia materials is usually less compared to the cost of classroom or seminar courses for large numbers of employees.

M-Learning

M-learning, or mobile learning, is still in its beginning stages. In this electronic learning mode, content typically delivered via the Internet to computers can be received via personal digital assistant devices (PDAs), therefore expanding the accessibility to a true anytime, anyplace level. Issues to consider are the type of device (small handheld versus tablet PC) and type of connectivity. Screens on a tablet PC are larger, permitting more information to be transmitted. Information can be downloaded from a PC to a mobile device and then accessed later away from the organization, or the device can be directly connected to the Internet via wireless connection. As with any form of e-learning, good instructional design is important. M-learning is not appropriate for very long courses with a great deal of material but might be appropriate for short updates.

Intensive Study Courses

Intensive study courses allow a great deal of material to be compressed into a small time frame. A common example is the weekend college, where students attend 10 to 12 hours per day on Saturday and Sunday. These courses are usually delivered on a college campus or at a hotel setting and require an overnight stay. This training method is suited for teaching special skills that can best be learned in a setting away from day-to-day operations. Examples of courses include cultural awareness, training in teamwork and **empowerment,** and management development.

A popular exercise is to take the organization's leadership team to an outdoor setting where they learn spirit and cooperation and the need to rely on others in order to overcome physical obstacles. The process builds trust to be transferred back to the work setting.

Check Your Understanding 25.3

Instructions: Answer the following questions on a separate piece of paper.

1. What factors should be considered in selecting a training method?

2. How is computer-based training as a learning method different from self-directed learning with textbooks?

3. When is it appropriate to deliver training in a classroom setting?

4. What training obstacles are reduced with e-learning?

5. How would a healthcare organization use its intranet to deliver training?

6. What topics are appropriate for intensive study training?

Workforce Retention

A 1998 study by Aon Consulting identified five factors that influence employee commitment to an organization (Odgers and Keeling 2000, p. 214). They include:

- A fearless corporate culture
- Job satisfaction
- Opportunities for personal growth
- Organizational direction
- The company's recognition of employees' need for work–life balance

Many employees leave organizations because of their need for flexibility. As personal lives become more complex, managers must learn to permit their employees more control over their own time if they are to gain their loyalty.

Turnover and Its Impact

Today's employees have different work expectations than their parents had. They want control of their careers and an employer that rewards them based on their performance. The "traditional" worker felt the employer was responsible for providing a career path and, in return, deserved the employee's long-term commitment to the job. Concerned with job security and stability, yesterday's worker preferred a predictable job, with some opportunity for growth, but desired direction with a small amount of creativity.

The "emerging" worker of the 21st century values growth over predictability, is concerned with opportunities for creativity, and understands that job security must be earned. Personal opportunity for growth, although it requires a job change, is preferred over remaining in a position that is stable but lacks opportunity for advancement.

The costs of hiring and training employees are quite significant. Therefore, organizations should try to minimize turnover by understanding what will retain employees.

Reasons that employees stay in organizations include:

- *Culture and work environment:* Employees prefer good communication and friendly workplace relationships.
- *Compensation:* Pay should be fair, based on performance and effort required for the job.
- *Training and development:* There should be opportunities for mentoring and career growth.
- *Role of the supervisor:* A supervisor should demonstrate high performance and good relationships with staff.
- *Growth and earnings potential:* There should be opportunities for new skill development and consequent financial rewards.

Organizations need to develop retention skills in managers. Pay should be fair, and job flexibility should be provided. Peer coaches may help employees work through difficulties that may cause them to leave. In addition, screening questions during the hiring process may help identify employees who have a high level of integrity and are less likely to suddenly resign.

Alternative Staffing Structures

A major resource of healthcare institutions is information. Electronic-based health information can be managed in places and at times and by people other than those physically located in the institution. As security and technology advance, new staffing arrangements will present both opportunities and challenges for the health information manager. This presents an opportunity to balance work and the personal lives of employees but will require knowledge of how to manage new legal, technical, and personal issues.

Flextime

Flextime generally refers to the employee's ability to work by varying his or her starting and stopping hours around a core of midshift hours, such as 10 a.m. to 1 p.m. Depending on their position and the institution, employees may have a certain degree of freedom in determining their hours. For example, an employee may be given flexibility to start any time between 6 a.m. and 8 a.m. and leave after having worked seven hours.

Compressed workweeks permit employees to work longer days and three or four days per week rather than the usual five eight-hour days. The advantages of this arrangement include increased productivity due to fewer start-and-stop periods, a reduction in commuting time, and additional days off for personal time. The disadvantages may include fatigue and a greater impact of absenteeism and tardiness.

Another option is **flex years.** With this option, employees may choose (at six-month intervals) the number of hours they work each month for the next year. Flex years are particularly attractive to parents of young children, who can work more hours during the school year and fewer hours during vacation periods, for example. In the HIM department, this may be a good option if an event such as an accreditation survey or the installation of a new computer system necessitates a heavier workload requiring more hours for a short period of time, but fewer hours later.

The advantages of flextime programs include a decrease in tardiness and absenteeism caused by taking time to handle personal matters, more productivity during the hours worked, the ability to adjust hours to the workload, and the opportunity to share limited resources across more employees and hours. Flextime programs also lessen the distinction between employees and supervisors and encourage the delegation of duties. However, such programs can be complex to administer and do not work well in situations where workers depend on the physical presence of others for interactive job responsibilities.

However, it is important to ensure that the flextime arrangement does not violate provisions of the Fair Labor Standards Act, the Occupational Safety and Health Act (OSHA), or antidiscrimination laws. To avoid problems, the facility's policy should be clear regarding the positions that are eligible for flextime; the work schedule should not be viewed as a reward for only certain employees. In addition, it is important to understand the impact of flextime on benefit plans, which may require employees to work a certain number of hours in a given time period. For example, nonexempt employees may have different regulations than exempt employees regarding overtime pay.

Even with its minor drawbacks, flextime appears to be a viable arrangement and, in most institutions, improves morale, encourages employee responsibility, and results in an overall increase in productivity.

Successful flextime programs have the following conditions in common:

- A person appointed to oversee the program, develop policies and procedures, and resolve differences between supervisors and employees
- A written policy that clearly states the positions that are open to flextime and those that are not
- An orientation program for supervisors when the program is first introduced or as part of a new supervisor's introduction to the organization
- A job function that will benefit from flexibility, for example, one that has high and low workloads at different time periods and one that permits the employee to work independently

Job Sharing

Job sharing is a work arrangement in which two or more people share one full-time job. For example, one employee may work mornings and another afternoons, but it also can mean working different days or weeks. A distinction must be made between job sharing and part-time work. In job sharing, one full-time job is split and all employees sharing the job may perform parts of the same project. Part-time jobs involve employees who work fewer than full-time hours and perform their jobs independently of others.

The main advantage of job sharing is that it enables organizations to attract employees who otherwise may not work because of personal responsibilities. This is an attractive option for parents and employees who want to attend school. The success of job sharing depends on the individuals in the job. They must be mature and cooperative and must want to work toward achieving the objectives of the job. Frequent communication is important regarding the status of projects or unplanned events that may alter the work requirements for a given day.

The disadvantages of job sharing include lack of continuity, particularly when one employee starts a task in the morning and another is responsible for completing it later in the day, and decreased productivity when the employees are not cooperative or fail to communicate well. Job sharing also may cause confusion for other employees or the public, who have to interact with several individuals rather than one.

Home-Based Work

Computer technology has created a new option for employees who work at home—**telecommuting.** HIM departments have seen an increase in the number of coders and medical transcriptionists who choose this option. Telecommuting provides an opportunity for employees who cannot travel from home for reasons such as physical or personal limitations to become employed and helps resolve the problem of shortages of qualified employees in critical job functions. It is an excellent alternative for physically challenged individuals. Individuals who choose this option are employees of the institution and are covered by the same policies and benefits as those who work on-site. The employer usually provides a computer and any networking hardware and software, and the employee is required to submit a detailed time sheet of hours worked.

The advantages of telecommuting include freedom from the time, expense, and physical requirements of commuting; the ability to work flexible hours; increased productivity; lack of distractions from other employees; and an increase in personal time. Moreover, the institution benefits from a reduced need for physical space and improved recruitment.

The disadvantages of telecommuting include employee difficulty in separating work and personal life and feelings of isolation. The "invisible" employee also creates unique challenges for the supervisor. One way to resolve this issue is to have the employee and the manager enter into a telecommuting agreement that defines the expectations of both parties regarding location, hours, equipment, and confidentiality. (See figure 25.7 for a sample agreement.) Suggested items to include in the agreement include work schedule, communication frequency and methods, goals, performance measures, confidentiality requirements, equipment maintenance responsibilities, and environmental safety requirements.

A particular issue for the HIM department is the confidentiality and security of personal health information transmitted over networks as records are sent for coding and dictation is sent for transcription. In addition, the information needs to be secured while in the employee's home, where it can be subject to physical damage or be viewed by the employee's family members or friends. The HIPAA security standards, in particular, provide specific requirements for remote access, including secure transmission, assurance of data integrity, and authentication methods.

As with flextime, clearly stated policies should be in place regarding who is eligible for telecommuting arrangements and their impact on benefit plans. Workers' compensation issues have not been fully resolved. If an employee trips in the home, for example, is this a workers' compensation injury? The answer appears to center on whether the individual was doing work at the time of the injury.

Although many issues still need answers, it appears that telecommuting will increasingly become an important option for HIM departments as a way to recruit and retain satisfied employees.

Figure 25.7.   Sample telecommuting agreement

Telecommuting Agreement

I have read and understand the attached Telecommuting Policy, and agree to the duties, obligations, responsibilities, and conditions for telecommuters described in that document.

I agree that, among other things, I am responsible for establishing specific telecommuting work hours, furnishing and maintaining my remote work space in a safe manner, employing appropriate telecommuting security measures, and protecting company assets, information, trade secrets, and systems.

I understand that telecommuting is voluntary and I may stop telecommuting at any time. I also understand that the company may at any time change any or all of the conditions under which I am permitted to telecommute, or withdraw permission to telecommute.

Note: The following elements are recommended specific to the situation.

1. Remote work location:

Address of employee residence or work premises

Work phone number, fax number, etc.

Description of work space at remote location

2. Telecommuting schedule:

On a weekly basis as follows

On a monthly basis as follows

No regular schedule (separate permission for each telecommuting day)

3. Regular telecommuting work hours:

From _____ to _____

Meal break/other breaks

4.   General description of the activities and functions to be completed by the telecommuter:

5.   Frequency of communication with company (that is, check voice mail, e-mail, etc.):

6.   Productivity requirements or expectations (if applicable):

7.   Company assets to be used at remote work location (description, ID numbers, and value):

8.   Company information systems to be accessed from remote work location (list):

9.   Noncompany services, equipment, software, and data to be used at remote work location (list):

10. Equipment and services to be provided by the telecommuter (list):

11. Security measures to be used by telecommuter and expectations (virus protection and frequency of program updates, use of personal firewalls for computer, shredding company documents, etc.):

12. Expectations for childcare for infants or young children during work hours:

13. Obligation to comply with company rules, policies, and procedures while telecommuting:

14. Other

This sample form was developed by AHIMA for discussion purposes only. It should not be used without review by your organization's legal counsel to ensure compliance with local and state laws.

Source: Dougherty and Scichilone 2002.

Outsourcing

In some cases, flexible job arrangements may not be an option for employees. Another solution to the problem of a shortage of qualified staff is **outsourcing.** In this arrangement, the institution contracts with an independent company with expertise in a specific job function. The outside company then assumes full responsibility for performing the function rather than just supplying staff. Thus, the health information manager's responsibility shifts from supervising employees to managing a vendor relationship.

Common functions that are candidates for outsourcing in the HIM department include transcription, release of information, and, most recently, coding. The outsourcing company may perform the functions either at the institution or partially or completely off-site. Advances in communication and security technology have resulted in many home-based workers being employed by such independent companies.

The advantages of outsourcing to the health information manager include the ability to complete work efficiently and with high quality while avoiding the problem of staff recruitment and supervision. With the increase in companies providing these services, outsourcing also can mean a reduction in cost because of competitive bidding. The advantages to the employees of outside companies include flextime and telecommuting—the ability to work varying hours, an increase in personal time, and increased morale. The disadvantages for the health information manager include less immediate control over the quantity and quality of the work, the need to know negotiation techniques, and the reliance on the vendor. HIPAA also requires special arrangements regarding security and confidentiality for outsourcing contractors.

Suggestions for successful outsourcing arrangements include:

- Seeking assistance from someone skilled in negotiation when developing the contract with the vendor
- Engaging legal counsel to review the language of the contract to ensure that it complies with the HIPAA requirements
- Requiring competitive bidding for each outsourced service at regular intervals
- Establishing expectations and performance standards for contractors
- Monitoring compliance with performance standards
- Performing periodic customer surveys to assess satisfaction with the service

Offshoring

Offshoring is a special case of outsourcing, where employees of the company are based overseas, most frequently in India, China, and the United Kingdom. The major benefits are cost savings and availability of a labor pool. Employees in foreign countries are generally paid much less than those in the United States and are extremely productive. There is also less turnover. HIM jobs such as transcription, coding, and insurance claims processing are very suited to these types of workers. Medical transcription is expected to grow from a $2.3 billion overseas market in 2004 to $4.2 billion by 2008. Jobs most suitable for offshoring have the following characteristics:

- No face-to-face customer service requirements
- High information content
- High wage differential with workers in the destination country
- Low social networking requirement
- Little management or interaction with others in the organization

Those countries with young populations that speak English are preferred. The country also should have reliable utilities and suitable digital and voice networks.

Quality control is an important issue. It is recommended that a service agreement be executed clarifying expectations. Tasks to be performed, acceptable turnaround times, quantity and quality standards, and how the performance measures will be tracked and reported should be spelled out. It is especially important to specify accountability for confidentiality because data are at risk when they are transmitted overseas. Finally, training requirements should be established, especially in English speaking and writing, as well as confidentiality.

Employee Development

In addition to the need to balance work and personal life, employees often look for opportunities for personal growth. By nature, they want to learn new skills and further their careers. A significant amount of training should be devoted to developing the ability of employees to help themselves, to realize that they are the ones responsible for their advancement.

Empowerment

Empowerment is the concept of providing employees with the tools and resources to solve problems themselves. In other words, employees obtain power over their work situation by assuming responsibility. Empowered employees have the freedom to contribute ideas and perform their jobs in the best possible way. The idea of empowerment actually began as part of total quality management programs, which many organizations initiated in order to improve the quality of service provided to customers and to increase their competitiveness in the marketplace. A high-quality organization strives to understand and improve work processes in order to prevent problems.

Healthcare organizations that empower their employees believe that all employees can perform—and truly want to perform—to their highest potential when given the proper resources and environment. Because they perform jobs on a regular basis, they are intimately familiar with the steps in the process. What the employees may lack are skills in analysis and problem solving. Training sessions in skills such as data analysis, use of control charts, or flowcharting will help employees to identify problems, develop alternatives, and recommend solutions.

To perform effectively, employees also need to be given responsibility, authority, and the trust to make decisions and act independently within their area of expertise. Figure 25.8 offers suggestions on how managers can empower their employees.

Empowered employees are less likely to complain or feel helpless or frustrated when they cannot resolve a problem on their own. Moreover, they are more likely to feel a sense of accomplishment and to be more receptive to solutions that they develop themselves. In addition, they tend to demonstrate commitment and self-confidence and to produce high-quality work.

One disadvantage that is frequently mentioned by managers is that empowerment involves too much time for meetings and discussion and takes employees away from the "real work." Actually, it is much more efficient to take the time necessary to prevent problems than to solve them after they occur. In the long run, empowered employees work more efficiently and productively.

Indeed, some managers are afraid to share power. They feel that they have worked hard to gain the power they have and are reluctant to give it up. But the manager who empowers others usually increases his or her own power because a high-performing unit reflects the manager's expertise.

An example of empowerment in the HIM department would be to train employees in the ROI function to solve a slow turnaround issue. The employees are probably more aware than the supervisor of problems that prevent them from filling requests for information (missing charts, insufficient fees, incomplete records). With proper training in brainstorming and flowcharting, as well as a supportive environment, the employees may be able to develop a procedure that can be performed differently to prevent delays.

Delegation

Delegation is the process of distributing work duties and decision making to others. To be effective, delegation should be commensurate with **authority** and responsibility. A manager must assign responsibility, which is an expectation that another person will perform tasks. At the same time, authority, or the right to act in ways necessary to carry out assigned tasks, must be granted. An employee cannot be expected to perform a job for which he or she is not given authority to obtain resources. Authority should equal responsibility when work is delegated. Finally, **accountability** must be created, which is the requirement to answer to a supervisor for results. An employee must be empowered to act, given the necessary tools and skills, and held accountable for the quality of his or her work.

Successful delegation includes:

- Assigning responsibility
- Granting authority
- Creating accountability

Guidelines for delegating are presented in figure 25.9. As an employee development tool, delegation can provide employees the opportunity to try new tasks previously performed by someone in a higher position and leads to empowerment because employees are given the opportunity to contribute ideas and fully utilize their skills. At the same time, the manager should remain available to provide assistance and support.

Sometimes managers have difficulty delegating because they feel that only they can do the job correctly. In other cases, they feel threatened by the idea that another employee can do their tasks and perhaps do them better. This thinking can lead to poor morale and result in talented employees leaving the organization. In addition, it can lead to managers being overburdened with work that could be done by others and to employees being denied opportunities to learn new skills.

In some situations, employees may be unwilling to accept delegated responsibilities when they feel that they are unqualified to do the tasks or that they are being dumped on. Dumping can involve assigning an employee unpleasant or unpopular work that seems to have little value or asking an employee to take on work in addition to an already demanding workload. This results in resentment or anger. Employees may feel this way when they have a poor working relationship with their supervisor, know that others have refused the same task, or have been taken advantage of in the past.

Figure 25.8. How to empower employees

- Get others involved in selecting their work assignments and the methods for accomplishing tasks.
- Create an environment of cooperation, information sharing, discussion, and shared ownership of goals.
- Encourage others to take initiative, make decisions, and use their knowledge.
- When problems arise, find out what others think and let them help design the solutions.
- Stay out of the way; give others the freedom to put their ideas and solutions into practice.
- Maintain high morale and confidence by recognizing successes and encouraging high performance.

Source: Schermerhorn 2005, p. 328.

Figure 25.9. Ground rules for effective delegation

- Carefully choose the person to whom you delegate.
- Define the responsibility; make the assignment clear.
- Agree on performance objectives and standards.
- Agree on a performance timetable.
- Give authority; allow the other person to act independently.
- Show trust in the other person.
- Provide performance support.
- Give performance feedback.
- Recognize and reinforce progress.
- Help when things go wrong.
- Don't forget *your* accountability for performance results.

Source: Schermerhorn 2005, p. 264.

To avoid these problems, employees should be selected who are either competent to perform the tasks or willing to undergo the necessary training. People are more willing to accept tasks that they understand, have a choice in doing, and recognize value added to the organization and their personal growth. Managers should set checkpoints, monitor how the delegate is doing, and allow the opportunity for questions and feedback.

Delegation is a skill that matches the right employee with the right task. It requires communication, support, and an environment that fosters risk taking. Effective delegation actually leads to a more efficient and productive department overall and mutually benefits the manager, the employee, and the institution.

Coaching and Mentoring

Both new employees and experienced employees who may be ready for a change can benefit from coaching or mentoring. As discussed earlier in this chapter, coaching is an ongoing process in which an experienced person offers performance advice to a less experienced person. However, coaching goes beyond teaching. A good coach is also a counselor, a resource person, a troubleshooter, and a cheerleader. Coaches deal with improving attitudes, morale, and career development in addition to giving instruction in specific tasks.

Effective coaches are dedicated leaders who display a high level of competence and are able to push or pull employees to their highest level of performance. They are role models who set a good example; show workers what is expected and how to get the job done well; provide praise or constructive feedback, where appropriate; and are ready to help with routine work alongside the employee, if necessary.

Coaching starts with orientation of the new employee and continues throughout his or her time with the organization. The more time the coach spends walking around observing and listening to employees, the more opportunities there will be to support, praise, and offer advice.

Helping employees should be done in a manner that encourages self-sufficiency. For example, when an employee comes forward with a problem, a good coach does not simply give the answer but, rather, asks the employee for suggestions. In other words, the coach's response should be "What do you think?" rather than "Here's what you should do."

Coaches defend and support their employees. They are facilitators who remove obstacles and obtain resources to enable and empower their staffs. It is important to praise performance above and beyond the expected, for example, when the employee completes a task ahead of schedule or offers to help a colleague. It is equally important to praise the worker who consistently meets objectives or improves in an area that was below standard, in other words, for doing what is expected. To be effective, both positive and negative feedback must be timely, specific, and in the right setting (privately or publicly depending on the circumstance). Good coaches direct negative feedback at the behavior they wish to correct, not at the person.

However, coaching can be done poorly. This happens when criticism is overused or praise is undeserved. In addition, the approach needs to be adjusted to the employee. Good coaching takes time to allow flexibility and encourage the employee to perform correctly without jumping in too quickly with advice.

Mentoring is a form of coaching. A mentor is a senior employee who works with employees early in their careers, giving them advice on developing skills and career options. Several employees may be assigned as protégés to the mentor, but contact is usually one-on-one. Through the mentoring relationship, employees have an advisor with whom they can solve problems, analyze and learn from mistakes, and celebrate successes. Many organizations have formal mentoring programs where protégés are matched with potential mentors. Other managers voluntarily offer to work with up-and-coming employees.

Mentors share their knowledge of management styles and teach prospective supervisors specific job or interpersonal skills. They may assign challenging projects that allow employees to explore real-life learning experiences while still under the guidance of an experienced teacher.

A recent use of mentoring is helpful in teaching diversity tolerance. In **reverse mentoring,** an employee from a minority group will provide mentoring to management staff, sharing their day-to-day perspectives and providing cultural awareness to the manager.

Successful mentoring depends on effective interaction between mentor and protégé. Mentors must be chosen who enjoy passing on their experience and knowledge to others.

Promotion

Promotion may be another tool to encourage employee development and commitment. When tied to training programs, it can become a powerful incentive. Promotion usually refers to the upward progression of an employee in both job and salary. However, it also can mean a lateral move to a different position with similar job skills or to a change within the same job as a result of completing higher education or credentialing requirements. To attract, retain, and motivate employees, organizations should provide a career development system that promotes from within.

When tied to promotion, career development programs offer an incentive to ambitious employees. Goals can be incorporated into the performance review process. In the HIM department, clerical employees can be encouraged to take classes that would lead to an associate's degree in health information technology or a bachelor's degree in health information administration, making them eligible for certification exams. In addition, employees may be encouraged to enter coding certificate programs and achieve coding certification.

The higher the status of the person in the organization, the more likely it is that promotion will work as a motivator. To improve employee performance, promotion should be awarded based on competence, not on seniority. In some organizations, union contracts emphasize seniority and thus restrict the organizations' ability to use competence as a sole criterion.

Promotion based on performance is usually measured by appraising past performance against standards. However, past performance does not always predict future potential. Some organizations use testing instruments to assess this capability.

Succession planning is a specific type of promotional plan in which senior-level position openings are anticipated and candidates are identified from within the organization. The candidates are given training through formal education, job rotation, and mentoring so that they can eventually assume these positions.

To be effective, promotion criteria should be published in a formal policy and procedure, which usually includes job postings of open positions, so that all employees have the opportunity to apply for consideration. When promotions appear to be given to favored employees, or when the procedure is shrouded in secrecy, promotion ceases to be attractive.

Incentive Programs

Voluntary employee turnover can be disruptive to an organization. Both high and low performers are more likely to leave than are average performers. It is important to try to retain high performers. The usual way to do this is through a **pay for performance** system. In order for these systems to be successful, it is important for the employee to make a connection between pay and performance. Incentive plan effectiveness is affected by differences in employee personalities and values. Each person is motivated by different needs, and they will not pursue rewards they do not find valuable. Therefore, an effective incentive program links effort directly to a reward, and the reward must be valued.

Rewards may be in the form of pay or other items, such as vacations, flexible work hours, prizes, or recognition on a plaque or bulletin board, or in a personal note. One reward system allows employees to select a reward from a catalog or Web site, allowing the employee to select something they value.

Incentives may be given based on the following structures:

- Pay for item completed (lines transcribed, charts coded)
- Pay based on success of a team achieving goals (this encourages collaboration, but high-performing individuals are not recognized)
- Pay based part on the individual and part on team performance
- Pay based on a standard rate plus premium if productivity exceeds the standard
- Merit pay given annually as a salary increase

An incentive plan may fail if it appears there is an emphasis on quantity without an associated focus on quality, or if the reward is not valued (such as increased pay given to an employee who would rather have time off). Finally, incentive programs must be accompanied with effective management.

The best incentive programs demonstrate that effort must be instrumental in obtaining the reward. Under the control of the employee, employees should support and value the plan, and employee goals should be SMART: specific, measurable, attainable, relevant, and timely.

Continuing Education

CE is a requirement of most professionals, including those in HIM. It usually requires a person to complete a certain number of hours of education within a given time period to maintain a credential or license status. Accrediting organizations, such as JCAHO, also include CE in their standards. The HIM field is changing rapidly, primarily in the areas of technology, e-HIM, and legal and regulatory requirements. It is important that credentialed professionals remain current in their knowledge of the profession so that they can provide high-quality skills to the organizations for which they work.

CE refers to keeping up with changes in the profession or to improving skills required to perform the same job. It is different from career development, which is geared toward preparing an individual for a new job. Sometimes this line is blurred. In HIM, management development programs may be essential for the current position when one is already a supervisor, for example. On the other hand, preparing a technical employee to assume a new management role would be considered career development. Some organizations have tuition reimbursement policies to encourage career development.

CE programs are most often provided by external organizations, such as the American Health Information Management Association (AHIMA) or its local chapters. Career development, by contrast, usually includes a combination of job rotation through progressively increasing job responsibilities in-house and externally taught formal classes and workshops.

As part of the formal performance appraisal process, CE goals should be set for all employees. A record should be kept in the employee's personnel file that indicates the number of CE hours earned as well as the topic, place, and person who provided the education. Management should support the individual's achievement by providing time off to attend workshops, flexible scheduling for formal classes offered at educational institutions, and financial reimbursement.

CE programs are delivered via many different formats to suit the individual learner. These include classroom as well as computer-based modules or Web-based courses that all employees can access, regardless of where they live or their personal or physical limitations. Continued skill development should be an important requirement for all HIM employees.

Instructions: Answer the following questions on a separate piece of paper.

1. Describe two techniques organizations can implement to reduce employee turnover.

2. In what work situations would an HIM department benefit from a flextime work arrangement?

3. What is one advantage to the employee of working compressed workweeks? To the department?

4. What potential problems with flextime should a manager be wary of? Give the possible solution to each problem.

5. What is the difference between job sharing and traditional part-time employment?

6. What items should be included in a telecommuting agreement?

7. What two functions does the HIM department commonly outsource?

8. What factors help ensure the success of an outsourcing arrangement?

9. Why are transcription jobs likely candidates for offshoring?

10. In what three ways can managers empower employees?

11. What two reasons might managers have for not empowering employees?

12. How are the concepts of delegation and empowerment related?

13. What three actions must be done for effective delegation?

14. When might an employee resist accepting delegated responsibilities?

15. What are the basic characteristics of effective coaches?

16. How does mentoring differ from coaching? How is it similar?

17. On what should promotion be based if it is to motivate?

18. Why do incentive programs fail?

19. Why do HIM professionals need continuing education?

Departmental Employee Training and Development Plan

Every healthcare organization and every HIM department have unique training needs. The level of education and experience of the employees, the tasks they perform, and the resources available will change the focus of training efforts. As table 25.1 (p. 707) shows, employee development is a continuum of concepts. The content, objectives, and frequency of a training program are all dependent on the specific situation that exists in an organization.

Training and Development Model

The following **training and development model** can be applied on various levels and will help an organization's HR department or a health information manager identify and fulfill the training needs of their employee group:

- *Step 1:* Perform a needs analysis.
- *Step 2:* Set training objectives.
- *Step 3:* Design the curriculum.
- *Step 4:* Determine the location and method of delivery.
- *Step 5:* Pilot the program.
- *Step 6:* Implement the program.
- *Step 7:* Evaluate the effectiveness of the program.

- *Step 8:* Make changes as needed.
- *Step 9:* Provide feedback to interested groups.

The plan should be approved and supported by upper management. Implementing a training program requires a substantial investment of time, money, and personnel. Developing a curriculum based on a systematic evaluation of needs is a much wiser investment than creating a program around the latest hot topic.

Perform a Needs Analysis

The needs analysis is critical to the design of the plan. This approach typically focuses on three levels: the organization, the specific job tasks, and the individual employee. The outcome of the needs analysis is an understanding of where training is needed in the organization (entry-level, remedial, or management development), based on the firm's strategic mission and goals. In addition, a list of the tasks to be learned at each level (based on the job description and the job specification, the specific skills and knowledge required) and an analysis of the deficiencies in knowledge and skills between the desired level and the current level of employees are completed.

This information can be obtained through observation, employee and manager interviews, surveys, tests, and task analysis of the job descriptions and job specifications.

Set Training Objectives

After the needs have been established, specific, measurable training objectives should be set. Objectives specify what the employee should be able to accomplish upon completion of the training program. These are based on the deficiencies that have been identified between the desired and current performance levels. It is important to set objectives before starting the program so that the results can be evaluated following completion of training.

Design the Curriculum

The curriculum is the subject content of the program that will be taught, including the sequence, activities, and materials. A budget needs to be prepared that identifies costs and available resources. Are there individuals within the organization who can develop and teach the program, or is it necessary to purchase an externally prepared program? Do materials such as videotapes or computer-based modules need to be produced? Do printed materials need to be developed and reproduced? Will the program be available over the Internet?

After these decisions are made, the curriculum must be organized into a program that supports adult learning and the stated objectives. All program elements need to be carefully prepared to ensure quality and effectiveness.

Determine the Location and Method of Delivery

Where and when the program should be delivered is an important part of the training plan. When space is available and the instructor and materials are available internally, a classroom setting might be suitable. On the other hand, when employees work over several shifts and days or in remote locations, computer-based CD-ROMs and/or Web-based delivery might permit the employee to more readily achieve the training objectives.

Pilot the Program

It is important to validate the program by introducing it to a test audience. When computer technology is part of the program delivery, all computer programs should be tested to make sure they work with a variety of hardware and/or Web browsers. Following completion of the program by a few employees, feedback should be obtained and the program revised, if necessary.

Implement the Program

The tested program now can be given to the entire audience for which it has been developed. When necessary, train-the-trainer workshops should be conducted for instructors who may not have formal training experience.

Evaluate the Effectiveness of the Program

Two issues should be addressed in evaluating training programs. The first is the method of evaluation; the second is the outcomes that will be measured.

Evaluation is most frequently assessed using a survey, such as the samples in figures 25.2 (p. 711) and 25.5 (p. 714). Opinions obtained immediately after the training, and again after a period of time, are valuable in assessing the effectiveness of the program for both trainees and managers. In addition, pretests and posttests help identify the level of knowledge or skill that has actually been learned.

When possible, an excellent method for evaluating the training program is to conduct a controlled experiment. A control group that receives no training is compared to a group that received training. Data are obtained from both groups both before and after training. It is then possible to determine the extent to which the training program caused a change in performance in the training group.

Four outcomes can be measured in evaluating effective training programs:

- *Reaction:* What is the reaction of the trainees immediately after the program? Are they excited about what they learned?
- *Learning:* What have the trainees actually learned? Can they now use a new software program?
- *Behavior:* Have supervisors noticed a change in employee behavior? Has morale improved?
- *Results:* How does the actual level of performance compare with the established objectives? Can the employees assign codes more accurately?

Make Changes as Needed

When the results of the evaluation show less-than-expected results, it is important to determine where changes may be helpful. This may include a change in the materials, the location or time of program delivery, or the subject content. In any case, it is important to adjust. A program that is not meeting the desired objectives is costly.

Provide Feedback to Interested Groups

After tallying the results of the evaluations and making any adjustments that are needed, it is important to provide feedback to the course developers, managers and supervisors of the involved departments, and the trainees. Communication is vital to maintaining interest and support for the training program. Feedback demonstrates a desire to respond to the needs of everyone involved in this important activity.

Laws and Regulations Affecting Training

In developing training programs, healthcare organizations must recognize that special accommodations may be required to address the needs of both a culturally diverse workforce and employees with disabilities. Employers need to understand the requirements affecting training that are included under Title VII of the 1964 Civil Rights Act, the 1991 Civil Rights Act, and the ADA. If completion of a training program is part of the selection process for a particular job, the organization must be able to demonstrate that the requirements are valid and do not discriminate against, or have a negative impact on, women, minorities, or disabled individuals. For example, the vocabulary in written documents used for training should match the level required for the job, and training equipment and locations should be accessible to individuals with mobility disabilities.

Employers can avoid liability for sexual harassment acts of their employees if they provide training to ensure that employees understand their rights and responsibilities. The courts interpret this as exercising reasonable care to prevent harassment.

Inadequate training exposes employers to potential liability for negligent training if they fail to train adequately and an employee harms a third party.

OSHA was passed to ensure safe working conditions. Among its many requirements is training to reduce unsafe acts. Hospitals are required to train employees in fire safety and other job-related safety measures. The training must be provided in the worker's native language, other than English, if necessary, and the worker must be able to demonstrate proficiency following the training.

The Allied Health Reinvestment Act of 2005 encourages individuals to seek and complete high-quality allied health education and training by providing funding for their studies. Grants are provided to healthcare organization for advertising campaigns and for partnerships between healthcare facilities and allied health educational programs. Scholarships may be given to applicants who agree to serve two years in a rural or other medically underserved area with allied health personnel shortages.

The ADA requires employers to provide reasonable accommodations for physical or mental limitations with regard to many employment-related functions, including training. This would require, for example, that accommodations be made to computer-based training to provide accessibility through voice recognition or screen readers, if necessary. The World Wide Web Consortium's Web Accessibility Initiative publishes information about ADA Compliance for Web sites (w3c.org/WAI).

Check Your Understanding 25.5

Instructions: Answer the following questions on a separate piece of paper.

1. What are the steps in a typical training and development plan?
2. What are three outcomes of a needs analysis?
3. What is the relationship between setting objectives and evaluating a training program?
4. What are three items to consider in designing a training program?
5. What are four outcomes that should be measured in program evaluation?
6. Discuss two laws that affect training programs and describe their impact.

Real-World Case

The employees of the HIM department in Midwest Community Hospital, a 100-bed facility located in the Chicago suburbs, have just returned from a meeting. Their director, Gary Smith, announced that the hospital was recently acquired by a large integrated delivery system, Hometown Health Systems. Hometown Health Systems has just implemented an electronic health record system and intends to ensure that the HIM department employees receive the necessary training to be prepared to assume their new e-HIM roles. Gary has been with the organization for 30 years and has indicated his intention to retire when the facilities merge, which is scheduled to occur in about six months. Hometown's corporate director of health information systems, Jane Winters, will assume responsibility for managing the department, with an assistant director to be appointed at Midwest who will assume day-to-day supervisory responsibilities.

Jane knows that three employees at Midwest might be qualified to assume the position and would like to fill it through promotion. All three candidates have positive and negative factors, some of which could be remedied with training. Gary and Jane plan to discuss the best approach to selecting the new supervisor, and Gary has been asked to assist in the process by preparing the selected employee for the transition. After returning from the meeting, Gary begins to review the three employees in his mind.

Bob has worked in the ROI area of the department for three years and recently obtained his RHIT credential after attending a local community college program. He is enthusiastic about working in the department and has frequently suggested new procedures, which has led to some friction with Gary, whose motto is "If it ain't broke, don't fix it!" He has been frustrated by the lack of available technology in the HIM department. Now that he has the credential, Bob has mentioned that he may want to begin looking elsewhere if his ideas are not appreciated at Midwest.

Sherry is a coder who has worked at Midwest for about one year. She began her employment at the hospital in the outpatient registration area. Six months after completing AHIMA's online coding program, she assumed the coding position in the HIM department. She is a single parent who is a self-proclaimed workaholic. In her spare time, she works at home as a coder for a physician's office to increase her income.

Linda currently works as the lead file clerk in the department. Of the three employees, she is the only one with supervisory experience, although she has had no formal management training. Gary had promoted her to the lead position because of her excellent attendance record and seniority. However, her employees have complained frequently to Gary that she "takes over" and corrects their work without explaining what they did wrong. Gary also knows that she does not feel comfortable disciplining employees and that she finds doing the job herself easier than working with the employee responsible for the job.

Gary will meet next Monday with Jane and is still unsure how to solve this dilemma.

Summary

Employees are the healthcare institution's most valuable asset. The decreasing availability of qualified employees means that responsibility for developing staff increasingly rests with the employer. Workforce development and retention must become part of the institution's strategic plan.

Training and development needs can be viewed on a continuum of five conceptual areas: orientation, training, in-service education, continuing education, and career development. Each healthcare organization's training program must be able to adapt to the different needs of its employees.

New employees need to be introduced to the rules and culture of the organization, the department, and the specific job duties they will be performing. This function is typically performed through a formal orientation program that provides employees with information regarding organizational policies and procedures, benefits, safety regulations, and an introduction to the work area. Finally, employees begin learning the duties and responsibilities of the specific jobs they will be performing. Preparing staff to carry out their specific job tasks should be an ongoing effort. Methods used to accomplish this include on-the-job-training, job rotation, and cross-training.

In-service education builds on basic skills provided during orientation and on-the-job training. It also is used when departments are restructured or when external requirements require employees to update their competency. This training needs to be available on a continuous basis and may be conducted by department managers in formal training sessions or through self-directed learning methods. AHIMA's e-HIM™ initiative, to promote the migration from paper to an electronic health information infrastructure, will require the training of HIM professionals in new competencies needed to fulfill future roles.

Future HIM professionals also will need training in diversity sensitivity, ethics, team building, and customer service skills as they prepare to carry out the e-HIM™ vision.

The techniques used to deliver training should be matched with the purpose of the training, the trainee's level of education and experience, location, and budget. Self-directed learning permits students to determine the pace of the learning. A number of CD-ROMs provide computer-based training for this purpose. Classroom lectures are useful for training large numbers of employees on factual knowledge in a short time period. E-learning methods overcome a number of obstacles of traditional training methods and provide anytime, anywhere instruction in a cost-effective mode. Some of these methods include electronic performance support systems, live teleconferencing, and synchronous or asynchronous Web-based courses.

Because training programs require a considerable investment of both time and money, the organization should encourage commitment to long-term employment. An important factor in maintaining job satisfaction is recognition by the company of employee needs for work–life balance. Alternative staffing arrangements permit employees to vary work hours and locations while still satisfying the organization's need for productivity. Options include flextime programs, job sharing, and telecommuting. For those who wish to work on a limited basis or for employers who cannot find qualified staff, outsourcing may be an option. Offshoring is a viable, cost-effective option for jobs with little face-to-face contact and high information content, including transcription, coding, and insurance claims processing.

Another factor that enhances employee job satisfaction is the opportunity for personal growth. Employees should be empowered with the tools and resources to solve problems themselves. Successful managers delegate effectively. Effective delegation leads to a more efficient and productive department and mutually benefits the manager, the employee, and the institution.

Employees just beginning their careers may benefit from mentoring. Mentors advise and teach specific job and interpersonal skills. Coaching is a process that begins in orientation and continues throughout the employee's time with the organization. Coaches act as role models, provide praise and constructive feedback, and help with routine work when needed.

Promotion can be a powerful incentive for employees when tied to career development programs. It should be awarded on competence, not seniority, and the criteria should be based on objective standards. Incentive programs that reward effort with something the employee values, such as pay, vacations, or other recognition, also may help reduce turnover and improve productivity.

Employees who hold professional credentials must complete CE requirements to remain current in their knowledge of the profession as it moves forward with its e-HIM™ vision. Continued skill development should be an important requirement for all HIM employees.

Because the training needs of every department are unique, it is important to develop a formal training and development plan. The plan begins with a needs analysis and the establishment of measurable objectives. A curriculum is then designed to meet those needs.

A successful and effective plan for employee training and development requires a substantial investment of time, money, and personnel. It should be approved and supported by upper management and based on a systematic evaluation of needs.

References

AHIMA e-HIM Task Force. 2003. Vision of the e-HIM future: A report from the AHIMA e-HIM Task Force. Supplement to *Journal of American Health Information Management Association*.

Dessler, G. 2005. *Human Resources Management*, 10th ed. Upper Saddle River, NJ: Pearson Prentice-Hall.

Dougherty, M., and R. Scichilone. 2002. Practice brief: Establishing a telecommuting or home-based employee program. *Journal of American Health Information Management Association* 73(7):72A–L.

Fottler, H., S. Hernandez, and C. Joiner, eds. 1998. *Essentials of Human Resource Management in Health Service Organizations*. Albany, NY: Delmar.

Keeling, B., and N. Kallaus. 1996. *Administrative Office Management*, 11th ed. Cincinnati, OH: South-Western.

Levenburg, N., and H. Major. 1998. Distance learning: Implications for higher education in the 21st century. Originally published in *The Technology Source*. Available online from technologysource.org/article/distance_learning__implications_for_higher_education_in_the_21st_century/.

Mondy, R., and R. Noe. 2005. *Human Resource Management*, 9th ed. Upper Saddle River, NJ: Pearson Prentice Hall.

O'Connor, B.N., M. Bronner, and C. Delaney. 2002. *Training for Organizations*, 2nd ed. Cincinnati, OH: South-Western.

Odgers, P., and B. Keeling. 2000. *Administrative Office Management*, 12th ed. Cincinnati, OH: South-Western.

Schermerhorn, J. 2005. *Management*, 8th ed. New York: John Wiley & Sons.

Workforce Management Magazine. 2001. Pros and cons of training modes. Available online from workforce.com/archive/article/22/13/14.php.

World Wide Web Consortium's Web Accessibility Initiative. w3c.org/WAI.

Chapter 26
Financial Management

Nadinia Davis, MBA, CIA, CPA, RHIA, FAHIMA

Learning Objectives

- To read, understand, and use balance sheets and income statements
- To explain the difference between financial accounting and managerial accounting
- To recognize the importance of accounting to nonfinancial managers
- To calculate and identify the components of basic financial ratios

- To understand the importance of internal controls and their role in financial management
- To describe the components of operational and capital budgets
- To discuss the impact of claims processing and reimbursement on financial statements
- To describe the financial management functions of HIM professionals

Key Terms

Accounting
Accounting rate of return
Accounts payable
Accounts receivable
Accrue
Acid-test ratio
Activity-based budget
Asset
Balance sheet
Bill hold
Budget cycle
Buildings
Capital budget
Cash
Charge description master (CDM)
Claims processing
Conceptual framework of accounting
Conservatism
Consistency
Contra-account
Corporation
Corrective controls
Cost accounting
Cost justification
Cost report
Credits
Current ratio
Debits
Debt ratio
Debt service

Depreciation
Detective controls
Direct costs
Direct method of cost allocation
Discharged, no final bill (DNFB)
Disclosure
Double distribution
Entity
Equipment
Expenses
Favorable variance
Financial Accounting Standards Board (FASB)
Financial data
Financial transaction
Fiscal year
Fixed budget
Fixed costs
Flexible budget
Forecasting
For-profit organizations
Fund balance
General ledger
Generally accepted accounting principles (GAAP)
Generally accepted auditing standards (GAAS)
Going concern

Government Accounting Standards Board (GASB)
Historical cost
Income statement
Indirect costs
Interim period
Internal controls
Internal rate of return (IRR)
Inventory
Journal entry
Liabilities
Liquidity
Long-term assets
Managerial accounting
Matching
Materiality
Mortgage
Net income
Net loss
Net present value
Not-for-profit organizations
Operational budget
Overhead costs
Owner's equity
Partnership
Payback period
Permanent budget variance
Preventive controls
Profitability index
Public Company Accounting Oversight Board (PCAOB)

Purchase order
Ratio analysis
Reliability
Request for proposal (RFP)
Retained earnings
Return on equity (ROE)
Return on investment (ROI)
Revenue
Securities and Exchange Commission (SEC)
Simultaneous equations method
Sole proprietorship
Stable monetary unit
Statement
Statement of cash flow
Statement of retained earnings
Statement of stockholder's equity
Step-down allocation
Temporary budget variance
Time period
Unallocated reserves
Unfavorable variance
Variable costs
Variance
Variance analysis
Zero-based budget

Introduction

A physician treats a patient. A hospital admits a woman in labor. A professional association offers continuing education for its members. All these are examples of organizations providing services for which they receive compensation. How organizations arrange to provide those services, determine compensation, and handle the flow of funds that these activities both require and generate is guided by financial management.

This chapter focuses on the concepts and tools associated with planning and controlling the financial resources required to operate a department or a work unit. It presents operations, labor, and capital budgeting processes and techniques; reviews organizational and departmental financial performance measures; and explores techniques for improving financial performance at the departmental level. Finally, the chapter acquaints readers with the language of financial and managerial accounting so as to enhance their understanding of the role of the HIM professional as a manager.

Theory into Practice

Olga Paluk is director of health information services (HIS) at a 540-bed urban acute care facility and, as such, is responsible for both the HIS and the patient registration departments. She reports to the chief financial officer (CFO), who is a certified public accountant. The inpatient census has been stable for the past three years and is expected to remain so. Further, the facility is stable financially but has only limited resources for improvements and expansion.

Olga has just received her budget instruction package from the CFO's office. She will use this package to request the resources that her departments will need in the coming year. There are two open positions: a patient registrar and an inpatient coder. An inefficient, incomplete chart system and a stand-alone encoder are accommodated with an extra file clerk and a dedicated data-entry clerk. Olga knows that if she is allowed to purchase a better incomplete chart system and interface the encoder with the main computer, she can

reorganize the staffing and promote from within the departments to fill the positions. She also knows that she will have to justify these actions to the CFO.

Olga will perform a cost analysis of the acquisition of the new equipment and the computer interface. She will compare these costs against the salaries of the eliminated positions. She will also compare the overall cost of using outsourced coding services on a regular basis with the cost of promoting from within. Olga knows that she will have to project the impact over three to five years to illustrate the long-term benefit to the organization.

Because Olga is familiar with the language of financial management and the facility's **capital budget** analysis process, she is able to justify the cost of the new equipment.

Healthcare Financial Management

The process of financial management involves various players within the organization's financial arena. Table 26.1 lists and describes the roles of the financial personnel who work in hospitals. However, healthcare financial management also involves a number of players outside the financial arena. For example, the process is of particular importance to health information management (HIM) professionals because they are immediately involved with the process of reimbursement.

HIM professionals are familiar with **financial data** as one of the components of a health record: the data related to payers and billing. To financial managers, financial data are the individual elements of organizational financial transactions. (The term *financial* refers to money and, as is discussed later, money is the measurement of financial transactions.) A **financial transaction** is the exchange of goods or services for payment or the promise of payment. Financial data are compiled into informational reports for users. The degree of detail that users require depends on their needs and is largely influenced by the relationship of the user to the originator of the transaction.

When financial transactions originate at the department level, the user may require specific details about them. For example, the pharmacy department will review its drug trans-

Table 26.1.   Financial personnel and their roles in a hospital

Position	Typical or Minimum Background	Financial Roles
Board of directors or trustees	Depends on the needs of the facility	Ultimate responsibility for the fiscal integrity of the organization
Chief executive officer (CEO)	Generally, master's-prepared in public administration, hospital administration, or business administration; occasionally, clinical background	Overall responsibility for administration of the organization
Chief financial officer (CFO)	Certified public accountant (CPA) or certified management accountant (CMA)	Overall responsibility for related departments, including patient accounts, internal auditing, and often HIM
Controller or accounting manager	CPA	Oversees accounting and cash disbursement, including payroll
Patient accounts manager	Bachelor's degree	Oversees claims processing

actions; the HIM department will review its purchases of supplies and services; and so on. On the administrative level, however, such detail is not usually required. Instead, informative summaries are often more useful. For example, an organization administrator does not usually need to know the number of cases of copier paper purchased in each department. Instead, he or she would look at the total office supply purchases and evaluate whether they were at appropriate and expected levels. Additional detail or explanation would not be required unless the purchases were unusual. The accumulation and reporting of financial data within an organization is an accounting function.

Accounting

Accounting is an activity as well as a profession. Just as there are many HIM roles and functions, so are there diverse accounting roles and functions. The accounting activity involves the collection, recording, and reporting of financial data. Accountants are both the individuals who perform these activities and many of those who use the reported data. Accounting is important because it is the language that organizations use to communicate with each other to effect transactions, determine investment strategies, and evaluate performance.

The **conceptual framework of accounting** underlies all accounting activity and is based on the following ideas:

- The benefits of the financial data should exceed the costs of obtaining them.
- The data must be understandable.
- The data must be useful for decision making. In other words, the data must be relevant, reliable, and comparable.

Although some of these requirements are similar to general data quality concerns, they are discussed specifically with financial data in mind. Figure 26.1 summarizes basic accounting concepts and principles.

Accounting Concepts

Six concepts define the parameters of accounting activity. These concepts are discussed in the sections below.

Entity

Financial data for different entities may not be mixed. An **entity** is a person or organization, such as a corporation or professional association. A business owner, for example, must not commingle business and personal data. This concept can be very difficult for small business owners, who may not understand why business receipts are not the same as personal income. It can be equally difficult for large corporations that own many different companies.

Going Concern

For the most part, organizations are designed to continue indefinitely. Therefore, unless otherwise stated, financial

Figure 26.1. Basic accounting concepts and principles

Basic Accounting Concepts
- *Entity:* The financial data of different entities are kept separate.
- *Going concern:* Organizations are assumed to continue indefinitely, unless otherwise stated.
- *Stable monetary unit:* Money is the measurement of financial transactions.
- *Time period:* Financial data represent a specified time period.
- *Conservatism:* Resources must not be overstated, and liabilities must not be understated.
- *Materiality:* The financial data collected by an organization are relevant to its goals and objectives.

Basic Accounting Principles
- *Reliability:* Amounts represent the transactions that occurred.
- *Cost:* Transactions are recorded at historical cost.
- *Revenue:* In order to record revenue, it must be earned and measurable.
- *Matching:* Expenses are recorded in the same period as the related revenue.
- *Consistency:* When an accounting rule is followed, all subsequent periods must reflect the same rule.
- *Disclosure:* Financial reports must be accompanied by helpful explanations, when necessary.

data are assumed to have long-range implications. When analysis of the data shows that the organization can continue to operate for the foreseeable future, the organization is considered a **going concern.** Assuming that a business is going to continue, projections of future activities can be made based on historical trends and assumptions about future conditions. The concept of going concern also places constraints on the organization to maintain sufficient financial and other resources to ensure future stability and growth.

Stable Monetary Unit

Every financial transaction must be quantified. For quantification to be meaningful, all of an entity's transactions must be quantified using a standard measurement. Money is the generally accepted standard measurement—the **stable monetary unit.** Organizations typically use the monetary unit of the country in which they are incorporated. In the United States, financial transactions are recorded in U.S. dollars and cents.

Time Period

Financial data represent transactions during a specified period of time: hour, day, week, month, quarter, year, and so on. The specific **time period** depends on the use of the data. The **fiscal year** (also called the financial year) is defined by the tax year. Individuals generally have a tax year that coincides with the calendar year. Organizations, on the other hand, use fiscal years that correspond to their business needs, usually their business cycle, which represents the total activities of the organization. For example, the U.S. government's fiscal year ends September 30.

For financial reporting purposes, a fiscal year is divided into quarters (three-month periods) and months. Because the months generally end on the last calendar day, the quarters can be of slightly different duration. For example, the first quarter of a fiscal year that begins April 1 includes April, May, and June: 91 days. The second quarter of that same fiscal year includes July, August, and September: 92 days. Figure 26.2 illustrates the extent of the difference in a nonleap year. Over time, it is common to compare similar quarters from year to year, particularly when the business cycle has predictable peaks and valleys.

Conservatism

Not all financial data represent completed transactions within the period represented. Sometimes estimates are involved, or transactions are completed between periods. When this occurs, **assets** and **revenue** can potentially be overstated and **liabilities** and **expenses** understated. Assets are resources of the organization such as cash, land, and buildings. They also include the payments due to the organization, such as **accounts receivable.** Liabilities are amounts owed by the organization, such as **accounts payable.** (Accounts receivable and accounts payable are discussed elsewhere in this chapter.) When amounts are estimated, efforts must be made to ensure that their use does not misrepresent the actual financial transaction. Therefore, financial data must comply with **conservatism** in that they fairly represent the financial results of the period.

Figure 26.2.   Impact of days in the month on fiscal quarter and semi-annual reporting (nonleap year)

Month	# of Days	Quarter	# of Days	Half	# of Days
January	31				
February	28				
March	31	Quarter I	90		
April	30				
May	31				
June	30	Quarter II	91	First Half	181
July	31				
August	31				
September	30	Quarter III	92		
October	31				
November	30				
December	31	Quarter IV	92	Second Half	184

Materiality

Materiality refers to the thresholds below which items are not considered significant. These thresholds may be a dollar value or a percentage of a dollar value. To a $100,000 professional association with $100,000 in income, $10,000 is a significant (material) amount. To a $100 billion oil company, $10,000 is not material. This issue arises when determining the significance of errors, potential liabilities, and the necessity for **disclosures** (discussed below).

Accounting Principles

Accounting principles support the quality of financial data. Because they are data, financial data must possess the same data quality characteristics, such as timeliness and validity, as any other type of data.

Reliability

In financial data, **reliability** refers to whether the data actually represent what occurred. Are the data free of material error both in the current period and over time?

Cost

Transactions are recorded at their **historical cost.** In other words, the measurement of any transaction takes place at the time of the transaction. For some transactions, such as the purchase of equipment or investment in marketable securities, there may be a change in the actual or perceived value of the underlying asset or liability. In those cases, adjustments or disclosures are made when reporting the financial data. Such adjustments or disclosures reflect measurements at the time of the adjustment or disclosure.

Revenue

Revenue consists of funds, goods, or services that increase the organization's assets as a result of its activities. For a hospital, reimbursement for healthcare services, donations of equipment, and donations of volunteer time are all revenue. Revenue may only be recognized when it has been earned and can be measured.

Matching

For an organization to generate revenue, it must incur expenses. Expenses may consist of payroll, rent, travel, raw materials, and so on. Therefore, expenses are recorded in the same period as the associated revenue, thereby **matching** the expenses and revenues.

Consistency

Some accounting rules include variations, and one of the most common variations is **depreciation.** Depreciation is the systematic adjustment to the historical cost of an asset, such as equipment, in order to match the expense of the asset with the revenue that it generates and to eliminate **variances** in expenses that large purchases in a single period can create. Organizations may choose whatever depreciation method best suits a particular asset. However, the principle of **consistency** requires that the method not change over the life of the asset. Thus, the financial data are prepared in the same way from one period to the next. In fact, organizations sometimes change their choices. Consistency then requires that financial data be restated to show the effect of the change applied to previous periods. Interestingly, some allowed financial accounting rules differ from tax accounting rules, producing different results.

Disclosure

Sometimes the financial data alone do not provide enough information for users of the data to make informed decisions. The impact of a building fire, a potential or ongoing lawsuit, or an expiring collective bargaining agreement cannot be reflected in the financial data when no financial transaction has occurred. Therefore, notes or disclosures that help the user to make informed decisions must accompany all financial data.

Authorities

Just as clinical data are organized and reported in predetermined formats for ease of communication, financial data also are organized and reported in specific ways. Theoretically, organizations can design their own accounting systems and reporting mechanisms. Internally, this is often the case, as will be seen with budgeting. However, organizations that want to borrow funds or attract investors must follow generally accepted rules that apply to their industry. Four major sources of accounting and reporting rules apply to healthcare organizations: the **Financial Accounting Standards Board** (FACB), the **Securities and Exchange Commission** (SEC), the Centers for Medicare and Medicaid Services (CMS), and the Internal Revenue Service (IRS).

Financial Accounting Standards Board

The FASB is an independent organization that sets accounting standards for businesses in the private sector. Its counterpart, the **Government Accounting Standards Board** (GASB), sets standards for accounting for government entities. The FASB promulgates the rules by which financial data are compiled and reported. These rules, which include the conceptual framework, are referred to as **generally accepted accounting principles** (GAAP) and **generally accepted auditing standards** (GAAS).

Securities and Exchange Commission

The SEC is a federal agency that regulates public and some private transactions involving the ownership and debt of organizations. The SEC sets standards regarding reporting financial data, disclosures, timing, marketing, and execution of these transactions. Public transactions take place through an exchange, such as the New York Stock Exchange (NYSE) or the National Association of Securities Dealers Automated Quotation System (NASDAQ).

Internal Revenue Service

The tax status of an organization plays a huge role in how the organization is administered. The IRS regulates and collects federal taxes. Healthcare organizations fall into one of two major tax categories: for-profit and not-for-profit. Within these categories are several legal structures, such as **sole proprietorship, partnership,** and **corporation.** A summary of legal structures is provided in table 26.2. The primary differences between for-profit and not-for-profit organizations are related to the level of accountability and the distribution of profits.

Public Company Accounting Oversight Board

Historically, the accounting profession has been largely self-regulated. FASB and GASB, although technically independent, have strong ties to the profession. Although IRS and SEC standards and regulations constrained the specific representation of financial activities, the accounting profession was free to accomplish its reporting and other activities without government intervention. However, that changed in 2002. The federal government responded to the collapse of ENRON, WorldCom, and others with the Sarbanes-Oxley Act, which restricted the professional services of independent auditors of public companies and, among other things, created the **Public Company Accounting Oversight Board** (PCAOB). As of this writing, the PCAOB has issued three standards and three rules pertaining to auditing, independence, ethics, and technical issues. The impact of Sarbanes-Oxley has been significant with respect to the way that public accountants do business; however, the overall impact of the PCAOB remains to be seen.

Centers for Medicare and Medicaid Services

CMS (formerly called the Health Care Financing Administration [HCFA]) is the federal agency that administers the Medicare program and the federal portion of the Medicaid program. The federal government is the largest single payer of healthcare expenses in the United States. Although CMS does not set accounting rules, it enforces the federal regulations

Table 26.2. Common legal structures of nongovernmental organizations

Structure	Description	Healthcare Examples
Sole Proprietorship	One owner; all profits are owner's personal income	Solo practitioners
Partnership	Two or more owners; all profits are owners' personal income	Physician group practices
Corporation	One or many owners; profits may be either held or distributed as dividends. Dividends are income to the owners. May be public or private. "Owners" may be individuals, other organizations, or an interest group.	Hospitals, insurance companies

regarding the reimbursement for Medicare and the federal portion of the Medicaid program and sets standards for the documentation and reporting of transactions related to such reimbursement.

Financial Organization

The way an entity organizes itself depends on its financing, its leadership, and its tax status. The three basic forms of business organization are the sole proprietorship, the partnership, and the corporation. Other organizational entities, such as trusts, are beyond the scope of this discussion.

- *Sole proprietor:* An independent coding consultant who operates from home and has no employees may choose to operate as a sole proprietor. The owner, or proprietor, is the leader of the organization and is responsible for all aspects of the business. Income from the business flows through the owner's individual tax returns. If the consultant's business expands, employees or subcontractors can be added without changing the organizational structure.
- *Partnership:* Two or more consultants who want to be in business together may choose a partnership structure. Partners share in the responsibility for the business, and income still flows through the individuals' tax returns. Partners do not need to share equally in the financial or other business responsibilities. A partnership agreement details the contractual arrangement. Because a partnership is a separate legal and accounting entity from the individuals, a tax identification number is required for the partnership and the partnership may be required to file its own tax returns detailing the income allocated to each partner. Partnerships survive as entities only so long as the partners remain together. A change in ownership dissolves the original partnership and a new one must be created.
- *Corporation:* A corporation is a legal entity that exists separately from its owners. Corporations pay their own taxes and have their own legal rights and responsibilities. In fact, the owners of the corporation may have nothing to do with its leadership or day-to-day operations. A corporation is typically governed by a board, and the day-to-day operations are led by one or more administrators who report to the board. The corporation pays its own taxes, and the income after taxes may or may not be distributed in whole or in part to the owners. This after-tax distribution is a dividend and is taxable income to the owner.

The underlying purpose of the organization drives another consideration in the financial organization of the business. Is the purpose of the business to generate income for the owners, or is there a more altruistic foundation? The answer to this question helps to define the tax status the organization will be able to maintain.

For-Profit Organizations

For-profit organizations may be sole proprietorships, partnerships, or corporations. A simple way to think of profits is as the funds remaining after all current obligations have been met, including taxes. The leadership of the organization may distribute the profits to the owners or otherwise invest them as they see fit. The desire to generate profits is not the issue, although it is certainly a common ideology. For-profit organizations may be privately or publicly owned.

Private ownership may be by an individual, a group of individuals, or an organization. Physician practices, urgent care centers, and freestanding ancillary care organizations are often privately owned. The distribution of profits from a privately owned organization is at the discretion of the owners or as defined by contract among owners.

Public ownership means that the ownership interest in the organization may be bought and sold in the financial marketplace. For example, Hospital Corporation of America (HCA) is a publicly held organization with hospitals in numerous states. Its stock is traded on the NYSE under the symbol *HCA*. A publicly held organization's board of directors determines the distribution of profits. Boards are constrained in these determinations by contractual obligations, such as mortgage contracts and preferred stock obligations, stockholder expectations, and strategic organizational goals.

Not-for-Profit Organizations

Not-for-profit organizations are not owned but, instead, are held in trust for the benefit of the communities they serve. Many hospitals fall into this tax category. Other not-for-profit organizations include professional associations such as the American Health Information Management Association (AHIMA) and charitable organizations such as the American Red Cross. There are two major categories of not-for-profit organizations: 501(c)(6) and 501(c)(3).

501(c)(6)

Most professional associations are organized under 501(c)(6), which gives them some tax benefits and the freedom to engage in some activities unrelated to their organizational purpose. For example, organizations under 501(c)(6) may lobby and sell goods and services but are largely involved in activities that benefit their major interest group, which may be defined as paid membership.

501(c)(3)

On the other hand, 501(c)(3) organizations are largely exempt from taxes but must confine their activities to the public benefit. Donations to 501(c)(3) organizations are tax deductible to the extent that no goods or services have been received in return. For that reason, charities are generally 501(c)(3) organizations and many 501(c)(6) organizations have charitable components that are separately incorporated. For example, AHIMA is a 501(c)(6) organization that has a 501(c)(3) component, the Foundation on Research and Education (FORE). Table 26.3 summarizes these common not-for-profit organizations.

Table 26.3. Common not-for-profit tax status

Not-for-Profit	Description	Healthcare Examples
501(c)(3)	Largely exempt from taxes, donations to these organizations can be tax-deductible. Underlying purpose of the organization must be charitable or educational.	Charities, AHIMA's Foundation on Research & Education
501(c)(6)	Partially exempt from taxes. May lobby and sell goods and services. Underlying purpose must benefit the interest group/public.	Professional associations, some hospitals

Tax Status Issues

It is important to understand the underlying tax status of an organization because tax status affects the organization's business decision making and long-term strategies. Undistributed profits from a for-profit organization may stay in the business and be available for investment or future distribution. There is no necessity to identify the future use for these funds, although stockholders may ultimately press for distribution when undistributed profits appear excessive. Occasionally, portions of undistributed profits are held in reserve for specific uses.

On the other hand, profits from a not-for-profit organization stay in the business. Because all such profits must be used for the benefit of the community the organization serves, the future use of these profits should be clearly defined. For further information about tax exemptions of organizations, see IRS Publication 557 (IRS 2004).

Sources of Financial Data

Just as a health record is built of the data collected into it, so financial records are composed of data. Health records are built on medical decision making; financial records originate with financial decision making, the smallest component of which is the transaction.

Transactions

Virtually every financial transaction consists of three fundamental steps:

1. Goods and/or services are provided.
2. A transaction is recorded.
3. Compensation is exchanged.

Each step may require a number of additional steps, depending on the service and the industry. In addition, the steps are not always performed in the same order. Independent contractors that perform hospital coding represent a simple example. The contractor codes the charts, submits an invoice, and receives a check from the hospital. In this case, four specific steps may be needed to support the transaction: keeping a log to track the charts that have been coded, preparing an invoice to bill the hospital, keeping a list of the invoices sent, and checking the invoices off when they are received.

In a hospital, multiple individuals and departments perform services and provide administrative support for financial transactions. Four areas are of particular concern in the context of this discussion: clinical services, patient accounts, health information management, and administration.

Clinical Services

Just as contract coders keep track of the records they have coded, so do clinical, or patient care, services providers keep track of the services they perform. The documents of original entry or source documents enable the healthcare facility to verify that the services were provided and to communicate to supporting departments that a transaction has been initiated. The source document includes two elements: the clinical documentation and the billing documentation.

The clinical documentation is the source document. Clinical documentation is a record of who has seen the patient and why and what tests or treatments were performed, in other words, everything clinically relevant that happened to the patient during his or her interaction with the organization.

Concurrent with the recording of this source document is the capture of the associated billing information. Regardless of the reimbursement system (discussed in chapter 14), the organization must capture the billable event in such a way that the financial transaction can be completed. Therefore, when a medication is administered to a patient, the clinical record reflects the medication, dosage, time, date and route of administration, and the clinical personnel who administered it. At the same time, the charge for the drug must be communicated to patient accounts. This detailed tracking of billable events also supports the cost accounting function, which is discussed later in this chapter.

Patient Accounts

The patient accounts department is responsible for collecting recorded transactions, billing the payer, and ensuring the correct receipt of reimbursement. This department depends on the reliable recording of services. This means that the capture of billing information must be timely and accurate in order to complete the financial transaction efficiently. In addition to the clinical support staff and departments, the patient accounts department relies on the HIM department for coded data.

Health Information Management

The HIM department is responsible for, among other things, identifying and recording the appropriate clinical codes to describe the patient's interaction with the organization. (See chapters 4 and 5.) In some cases, this coding drives the reimbursement to the facility; in other cases, it is used to support the billing.

Increasingly, the reimbursement requirements mandated by CMS and other plans and payers are commingling clinical data with the coding data that describe them. For example, the Minimum Data Set used in long-term care combines the clinical data with the codes. The HIM department should be responsible for assigning or ensuring the accuracy of the codes.

In addition to the coding activity, the HIM department is responsible for aggregating and maintaining the documentation that supports the reimbursement.

Administration

Financial transactions occur throughout the facility. Employees are paid, equipment and supplies are purchased, and departments perform services for each other. The finance department accumulates and analyzes all of the financial data. Ultimately, the entire management team participates in the review and analysis of financial data.

Uses of Financial Data

Financial data are generated virtually everywhere in a healthcare facility. Managerial and supervisory personnel use these data for four key purposes: to track reimbursement, to control costs, to plan future activities, and to forecast results.

Healthcare facilities are service organizations that derive almost all their income from clinical activities. Therefore, a key use of financial data is to track reimbursement and ensure that the desired amount of profit is generated. In the current environment of managed care, where payers often dictate the amount of reimbursement, the provider is increasingly unable to set reimbursement levels. Therefore, the cost of providing services has become the only controllable factor.

Controlling costs is best done at the departmental level. For example, the CEO of a hospital does not shop around for the best price on copier paper, and the CFO does not monitor employee productivity in the food services department. Each department is charged with responsibility for ensuring prudent management of financial and other resources. Departments are given this charge through the budget process, which is one of the outcomes of administrative planning.

Administrative planning reflects the organization's mission. From that mission, goals and objectives are derived that help move the organization toward meeting its mission. Financial data are used to analyze trends, develop budgets, and plan for the future. Planning cannot be accomplished by using historical data alone because the industry changes, sometimes very rapidly. Therefore, the administration must forecast future scenarios.

Forecasting is the prediction of future behavior based on historical data as well as environmental scans. It can be as simple as predicting the profits of an organization on the basis of anticipated changes in reimbursement. It also can involve complicated predictions of consumer behavior based on market research and news reports.

Check Your Understanding 26.1

Instructions: Answer the following questions on a separate piece of paper.

1. If an insurance company representative were to contact the HIM department about a claims audit, which financial personnel should he or she be directed to and why?

2. Given that DRG payments are predetermined, why would a hospital not record revenue on the basis of the working DRG?

3. Big Medical Center earned a lot more revenue than expected this year but does not expect to earn as much next year. To make the financial reports more consistent, a junior accountant suggests that the hospital record some of next year's expenses this year. Would you agree or disagree that this is a good strategy? Why?

4. What role does CMS play in a hospital's financial management?

5. If a hospital's HIM department has excess coding or transcription staff, can the hospital sell coding or transcription services to other hospitals (based on what has been covered so far in this chapter)? Why or why not?

Basic Financial Accounting

A basic understanding of the mechanics of financial accounting helps department managers to understand the impact of their financial transactions on the overall organization. The system of recording financial transactions is based on balancing the *purpose* of the transactions with their impact on the organization. For example, a facility purchases drugs with the purpose of ensuring that sufficient and appropriate drugs are on hand to treat patients. The purchase of the drugs increases the facility's pharmaceutical **inventory.** The impact of that purchase is the outlay of cash. After the cash is spent on drugs, it cannot be spent on something else. Recording both the increase in inventory and the outlay of cash enables the organization to understand and communicate information about its activities. Fundamental to this communication is an understanding of the components of financial data and their relationship to each other.

Assets

An asset is something that is owned or due to be received. In a transaction, the compensation that has been earned by providing goods or services becomes an asset as soon as it has been earned. Examples of assets include **cash,** inventory, accounts receivable, buildings, and equipment.

Cash

Cash consists of monetary instruments and those instruments that can be converted into cash quickly. The latter are often referred to as cash equivalents. Included in cash are funds that are maintained in bank accounts. It is important to remember that, for accounting purposes, currency and bank accounts are both considered cash. At the point of sale, such as purchasing lunch in the cafeteria, currency may be tendered. CMS, on the other hand, does not deliver reimbursement to a hospital in truckloads of currency; instead, it wires funds between financial institutions. Nevertheless, both are considered cash to the hospital. Cash is only an asset when it has been received.

Inventory

An organization has inventory if it maintains goods on hand that it intends to sell to a client. Drugs are part of a hospital's pharmaceutical inventory because they are effectively on hand to be sold to patients. It is important to distinguish between goods that are available for sale and goods that are used by the organization in other ways. Photocopy paper is inventory to the office supply store. To the hospital, it is used for general business purposes. In this case, the hospital is the client (the consumer of the goods). Because hospitals are primarily service organizations, and the provision of goods is incidental to the services provided, hospitals tend not to have a great deal of inventory.

Accounts Receivable

When an organization has delivered goods and/or services, payment for same is expected. Remember that the second step in a transaction is to record the transaction. Because the revenue has been earned upon delivery or provision of the goods and/or services, the organization must have some way to keep track of what is owed as a result. Organizations account for these amounts owed by listing their accounts receivable. Accounts receivable then is merely a list of the amounts due from various customers (in this case, patients). Payment on the individual amounts is expected within a specified period. A schedule of those expected amounts is prepared in order to track and follow up on payments that are overdue (late). Figure 26.3 shows one way to prepare a simple aged accounts receivables report. This list also could be sorted by discharge date and the amounts subtotaled.

Figure 26.3. Aged accounts receivable

	D/C	0–30 days	31–60 days	61–90 days	91–120 days	>120 days	Total A/R
46153153	04/15/05					149	149
46160492	07/06/05				25		25
46162518	07/31/05			10			10
46162874	08/31/05			30			30
46163484	08/07/05					165	165
46162580	07/30/05				114		114
46125122	06/19/04					16	16
46160520	07/06/05				50		50
46169245	10/09/05	175					175
46165628	09/30/05		266				266
46163713	08/12/05			52			52
46166048	09/04/05		280				280
46161964	07/23/05				94		94
46162506	07/30/05				94		94
46164953	08/25/05			52			52
46169231	10/09/05	25					25
46157104	05/30/05					50	50
46124652	06/15/04					84	84
46126673	07/09/04					148	148
46122161	05/20/04					207	207
Total Amounts		**$200**	**$546**	**$144**	**$377**	**$819**	**$2,086**
Total Number of Accounts		**2**	**2**	**4**	**5**	**7**	**20**

Source: Adapted from Schraffenberger 2005, p. 298.

Building

Many organizations own the **buildings** in which they reside. These buildings are assets to the organization because they are part of its physical plant, its infrastructure. If an organization leases space for its operations, that space is not considered an asset because the organization does not own it. Buildings are considered **long-term assets** because they are typically owned for many years.

Equipment

Equipment is another long-term asset. Hospitals include CT scanners, computers, and vehicles in this category. Each organization decides what items are relevant to this category, depending on industry conventions and materiality. For example, a large hospital would rarely consider a $500 computer to be equipment whereas an independent coding consultant might view it as a significant, long-term investment.

Purchase Price

In acquiring a piece of equipment (and certain other assets), the transaction is recorded at the purchase price. For example, the hospital purchases digital mammography equipment for $200,000. The hospital then would have a $200,000 asset in equipment. However, the equipment gradually wears out from use over time. That $200,000 asset is not worth $200,000 four years after it was purchased. To provide better information about the financial value of its equipment, the organization provides an estimate of this decrease in value every year. This estimate is called depreciation.

Depreciation

Depreciation is an example of a **contra-account.** This estimate of the cumulative decrease in value of an asset actually reduces the value of the underlying asset. Thus, the mammography equipment purchased for $200,000 may have accumulated a depreciation of $75,000 after two years. At that point, its value to the organization is $125,000. The cumulative or accumulated depreciation is associated with its underlying assets when the value of those assets is being reported.

Liabilities

Liabilities are essentially debts. They are amounts that are owed, often due to the acquisition of an asset.

Accounts Payable

Accounts payable is a liability that is created when the organization has received goods or services but has not yet remitted the compensation. Going back to the accounts receivable discussion, the provider of the goods and/or services records a receivable when payment is not received at the point of the sale. On the other side of that transaction is the organization for which the goods and/or services were provided. When the recipient of the goods and/or services does not intend to pay immediately, the amount is recorded in accounts payable. The recipient also records either the acquisition of an asset or the expense (discussed next).

Mortgage

A **mortgage** is a liability that is created when the organization borrows money and uses a physical asset, such as a building, as collateral.

Equity/Fund Balance

All financial accounting is based on an equation that pictures the organization holistically, balancing what is owned against what is owed: assets versus liabilities. **Owner's equity** is the difference between assets and liabilities. In a not-for-profit environment, the difference between assets and liabilities is referred to as the **fund balance.** These relationships can be expressed in the following equation:

$$\text{Assets} - \text{liabilities} = \text{owner's equity}$$

The purchase of a house illustrates this equation. The purchase of a house typically involves a deposit of cash and an assumption of a mortgage. The house is an asset whose value is, historically, the price that was paid at the time of the purchase. The mortgage is a liability. As mortgage payments are made, the amount of the mortgage owed declines. The deposit of cash is the owner's equity in the house. As mortgage payments are made, the amount of owner's equity in the house increases. For example, Dr. James purchases an office building for $200,000. She makes a down payment (or deposit) of $50,000 and assumes a mortgage of $150,000. As the mortgage is paid over 30 years, the historical value of the house remains the same, the amount of the mortgage decreases, and the owner's equity in the property increases. When the mortgage is completely paid, the owner's equity in the house equals the historical value of the house, as shown in the table below:

	Assets		Liabilities		Equity
At purchase	$200,000	−	$150,000	=	$ 50,000
After 10 years	$200,000	−	$100,000	=	$100,000
After 20 years	$200,000	−	$ 50,000	=	$150,000
After 30 years	$200,000	−	- 0 -	=	$200,000

Earlier, it was stated that the equation balances what is owned and what is owed. Therefore, another way to look at the accounting equation is:

$$\text{Assets} = \text{liabilities} + \text{owner's equity}$$

Using the previous mortgage example, the second version of the equation proves very useful. At every step in the following calculation, the equations balance:

	Assets		Liabilities		Equity
At purchase	$200,000	=	$150,000	+	$ 50,000
After 10 years	$200,000	=	$100,000	+	$100,000
After 20 years	$200,000	=	$ 50,000	+	$150,000
After 30 years	$200,000	=	- 0 -	+	$200,000

Assets, liabilities, and equity/fund balance are the components of the **balance sheet** (discussed later in this chapter). Before that, however, it is important to understand the compensation components of financial information.

Revenue

Revenue consists of earned, known amounts. It is the compensation that has been earned by providing goods and services to the client/patient as well as amounts received or earned from other sources.

Sources of Revenue

Patient services is the main source of revenue for a healthcare facility. Indeed, depending on the nature of the facility, patient services may be its only source of revenue. Examples of nonclinical services include employee food services, donated services, monetary donations, and copy fees.

Categories of Revenue

How an organization describes its revenue depends on industry convention, materiality, and whether the revenue is recurring or unusual. Most organizations can group their revenue sources into at least two categories: operating and nonoperating.

Operating Revenue

A hospital considers patient services revenue to be operating revenue. Because the hospital is in the business of serving patients, patient services is its main source of revenue and thus falls under the heading of operating revenue. Consider food services. Inpatients must be fed, so food services comes under patient services and thus operating expenses. The employee cafeteria also generates revenue, but the revenue it generates is unrelated to patient services.

Another dilemma is investment income. A hospital with a large endowment that generates significant income may want to highlight this investment revenue in a separate category.

Nonoperating Revenue

Investment income is one example of nonoperating income. Other examples include gift shop sales and unrestricted monetary donations.

Revenue from any source increases equity. A coding consultant works for a week at a client hospital and earns $1,500. He receives a check from the hospital and deposits it in his bank account. This increases his asset by the amount of the deposit: $1,500. The increase in the asset, absent an associated liability, increases equity by the same amount:

Assets	–	Liabilities	=	Equity
$1,500	–	- 0 -	=	$1,500

To this consultant, the increase in cash is directly reflected as an increase in equity. Thus, revenue increases equity.

Expenses

It is unlikely that the generation of revenue is without any reduction of cash or liability being incurred. The consultant coder in the previous example must purchase codebooks and/or coding software, travel from home to client and back, and engage in continuing education (CE). Expenses, then, represent the utilization of resources by the organization in order to generate revenue. The consultant coder uses cash to purchase a codebook. The codebook helps to generate revenue for one year, at which time it expires. Therefore, the price of the codebook is an expense to the coder.

October Activity						
	Assets	–	Liabilities	=	Equity
Beginning balance	$1,500	–	- 0 -	=	$1,500
Purchase codebook	<100>	–		=	<100>
Pay health insurance	<100>	–		=	<100>
Receive payment from client	$1,200	–		=	$1,200
Purchase computer (on credit)	<200>	–	800	=	<1,000>
Receive payment from client	$1,300	–		=	$1,300
Attend CE session	<80>	–		=	<80>
Ending balance	$3,520	–	800	=	$2,720

This simple example illustrates the impact on the accounting equation of the financial transactions discussed thus far. Notice that increasing a liability reduces equity in the same manner that decreasing an asset does.

Purchasing

The types of expenses incurred by an organization depend on its business. A hospital's largest expenses are generally related to human resources: salary and fringe benefits. Similarly, an independent consultant's largest expense may be health insurance. Because expenses offset revenue, expenses reduce equity. As previously stated, healthcare organizations typically cannot affect revenue by raising prices. Therefore, they must attempt to control expenses as much as possible. One way to do this is through the purchasing function.

Organization

Organizations handle the purchasing function differently, depending on their size and needs. Large organizations tend to maintain a central purchasing and distribution department that is responsible for the acquisition of supplies and equipment.

Significant savings can be obtained by purchasing supplies in bulk and distributing them as needed to departments. Central purchasing also has the benefit of minimizing the space required for storage of items on hand. Central purchasing systems should be designed to minimize the risk of loss due to misappropriation of stored items. The periodic inventory of items on hand and the itemized distribution of stored items can assist in this process.

In order to obtain the benefits of purchasing in large quantities, some facilities combine their purchasing efforts. Hospital associations, for example, may offer coordinated purchasing on behalf of multiple facilities. Nevertheless, the control over the use of the items remains with the department.

Maintaining a central purchasing and distribution department results in direct administrative costs to the organization (for example, salary, facility maintenance, and administrative processing). Therefore, the control benefits of centralized purchasing must be weighed against the cost of such operations. Savings also can be obtained by limiting the source of supplies to one or two key vendors who offer discounts to the organization. In this scenario, managers would order items as needed, but only from approved vendors.

Finally, an organization may choose to allow individual departments to make purchases independently. Although this can result in additional supply and equipment costs, there may be overall savings in not maintaining a central purchasing department. The major disadvantages of independent, or decentralized, purchasing are the need for operational areas in which to store supplies and the allocation of managerial resources to purchasing.

Regardless of the purchasing system used, controls must be in place to ensure the efficient execution of approved transactions. **Purchase orders,** shipping/receiving documents, and invoices are the key controls over the purchase process.

Purchase Orders

The purchase order system ensures that items purchased have been properly authorized prior to ordering. Authorization is often tied to dollar limits and/or the budget process. In a paper environment, a purchase order is a paper form on which all details of the intended purchase are reported. Purchase orders for routine, budgeted items often require only the authorization of a supervisor or manager. For large-dollar items, as specified in the organization's policy and procedure manual, additional authorization may be required. In a computer-based system, there may be no physical form; however, authorization levels are still required.

The purchase order shows that the appropriate individual with the appropriate authorization ordered the specific items. The order is then forwarded to the vendor. The originator of the order keeps a copy, and another copy is sent to the accounts payable department. When there is a central receiving department, that department also should receive a copy of the order.

Shipping/Receiving Documents

Items received from a vendor contain a packing slip, also known as a shipping document. This document lists the quantities and descriptions of the items sent from the vendor, but not the price. The recipient of the items must verify that the items received match the ones that were ordered.

The verified shipping/receiving document is forwarded to accounts payable.

Invoices

The vendor sends an invoice (bill or request for payment) directly to accounts payable. The accounts payable department matches the invoice to the shipping/receiving document and the purchase order on file. When all the documents match, the invoice can be processed and payment scheduled.

Statements

A **statement** is merely a list of outstanding invoices the vendor has sent, but for which no payment has been received. Some companies send statements that include all activity for the period, including payment. The statement is one way the vendor lets the customer know that payments are late. Statements are not payable without supporting documentation. When there is no purchase order, receiving document, and invoice, accounts payable will not remit payment.

Statements received for which there is no underlying documentation should be treated as suspicious. Purchases may have been made without proper authorization. Additionally, there are unscrupulous organizations that send only statements when no transaction has taken place in the hope that the receiving organization's controls are lax and payment will be made. This is particularly true of certain fraudulent subscriptions and advertising schemes.

Inventory Slips

In a centralized purchasing system, some mechanism must be in place to track the distribution of items to other departments. Frequently paper based, a form is completed requesting items and verifying their receipt. These systems are purely internal because items are on hand. The financial transaction consists of moving the responsibility for the expense of the items from the purchasing department to the requesting department.

Table 26.4 shows some common accounts and what they represent.

Documents of Original Entry

As previously discussed, financial transactions begin with the documents of original entry or source documents. Whether the organization's transactions are recorded on paper or via computer, there must be a way to determine the origination of the transaction. The originating document details the parties involved in the transaction, the amount of the transaction, the type of financial impact involved (revenue/expense, asset/liability, and the individual responsible for the transaction.

Double-Entry Bookkeeping

All financial transactions are recorded with the accounting equation in mind. To simplify the recording of transactions, accountants use special terminology to reflect the maintenance of a balanced equation.

Debits and Credits

Visually, transactions have two sides: left and right. **Debits** are shown on the left; **credits** are shown on the right. Each account has two sides: increase and decrease. In asset accounts, the left-hand debit side represents the natural balance of the account and debits increase the account. Conversely, credits decrease an asset account. Obviously, for the accounting equation to balance, the opposite is true of liabil-

ity and equity accounts. The right-hand credit side of liability and equity accounts represents the natural balance, and credits increase the accounts. Instead of using minus signs or brackets to represent the increases and decreases, debits and credits provide an additional safeguard against clerical error because every transaction must balance.

Look at the coding consultant example again, using debits and credits.

October Activity								
	Assets		−	**Liabilities**		=	**Equity**	
	Debit	**Credit**		**Debit**	**Credit**		**Debit**	**Credit**
Beginning balance	$1,500		−	- 0 -		=		$1,500
Purchase codebook		100	−			=	100	
Pay health insurance		100	−			=	100	
Receive payment from client	$1,200		−			=		$1,200
Purchase computer (on credit)		200	−		800	=	1,000	
Receive payment from client	$1,300		−			=		$1,300
Attend CE session		80	−			=	80	
Ending balance	$3,520		−		800	=		$2,720

Table 26.4.　Common accounts

Account	Description	Example
Assets		
Cash	Money. Typically, money is represented by several accounts, depending on how the money is stored (for example, in different banks).	Bank account
Inventory	Goods that are available for sale.	Pharmaceuticals
Accounts receivable	Amounts owed the organization for goods and services.	Claims to payers that have not yet been paid
Building	Permanent structures. The land on which they are built is often listed separately.	Office building
Equipment	Represents items that are used to generate revenue or to support the organization during more than one business cycle.	Photocopier CT scanner
Liabilities		
Accounts payable	Amounts the organization owes but has not yet paid.	Supplies purchased on credit
Loans payable	Amounts the organization has borrowed that will be paid over more than one business cycle.	Bank loan
Mortgage payable	Amounts the organization has borrowed to finance the purchase of buildings and equipment.	Building mortgage
Equity		
Capital/stock/fund balance	In a sole proprietorship or partnership, capital is the owner's equity in the organization. In a corporation, stock is the amount invested by owners in the corporation. In a not-for-profit organization, the fund balance is the amount represented by the difference between assets and liabilities.	
Retained earnings/ reserves	In a corporation, retained earnings are profits that have not been distributed. Reserves are amounts that have been designated for a specific purpose.	
Revenue	Temporary account that captures amounts earned by the organization in the current fiscal year.	The difference between revenue and expenses is net income (profits or losses). These accounts are closed at the end of every fiscal year and the net income is moved to Retained Earnings/Reserves.
Expenses	Temporary account that captures amounts disbursed by the organization in the current fiscal year to support the generation of revenue.	

Impact on Individual Accounts

Assets involve multiple accounts as described previously: cash, accounts receivable, and building. Similarly, liabilities have their own accounts. Revenues and expenses fall into the equity section. This system of debits and credits enables us to understand immediately whether a transaction increases or decreases a particular account. Individual accounts increase and decrease in value; however, the overall equation always remains in balance.

Recording Transactions

Financial transactions are recorded, or posted, to the accounts described above according to a system of journal entries.

Journal Entry

Each **journal entry** contains at least one debit and one credit, and the dollar value of all the debits and all the credits are the same. Ensuring that the debits and credits equal is one aspect of ensuring the accuracy of financial data. Other aspects include posting to the correct accounts and in the correct time period. The following tabulation illustrates the purchase of supplies on credit. The supplies are delivered on February 24, and the supplier's invoice is paid on March 15. Note that no financial transaction is recorded until the supplies are received.

Date	Description	Debit	Credit
2/24	Supplies expense	$300	
	Accounts payable		$300
	Purchase office supplies		
3/15	Accounts payable	$300	
	Cash		$300
	Pay 2/24 office supply invoice		

The accounts payable amount is eliminated when the invoice is paid. It is common business practice to record, or **accrue,** liabilities as they are incurred. This accrual basis of accounting enables organizations to understand their total liabilities continuously and to match expenses with the associated revenue. Some organizations, such as small professional associations and sole proprietorships, only record transactions when the cash is paid or received. This cash basis of accounting is analogous to the way individuals handle their private transactions.

In the preceding tabulation, the supplies expense entry is a debit to increase that account. Expenses are temporary equity accounts that close annually. Revenue increases net income; expenses reduce net income. Therefore, revenue accounts have a natural credit balance and expenses have a natural debit balance.

It should be noted that all the financial accounting examples in this chapter relate to corporate and not-for-profit accounting. Government accounting activity, although a system of debits and credits, is significantly different in some respects. For example, a supply purchase would be recorded (encumbered) at the time the supplies were budgeted and then reduced at the time they were ordered.

General Ledger

In a paper-based accounting system, journal entries are listed chronologically in a general journal and their components are posted to the individual accounts. The list of all the individual accounts is referred to as the **general ledger.** In a computer-based environment, only the original journal entry is posted. The computer stores the entries and generates summaries of the individual accounts on request. This system is similar to a computer-based incomplete chart system in which the deficiencies are recorded only once but can be summarized and printed in a variety of ways, on demand.

The example in figure 26.4 is based on this chapter's original description of a financial transaction. The result of this completed transaction is an increase in cash and an increase in equity (revenue). Note that the amount in accounts receivable is eliminated when the reimbursement is received.

Nonfinancial managers are rarely required to make actual journal entries to record financial transactions. However, they do initiate the transactions and receive reports that detail them. Often the reports only show the department's side of the transaction. For example, a purchase of supplies would appear to the manager on a list of expenses and be added to a summary of all supply expenses on another report. The cash and accounts payable portions of the transaction would not show because they are controlled by the accounting department. Managerial reporting activity is discussed later is this chapter.

Financial Statements

At the departmental level, individual financial transactions are reviewed for data quality and compliance with policies and procedures. On an administrative level, the overall

Figure 26.4.   Example of a financial transaction

> **Service provided:**
> Physician sees in the office a new patient, whose chief complaint is an itchy rash.
>
> **Transaction recorded:**
> Clinical record: History and physical/progress note reflect examination of rash and notation that the patient encountered poison ivy while weeding his garden. OTC topical ointment prescribed, and free sample distributed with instructions.
>
> Billing record: Encounter form—office visit code 99201 and ICD-9-CM code 692.6 circled.
>
> Journal entry:
>
> | | Debit | Credit |
> |---|---|---|
> | Accounts Receivable—Patient X | 60 | |
> | Patient Service Revenue | | 60 |
>
> **Reimbursement received:**
> Journal entry:
>
> | | Debit | Credit |
> |---|---|---|
> | Cash | 60 | |
> | Accounts Receivable—Patient X | | 60 |

impact of transactions is generally of more interest than the individual transactions; therefore, summary reports are prepared. These summaries also are used to communicate with lending institutions, potential investors, and regulatory agencies. A variety of summaries are useful for analyzing an organization's financial activities. The two most common reports are the balance sheet and the **income statement.**

Balance Sheet

The balance sheet is a snapshot of the accounting equation at a point in time. Because every financial transaction affects the equation, theoretically, the balance sheet will look different after every transaction. To ensure a meaningful evaluation, the balance sheet is typically reviewed on a periodic basis (monthly, quarterly, semiannually, and/or annually). It is often compared to balance sheets from previous fiscal years in order to analyze changes in the organization.

The balance sheet lists the major account categories grouped under their equation headings: assets, liabilities, and equity/fund balance. Figure 26.5 shows a sample balance sheet. The dollar amount shown next to each account category is the total in each category on the date listed at the top of the report.

Income Statement

The income statement summarizes the revenue and expense transactions during the fiscal year. Like the balance sheet, the income statement can be reviewed at any point in time. Unlike the balance sheet, which represents all account balances at a point in time, the income statement contains only income and expense accounts and reflects only the activity for the current fiscal year.

The difference between total revenue and total expenses is **net income.** When total expenses exceed total revenue, net income is a negative number, or a **net loss.** Net income increases owner's equity; net loss decreases owner's equity.

Figure 26.6 shows the relationship between the balance sheet and the income statement.

Income statement accounts are not listed on the balance sheet because the effect of their activity is reflected in the fund balance shown on the balance sheet. At the end of the fiscal year, all income statement accounts are closed and the net results are added to, or subtracted from, the appropriate fund balance. For the purposes of periodic reporting, fund balances are adjusted in this manner every time the balance sheet is prepared. However, at the end of the fiscal year, the income and expense accounts are actually closed so that the new fiscal year begins at zero.

Analysis Statements

A number of other types of summary statements are required by users to analyze an organization's financial activity and position. Depending on the organization and their use, the additional financial statements may be required by GAAP as part of a complete financial summary report. Figure 26.7 (p. 750) shows a two-year comparative balance sheet and three very simple examples of statements that help to explain the changes from one year to the next. These statements are

Figure 26.5.   Sample balance sheet

Balance Sheet as of 12/31/05			
Assets		**Liabilities**	
Cash	$ 500,000	Accounts payable	$ 600,000
Accounts receivable	600,000	Mortgage	2,000,000
Inventory	400,000	Total liabilities	$2,600,000
Building	2,500,000		
		Fund Balance	
		Restricted funds	$1,000,000
		Unrestricted funds	400,000
		Total fund balance	$1,400,000
Total assets	$4,000,000	Total liabilities + Fund balance	$4,000,000

Figure 26.6.   Relationship between the balance sheet and the income statement

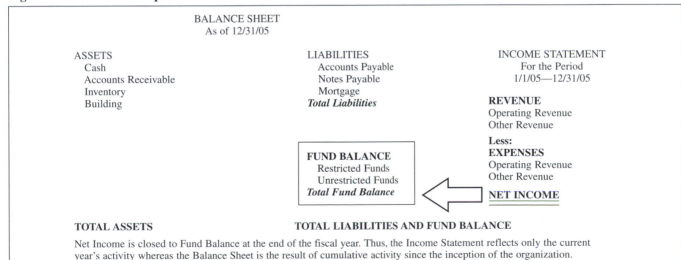

Figure 26.7. Two-year comparative balance sheet with analytical statements

Comparative Balance Sheet		
	12/31/05 (000)	12/31/04 (000)
Assets		
Cash	$ 500	650
Accounts receivable	600	700
Inventory	400	350
Building	2,500	2,250
Total assets	$4,000	$3,950
Liabilities		
Accounts payable	600	550
Mortgage	2,000	2,100
Total Liabilities	$ 2,600	$ 2,600
Fund Balance		
Restricted funds	400	400
Unrestricted funds	1,000	900
Total Fund Balance	$1,400	$1,300
Total Liabilities & Fund Balance	$4,000	$3,900

Statement of Changes in Unrestricted Fund Balance as of 12/31/2005

	(000's)
Balance at 1/1/05	900
Excess of revenues over expenses	100
Balance at 12/31/05	1,000

Statement of Revenues and Expenses 1/1/2005—12/31/2005 (in thousands)

Revenues	
Net patient service revenue	$650,000
Unrestricted gifts	40,000
Other	95,000
Total Revenue	$785,000
Expenses	
Salaries and wages	$340,000
Fringe benefits	95,000
Supplies	175,000
Total expenses	$700,000
Income from operations	$85,000
Nonoperating gains	
Unrestricted gifts	$15,000
Excess of revenues over expenses	$100,000

Cash Flows from Operating Activities 1/1/2005–12/31/2005 (in thousands)

Revenue in excess of expenses	100
Decrease in accounts receivable	100
Increase in inventory	−50
Increase in account payable	50
Net cash provided by operating activities	200
Cash flows from investing activities	
Purchase of property, plant, and equipment	−250
Net cash used by investing activities	−250
Cash flows from financing activities	
Repayments of long-term debt	−100
Net cash used by financing activities	−100
Net increase (decrease) in cash	-150
Cash at beginning of year	650
Cash at end of year	500

included for completeness of discussion and are not statements that HIM professionals generally need to analyze.

Cash Flow

The **statement of cash flow** (also called the statement of changes in financial position) details the reasons that cash changed from one balance sheet period to another. It shows the analyst whether cash was used to purchase equipment or to pay down debt and whether any unusually large transactions took place.

Retained Earnings

The **statement of retained earnings** expresses the change in retained earnings from the beginning of the balance sheet period to the end. Retained earnings are affected, for example, by net income/loss, distribution of stock dividends, and payment of long-term debt.

Stockholders' Equity

The **statement of stockholders' equity** (also called the statement of fund balance) details the reasons for changes in each of the stockholder's equity accounts, including retained earnings.

Ratio Analysis

After the financial statements have been prepared, they are ready for **ratio analysis.** Financial analysts can use financial statements, particularly the balance sheet, to determine whether an organization is using its resources similarly or differently from other organizations in the same industry. In retail sales, analysts compare inventory turnover; that is, how quickly inventory is sold. In any industry, one of the most common reasons to analyze financial statements is to lend money to the organization or to invest in it. Thus, the organization's use of assets compared to its liabilities is extremely important.

Ratios are only meaningful within the context of the organization's industry. It is not useful to compare a ratio for a hospital against a ratio for an automobile manufacturer, except to state that one would expect the ratios to be different. Whether an organization's particular ratio is good or bad depends on expected ratios for similar organizations in that industry.

The Healthcare Financial Management Association publishes industry ratio medians annually as a member service. Some state hospital associations also publish ratio information.

Liquidity and Debt Service

A key issue to lenders and investors is the organization's ability to discharge its financial obligations. **Liquidity** refers to the ease with which assets can be turned into cash. This is important because payroll, loan payments, and other financial obligations are typically paid in cash. **Debt service** is the extent to which those financial obligations are loans.

Current Ratio

An organization's ability to pay current liabilities with current assets is very important to lenders. Current assets include cash, short-term investments, accounts receivable, and inventory. Current assets implicitly will be (or could be) converted to cash at some point within a year, through either collections, sales, or other business activity. Current liabilities include accounts payable and the current portion of loan obligations. Again, the term *current* implies that the liability will be discharged within a year. The **current ratio** compares total current assets with total current liabilities:

$$\frac{\text{Total current assets}}{\text{Total current liabilities}}$$

From the balance sheet in figure 26.5, one can take the current assets (cash plus accounts receivable plus inventory) and divide them by the current liabilities (accounts payable) to determine the current ratio:

$$\frac{1,500,000}{600,000} = \frac{15}{6} = \frac{2.5}{10}$$

The current ratio indicates that for every dollar of current liability, $2.50 of current assets could be used to discharge the liability, which even common sense tell us is good.

Acid-Test Ratio

Inventory is a current asset because it is presumed that inventory will be sold, or turned over, within one fiscal year. However, inventory can become obsolete very quickly (for example, in the fashion and computer industries). Pharmaceuticals can expire before they are used. For expensive items such as motor vehicles, saleable merchandise may be retained in inventory longer than expected or desirable. Therefore, a stricter measure of an organization's ability to pay current liabilities is needed. The **acid-test ratio** compares current liabilities to the current assets that are truly liquid, that is, able to be turned into cash quickly:

$$\frac{(\text{Cash} + \text{short-term investments} + \text{net current receivables})}{\text{Total current liabilities}}$$

Short-term investments include money market funds, certificates of deposit, and treasury bills, for example. Using the balance sheet in figure 26.5 again, the acid-test ratio is:

$$\frac{1,100,000}{600,000} = \frac{1.1}{6.0} = \frac{1.83}{1.00}$$

In this example, the acid-test ratio reveals that for every dollar of current liabilities, 1.83 dollars of current assets could be used immediately or sold quickly to discharge the liabilities.

Debt Ratio

Looking back to the mortgage example, the organization's building asset was purchased using 10 percent cash and 90 percent mortgage. Ninety percent of that asset was financed with debt. Looking at all the liabilities and all the assets together gives the analyst an overall picture of how the assets were acquired. The **debt ratio,** therefore, is total liabilities divided by total assets.

It is important to remember that all ratio analysis is industry specific and varies somewhat depending on the economic environment. Therefore, ratio analysis can be used to compare similar organizations at a specific point in time or the same organization at different points in time. However, a hospital ratio would never be compared with a professional association ratio.

Profitability

The above examples illustrate how organizations can evaluate their ability to pay their bills. Another measure of an organization's health is its profitability. Profitability refers to an organization's increase in value: how well does it invest its assets? As with other ratios, profitability measures are only meaningful as benchmarks against like organizations or in trending a single organization over time.

Return on Investment

Return on investment (ROI) measures the increase in the value of an asset. In a savings account, this increase is measured as the amount of interest received in a period. The beginning balance in the account is the measurement of the asset. Interest received in the period is the return. Thus:

$$\text{ROI} = \frac{\text{Interest earned in the period}}{\text{Asset value at the beginning of the period}}$$

Return on individual investments can be calculated in this manner. For an entire organization, interest earned is replaced by earnings, usually after taxes. Asset value is replaced by total assets

$$\text{ROI} = \frac{\text{Earnings (after taxes)}}{\text{Total assets}}$$

Return on Equity

ROI does not tell the whole story because it only indirectly measures the liabilities incurred in order to acquire or generate the asset. Generating sufficient overall profits to ensure ongoing operations, as well as maintaining and upgrading assets, is especially of interest to users of financial information. An organization may use several profitability ratios to gauge overall performance. **Return on equity (ROE)** is an important indicator for determining an organization's efficiency or profitability level. It measures the excess of revenue over expenses (net income) for an accounting period compared to the total fund balance (equity)

To illustrate, examine the acquisition of technology to generate income.

Purchase: $100,000 (invest in transcription system)
Liability: $90,000 (long-term loan from bank)
Net income: $30,000 (after taxes)

$$ROI = \frac{\$30,000}{\$100,000} = 30\%$$

$$ROE = \frac{\$30,000}{\$10,000} = 300\%$$

Additional measures of return are discussed later in the section on capital projects.

Check Your Understanding 26.2

Instructions: Answer the following questions on a separate piece of paper.

1. List three assets and three liabilities.

2. Why are revenue and expense accounts part of owner's equity?

3. What inventory does a hospital have?

4. What is the difference between a debit and a credit?

5. Why is knowledge of accounting important to nonfinancial managers?

6. A lender wants to know how quickly a borrower would be able to repay a debt. What is the best ratio to use for this analysis? Why?

Cost Accounting

To obtain appropriate compensation for goods and services provided, the organization must understand and measure the resources used to manufacture, acquire, or otherwise produce those goods and services. The measurement of those resources is monetary and is referred to as their cost. In manufacturing and other goods-oriented businesses, sales are compared to the cost of goods sold, which are composed of raw materials and other manufacturing costs. In a service industry, the underlying costs consist largely of human resources.

Types of Costs

Cost accounting is the discipline of identifying and measuring costs and is a unique subset of the accounting profession. However, a general understanding of the terminology helps nonfinancial managers participate in and support the process.

There are numerous categories of costs, but the most important for purposes of this discussion are discussed below.

Direct Costs

Direct costs are traceable to a specific good or service provided. To a hospital, the cost of a specific medication can be matched to the specific patient to whom it was administered. Similarly, to a consulting firm, the hours that a consultant coder spends coding are directly linked to the records that are coded.

Indirect Costs

Indirect costs are incurred by the organization in the process of providing goods or services; however, they are not specifically attributable to an individual product or service. The cost of providing security services at a hospital or clerical support at the switchboard are indirect costs with respect to patient care. To the consulting firm, the cost of CE for its coding staff is an indirect cost of providing services to a particular client.

The classification of costs as direct or indirect depends on the relationship of the cost to the client, department, product, service, or activity in question. Payroll in the security department is an indirect cost to patient care, but it is a direct cost to the security department. Therefore, the distinction between direct and indirect costs is important in understanding the broader financial impact of activities within the facility. In developing capital projects (discussed later in this chapter) such as the development and implementation of an electronic health record, an understanding of the associated costs (and, conversely, the cost savings) is crucial in making realistic financial estimates and projections.

Fixed Costs

For planning and analysis, it is useful to classify costs as fixed or variable. **Fixed costs** remain the same, despite changes in volume. For example, a manager's base salary does not change, regardless of patient volume or other changes in activity. Mortgage payments also are not dependent on activity.

Variable Costs

Variable costs are sensitive to volume. Medication is a good example. The more patients are treated, the more medication is used. Paper medical record documentation is another example. The larger the volume of patients, the more paper is used.

Costs may behave in a combination of fixed and variable ways and volume is not the only change agent. (For a detailed discussion of cost classifications, see Cleverley and Cameron, chapter 11.)

Cost Reports

Prior to implementation of prospective payment systems (PPSs), Medicare reimbursement to hospitals was related directly to the costs incurred by the facilities. Individual facility **cost reports** were submitted to Medicare, identifying the direct and indirect costs of providing care to Medicare patients. Direct costs include nursing and radiology; indirect costs include medical records and information systems. Preparation of cost reports requires the definition of products or services, establishment of cost centers, and identification of service units (Dunn 1999, pp. 64–65). The expense of nonrevenue-producing cost centers is allocated to revenue-producing cost centers in order to fully understand the cost of providing services.

Allocation of Overhead

The attribution of indirect or **overhead costs** to revenue-producing service units illustrates the budget concept that all activities must support the mission of the organization. There are four methods of allocation of overhead:

- The **direct method of cost allocation** distributes the cost of overhead departments solely to the revenue-producing areas. Allocation is based on each revenue-producing area's relative square footage, number of employees, or actual usage of supplies and services. (See figure 26.8.)
- **Step-down allocation** distributes overhead costs once, beginning with the area that provides the least amount of nonrevenue-producing services.
- **Double distribution** allocates overhead costs twice, which takes into consideration the fact that some overhead departments provide services to each other.
- The **simultaneous equations method** distributes overhead costs through multiple iterations, allowing maximum distribution of interdepartmental costs among overhead departments.

The last three methods of cost allocation above assume that overhead cost centers such as housekeeping perform services for each other as well as for revenue-producing areas. Therefore, overhead costs are distributed among overhead cost centers as well as revenue-producing areas.

Although each of these methods may produce slightly different results, the ultimate goal is to allocate overhead costs appropriately. Appropriate allocation enables the facility to express the full cost of providing services.

Impact on Reimbursement

Although cost reporting is no longer used to directly determine Medicare reimbursement, some payers still use cost reports to make reimbursement decisions. In addition, CMS uses cost reports to help determine facility-specific and regional cost adjustment factors for healthcare PPSs.

Charge Description Master

Chapter 14 discusses the various types of reimbursement to healthcare providers. Regardless of the reimbursement method, however, the facility must be able to evaluate the underlying cost of providing services and to compare its actual reimbursements to the potential reimbursements based on charges. To do this, all individual patient charges are captured in the patients' accounts. The charges themselves and the underlying costs of the services provided are maintained in a database called the **charge description master** (CDM). (Several alternative terms are used for the database, such as charge data master and chargemaster.) Using the individual patient charges and the associated clinical codes, the patient accounts department is able to prepare reimbursement claims.

The CDM collects information on all the goods and services the facility provides to its clients. Responsibility for maintaining the database varies among facilities, and multiple departments contribute to the data. Because many of the charges are associated with CPT/HCPCS codes, the HIM department is usually involved in the routine maintenance of this database.

The purpose of the CDM is to facilitate charge capture by centralizing and standardizing charge data within the

Figure 26.8. Direct allocation versus step allocation

	NonRevenue-Producing Department		Revenue-Producing Department	
	HIM Department	Business Office	Medicine	Laboratory
Direct method:				
Overhead costs before allocation	$360,000	$240,000	$400,000	$250,000
Allocation				
HIM (# discharges processed)	($360,000)		$340,000	$20,000
Business office (# labor hours used)		($240,000)	$80,000	$160,000
Total overhead after allocation	$0	$0	$820,000	$430,000
Step method:				
Overhead costs before allocation	$360,000	$240,000	$400,000	$250,000
Allocation				
HIM (# discharges processed)	($360,000)	$50,000	$300,000	$10,000
Business office (# labor hours used)		($290,000)	$90,000	$200,000
Total overhead after allocation	$0	$0	$790,000	$460,000

facility. Grocery stores do this by linking UPC symbols to the price and description of grocery items. The customer sees the evidence of this activity on the grocery bill but does not see that the database also contains the cost of the item, the vendor, and the underlying general ledger information. Similarly, the CDM enables the facility to capture and record patient charges as they are incurred. For the charges to be captured accurately, the CDM must be updated routinely as new services emerge, costs change, and CPT code descriptions change. Use of a properly updated CDM also helps the facility administratively by enabling the statistical reporting of charge-related activities.

The components of the CDM vary, depending on the needs of the healthcare organization. At a minimum, the fields for each record include (Schraffenberger 2005, p. 135):

- *Charge code:* The facility's internal tracking number
- *Item description:* The facility's description of the item
- *General ledger (GL) key:* The reference to the facility's accounting system
- *Revenue code:* The three-digit Medicare billing reference
- *Insurance code mapping:* Multiple fields to reference alternative billing codes for the item for different payers
- *Charge:* The charge for the item
- *Activity date/status:* Whether the item is currently being used

Figure 26.9 provides an example of a CDM and its components.

Maintenance of the CDM is a multidisciplinary activity. For example, the HIM department knows the clinical codes, the patient accounts department knows the general ledger codes, the pharmacy department knows the drugs and their costs, and the finance department knows the associated charge formulas. Pharmacy cannot realistically update radiology's data nor can finance update charges without knowledge of underlying costs.

To coordinate the update effort, a single department, usually finance, should be assigned responsibility for ensuring timely updates. The finance department then should enlist the assistance of other disciplines, including HIM. Update frequency depends on the data element to be updated, but certainly whenever underlying costs change. For example, pharmacy charges may be updated every time inventory is replenished. The entire CDM must be reviewed at least annually. Identification and substantiation of actual costs provide the foundation for the development of what an organization charges for its services. The subsections below follow those charges through the revenue cycle from here (even though they are not technically cost accounting topics).

Claims Processing

Claims processing involves accumulating charges for services, submitting claims for reimbursement, and ensuring that claims are satisfied. As this chapter has already discussed, this is the responsibility of the patient accounts department. However, the patient accounts department can only process what the service providers have accumulated and what HIM has coded.

Claims processing is often outsourced in nonhospital ambulatory care because physician offices and other small facilities often do not have the resources to perform this complex activity effectively. The activity of submitting a claim is often called dropping a bill. Because reimbursement for clinical services provided is the healthcare facility's largest source of revenue, timely, accurate claims processing is necessary.

Sometimes facilities adopt a **bill hold** policy. This policy dictates a waiting period between the patient's discharge date and claim submission (dropping the bill). Bill hold assumes that there will be a delay in accumulating the charges incurred by a patient. By incorporating this predicted delay into normal operations, the facility creates a preventive control to avoid underbilling or having to submit late charges to the payer.

Third-party payers generally will not reimburse a claim that does not include the clinical diagnostic and procedural codes. This is true whether the reimbursement is based on a PPS, actual charges, or some other method. For this reason, the patient accounts department cannot drop a bill until the patient record has been coded. Therefore, timely, accurate coding is critical to the reimbursement process and directly affects the facility's cash flow.

Accounts Receivable

During a patient's encounter with a healthcare provider, individual services are performed and associated charges are incurred. Each charge is recorded in a subledger for the specific patient account. Because each charge represents a completed transaction, the amount of the charge becomes revenue (earned and measurable) and receivable. However, from a practical standpoint, the claim to the payer is not rendered until after patient discharge, at which time the charges incurred by the patient during his or her stay are finalized. For example:

4/15	Accounts Receivable—Patient	$5,500
	Patient Services Revenue	$5500
	Total charges for account #0146589	

Cumulating charges and postdischarge billing work well for ambulatory care and most acute care encounters. For long-term care, however, interim billing is necessary. When an interim bill is dropped, the reimbursement received reduces the accounts receivable for that patient.

Posting the receivable and dropping the bill are two different activities. To monitor timely claims processing, a summary report of patient receivables is frequently generated. This summary report has no standard title. It is sometimes called DNFB, which stands for **discharged, no final bill,** or merely accounts receivable, or AR.

Figure 26.9. Sample charge description master

Charge Code	Item Description	CPT/HCPCS Code			Revenue Code	G/L Key	Activity Date
		INS CODE A	INS CODE B	INS CODE C			
2110410000	ECHO ENCEPHALOGRAM	76506	76506	Y7030	320	15	12/2/2001
2110410090	F/U ECHO ENCEPHALOGRAM	76506	76506	Y7040	320	15	12/2/2001
2110413000	PORT US ECHO ENCEPHALOGRAM	76506	76506	Y7050	320	15	12/2/2001
2120411000	ULTRASOUND SPINAL CONTENTS	76800	76800	Y7060	320	15	12/2/2001
2130401000	THYROID SONOGRAM	76536	76536	Y7070	320	15	1/1/2003
2151111000	TM JOINTS BILATERAL	70330	70330	Y7080	320	15	8/12/2002
2161111000	NECK LAT ONLY	70360	70360	Y7090	320	15	10/1/2001
2162111000	LARYNX AP & LATERAL	70360	70360	Y7100	320	15	10/1/2001
2201111000	LONG BONE CHLD AP	76061	76061	Y7110	320	15	8/12/2002
2201401000	NONVASCULAR EXTREM SONO	76880	76880	Y7120	320	15	10/1/2001
2210111000	SKULL 1 VIEW	70250	70250	Y7130	320	15	1/1/2003
2210112000	SKULL 2 VIEWS	70250	70250	Y7140	320	15	8/12/2002
2210114000	SKULL 4 VIEWS	70260	70260	Y7150	320	15	8/12/2002
2211111000	MASTOIDS	70130	70130	Y7160	320	15	1/1/2003
2212111000	MANDIBLE	70110	70110	Y7170	320	15	12/2/2001
2213111000	FACIAL BONES	70140	70140	Y7180	320	15	12/2/2001
2213114000	FACIAL BONES MIN 4	70150	70150	Y7190	320	15	12/2/2001
2214111000	NASAL BONES	70160	70160	Y7200	320	15	1/1/2003
2215111000	ORBITS	70200	70200	Y7210	320	15	1/1/2003
2217111000	PARANASAL SINUSES	70220	70220	Y7220	320	15	1/1/2003

Source: Schraffenberger 2005, 136.

Components of Accounts Receivable

The individual charges for a patient's account are collected in a database. The actual components of the database vary, depending on the needs of the facility. Patient identifying data and financial data collected at registration are components of the database. Individual charges incurred also are collected. Maintenance of patients' accounts in a database enables the facility to analyze these financial data in a number of ways.

Review and Analysis of Accounts Receivable

Department managers review the patient account database for different reasons. The pharmacy department may request a listing of all pharmaceutical charges in order to compare the posted charges with its records. This detective control enables the pharmacy department to ensure that all dispensed medications are charged. The chief financial officer (CFO), on the other hand, may target one number: total charges for patients who have been discharged, but for whom no final bill has been dropped. When the total charges exceed a predetermined threshold, the CFO will require an explanation from the patient accounts department.

A predetermined threshold may be a dollar amount and/or a time period, such as days in accounts receivable. For example, an acceptable level of unbilled charges may be $1,000,000. A dollar threshold would be determined taking into consideration the cash flow needs of the facility as well as the facility's historical experience in accurate billing.

An alternative or concomitant threshold would be days in accounts receivable, which refers to the number of days an invoice has been outstanding after it has been billed. Of course, the first step is to mail out the final bill. Because one common reason for no final bill is the lack of clinical codes, the HIM department may be involved in delivering the explanation. Figure 26.10 provides an example of an accounts receivable report.

The HIM department participates in ensuring timely claims processing by timely coding of the clinical records. Therefore, effective coding management includes the routine analysis of the DNFB. Figure 26.10 illustrates a portion of a DNFB. Notice that the report lists the outstanding charges by the patient's last name. The patient's medical record number and discharge date enable the HIM department to locate the patient's clinical record. The sample report indicates that patient number 124785 was discharged 13 days before the report was prepared and that the accumulated charges are $18,139.45. The reason listed for failure to drop the bill is "no final diagnosis." Seeing this, the HIM department manager would have located the record, determined why it had not been coded, and taken action to solve whatever problem had prevented its coding. Typical problems include lack of a pathology report, uncertainty as to principal diagnosis, and backlog in the coding function. Table 26.5 (p. 758) lists some common coding delays and actions that can be taken to solve the underlying problem.

Because the patients' account data are maintained in a database, theoretically, they can be retrieved in whatever format is useful to the manager. Many facilities' computer systems include sophisticated report-writing functions that enable managers to query the database for the desired data and retrieve a report in the desired format, as needed. Of course, this situation is ideal; other systems do not provide this capability. The facility's information systems (IS) department should be able to provide the manager with a customized report routinely.

The frequency with which managers review the accounts receivable data depends on the facility's policies and procedures as well as on the impact on claims processing. To proactively manage the outstanding receivables, some HIM managers review the data daily and take action on large-dollar accounts. Because the entire AR report may contain hundreds of accounts, the manager may request a report of all accounts with an amount over $10,000 that were discharged over two days ago. Even with a bill-hold policy of three or four days, a targeted report enables the HIM department to prioritize the processing of high-dollar accounts quickly.

The priority of coding high-dollar accounts quickly must be balanced against the need to maintain the even distribution of workload and orderly processing of all records in the HIM department. Ten $5,000 accounts are financially equivalent to one $50,000 account. Failure to process those 10 accounts because the routine was disrupted in order to process one account is not good financial management. Therefore, routine, timely processing of all records can obviate prioritization by dollars.

Impact of Accounts Receivable on Financial Statements

Accounts receivable represents a current asset. Delays in processing claims cause receivables to age. Aged receivables can negatively affect a facility's ability to borrow money. Failure to claim and collect receivables affects cash, which in turn negatively affects the facility's ability to discharge its current liabilities, the largest of which is payroll. Therefore, in a facility for which reimbursement is the largest revenue item and payroll is the largest expense, there is a direct relationship between getting paid and paying employees. Thus, the role of HIM becomes a critical component of maintaining the facility's fiscal integrity.

Internal Controls

In any industry, **internal controls** must be in place to safeguard assets and to ensure compliance with policies and procedures. Internal controls may be designed to prevent the theft of cash or to ensure that a patient receives the correct medication. The three major categories of internal controls are preventive, detective, and corrective controls.

Figure 26.10. Example of an accounts receivable report

Anyplace Health Systems

Accounts Not Selected for Billing—Inpatients

Patient Financial Services Version

Patient Name	Acct. #	Med Rec #	Status	Unbilled Charges	Days Since Disch.	Pt. Type	Insurance Verification			Final Dx	DRG	Open Orders	Fin. Class
							Ins. 1	Ins. 2	Ins. 3				
Axxxxxx, Rxxx	1452585	124785	Discharged	18,139.45	13	E-Inpt	Yes	Yes	Yes	No	000	No	J
Bxxxx, Vxxxx	4568972	258564	Discharged	1,173.75	26	Inpt	No	No	No	Yes	466	No	T
Cxxxx, Axxxx	7456594	256632	Discharged	10,286.70	5	E-Inpt	Yes	Yes	Yes	Yes	277	Yes	Q
Fxxxx, Txxxxx	7458961	148965	Discharged	3,425.45	15	Inpt	No	Yes	Yes	No	000	Yes	F
Plxxxxx, Gxxxxx	8585964	745321	Discharged	15,452.25	8	Inpt	Yes	Yes	Yes	Yes	321	Yes	J
Zxxx, Mxxxxxxx	7458946	147589	Discharged	25,584.55	20	E-Inpt	Yes	Yes	Yes	No	000	No	B
Totals	I/P Discharged 6			74,062.15									
							Reason for Rejection	Insurance Not Verified 4		No Final Dx 4		Open Orders 4	
								Open Orders 0		Invalid DRG 0			

Anyplace Health Systems

Accounts Not Selected for Billing—Outpatients

Patient Financial Services Version

Patient Name	Acct. #	Med Rec #	Status	Unbilled Charges	Days Since Disch.	Pt. Type	Insurance Verification			Final Dx	DRG	Open Orders	Fin. Class
							Ins. 1	Ins. 2	Ins. 3				
Cxxxx, Jxxx	5869751	586462	O/P – Recur.	1,377.50	34	Recur.	No	Yes	Yes	Yes	131	No	T
Dxxx, Axxx	7469832	154783	O/P – Surg	10,850.40	16	Surgical	Yes	Yes	Yes	Yes	479	Yes	L
Gxxx, Dxxxxx	7459831	852697	O/P	12,587.75	4	Out	Yes	Yes	Yes	No	000	No	Q
Totals	Recurrent Outpatients 1			1,377.50			Reason for Rejection	Insurance Not Verified 1		No Final Dx. 2			
	Outpatient Surgical 1			10,850.40				Open Orders 1		Invalid DRG 0			
	Outpatient General 1			12,587.75									

Preventive

Preventive controls are implemented prior to the activity's taking place because they are designed to stop an error from happening. In financial management, pretransaction supervisory review and authorization is a preventive control. Computer data-entry validation is another preventive control. Data-entry validation prevents the user from entering "64," for example, as a day of the month. Preventive controls are sometimes more costly than their effect warrants. In those cases, controls must be put in place to find and correct errors.

Detective

Detective controls are designed to find errors that have already been made. Detective controls tend to be less expensive than

preventive controls and can be implemented at many levels. Quantitative record reviews and computer validity edits are examples of detective controls. In accounting, the summing of debits and credits is a detective control because the two sums must always be equal. Footing and cross-footing financial reports is another detective control. (See figure 26.11.)

Corrective

When an error or other problem has been detected, action must be taken to correct the error, solve the problem, or design controls to prevent future errors or problems. The error or problem must be analyzed to determine the cause. When a correction can be made, it is documented and implemented. However, some errors, such as amputation of an incorrect

Table 26.5.   Remedies for common coding delays

Reason for Failure to Code	Underlying Issue(s)	Possible Actions
Lack of pathology report	Pathology department may not have completed the analysis.	Ask the pathology department for an estimated completion date and a STAT dictation.
	Pathologist may not have dictated the report.	Ask the pathology department for a STAT dictation or a verbal confirmation of the pathology diagnosis.
	Pathology reports may not have been in the charts.	Search the reports for the missing one. In a computer-based environment, coders should have the ability to search for the reports online.
Uncertain principal or additional diagnosis	Waiting for a response to a physician query	Elevate the query to the managerial level. Meet the physician on the nursing unit during morning rounds, if necessary.
Coding backlog	Coder(s) out sick	Prioritize coding by receivable size instead of discharge date.
	Coder(s) on vacation	Consider overtime pay for staff to fill in.
	Coding function understaffed	Assign qualified supervisory personnel to assist and/or support coders.
		Plan vacation coverage in advance to avoid affecting the facility's cash flow.
		Long-term understaffing can impair coding quality. Outsourcing should be considered. Coding quality and DNFB impact are typical justifications for approving additional coding staff.

Figure 26.11.   Footing and cross-footing financial reports

SUMMING OF DEBITS AND CREDITS

Cash	$1,345	
Photocopy paper		$974
Toner		$362

In this journal entry, the debit ($1,345) does not match the credits ($1,336). This means that an error has been made. Reference back to the original documentation will reveal that the sales tax on the items was not accounted for.

FOOTING AND CROSS-FOOTING

	January	February	March	Year-to-date (Cross-foot)
Payroll	20,000	20,000	20,000	60,000
Benefits	6,000	6,000	6,000	24,000
Office supplies	1,000	1,000	1,000	3,000
Equipment service	400	500	600	500
				87,500?
Monthly Totals	27,400	27,400	27,400	82,200?
	(Foot)			

The foot is the sum of the columns; the cross-foot is the sum of the rows. Notice that in this example the sums do not match. Footing and cross-footing reports that are supposed to represent arithmetic totals is a very useful detective control, particularly with manually prepared or PC-prepared reports. A simple error in creating a formula in a spreadsheet program can cause an entire report to be wrong.

limb, cannot be corrected. In these cases, analysis of the root cause is important so that the error can be prevented in the future. In financial management, very few errors cannot be corrected. Typical errors include posting transactions to an incorrect account, posting transactions that have not been completed, and posting incorrect amounts. Even financial statement errors can be corrected and the reports redistributed. Problems that cannot always be corrected include theft of assets and failure to invest funds on a timely basis. These problems require analysis and development and implementation of controls for the future.

Corrective controls are designed to fix problems that have been discovered, frequently as a result of detective controls. Many errors and problems occur routinely, such as failing to complete forms, making computation errors, and wrongly posting transactions. Therefore, procedures must be in place to ensure the timely and accurate correction of the error or solution to the problem. In the HIM department, the incomplete chart system is a corrective control. Incomplete charts have been detected, the source of the error identified, and the responsible individual contacted for completion of the chart. In financial management, supervisory review of transactions is typically used to detect errors and problems. The ability to correct errors in journal entries is essential.

Internal controls may be present at every level of the organization. In a service organization, such as a hospital, controls over expenditures are some of the most important responsibilities of individual managers. Two key methods of exerting such controls are through purchasing and analysis of variances.

Basic Managerial Accounting

Managers must have some understanding of **managerial accounting** in order to control the financial aspects of their departments' operations. As stated earlier, managers must work within budgets that have been developed based on their organization's goals and objectives. Therefore, it is not sufficient for a manager merely to review for accuracy the financial transactions generated by the department during the period. Rather, the transactions must be compared to the expected or budgeted transactions to ensure that the goals and objectives of both the department and the organization are being met. The development, implementation, and analysis of systems that track financial transactions for managerial control purposes is called managerial accounting. Managerial accounting includes both budget and cost analysis systems.

Types of Budgets

In addition to the most familiar budgets, operating and capital budgets (discussed next), organizations develop and monitor other budgets, including financial budgets, cash flow budgets, and incremental budgets. These budgets are the responsibility of the finance department.

The development and monitoring of budgets is guided by the facility's policy and procedures manual and the management styles of the administrative and departmental management team. Therefore, it is extremely important for department managers to understand the facility's budgeting methods, including how administration uses budgets.

At best, a budget is a manager's best guess at the outcomes of future financial transactions. Unexpected events that influence those transactions, such as declining census, increase in interest rates, and staffing changes, create budget variances. Some budgets are specifically designed to take these fluctuations into consideration. A budget can represent virtually any projected set of circumstances. Therefore, there are many different types of budget methodologies. Common methodologies include fixed, flexible, activity-based, and zero-based budgets.

The most common type of budget is a **fixed budget.** Budget amounts are based on expected capacity. Fixed budgets do not change when expected capacity changes. For example, the HIM department would budget file folder expense on the basis of the estimated number of discharges and the historical need to replace worn folders. When the number of discharges materially increases or declines, the file folder expense will increase or decrease, thus creating a budget variance.

Flexible budgets are based on projected productivity. In this case, the HIM department would budget file folder expense at several levels of discharges. As the actual discharges become known, the budget reflects the estimate at that level of activity. Used primarily in manufacturing, this method of budgeting also is useful for projecting personnel budgets in service areas, such as nursing units, where increased activity has a direct impact on staffing and supplies.

Activity-based budgets are based on activities or projects rather than on departments. Typically used for construction projects, an activity-based budget can be useful for any project that spans multiple budget lines or departments and for projects that span more than one fiscal year. Computer system installation and implementation should be controlled using an activity-based budget.

Different budget methodologies are developed to meet the needs of the organization. Fixed and flexible budgets are characteristic of operating budgets. Activity-based budgets are more often used for capital projects. All three types of budgets can be used by virtually any organization. **Zero-based budgets,** on the other hand, apply to organizations for which each budget cycle poses the opportunity to continue or discontinue services based on the availability of resources. Every department or activity must be justified and prioritized annually in order to effectively allocate the organization's resources. Professional associations and charitable foundations, for example, routinely use zero-based budgeting.

Operational Budgets

The purpose of an **operational budget** is to allocate and control resources in a manner consistent with the organization's goals and objectives. These goals and objectives are tied to the organization's mission. Each department also should have its own mission, goals, and objectives that identify how it contributes to the organization's overall mission. Every item in the operational budget should have a direct relationship to a departmental goal that supports an organizational goal.

The budget process begins with the board of directors/trustees, who approve the fiscal assumptions for the upcoming year. Those assumptions are quantified and communicated to the department managers, who develop budgets based on those assumptions. Typical assumptions include the desired growth in revenue and/or target cost reductions.

Budget Cycle

The operational **budget cycle** generally coincides with one fiscal year. The purpose of the operational budget is the quantification of the projected results of operations for the coming fiscal year. This process begins three to four months before the end of the current fiscal year. Projected budgets should be collected, compiled, reviewed, and approved prior to the start of the new fiscal year.

Fiscal Period

An organization's budget year coincides with its fiscal year on file with the IRS. Although the actual operational budget generally only applies to one fiscal year, financial managers often project multiple years of budgets with a variety of scenarios in order to test the financial impact of current decision making.

Interim Periods

In a computerized environment, it is relatively easy to generate financial reports as frequently as needed by management. However, monthly budget reporting is most common. Any period that represents less than an entire fiscal year is an **interim period.** Figure 26.12 provides a sample budget report for an HIM department for May. The budgeted amounts for each item are listed next to the actual amounts for the month. As is common, the year-to-date (in this case, January through May) budget and actual amounts also are included. It is very useful for budget reports to show the differences between budgeted and actual amounts. Such differences are called variances. Many budget reports also show the percentage variance for each item, based on the budget. Managers may be required to explain variances that exceed a particular dollar value or a specified percentage.

In the budget report shown in figure 26.12, there is a large variance in May's budgeted expense for printer paper. By following that line item across to the year-to-date amount, it is evident that there is no year-to-date variance in the budget. This illustrates a timing difference between the expected expense and the actual expense. The budget may have placed that expense in April, even though the actual expense occurred in May. These types of temporary variances are the result of normal business activities, and although they may require explanation, they are usually not of concern.

Budget Components

The components of an operational budget generally follow the format of the income statement and list revenue items and expense items. Every department is different, depending on its unique activities. However, budget reports tend to be uniform throughout the organization. Therefore, line items that do not apply to a particular department are likely to be listed with zero values rather than be omitted.

Revenues

In the HIM department, there is little, if any, revenue. Occasionally, a facility with excess capacity will contract out transcription services. Copy fees are another potential source of revenue; however, because such fees are cost based, they are probably more appropriately considered a reimbursement (reduction of expenses).

Expenses

The HIM department budget consists primarily of expenses. Expenses may be incurred as a result of financial transactions outside or within the organization. Some departments, such as housekeeping and facilities maintenance, perform services for other facility departments. Therefore, charges from these departments may appear on the budget. Such charges are generally carried forward through the budget allocation process and usually are not estimated by individual managers.

Figure 26.12.   HIM department budget report for May

Description	May Budget	May Actual	May Variance	YTD Budget	YTD Actual	YTD Variance
Payroll	$25,000	$22,345	$2,655	$125,000	$110,321	$14,679
Fringe benefits	$8,000	$7,360	$640	$40,000	$37,870	$2,130
Contract services	$5,000	$8,000	($3,000)	$25,000	$40,000	($15,000)
Office supplies	$150	$145	$5	$750	$975	($225)
Printer paper	$100	$250	($150)	$500	$500	—
Postage	$95	$97	($2)	$475	$456	$19
Travel	$0	$0	—	$0	$0	—
Continuing education	$0	$0	—	$0	$45	($45)

Ordinarily, the single largest expense in a healthcare facility is payroll. This is typical for service organizations. Payroll can be a difficult expense to project because employees have different anniversary dates and different salary increases.

The cost of employee benefits is part of payroll but is often listed separately. Facilities rarely expect department managers to calculate benefits budgets because this is a human resources–controlled line item. The cost of benefits tracks with payroll.

The next largest expense account is often supplies. Clinical supplies are a substantial item on the cardiology or radiology department budget, whereas office supplies might be a large item for health information management.

Cost of goods sold is a manufacturing concept that refers to the underlying cost of making the finished goods. This concept applies to healthcare providers in the sense that there is a cost basis for providing services. For every inpatient treated, there are payroll, utility, office supplies, pharmaceutical, and equipment costs that the facility incurred. Unlike manufacturing, in which the cost of producing items is tracked very closely, healthcare facilities historically have not been good at tracking the underlying costs of providing services to individual patients. The costs of providing care are often analyzed in the aggregate.

Management of the Operating Budget

When the operating budget has been developed and approved, it is the responsibility of the department management to ensure that the budget goals are met. As a general rule, in meeting goals, revenue should meet or exceed budget and expenses should meet or be less than budget. However, because expenses support revenues, an increase in revenues (perhaps due to unexpected volume) may signal an expected increase in expenses, such as variable expenses. This is particularly true when the patient census exceeds expectations. Despite the logical and expected nature of these results, managers are required to investigate and explain differences between budgeted and actual amounts on a regular basis.

Identification of Variances

A variance is the arithmetic difference between the budgeted amount and the actual amount of a line item. **Variance analy-**sis places accountability for financial transactions on the manager of the department that initiated the transaction.

Variances are often calculated on the monthly budget report. The organization's policies and procedures manual defines unacceptable variances or variances that must be explained. In identifying variances, it is important to recognize whether the variance is favorable or unfavorable and whether it is temporary or permanent.

Timing
The problems identified by variance analysis and the action that must be taken depend largely on whether the variance is temporary or permanent. Temporary variances are generally self-limiting.

Temporary budget variances are not expected to continue in subsequent months. For example, a department may budget for a large purchase of file folders in May. When that purchase does not actually take place until July, there will be a temporary variance in the May and July monthly report and a temporary variance in the May and June year-to-date numbers. Figure 26.13 illustrates this point. In this example, the HIM department budgeted $260 per month for department supplies, plus an additional $9,750 in May for file folders. Because of an unexpectedly low census, the file folders were not needed until July. This created a temporary, favorable variance in expenditures in May and June.

In contrast, **permanent budget variances** do not resolve during the current fiscal year. In the preceding example, a variance still would have existed at the end of December (the close of the fiscal year) if the file folders had been budgeted in November. The department supplies variance then would be a permanent variance during the current fiscal year and would be budgeted as an expenditure for the following year in January.

Impact
In addition to identifying whether timing is an issue, the variance analysis is expected to identify whether the variance is favorable of unfavorable. This is often obvious from the budget report but should be stated clearly when discussing the variance.

Figure 26.13. Examples of budget variances

May Budget Report						
	May Budget	**May Actual**	**May Variance**	**YTD Budget**	**YTD Actual**	**YTD Variance**
Department supplies	10,000	250	9,750	11,000	1,250	9,750

June Budget Report						
	June Budget	**June Actual**	**June Variance**	**YTD Budget**	**YTD Actual**	**YTD Variance**
Department supplies	250	250	0	11,250	1,500	9,750

July Budget Report						
	July Budget	**July Actual**	**July Variance**	**YTD Budget**	**YTD Actual**	**YTD Variance**
Department supplies	250	10,000	−9,750	11,500	11,500	0

Favorable variances occur when the actual results are better than budget projections. Actual revenue in excess of budget is a favorable variance. **Unfavorable variances** occur when the actual results are worse than what was budgeted. Actual expenditure in excess of budget is an unfavorable variance. Note that the terms *favorable* and *unfavorable* refer to the impact on the organization rather than to the magnitude or direction of the variance. Sometimes the terms *negative* and *positive* are used instead. This can be confusing because a negative expense variance is favorable. Therefore, it is extremely important to ensure that the manager understands and correctly uses the language of the organization.

Explanation of Variances

The analysis of budget variances is a financial management control. Administration may review the monthly budget report first and then ask questions of the appropriate manager. In other instances, the department managers are automatically required to respond to certain variances.

In general, the reason for a temporary budget variance is the timing of the transaction. Looking back to the department supplies/file folder example in figure 26.13, there is a very simple explanation for the temporary variance. In wording the explanation to administration, the department manager should state:

- The nature of the variance (favorable or unfavorable, temporary or permanent)
- The exact amount of the variance
- The cause of the variance
- Any ameliorating circumstances or offsetting amounts

Amount

In the analysis of variance, materiality is an issue. Rarely will a manager be required to explain a $5 variance. Clearly, the cost of a manager's time to explain such an insignificant amount far exceeds the benefit of knowing why the variance has occurred. In fact, because budgets are largely estimates, it would be quite odd if the actual amounts always matched the budgeted amounts. Therefore, dollar and/or percentage limits are set in the organization's policies and procedures manual. Variances that exceed these limits must be explained in detail.

Cause

For the folder example, the explanation might be something like the following: "In department supplies, the favorable, temporary variance of $9,750 will resolve in July when the budgeted expenditure for file folders is processed." For such a temporary variance, no additional explanation is necessary; however, the administration may prefer more detail. In that case, the relationship between low census and the need for file folders could be added to the explanation.

Temporary variances are not typically of serious concern to administrations. However, permanent variances can be a problem because management of departmental budgets

is an important indicator of the competence of department managers.

Whether a variance is temporary or permanent depends on the answers to two questions:

- Are the subsequent transactions that will balance the variance likely to occur within the same fiscal year?
- Is it reasonably certain the transactions will occur as predicted?

If the balancing transactions are unlikely to take place during the current fiscal year, the result is a permanent variance in the current budget report. Sometimes the manager may not know when—or if—the transactions will actually take place. For example, the manager may have budgeted $2,000 for attendance at an unspecified CE conference in June. A conflict with the JCAHO survey prevented the manager from attending the conference, creating a favorable expense variance. As long as the manager believes the amount will be spent appropriately at some time during the fiscal year, the variance is temporary. For example, the manager may be able to attend a conference later in the year. However, if the manager knows that there is no chance of attending a conference and appropriately spending the budgeted amount, the variance should be explained as permanent.

Additional explanation is probably necessary for a permanent variance. An expenditure that must be deferred until the next fiscal year is particularly important. In that case, the explanation might be as follows: "In department supplies, there is a favorable, permanent variance of $9,750. Because of an unexpectedly low census, the purchase of additional file folders for discharged patient records was not necessary this year. This amount is included in next year's budget."

Circumstances

Managers may have the opportunity to utilize favorable variances in one line item to offset unfavorable variances in another line item. For example, unused travel budget may be used for CE. The explanation of these circumstances will generally be carried forward through all remaining variance analyses for the remainder of the fiscal year.

The ability to work with the departmental budget as a whole as opposed to justifying line items is entirely dependent on the administration of the budget process. One typical example of offsetting variances occurs when an employee leaves and cannot be replaced immediately. Several things may happen. The vacancy may cause a favorable variance in payroll expense until the position is filled or an unfavorable variance in payroll expense if other employees are paid overtime to help fill the vacancy. Both these variances may be permanent. Finally, the vacancy may cause a favorable variance in payroll expense and an unfavorable variance in consulting expenses when the vacant position is outsourced. In the latter case, the two variances at least partially offset each other, which must be explained in the monthly variance report.

Capital Budget

Unlike the operational budget, which looks primarily at projected income statement activity for the next fiscal year, the capital budget looks at long-term investments. Such investments are usually related to improvements in the facility infrastructure, expansion of services, or replacement of existing assets. Capital investments focus on either the appropriateness of an investment (given the facility's investment guidelines) or choosing among different opportunities to invest. The capital budget is the facility's plan for allocating resources over and above the operating budget.

Funding for the capital budget may come from diverse sources. For example, donations or grants may fund a building project or **retained earnings** or **unallocated reserves** may fund equipment purchases. Federal and state government funds may be available to offset the cost of capital investments. Regardless of the source of the funds, capital investments are defined by facility policy and selected using financial analysis techniques.

Large-Dollar Purchases

From a departmental perspective, capital budget items are large-dollar purchases, as defined by facility budget policies and procedures. Capital budget items usually have a useful life in excess of one fiscal year, making them long-term assets, and a dollar value in excess of a predetermined amount, often $500 or $1,000. The most common HIM department capital budget items include shelving, office furniture, photocopying equipment, and computer equipment. Computer software, and even some computer hardware, has a limited useful life and is often included in the operating budget. Some organizations maintain a separate capital budget and process for computer-related equipment and software. In addition, in such cases, control over the acquisition of the related long-term assets may rest with the information technology or information systems department.

Acquisitions

The acquisition of long-term assets may be controlled by the purchasing department. The purchasing department may already have a contract with a specific vendor to provide certain types of equipment or furniture. In the absence of an existing contract, it may still be the purchasing department's responsibility to ensure the appropriate acquisition of assets through the **request for proposal** (RFP) process. The RFP process is a preventive control designed to eliminate bias and to ensure competitive pricing in the acquisition of goods and services.

Cost-Benefit Analysis

An old photocopying machine breaks down at least once a week. Repair of the machine takes up to two days and is increasingly expensive. During the downtime, ROI clerks must use a machine located two floors below the HIM department and shared by three other departments. It seems obvious to HIM department personnel that a new machine is needed. Including a new machine in the HIM department's capital budget request is certainly warranted. However, funding for a new machine is based on specific, detailed **cost justifications** and is weighed in comparison to all departments' requests. Facility administration may be forced to choose between a new copier for the HIM department and several new computers for the patient accounts department. All other factors being equal, increased efficiency and productivity in claims processing is likely to be chosen over increased efficiency in release of information.

Depreciation

As discussed earlier, certain long-term assets, such as equipment and furniture, wear out over time and must be replaced. Such assets contribute to revenue over multiple fiscal periods. Therefore, the cost of these assets is not booked as an expense at the time of purchase. Rather, the current asset, cash, is exchanged for a long-term asset, equipment. A portion of the historical cost of equipment then is moved from asset into expense each fiscal year and cumulated into the contra-account: accumulated depreciation. Eventually, the cost of equipment has been expensed and equipment is zero. The purpose of depreciation is to spread the cost of an asset over its useful life. (See tables 26.6 [p. 764] and 26.7 [p. 765].)

Note that the depreciation of long-term assets does not have a direct relationship to the activity of actually using the asset. It is not unusual to depreciate an asset over five years and then continue to use it for another five. For example, a facility whose equipment is fully depreciated and whose current assets are heavily financed with debt obligations may be unable to reinvest in new equipment. Thus, the capital budget is critical for the facility's continuing operations.

Capital Projects

A facility's ability to invest in capital projects is very important to the continued success of its operations. Because buildings deteriorate, equipment wears out, and new technology is important to healthcare delivery, capital improvements must be implemented. Individual departments request equipment purchases and facility improvements as the needs arise. Facility administration must choose among the suggested projects to optimize use of its resources.

In addition to capital improvements, facilities may make capital investments that improve operational efficiency. Some of these capital investments require broader analysis than the cost of the equipment. Replacing a manual incomplete tracking system, for example, with a computer-based system involves an analysis of employee time and departmental space allocations as well as the associated equipment and software costs.

Facility administration looks at capital projects differently than it reviews operational activities. Theoretically, operational activities contribute to the generation of revenue for the facility. For example, all hospital activities either provide healthcare services or in some way support departments that provide healthcare services. A hospital may elect to perform its own printing rather than outsource the printing function; however, it is unlikely to provide printing services to the general public. Printing forms supports clinical and administrative services internally; running a printing business does not. Therefore, the justification for operational budget amounts generally rests on the extent to which the underlying activities support the mission of the facility at the projected productivity levels.

Finally, budgeted capital funds generally must be expended in the time period for which they were approved. Even when allocated, capital budget items may be prioritized and timed so that purchases are made only with administrative approval. This is often the case when actual funding does not meet anticipated levels or when unforeseen circumstances change administrative priorities.

For capital budgets, supporting the mission of the facility is not sufficient justification. Capital projects also must satisfy predetermined levels of return on the projected investment.

Cost Justification

All departments in a facility compete for finite facility resources. Therefore, department managers must be famil-

iar with cost justification techniques and with their facility's method of analyzing capital projects. Typical cost justifications are based on increased revenue, increased efficiency, improved customer service, and reduced costs. The analysis of a capital project is based on the estimated ROI, including the weight of costs versus the benefits to be derived from the project. The specific cost-benefit analysis method used by facility administration depends on the characteristics of the project as well as the preferences of the analyst. When no specific cash inflows are expected, return may be based on depreciation or other cost savings. Sometimes the capital budget includes the allocation of resources for assets whose acquisition will attract or retain valuable personnel or physician relationships. Even in such cases, the acquisition should be analyzed financially, not just politically.

Payback Period

The **payback period** is the time required to recoup the cost of an investment. Mortgage refinancing analysis frequently uses the concept of payback period. Mortgage refinancing is considered when interest rates have dropped. Refinancing may require up-front interest payments, called points, as well as a variety of administrative costs. The payback period is the

Table 26.6. Sample depreciation methods

Straight Line	The cost of the asset is expensed equally over the expected life of the asset. The estimated sale value of the asset at the end of its useful life is called the residual value and is subtracted from the cost prior to depreciation.	$\dfrac{\text{Cost} - \text{residual value}}{\text{\# of years (useful life)}}$
	Example: Copy machine purchased at a cost of $5,000 Useful life = 4 years Residual value = $200 Annual depreciation = $\dfrac{\$5,000 - \$200}{4}$ = $1,200 per year	
Units of Production	The cost of the asset is expensed over the expected life of the asset, measured in usage. In this case, usage would a number of copies.	$\dfrac{\text{Cost} - \text{residual value}}{\text{\# of copies (useful life)}}$
	Example: Copy machine purchased at a cost of $5,000 Useful life = 100,000 copies Residual value = $200 Depreciation rate = $\dfrac{\$5,000 - \$200}{100,000}$ = $0.048 (4.8 cents) per copy Annual depreciation = $0.048 times the number of copies actually made	
Accelerated	There are several accelerated depreciation methods, all of which are designed to expense more of the asset's value early in its useful life. One such method is called double declining balance (DDB). DDB expenses the asset at double the straight-line method, based on the book value rather than on the historical cost.	Book value times twice the straight line rate Straight line rate = $\dfrac{\text{annual depreciation}}{\text{cost} - \text{residual value}}$
	Example: Copy machine purchased at a cost of $5,000 Useful life = 100,000 copies Residual value = $200 Straight line rate = $1,200/$4,800 = 25% Annual depreciation = Book value times 50%	

Note: These examples of depreciation methods are just a few of the acceptable methods in use today for various purposes. The reader should be aware that there are other methods and that not all methods are acceptable for income tax purposes or for GAAP. Accounting for income taxes is beyond the scope of this discussion.

time it takes for the savings in interest to equal the cost of the refinancing.

The advantage of using a payback period to analyze investments is that it is relatively easy to calculate and understand. For example, a payback period can be used to describe the time it takes for the savings in payroll costs to equal the cost of productivity-enhancing equipment. In the previous photocopy machine example, the payroll costs would be calculated based on downtime incurred when using a copier in another area of the building.

The disadvantage of a payback period is that it ignores the time value of money. Because the funds used for one capital investment could have been invested elsewhere, there is always an inherent opportunity cost of choosing one investment over another. Hence, there is an assumed rate of return against which investments are compared and a benchmark

rate of return under which a facility will not consider an investment.

Accounting Rate of Return

Another simple method of capital project analysis is the **accounting rate of return.** This method compares the projected annual cash inflows, minus any applicable annual depreciation, divided by the initial investment. Consider the purchase of a CT scanner. Reimbursement from use of the machine is the cash inflow. Depreciation is easily calculated, based on the initial investment.

Accounting rate of return is another example of a simple method of capital project analysis. However, it also ignores the time value of money. In addition, accounting rate of return is based on an estimate. If the analyst incorrectly projects annual cash inflows, the projected rate of return will be incorrect.

Table 26.7. Sample depreciation schedule

Copy machine purchased at a cost of $5,000
Useful life = 100,000 copies
Residual value = $200

Straight Line-Depreciation (25% of Cost minus Residual Value annually)

	Book Value at Beginning of Year	Depreciation	Accumulated Depreciation	Book Value at End of Year
Year 1	$5,000	$1,200	$1,200	$3,800
Year 2	3,800	1,200	2,400	2,600
Year 3	2,600	1,200	3,600	1,400
Year 4	1,400	1,200	4,800	200
Year 5	200			

Units of Production (4.8 cents per copy annually)

	Book Value at Beginning of Year	Number of Copies Used	Depreciation	Accumulated Depreciation	Book Value at End of Year
Year 1	$5,000	20,000	$960	$960	$4,040
Year 2	4,040	20,000	960	1,920	3,080
Year 3	3,080	22,000	1,056	2,976	2,024
Year 4	2,024	25,000	1,200	4,176	824
Year 5	824	25,000	624	4,800	200

Notice that in units of production the useful life is based on the number of copies used—not on the time in service. In this example, the copier does not become fully depreciated until year 5. Also, the depreciation cannot exceed the cost less the residual value; therefore, the depreciation in year 5 is only $624.

Double Declining Balance (50% of book value annually)

	Book Value at Beginning of Year	Depreciation	Accumulated Depreciation	Book Value at End of Year
Year 1	$5,000	$2,500	$2,500	$2,500
Year 2	2,500	1,250	3,750	1,250
Year 3	1,250	625	4,375	625
Year 4	625	425	4,800	200
Year 5	200			

Notice that in DDB, the final depreciation entry in year 4 reduces the book value to the residual value (50% of $625 is really $375.50, but we added $49.50 to make the depreciation 425 so that book value drops to $200 at the end of year 4).

Return on Investment

ROI is most frequently used to analyze marketable securities retrospectively. The increase in market value of the securities divided by the initial investment is the ROI. When an income stream is associated with the investment, the income stream is added to the market value of the securities in calculating return. In comparing the ROI among different securities, the tax implications must be considered. Long-term gains are taxed differently than short-term gains. Tax-exempt investments result in different returns than taxable investments.

With respect to capital investments, the equation is similar. Divide the controllable operating profits by the controllable net investment. Operating profits are the cash inflow minus the direct costs of operation.

As with accounting rate of return and payback period, ROI is easy to calculate and understand. Similarly, it does not consider the time value of money.

Net Present Value

To take into consideration the time value of money, the analyst must establish an interest rate at which money could have otherwise been invested. From that implied interest rate and the projected future cash inflows of the investment, the present value of the cash inflows is calculated. Present value is the current dollar amount that must be invested today in order to yield the projected future cash inflows at the implied interest rate. **Net present value** is the calculated present value of the future cash inflows compared to the initial investment.

The advantage of using net present value to analyze investments is that it considers the time value of money. When choosing among like investments, net present values can be reliably compared to determine the financial advantages of the investment.

As with other analysis tools, analysts may have to estimate the projected cash flows. However, the main disadvantage of net present value is that the interest rate is subjective. Therefore, it is best used to compare multiple investment opportunities rather than to analyze one investment alone. Another disadvantage of using net present value is that it requires some knowledge of mathematics to accept its validity and understand its relevance. Fortunately, financial calculators and computer programs have made the calculation of net present value relatively simple.

Internal Rate of Return

Internal rate of return (IRR) is the interest rate that makes the net present value calculation equal zero. In other words, it is the interest rate at which the present value of the projected cash inflows equals the initial investment. IRR considers the time value of money. Both individual and multiple investments can be evaluated. As with net present value, a knowledge of mathematics is helpful. The main disadvantage is that a project may have multiple IRRs.

Profitability Index

Facilities cannot automatically invest in seemingly profitable projects. For example, a $500,000 radiology equipment investment may have a present value of cash inflows of $1,500,000, for a net present value of $1,000,000. At the same time, a $10,000 pharmacy computer system yields a net present value of $30,000. This seems to be a great investment; however, the facility's capital budget may be limited to $100,000. In this case, a **profitability index** helps the organization prioritize investment opportunities. For each investment, divide the present value of the cash inflows by the present value of the cash outflows. In this example, the pharmacy system has a higher profitability index, as illustrated below:

Radiology		Pharmacy
$1,500,000	Present value of cash inflows	$40,000
$500,000	Present value of cash outflows	$10,000
3	Profitability index	4

Check Your Understanding 26.3

Instructions: Answer the following questions on a separate piece of paper.

1. Compare and contrast financial accounting and managerial accounting.

2. Compare and contrast operational budgets and capital budgets.

3. A not-for-profit organization offers a variety of programs and services. Each functional department in the organization plays some role in delivering all these programs and services. What type of operational budget would be most effective in this environment? Why?

4. Why would an organization choose a fiscal year that does not coincide with the calendar year?

5. The HIM department has a YTD budget for a payroll of $100,000. The actual YTD amount is $98,000. Is this a favorable or an unfavorable variance?

Real-World Case

Bright Hospital is a 270-bed, not-for-profit community hospital. Its largest percentage of patients consists of mothers and newborns, followed by a mix of cardiovascular-related admissions. It has an emergency department staffed by hospital employees. Bright's fiscal year follows the calendar year, ending December 31. In August, Bright began its year-end budget process by establishing its financial assumptions for the following two years. Bright assumed that revenue would remain constant, that it would continue its existing contracts with payers, that its Medicare population percentage would not change, and that no major infrastructure maintenance would be required in the upcoming fiscal year. No major capital projects were anticipated. In its operational budget, administration plans to include resources for a JCAHO steering committee and related activities to prepare for the anticipated accreditation visit in the subsequent year. Administration distributed operational and capital budget compilation packages to department managers for completion and return by September 30.

Bright Hospital does not have a large marketing department. It has one marketing professional on staff whose responsibilities include the development and publishing of brochures and coordination of patient satisfaction surveys, which are compiled and analyzed by an outside vendor. In the past two years, there has been a slight, but continuing, decline in patient satisfaction among maternity patients. Suggestions for improvement have varied, but common complaints center on the lack of soothing ambiance in labor and delivery and the hospital policy prohibiting overnight visitors.

The maternity and newborn departments have been very concerned about declining patient satisfaction. They are worried that the current year's slight decline in maternity admissions is the result of that dissatisfaction and that patients are traveling a little further to give birth at a neighboring medical center, at which some of their physicians also have privileges. The departments would like to renovate the maternity and newborn wing, forming a women's center with increased emphasis on wellness and ancillary services. This would be a two-year capital project that would require marketing support and some minor disruption of services during construction.

The cardiology department is very excited. It has just learned that a well-respected cardiologist has retired to the area and is exploring the idea of opening a small consulting practice. The cardiologist has not yet applied for privileges at any area hospitals, but it is known that she is used to working in a facility with its own cardiac catheterization lab. Because the current chief of the medical staff at Bright is a personal friend of the cardiologist, the cardiology department believes that she could be lured on staff if the hospital had its own lab. Based on the volume of patients that Bright currently sends out to another facility for cardiac catheterization, the cardiology department believes that patient care would be facilitated by the expansion and that the increased revenue would help justify the cost.

The HIM department has recently lost several employees to retirement and promotions within the facility. It is currently down two coders and a file clerk, and has reduced its weekend coverage to one person, day shift only. Transcription is handled largely by the department, with an outside service processing any overflow. The HIM department would like to outsource all of its transcription and move to a Web-based coding system that would allow the coders to telecommute. This plan would improve productivity, decrease transcription and coding delays, and shorten billing time. In addition, the computer-based storage of documents involved in these changes would facilitate release of information. All three departments submitted capital budget requests for the projects described.

Summary

Management roles in any healthcare facility require some knowledge of accounting and financial management. The ability to read, understand, and interpret pertinent financial reports is a desirable business skill. Because of the close ties between reimbursement and HIM, this basic skill is even more important. Although the financial accounting methodologies of compiling and analyzing financial statements may not be needed routinely, the managerial accounting skills involving budget preparation and analysis are critical. Also important is an awareness of the preventive, detective, and corrective controls that managers must implement to ensure the accuracy of financial data.

Operational budgets are developed annually to allocate resources for the normal functioning of the facility, according to its mission. Operational budgets focus on revenues and expenses. Capital budgets separately identify and analyze long-term asset acquisitions that are designed to maintain and improve the facility's infrastructure, improve operational efficiency, or expand business, for example. Capital budget requests are analyzed for their cost versus benefit as well as return on investment.

Efficient claims processing has a direct impact on the ability of a facility to fund its operations, including paying its bills and meeting payroll obligations. HIM plays a direct role in ensuring efficient claims processing by participating in charge description master review, participating in the analysis and minimization of the AR totals, and ensuring efficient and accurate coding of records.

References

Cleverley, W., and A. Cameron. 2003. *Essentials of Health Care Finance*, 5th ed. Sudbury, MA: Jones and Bartlett.

Dunn, R. 1999. *Finance Principles for the Health Information Manager.* Chicago: AHIMA.

Schraffenberger, L.A., ed. 2005. *Effective Management of Coding Services*, 2nd ed. Chicago: AHIMA.

Chapter 27
Project Management

Patricia B. Seidl, RHIA, CCDM

Learning Objectives

- To understand how a project differs from an organization's daily operations
- To describe the components of a project
- To discuss reasons for project success versus project failure
- To describe different project team structures
- To understand the responsibilities of the project manager
- To understand the project management process and to recognize the technical and people skills involved
- To identify the components of a project proposal document
- To understand the steps in planning and organizing a project
- To estimate work, duration, and resource requirements
- To understand how to anticipate and manage project risk
- To understand how to track a project's progress and analyze variances
- To describe the types of plan revision
- To understand the concept of scope management
- To recognize the components of a communication plan

Key Terms

Assumptions
Baseline
Change control
Contingency
Critical path
Dependency
Duration
Issue log
Predecessor
Project charter
Project components
Project definition
Project deliverables
Project management life cycle
Project management software
Project network
Project office
Project plan
Project schedule
Project scope
Project team
Resources
Risk
Roles and responsibilities
Scheduling engine
Scope creep
Sponsor
Stakeholders
Statement of work
Subprojects
Successor
Task
Variances
Work
Work breakdown structure
Work products

Introduction

Although health information management professionals practice in many diverse healthcare delivery systems and domains, there is a common responsibility across all lines of business: leading or participating in projects. It is important to understand the concepts and best practices of project management in order to engage fully and effectively as a project team member. Although there are many different types, all projects have similar attributes: Their objectives are of benefit to the organization, they all follow the project management process, the same characteristics of the project manager are needed, they all involve a project team, and they all result in some type of outcome.

Projects consist of organizational and behavioral components. Organizational or structural components guide the team toward its end goals. Behavioral components include the concepts of leading, motivating, politics, and interpersonal communication.

This chapter describes the different elements of a project and the different types of projects that healthcare organizations might undertake. It also focuses on how projects are managed and tracked to ensure their success.

Theory into Practice

A healthcare facility is due for a Joint Commission on Accreditation of Healthcare Organizations (JCAHO) survey later this year. The facility has strived to make compliance with JCAHO standards part of its normal operational processes and has decided to perform an assessment to ensure that any new or revised standards have been incorporated into its practices.

The facility first forms a multidisciplinary team and assigns a project manager. The project manager spearheads, and the team contributes to, preparing a plan that details the **tasks** that need to be accomplished. Team members are assigned tasks and decide to meet every two weeks to discuss their progress.

The team then begins the assessment. Each department conducts a review of the JCAHO standards, comparing them to the department's policies and procedures to ensure that all the standards are being met. The departments pay special attention to new standards to ensure that they are interpreting the standards correctly. When necessary, team members seek out colleagues who have recently undergone a survey to answer questions on the standards. When a deficiency is found, it is logged and assigned to the appropriate department personnel for resolution and given a resolution due date.

After all the deficiencies have been documented, the team monitors the list and updates it regularly with the progress of the policy and procedure revisions. If the policy and procedure revisions are not occurring in a timely manner, the project manager needs to refer the issue to the project's sponsor.

After all the deficiencies have been addressed through updated policies and procedures, each department conducts employee educational sessions to incorporate the revisions into its daily operations.

Finally, the facility conducts a mock survey. It also prepares and executes a training program for the entire institution so that all employees know what to expect when the JCAHO surveyors arrive.

As the JCAHO survey date draws near, each team member prepares a list of items that the surveyors may request. This will help the facility to respond quickly to the requests during the actual survey.

After the JCAHO survey has been conducted and the results received by the facility, the team's final responsibility is to follow up on the survey recommendations.

The Project

An organization undertakes a project because it has determined the need for some type of change. This need may be the result of a company's strategic agenda, such as implementation of a new computer system, or it may be in response to passage of a new government regulation. After the need for the project has been acknowledged, the project enters the project management life cycle or process.

Every project has an identified sponsor. The **sponsor** is the facility employee with the most vested interest in the project's success. It is a good practice to select someone who has responsibility for the organization's departments, divisions, and personnel that will be affected by the project. The project will open up many issues that, in some situations, must be resolved by an authority figure. It is much easier to obtain a decision or consensus when the sponsor already has established control over the areas involved in the project. The sponsor often approves the budget for the project and is ultimately responsible for the project expenditures.

The project also has **stakeholders.** A stakeholder is anyone in the organization who is affected by the project product. Stakeholders include personnel who are on the project team, personnel whose daily work will be changed because of the project's product, and the managers and executives for those departments involved in the project. Each stakeholder has different concerns relative to the project's objectives and goals. The **project team** wants to produce a high-quality product. Departmental personnel worry about their ability to adapt to the procedures and skills required by the new or changed product. Department managers and executives must support the functional changes that may be needed as a result of the project. Each stakeholder will evaluate the project's success based on these concerns and the expectations they hold for how the project will benefit them.

Definition of a Project

A Guide to the Project Management Body of Knowledge (PMBOK Guide) describes a project as "a temporary endeavor undertaken to create a unique product or service"

(Project Management Institute 2004, p. 5). A project has the following characteristics:

- Specific objectives or goals to be achieved
- A defined start and end date
- A defined set of resources assigned to perform the required work
- Specific deliverables or work products
- A defined budget or cost

A project differs from the day-to-day operations of an organization. Operations are concerned with the everyday jobs needed to run the business. The personnel involved in the operational aspects of the business perform the same functions on a routine basis. This work does not end. In contrast, a project has a precise, expected result produced by defined **resources** within a specific time frame.

Project Parameters

A well-defined project has specific objectives. After the project's objectives have been defined, all project activities should be focused on meeting them. The project activities result in project deliverables or **work products.** When the project activities have concluded and the project deliverables have been completed, the project ends.

The process of documenting project parameters is discussed later in this chapter.

Project Components

Lewis writes that a project's objectives include cost, performance, time, and scope. Cost is the project budget, performance relates to the quality of the project work, time is the schedule, and **project scope** is the magnitude of the work to be done. He illustrates the relationship with the expression "Cost is a function of Performance, Time, and Scope." Should the cost, performance, or schedule variable change, the relationship dictates that the scope will change (Lewis 1998, pp. 61–62). The project manager and the sponsor must acknowledge this relationship and be willing to make the trade-offs that will be needed when the variables change.

When developing the **project plan,** the project manager translates the objectives into three **project components:** scope, resources, and schedule. These components have a strong dependency. Again, if one of the three changes, one of the other two parameters must change as well. This is often illustrated as a triangle. (See figure 27.1.)

Project resources are not just people. A resource is any physical asset needed to complete a task. This includes facilities, equipment, materials, and supplies. Resources also can include individuals from outside organizations, such as suppliers or vendors.

One reason why many projects fail to meet their objectives within the expected time frame and budget is that their scope begins to grow as they progress. For example, new functions or features are added to a software implementation. This is commonly known as **scope creep.** The requestor

Figure 27.1.   Illustration of project components

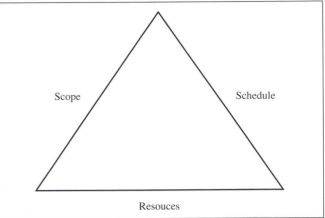

presents each change as a small revision with low impact on time line or cost. However, several minor changes soon add up to a more significant modification to the original work or cost estimate. The project manager must be diligent to prevent scope creep. (This topic is discussed in detail later in this chapter.)

Project Assumptions

Assumptions are scope-limiting parameters. They provide constraints on what is and is not included in the project. For example, if the project is to implement a lab results-reporting system on the clinical units, one of the assumptions may be that the clinical personnel will look up results online, therefore, printers are not included in the project budget.

Assumptions define answers to unknown questions. For instance, at the beginning of the project, the project manager may not know what personnel will be assigned to the project and thus will not know the skill set that will be available. One assumption might be that a project team member from a particular department on a cross-departmental project is a decision maker. In other words, when the project team meets to design the user interface for a software implementation, the decisions can be made in that meeting and will not be deferred to a person outside the team. If this assumption does not prove to be true, the project manager is faced with a potential delay because the process required for decision making was not accounted for in the **project schedule.**

Assumptions directly affect the project estimates for the resource and time line requirements. Therefore, it is critical that the project manager obtain agreement from the sponsor and the stakeholders on all assumptions. A lack of buy-in by all the project participants puts the objectives at **risk.** Many projects immediately start down the path of failure because the assumptions were not addressed adequately at the project start.

Types of Projects

There are many different types of projects. Although they share some attributes, projects can be vastly different in several aspects. Some projects are short term and completed in the span of weeks; other projects take years to complete. One project may involve only a single department; another may require participation across the facilities in an integrated delivery system (IDS).

Following are types of projects in which health information management (HIM) professionals may be involved:

- Instituting new or revised procedures to address new regulations
- Conducting a chargemaster review
- Preparing for a JCAHO survey
- Implementing a new dictation system
- Merging two HIM departments
- Creating a new employee orientation program
- Implementing a new business procedure or process

A complex project may comprise several **subprojects.** The subprojects share common milestones and objectives but may be managed by different project managers. Subproject information may be compiled into one report to show information across all associated projects.

Project Risk versus Project Value

Projects are undertaken to specifically incorporate some requirement or business need. Although the organization certainly expects a positive outcome, there are always some risks to the organization as well. One of the project manager's responsibilities is to mitigate risk. However, the organization will need to weigh the cost of potential risks against the perceived value to be gained.

Project risk can take many forms and be of either a technical or psychological nature. For example, implementing a state-of-the-art computer system may provide leading-edge technology that sets the organization apart from its competitors. However, the availability of personnel who can provide support for new technology may be limited.

Another example would be a project that introduces a significant change to a department employee's responsibilities. However, the change positions the employee out of his or her comfort zone. Before the project begins, an employee may be considered an expert in his or her job responsibilities. At the conclusion of the project, the same employee may have new duties and will not have the same proficiency in them. This could cause self-esteem problems. It is not uncommon for employee turnover to occur during a project because of this threat to job security.

Check Your Understanding 27.1

Instructions: Answer the following questions on a separate piece of paper.

1. Why does an organization start a project?
2. What are the similar responsibilities of the project's sponsor and stakeholders? What are examples of different responsibilities?
3. How do projects and organizational processes differ?
4. What is scope creep?

Project Management

The *PMBOK Guide* defines project management as "the application of knowledge, skills, tools, and techniques to project activities to meet project requirements" (Project Management Institute 2004, p. 8). Project management is concerned with completing a project within the expected cost and time line with high-quality results. This is not easy to accomplish and, as a consequence, interest in project management best practices is very high. Many organizations are starting to stress the importance of solid project management methodologies and are establishing project offices to support the organization's project managers. A **project office** is responsible for defining project management procedures, conducting risk analyses on projects, and mentoring project managers.

Overview of Project Management

The discipline of project management has emerged as organizations have come to realize that projects cannot succeed without it. As Kliem and Ludin point out, project management has traditionally focused on project cost, schedule, and quality. They consider this to be the classical approach to project management. Their belief is that project management is now taking a more behavioral approach by viewing the project as a total system, emphasizing the project's human aspects (Kliem and Ludin 1998, p. 6).

Projects have customarily been deemed successful when they meet their objectives but do not exceed their approved cost and estimated schedule. Kliem and Ludin break down the reasons for project success and failure based on the classical or behavioral approach. These reasons are listed in table 27.1.

Lewis also proposes a different definition of project success. He challenges the commonly held belief that a project has failed when it does not meet its cost, performance, time, or scope targets by questioning how these targets were established. The targets may have been unrealistic and thus impossible to meet. By citing several studies, Lewis concludes that it is how closely the project outcomes align with the perceptions held by the key project personnel that determines project success (Lewis 1998, pp. 39–43). As an example, if a project comes in under budget but ends up solving the wrong problem, is it successful? A project may meet the schedule but have unexpected and undesirable consequences. As Thomas K. Connellan, a speaker, trainer, consultant, and senior principal of a customer relationship management consulting firm, once said, "There is no point in doing well that which you should not be doing at all."

The Project Management Life Cycle

Every project follows a **project management life cycle** regardless of its size or duration. Each process in the life cycle has its own importance. Any one of the processes cannot be eliminated or minimized without endangering the success of the project. The project management life cycle consists of a number of processes. (See table 27.2.) Each process is discussed in more detail later in this chapter.

Table 27.1.   Reasons for project success and failure

Project Success	
Classical	**Behavioral**
Well-defined goals and objectives	Agreement on goals and objectives
Detailed work breakdown structure	Commitment to achieving goals and objectives
Clear reporting relationships	High morale
Formal change management disciplines in place	Good teaming
Channels of communication exist	Cooperation among all participants
Adherence to scope	Receptivity to positive and negative feedback
Reliable estimating	Receptive culture to project management
Reliable monitoring and tracking techniques	Realistic expectations
Clear requirements	Good conflict resolution
Reasonable time frame	Executive sponsorship
Broad distribution of work	Good customer–supplier relationship
Project Failure	
Classical	**Behavioral**
Ill-defined work breakdown structure	Inappropriate leadership style
High-level schedule	No common vision
No reporting infrastructure	Unrealistic expectations
Too pessimistic or optimistic estimates	Poor informal communications and interpersonal relationships
No change management discipline	No buy-in or commitment from customer or people doing work
Inadequate formal communications	Low morale
Inefficient allocation of resources	Lack of training
No accountability and responsibility for results	Poor teaming
Poor role definition	Culture not conducive to project management
Inadequacy of tools	Lack of trust among participants
Ill-defined scope	False or unrealistic expectations
Unclear requirements	No or weak executive sponsorship
Too high, too long, or too short time frame	Mediocre knowledge transfer

Source: Reprinted from *Project Management Practitioner's Handbook*. Copyright © 1998 Ralph L. Kleim and Irwin S. Ludin. Used with permission of the publisher, AMACOM, a division of American Management Association, New York, NY. All rights reserved. *http://www.amanet.org.*

The Project Team

By definition, a project results in an end product through the completion of task activities. The execution of these task activities is the responsibility of the project team. A project team is composed of individuals who possess the knowledge and skill set to produce the project deliverables and work products.

The type of project determines the size of the project team and the originating location of the resources. A project that affects only one department will typically have project team members from only that department. A project with organization-wide objectives will have a cross-departmental team, whereas a project for an IDS will include representatives from all the system's facilities.

There are three types of project team structure: functional, projectized, and matrixed (Project Management Institute 2004, pp. 28–32).

Functional Team Structure

In a strictly functional organization, the project is thought to affect only one department. The functional manager may assume responsibility for managing the project. The team members are primarily from the functional department, and the functional manager confers with other functional managers on any issues affecting those departments.

Projectized Team Structure

The projectized organization has dedicated resources that are involved only in project work. Team members report to the project manager not only on project assignments, but also as their direct manager.

Matrixed Team Structure

The matrixed organization maintains the functional organization. Team members report to a functional manager and

Table 27.2.   Project management life cycle

Project definition	This process will determine the project objectives, activities, assumptions, high-level cost estimate, and anticipated schedule.
Planning and organization	A detailed project plan is developed that delineates the tasks to be performed, the resources necessary for each task, and the estimated task duration, start, and finish. The project team is assembled.
Tracking and analysis	By tracking project progress and analyzing it against the original plan, the project manager is able to determine when the project is not moving forward as planned.
Project revisions	When the analysis reveals project deviations, the plan may need to be modified in order to still meet the project objectives.
Change control	This is the process of managing change requests to the original project definition.
Communication	This process occurs throughout the project life cycle. Project information is collected from, and disseminated to, all stakeholders.

remain employees of that department. The team members receive their project assignments from the project manager.

In a matrixed organization, assigning the members of the project team can pose a dilemma for the stakeholders and the project manager. Typically, the best people to have on a project team are the ones who most intimately understand the processes and procedures affected by the project. However, these people have operational responsibilities in their respective departments that do not disappear while the project is in progress. Depending on the scope of the project, the time commitment required of the project team can be quite significant.

It is important to define the **roles and responsibilities** of the project team. In a matrixed organization, the project team members do not report to the project manager in an organizational structure. However, the project manager holds team members accountable for their tasks.

Check Your Understanding 27.2

Instructions: On a separate piece of paper, prepare a grid that lists examples of the types of projects an HIM professional may be involved in. For each project list the following:

- The project objectives
- The factors that will be used to measure project success
- The factors that may contribute to project failure
- The members of the project team

The Project Manager

The project manager is the individual with responsibility for directing the project activities from initiation through closure. Depending on the size of the project, the project manager may be a dedicated resource or may be performing these duties along with other operational assignments. For example, for a project confined to a single department, an assistant director may be asked to manage the project while the department director takes on the sponsor role. In other situations, one of the team members may be asked to be the project leader while still performing specific task assignments for the project.

In circumstances where the project manager is not fully devoted to the project, it is easy for the project management duties to fall by the wayside, especially because many of these may produce intangible results. (The functions of the project manager are discussed in a subsequent section of this chapter.) The project sponsor must ensure that an adequate percentage of the resource's time is allocated to these responsibilities.

Competencies and Skills

A project manager must possess both functional and behavioral skills. Some of his or her responsibilities are purely operational, for example, preparing a project plan. However, several skills are required that touch on the human side of projects. All projects result in a change in the organization. Facilitating an organization through the impact of these changes requires attributes that are described as "soft skills."

Project managers are very often in the position of having great responsibility, but little authority, because the project team members do not report to them from an organizational perspective. Thus, project managers must get results from the team members through leadership and influence.

Project managers should possess the following skills:

- General management skills of planning, directing, organizing, and prioritizing
- Leadership skills of influencing, motivating, providing vision, and resolving conflict
- Communication skills of being able to interact with all levels of an organization and of being able to understand different communication styles and mediums
- Facilitation skills, including negotiation, consensus building, and meeting management
- Analytical skills, including innovative thinking, problem solving, and decision making

Functions

The project manager performs several functions over the course of the project management life cycle. These functions are described in table 27.3.

The Project Management Process

A project follows a defined process regardless of size, type, or industry. The process is scalable, meaning that the depth to which a particular process is performed may vary according to project length, scope, or other parameters. However, to ensure the success of the project, all these processes must be performed to some degree.

Project Definition

Project definition sets the expectation for the what, when, and how of the project. As noted under the project parameters section of this chapter, every project comprises three components: What is to be done (scope), the resources needed to accomplish the objectives, and the amount of time required to complete the project. The project definition process formally documents these variables for the project. This process is important for several reasons. First, it provides all project stakeholders, team members, and other personnel with the same information about the project—what it will accomplish, when it will be done, and what resources it will require. Second, it is then used as the basis for understanding when requested changes are out of the project's scope.

Determine Project Scope and Define Project Deliverables

The definition of the project starts with determining its goals. The project's goals or objectives should be measurable. If they are not, it will be impossible for the project manager and the stakeholders to determine whether the project is successful. (Examples of objectives are shown in table 27.4.)

Table 27.3.   Functions of the project manager

Set the project expectations.	As noted earlier, project success is tied to the perception that the project met the objectives. The project manager has responsibility for properly setting the project expectations and continually resetting them as the project progresses.
Create the project plan and recruit the project team.	The project manager generates a project schedule with the estimated work effort. The project team is organized, with each team member understanding his or her roles and responsibilities. The project manager leads team development efforts to form an effective, motivated team. He or she uses interpersonal skills to establish a rapport with team members.
Manage project control.	When the project is under way, the project manager must have a clear understanding of its status. Informal and formal communication methods are used to determine project progress. The project manager maintains the project plan to perform variance analysis. The project manager works with the project team to bring tasks to closure by facilitating decision-making and issue resolution. The project manager facilitates the removal of any obstacles that prevent the team from producing the project deliverables.
Recommend plan revisions.	If a plan is not progressing as scheduled, the project manager must determine what actions need to be taken to put the project back on track. He or she gains consensus on the changes from the sponsor and the stakeholders, and monitors any new risks to the plan.
Execute change control.	The project manager institutes a policy and procedure for managing change requests. He or she keeps everyone focused on the end goal.
Prepare, document, and communicate project information.	Project documentation is a key facet of project communication. The project manager creates the communication plan that will be used to determine when, how, and what information is to be gathered and distributed. He or she facilitates the dissemination of information throughout the organization. Although the project team members create much of the documentation through the project deliverables, the project manager is responsible for ensuring that documentation exists and is available.

The next step in defining the project is to determine the tangible end results of the project. These are typically called **project deliverables.** The project deliverables indicate when the project activities have been completed. Typical deliverables for a software implementation include:

- System requirements
- User interface design document
- Test plans
- Training and procedure manuals
- Production software

Estimate the Project Schedule and Cost

The next step in project definition is to estimate how long the project will take and how much it will cost. At this point in the process, the project may not have been approved, so this information is needed in order for the stakeholders to make an informed decision. This also poses a dilemma for the project manager. He or she may not have enough detailed information about the project to make an estimate. (A detailed analysis occurs in the project planning phase.)

In this case, the project manager has a few options. One is to evaluate a past project that is similar in scope and to extract pertinent information from it that can be used in estimating the new project. A second option is to confer with professional colleagues who have experience in the proposed project. If a similar project is unavailable for analysis, a third alternative is for the project manager to use his or her expert judgment and intuition based on other professional experiences. Another opportunity would be available if the project manager were working with a vendor. The vendor would likely have experience in these types of projects and could assist the project manager in formulating estimates.

Prepare the Project Proposal

As stated above, one of the purposes of the project definition phase is to set project expectations. The project manager now should be ready to record the project objectives, scope, deliverables, expected time line, and anticipated cost in a written document. This document is known by various names. Typical names include **project charter, statement of work,** and project definition document or business plan.

The project proposal contains several topics. The following information should be included:

- *Summary:* The summary provides an overview of the project and can provide any relevant background history and reasons why the project is being proposed.

Table 27.4.   Examples of measurable and nonmeasurable objectives

Type of Project	Nonmeasurable Objective	Measurable Objective
Implementation of a patient accounting system	Improve communication between the HIM department and the patient accounting department	Decrease discharged, not-final-billed accounts from 10 days after discharge to 3 days
Implementation of a document imaging system	Increase availability of patient records	Decrease the number of chart requests by 50%
Institute a home coding program	Improve coder satisfaction	Decrease staff turnover by 20%

- *Objectives:* The objectives state the project's goals.
- *Project activities:* This section is a high-level description of the major project tasks and maps out how the project will produce the project deliverables. These activities will be detailed during the project planning phase.
- *Assumptions:* Assumptions provide input on the estimates for the resource and time line requirements. Inclusion of the assumptions in the project definition document sets the stage for their acknowledgment and agreement. Assumptions may or may not prove to be true as the project progresses. The importance of identifying assumptions is that when one does not prove to be true, one of the project components will likely need to be altered.
- *Roles and responsibilities:* This section defines the types of resources needed on the project and delineates who does what. Its concept is not dissimilar to defining a department's organizational structure. The purpose is to ensure that everyone is aware of everyone's duties and the lines of authority. It is a good idea to include a project organization chart. The project manager usually does not have management authority over the team, so documenting the roles is crucial in order to understand how the team will function.
- *Schedule/cost:* Schedule and cost information is provided at a very high level because it will be further refined during the project planning phase. Cost estimates will include those for personnel, equipment, and supplies. If an external company will be providing some project services, this section should indicate whether the engagement is based on time and materials or fixed-fee pricing.
- *Deliverables:* The discussion of deliverables is another component of setting expectations. By documenting the tangible output from the project, everyone will understand when the project tasks are complete. This section can be specific by including the following types of information for each deliverable:
  —Type (for example, Microsoft Word)
  —Expected length or size
  —Number of copies provided
  —Mode of delivery (for example, through e-mail)

Check Your Understanding 27.3

Instructions: On a separate piece of paper, prepare a project proposal document for one of the projects you listed in Check Your Understanding 27.2. Include the project objectives, deliverables, high-level project activities, assumptions, and roles and responsibilities. What needs to be considered when estimating the project cost?

Project Planning

After a project has been approved, it moves into the planning phase. The purpose of this phase is to further refine the project work effort, time line, and cost. During the project planning phase, the project manager creates a project plan that details the tasks to be performed, the resources needed to perform each task, the estimated work effort, and the estimated start and finish dates.

The project manager may use **project management software** to aid this process. Also known as a **scheduling engine,** project management software can provide the tools to automate some of the functions the project manager must perform. However, a software tool cannot perform the behavioral roles required of the project manager. Beware of software product literature promising a successful project simply by using it!

Identify Project Activities

When a project is initiated, the project manager is faced with the question, How do we complete the project objectives and produce the project deliverables? Creating a project plan that lists each activity provides the road map to answer this question. For example, when a person decides to go on a vacation, he or she does not simply go to the airport. First, he or she has to decide where to go and how to get there and then make the appropriate reservations and so on.

A project plan starts with a **work breakdown structure** (WBS), or task list. The WBS is a hierarchical list of steps needed to complete the project. This structure provides levels that are similar to the concept of a book outline. Each level drills down to more detail. The lowest level is the task level, which is the level to which resources are assigned and work effort estimates are made.

A good place to begin in building the WBS is with the deliverables. Every deliverable should have a set of corresponding tasks to produce it. After every deliverable has been covered, the next area to address is the tasks that do not produce deliverables per se. What kind of tasks are they? One such task would be project management. Although project management tasks certainly produce plenty of documentation, the output is not a deliverable for the project itself, meaning that it does not contribute to the project objectives.

When creating the WBS, the project manager is faced with determining the level of task detail to be included. When the task level is not itemized enough, it will be difficult to assess the progress on the task. Having too much detail presents its own problems if the project manager is using project management software because he or she will spend too much time managing the project plan instead of doing the actual project. The level of detail directly correlates to the project manager's ability to control the project. He or she must determine the level of detail that provides this control.

Table 27.5 is an illustration of too much detail in a project plan. The list on the left represents steps, not tasks. The project plan should not be thought of as a to-do list. The list on the right represents a more manageable level of detail.

Construct the Project Network

When all the tasks have been defined, the next step is to determine the **dependency** among tasks. The tasks in the project plan cannot all start at the same time. For example, training on a new computer system cannot begin until the training materials have been completed and the system has been thoroughly tested.

The definition of dependencies among the project tasks is the first step in scheduling the project. The purpose of the project schedule is to provide information on when the particular tasks can begin and when they are scheduled to end. The overall **project network** is defined through these dependencies.

Figure 27.2 shows an example of a project schedule for the JCAHO project described in the theory into practice section.

There are a few types of dependencies:

- *Finish-to-start:* This means that the first, or **predecessor,** task must finish before the dependent, or **successor,** task can start. Finish-to-start is the most common type of dependency.
- *Start-to-start:* This states that the successor task cannot start until the predecessor task begins. An example of this relationship would be in a computer system conversion. The user workstation hardware for the old system cannot be swapped out with the hardware for the new system until the old system is taken off-line when the conversion process begins.

- *Finish-to-finish:* In this definition, the successor task cannot finish until the predecessor task finishes. An example of this dependency would be completing training materials when the system testing for a computer system is complete. The materials cannot be finished until the project manager is assured, via testing, that all modifications to the software have been completed.

Estimate Activity Duration and Work Effort

After the tasks have been defined, the project manager determines who will perform each task (resources), the amount of effort it will take to complete the task (work), and how long it will take to finish the task (duration). **Work** and **duration** are two different values. For example, if Emily is assigned to a task for 24 hours of work effort, how long will it take her to complete the task? It depends on how much of Emily's overall workday she devotes to this particular task. If she spends 100 percent of her day on this task and the assumption is that she is scheduled to work eight hours a day, she can complete the task in three days. If she can only dedicate 50 percent of her time to the task, she will complete the task in six days.

This calculation is shown in table 27.6 (p. 778). If multiple resources can be assigned to the task, the task duration can be reduced.

Estimating the work effort for tasks is difficult and can be time-consuming, especially if the organization does not have much experience in the type of project being performed. (Various methods for estimating work were discussed earlier in the chapter.)

It is best to get estimates from the people who will be performing the work. If the team has not been assigned, the functional manager of the area may be called on to provide this information. Either way, the project manager may still encounter unrealistic values because people tend to underestimate the effort in those instances where historical information

Table 27.5.   Illustration of steps versus tasks

Steps	Tasks
Invitations	**Invitations**
Shop for Invitations	Select and Purchase Invitations
Choose Invitation	Mail Invitations
Purchase Invitations	
Address Invitations	
Purchase Stamps	
Mail Invitations	

Figure 27.2.   Example of a project schedule

Task Name	Duration	F	S	S	M	T	W	T	F	S	S	M	T	W	T	F	S
⊟ **Readiness Assessment**	**3 days**																
Conduct assessment	1 day																
Update policies and procedures	1 day																
Conduct employee education	1 day																
⊟ **Prepare for Survey**	**3 days**																
Conduct mock survey	1 day																
Correct problem areas	1 day																
Conduct institutional training program	1 day																
Prepare list of survey requests	1 day																
⊟ **JCAHO Survey**	**2 days**																
Estimated survey date	0 days																
Review survey recommendations	1 day																
Implement plan to address recommendations	1 day																

is unavailable. Some people overcompensate in their estimate if they do have experience in projects, knowing that unforeseen circumstances can come up.

And, unfortunately, Parkinson's Law, which says that "Work expands to fill the time," complicates the estimating situation. Typically, if a resource is told that 16 hours of work effort are allocated for a task, he or she will expend all 16 hours.

The assumptions for the project also play a role in defining the estimates. For example, if an assumption is that a software engineer knowledgeable in the applicable software language will be assigned to the project, the work estimates will be lower than if the assumption is that an inexperienced resource will be assigned.

After the work effort values have been determined and the task durations calculated, the project network reflects a more realistic time frame. The project finish date is calculated based on the task dependencies and task durations. Figure 27.3 shows how the project tasks from figure 27.2 are now scheduled.

If a project manager is using project management software, the **critical path** for the project can be determined. The critical path is the series of specific tasks that determine the overall project duration.

The critical path is important for the project manager to understand because any change in the start or finish of one of the tasks on the critical path means the expected project finish date will change. Changes to the critical path can happen in a variety of ways, including:

- The duration of a task may change because the work effort or resource availability changes.
- The expected start date for the task changes because the finish date for a predecessor task changes.
- The finish date for a task changes because a resource's availability is changed. Perhaps a person schedules vacation or training for a week or his or her availability for the project changes because he or she is assigned additional duties outside the project.

The project manager also can use the critical path to determine how to shorten the overall project schedule. It is typical for the stakeholders of a project to already have a predetermined expected finish date for the project when it is

Table 27.6.   Calculation of duration based on work and percentage of day

Situation	Resources	Work	Percentage of Day	Duration
Emily is the only resource assigned to a task and will focus on that task until it is complete.	Emily	40 hours	100%	5 days
Emily is the only resource assigned to a task and can only dedicate half of her time to the task.	Emily	40 hours	50%	10 days
Emily and John are assigned to a task and can share the responsibilities. They will focus on this task until it is complete.	Emily John	20 hours 20 hours	100%	2.5 days
Emily and John are assigned to a task and can share the responsibilities. They can dedicate half of their time to this task.	Emily John	20 hours 20 hours	50% 50%	5 days

Figure 27.3.   Example of a revised project schedule

proposed. It is not uncommon for this date to be earlier than the project finish date calculated by the scheduling engine software. The project manager is faced with the situation of fitting the tasks into this predetermined schedule. The way to do this is to look at the critical path tasks to determine how they could be accomplished sooner.

A project plan for an office move is displayed in figure 27.4. Each task is flagged as to whether or not it is on the critical path. It is easy to see in this illustration that if the start or finish of task 10 (Order office furniture) changes, it will not affect the project end date. However if the dates for task 6 changes (Finalize lease on office space), there will be an impact on the overall finish date.

Conduct Risk Analysis

With the project network calculated, the project manager has a plan for the project schedule, work effort, and cost. However, it is a very ideal project; it assumes that all the tasks will occur as scheduled and estimated. For example, as soon as a predecessor task finishes, the successor task begins. It also assumes that the resources will be available on the exact day the task is scheduled to begin. At this point, the project is not accommodating delays such as illness, a delay in hardware acquisition, or the learning curve encountered when using a new technology.

If one thing can be accurately predicted about a project, it is that it will not progress as scheduled. To account for the inevitable changes, the project manager should perform a risk analysis and adjust the project schedule, work effort, or cost projections to incorporate any anticipated risk.

To conduct a risk analysis, the project manager first documents the types of risks that may occur. He or she then assigns a probability factor and an impact factor. The probability factor indicates the odds of the particular risk occurring. The impact factor designates the effect the risk will

have on the project if it does occur. These two factors are then multiplied together to calculate the risk factor.

A **contingency** should be put in place for any risk with a high-risk factor. The contingency describes what the project team will do if the risk is realized. For example, to mitigate the risk of losing a key project team member, the project manager would ensure that the project documentation is kept up-to-date. The impact of the contingency should be reflected in the project plan. For the example cited, the project manager would make sure that a task is in the project plan for updating project documentation.

An example of a risk analysis can be illustrated by using a situation you may be familiar with—planning a vacation. (See table 27.7.) For this example, the vacation will be to a Caribbean island in November, which happens to be during hurricane season.

As with assumptions, the project manager should obtain consensus from the project team, project sponsor, and stakeholders for the contingency plans. After the initial risk assessment is documented, a synopsis can be included in the project manager's status report. This synopsis could include any changes to the risk factors, realized and unrealized risks, and changes to contingency plans. After the threat of the risk is over, it can be removed from the report.

Check Your Understanding 27.4

Instructions: Prepare a work breakdown structure for the project you initiated in Check Your Understanding 27.3. Include the following for the tasks: task name, predecessor task(s), associated deliverable(s), and a list of the team members who will work on the task. Then answer the following questions on a separate piece of paper.

1. What methods can be used to estimate the work effort for a task?

2. What are some potential risks to the project you selected in Check Your Understanding 27.3? What contingencies can be put in place to mitigate this risk?

Figure 27.4.   Example of a project plan with critical path shown

ID	Task Name	Start	Finish	Critical	January	February	March
1	**Office Move**	**Jan 3**	**Mar 8**	**Yes**			
2	**Office Space**	**Jan 3**	**Mar 8**	**Yes**			
3	Identify requirements for new office space	Jan 3	Jan 5	Yes			
4	Identify potential office sites	Jan 6	Jan 12	Yes			
5	Make final decision on office space	Jan 13	Jan 21	Yes			
6	Finalize lease on office space	Jan 24	Jan 27	Yes			
7	Design office space	Jan 28	Mar 1	Yes			
8	Assign office space	Mar 2	Mar 8	Yes			
9	**Office Equipment**	**Jan 24**	**Mar 4**	**No**			
10	Order office furniture	Jan 24	Jan 26	No			
11	Order new office equipment	Mar 2	Mar 4	No			
12	Order phone system	Mar 2	Mar 2	No			
13	**Moving Companies**	**Jan 28**	**Feb 16**	**No**			
14	Select the move day	Jan 28	Jan 28	No			
15	Obtain estimates from moving companies	Jan 31	Feb 15	No			
16	Hire movers	Feb 16	Feb 16	No			

Table 27.7.   Example of risk analysis

Risk Description	Probability Factor Low = 1 Medium = 3 High = 5	Impact Factor Range is 1–10 Low = 1 High = 10	Risk Factor (Probability × Impact)	Contingency
Forget to pack an item	5	3	15	Prepare a packing list
Traffic congestion on the way to the airport	1	10	10	Check road construction hotline and radio traffic reports; allow extra travel time
Rain during the vacation	3	8	24	Plan some indoor activities
Luggage doesn't make it to the destination	1	10	10	Purchase additional baggage insurance
Hurricane strikes the resort	5	10	50	Purchase trip cancellation insurance

Project Implementation

When the project planning is complete, the organization is ready to begin the project. The project manager has prepared the project schedule, identified the work effort requirements, and anticipated potential delays. Before the project begins, he or she will capture a **baseline** of the project schedule and work effort. The baseline is a copy of the original estimates for the project. It is captured so that the progress of the project can be compared to the original plan. This comparison is discussed in further detail later in this chapter.

Hold a Project Kickoff Meeting

It is customary to hold a project kickoff meeting when the project gets under way. This meeting sets the tone for the project and helps everyone understand its importance. A typical agenda for the meeting includes the following items:

- Executive presentation, during which the sponsor or key stakeholder presents the background on the project with a particular emphasis on why the organization is embarking on this endeavor
- Project objectives
- Project organization chart
- Team roles and responsibilities
- High-level WBS (approach)
- Project schedule
- Key assumptions and constraints
- Project control and communication, including project tracking, meeting schedule, project documentation, change control procedure, and issue tracking

Perform Project Tasks and Produce Deliverables

The project team now has responsibility for performing the scheduled tasks and producing the project deliverables. The project manager has responsibility for ensuring that all participants understand what is to be done and when.

At this point in the project, the team may become bogged down in indecisiveness, resistance to change, and bureaucracy. The project manager works with the team, the stakeholders, and the project sponsor to keep the project moving by getting issues resolved and decisions made. The project manager may use various problem-solving and decision-

making techniques to facilitate this process. (See chapter 21 for more information on this subject.)

Track Progress and Analyze Variance

When the project is under way, the project manager needs to follow how it is progressing. He or she must be able to provide the following information to the stakeholders and the project team:

- Will the project be completed on time?
- Will the project cost more than planned?
- Will the project objectives be met?

The project manager can answer these questions only by actively tracking the project's progress and analyzing its progress against the original plan.

Project Tracking

The project is tracked through the process of collecting actual progress and remaining effort from the project team members. Each team member should provide information on a periodic basis. The frequency of progress information depends on the duration of the project. For a short project of less than two months in duration, updates may be needed more than once a week. Longer projects may require a weekly progress report. In determining tracking frequency, the project manager should consider the effort of obtaining the information and updating the project plan against the level of information needed to perform the variance analysis and, more important, should be able to adequately respond to required plan revisions when a project is in trouble.

Each project team member should report the following information for each task:

- Actual start date or new scheduled start date (when the task was not started on time)
- Percentage of complete or actual work
- Remaining work or expected finish date
- Actual and remaining cost
- Actual finish date (for completed tasks)
- Issues

It is usually difficult to obtain actual progress from the project team members. There are both procedural and psychological reasons for this. With regard to procedural reasons, the project manager has to set up a mechanism for getting the information. This may be a hard-copy report, or it may be automated through project management software. Unfortunately, the process of getting the information can be tedious and project managers often neglect it to pursue other project management processes that they deem to be more important.

With regard to psychological reasons, people are inclined to overestimate their progress. They tend to tell someone what they believe that person wants to hear rather than report true progress. People also may become defensive about their progress, especially in situations where they are behind schedule or over budget. Although some personal accountability may be involved, often the reason for the delay or overrun is not directly within the team member's control. The project manager can set the right tone for the data collection process by letting the team know how the information will be used. Honesty from team members should not result in punitive measures, unless an individual has been consistently negligent in his or her project responsibilities. When a project team member is not performing as needed, the project manager needs to address this issue. (Refer to chapter 21 for management strategies that can be used to resolve this situation.)

Variance Analysis and Project Revision
After updating the project schedule with the task progress, the project manager compares the task start date, expected finish date, estimated work effort, estimated cost, and estimated duration to what was originally planned. As stated above, all projects do not progress as originally planned. The project manager must concentrate on those **variances** that are substantially affecting the project's time line, budget, and objec-tives. For example, a task may start later than planned, but if it is not on the project's critical path, the delay will not affect the project finish date. However, if the task is on the critical path, the project manager must determine how to make up the delay and still complete the project on schedule. A task may have started on time but consume a higher work effort than originally estimated. Unless other tasks in the plan consume less than the original estimate, the overall project will exceed the work estimates and thus the cost estimate.

Figure 27.5 shows a report for the office move project plan that can be used to assess the variances. The work and cost variances are shown directly to the right of the task name. The right side of the report is known as a Gantt chart. The Gantt chart was developed by Henry L. Gantt as a method to illustrate the time needed for each task. On the figure 27.5 report, there are two bars for each task. The top bar shows the start and finish dates as they have been rescheduled based on tracking information. The bottom bar shows the baseline dates. The report shows that due to the fact that task 5 will not finish according to the original schedule, tasks 6 and 7 also will be delayed. These tasks are on the critical path; therefore, the delay must be addressed if the project is to remain on schedule. (Refer to figure 27.4, p. 779.)

To get the project back on track, the project manager must evaluate the available options. All these options are a variant of the variables that make up the project parameters: scope, performance, cost, and time line. The project manager needs to clearly document the options and ramifications of each and present the documentation to the project's stakeholders. The sponsor and the stakeholders will make the decision based on what is most important to the success of the project. For example, in a software implementation, it may be more

Figure 27.5.   Example of project plan with information to assess variances

important for the new system to contain all the desired functionality than it is for the implementation to meet the budget. The sponsor may be willing to do this to obtain department satisfaction and compliance with the new system.

Table 27.8 shows the types of plan revisions the project manager may propose and the risks involved in using each option.

Establish Change Control

In addition to proposing project revisions to keep the project on track, the project manager is usually faced with requests for changes to the original project scope. These requests can be the result of any of the following:

- A change in a departmental procedure
- A new or revised organizational initiative
- A new or revised regulatory requirement
- A desired change in the design of a system function

Changes to project scope are inevitable and should not be automatically considered a form of project failure. It is the way project changes are handled that can have a negative impact on the success of the project. The most important factor in scope change is for the stakeholders to understand the impact of the requested change and, if approved, be willing to accept the ramifications the change will have on the project's schedule and cost. In other words, the project manager must be in control of the changes. Just as in plan revision, all changes to the plan will affect the final project outcome in terms of scope, work, time line, or cost. When the project manager, sponsor, and other stakeholders do not acknowledge the impact of the change by approving a corresponding modification to one of the other variables, the quality of the project suffers.

The procedure for **change control** should be established at the beginning of the project in order to set the proper expectations for how scope modifications will be handled. The process should be as follows:

1. The requestor completes a change request form.
2. An impact analysis is performed. Its purpose is to determine the effect the change will have on the project.

Table 27.8.   Potential risks in revising project plans

Options for Plan Revision	Potential Risks
Decrease the scope of work by removing some of the project requirements. Requirements may be eliminated or deferred to a subsequent project.	Project objectives may be compromised.
Eliminate the nice-to-have features of the project to decrease the scope of work.	Project objectives may be compromised.
Add more resources to get the work done faster.	Project cost may be compromised.
Ask team members to get the work done by putting in extra time.	Project cost may be compromised.
Evaluate the project plan to determine whether some tasks can start sooner. Look for finish-to-start dependencies to determine whether the tasks can overlap.	Quality may suffer when shortcuts are taken to shorten the schedule.

For example, there may be a positive impact on the relationship to the system's objectives, but the request may increase the work effort.

3. The request is presented to the stakeholders for approval. If the change is approved, the stakeholders have indicated they are willing to accept the ramification on the project time line or cost. In other words, the benefits of the change outweigh the goal to stay within the original project budget.

Communicate Project Information

One of the success factors for a project is good project communication. All involved parties need to be kept apprised of the project's progress, understand any outstanding issues, understand the change control requests, and understand the project politics. Several forms of project communication are used during the project: project status meetings, project status reports, **issue logs,** and project plans.

Project Status Meetings

A project status meeting is a formal meeting attended by the project team members. Its purpose is to report accomplishments, to review the status of in-progress project tasks, and to discuss issues that are impeding the completion of any tasks.

There are a few cautions for the project manager when conducting the meeting. The first is that project team members may feel pressure to report a rosy picture of the task progress because they are among their peers. A task may be behind schedule to the point that it will most likely delay the overall project schedule, but a team member may be reluctant to report this to avoid being held accountable for the entire project missing its target finish date. Although formal status meetings are important for a project, the informal status reporting from the team members is just as important. The project manager should spend time with team members outside the meeting where the team member may feel that the environment is more conducive to an honest appraisal of the task progress.

The second problem with some status meetings is that participants become bogged down in discussions that cannot be resolved in the meeting. For example, team members may be discussing an issue in terms of what it is instead of actually resolving it. Although everyone must understand all project issues, it is not good use of the status meeting time to discuss the issue unless all the decision makers are in the room. Generally, issues should be handled in separate meetings outside the project status meeting.

Project Status Reports

A project status report is the formal documentation of the project progress. Again, although formal documentation is a required component of the project, the project manager should supplement this reporting with ad hoc conversations with the team members and stakeholders. This informal reporting, sometimes referred to as "walk-around" status reporting, can elicit information on the politics, conflicts, personality disputes, and bureaucracy that tend to impede task progress.

The frequency of status reports varies depending on the overall project duration. A short project may require weekly reporting whereas a long project may require monthly reporting. Whatever frequency is selected, it should support the project manager's ability to react to changes, delays, and issues.

Topics to be included in a status report include:

- Objectives for the period
- Accomplishments during the period
- Explanation of any differences
- Objectives for next period
- Issues

When the task-tracking procedure and the formal status report follow the same frequency schedule (for example, both are completed on a weekly basis), the project manager may choose to collect this information on the same form. The feasibility of this also depends on the method selected for tracking. When task tracking is automated via project management software, the ability to also collect task status information may or may not be supported.

Issue Log

Issues are items that prevent the completion of a project task. Because all projects introduce some type of change, it is inevitable that issues will arise. The purpose of the issue log is to document the issues so that the project manager can ensure that they are resolved in a timely manner. The issue log should include:

- A description of each issue
- Name of the team member assigned to resolve the issue
- Priority (for example, high, medium, low)
- Date the issue was opened
- Status (open, deferred, or closed)
- The required resolution date
- A descriptive status of the issue
- Resolution date and description of the resolution

After the issue log is established, the team needs to actively be working the issues toward resolution. This is where the skills of negotiation, conflict management, and innovative thinking are critical. Consensus among the affected parties is always the best solution in any issue, but in some situations the project sponsor must be called on to end a deadlock.

The issue log also can be used to capture ideas and topics that are not either specifically pertinent to the project or within its scope. These topics are often referred to as "parking lot" items. Placing them on the issue log (with a separate priority or status) is a good time management technique that ensures that the ideas will not be forgotten.

Project Plans

Reports generated from the project plan can provide information on the status of the project tasks. These reports are usually produced for the stakeholders to provide a snapshot of the project. When the project manager is using project management software, it is able to produce a variety of reports, including:

- Gantt chart that visually displays the task start and finish dates along with the percent of progress completed
- Tasks that are behind schedule
- Task list displaying the critical path tasks
- Tasks exceeding the original work estimate
- Resource reports showing the estimated work for each resource broken down by week or month

An example of a resource report is shown in figure 27.6 (p. 784).

Prepare the Final Report

When the project has been concluded, it is good practice to produce a final project report. The purpose of the report is to bring closure to the endeavor by documenting the project's final outcome. The topics to be included in the report include:

- A list of the project objectives with a description of how each objective was accomplished
- A list of the project deliverables
- The final project budget, detailing the comparison of the original estimate to the actual cost
- The final project schedule, detailing the comparison of the original dates to the actual dates

Celebrate Success

Projects can be very stressful to an organization. Therefore, it is important for the stakeholders and the project manager to provide the leadership to motivate team members and departments throughout the project duration. One of the ways this can be accomplished is by emphasizing the project's importance by celebrating accomplishments. For example, several social events might be held during the project to honor key project milestones. The project stakeholder could thank project participants for the effort expended thus far and encourage the same level of commitment for the remaining project activities.

After the project is completed, a more formal celebration may take place. All project contributors should be invited and recognized for their efforts.

Check Your Understanding 27.5

Instructions: Answer the following questions on a separate piece of paper.

1. What project progress information should project team members provide to the project manager?

2. What are some of the barriers to obtaining accurate progress information from team members?

3. What is change control?

4. What are some of the problems with formal project communications methods?

Figure 27.6. Example of a resource report

ID	Resource Name	Work	Details	January	February	March	April
1	Chief Relocation Officer	30 hrs	Work	30h			
	Identify requirements for new office space	20 hrs	Work	20h			
	Make final decision on office space	5 hrs	Work	5h			
	Finalize lease on office space	5 hrs	Work	5h			
2	Office Manager	257 hrs	Work	64.87h	137.78h	54.35h	
	Identify potential office sites	20 hrs	Work	20h			
	Design office space	100 hrs	Work	8.7h	86.95h	4.35h	
	Assign office space	10 hrs	Work			10h	
	Order office furniture	30 hrs	Work	30h			
	Order new office equipment	30 hrs	Work			30h	
	Order phone system	10 hrs	Work			10h	
	Select the move day	2 hrs	Work	2h			
	Obtain estimates from moving companies	50 hrs	Work	4.17h	45.83h		
	Hire movers	5 hrs	Work		5h		

Real-World Case

Reimbursement rules require that the chargemaster drive a facility's charges. To receive the optimal reimbursement for services rendered, the chargemaster must be up-to-date and all-inclusive and must meet any payer rules and regulations.

The facility has decided to undergo a review of its chargemaster to ensure that it meets the above criteria. In addition to the comprehensive evaluation, one of the other objectives of the project will be to institute the procedures to ensure that all additions, revisions, and deletions meet the chargemaster standards.

Summary

The art of project management encompasses a wide variety of responsibilities and skills. Project management does not just involve the creation and maintenance of a project plan. Organizations need to realize that good project management does not just happen. The concepts of project management must be understood and embraced at all levels of the organization. When the organization's executives do not support good project management methodology, the risk of project failure will outweigh any perceived benefits.

When a project is started, all parties must understand its objectives. The lack of a common vision for what the project will achieve is the first opportunity for the project to fail. All stakeholders must be willing to commit the required resources to the project and to support the procedural changes that will inevitably occur as a result of the project. All project personnel also can contribute to the success of the project by keeping proposed project changes to a minimum.

A project adheres to the project management life cycle. Depending on the size and type of project, each process is scalable. In other words, the extent to which each process is performed may vary, but all processes should be included in every project.

The project manager is in a unique position in situations where a project crosses departmental boundaries. He or she has responsibility for the project success, but generally little authority over the members of the project team. The project manager must possess technical, functional, and analytical skills as well as leadership, influential, and motivational abilities.

References

Kliem, R.L., and I.S. Ludin. 1998. *Project Management Practitioner's Handbook.* New York: AMACOM.

Lewis, J.P. 1998. *Mastering Project Management.* New York: McGraw-Hill.

Project Management Institute. 2004. *A Guide to Project Management Body of Knowledge.* Newtown Square, PA: PMI.

Chapter 28
Strategic Management: Shaping and Leading Change

Linda L. Kloss, MA, RHIA

Learning Objectives

- To define and describe strategic management as an essential set of skills for leading health information management (HIM) services
- To explore the skills that strategic health information managers possess
- To distinguish strategic management from strategic planning
- To understand how strategic management complements other management tools and approaches
- To describe the benefits of strategic management and relate these to leadership and management principles and to the change management process
- To describe techniques for considering future HIM challenges and identifying strategic options
- To identify examples of strategic management as applied to HIM practice
- To understand how HIM strategies fit into broader information strategies and the overall strategy of the organization
- To describe the qualities and attributes of a strategic leader in health information management

Key Terms

Brainstorming
Coalition building
Environmental scanning
Forecasting
Kolb's "Learning Loop"
Nominal group technique
Paradigm
Scenarios
Storytelling
Strategic management
Strategic planning
Strategy
Strategy map
Tactic
Vision

Introduction

Setting **strategy** is often viewed as the work of senior managers and boards of trustees. Strategy is thought of as being handed down from on high, embodied in slogans and generally not very relevant to the day-to-day work of most employees in the organization. Sometimes strategy is detailed in a three- to five-year strategic plan that lays out goals and key actions to meet the organization's goals. But strategy is no longer the sole purview of senior managers, planning departments, or consultants. The ability to develop effective strategies is a key attribute of successful managers at all levels in today's organizations. Employers cite **strategic management** and change leadership as competencies they look for in health information management (HIM) professionals (AHIMA 2004, p. 6).

Simply stated, a strategy is a course of action designed to produce a desired outcome. Strategy requires making choices about what to do and what not to do. Strategic management is not the same as operations improvement. Operations improvement focuses on improving how existing programs and services are carried out. By definition, it is internally focused. Strategy development is a search for new programs and services that will improve the organization's fit with the external world.

Management theories about the importance of strategy and how to set strategy are changing. This reconsideration is a reflection of the speed of change in every facet of contemporary life including healthcare.

This chapter explores the importance of strategy to effective management and describes approaches to making and communicating strategic choices. It discusses the importance of strategic management for organizational learning and illustrates how HIM professionals use strategy to shape and effect change.

Theory into Practice

A large multispecialty group practice clinic has just hired a registered health information administrator (RHIA) to manage its transition to an electronic health record (EHR). The clinic's director of information technology (IT) suggested the need for an RHIA because in his last job, the HIM and IT teams worked very closely to implement an EHR and he believed that the HIM competencies were a key ingredient in that successful implementation. The IT director knows that the transition will be more successful with an RHIA to oversee the project, manage all issues relating to the transition from paper to electronic records, handle the design of new policies and procedures for e-records, and manage user education. The clinic's senior management envisions a system that will allow physicians to access information from satellite clinics and other remote sites and to provide information to patients through a personal health record (PHR) view into the EHR.

Early in her tenure, the new project director discovered that senior management and IT's understanding of the need for health information system improvements was not shared by most other clinical staff, physicians and nonphysicians alike. In part, this was because external factors such as new pay-for-performance plans had not yet come to the community and the clinic was somewhat insulated from industrywide efforts to transition from paper to electronic records within 10 years. Moreover, there was no shared vision of what benefits could accrue to the clinic, its associates, staff, and patients if IT were used to support patient care processes.

The project director decided to approach change on two fronts at the same time. One front would center on delivering short-term benefits to physicians that would improve their efficiency through easier access to information. These benefits also would enable physicians to use technology for some routine tasks relating to maintaining records. For example, handheld devices were implemented to allow access to scheduling information and to lab and medication information on patients. Next, electronic prescribing software was added along with electronic signature capability. Dictation systems also were upgraded. Improvements in these functions would increase everyone's confidence in the director's abilities and would garner her support for the tougher projects of implementing full electronic records and PHRs.

While the project phase of improving productivity through selected tools was being implemented, the project director convened a series of cross-departmental sessions to design a **vision** for the clinic's EHR and PHR systems. Given the need to expand physician and staff understanding of the benefits of the EHR/PHR, these visioning sessions were used to educate staff about the systems' possibilities. The sessions also allowed the RHIA to learn more about practice management styles and the work processes that need to be redesigned before EHR/PHR implementation. This information was essential in developing specifications for acquiring the EHR solution that would best fit the clinical staff's needs.

Additionally, the visioning meetings allowed the project director to establish rapport with staff throughout the organization. She knows how essential this is to successful implementation of the EHR/PHR down the road. She begins to identify allies in this change and likely opponents. She also learns how decisions are made and whether EHR/PHR implementation can be a top-down decision or whether she should advise senior management that the decision must come about through consensus-building approaches. Consensus may take longer, but it may be the style that fits best with the clinic's culture. As a new employee, the project director needs to assess all these factors for herself as they will be essential in managing the political and cultural aspects of converting the clinic to an EHR/PHR system.

Skills of Strategic Managers

The definition of strategy is straightforward, but the skills for setting and executing strategy are far from simple. HIM professionals must take advantage of opportunities to learn and develop skills for strategic management, including:

- Monitoring trends in healthcare and information management
- Reflecting on how trends can affect the future
- Considering how changes in one area can affect others in the organization
- Considering how a course for change is set
- Helping others visualize the need for change and recruiting them as partners in moving a change agenda
- Implementing plans effectively
- Questioning the status quo on an ongoing basis
- Being self-reflective and a lifelong learner

Strategy is no longer a management domain reserved for senior managers. Today, all managers must develop skills and competencies that enable them to think and act strategically. These skills include sharpening one's ability to *observe the world around you*. Strategic managers watch for changes in the larger environment beyond the healthcare industry, including political, economic, social, and technological changes. Such changes may involve staff attitudes, public policy, ethics, or inventions and innovations. Managers must consider how these changes are affecting—or might affect—healthcare and the organizations in which they work. For example, shifts in public attitudes regarding the value placed on personal privacy have implications for health information policies and practices regarding patients who request access to their records.

Strategic managers develop skills in reflecting on *the implications and opportunities* afforded by trends. Whether reading a journal or discussing new ideas with others, strategic managers are always testing new ideas, identifying those that have merit and discarding those that do not. They are making linkages between the trends and the value-adding actions they can take. For example, federal programs to adjust physician reimbursement on the basis of certain quality parameters suggest a need to elevate organizational standards for data integrity so that pay-for-performance determinations are accurate and fair.

Effective strategic managers are creative in how they make associations among trends, ideas, and new opportunities. These associations are not always direct as in the examples about privacy and public policy or data quality and pay for performance. Making strategy choices may be the result of drawing lessons from analogous situations. When faced with an unfamiliar problem or opportunity, experienced managers often learn from similar situations they have seen or heard about and apply what they have learned to current situations (Gavetti and Rivkin 2005, pp. 54–63). For example, faced with an intractable shortage of trained coders, the HIM director institutes a coder-training program sponsored by her healthcare organization and modeled on a similar program used to address the shortage of nurses in the community.

Strategic managers also *continually look for opportunities to improve on the status quo*. They do not accept the old adage, "If it's not broken, don't fix it." They always look for ways to make things better and are willing to take some risks and evaluate new approaches through trial and error. They know that standing still is really moving backward. They understand that no action may be less tolerable than trying something even if does not fully succeed. For example, the quality of coded data for inpatient services is at 94 percent and the data quality manager thinks that adjusting staff assignments may make better use of staff skills and improve performance.

New managers may lack the confidence to initiate change and may have few analogous experiences to draw on. Still, they should guard against accepting or perpetuating artificial barriers to creativity characterized by common squelchers, such as "We've never done that before," "We have always done it that way," or "That's not my job." Confidence comes from experience, and experience requires action and thoughtful reflection on what did and did not work.

Finally, strategic managers learn to help others contribute to new thinking and new ideas. They know that the best solutions represent the best thinking of all the stakeholders. Thus, strategic managers learn techniques to bring out the best thinking of all staff, superiors, colleagues, and other constituents for their change agenda. As Drucker says, "the only definition of a leader is someone who has followers" (Drucker 1996, p. xii). For example, in pursuit of a goal to decrease the amount of printing being done by physicians from electronic records, the health information manager knew that support from nursing and other staff in the patient care units was essential for success. He oversaw implementation of a multifaceted plan to reduce the rate of printing on the units and shared credit with nursing when the print rate began to decline.

The skills of the strategic manager are learned. Learning begins by recognizing the importance of strategy to today's successful managers. For HIM professionals, the learning begins with their professional course work and directed learning experiences. Skills are learned and subsequently honed through work experience, particularly opportunities to be part of—and to lead—change management projects.

From Strategic Planning to Strategic Management

Strategic planning was described in the management literature in the 1960s and the decades that followed. It was a prominent and highly touted organizational function. Early applications were characterized by rigorous and formal analysis of data to deduce a desired future and the steps to achieve it. In large corporations, departments of planners prepared forecasts with the aid of computer analysis. The complex reports were delivered to senior managers who were largely uninvolved in the process.

These approaches have fallen out of favor for several key reasons. First, **forecasting** the future, particularly in such volatile times, is a near impossibility. Also, by the time a complex three- to five-year plan is finalized and delivered to senior managers, it is undoubtedly out-of-date. Finally, if senior managers are not involved in strategy development, the plan is unlikely to be seen as relevant and unlikely to be implemented.

No one phrase is the accepted successor for this type of strategic planning. In fact, today you are likely to still hear the activity referred to as strategic planning in many organizations. However, it is important to get beneath the words to understand the process being followed. It may be called strategic planning, but it may embody many of the newer concepts that often are called strategic management. For example:

- It is framed by organizational values, vision, and mission.
- It takes into account possible futures, rather than trying to forecast the future.
- It is truly the work of management, even when guided by consultants, and has broad input and participation.
- It is action oriented, with a commitment to bringing about change.
- It results in organizational learning.

Strategic management is a way of introducing innovation into decision making and engaging others in the change process. With the very rapid changes in HIM practice, this discussion of strategic management is not academic. Strategic management should be viewed as a component of each of the five functions of management discussed in chapter 21. Every aspect of management involves a strategic management component, as described below.

With organizational learning as a centerpiece, this approach unifies change management, strategy development, and leadership. In all three, we learn by observing and reflecting on the results of our experiences. This concept is best depicted in **Kolb's "Learning Loop,"** shown in figure 28.1 (Kolb 1988, pp. 68–88).

To undertake deliberate change, we reflect on our experiences and become aware of new patterns and trends that we did not perceive before. We form new ways of looking at the

opportunities and the implications of our experiences. We evaluate new theories about what can and should be, and then apply these theories and test their implications. We observe and reflect on the results of our experiences, thus beginning the loop again.

Elements of Strategic Management

As shown in figure 28.2, strategic management is a logical process that comprises a number of steps that may be explicit or implicit. It begins with a vision of how you would like things to be. For example, the vision for a managed care health plan might be to have fully engaged patients who are full partners with the health plan in maintaining their health. Obviously, many strategic issues need to be addressed for this vision to be realized and these must be identified and understood. Some of the issues might involve lack of incentives for patients to engage in wellness activities, cultural diversity, lack of electronic PHRs, and computer and health literacy issues.

Major goals to move toward the vision are described. These become more precise than the overall vision. For example, providing all citizens with access to lifetime electronic PHRs might be a goal to achieve the vision of empowered consumers. The vision and goals describe where you want to go, and the issues describe what must be addressed to get there. The strategies are how you intend to pursue the vision and achieve the goals. The **tactics** are the specific plans to implement strategies.

Although depicted as a linear process, overall strategic management is never so neat and organized and the best strategies may emerge from trial and error. But effective strategy will not emerge without a clear idea of where you want to lead your organization and a realistic assessment of the issues to overcome. Moreover, strategic management will not happen

Figure 28.1.   Kolb's "Learning Loop"

Source: Kolb 1988.

Figure 28.2.   Elements of strategic management

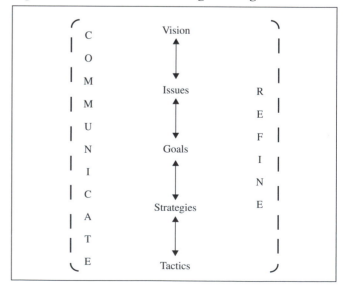

in isolation. Stakeholders, whether staff, customers, patients, or senior managers, must be engaged in each phase of the process.

Each step involves learning, which in turn enables plans to be improved upon making subsequent efforts more effective. Thus, experience sharpens and clarifies our understanding of the issues, allowing us to be more precise in goal setting. Strategies and tactics are continually modified with experience. Strategic management, like Kolb's "Learning Loop" is a process that leads to organizational learning and improvement over time.

In contrast to traditional strategic planning, where all steps are neatly outlined before implementation is begun, strategic management requires a willingness to learn and change as you go along.

Check Your Understanding 28.1

Instructions: On a separate piece of paper, answer the following questions relating the example described in the Theory into Practice section with the introductory content and the discussion on the elements of strategic management.

1. Would you conclude that "a system that allows the physicians to access information from satellite clinics and other remote sites..." is a goal, a strategy, or a tactic?

2. Write a two-sentence vision statement describing what the clinic's senior management wants the project director to achieve regarding the electronic health record.

3. List the two skills of a strategic manager that were best exhibited in the way the new RHIA project manager worked out a plan to move forward.

Begin with a Vision

According to Kouzes and Posner, "A vision describes a bold and ideal image of the future" (1995, p. 94). It is the catalyst for change. As Kouzes and Posner state, "if leaders are going to take us to places we've never been before, constituents of all types demand that they have a sense of direction" (1995, p. 95).

A vision states the direction for change and helps motivate people to take action. In 2003, the American Health Information Management Association (AHIMA) convened an interdisciplinary panel of experts to craft a vision for electronic health information management (e-HIM):

> Electronic health information management is the body of knowledge and practice that assures the availability of health information to facilitate real-time healthcare delivery and critical health-related decision making for multiple purposes across diverse organizations, settings, and disciplines.

This vision statement describes features of electronic health information management that work in real time to support critical decision making across healthcare. The vision reflects a more diverse field with a critical charge. It has been used to help catalyze the field to embrace e-HIM™ as a change strategy.

In 2005, AHIMA's board of directors again looked to the future to consider how the field of HIM is changing and the impact of the changes on the profession and on the professional association. It reaffirmed the vision crafted in 2003 and articulated new insights about strategies that would secure a strong future for the profession.

Designing a compelling vision requires a solid understanding of the internal and external environment. It also requires the ability to break free of the current **paradigm** and to think creatively about a new reality for the future.

Following are examples of vision statements for health information management. A director of HIM services for a health system envisions services that make the fullest use of technology to provide high-quality, cost-effective information to authorized users. He expressed this idealized vision as follows:

> It is our goal to utilize state-of-the-art information technology and best practices grounded in applied research in every phase of our operation so that we are able to deliver accurate information in digital form to support patient care and healthcare operations. This ambitious goal will require us to become more externally focused, to gain a deeper understanding of user needs, and to work closely with others within and outside our organization. It will also require health information services staff to work together to question all current practices and be willing to try new approaches even if they are not all successful.

This vision lays out a very substantial challenge, yet it provides focus. First, the overarching vision is to be able to deliver all information to all users of HIM services in digital form. It acknowledges that technology is only as good as the enabling processes; therefore, it promises use of best practices. These practices are not to be just what we might think are best but, rather, are practices substantiated by applied research that demonstrates their validity. The vision statement acknowledges that achieving this vision will require new ways of working. First, success will require gaining a deeper understanding of the needs of those who rely on the information and of those whose collaboration is needed to achieve the vision. Second, it will require effective teamwork among HIM staff who must become more comfortable with change and with risk taking.

In another example, an HIM consultant for a long-term care system was having difficulty gaining support for her vision of what an EHR could contribute to the residents, staff, and the overall organization. She developed the following description of her vision:

> All members of the care team have immediate access to complete and accurate information for each resident. This information recaps care delivered and presents the status of all health, social, ADL, and other resident-specific issues being managed. Information needs to be entered just once and is available for a variety of patient care, quality improvement, and administrative uses. Summary reports are used as the basis for shift change briefings and for periodic care conferences. The information system prompts caregivers to actions that need to be taken and alerts them to changes in status that require special vigilance. Data entered into the system summarizing observations, care given, orders, and activities produce a record of care that meets licensing and other external requirements. The system also automatically accumulates the information needed for care and operations management and for external reporting.

This vision highlights the benefits of implementing an EHR from the perspective of improving management of the care process every day. It underscores the fact that information for management and internal and external reporting should be a byproduct of the system, thereby reducing the redundant paperwork that currently requires so much staff time. A careful parsing of the vision reveals the major features and functions required of a system. For example, the system must be capable of producing a change-of-shift summary report recapping care processes and the status of all resident problems being managed. It also must accumulate the data needed for MDS (Minimum Data Set) and other reporting. The vision serves as a starting point for creating a more detailed set of specifications and evaluating potential system vendors.

Visions also can be more narrowly focused on a particular project. For example, a data quality manager for a multispecialty group practice clinic prepared the following vision statement to help the physicians and coding staff rally around a proposed project to improve the timeliness and accuracy of billing processes through the use of computer-assisted coding tools:

> During each patient visit, the physician enters problems, treatments, orders, and follow-up plans into his or her handheld personal assistant device (PDA). PDA data are periodically uploaded to the clinical data repository throughout the day and data are combined there with other patient-specific reports and information. Codes are auto-assigned by the systems and missing data are flagged. Clinical data analysts review each visit record to check the accuracy of the auto-generated codes and determine whether the information substantiates the codes assigned. A visit record is either marked for billing or flagged as incomplete with supplementary information requested from the physician or referred service. Ninety percent of visits are billed within one business day, 95 percent within three business days, and the balance within five business days.

This vision statement has three major elements. First, it sets an aggressive goal of billing 90 percent of visits on the day of service. To do so, physicians must initiate the process using electronic tools to eliminate time-consuming handling of handwritten information. The new role of clinical data analyst is introduced, reflecting the role of coding specialists with advanced data quality and compliance management skills.

These vision statements relate to HIM challenges. However, it is important that the HIM vision complement the organization's overall vision and mission. For example, the organization's vision is to be known for its advanced clinical services in cardiac and oncology care. To achieve this vision, the organization is pursuing a strategy of attracting clinical talent with national reputations and expanding clinical research programs. This overall vision and these strategies should be accounted for in crafting the HIM vision and strategies.

Strategic managers understand the overall organizational goals and take them into account when crafting their own plans. First, they seek ways to support and further the overall goals of the organization through the priorities they set for their areas of responsibility. For example, will the cancer registry program need to be upgraded to support the more sophisticated information needs of a world-class oncology service? As a practical matter, it is hard to sell a plan that is out of step with priorities. Advancing the organization's goals through your efforts is the mark of a successful manager.

Creating a Commitment to Change

The organization's vision sets the broad directional strategy leaving the details to be worked out. Kotter explains that an effective vision statement has the following characteristics (2002, p. 72):

- It conveys a picture of what the future will look like.
- It appeals to the long-term interests of the stakeholders.
- It sets forth realistic and achievable goals.
- It is clear enough to provide guidance in decision making.
- It is flexible so that alternative strategies are possible as conditions change.
- It is easy to describe and communicate.

Remember that visions are pictures of the *desired* future. You may never realize a vision in its entirety. Today's technology may not yet support lifetime PHRs or auto-coding of 100 percent of cases, but that does not mean these bold pictures should not be sketched. All health information may never be in digital form, but that does not mean this should not be our vision. Visions must be important and worth pursuing; otherwise, why would others become engaged?

Visions should evoke a sense of excitement and urgency from those closest to the process. If the designers are not getting excited about the possibilities the vision presents, you are not likely to generate excitement from others. A sense of urgency is essential to overcome the forces that protect the status quo.

Check Your Understanding 28.2

Instructions: Based on an expanded understanding of the elements of a vision statement, improve on the two-sentence vision you prepared in exercise 28.1. On a separate piece of paper, revise and expand the statement so that it meets the elements of an effective vision statement as outlined by Kotter.

Understanding the Environment

Knowledge of the environment is essential to vision and strategy formulation. Sometimes called **environmental scanning,** this data-intensive process is the continuous process of gathering and analyzing intelligence about trends that are—or may be—affecting HIM. It is both internally focused on the healthcare organization and HIM and externally focused on industry and societal trends. Internal environmental assessment as adapted from the work of Bryson (1995, pp. 90–92) includes analysis of:

- *Performance indicators:* Budget targets and results, performance and productivity measures, staff and customer feedback

- *Resources:* Budgeted staff, information technology, and educational resources, programs, competencies, organizational culture
- *Present strategy:* Organization-wide strategy and priorities, information management strategy, information systems plans and priorities, compliance programs, products and services, business processes

External environmental assessment as adapted from Bryson (1995, pp. 87–89) includes analysis of:

- *Forces and trends:* Political, economic, demographic, social, technological, and educational
- *Resource constraints:* Healthcare reimbursement systems, patient and customer trends, regulators, competitors
- *Collaborators:* Current and potential collaborators

An HIM manager who focuses exclusively on his or her own area of responsibility, whether managing a department, a service, or a project, will have a difficult time succeeding as a strategic manager. Understanding the environment provides the context for the tough decisions involved in setting direction, designing strategy, and leading change. Some ways to be in touch with the environment include:

- Taking inventory of your sources of internal and external information to identify and fill information gaps
- Building performance measures to gain perspective on trends over time
- Becoming involved in projects and task forces at your organization to interact with a wide range of coworkers
- Developing your personal reading list to follow the thinking of experts in the field
- Reading what futurists are saying about how things will change
- Becoming active in your professional association, AHIMA, and other groups
- Building your network of professional colleagues
- Making full use of the information resources that AHIMA and other organizations make available
- Contributing to the professional body of knowledge when you develop new HIM practice solutions

Environmental Trends

Analyzing the changing environment and envisioning the future is at the same time an analytic and a highly creative activity. Understanding trends requires analysis of:

- The relationships between trends
- The sequence of events
- Causes and effects
- Priority among items

To bring out the best thinking of a team or work group, it is often helpful to use techniques that help participants consider factors from different perspectives. A number of group process techniques such as **brainstorming, nominal group technique,** and others help unleash each individual's creative talent.

Storytelling is another such technique. Telling stories about the future suggested by the trends has a number of advantages, including:

- Most people are comfortable with this approach.
- Findings are presented in an understandable and real-world context.
- Stories are memorable, making it easier for others to remember essential points.
- Stories generate excitement and are fun to develop.

One storytelling technique that is used in more sophisticated strategy planning is that of **scenarios.** The word *scenario* literally means a script of a play or story, or a projected sequence of events. Scenarios are defined as "focused descriptions of fundamentally different futures presented in coherent script-like or narrative fashion" (Schoemaker 1993, 193–213). They are plausible stories about how the future might unfold. They are not meant to predict but, rather, simply to interpret and clarify how environmental trends may play out.

Scenarios are based on analysis and interaction of environmental variables. Environmental scanning is an important preparatory step in scenario development. Based on study of the environment, three or four scenario themes reflecting alternate possible futures are developed. Stories are constructed that describe how each of these themes might be played out. These stories are refined through input and further study until they reflect the group's best thinking about what futures might be in store for the organization under various circumstances.

To understand how the clinical coding function might change in the future, an AHIMA task force studied environmental trends and developed four scenarios, each highlighting a slightly different, but plausible, future (Johns 2000, pp. 26–33):

- The first scenario described the impact on coding if a breakthrough technology became available that would automate a great deal of the coding that is now being done manually or with the help of encoders.
- The second scenario described the impact on coding functions if healthcare organizations were strategically committed to using information to improve the quality of care information and hence the organization's strategic positioning.
- The third scenario involves the role of coding in an increasingly regulatory environment in which healthcare spending is ratcheted down and investments in technology are constrained.
- The fourth scenario involves greater consumer involvement in making healthcare decisions and maintaining personal health information.

One can quickly see that all are plausible scenarios. The future of coding will be affected by all these factors, but one or more may have a greater impact than others. Strategic managers would develop contingency plans to account for the variables that may shape the future.

AHIMA also used scenarios to consider how medical transcription would be affected by technology (AAMT and AHIMA 2005). The steering group for this future project also prepared four likely future scenarios concerning medical transcription practice and a set of strategic actions to ensure that the field is well prepared to adapt regardless of which of the scenarios actually proves true (Fuller and Dennis 2005, pp. 48–51).

Build a portfolio of techniques that you can use to bring out the best thinking of others. Peruse the business shelves of major bookstores for guidebooks containing exercises and techniques to improve group process. Observe techniques used by facilitators to improve how groups work and think together. Keep a notebook or computer file of such techniques and practice them whenever you have the opportunity. Effective strategic managers know how to facilitate groups to help them think and work well together.

Check Your Understanding 28.3

Instructions: Answer the following questions on a separate sheet of paper.

1. List four ways that you do external "environmental scanning" in your everyday life (for example, read the Sunday newspaper, belong to list-servs, and so on).

2. Explain how—and how well—you stay in touch with new developments and trends in each of the following sectors:

   - Your community
   - The healthcare industry
   - The nation
   - The world

3. Identify two additional "external scanning" activities that you can incorporate into your life that would help you improve your rating in the exercise above by improving your grasp of the external environment.

4. In groups of four to six, reach consensus on the three most important ways that a new HIM professional can stay current with practice trends in HIM. You will need a flip chart and markers for this exercise.

   In your small group:

   - First, work quietly for five minutes to construct a group list. Write the best ideas on a piece of paper.

   - Allow each member of the group to contribute one idea. Write each idea on the flip chart. Go around the group until all ideas have been contributed. Do not repeat identical ideas.

   - When all ideas have been contributed, ask the group to rate the importance of each idea using the following scale: 5 points for very important, 3 points for somewhat important, 1 point for minimally important, and 0 points for those suggestions you do not think are at all important.

   - Tally the scores of each rater to produce a total score per idea. Rewrite the ideas in order of the most to least important based on the group's ratings.

Note: The group process technique used in this exercise is called the nominal group technique. Begin your facilitator's notebook with this technique.

From Vision to Strategy

As defined earlier, a strategy is an action or set of actions that moves the organization toward its vision. Strategic management is about pursuing a new set of activities or new ways of carrying out current activities that move the organization toward its vision. It may take the form of new or redesigned programs or services. It may involve implementing new systems, outsourcing certain operations, or merging functions with another organizational entity. It also may entail phasing out an outdated program or adopting new technologies. Finally, it may be aimed at bringing an organization into compliance with new regulations or finding new ways to reduce operating costs.

It is important to remember that strategic management is not the same as operations improvement. Operations improvement is internally focused whereas strategic management seeks to improve the position of the organization in the broader world in which it operates.

Techniques such as scenario development and environmental scanning are useful in formulating strategy because they shift the focus from internal to external. However, do not expect to identify exciting new strategies by looking at the past or looking inward. Look outside the organization and look to the future in formulating strategy.

To illustrate the thought process involved in moving from vision to strategy, consider the sample shown in figure 28.3 based on the vision statement presented on page 790 to move from a predominantly paper record to a digital record.

The next step is to prepare a detailed tactical plan to carry out each strategy. For example, implementing the strategy "Acquire and implement electronic signature software" requires research about technology vendors that offer software compatible with the clinical data repository. It requires budgeting for this technology, securing support for your plan, issuing an RFP, checking references, and so on.

Figure 28.3.   Issues to strategies: Digital information for patient care and healthcare operations

Strategic Issue #1: Transcribed reports currently become part of the EHR through scanning only; content is not in digital form.	
Goals	**Strategies**
Physicians are able to review and modify dictated reports online.	1. Implement electronic signature software. 2. Design and pilot test a process whereby physicians can authenticate, make changes to, and reassign a transcribed report online. 3. Design a phased plan for implementation of online physician review that is coordinated with the availability of online access to electronic reports.
Voice recognition converts dictated reports to digital information for storage in the EHR.	1. Implement voice recognition in the emergency, cardiac cath, and imaging departments. 2. Upgrade the EHR to accept input from voice recognition in structured reports. 3. Design and pilot test a plan for storing output in the EHR.

Building a strategy grounded in a vision provides a context to continually assess whether you are on track and whether you are making progress. The AHIMA board of directors identified six key strategies in its 2005 future visioning session that were supported by the e-HIM vision and a deep understanding of the external environment. They were cast as transformative "from-to" statements, reflecting the key changes that AHIMA must lead over the next decade:

- From variable health record content and formats to standardization
- From passive responsiveness to vendors to system-building certification of offerings
- From exclusivity to inclusive membership driven by role, aspirations, and interests
- From academic only to academic and performance-based certification
- From autonomy and self-sufficiency to working alliance with like-minded bodies
- From traditional leadership to governance adept at advancing change

For each key area for strategic action, a **strategy map** was designed that began with a brief description of the current state in 2005 and a desired state in 2015. A set of short-term actions to be undertaken in 2005–2006 was determined along with future milestones that should be met along the way to 2015. A sample map is shown in figure 28.4. Depicting change as a sort of road map is a useful way to help others understand the goals and the course of change.

Check Your Understanding 28.4

Instructions: Complete the following steps on a separate piece of paper.

1. Prepare a template for the strategic issue worksheet shown in figure 28.3 using your PC word-processing or presentation software (Microsoft Word, Microsoft PowerPoint).

2. Select one of the three vision statements on pages 789–790 and analyze the vision to identify one strategic issue. Then describe the strategic issue in one or two sentences on the form.

3. In the space provided on the form, write at least two goals that would need to be pursued to address the issue.

4. Identify one or more strategies that would need to be implemented to move toward each goal.

5. Finally, describe the logic you followed in determining the strategic issue, setting goals, and developing strategies.

Strategic Management in Practice

Porter advises that the "essence of strategy is deciding what not to do" (1996, pp. 61–78). He urges managers to view strategy as a series of trade-offs. Major change will impact current activities and may well require their modification or even elimination. No organization has the resources to take on major new programs without considering their impact on current programs. Making trade-offs is difficult for most managers. Letting go of even a marginal program may produce a backlash. However, resources must be reallocated to those programs that will enable the organization to operate at a new plane.

Figure 28.4. Strategy map: From variable health record content and formats to standardization

It is important to look at the range of strategies being pursued to be clear about priorities, identify opportunities for synergy and integration, and identify strategies that no longer add value. The strategy map provides a visual framework for integrating the four perspectives of a balanced scorecard (Kaplan and Norton 2004, p. 55).

The balanced scorecard is a technique for measuring organizational performance across the following four perspectives (Kaplan and Norton 2004, p. 31):

- *Financial perspective:* How must we be financially responsible to the organization as a whole?
- *Customer perspective:* To achieve our vision, how should we appear to our customers, internal and external?
- *Internal process perspective:* To satisfy our customers, which operational processes must we excel at?
- *Learning and growth perspective:* How will we improve our ability to change and improve?

The strategy map enables examination of the cause-and-effect relationships among the above perspectives. Figure 28.5 shows a strategy map for improving the real and perceived value of HIM services.

Tactical Planning

Strategy should not be confused with tactics. Often "strategic plans" are written at a tactical rather than a strategic level. Tactics describe how you will carry out the strategy. For example, if the strategy is to reduce the accounts receivable days attributable to coding backlogs, tactics may include authorizing overtime, hiring contract coders, and redesigning the record completion processes. When formulating strategies, question whether you are getting too deeply into how you will do something. Remember that strategy is *what* you are going to do; tactics are *how* you plan to do it.

Support for the Change Program

Sound change strategies and tactics alone do not ensure success. Success depends on great execution, including securing support for your change effort. Healthcare organizations are highly complex with many competing priorities. Gaining approval, even for the best-designed efforts, may be difficult.

An experienced HIM director with support from the IT director tried for three consecutive budget cycles to get funding for a document-imaging program. The request was accompanied by a solid return on investment (ROI) picture in terms of reductions in full-time equivalents, cost of storage, and increased productivity. In year four, the director tied the request not merely to how change would affect the HIM service, but also how it would support improved access to health information, reduce errors caused by illegibility, and improve communication among caregivers. In light of the JCAHO's new patient safety goals, the HIM director enlisted the help of nursing leadership to make the budget case. Nursing spoke to how this solution would improve access to information at the patient care bedside and would help link various electronic documentation systems already in place. The caregivers stressed the need to link the systems to help them do their jobs better. By taking this approach, the document-imaging system was presented to the board of directors, by the organization's Patient Safety Council chairperson and was approved by the board without hesitation.

Take a Systems Approach

According to Tichy, "the development of change strategy involves simultaneous attention to three [organizational] systems—technical, political, and cultural" (1983). The technical systems are concerned with the business we are in and how we conduct that business (for example, the process we

Figure 28.5.   Strategy map: Improving the value of HIM services

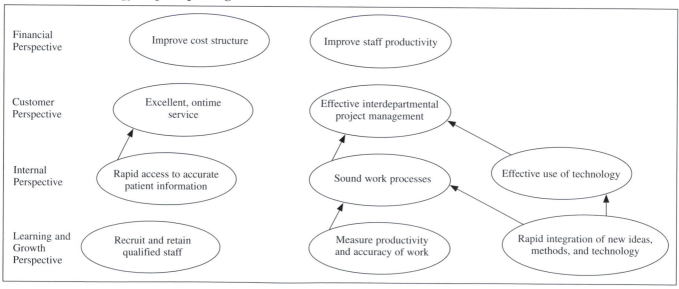

use to manage patient information). Political systems involve the distribution of power and influence in the organization (for example, the authority of the medical staff, the approval and decision-making processes). Cultural systems are the style and values that define how the organization typically operates.

Major change throws the organization into chaos as existing systems are deliberately unglued. This is a time of great vulnerability, and managers must be vigilant, watching for and thoughtfully addressing unintended effects that could make it difficult to achieve realignment. Managers must be sensitive to the very real emotional relationships among individuals in a group and how change will affect relationships between individuals and between the manager and others. Times of change are times of high stress and anxiety. This may play out in a number of ways. For example, in times of great change, employees may be more inclined to look for other employment opportunities as it is threatening and unsettling to go through change. Some turnover in staff may be an acceptable and unavoidable result, but the manager should be attentive and sensitive so that turnover does not derail the ability to carry out the project.

The technical, political, and cultural systems are highly interdependent, and any change will have intended and unintended impact on all three systems. For example, when implementing new technology such as EHRs or other major systems, the focus is often on features and functions of the system. Securing the right champions for the system and understanding how it affects the work and formal and informal interactions of staff is more challenging and important to successful implementation than features and functions. The successful strategic manager leading wide-scale technology change will be the one who excels at helping people get behind and become involved in the change. The manager who focuses only or primarily on installing the hardware and software will not succeed.

Managers should not let these challenges keep them from pursuing the strategies their organization needs. But success will depend on how well change is managed from a systems perspective. The manager must attend to all three system aspects throughout the implementation process. He or she also should be aware that implementation is not complete until all three systems are back in a new alignment after the changes are in place.

Manage the Politics of Change

Organizational change is a political process. Change leadership requires the courage to persevere even in the face of criticism; however, plowing ahead without considering the political implications may be folly. According to Bryson, managing the politics of change requires "finding ideas (visions, goals, strategies) that people can support and that further their interests . . . and making deals in which something is traded in exchange for that support" (1995, p. 225).

Political savvy entails skill in mediating and shaping conflicts that are inevitable when people are offered real choices with real consequences. Deliberately enlist the support of thought and opinion leaders. Reach out to those who may be most threatened by the proposed change; do not wait for them to come to you. Early engagement may turn potential resisters into supporters. At the very least, it will help change leaders build their arguments and communication plan to address the concerns of those who oppose the change.

Coalition building is one technique for managing the political dimensions of change. Change may threaten to shift the balance of power, and employees or coworkers who feel threatened may react by joining together to increase their own power so as to influence the course of events. Coalitions can be a force for thwarting change, or leaders can use coalition building as a way to build support for change. The example of the manager who gained the support of nursing to move ahead on the document management system project illustrates the power of coalition building.

The first step in building a coalition is to honestly assess subgroups in terms of how they will view the proposed change. Before embarking on a major change, consider the following questions carefully:

- Who will be most affected by the change?
- What benefits (for example, power) might these individuals perceive they will lose?
- Are their fears real? If so, what options are available to help overcome their fears?
- Does the change have the potential to create new benefits for these individuals?
- Can a negative reaction be avoided by engaging individuals or groups in the process?
- If you are not successful in getting them on your side, is their influence likely to be strong enough to derail the change plan?

Even when you are not successful in getting resisters on your side, you will have better information about the strength of their feelings and their resolve to oppose change. At the same time, you are working to diffuse potential resistance and to focus on building support for the change.

Create a Sense of Urgency

Kotter asserts that "by far the biggest mistake people make when trying to change organizations is to plunge ahead without establishing a high enough sense of urgency" (1995, pp. 59–67). Leaders may overestimate the extent to which they can force change on the organization.

To increase the sense of urgency, leaders must remove or minimize the sources of complacency. Some examples of how this might be done include:

- Engaging employees, customers, and coworkers in a dialogue about change through a series of meetings

- Convening a project steering committee with representatives from all stakeholder groups
- Identifying opinion leaders and securing their support early on
- Presenting believable stories or scenarios that illustrate the potential futures that might occur if action is not taken
- Creating new vehicles for communication, such as a project newsletter

Communicate, Communicate, Communicate

Communication is key to engaging others in the vision and change process. DePree sums it up by saying that "if you're a leader and you are not sick and tired of communicating you probably aren't doing a good enough job" (1992, p. 100).

A benchmarking study of how companies have successfully communicated change showed that communication is critical at three stages of the change process: as it is being planned, throughout implementation, and after it is complete (Powers 1997, pp. 30–33). Effective communication was shown to be critical at each stage, even to the point of releasing partial information when details are incomplete.

At the planning stage, leaders should communicate the need for change and the vision. Remember, if followers do not accept the vision, the rest of the change process is likely to be very rocky. Communicating results, even when they are incomplete, is an important reinforcement. It makes the change real and maintains the necessary momentum.

Communication is most effective if the message is tailored to the recipient. Identify needs and opportunities to customize your message to subgroups that have a particular set of issues. For example, the message to the medical staff will be different from the message to staff in health information services. Before implementing the use of report templates to expedite dictation, the manager may design a tactical plan that details all the elements of the communication plan for each of the constituent groups affected by, or with an interest in, the project.

The communication plan must offer groups the opportunity to "talk back." Kotter reminds us that the "downside of two-way communication is that feedback may suggest that you are on the wrong course and that the vision and plans need to be reformulated. But in the long run, swallowing your pride and reworking the vision and plan is far more productive than heading off in the wrong direction—or in a direction that others won't follow" (2002, p. 100).

Kotter also reminds us that communication comes in two forms—words and actions—and that the most effective communication is characterized by deeds. "Behavior from important people that is inconsistent with the vision overwhelms other forms of communication" (2002, p. 90). Leaders become the symbols for the change. Their motivations may be questioned and their actions scrutinized. Others will watch the leaders' actions for signals of commitment to the course of action and rightly insist on their integrity.

Ethics and integrity must be front and center all the time, but particularly during times of important change. At these times, the political, cultural, and technical systems are out of alignment. There is opportunity for events to take unexpected turns. Leaders' actions are closely scrutinized and their motives may be suspect.

How to Implement Strategic Change

Your vision and strategies are designed, the change management team is in place, and the guiding coalitions are organized. Now comes the hard work. Implementation requires all the managerial skills described in chapter 21, including planning, budgeting, monitoring, and producing results.

Create and Communicate Short-Term Wins

Major change takes time. Your vision may be compelling and your strategies right on target, but if short-term results cannot be demonstrated, you may lose support and the momentum for change may begin to erode. The best way to sustain your change effort is to sequence the implementation plan in such a way that short-term successes are clearly demonstrated and celebrated. For example, in implementing a new compliance plan, the data quality manager for a group practice reported statistics to the chiefs of service showing the monthly claims rejection rate. As this rate began to decline, the manager organized special events such as a dessert party and flowers for office managers at each improvement milestone. These touches garnered attention and maintained momentum for the project.

Deliberately seed your implementation plan with a number of short-term projects that have a high likelihood of success. This tactic enables the implementation team to work together to assess how much effort and how many resources will be required for later phases. It demonstrates that the program of planned change is real and not just talk. Moreover, it strengthens the courage and commitment of the leaders and the guiding coalitions.

Get new programs launched quickly by using techniques such as rapid prototyping, demonstration projects, or pilot tests. The details do not always need to be fully worked out to create visible demonstrations. You do not need to secure approval for full implementation as you are testing an approach to see its value. In test mode, all operational details do not need to be worked out before "going live." You need not anticipate all the intricacies up front; just begin the journey and adjust as you go. Prototyping and pilot tests also offer a way to show others how redesigned processes or new technology might work when it is fully implemented.

Pace and Refine Change Plans

Implementation requires managing interdependent projects at various stages of design, development, and deployment. One of the most difficult implementation challenges is deciding what phases should be advanced first and how fast or slow to move through them. Sequencing and pacing change requires thorough knowledge of your organization and its capacity for change. Again, consider all organizational components—cultural, political, and technical—and the available financial and managerial resources.

The higher the stakes, the more likely it is that a proposed change will be controversial. If the only viable approach is likely to meet with resistance, more time and effort are needed up front to gain acceptance before the approach is implemented. The importance of two-way communication throughout the process cannot be overemphasized.

The timing of change is critical. Change leaders can cite examples of projects that moved too quickly and projects that moved too slowly. Lawrence sums up this challenge: "I have become convinced that the real art of leadership lies in careful pacing. Pacing means moving simultaneously in a variety of areas and keeping each area progressing so that the combined cadence does not tear the organization apart. I'm positive that nobody gets timing 100 percent right. But the winners do it less wrong" (1998, pp. 291–308).

Implementation is a process of guiding, adjusting, and improving as you go. According to Walton, "Invariably, the organizational, strategic and leadership choices made during the earlier phases are only partially informed. As experience and events provide feedback to the organization, adjustments are almost always called for" (1998, pp. 347–66).

Implementing change is a highly iterative process. Expect that your plans and tactics will need to be modified as you gain experience. Create budgets and timetables that permit frequent course corrections.

Maintain Momentum and Stay the Course

Because leading change is a process of learning and adjusting, change leaders must learn to tolerate—and even enjoy—uncertainty. Change sponsors are eager to see their well-crafted strategies take hold and inevitably feel discour-

aged by a lengthy process. In addition to celebrating short-term wins, other ways to maintain momentum and keep moving include:

- Working quickly to resolve the thorny issues.
- Reiterating what will happen if change either does not occur or is watered down by compromise. If possible, focus on the consequences due to external trends.
- Keeping your eyes on the prize. Put every action in context. Regularly revisit the vision, goals, and strategies to regenerate a sense of purpose. Help others by making the goals as tangible as possible.
- Remembering that resistance to change is natural. Do not take it personally.
- Rethinking the tactics, sequence, and pace regularly to keep from getting bogged down. If you do get bogged down, institute some actions that will produce short-term gains. Keep moving.
- Maintaining the sense of urgency. Although you should celebrate short-term wins, do not let these celebrations mitigate the sense of urgency you have created. Also, do not let intermediate gains be mistaken for the bigger goals.

For maximum and sustained impact, the change you have introduced must become part of the fabric of your organization. It must become the way the organization operates, thinks, and behaves. At some point, it must become part of the culture. Even after change is implemented, there often continues to be a tug backward to the old reality. So strong is the effect of culture, leaders should be on the lookout for signs of slippage and for opportunities to reinforce the value of the new reality. To ensure that change is lasting and to prepare the organization for more change, leaders should:

- Quantify the impact, benefits, and value of the changes and use data to identify the direction for future change
- Continue intensive communication on issues facing HIM and the organization
- Integrate change competencies and behaviors into performance appraisal and management development programs
- Approach strategy, change, and organizational development as a continuous process

Measure Your Results

Environmental scanning was shown to be an important prerequisite to launching major change. It is also the way to measure the impact of change and to determine what further change is needed. Any time strategic change is undertaken, the measures by which its success will be judged should be made part of the performance measures data set. Environmental scanning must become a core competency of the organization and part of its routine work. It need not be an elaborate system, but it should be systematic and ongoing and it must include information on performance, trends, attitudes, and satisfaction.

Real-World Case

According to coverage in the *Journal of the American Health Information Management Association,* consumer-maintained or accessible personal health records is a trend that is gaining momentum and is an important component of the national health information strategy. Some healthcare systems already offer personal health record views into their electronic health record systems. As consumers become more knowledgeable about healthcare matters, they seek access to more information about their own and their family members' health and healthcare. The employer- and insurance-sponsored consumer-directed health plans also are encouraging patients to become more knowledgeable about health and healthcare.

This trend is expected to affect health information management as practitioners become not only patient advocates in the emerging e-world, but also knowledge and content experts. One of the experts interviewed by the journal described the impact of this trend on HIM as a "sea change." This is a way of describing a profound change from which there is no turning back. AHIMA now sponsors a consumer Web site, MyPHR.com, and a consumer education campaign.

Although great change is forecast, just what form it will take is not at all clear. This presents a real-life strategic challenge for HIM professionals who must consider plausible alternate futures when constructing visions and formulating strategies.

Summary

Health information management (HIM) is a dynamic profession that offers great opportunities to advance and contribute in a variety of important roles. Professional course work has required that you consider the attributes of a professional and the responsibilities of professionalism. You have learned about managing systems, resources, and people. This chapter has introduced you to the HIM professional as a strategic leader, a role that probably does not feel very comfortable to you now.

In truth, it will require experience to perfect the skills of strategic management and it will require a commitment to lifelong learning. One of the first ways to apply the lessons of this chapter is in evaluating your options for your first position as an HIM professional.

In the course of interviewing for positions, look closely at the organizational environment to identify evidence that constructive change is valued. What is the organization's strategic focus? Does its culture value idea sharing and innovation? What is the vision for HIM services? How is the political environment and how are decisions made? Are there any examples of change projects that have been very successful? Have any change projects failed? What lessons were learned from successful or failed projects?

Even seasoned managers are learning and improving their abilities every day. There is no such thing as a master manager who knows it all. What is important is to keep the lessons in mind as one gains experience and grows in confidence as a strategic manager. This chapter has explored the following five lessons (Bryson 1995, p. 225):

Lesson 1. Leading change is more than a process to be managed, it is a way of thinking and acting.

Managing change is a central strategic challenge for all organizations. The challenge may be even greater in healthcare organizations because their cultures tend to be averse to change and their governance structures and decision-making processes are more complicated than those of the typical business organization. Leading change requires a vision, and it often requires building new organizational capabilities, such as environmental scanning, creative group process, and a more external focus.

Lesson 2. Leading change must be approached as a central and fundamental role of all managers.

The best way to learn how to become more strategic is just to begin. Leading change requires creativity and imagination grounded in good information, managerial competence, and effective decision making. Do not expect to get it exactly right the first time, the second time, or any time. It is better to make mistakes than to take no risks. As lessons are learned, they should be chronicled so that the "learning loop" helps improve future decisions.

Lesson 3. Effective change happens only after others are engaged in a meaningful and personal way and earn their acceptance.

All change is ultimately about increasing effectiveness. To be successful, you must first understand what your "customers" want and need and how to deliver real value. This requires information and continuous two-way communication about issues, ideas, and trends. Acceptance for change strategies must be earned. Leaders must be politically savvy, learning to communicate the rationale for change, the expected results, and the consequences of nonaction. They must be sensitive to the fact that it takes time to disseminate a change message and for the message to be assimilated at a personal level. Change projects should move at a deliberate pace, but a pace that takes the needs of others into account.

Lesson 4. Successful organizations will have a bias for action because learning to lead change is a byproduct of leading change while knowing how to be successful

A bias for preserving the status quo is strong in most organizations. This must be replaced with a bias for action. Leading change is a learning process, and success increases the sense of possibility and the excitement to tackle the next challenge. Organizations that are on the move are energized, and this energy will be felt by their employees, coworkers, superiors, and customers. Learning to lead change is an essential skill in today's fast-paced world of work.

Lesson 5. There is great opportunity for HIM professionals who understand that leadership, change, and learning are intertwined.

Our society talks a lot about leadership, change, and learning. What is only now becoming clear is that these concepts are really intertwined. As Beer, Eisenstat, and others state, "One cannot contemplate dramatic change occurring within an organization without the exercise of some leadership. And the organization does not change fundamentally without significant reorientation and learning by its leaders and members. Without learning, the attitudes, skills, and behavior needed to formulate and implement a new strategic task will not develop" (1993, p. 217). The goal is to reorient your organization to value innovation and change. This takes time, perseverance, and courage. Nonetheless, this is the goal strategic managers should have for the organizations they are privileged to lead.

References

American Health Information Management Association. 2004 (June). Study: Employment of HIM professionals in the U.S.: Current patterns and future prospects. Chicago: AHIMA.

Beer, M., R.A. Eisenstat, et al. 1993. Why change programs don't produce change. In *The Learning Imperative: Managing People for Continuous Innovation,* edited by R. Howard. Boston: Harvard Business School Press.

Bryson, J.M. 1995. *Strategic Planning for Public and Nonprofit Organizations,* rev. ed. San Francisco: Jossey-Bass.

DePree, M. 1992. *Leadership Jazz.* New York: Dell Publishing.

Drucker, P. 1996. Not enough generals were killed. In *The Leader of the Future,* edited by F. Hesselbein and M. Goldsmith. San Francisco: Jossey-Bass.

Fuller, S.R., and J. Callahan Dennis. 2005 (July–August). Transcription's future(s): AAMT and AHIMA outline scenarios for the years ahead. *Journal of American Health Information Management Association* 76(7):48–51.

Gavetti, G., and J.W. Rivkin. 2005. How strategists really think: Tapping the power of analogy. *Harvard Business Review* 83(4):54–63.

Johns, M. 2000. A crystal ball for coding. *Journal of American Health Information Management Association* 71(1):26–33.

Kaplan, R.S., and D.P. Norton. 2004. *Strategy Maps: Converting Intangible Assets into Tangible Outcomes.* Boston: Harvard Business School Press.

Kolb, D.A. 1988. Integrity, advanced professional development, and learning. In *Executive Integrity,* edited by S. Srivastra. San Francisco: Jossey-Bass.

Kotter, J.P. 2002. *Heart of Change: Real-Life Stories of How People Change Their Organizations.* Boston: Harvard Business School Press.

Kotter, J.P. 1995. Leading change: why transformation efforts fail. *Harvard Business Review* 73(2):59–67.

Kouzes, J.M., and B.Z. Posner. 1995. *The Leadership Challenge: How to Keep Getting Extraordinary Things Done in Organizations.* San Francisco: Jossey-Bass.

Lawrence, D.M. 1998. Leading discontinuous change: Ten lessons from the battlefront. In *Navigating Change,* edited by D.C. Hambrick, D.A. Nadler, and M.L. Tushman. Boston: Harvard Business School Press.

Porter, M.E. 1996. What is strategy? *Harvard Business Review* 74(6):61–78.

Powers, V.J. 1997. Benchmarking study illustrates how best-in-class achieve alignment, communicate change. *Communication World* 14(2):30–33.

Schoemaker, P.J.H. 1993. Multiple scenario development: Its conceptual and behavioral foundation. *Strategic Management Journal* 14:193–213.

Tichy, N.M. 1983. *Managing Strategic Change: Technical, Political and Cultural Dynamics.* New York: John Wiley & Sons.

Walton, E. 1998. Senior leadership and discontinuous change. In *Navigating Change,* edited by D.C. Hambrick, D.A. Nadler, and M.L. Tushman. Boston: Harvard Business School Press.

Appendices, Glossary, and Index

Appendix A
Sample Documentation Forms

Figure A.1a.   Admission record (Face Sheet) in paper format

University of Anystate Hospitals

ADMISSION RECORD

PATIENT LABEL

	Health Record #	Admission Date/Time	Discharge Date/Time	Service	Station	Room #	Patient Type	Financial Class.	BL/Account #

Patient

Location(s)					Language	Sex	Race	Marital Status	Date of Birth	Age

| Patient Name and Address | SSN

Primary Telephone # | Patient Employer | Telephone # |
|---|---|---|---|

Employers

Guarantor

| Guarantor Name and Address | SSN

Relationship | Guarantor Employer | Telephone # |
|---|---|---|---|

Insurance

Insurance 1	Insurance 2

Miscellaneous

Emergency Contact	Spouse
Home: Work:	Home: Work:

Admission Dx/Presenting Complaint	Arrival Mode	Admission Type/Source

Admitting Physician	Attending Physician	Referring Physician	Primary Care Physician

Alerts	Previous Admission Date

For Emergency Department Use Only
Allergies   LMP   T   R   P   BP   Time   Signature

Diagnoses/Procedures	DRG/Code(s)
Principal Diagnosis:	
Other Diagnoses:	
Principal Operation/Procedure:	
Other Operation(s)/Procedure(s):	

Physician Signature: _____   Date: _____

ADMISSION RECORD
000001 (11/2002)

Figure A.1b.   Admission record in electronic format

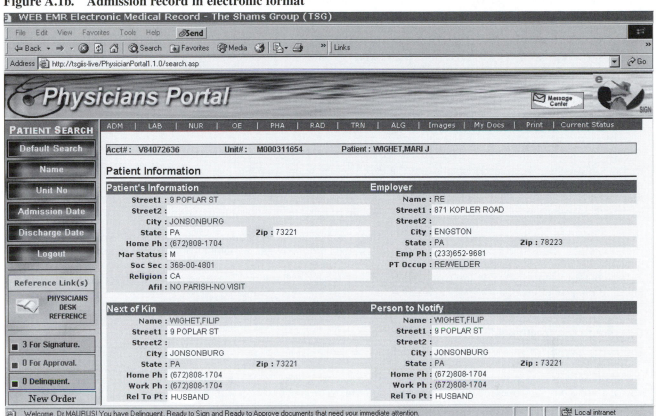

Figure A.2. Combined consent to treatment and consent to the use and disclosure of protected health information

---

University of Anystate Hospitals

**CONSENT FOR TREATMENT AND DISCLOSURE
OF PROTECTED HEALTH INFORMATION**
PAGE 1 OF 2

PATIENT LABEL

To the Patient (or his/her parent, guardian, or legal representative):

Before University of Anystate Hospitals and Clinics or any of its departments can provide inpatient or outpatient services to you, you will need to understand the services you are to receive, give the hospital your consent to perform those services, and agree to pay for them. You will also need to understand the ways the hospital uses the information in your health record and agree to allow the hospital to use that information.

Part I of this form covers your consent to treatment and explains other important matters related to your healthcare. Part II explains the use of your personal health information. You may ask a member of the admissions staff to read this form to you, and we encourage you to ask any questions you may have about it. When you fully understand the form's content, please sign it in the place indicated on the back of the form. Thank you very much for helping us to fulfill the hospital's responsibility to you and the rest of the community we serve.

Part I: Treatment-Related Information

Consent to the Treatment

You authorize your physician and/or other qualified medical providers to perform medical treatments and services on your behalf. You also consent to all of the hospital medical and/or diagnostic services ordered for you during your outpatient visit or inpatient stay in the hospital. This consent includes testing for infections such as hepatitis B and HIV and providing blood or body fluids for such tests in order to protect you and/or those who care for you.

Payment for Services and Insurance

You are directly responsible for paying for the services provided during your hospital visit or stay. The hospital will work directly with the third parties who provide coverage of your medical expenses, including health insurance companies, Medicare, Medicaid, Workers' Compensation, and various types of liability, accident, and disability insurance providers. By signing this form, you attest that your insurance coverage is current, valid, and effective and that you will promptly pay any required copayment amounts and unpaid deductibles. If your stay qualifies for Medicare coverage, the benefits you will receive include coverage for the physician services that were performed as part of your hospital care.

You guarantee payment to the hospital for all noncovered services and any unpaid, billed amounts not covered by insurance benefits when your insurance plan allows the hospital to bill you for any unpaid balances. You understand and accept that your physician's orders may include services not paid by insurance plans but will be provided to you by the hospital. Also, you accept that insurance plans may deny payment for what you believed were covered services, resulting in your responsibility for paying for these services. You may be billed for the professional component of any hospital services, such as the professional component for clinical laboratory tests.

Valuables

You accept full responsibility for your valuables, especially money or jewelry. The hospital does not accept any liability for your valuables. The hospital expects you will entrust any valuables to family or friends for safekeeping. Alternatively, you may deposit them in the safe that the hospital provides for that purpose. This is especially important when you are an inpatient, but this responsibility also extends to when you are an outpatient and must change into a hospital gown, remove jewelry, or undergo sedation during a medical procedure.

Special Note for Medicare or CHAMPUS Beneficiaries

You acknowledge and certify by your signature that all of the information you have provided to the hospital for Medicare or CHAMPUS benefits is correct. You also agree to allow the hospital or others who have information on your Medicare or CHAMPUS benefits claim to provide this information to Medicare or CHAMPUS or their agents in order for them to determine your eligibility for benefits. To carry out this activity, the hospital may use a copy rather than the original of this consent form. You also acknowledge that you have received a copy of the *Important Message from Medicare* or the *Important Message from CHAMPUS* form. This acknowledgement does not waive your rights for a review or make you liable for payment.

Figure A.2.   (Continued)

University of Anystate Hospitals

**CONSENT FOR TREATMENT AND DISCLOSURE
OF PROTECTED HEALTH INFORMATION**
PAGE 2 OF 2

PATIENT LABEL

Part II: Health Record-Related Information

Consent to the Use and Disclosure of Protected Health Information

You agree to honestly, completely, and correctly provide all requested information. You also agree to permit the hospital to share your health record as applicable under the law with your physician, your insurers, Medicare, Medicaid, or their designated agents. They may review your record and copy it in full or in part in order to obtain billing and payment information. Insurers (private or government) may also use your health record to determine whether they cover your services. You agree to allow the hospital to use the record created during this visit to meet any reporting requirements related to your care and to collect payment for the services you received. You agree to allow your physicians to send copies of your health records to other physicians, hospitals, and healthcare facilities as they deem necessary for continuity of care. You also agree to have your name posted on scheduling boards and outside your hospital room.

Specific Uses of Your Protected Information

The hospital originates and maintains health records describing your health history, symptoms, examination and test results, diagnoses, treatment, and any plans for future care or treatment. This information serves as:

- The basis of care planning and treatment

- A means of communication among the many healthcare professionals who contribute to your care

- A source of information for applying diagnosis and surgical information to your bill

- A means by which a third-party payer (usually your insurance company or a government healthcare program) can verify that the services billed were actually provided

- A tool for routine healthcare operations, such as assessing quality and reviewing the competence of healthcare professionals

Your signature acknowledges that you received the *Notice of Information Practices,* which provides a description of information uses and disclosure practices. You accept and understand that:

- You have the right to review the notice prior to signing this consent.

- The hospital reserves the right to change the notice and its information practices, for past, current, or future information. The new notice will contain the effective date on its first page and be made available on our Web site.

- You have the right to object to the use of your health information for the hospital's patient directory.

- You have the right to request restrictions on the use or disclosure of your health information to carry out treatment, payment, or healthcare operations and to correct error(s) in your record. The hospital, however, is not required to agree to the restrictions requested.

- You may revoke in writing the consent that you provide to the hospital. The revocation does not apply to any uses of your information made by the hospital in reliance upon this consent form and on the belief that your consent was still effective.

I certify that I have read (or had read to me) both parts of this form and fully understand and agree to the content.

Patient/Agent: _____   Date: _____

If you are signing as the patient's agent, please state your relationship to the patient (parent, guardian, or legal representative): _____

Witness (when form is accepted verbally,
by telephone, or by electronic means): _____   Date: _____

CONSENT FOR TREATMENT AND DISCLOSURE
000002 (11/2002)

Figure A.3. Acknowledgment of notice of privacy practices

Anytown Community Hospital

**ACKNOWLEDGMENT OF NOTICE
OF PRIVACY PRACTICES**

PATIENT LABEL

I understand that as part of my healthcare, this organization originates and maintains health records describing my health history, symptoms, examination and test results, diagnoses, treatment, and any plans for future care or treatment. I understand that this information serves as:

• A basis for planning my care and treatment

• A means of communication among the many health professionals who contribute to my care

• A source of information for applying my diagnosis and surgical information to my bill

• A means by which a third-party payer can verify that services billed were actually provided

• And a tool for routine healthcare operations such as assessing quality and reviewing the competence of healthcare professionals

I understand and have been provided with a *Notice of Information Practices* that provides a more complete description of information uses and disclosures. I understand that I have the right to review the notice prior to signing this consent. I understand that the organization reserves the right to change their notice and practices and prior to implementation will mail a copy of any revised notice to the address I've provided. I understand that I have the right to object to the use of my health information for directory purposes. I understand that I have the right to request restrictions as to how my health information may be used or disclosed to carry out treatment, payment, or healthcare operations and that the organization is not required to agree to the restrictions requested. I understand that I may revoke this consent in writing, except to the extent that the organization has already take action in reliance thereon.

☐ I request the following restrictions to the use or disclosure of my health information:

_____

_____

_____
Signature of Patient or Legal Representative   Date

_____
Witness   Date

_____
Notice Effective Date or Version

☐ Accepted   ☐ Denied

_____   _____ _____
            Signature   Title   Date

ACKNOWLEDGMENT OF PRIVACY NOTICE
100093 (1/2002)

Figure A.4.   Discharge order in paper format

University of Anystate Hospitals

PHYSICIAN ORDERS

PATIENT, PETUNIA P.
000000001
DOB: 08/14/1949

Drug Allergies: *Codeine*

Date/Time	RN Signature	Physician Order/Physician Signature
10/11/04 **6:00 a.m.**	**Claire Barton, RN**	*(1) Admit via surgery (2) NPO* *(3) CBC, urinalysis (4) BCP 8* *(5) Prothrombin time, PTT (6) Type and screen* *(7) PA chest X-ray* *(8) EKG* *(9) Prep abdomen* *(10) Start IV fluids: 1000 cc D5LR at 125 cc/h via 18g Jelco* *(11) Mefoxin 2 g IV at 7:45 a.m.* Myron P Gynsurg MD 10/11/04
10/11/04 **10:00 a.m.**	**Claire Barton, RN**	*(12) Morphine sulfate 2 mg PCA IV RR q.1.0–1.5.h.* *(13) Mefoxin 2 g IV in 8 h then discontinue* *(14) D5LR 1000 cc at 125 cc/h (15) Liquid diet* *(16) Bed rest* *(17) Vital signs every 4 h* Myron P Gynsurg MD 10/11/04
10/11/04 2:00 p.m.	Nancy Nurse, RN	Telephone order from Dr. Gynesurg: (18) Morphine sulfate 2 mg IV push Myron P Gynsurg MD 10/12/04
10/11/04 3:00 p.m.	Nancy Nurse, RN	Telephone order from Dr. Gynesurg: (19) Temporarily discontinue PCA pump until vital signs return to normal (20) Vital signs every hour Myron P Gynsurg MD 10/12/04
10/12/04 12:05 p.m.	Nancy Nurse, RN	(21) Remove Foley (22) Begin to ambulate (23) Soft diet (24) Vital signs every 4 h Myron P Gynsurg MD 10/12/04
10/13/04 12:15 p.m.	Nancy Nurse, RN	(25) Discontinue morphine (26) Darvacet-N 100 mg, one or two tablets q.4h. as needed for pain (27) Solid diet Myron P Gynsurg MD 10/13/04
10/14/04 8:00 a.m.	Nancy Nurse, RN	(28) Discontinue IVs (29) Discharge to home—see discharge instruction sheet Myron P Gynsurg MD 10/14/04

PHYSICIAN ORDERS
000010 (11/2002)

Figure A.5.   Obstetric admission record in paper format

Anytown Community Hospital

OBSTETRIC ADMITTING RECORD
PAGE 1 OF 2

PATIENT LABEL

Admission Date ____ / ____ / ____   Time_____
☐ Ambulatory   ☐ Stretcher   ☐ Oriented to Unit
☐ Wheelchair   ☐ Transfer from _____   ☐ Safety/Security

G	T	Pt	A	L	LMP	EDD	Weeks
					/ /	/ /	
					EDD by Fetal Assessment / /		

Race/Ethnicity _____ Age _____
Advance Directives ☐ None ☐ Living Will
                    ☐ Medical Power of Attorney
Organ Donor ☐ Yes ☐ No
Pain ☐ No ☐ Yes (site: _____)
      Intensity   0 _____10
                   None   Highest
Last Oral Intake
      Fluids ____ / ____ / ____ Time _____
      Solids ____ / ____ / ____ Time _____

Allergy/Sensitivity ☐ None ☐ Latex
☐ Other: _____

Reasons for Admission
☐ Onset of Labor
☐ Induction of Labor
☐ Spontaneous Abortion
☐ Cesarean Section
   ☐ Primary ☐ Repeat
   (Reason for primary: _____)
☐ Tubal Ligation
☐ Vaginal Bleeding
☐ ROM ☐ Premature ☐ Prolonged
☐ Preterm Labor
Reasons for Admission: _____
_____

Observation Evaluation
☐ Fetal Status
☐ Ultrasound
☐ Amniocentesis
☐ NST ☐ CST
☐ Medical Complications
_____
☐ Obstetric Complications
_____

Medications ☐ None
Type/Dose   Last Taken   With Patient   Disposition
                                   No   Yes
_____   _____   ☐   ☐   _____
_____   _____   ☐   ☐   _____
_____   _____   ☐   ☐   _____

MD/CDM   Phone # | Support Person/Relationship Phone #:

| Personal Effects | | Disposition | | |
Item	With Patient	With Support Person	Other (Describe)

Patient Triage Data
Contractions ☐ None ☐ Palpation ☐ Tocotransducer
Frequency _____ Duration _____ Intensity _____
Began on ____ / ____ / ____ Time_____
Pain intensity   0 _____10
                 None   Highest
Membranes ☐ Intact ☐ Bulging
               ☐ Ruptured (date ____ / ____ / ____ Time _____)
               ☐ Nitrazine test   ☐ pos ☐ neg   ☐ Sterile speculum exam
               ☐ Fern test   ☐ pos ☐ neg   (findings: _____)

Fluid ☐ Clear ☐ Bloody ☐ Meconium stained
           ☐ Foul odor ☐ No foul odor ☐ None observed
Vaginal Bleeding ☐ None ☐ Normal show
                      ☐ Bleeding (describe: _____)
Cervical Exam By: _____
    Station _____ Effacement_____ Dilatation _____cm
    Presentation ☐ Vertex   ☐ Transverse lie
                  ☐ Face/brow   ☐ Compound
                  ☐ Breech   ☐ Unknown
                  (type: _____)

Physical Assessment

Height	Weight Pregrav/Grav	T	P	R	BP

Detail Abnormal Findings

System	Normal	Abnormal		Normal	Abnormal
HEENT	☐	☐	Respiratory	☐	☐
Neurologic	☐	☐	Abdomen	☐	☐
Skin	☐	☐	Gastrointestinal	☐	☐
Breasts	☐	☐	Urinary	☐	☐
Extremities	☐	☐	Genitalia	☐	☐
Cardiovascular	☐	☐			

Initial Problems Identified ☐ None   Plan
1. _____
2. _____
3. _____

Fetal Evaluation Data   Multiple Gestation ☐ No ☐ Yes
Fundal Height _____ cm
Fetal Weight (est.) _____   Presentation   Position
FHR _____   1. _____   _____
☐ Fetoscope ☐ Fetal Monitor   2. _____   _____
☐ Doppler   ☐ Other: _____   3. _____   _____

Specimens Obtained (Check all that apply)

Urine Test	Time	Results	Blood Test	Time	Results
☐ Urinalysis			☐ Hgb		
☐ C+S			☐ Hct		
☐ Glucose			☐ VDRL/RPR		
☐ Albumin			☐ Type/Screen		
☐ Ketones			☐		
☐ pH			Cervical Culture		
☐ Blood			☐ GBS		
☐ Toxicology			☐		
Admitting Signature	Date/Time		Examiner Signature		Date/Time

Figure A.5.   (Continued)

Anytown Community Hospital

OBSTETRIC ADMITTING RECORD
PAGE 2 OF 2

PATIENT LABEL

Significant Prenatal Data

Prenatal Records Available on Admission

☐ No ☐ Yes Source _____

First Visit by 13 Weeks ☐ Yes ☐ No

Regular Care ☐ Yes ☐ No

Prenatal Classes ☐ Yes ☐ No

Pediatric Provider

General Health ☐ Healthy

☐ Functional Deficit (Type_____)

☐ Recent Exposure to Communicable Disease

   Type/Date _____ ____ / ____ / ____

   ☐ Illness (≤14 days prior to admission)

   Type/Treatment _____

☐ Chronic Condition _____

Nutritional Status ☐ Well-nourished ☐ Malnourished ☐ Obese

☐ Special Diet _____

Eating Disorder ☐ None ☐ Identify _____

Nutritional Problems ☐ None ☐ Identify _____

Lab Findings

☐ None

Blood Type
& Rh _____

Rubella
Titer _____

Serology _____

HBsAg _____

HIV _____

GBS _____

_____ _____

Fetal Assessment Tests

☐ None

Date	Test	Result
/		
/		
/		
/		

Hospitalizations ☐ None

1. ___/___/___ Reason _____

2. ___/___/___ Reason _____

Plans for Birth and Hospital Stay ☐ Birth Plan Attached

Support Person Present in L&D ☐ No ☐ Yes _____

Other Family Members in L&D ☐ No ☐ Yes _____

Anesthesia ☐ None ☐ Local ☐ Epidural ☐ Spinal ☐ General

Delivery Site/Position _____

Personal Requests _____

Adoption ☐ No ☐ Yes Contact with Infant ☐ No ☐ Yes

Adoption Contact _____

Feeding Preference ☐ Breast ☐ Bottle

☐ Tubal Ligation Authorization Signed ☐ Yes ☐ No

☐ Circumcision Authorization Signed ☐ Yes ☐ No

Problems Identified ☐ None

	Active	Resolved
1. _____	☐	☐
2. _____	☐	☐
3. _____	☐	☐
4. _____	☐	☐

Psychosocial Data ☐ See Prenatal Records

Emotional Status ☐ Happy ☐ Ambivalent ☐ Concerned

☐ Depressed ☐ Angry ☐ Other _____

Communication Barriers ☐ None

☐ Language ☐ Interpreter _____

☐ Vision ☐ Reading ☐ Writing ☐ Hearing

☐ Speech ☐ Other _____

Support System

Marital Status S M Sep D W Father involved ☐ Yes ☐ No

Other Support ☐ None ☐ _____

Occupation _____

Religion ☐ N/A ☐ _____

Personal/Cultural/Religious Customs Affecting Care and/or Learning

☐ None ☐ Identify _____

_____

Basic Needs Met   Yes No   If No, Explain

Food ☐ ☐

Clothing ☐ ☐

Housing ☐ ☐

Transportation ☐ ☐

Finances ☐ ☐

Life Stress	No	Yes	If Yes, Explain
Physical Abuse	☐	☐	
Emotional Abuse	☐	☐	
Major Change	☐	☐	
Self-Care Needs	☐	☐	
Serious Illness	☐	☐	
Other _____	☐	☐	

Substance Abuse	No	Yes	If Yes, Amount/Day, Last Use
Tobacco	☐	☐	_____
Alcohol	☐	☐	_____
Prescribed Drugs	☐	☐	_____
Illicit Drugs	☐	☐	_____

Educational Needs	Mother	Support Person	Comments
Stages/Phases of Labor	☐	☐	
Coping Techniques	☐	☐	
Infant Feeding	☐	☐	
Infant Care	☐	☐	
Other _____	☐		

Preferred Learning Methods	Yes	No
One-on-One Instruction	☐	☐
Group Instruction	☐	☐
Written Information	☐	☐
Audio/Visual Information	☐	☐
Demonstration/Practice	☐	☐

Discharge Planning Data   Planned Length of Stay _____ Days

Home Setting

	Yes	No
Heat, running water, refrigeration	☐	☐
Infant Care Supplies/Car Seat	☐	☐
Phone in home	☐	☐
Transportation available	☐	☐
Adult assistance available	☐	☐

Referrals

☐ RN Case Manager ☐ Utilization Review ☐ Other _____

☐ Home Care RN ☐ Social Service

☐ Nutritionist/Dietitian ☐ Pediatric Provider

MD/CNM

Notified by _____ Date/Time _____

Admitting

Signature _____ Date/Time _____

OBSTETRIC ADMITTING RECORD
200305 (06/2003)

Figure A.6. Consultation report

Anytown Community Hospital

CONSULTATION REPORT
PAGE 1 OF 2

PATIENT, BLUTO P.
070095111
DOB: 04/01/1930

I was asked by Dr. Doctor to evaluate Mr. Patient for consideration of left VATS talc pleurodesis.

CHIEF COMPLAINT: Shortness of breath

HISTORY OF PRESENT ILLNESS: Mr. Patient is a 73-year-old male who has a history of metastatic pancreatic cancer. He was found to have left pleural effusion and underwent thoracentesis. He returned with a recurrent effusion. He was admitted on 05/12/2003 and underwent left chest tube thoracostomy and an attempt at talc pleurodesis through the chest tube. He has had residual pneumothorax and continues to drain from the left chest tube. He was referred for the purpose of left VATS talc pleurodesis.

PAST SURGICAL HISTORY: His past surgical history is remarkable for Whipple procedure.

PAST MEDICAL HISTORY: His past medical history is remarkable for prostate cancer and pancreatic cancer.

MEDICATIONS: Avalide and pancrease

ALLERGIES: He has no known drug allergies.

FAMILY/SOCIAL HISTORY: Remarkable for being married. He drinks socially.

REVIEW OF SYSTEMS: Remarkable for no history of seizure or stroke, no history of previous pneumonia, no history of previous myocardial infarction, no history of previous liver failure, renal failure. He has had no swelling in his legs.

PHYSICAL EXAMINATION: He is 5 feet 6 inches tall. He weighs 158 pounds. His blood pressure is 126/70. His pulse is 62. His respiratory rate is 20. His temperature is 97.1. His neurological exam is remarkable for a normal affect. He is oriented × 3. His gross motor examination is 5/5 in all four extremities. His head and neck exam is remarkable for no icteric sclerae. He has no oral lesions. His neck demonstrates no cervical or supraclavicular adenopathy. He has no carotid bruits. His chest exam is remarkable for no use of accessory muscles, no dullness to percussion. He has a left chest tube in place with no air leak. He has serous-appearing drainage from his left chest tube. His breath sounds are remarkable for a slight decrease in breath sounds in the left lateral lung. His cardiovascular exam is remarkable for no lift, heave, or thrill. He has a normal S1, S2 without murmurs. Abdomen is remarkable for well-healed Whipple incision. His abdomen is nontender, nondistended without evidence of masses or organomegaly. His extremities are without clubbing, cyanosis, or edema.

His chest CT shows a loculated left pneumothorax with small residual effusion. He has chest tube in place. This is a small caliber tube. His chest X ray shows loculated left pneumothorax.

Figure A.6. (Continued)

Anytown Community Hospital **CONSULTATION REPORT** PAGE 2 OF 2	PATIENT, BLUTO P. 070095111 DOB: 04/01/1930

His laboratory studies are further remarkable for urinalysis that is normal, an EKG that is normal sinus rhythm, sodium of 133, potassium 3.8, chloride 95, BUN 19, creatinine 1.1, PPTT of 11.8, INR of 0.9, PTT of 29.

My impression is that Mr. Patient is a 73-year-old male with metastatic pancreatic cancer status post Whipple. He has a recurrent left pleural effusion. He has undergone previous tube thoracostomy and pleurodesis and now has a residual left pneumothorax and residual chest tube drainage from his malignant effusion.

I have recommended to Mr. Patient that we proceed with left VATS talc pleurodesis today. He understands that his risks include, but are not limited to, death (1–2%), bleeding requiring blood transfusion, infection, prolonged air leak from the cut surface of his lung, and a 30% chance of recurrent effusion. Understanding these risks as well as the alternative of continued drainage, he wishes to proceed today with left VATS talc pleurodesis.

Thank you very much for allowing me to participate in his care.

Signature:

James W. Medman, MD

Date: 5/17/03

d: 05/17/2003
t: 05/20/2003
JWM, MD/mc

Figure A.7.   Initial nursing assessment

Midwest Medical Center

INITIAL NURSING ASSESSMENT

PATIENT LABEL

Baseline Information

| Date: | Time: | Age: | Arrived: AMB   WC   Stretcher   EMS   Carried   Other: | Primary MD: |

Initial/Chief Complaint/History of Present Illness:

| T:
PO   R   TM | P: | R: | BP: R   L | ⊕ O₂
Sats   % | Sex:
M   F | Height: | Weight: Actual:
Stated: |

⊕ Tetanus/Immunizations: | Pneumococcal Vaccine ☐ No   ☐ Yes   Most Recent Date:

⊕ Pregnant   ☐ No   ☐ Yes   LNMP: | Influenza Vaccine   ☐ No   ☐ Yes   Most Recent Date:

Allergies: ☐ None   ☐ Medications   ☐ Latex   ☐ Food   ☐ Anesthesia   ☐ Other

List Names and Reactions:

TB Assessment (Initiate airborne isolation if 4 or more criteria are checked yes)

Persistent Cough > 2 weeks ☐ No ☐ Yes	Abnormal Chest X-Ray	☐ No ☐ Yes	Respiratory Isolation
Fever > 100.4 (night sweats) ☐ No ☐ Yes	Physician Order for AFB (smear/culture)	☐ No ☐ Yes	Ordered ☐ No ☐ Yes
Unexplained Weight Loss ☐ No ☐ Yes	Recent Exposure to Person with Suspected TB or +PPD	☐ No ☐ Yes	

RN/LPN Signature: _____

☐ See Home Medication Orders   Medication/Over the Counter/Herbal History   ☐ Investigation Drugs/Devices

Medication	Dose	Freq	Last Dose	Medication	Dose	Freq	Last Dose

Hospitalizations/Surgeries:

Medical History

Neurological	☐ No	☐ Yes		Sensory Impairment	☐ No	☐ Yes	
Cardiovascular	☐ No	☐ Yes		Endocrine	☐ No	☐ Yes	
Hypertension	☐ No	☐ Yes		Blood Disorder	☐ No	☐ Yes	
Respiratory	☐ No	☐ Yes		Cancer	☐ No	☐ Yes	
Gastrointestinal	☐ No	☐ Yes		Psychological	☐ No	☐ Yes	
Renal/Urological	☐ No	☐ Yes		Tobacco Use	☐ No	☐ Yes	
Gynecological	☐ No	☐ Yes		Alcohol/Drug Use	☐ No	☐ Yes	
Musculoskeletal	☐ No	☐ Yes		Infectious Disease	☐ No	☐ Yes	
Integumentary	☐ No	☐ Yes		Cough/Cold Past 2 Weeks	☐ No	☐ Yes	
EENT	☐ No	☐ Yes		Anesthesia	☐ No	☐ Yes	

Source of Information   ☐ Patient   ☐ Family   ☐ Unable to Obtain   ☐ Other   ☐ Medications Sent Home with Patient: _____

| Arrival Date: | Arrival Time: | T:
PO   R   TM | P: | R: | BP: R   L | O₂ Sats   %:
(If applicable) |

RN Initial: _____ **RN Signature:** _____ **Date:** _____ **Time:** _____ **Unit:** _____

RN Initial: _____ **RN Signature:** _____ **Date:** _____ **Time:** _____ **Unit:** _____

INITIAL NURSING ASSESSMENT
000039 (10/2002)

Figure A.8.   Patient care plan

University of Anystate Hospital

PATIENT CARE PLAN
PAGE 1 OF 2

PATIENT LABEL

Admitting Physician:

Admission Date: | Diagnosis: | Isolation:

Operative/Special Procedures: | Date: | Allergies:

Vital Signs	**Activity**	**Bladder/Bowel**	**Treatments**
☐ TPR _____	☐ Bedrest _____	**Bladder:**	☐ S&A _____
☐ BP _____	☐ BRP _____	☐ Strain Urine	☐ Self _____
☐ Neuro checks _____	☐ Up in Chair _____	☐ Check Voiding _____	☐ NG _____
☐ Circ. checks _____	☐ Ambulate _____	☐ Cath PRN _____	☐ Gomco _____
☐ Weight _____		☐ Foley Cath	☐ Clamp _____
☐ Telemetry _____	☐ Up Ad Lib _____	☐ Date Inserted_____	☐ Irrigate _____
☐ Transport S Tele _____	☐ Head of Bed _____	☐ S.P. Cath	☐ Chest Tube _____
Diet and Fluids	☐ Foot of Bed_____	☐ Condom Cath	☐ Wound _____
Diet:	☐ TCDB _____	☐ Irrigate Cath q. ___ h.	
☐ NPO _____	☐ Leg Exercises_____	with: _____	☐ Others: _____
☐ Regular _____	☐ Others_____	☐ Bladder Irrigation _____	
☐ Other _____		☐ IDEO Conduit_____	**Respiratory**
☐ Snack _____	**Hygiene**	☐ Incontinent _____	☐ Ventilator _____
☐ Tube Feedings _____	☐ Self	**Bowel:**	
☐ Supplemental _____	☐ Assist	☐ Check BMs _____	☐ O₂
☐ Restrict _____	☐ Complete	☐ Suppository _____	☐ Mask
☐ Force _____	☐ Tub/Shower		☐ Nasal Cannula
☐ Ice Chips _____	☐ Mouth/Denture Care	☐ Enema _____	☐ AMT
Fluids:		☐ Ostomy _____	☐ Suction
☐ Intake _____	☐ Shampoo _____	☐ Incontinent _____	☐ Triflow
☐ Output_____	☐ Skin Care _____	☐ Others _____	☐ IPPB/HHN _____
☐ Others_____	☐ Others_____		☐ Others _____

Tube Feeding

Type of Tube	Type and Strength of Feeding	Rate	Count	Irrigation	Bag ▲

Safety Measures

☐ Siderails
  ☐ Upper _____
  ☐ Lower _____
☐ Restraints
☐ Seizure Precautions
☐ High Risk for Falls
☐ Self-Injury Precautions

IV Therapies

#	Solution	Additives	Rate	Count

Site Care/Tubing Change

Start/Date				
Type/Size				

Blood Transfusions

Figure A.8.   (Continued)

University of Anystate Hospital

PATIENT CARE PLAN
PAGE 2 OF 2

PATIENT LABEL

Date	Daily Lab Work	Date	Lab Work	Date	X-Ray/Special Procedures

Date	Preps for Procedures

Special Equipment	Miscellaneous
☐ Traction _____	
☐ Trapeze _____	
☐ _____ Bed	
☐ _____ Mattress	
☐ Sheepskin	
☐ Crutches	
☐ Walker	
☐ Teds	
☐ Others _____	
_____	
Therapies	
☐ Physical _____	
☐ Speech _____	
☐ OT _____	
Transportation	
☐ Wheelchair	
☐ Stretcher	
☐ Ambulatory	
☐ Bed	
Consultations	
_____	
_____	
_____	

PATIENT CARE PLAN
000072 (10/2002)

Figure A.9.   Clinical pathway

University of Anystate Hospitals

CLINICAL PATHWAY:
CESAREAN SECTION DELIVERY
PAGE 1 OF 3

This document should be considered a *guideline.* Outcomes will vary depending on the patient's severity of illness and other factors/conditions that affect or alter expected outcomes.

Key: Fill in appropriate location for nursing unit. Initial completed intermediate and discharge outcomes. Circle any variances and document on variance log. Once variance is resolved, date and inital clinical pathway.

Expected Discharge Outcomes	Preop Date _____ Time _____	Operative/Recovery Date _____ Time _____
	Nursing Unit _____	Nursing Unit _____

Cardiovascular
• Hemodynamically stable
• Chest clear to auscultation bilaterally
	Stable BP (< 140/90 or no increases
	  > 30 mm systolic or
	  > 15 mm diastolic) _____
	Chest clear _____
		Stable BP (< 140/90 or no increases
		  > 30 mm systolic or
		  > 15 mm diastolic) _____

Gastrointestinal • Bowel sounds present • Tolerates regular diet • Passing flatus	NPO	
Genitourinary • Normal bladder function		Foley patent, draining clear yellow urine _____ UOP ≥ 30 cc/h _____

Reproductive
• Delivery of well newborn
• Involution progressing
• Minimal physical discomfort
• Breast: Skin and nipples intact
	Adequate prenatal care _____
	Reassuring father _____
	No signs/symptoms of
	  uterine/vaginal bleeding _____
		Fundus firm, lochia small
		  to moderate _____
		Pain control initiated _____
		EBL ≤ 1000 cc _____
		Delivery of well newborn _____

Integumentary • Incision intact with evidence of healing • No signs/symptoms of infection		Abdominal dressing dry and intact _____
Psychosocial • Patient/family demonstrates adjustment to parental role		

Education
• Patient/family able to identify problems
  that require immediate medical attention
• Patient/family able to verbalize under-
  standing of care needs (wound, etc.)
	States/understands
	plan of care _____	

Discharge Planning
• Patient/family able to verbalize support
  system(s) and/or support system for
  home care established
• Patient/family able to manage
  continuing care needs
• Patient discharged
	Patient/family identifies
	support system
	for home care _____	

Date	Initials	Signature	Date	Initials	Signature	Date	Initials	Signature

Figure A.9.   (Continued)

University of Anystate Hospitals

CLINICAL PATHWAY:
CESAREAN SECTION DELIVERY
PAGE 2 OF 3

PATIENT LABEL

This document should be considered a *guideline*. Outcomes will vary depending on the patient's severity of illness and other factors/conditions that affect or alter expected outcomes.

Key: Fill in appropriate location for nursing unit. Initial completed intermediate and discharge outcomes. Circle any variances and document on variance log. Once variance is resolved, date and inital clinical pathway.

Expected Discharge Outcomes	Postoperative Day Date _____ Time _____	Postop Day #1 Date _____ Time _____
	Nursing Unit _____	Nursing Unit _____
Cardiovascular • Hemodynamically stable	Able to turn, cough, and deep-breathe every 2 h _____ Chest clear _____	Ambulates with assistance _____ Chest clear _____
Gastrointestinal • Bowel sounds present • Tolerates regular diet • Passing flatus	Tolerates clear liquids, no nausea or vomiting _____	Bowel sounds present _____ Tolerates regular diet _____
Genitourinary • Normal bladder function	Foley patent, draining clear yellow urine _____ UOP > 240 cc/8 h _____	Normal bladder function _____ UOP < 240 cc/8 h _____

Reproductive
• Delivery of well newborn
• Involution progressing
• Minimal physical discomfort
• Breast: Skin and nipples intact
	Fundus firm, lochia small
	   to moderate _____
	Pain controlled _____
		Fundus firm, lochia small
		   to moderate _____
		Pain controlled _____

Integumentary
• Incision intact with evidence of healing
• No signs/symptoms of infection
	Abdominal dressing dry
	   and intact _____
	Afebrile (<100.4ºF) _____
		Wound edges approximated,
		   no signs/symptoms
		   of infection _____
		Afebrile (<100.4ºF)

Psychosocial
• Patient/family demonstrate adjustment
   to parental role
	Demonstrates appropriate
	   parent/infant interaction _____
		Demonstrates appropriate
		   parental/infant interaction_____

Education
• Patient/family able to identify problems
   that require immediate medical attention
• Patient/family able to verbalize under-
   standing of care needs (wound, etc.)
	States/understands postop
	   plan of care _____
	Initiates breast-feeding _____
		Establishes infant feeding _____

Discharge Planning
• Patient/family able to verbalize support
   system(s) and/or support system for
   home care established
• Patient/family able to manage continu-
   ing care needs
• Patient discharged
		Discusses plan for discharge_____

Date	Initials	Signature	Date	Initials	Signature	Date	Initials	Signature

Figure A.9.   (Continued)

University of Anystate Hospitals

CLINICAL PATHWAY:
CESAREAN SECTION DELIVERY
PAGE 3 OF 3

This document should be considered a *guideline.* Outcomes will vary depending on the patient's severity of illness and other factors/conditions that affect or alter expected outcomes.

Key: Fill in appropriate location for nursing unit. Initial completed intermediate and discharge outcomes. Circle any variances and document on variance log. Once variance is resolved, date and inital clinical pathway.

Expected Discharge Outcomes	Postop Day #2 Date _____ Time _____	Postop Day # 3/Discharge Outcomes Date _____ Time _____
	Nursing Unit _____	Nursing Unit _____

Cardiovascular
• Hemodynamically stable
	Participates in self-care _____
	Ambulates in hall _____
	Chest clear _____
	Stable BP (<140/90 or no
	   increases > 30 mm systolic
	   or > 15 mm diastolic _____
		Responsible for self-care _____
		Vital signs within normal _____
		Chest clear _____

Gastrointestinal • Bowel sounds present • Tolerates regular diet • Passing flatus	Active bowel sounds _____ Passing flatus _____ Tolerates regular diet _____	Active bowel sounds _____ Passing flatus _____ Tolerates regular diet _____
Genitourinary • Normal bladder function	Bladder function normal _____ UOP >240 cc/8 h _____	Normal bladder function _____
Reproductive • Delivery of well newborn • Involution progressing • Minimal physical discomfort • Breast: Skin and nipples intact	Fundus firm, lochia small to moderate _____ Pain controlled _____	Delivery of well newborn _____ Involution progressing _____ Minimal physical discomfort _____ Breasts and nipples intact _____

Integumentary
• Incision intact with evidence of healing
• No signs/symptoms of infection
	Wound edges approximated,
	   no signs/symptoms
	   of infection _____
	Remains afebrile (<100.4ºF) _____
		Incision intact with evidence
		   of healing _____
		No signs/symptoms
		   of infection _____

Psychosocial
• Patient/family demonstrates adjustment to parental role
	Parental adjustment
	   progressing _____
	Demonstrates appropriate
	   parental–infant interaction _____
	Patient/family verbalizes thoughts/
	   feelings about childbirth _____
		Patient/family demonstrates
		   adjustment to parental role _____

Education
• Patient/family able to identify problems that require immediate medical attention
• Patient/family able to verbalize understanding of care needs (wound, etc.)
	Verbalizes/demonstrates
	   self-care knowledge
	   and skills _____
	Demonstrates infant
	   feeding _____
		Patient/family able to identify
		   problems that require immediate
		   medical attention _____
		Patient/family able to verbalize
		   understanding of care needs
		   (wound, infant feeding) _____

Discharge Planning
• Patient/family able to verbalize support system(s) and/or support system for home care established
• Patient/family able to manage continuing care needs
• Patient discharged
	Support system for home
	care established _____
		Patient/family able to verbalize support
		   system(s) and/or support system
		   for home care established _____
		Verbalizes understanding
		   of follow-up care _____
		Discharged home _____

Date	Initials	Signature	Date	Initials	Signature	Date	Initials	Signature

CLINICAL PATHWAY: C-SECTION
300111 (5/2004)

Figure A.10a.   Graphic vital signs

Figure A.10b.   Vital signs in electronic format

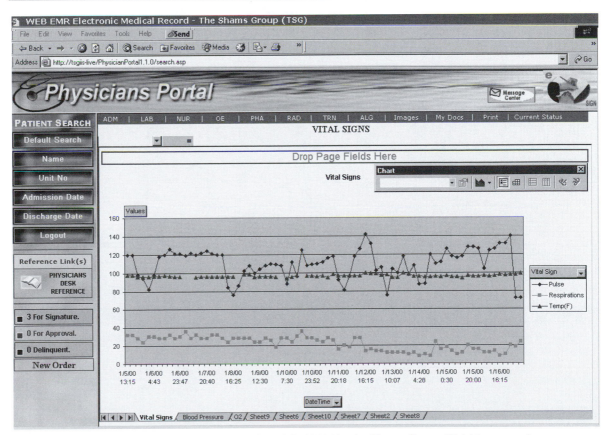

Figure A.11a.   Medication administration record

University of Anystate Hospitals and Clinics

MEDICATION ADMINISTRATION RECORD

PATIENT LABEL

Site Codes: A = L upper arm   IV Site Codes: 1 = L extremity
　　　　　　B = R upper arm　　　　　　　　　　2 = R extremity
　　　　　　C = L hip　　　　　　　　　　　　　3 = Central line
　　　　　　D = R hip　　　　　　　　　　　　　4 = Other
　　　　　　E = L thigh
　　　　　　F = R thigh　　Reasons Doses Not Given:　Ⓝ = NPO　　Ⓡ = Refused　　Ⓢ = Sleeping
　　　　　　G = Abdomen　　　　　　　　　　　　Ⓟ = On pass　　Ⓞ = Other
　　　　　　H = Chest　　　　　　　　　　　　　Ⓣ = Testing　　ⒹⒸ = Discontinued

Drug/Dose/Route	Order #	Scheduled	Start	Stop	7–3	3–11	11–7

Stat/One-Time Medications	Date	Time	Site	Initials

Initials	Signature	Initials	Signature	Initials	Signature

MEDICATION ADMINISTRATION RECORD
000028 (11/2002)

Figure A.11b.   Medication administration record in electronic format

Figure A.12a.   Laboratory report

Midwest Medical Center

LABORATORY SERVICES REPORT:
COAGULATION

PATIENT, WYLIE C.	
090241237	
DOB: 10/10/1918	

ADMISSION DATE: 05/14/03

ADMITTING PHYSICIAN: M. D. Doctor

SPECIMEN DATE: 05/20/03

COLLECTED TIME: 4:55 p.m.

WEEKDAY: Tuesday

——ROUTINE COAGULATION——		UNITS	REFERENCE	
PT	**17.6 H**	SEC	11.2–13.8	
INR	1.9			(1)
PTT	32.0	SEC	22.1–32.5	(2)

H = High

Footnotes

(1) The INR therapeutic range (1.5–4.0) for patients on warfarin therapy will depend on the clinical disorder being treated.

(2) Effective August 19, 2002, the suggested therapeutic range may vary from 40.9–68.3 sec for inpatients on heparin therapy.

Figure A.12b. Laboratory report in electronic format

Figure A.13.   Echocardiographic report

Anytown Community Hospital

ECHOCARDIOGRAPHIC REPORT

TEST, PATIENT
009999999
DOB: 04/01/1930

DATE: 06/02/2003

REFERRING PHYSICIAN: Dr. Doctor

INDICATION FOR STUDY: Murmur

TAPE: House 528

Outpatient Study

Two-dimensional and M-mode echocardiograms were performed

The left atrium is at the upper limits of normal size at 3.7 cm compared to an aortic root diameter of 2.9 cm. The left ventricle is at the upper limits of normal size with a normal internal dimension of 5.6 cm in diastole and 3.3 cm in systole. There is normal wall thickness. There is hyperdynamic left ventricular systolic performance. The ejection fraction is estimated at greater than 70%. No specific regional wall motion abnormalities were identified. The cardiac valves appear structurally normal. No intracardiac masses were identified and a pericardial effusion was not visualized.

Conventional as well as color-flow Doppler imaging was performed. There are findings of mitral regurgitation which is estimated to be at least moderate to severe, if not severe. There is tricuspid regurgitation with peak right ventricular systolic pressure of 31 mmHg. No other significant valvular stenoses or regurgitation were identified.

IMPRESSION:

1. The left atrium and left ventricle at the upper limits of normal size with a hyperdynamic left ventricular systolic performance.

2. There is evidence of mitral regurgitation which is at least moderate to severe. Would consider transesophageal echocardiography to further assess the severity of the mitral regurgitation as well as potentially its etiology.

Signature:

Philip Default

Philip Default, MD

6/2/03

Date

d: 06/02/2003
t: 06/02/2003

Figure A.14.   Electrocardiograph report

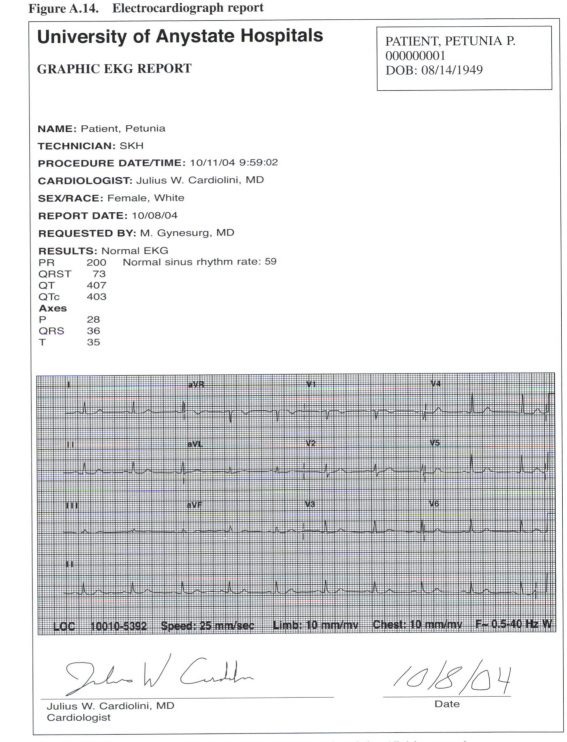

University of Anystate Hospitals

GRAPHIC EKG REPORT

PATIENT, PETUNIA P.
000000001
DOB: 08/14/1949

NAME: Patient, Petunia

TECHNICIAN: SKH

PROCEDURE DATE/TIME: 10/11/04 9:59:02

CARDIOLOGIST: Julius W. Cardiolini, MD

SEX/RACE: Female, White

REPORT DATE: 10/08/04

REQUESTED BY: M. Gynesurg, MD

RESULTS: Normal EKG
PR   200   Normal sinus rhythm rate: 59
QRST   73
QT   407
QTc   403
Axes
P   28
QRS   36
T   35

LOC   10010-5392   Speed: 25 mm/sec   Limb: 10 mm/mv   Chest: 10 mm/mv   F~ 0.5-40 Hz W

Julius W. Cardiolini, MD
Cardiologist

10/8/04
Date

Figure A.15.   Informed consent for operation with blood products

University of Anystate Hospitals

**INFORMED CONSENT FOR OPERATION/
PROCEDURE/ANESTHESIA INCLUDING
BLOOD AND BLOOD PRODUCTS**

PATIENT LABEL

1. I give permission to Dr.(s) _____ to perform
   the following procedure(s): _____

   _____

   _____ on _____ (patient's name).

2. I understand that during the procedure(s), new findings or conditions may appear and require an additional procedure(s) for proper care.

3. My physician has explained the following items:
   - the nature of my condition
   - the nature and purpose of the procedure(s) that I am now authorizing
   - the possible complications and side effects that may result, problems that may be experienced during recuperation, and the likelihood of success
   - the benefits to be reasonably expected from the procedure(s)
   - the likely result of no treatment
   - the available alternatives, including the risks and benefits
   - the other possible risks that accompany any surgical and diagnostic procedure (in addition to those already discussed). I acknowledge that neither my physician nor anyone else involved in my care has made any guarantees or assurances to me as to the result of the procedure(s) that I am now authorizing.

4. I know that other clinical staff may help my physician during the procedure(s).

5. I understand that the procedure(s) may require that I undergo some form of anesthesia, which may have its own risks.

6. Any tissue or specimens taken from my body as a result of the procedure(s) may be examined and disposed of, retained, preserved, or used for medical, scientific, or teaching purposes by the hospital.

7. I understand that my procedure(s) may be photographed or videotaped and that observers may be present in the room for the purpose of advancing medical care and education.

8. I understand that during or after the procedure(s) my physician may find it necessary to give me a transfusion of blood or blood products. My physician has explained the alternatives to, and possible risks of, transfusion.

9. I understand what my physician has explained to me and have had all my questions fully answered.

10. Additional comments: _____

    _____

After talking with my physician and reading this form, I give my consent to the procedure(s) described above.

Signature of Patient or
Legal Representative: _____ Date: _____ Time: _____

If Legal Representative, Relationship to Patient: _____

Witness: _____

Verbal or Telephone Consent

Name of Legal Representative: _____ Date: _____ Time: _____

Relationship to Patient: _____

Witness: _____ Witness: _____

I have explained the risks, benefits, potential complications, and alternatives of the treatment to the patient and have answered all questions to the patient's satisfaction, and he/she has granted consent to proceed.

Physician Signature: _____ Date: _____ Time: _____

INFORMED CONSENT FOR OPERATION
000015 (11/2002)

Figure A.16.   Anesthesia record

University of Anystate Hospitals

ANESTHESIA RECORD
PAGE 1 OF 2

PATIENT LABEL

Date: _____   Time: _____
Age: _____ Sex: _____ Height: _____ Weight: _____ BP: _____ P: _____ R: _____ T: _____
Lab: _____ Status: _____
Allergies: _____ Last Intake: _____
Premedication: _____

☐ **Patient reassessed immediately prior to induction. Condition satisfactory for planned anesthesia.**

Vital Signs

Time	

Machine Check
Initials
Patient Position

☐ General
☐ Regional
☐ Local
☐ Monitored
☐ IVs (spinal/EPI needle)

Position
Prep
Site
Agent
Paresthesia
Catheter
Sensory Block TO

☐ Heat/Moisture Exchanger
☐ Warming Blanket
☐ Fluid Warmer
☐ Bair Hugger

Endotracheal Tube
Cuff Inflated
Laryngoscope Blade
Stylet
Direct Vision
Blind

Systolic
∨
Diastolic
∧
Pulse
/\·/\·
Respiration
○
Spon
●
Assist
⊙
Controlled

Surgery Start/End
⊗
Anesthesia Start/End
X

Anesthesia Start
_____
Anesthesia End

240
220
200
180
160
140
120
100
80
60
40
20
15
10
5

Figure A.16.   (Continued)

University of Anystate Hospitals

ANESTHESIA RECORD
PAGE 2 OF 2

Monitors
- ☐ NIBP   ☐ R   ☐ L
- ☐ APB   ☐ R   ☐ L
- ☐ T (site): _____
- ☐ Pulse oximeter (site): _____
- ☐ ECG (lead): _____
- ☐ Airway gas monitor
- ☐ FiO$_2$ analyzer
- ☐ Pulmonary artery
- ☐ CVP
- ☐ EEG
- ☐ Stethoscope (site): _____
- ☐ SSEP
- ☐ Peripheral nerve stimulator
- ☐ Capnography

Remarks

Fluid		Fluid		Fluid		Fluid		Fluid		Fluid	
Start	Finish	Start	Finish	Start	Finish	Start	Finish	Start	Finish	Start	Finish

Operation		Recovery Room Time: _____
		BP
Surgeon	Anesthesiologist Date	P T °F Endotracheal In ☐ Out ☐
		Condition SpO$_2$ %

Preanesthesia Evaluation

Review of Clinical Data

- ☐ Yes   ☐ No   Patient Medical History Reviewed
- ☐ Yes   ☐ No   Current Medications Reviewed
- ☐ Yes   ☐ No   Allergies Reviewed
- ☐ Yes   ☐ No   ☐ N/A   Lab Results Reviewed
- ☐ Yes   ☐ No   ☐ N/A   CXR Results Reviewed
- ☐ Yes   ☐ No   ☐ N/A   EKG Results Reviewed

Pertinent Physical Exam

	Normal	Abnormal	Comments
EENT			
Respiratory			
Cardiac			
Mental Status			

Anesthesia History

- ☐ Yes   ☐ No   Past Hx of Anesthesia Complications
- ☐ Yes   ☐ No   Family Hx of Anesthesia Complications
- ☐ Yes   ☐ No   History of Malignant Hyperthermia

ASA Classification

1   2   3   4   5   E

Airway Evaluation

Dentures:	☐ None ☐ Upper ☐ Lower
Capped Teeth:	☐ None ☐ Yes
Condition of Teeth:	☐ Good ☐ Fair ☐ Poor

Estimated Intubation Difficulty:

☐ Normal   ☐ Moderately Difficult   ☐ Difficult

Anesthesia Plan

- ☐ General   ☐ Rapid Sequence Intubation
- ☐ Spinal   ☐ MAC
- ☐ Epidural   ☐ Epidural for POPM
- ☐ Regional Block

☐ Alternatives, risks of anesthesia, and potential complications were discussed. Patient and/or guardian state understanding and acceptance of anesthesia plan.

Comments:

_____
Anesthesiologist   Date

ANESTHESIA RECORD
000017 (11/2002)

Figure A.17a.   Operative report

Midwest Medical Center

OPERATIVE REPORT
PAGE 1 OF 2

PATIENT, TWEETY PYE
00555066
DOB: 02/18/1948

DATE: 06/02/2003

SURGEON: Douglas Default

ASSISTANT: Stanley Cutter

ANESTHETIC: Spinal

PREOPERATIVE DIAGNOSES:

1.   Intrauterine pregnancy, term, previous cesarean section, voluntary repeat cesarean section

2.   Multiparity, voluntary sterilization

POSTOPERATIVE DIAGNOSES:

1.   Intrauterine pregnancy, term, previous cesarean section, voluntary repeat cesarean section

2.   Multiparity, voluntary sterilization

3.   Delivery of viable unengaged 6 pound 2 ounce female, APGAR 8–9

OPERATION:

1.   Low-segment transverse cesarean section

2.   Bilateral partial salpingectomy

COMPLICATIONS: None

DRAINS: One Foley catheter in urinary bladder

ESTIMATED BLOOD LOSS: Approximately 500 to 600 cc

PACKS: None

DESCRIPTION OF OPERATION: After satisfactory level of spinal anesthesia was obtained, the patient was placed in the dorsal supine position with mild left lateral uterine displacement. The lower abdominal skin tissues were prepped with a Hibiclens solution. She was then draped with sterile drapes in a sterile manner.

There was a previous transverse skin scar on the lower abdominal skin. A repeat transverse skin incision was made very carefully with sharp dissection. The fascia of the anterior abdominal wall was incised in a lateral crescentic manner exposing the rectus muscles, which were then bluntly divided in the midline exposing the peritoneum, which was then carefully incised in a vertical manner. There was a wetting amount of peritoneal fluid. The peritoneum reflection over the lower anterior uterine segment was then incised in a superficial transverse manner, and the "bladder flap" was gently pushed off the lower segment without difficulty.

Figure A.17a.   (Continued)

Midwest Medical Center

OPERATIVE REPORT
PAGE 2 OF 2

PATIENT, TWEETY PYE
00555066
DOB: 02/18/1948

A transverse uterine incision was made very carefully with both sharp and blunt dissection. The myometrium was noted to be only 2 to 3 mm in thickness. The amniotic fluid was clear. The unengaged vertex was delivered through the uterine and abdominal incision without difficulty. The nasal and oropharynx were suctioned with bulb suction prior to the newborn's initial inspiration. The remainder of the delivery was accomplished without difficulty. The cord was clamped and severed, and the newborn was handed crying and in good condition to the awaiting nursery personnel.

The placenta was then manually removed from a fundal location showing a central insertion of a three-vessel cord. There were no visible extensions of the uterine incision. Both tubes and ovaries appeared normal for pregnant state. The uterine incision was then closed with a running interlocking #1 chromic suture.

With the patient's strong desire for permanent sterilization, approximately 1 to 1.5 cm segment of the isthmic portion of each fallopian tube was isolated with Babcock clamps, doubly ligated and excised, and sent to the laboratory labeled as portion of left and right fallopian tube, respectively. Hemostasis was deemed adequate. Both tubes appeared occluded.

The abdominal cavity was irrigated with copious amounts of warm normal saline. The first sponge, needle, and instrument counts were correct. The parietal peritoneum was then closed with a running 0 chromic suture. Hemostasis was deemed adequate in the subfascial space. The fascia was then approximated with running 0 PDS suture. Hemostasis was deemed adequate in the subcutaneous tissue. The skin was then approximated with running 3-0 Vicryl subcuticular suture. Sterile dressing was placed upon the incision.

The patient tolerated the procedure quite well and was sent to the recovery room in good condition. The newborn was taken to the nursery by the nursery personnel in good condition. The second and third sponge, needle, and instrument counts were corrected.

Signature:

Douglas D Dwitt _____   6/2/03 _____

Douglas D. Default, MD   Date

d: 06/02/2003
t: 06/04/2003
DDD, MD/sf

Figure A.17b.   Operative report in electronic format

WEB EMR Electronic Medical Record - The Shams Group (TSG)

File   Edit   View   Favorites   Tools   Help   *Send*

Back   •   •   Search   Favorites   Media

Address   http://tsgiis-live/PhysicianPortal1.1.0/search.asp   Go

Physicians Portal

Message Center

| PATIENT SEARCH | ADM | LAB | NUR | OE | PHA | RAD | TRN | ALG | Images | My Docs | Print | Current Status |

Default Search

Name

Unit No

Admission Date

Discharge Date

Logout

Reference Link(s)

PHYSICIANS DESK REFERENCE

■ 3 For Signature.

■ 0 For Approval.

■ 0 Delinquent.

New Order

Acct#: V84072636   Unit#: M000311654   Patient: WIGHET,MARI J

Patient: V84072636 - WIGHET,MARI J
    Unit#: M000311654   Age / Sex: 62/F   LOC: ST1 --
    Status: IN   Reg: 05/15/2001   DIS:

OPERATIVE REPORT

PREOPERATIVE DIAGNOSIS: Right Carotid Stenosis ICA, 99%.

POSTOPERATIVE DIAGNOSIS: Right Carotid Stenosis ICA, 99%.

SURGEON: N. PETERS, M.D.   ASSISTANT: Dr. ELASGHAT

DATE: 66-66-99

OPERATION: Right Carotid Endarterectomy.

ANESTHESIA: Cervical Block Supplemented with General Anesthesia.
ESTIMATED BLOOD LOSS: Negligible. Clamped times 12 minutes.

GROSS FINDINGS: DESCRIBE ALL PATHOLOGICAL FINDINGS AND ALL ORGANS EXPLORED,
                NORMAL AND ABNORMAL.

Patient brought to the operating room and identified by me. Prepped and draped in the
usual fashion. After cervical block and general anesthesia, incision made in the right
neck, deepened through the platysma. Sternomastoid muscle retracted laterally. The
internal jugular vein was retracted laterally. The _____ vein was divided and
ligated with silk ties and common carotid artery was exposed and then the resection
proceeded superiorly to expose the bifurcation which was infiltrated with 1% Lidocaine.
Vascular loops are fastened around the common ECA and then the ICA without any difficulty.
Resection in the ICA proceeded beyond the block. Following this, systemic Heparinization
of 6000 units of IV Heparin push given and was also crossclamped. Arteriotomy made and
extended well into the ICA beyond the block. The block was removed from the common ECA and
the ICA in one block. External back bleeding was noted in the ICA as well as ECA.
Arteriotomy site was flushed with Heparinized saline, closed in routine fashion utilizing
6-0 Prolene sutures from either direction and the circulation was established into the ECA
first and then into the ICA. Arteriotomy site was hemostatically adequate. Wound closure

Figure A.18a.   Surgical pathology report

Midwest Medical Center

SURGICAL PATHOLOGY CONSULTATION

PATIENT, SWEETPEA C.
007770021
DOB: 12/18/1931

ADMITTING PHYSICIAN: M. D. Doctor

CONSULT PHYSICIAN 1:

CONSULT PHYSICIAN 2:

ACCESSIONED IN LAB: 05/20/2003

ACCESSION #: S-03-010101

DATE OF SURGERY: 5/20/2003

SPECIMEN: A-Vag Mucosa

CLINICAL DATA: Cystocele/rectocele, stress incontinence

GROSS: Received are four wrinkled, variegated, pink/tan portions of vaginal mucosa, which are $7 \times 6 \times 1$ cm in aggregate dimension. Representative portions of each are submitted for microscopic evaluation. M/1/pg.

MICROSCOPIC COMMENT: Sections are of squamous mucosa. There are no atypia.

DIAGNOSIS: Squamous mucosa, multiple portions exhibiting no atypia (vaginal)

Signature:

Walter Q. Pathman, MD

5/20/03

Date

d: 05/20/2003
t: 05/23/2003
WQP, MD/jt

Figure A.18b.   Surgical pathology report in electronic format

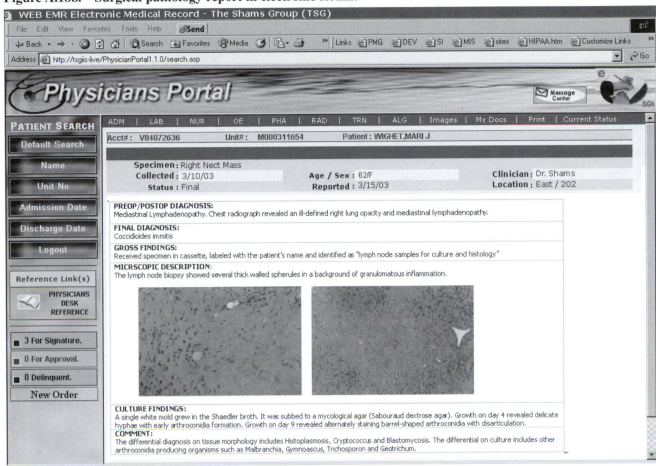

Figure A.19a.   Discharge summary

Midwest Medical Center

DISCHARGE SUMMARY

SAYLORMEN, POPEYE T.
333333333
DOB: 02/09/1961

PHYSICIAN/SURGEON: Philip P. Heartstopper, MD

DATE OF DISCHARGE: 05/18/2003

PRINCIPAL OPERATION AND PROCEDURE: OPCAB × 3, left internal mammary artery of the LAD, saphenous vein graft to D-1, and saphenous vein graft to OM-1

HISTORY OF PRESENT ILLNESS: Mr. Saylormen was seen at the request of Dr. Doctor regarding surgical treatment of ischemic heart disease. He is a 42-year-old male with a family history of coronary artery disease. He smokes a pipe and had a previous myocardial infarction approximately three years ago. His current status is postangioplasty. While working on a construction project, he developed anginal-type symptoms and was seen in the emergency room and then admitted to the hospital for further evaluation.

ADMITTING DIAGNOSIS: Coronary artery disease

HOSPITAL COURSE: The patient underwent cardiac catheterization and was found to have significant three-vessel coronary artery disease. It was felt that he would benefit from undergoing an OPCAB procedure. On 05/14/03, the patient underwent OPCAB × 3 as described above. The patient tolerated the procedure well and returned to the Cardiothoracic Intensive Care Unit hemodynamically stable. On postoperative day one, he was weaned from mechanical ventilation, extubated, and transferred to the Cardiothoracic Step-Down Unit, where he continued on a progressive course of recovery. On postoperative day four, he was up and about in his room and the halls without difficulty. Upon discharge, he was tolerating his diet well. His lungs were clear. His abdomen was soft, and his incisions were unremarkable. His vital signs were stable. He was in normal sinus rhythm. His heart rate was in the 70s and 80s. Blood pressure had been running consistently in the low 110s/60s. He was afebrile. Oxygen saturations on room air were reported at 97%.

LABORATORY DATA AT DISCHARGE: BUN 14, Creatinine 0.9, H&H 8.8 and 25.4

MEDICATIONS AT DISCHARGE: Lisinopril 5 mg q.d.; Lipitor 80 mg q.d.; metoprolol 50 mg q.d.; aspirin 81 mg q.d.; Darvocet-N 100—one to two tablets every 4–6 hours as needed for pain; iron sulfate 325 mg q.d. × 30 days; and Colace 100 mg b.i.d. × 30 days

DIET: He may follow a regular diet.

FINAL DIAGNOSIS: Coronary artery disease

DISPOSITION: No lifting greater than 10 pounds. No driving for 4–6 weeks. He may shower but he should not take a tub bath. Follow up with Dr. Doctor in 1–2 weeks.

_____   5/18/03
Philip P. Heartstopper, MD   _____
                                                                      Date

d: 05/18/2003
t: 05/19/2003
PPH, MD/mb

Figure A.19b.   Discharge summary in electronic format

Figure A.20. Physician's order sheet in paper format

University of Anystate Hospital

PHYSICIAN ORDERS

PATIENT LABEL

Drug Allergies

Date and Time	RN Signature	

PHYSICIAN ORDERS
000122 (02/2003)

Figure A.21.   Example of a HIPAA-compliant authorization form

Midwest Medical Center

CONSENT FOR DISCLOSURE
OF HEALTH INFORMATION

PATIENT LABEL

(1)   I hereby authorize (name of provider) to disclose the following information from the health records of:

Patient Name: _____   Date of Birth: _____

Address:_____

Telephone: _____   Patient Number: _____

Covering the period(s) of healthcare:

From (date) _____   to (date) _____

From (date) _____   to (date) _____

(2)   Information to be disclosed:

☐ Complete health record(s)

   ☐ Discharge summary   ☐ Progress notes

   ☐ History and physical examination   ☐ Laboratory test results

   ☐ Consultation reports   ☐ X-ray reports

☐ Photographs, videotapes, digital or other images

☐ Other (please specify) _____

I understand that this will include information relating to (check if applicable):

☐ AIDS (acquired immunodeficiency syndrome) or HIV (human immunodeficiency virus) infection

☐ Psychiatric care

☐ Treatment for alcohol and/or drug abuse

(3)   This information is to be disclosed to _____ for the purpose of

_____.

(4)   I understand this authorization may be revoked in writing at any time, except to the extent that action has been taken in reliance on this authorization. Unless otherwise revoked, this authorization will expire on the following date, event, or condition: _____

_____

(5)   The facility, its employees, officers, and physicians are hereby released from any legal responsibility or liability for disclosure of the above information to the extent indicated and authorized herein.

_____   _____
Signature of Patient or Legal Representative   Date   Signature of Witness   Date

CONSENT FOR DISCLOSURE OF HEALTH INFORMATION
000089 (9/2001)

Figure A.22.   Example of a request for accounting of disclosures

Anytown Community Hospital

REQUEST FOR ACCOUNTING OF DISCLOSURES

Date of Request:_____

Patient Name: _____

Date of Birth:_____ Health Record Number: _____

Patient Address: _____

Address to Send Disclosure Accounting (if different from above):

_____

Dates Requested

I would like an accounting of all disclosures for the following time frame.

From:_____ To: _____

(Please note: The maximum time frame that can be requested is six years prior to the date of request.)

Fees

First request in a 12-month period: Free

Subsequent requests: (Insert cost-based fee per entity)

The fee for this request will be: _____

I understand that there is a fee for this accounting and wish to proceed. I also understand that the accounting will be provided to me within 60 days unless I am notified in writing that an extension of up to 30 days is needed.

_____   _____
     Signature of Patient or Legal Representative   Date

For Healthcare Organization Use Only:

Date Received: _____ Date Sent:_____

Extension Requested: ☐ No   ☐ Yes, Reason _____

Patient Notified in Writing on This Date:_____

Staff Member Processing Request: _____

REQUEST FOR ACCOUNTING OF DISCLOSURES
300252 (10/2002)

Appendix B
Sample Position Descriptions

The following position descriptions and related articles may be found in the AHIMA Web site at ahima.org. In some cases, access is restricted to AHIMA members. (Some descriptions are included in more than one category.) The Web site is regularly updated to reflect current and emerging practice areas.

Role	Job Title
Compliance	Compliance and Privacy Officer—eHealth Compliance Director Compliance Officer Compliance Specialist HIPAA Compliance Coordinator
Consulting	*See: Starting a consulting business*
Data management	APC Coordinator Cancer Registrar Clinical Coding Specialist Clinical Data Specialist Data Quality Manager Data Resource Administrator Decision Support Specialist DRG Coordinator HIM Clerk Information Security Manager Information Services Manager MPI Manager Patient Information Coordinator Research Data Analyst
EHR	Clinical Analyst Clinical Applications Coordinator Clinical Project Manager, Senior Project Manager Clinical Research Associate Clinical Vocabulary Manager Compliance and Privacy Officer—eHealth Enterprise Applications Specialist Health Systems Specialist Health Information Services Department Technician Information Privacy Coordinator Integration Architect (Implementation) Optical Imaging Coordinator Process Improvement Engineer Records and Information Coordinator Risk Management Specialist Senior Document Coordinator Solution Analyst Solution Consultant Systems Analyst *See: EHR career opportunities: Sample HIM job descriptions*

Role	Job Title
Emerging roles	Clinical Data Specialist Data Quality Manager Data Resource Administrator Health Information Manager for Integrated Systems Information Security Manager Patient Information Coordinator Research and Decision Support Specialist *See: Evolving HIM careers: Seven roles for the future*
General	Educator Health Information Management Director HIM Domain Manager Medical Staff Coordinator Patient Information Coordinator Risk Manager Utilization Management Director
Privacy & security	Compliance and Privacy Officer—eHealth Compliance and Regulatory Management Officer Compliance Manager, Director, Officer Copy Service Manager Corporate Compliance Director Disclosure Coordinator Information Officer, Chief Information Officer Information Security Manager Information Services Manager Medical Records Manager Patient Accounts Manager Privacy Officer, Chief Privacy Officer Release of information Coordinator Security Manager, Director, Officer *See: Success at every level: A career ladder for privacy officers*
Quality	Quality Improvement Director

Appendix C
Sample Notice of Health Information Practices

This notice describes how information about you may be used and disclosed and how you can get access to this information. Please review it carefully.

Understanding Your Health Record/Information

Each time you visit a hospital, physician, or other healthcare provider, a record of your visit is made. Typically, this record contains your symptoms, examination and test results, diagnoses, treatment, and a plan for future care or treatment. This information, often referred to as your health or medical record, serves as a:

- basis for planning your care and treatment
- means of communication among the many health professionals who contribute to your care
- legal document describing the care you received
- means by which you or a third-party payer can verify that services billed were actually provided
- tool in educating health professionals
- source of data for medical research
- source of information for public health officials charged with improving the health of the nation
- source of data for facility planning and marketing and
- tool with which we can assess and continually work to improve the care we render and the outcomes we achieve.

Understanding what is in your record and how your health information is used helps you to:

- ensure its accuracy
- better understand who, what, when, where, and why others may access your health information
- make more informed decisions when authorizing disclosure to others.

Your Health Information Rights

Although your health record is the physical property of the healthcare practitioner or facility that compiled it, the information belongs to you. You have the right to:

- request a restriction on certain uses and disclosures of your information as provided by 45 CFR 164.522

- obtain a paper copy of the notice of information practices upon request

- inspect and copy your health record as provided for in 45 CFR 164.524

- amend your health record as provided in 45 CFR 164.528

- obtain an accounting of disclosures of your health information as provided in 45 CFR 164.528

- request communications of your health information by alternative means or at alternative locations

- revoke your authorization to use or disclose health information except to the extent that action has already been taken.

Our Responsibilities

This organization is required to:

- maintain the privacy of your health information

- provide you with a notice as to our legal duties and privacy practices with respect to information we collect and maintain about you

- abide by the terms of this notice

- notify you if we are unable to agree to a requested restriction

- accommodate reasonable requests you may have to communicate health information by alternative means or at alternative locations.

We reserve the right to change our practices and to make the new provisions effective for all protected health information we maintain. Should our information practices change, we will mail a revised notice to the address you've supplied us.

We will not use or disclose your health information without your authorization, except as described in this notice.

For More Information or to Report a Problem

If you have questions and would like additional information, you may contact the Director of Health Information Management at (444)111-1111.

If you believe your privacy rights have been violated, you can file a complaint with the Director of Health Information Management or with the Secretary of Health and Human Services. There will be no retaliation for filing a complaint.

Examples of Disclosures for Treatment, Payment and Health Operations

We will use your health information for treatment. For example: Information obtained by a nurse, physician or other member of your healthcare team will be recorded in your record and used to determine the course of treatment that should work best for you. Your physician will document in your record his expectations of the members of your healthcare team. Members of your healthcare team will then record the actions they took and their observations. In that way the physician will know how you are responding to treatment.

We will also provide your physician or a subsequent healthcare provider with copies of various reports that should assist him/her in treating you once you're discharged from this hospital.

We will use your health information for payment. For example: A bill may be sent to you or a third-party payer. The information on or accompanying the bill may include information that identifies you, as well as your diagnosis, procedures and supplies used.

We will use your health information for regular health operations. For example: Members of the medical staff, the risk or quality improvement manager, or members of the quality improvement team may use information in your health record to assess the care and outcomes in your case and others like it. This information will then be used in an effort to continually improve the quality and effectiveness of the healthcare and service we provide.

Other Uses or Disclosures

Business Associates: There are some services provided in our organization through contacts with business associates. Examples include physician services in the Emergency Department and Radiology, certain laboratory tests, and a copy service we use when making copies of your health record. When these services are contracted, we may disclose your health information to our business associate so that they can perform the job we've asked them to do and bill you or your third-party payer for services rendered. So that your health information is protected, however, we require the business associate to appropriately safeguard your information.

Directory: Unless you notify us that you object, we will use your name, location in the facility, general condition, and religious affiliation for directory purposes. This information may be provided to members of the clergy and, except for religious affiliation, to other people who ask for you by name.

Notification: We may use or disclose information to notify or assist in notifying a family member, personal representative, or another person responsible for your care, your location, and general condition.

Communication with Family: Health professionals, using their best judgement, may disclose to a family member, other relative, close personal friend, or any other person you identify health information relevant to that person's involvement in your care or payment related to your care.

Research: We may disclose information to researchers when their research has been approved by an Institutional Review Board that has reviewed the research proposal and established protocols to ensure the privacy of your health information.

Funeral Directors: We may disclose health information to funeral directors consistent with applicable law to carry out their duties.

Organ Procurement Organizations: Consistent with applicable law, we may disclose health information to organ procurement organizations or other entities engaged in the procurement, banking, or transplantation of organs for the purpose of tissue donation and transplant.

Marketing: We may contact you to provide appointment reminders or information about treatment alternatives or other health-related benefits and services that may be of interest to you.

Fund Raising: We may contact you as part of a fund-raising effort.

Food and Drug Administration (FDA): We may disclose to the FDA health information relative to adverse events with respect to food, supplements, product and product defects, or postmarketing surveillance information to enable product recalls, repairs, or replacement.

Workers Compensation: We may disclose health information to the extent authorized by law and to the extent necessary to comply with laws relating to workers compensation or other similar programs established by law.

Public Health: As required by law, we may disclose your health information to public health or legal authorities charged with preventing or controlling disease, injury, or disability.

Correctional Institution: Should you be an inmate of a correctional institution, we may disclose to the institution, or agents thereof, health information necessary for your health and the health and safety of other individuals.

Law Enforcement: We may disclose health information for law enforcement purposes as required by law or in response to a valid subpoena.

Federal law makes provision for your health information to be released to an appropriate health oversight agency, public health authority, or attorney provided that a workforce member or business associate believes in good faith that we have engaged in unlawful conduct or have otherwise violated professional or clinical standards and are potentially endangering one or more patients, workers, or the public.

My signature below indicates that I have been provided with a copy of the notice of privacy practices.

_____

Signature of Patient or Legal Representative

Date _____

If signed by legal representative, relationship to patient_____

Effective Date: _____

Distribution: Original to provider; copy to patient

The above form is not meant to encompass all the various ways in which any particular facility may use health information. For example, those who use protected health information for fundraising or marketing will want to add those types of disclosures. It is intended to get the reader started developing their own notice. As with any form of this nature, the document should be reviewed and approved by legal counsel prior to implementation.

Source: AHIMA. 2002 (November). Practice brief (updated): Notice of information practices. *Journal of American Health Information Management Association.* Available online from ahima.org.

Appendix D
Web Resources

American Health Information Management Association (AHIMA)
ahima.org
AHIMA is a professional association representing more than 50,000 specially educated health information professionals who work throughout the healthcare industry. This site includes *Journal of AHIMA* indexes and articles, position statements, practice briefs, frequently asked questions, member forums, job board, hot topics, legislative issues, the fellowship program, and many other resources for HIM professionals.

AHIMA Communities of Practice
ahimanet.org/COP
AHIMA Communities of Practice were launched in 2001, providing a virtual connection for AHIMA members in similar healthcare settings or with similar interests or concerns.

Accreditation Association for Ambulatory Health Care (AAAHC)
aaahc.org
AAAHC is committed to advocating high-quality health services in ambulatory healthcare organizations through the development of standards and survey and accreditation programs.

Accredited Standards Committee—X12N
x12.org
ASC X12, comprised of cross-industry representation, delivers the most widely implemented electronic data interchange (EDI) standards that interact with a multitude of e-commerce technologies and serves as the premier source for integrating electronic applications.

Agency for Healthcare Research and Quality (AHRQ)
ahrq.gov
Home page for the government association for research to increase quality healthcare.

American Accreditation HealthCare Commission/URAC
urac.org
A nonprofit organization that establishes standards for the managed care industry.

American Association for Medical Transcription (AAMT)
aamt.org
AAMT represents and advances the profession of medical transcription and its practitioners.

American Association of Health Plans (AAHP)
aahp.org
A national trade association representing health maintenance organizations, preferred provider organizations, point-of-service plans, and other health plans.

American Association of Preferred Provider Organizations (AAPPO)
aappo.org
A national association of network-based preferred provider organizations and affiliate organizations.

American College of Healthcare Executives (ACHE)
ache.org
An international society of healthcare executives, ACHE offers credentialing and educational programs.

American Hospital Association (AHA)
aha.org
Members of the American Hospital Association are grouped into three categories: institutional (short-term hospitals, long-term hospitals, headquarters of healthcare systems, nonhospital preacute and postacute facilities, and hospital-affiliated education programs), associate, and personal.

American Hospital Association Research Data
ahadata.com
Detailed hospital research databank and resource for healthcare provider information.

American Health Lawyers Association
healthlawyers.org
Organization for lawyers associated with the health field.

American Medical Association (AMA)
ama-assn.org
AMA's strategic agenda remains rooted in its historic commitment to standards, ethics, excellence in medical education and practice, and advocacy on behalf of the medical profession and the patients it services.

American Medical Informatics Association (AMIA)
amia.org
AMIA is a nonprofit membership organization of individuals, institutions, and corporations dedicated to developing and using information technologies to improve healthcare.

American National Standards Institute (ANSI)
web.ansi.org
This Web site includes a public forum for the voluntary coordination of healthcare informatics standards among all U.S. standard-developing organizations.

American Nursing Informatics Association (ANIA)
ania.org/
ANIA is a nonprofit membership organization of individuals dedicated to promoting the field of nursing informatics and offering its members resources that enrich their roles in the field of nursing informatics.

American Society for Testing and Materials (ASTM)
astm.org
An organization that sets technical standards for industries.

America's Health Insurance Plans (AHIP)
ahip.org/
A trade association representing the private healthcare system that provides health, long-term care, dental, disability, and supplemental coverage to consumers.

Association for Electronic Health Care Transactions (AFEHCT)
afehct.org
Supports the use of EDI to improve and reduce the cost of healthcare.

Association of State and Territorial Health Officials (ASTHO)
astho.org
A nonprofit organization representing the state and territorial public health agencies of the United States, U.S. territories, and the District of Columbia.

Canada's Health Informatics Association
coachorg.com
An organization of individuals representing the full range of healthcare-related organizations and agencies, including government and nongovernment telecommunications technologies, and educational institutions, which is dedicated to promoting a clear understanding of health informatics within the Canadian health system.

Canadian Health Information Management Association (CHIMA)
chra.ca
CHIMA home page.

Canadian Institute for Health Information
http://secure.cihi.ca
A nonprofit organization that provides Canadians with essential statistics and analysis about their health and their healthcare system.

CCH Internet Research Network
health.cch.com/network
Links to many federal laws, regulations, and programs: Balanced Budget Act, APCs, home health agency licensure, Medicare and Medicaid, OASIS, and PPS.

The Center for Health Transformation
healthtransformation.net.
A unique collaboration of national leaders dedicated to accelerating the adoption of transformational ideas, policies, and technologies to create a healthcare system characterized by better outcomes and more choices at lower cost.

Centers for Disease Control and Prevention (CDC)
cdc.gov
CDC home page.

Centers for Medicare and Medicaid Services (CMS)
cms.gov
A federal agency that administers Medicare, Medicaid, and the State Children's Health Insurance Program.

The Certification Commission for Healthcare Information Technology
cchit.org
A voluntary, private-sector initiative to certify HIT products

Code of Federal Regulations (CFR)
www.gpoaccess.gov/cfr/index.html
The CFR is a codification of the general and permanent rules published in the Federal Register by the executive departments and agencies of the federal government.

College of Healthcare Information Management Executives (CHIME)
cio-chime.org
CHIME was formed with the dual objective of serving the professional development needs of healthcare CIOs and advocating the more effective use of information management within healthcare.

Connecting for Health
connectingforhealth.org
A public-private collaborative designed to address the barriers to development of an interconnected health information infrastructure. Established by the Markle Foundation, it receives additional funding and support from the Robert Wood Johnson Foundation.

Department of Health & Human Services (HHS)
hhs.gov
The Department of Health and Human Services is the U.S. government's principal agency for protecting the health of all Americans and providing essential human services, especially for those who are least able to help themselves.

Disease Management Association of America (DMAA)
dmaa.org
A nonprofit organization representing the disease management community.

e-Health Initiative
ehealthinitiative.org
The eHealth Initiative is a corporate membership organization. It, and the Foundation for eHealth Initiative, are independent, nonprofit affiliated organizations whose missions are the same: to drive improvement in the quality, safety, and efficiency of healthcare through information and information technology.

Federation of American Hospitals (FAHS)

fahs.com

Represents owned and managed hospitals and health systems that offer traditional care, ambulatory care, psychiatric and rehabilitative care, and allied companies involved in health insurance and healthcare systems.

Health Care Compliance Association (HCCA)

hcca-info.org

HCCA is a forum for healthcare professionals involved in compliance serving all segments of the healthcare industry.

Health Internet Ethics

hiethics.org

A coalition of health sites supporting high ethical standards.

Health Level Seven (HL7)

hl7.org

One of the ANSI-accredited standards-developing organizations operating in the healthcare area, producing standards for particular healthcare domains such as pharmacy, medical devices, imaging, and insurance transactions.

Health on the Net Foundation (HON)

hon.ch

Dedicated to realizing the benefits of the Internet and related technologies in the fields of health and medicine.

Health Privacy Project

healthprivacy.org

Cites, summarizes, and provides links to federal and state disclosure laws and provides articles covering privacy issues.

Health.gov

health.gov

This site is a portal to the Web sites of a number of multi-agency health initiatives and activities of the U.S. Department of Health and Human Services and other federal departments and agencies.

Healthcare Billing and Management Association (HBMA)

hbma.org

Founded in 1993, the HBMA is the only trade association representing third-party medical billers.

Healthcare Information and Management Systems Society (HIMSS)

himss.org

HIMSS is a trade association driving the adoption of strategic information management and technology in the health industry.

Healthcare Cost and Utilization Project (HCUP)

ahrq.gov/data/

National statistics, trends, and selected state statistics about hospital stays.

Healthcare Financial Management Association (HFMA)

hfma.org

Professional association for financial management professionals working in healthcare.

National Association for Home Care and Hospice (NAHC)

nahc.org

An organization supporting the home care side of the health industry.

Human Anatomy Online

innerbody.com

Each anatomy topic has animations, hundreds of graphics, and thousands of descriptive links.

International Medical Informatics Association (IMIA)

imia.org

IMIA home page.

Internet Healthcare Coalition (IHC)

ihealthcoalition.org

Healthcare resources on the Internet; affiliations include publishers of professional and consumer health information.

The IPA Association of America (TIPAAA)

tipaaa.com

Assists independent/integrated physician associations by providing services that lead to decisions that will contribute to the implementation of appropriate operational systems, resulting in greater efficiency.

Joint Commission on the Accreditation of Healthcare Organizations (JCAHO)

jcaho.org

Evaluates and accredits healthcare organizations and programs in the United States.

Journal of the American Medical Informatics Association (JAMIA)

jamia.org

Articles and abstracts from JAMIA.

Kaiser Foundation

statehealthfacts.kff.org

Provides individual state healthcare profiles and comparative healthcare data for all 50 states.

Leapfrog Group Outcomes Data

healthgrades.com

Leapfrog outcomes data for hospitals across the country.

Mayo Clinic

mayoclinic.com

The Mayo Clinic home page.

Medical Group Management Association (MGMA)

mgma.com

MGMA strives to improve the effectiveness of medical group practices and the knowledge and skills of those who manage and lead them.

Medical Transcription Industry Alliance (MTIA)

mtia.com

A nonprofit membership association serving the needs of medical transcription companies and health information management professionals.

MEDLINE

medlineplus.gov

A subservice of the National Library of Medicine.

Merck Manual Home Edition

merck.com/pubs/mmanual/

Medical reference book.

NANDA International
nanda.org
NANDA International is a member driven, grassroots organization committed to the development of nursing diagnostic terminology.

National Alliance for Health Information Technology (NAHIT)
nahit.org
The mission of the NAHIT is to improve quality and performance through standards-based information systems.

National Association for Healthcare Quality (NAHQ)
nahq.org
Web site for the organization for healthcare quality professionals.

National Association of Health Data Organizations (NAHDO)
nahdo.org
Membership organization dedicated to strengthening the nation's health information system by bringing together a network of state, federal, and private sector technical and policy leaders and consultants to expand health systems development and shape responsible health information policies.

National Center for Health Statistics (NCHS)
cdc.gov/nchs/
The federal government's principal vital and health statistics agency; part of the Centers for Disease Control and Prevention.

National Committee for Quality Assurance (NCQA)
ncqa.org
An independent, nonprofit organization that evaluates and reports on the quality of the nation's managed care organizations.

National Committee on Vital and Health Statistics (NCVHS)
ncvhs.hhs.gov
Home page for NCVHS.

National Health Information Infrastructure (NHII)
aspe.hhs.gov/sp/nhii
U.S. Department of Health and Human Services Web page for NHII.

National Technical Information Service (NTIS)
ntis.gov
NTIS acts as the central source for U.S. government scientific, technical, and business information. This growing collection, including millions of publications as well as audiovisual materials, computer data files, and software, originates from U.S. federal agencies, industry and university contractors with the federal government, and a worldwide compendium of research and development organizations.

National Institutes of Health (NIH)
nih.gov
Home page for NIH.

National Library of Medicine (NLM)
nlm.nih.gov/nlmhome.html
A biomedical library.

National Uniform Billing Committee (NUBC)
nubc.org
An organization created to meet the goals of administrative simplification as outlined in the Health Insurance Portability and Accountability Act of 1996.

National Uniform Claim Committee (NUCC)
nucc.org
Develops a standardized data set for use by noninstitutional healthcare communities to transmit claim and encounter information to and from all third-party payers.

Office of the National Coordinator for Health Information Technology (ONC)
hhs.gov/healthit/
Homepage for ONC

Physicians' Desk Reference (PDR)
pdr.net
Online home of the Physicians' Desk Reference.

International Association of Privacy Professions (IAPP)
privacyassociation.org
An organization for privacy officers in North America.

Professional Association of Health Care Office Management (PAHCOM)
pahcom.com
Provides a support system to the managers of group and solo physician practices.

PubMed
ncbi.nlm.nih.gov/entrez/query.fcgi?DB=pubmed
PubMed is a service of the National Library of Medicine that includes over 15 million citations from MEDLINE and other life science journals for biomedical articles dating back to the 1950s. PubMed includes links to full text articles and other related resources. (See AHIMA article: Getting to know PubMed: An overview.)

Quality Interagency Coordination Task Force (QuIC)
quic.gov
Federal agencies that purchase, provide, study, or regulate health services and collaborate toward the common goal of high quality and efficient healthcare systems.

The Rehabilitation Accreditation Commission (CARF)
carf.org
A nonprofit organization offering accreditation to programs and services in rehabilitation, behavioral health, and other areas.

Systematized Nomenclature of Medicine (SNOMED)
snomed.org
Web site for the division of College of American Pathologists that oversees the direction and scientific maintenance of the Systematized Nomenclature of Medicine, better known as SNOMED.

U.S. Government Printing Office
gpo.gov
Government publications.

Workgroup for Electronic Data Interchange (WEDI)
wedi.org
A resource for electronic connectivity in the healthcare industry.

Appendix E
2004 American Health Information Management Association Code of Ethics

Preamble

The ethical obligations of the health information management (HIM) professional include the protection of patient privacy and confidential information; disclosure of information; development, use, and maintenance of health information systems and health records; and the quality of information. Both handwritten and computerized medical records contain many sacred stories—stories that must be protected on behalf of the individual and the aggregate community of persons served in the healthcare system. Healthcare consumers are increasingly concerned about the loss of privacy and the inability to control the dissemination of their protected information. Core health information issues include what information should be collected, how the information should be handled, who should have access to the information, and under what conditions the information should be disclosed.

Ethical obligations are central to the professional's responsibility, regardless of the employment site or the method of collection, storage, and security of health information. Sensitive information (genetic, adoption, drug, alcohol, sexual, and behavioral information) requires special attention to prevent misuse. Entrepreneurial roles require expertise in the protection of the information in the world of business and interactions with consumers.

Professional Values

The mission of the HIM profession is based on core professional values developed since the inception of the Association in 1928. These values and the inherent ethical responsibilities for AHIMA members and credentialed HIM professionals include providing service; protecting medical, social, and financial information; promoting confidentiality; and preserving and securing health information. Values to the healthcare team include promoting the quality and advancement of healthcare, demonstrating HIM expertise and skills, and promoting interdisciplinary cooperation and collaboration. Professional values in relationship to the employer include protecting committee deliberations and complying with laws, regulations, and policies. Professional values related to the public include advocating change, refusing to participate or conceal unethical practices, and reporting violations of practice standards to the proper authorities. Professional values to individual and professional associations include obligations to be honest, bringing honor to self, peers and profession, committing to continuing education and lifelong learning, performing association duties honorably, strengthening professional membership, representing the profession to the public, and promoting and participating in research.

These professional values will require a complex process of balancing the many conflicts that can result from competing interests and obligations of those who seek access to health information and require an understanding of ethical decision-making.

Purpose of the American Health Information Management Association Code of Ethics

The HIM professional has an obligation to demonstrate actions that reflect values, ethical principles, and ethical guidelines. The American Health Information Management Association (AHIMA) Code of Ethics sets forth these values and principles to guide conduct. The code is relevant to all AHIMA members and credentialed HIM professionals and students, regardless of their professional functions, the settings in which they work, or the populations they serve.

The AHIMA Code of Ethics serves six purposes:

- Identifies core values on which the HIM mission is based.
- Summarizes broad ethical principles that reflect the profession's core values and establishes a set of ethi-

cal principles to be used to guide decision-making and actions.

- Helps HIM professionals identify relevant considerations when professional obligations conflict or ethical uncertainties arise.
- Provides ethical principles by which the general public can hold the HIM professional accountable.
- Socializes practitioners new to the field to HIM's mission, values, and ethical principles.
- Articulates a set of guidelines that the HIM professional can use to assess whether they have engaged in unethical conduct.

The code includes principles and guidelines that are both enforceable and aspirational. The extent to which each principle is enforceable is a matter of professional judgment to be exercised by those responsible for reviewing alleged violations of ethical principles.

The Use of the Code

Violation of principles in this code does not automatically imply legal liability or violation of the law. Such determination can only be made in the context of legal and judicial proceedings. Alleged violations of the code would be subject to a peer review process. Such processes are generally separate from legal or administrative procedures and insulated from legal review or proceedings to allow the profession to counsel and discipline its own members although in some situations, violations of the code would constitute unlawful conduct subject to legal process.

Guidelines for ethical and unethical behavior are provided in this code. The terms "shall and shall not" are used as a basis for setting high standards for behavior. This does not imply that everyone "shall or shall not" do everything that is listed. For example, not everyone participates in the recruitment or mentoring of students. A HIM professional is not being unethical if this is not part of his or her professional activities; however, if students are part of one's professional responsibilities, there is an ethical obligation to follow the guidelines stated in the code. This concept is true for the entire code. If someone does the stated activities, ethical behavior is the standard. The guidelines are not a comprehen-

sive list. For example, the statement "protect all confidential information to include personal, health, financial, genetic and outcome information" can also be interpreted as "shall not fail to protect all confidential information to include personal, health, financial, genetic, and outcome information."

A code of ethics cannot guarantee ethical behavior. Moreover, a code of ethics cannot resolve all ethical issues or disputes or capture the richness and complexity involved in striving to make responsible choices within a moral community. Rather, a code of ethics sets forth values and ethical principles, and offers ethical guidelines to which professionals aspire and by which their actions can be judged. Ethical behaviors result from a personal commitment to engage in ethical practice.

Professional responsibilities often require an individual to move beyond personal values. For example, an individual might demonstrate behaviors that are based on the values of honesty, providing service to others, or demonstrating loyalty. In addition to these, professional values might require promoting confidentiality, facilitating interdisciplinary collaboration, and refusing to participate or conceal unethical practices. Professional values could require a more comprehensive set of values than what an individual needs to be an ethical agent in their personal lives.

The AHIMA Code of Ethics is to be used by AHIMA and individuals, agencies, organizations, and bodies (such as licensing and regulatory boards, insurance providers, courts of law, agency boards of directors, government agencies, and other professional groups) that choose to adopt it or use it as a frame of reference. The AHIMA Code of Ethics reflects the commitment of all to uphold the profession's values and to act ethically. Individuals of good character who discern moral questions and, in good faith, seek to make reliable ethical judgments, must apply ethical principles.

The code does not provide a set of rules that prescribe how to act in all situations. Specific applications of the code must take into account the context in which it is being considered and the possibility of conflicts among the code's values, principles, and guidelines. Ethical responsibilities flow from all human relationships, from the personal and familial to the social and professional. Further, the AHIMA Code of Ethics does not specify which values, principles, and guidelines are the most important and ought to outweigh others in instances when they conflict.

Code of Ethics 2004

Ethical Principles: The following ethical principles are based on the core values of the American Health Information Management Association and apply to all health information management professionals.

Health information management professionals:

   I. *Advocate, uphold and defend the individual's right to privacy and the doctrine of confidentiality in the use and disclosure of information.*

   II. *Put service and the health and welfare of persons before self-interest and conduct themselves in the practice of the profession so as to bring honor to themselves, their peers, and to the health information management profession.*

   III. *Preserve, protect, and secure personal health information in any form or medium and hold in the highest regard the contents of the records and other information of a confidential nature, taking into account the applicable statutes and regulations.*

   IV. *Refuse to participate in or conceal unethical practices or procedures.*

   V. *Advance health information management knowledge and practice through continuing education, research, publications, and presentations.*

   VI. *Recruit and mentor students, peers and colleagues to develop and strengthen the professional workforce.*

   VII. *Represent the profession accurately to the public.*

   VIII. *Perform honorably health information management association responsibilities, either appointed or elected, and preserve the confidentiality of any privileged information made known in any official capacity.*

   IX. *State truthfully and accurately their credentials, professional education, and experiences.*

   X. *Facilitate interdisciplinary collaboration in situations supporting health information practice.*

   XI. *Respect the inherent dignity and worth of every person.*

How to Interpret the Code of Ethics

The following ethical principles are based on the core values of the American Health Information Management Association and apply to all health information management professionals. Guidelines included for each ethical principle are a noninclusive list of behaviors and situations that can help to clarify the principle. They are not to be meant as a comprehensive list of all situations that can occur.

   I. *Advocate, uphold, and defend the individual's right to privacy and the doctrine of confidentiality in the use and disclosure of information.*

Health information management professionals **shall:**

   1.1.   Protect all confidential information to include personal, health, financial, genetic, and outcome information.

   1.2.   Engage in social and political action that supports the protection of privacy and confidentiality, and be aware of the impact of the political arena on the health information system. Advocate for changes in policy and legislation to ensure protection of privacy and confidentiality, coding compliance, and other issues that surface as advocacy issues as well as facilitating informed participation by the public on these issues.

   1.3.   Protect the confidentiality of all information obtained in the course of professional service. Disclose only information that is directly relevant or necessary to achieve the purpose of disclosure. Release information only with valid consent from a patient or a person legally authorized to consent on behalf of a patient or as authorized by federal or state regulations. The need-to-know criterion is essential when releasing health information for initial disclosure and all redisclosure activities.

   1.4.   Promote the obligation to respect privacy by respecting confidential information shared among colleagues, while responding to requests from the legal profession, the media, or other nonhealthcare-related individuals, during presentations or teaching and in situations that could cause harm to persons.

   II. *Put service and the health and welfare of persons before self-interest and conduct themselves in the practice of the profession so as to bring honor to themselves, their peers, and to the health information management profession.*

Health information management professionals **shall:**

   2.1.   Act with integrity, behave in a trustworthy manner, elevate service to others above self-interest, and promote high standards of practice in every setting.

2.2.   Be aware of the profession's mission, values, and ethical principles, and practice in a manner consistent with them by acting honestly and responsibly.

2.3.   Anticipate, clarify, and avoid any conflict of interest, to all parties concerned, when dealing with consumers, consulting with competitors, or in providing services requiring potentially conflicting roles (for example, finding out information about one facility that would help a competitor). The conflicting roles or responsibilities must be clarified, and appropriate action must be taken to minimize any conflict of interest.

2.4.   Ensure that the working environment is consistent and encourages compliance with the AHIMA Code of Ethics, taking reasonable steps to eliminate any conditions in their organizations that violate, interfere with, or discourage compliance with the code.

2.5.   Take responsibility and credit, including authorship credit, only for work they actually perform or to which they contribute. Honestly acknowledge the work of and the contributions made by others verbally or written, such as in publication.

Health information management professionals **shall not:**

2.6.   Permit their private conduct to interfere with their ability to fulfill their professional responsibilities.

2.7.   Take unfair advantage of any professional relationship or exploit others to further their personal, religious, political, or business interests.

III.   Preserve, protect, and secure personal health information in any form or medium and hold in the highest regards the contents of the records and other information of a confidential nature obtained in the official capacity, taking into account the applicable statutes and regulations.

Health information management professionals **shall:**

3.1.   Protect the confidentiality of patients' written and electronic records and other sensitive information. Take reasonable steps to ensure that patients' records are stored in a secure location and that patients' records are not available to others who are not authorized to have access.

3.2.   Take precautions to ensure and maintain the confidentiality of information transmitted, transferred, or disposed of in the event of a termina-

tion, incapacitation, or death of a healthcare provider to other parties through the use of any media. Disclosure of identifying information should be avoided whenever possible.

3.3.   Inform recipients of the limitations and risks associated with providing services via electronic media (such as computer, telephone, fax, radio, and television).

IV.   Refuse to participate in or conceal unethical practices or procedures.

Health information management professionals **shall:**

4.1.   Act in a professional and ethical manner at all times.

4.2.   Take adequate measures to discourage, prevent, expose, and correct the unethical conduct of colleagues.

4.3.   Be knowledgeable about established policies and procedures for handling concerns about colleagues' unethical behavior. These include policies and procedures created by AHIMA, licensing and regulatory bodies, employers, supervisors, agencies, and other professional organizations.

4.4.   Seek resolution if there is a belief that a colleague has acted unethically or if there is a belief of incompetence or impairment by discussing their concerns with the colleague when feasible and when such discussion is likely to be productive. Take action through appropriate formal channels, such as contacting an accreditation or regulatory body and/or the AHIMA Professional Ethics Committee.

4.5.   Consult with a colleague when feasible and assist the colleague in taking remedial action when there is direct knowledge of a health information management colleague's incompetence or impairment.

Health information management professionals **shall not:**

4.6.   Participate in, condone, or be associated with dishonesty, fraud and abuse, or deception. A noninclusive list of examples includes:

- Allowing patterns of retrospective documentation to avoid suspension or increase reimbursement

- Assigning codes without physician documentation

- Coding when documentation does not justify the procedures that have been billed

- Coding an inappropriate level of service

- Miscoding to avoid conflict with others

- Engaging in negligent coding practices

- Hiding or ignoring review outcomes, such as performance data

- Failing to report licensure status for a physician through the appropriate channels

- Recording inaccurate data for accreditation purposes

- Hiding incomplete medical records

- Allowing inappropriate access to genetic, adoption, or behavioral health information

- Misusing sensitive information about a competitor

- Violating the privacy of individuals

V. Advance health information management knowledge and practice through continuing education, research, publications, and presentations.

Health information management professionals **shall:**

5.1. Develop and enhance continually their professional expertise, knowledge, and skills (including appropriate education, research, training, consultation, and supervision). Contribute to the knowledge base of health information management and share with colleagues their knowledge related to practice, research, and ethics.

5.2. Base practice decisions on recognized knowledge, including empirically based knowledge relevant to health information management and health information management ethics.

5.3. Contribute time and professional expertise to activities that promote respect for the value, integrity, and competence of the health information management profession. These activities may include teaching, research, consultation, service, legislative testimony, presentations in the community, and participation in their professional organizations.

5.4. Engage in evaluation or research that ensures the anonymity or confidentiality of participants and of the data obtained from them by following guidelines developed for the participants in consultation with appropriate institutional review boards. Report evaluation and research findings accurately and take steps to correct any errors later found in published data using standard publication methods.

5.5. Take reasonable steps to provide or arrange for continuing education and staff development,

addressing current knowledge and emerging developments related to health information management practice and ethics.

Health information management professionals **shall not:**

5.6. Design or conduct evaluation or research that is in conflict with applicable federal or state laws.

5.7. Participate in, condone, or be associated with fraud or abuse.

VI. Recruit and mentor students, peers and colleagues to develop and strengthen professional workforce.

Health information management professionals **shall:**

6.1. Evaluate students' performance in a manner that is fair and respectful when functioning as educators or clinical internship supervisors.

6.2. Be responsible for setting clear, appropriate, and culturally sensitive boundaries for students.

6.3. Be a mentor for students, peers and new health information management professionals to develop and strengthen skills.

6.4. Provide directed practice opportunities for students.

Health information management professionals **shall not:**

6.5. Engage in any relationship with students in which there is a risk of exploitation or potential harm to the student.

VII. Accurately represent the profession to the public.

Health information management professionals **shall:**

7.1   Be an advocate for the profession in all settings and participate in activities that promote and explain the mission, values, and principles of the profession to the public.

VIII. Perform honorably health information management association responsibilities, either appointed or elected, and preserve the confidentiality of any privileged information made known in any official capacity.

Health information management professionals **shall:**

8.1. Perform responsibly all duties as assigned by the professional association.

8.2. Resign from an association position if unable to perform the assigned responsibilities with competence.

8.3. Speak on behalf of professional health information management organizations, accurately representing the official and authorized positions of the organizations.

IX. *State truthfully and accurately their credentials, professional education, and experiences.*

Health information management professionals **shall:**

9.1. Make clear distinctions between statements made and actions engaged in as a private individual and as a representative of the health information management profession, a professional health information organization, or the health information management professional's employer.

9.2. Claim and ensure that their representations to patients, agencies, and the public of professional qualifications, credentials, education, competence, affiliations, services provided, training, certification, consultation received, supervised experience, and other relevant professional experience are accurate.

9.3. Claim only those relevant professional credentials actually possessed and correct any inaccuracies occurring regarding credentials.

X. *Facilitate interdisciplinary collaboration in situations supporting health information practice.*

Health information management professionals **shall:**

10.1. Participate in and contribute to decisions that affect the well-being of patients by drawing on the perspectives, values, and experiences of those involved in decisions related to patients. Professional and ethical obligations of the interdisciplinary team as a whole and of its individual members should be clearly established.

XI. *Respect the inherent dignity and worth of every person.*

Health information management professionals **shall:**

11.1. Treat each person in a respectful fashion, being mindful of individual differences and cultural and ethnic diversity.

11.2. Promote the value of self-determination for each individual.

Acknowledgement

Adapted with permission from the Code of Ethics of the National Association of Social Workers.

Resources

National Association of Social Workers. "Code of Ethics." 1999. Available online from www.socialworkers.org/pubs/code/code.asp.

Harman, L.B., ed.. 2001. *Ethical Challenges in the Management of Health Information.* Gaithersburg, MD: Aspen.

AHIMA Code of Ethics, 1957, 1977, 1988, and 1998.

Revised & adopted by AHIMA House of Delegates—July 1, 2004

Appendix F
Answers to Check Your Understanding Exercises

Chapter 2

Check Your Understanding 2.1
1. b Greeks
2. d American Medical Association
3. d License
4. a Nurses
5. c Registered nurses
6. c Patient outcomes
7. a Accreditation
8. b Allied health

Check Your Understanding 2.2
1. b Authorized grants for states to construct new hospitals
2. g Required extensive changes in the Medicare program to control the rising cost of providing healthcare services to Medicare beneficiaries (PPS general implementation)
3. a Amendments to the Social Security Act that brought Medicare and Medicaid into existence
4. d Required hospitals to conduct continued-stay reviews for Medicare and Medicaid patients
5. h Instituted the Agency for Healthcare Policy
6. c Required concurrent review for Medicare and Medicaid patients
7. e Established the National Practitioner Data Bank
8. f Required peer review organizations to report actions taken against physicians to state medical boards and licensing agencies

Check Your Understanding 2.3
1. a Part of this organization's mission is to "enhance healthcare leadership and management excellence."
2. b This organization was originally called the Association of Hospital Superintendents.
3. f This organization's mission is to promote the art and science of medicine and to improve public health.
4. e Part of this organization's mission is to work for the improvement of health standards and the availability of healthcare services.
5. d This association was founded in 1928 under the name the Association of Record Librarians of North America.
6. c This organization was originally a commission instituted by the AHA in 1929.

Check Your Understanding 2.4
1. T
2. T
3. T
4. T
5. T
6. T
7. T
8. F
9. T
10. T

Check Your Understanding 2.5
1. c Subacute care
2. d Accessibility
3. d Quality improvement
4. c Managed care
5. a Population groups
6. b Patient-focused care
7. c Rehabilitation facilities
8. b Computers

Check Your Understanding 2.6

1. c   Represents a reversal in the balance between institutional and community care
2. e   Has an analysis and leadership role for health promotion and disease prevention.
3. a   Fastest-growing sector of Medicare
4. h   Care provided mainly in the home to the terminally ill and their families
5. j   Healthcare rendered in a nonacute care facility to patients who require inpatient nursing and related services for more than 30 consecutive days
6. f   Provides healthcare and healthcare planning services usually at the local level and to low-income patients
7. d   Are designed to meet patients' daily living, schooling, recreational, socialization, and routine medical care needs
8. g   Provides alternatives to inpatient care or serves as transition from inpatient to outpatient care or discharge
9. i   Care provided by different caregivers at several different levels of the healthcare system
10. b   Provides emergency services and urgent care for walk-in patients

Check Your Understanding 2.7

1. T
2. T
3. T
4. F
5. T
6. T
7. T
8. T

Chapter 3

Check Your Understanding 3.1

1. Informatics applies information management in the context of computer-based systems that are designed to support specific types of users in performing their work (for example, decision-making support). Information management, however, is a more generalized discipline with similar aims that are applied in both paper-based and computer-based environments.
2. Healthcare professionals use data and information constantly throughout their day to perform work for patients. They need to review previous and current clinical, financial, and demographic patient data and information as well as document new findings. Patient information is crucial for sharing and planning patient care with the healthcare team of professionals, for proper consultation and appropriate referrals, and for appropriate patient interaction from patient visits to patient billing.
3. Due to the ease and availability of Web-based commerce, online banking, ATMs, and other technologies, healthcare appears to lag behind. The healthcare industry is just beginning to adopt Web-based services for patients such as appointment scheduling, demographic and insurance updates, and e-mail contact with physicians or clinicians. This perception may be changed by informing healthcare consumers of the advances in healthcare technology, the importance of privacy and standards when sharing patient information, and the subjectivity of clinical practice, which makes healthcare different from other industries.

Check Your Understanding 3.2

1. The goal of healthcare informatics is to understand the structure, dynamics, and design of information systems, which are composed of people, technology, and organizational factors. This understanding allows optimum flow and use of information for every task in every context for every user. The healthcare informatics discipline focuses on the development of computer-based applications that are specifically designed to support different types of users in performing their work or meeting their needs. Healthcare informatics makes it possible for organizations to improve communications, achieve better outcomes, improve processes, and make administration more efficient.
2. The Institute of Medicine (IOM) released a report in 1991 (and rereleased it in 1997) based on the work of the IOM's Committee on Improving the Patient Record in Light of Technology. This report championed the computer-based patient record. Two additional IOM reports, one released in 1999 and the second in 2001, were based on the work of the IOM's Committee on the Quality of Healthcare in America, which identified major issues associated with deaths attributable to preventable medical errors and called for a transformation of healthcare delivery in the United States. The IOM's third and fourth reports were also from the IOM's Committee on the Quality of Health Care in America. The 2002 report argued that the federal government should lead the development of clinical standards for measuring care, and called for financial incentives for organizations that improve quality. The 2003 report proposed the Consolidated Health Informatics (CHI) initiative in which the DHHS, DoD, and VA work with the NCVHA to identify appropriate clinical data standards. This report mandated that EHRs operate as a part of a national network of health information accessible by

all healthcare organizations. In all these landmark reports, information technology (IT) needs and benefits were included in the call to action.

3. The National Health Information Network (NHIN) is a government-sponsored initiative also referred to as the "Medical Internet." The purpose of this initiative is to provide a comprehensive view of a patient's health information at the point of care through the development of a interconnected, knowledge-based network of interoperable information systems. Providers of care will be able to electronically exchange information among all electronic health records so that a complete EHR can be assembled whenever and wherever a patient presents for care.

4. Barriers include a current lack of standards, which are necessary for interoperability and data sharing; insufficient funding; a lack of ongoing economic incentives, which are needed to sustain infrastructure operations; and public concern over privacy.

5. This approach is not fully integrated; rather, it consists of distinct, distributed, disparate, and decentralized databases. Centralization only occurs with an EMPI for demographic data. This approach is favored because it does not require a unique national patient identifier, it allows contributing organizations to retain ownership and control of their data, and new computer systems are not required, which allows for an easier transition to the regional EHR. Drawbacks include the lack of a centralized database, standardization, and a unified data model. The lack of these things makes decision support and reporting difficult.

Check Your Understanding 3.3

1. Structured data include laboratory test results; demographic data such as name, address, and birth date; financial data such as dollar amounts charged for services; and codes that represent case-mix types. Unstructured data include transcribed radiology reports and histories and physicals.

   The term *discrete data* is another term for structured data and includes, for example, ICD-9-CM codes, patient weight and height measurements, and dollar amounts. Examples of free text data include handwritten progress notes and transcribed pathology reports

2. When a healthcare professional searches for discrete data or structured data, the database search engine can easily find, retrieve, and manipulate the data element. Free-text data, or unstructured data, cannot be easily retrieved or manipulated.

3. Both diagnostic images and document images are bit-mapped data. All document images and some diagnostic images are based on analog documents (paper or photographic film) that must be scanned to digitize

the data for electronic storage. However, some diagnostic images are based on digital modalities, such as images resulting from computed radiography (CR), magnetic resonance (MR), and computed tomography (CT).

4. Examples of real audio include digital heart sounds, voice annotation, and voice recognition. Cardiac catheterizations, ultrasounds, and echocardiograms are examples of motion or streaming data. Examples of signal or vector data include fetal heart monitor, ECGs (electrocardiograms), and EEGs (electroencephalograms).

5. Possible answers:

   a. Speech recognition technology employs basic natural language processing capabilities as it translates spoken words (natural language voice bytes) into text. However, speech recognition technology does not yet employ the advanced capabilities of natural language processing; for instance, speech recognition technology is not yet capable of taking two sound-alike terms (such as ileum and ilium) with different meanings and then selecting the correct term based on an analysis of the context.

   b. Natural language processing technology and Boolean searching differ from each other in that the former considers sentence structure (syntax), meaning (semantics), and context to accurately extract data from free text. For example, "no shortness of breath, chest pain aggravated by exercise" and "no chest pain, shortness of breath aggravated by exercise" look the same to a Boolean word search engine when it identifies occurrences of "chest" and "pain" in the same sentence. Natural language processing technology, however, would discern the syntactical and semantic differences between these two phrases.

Check Your Understanding 3.4

1. Bar coding is commonly used in healthcare; examples include labels, patient wristbands, specimen containers, and medication packets. Optical character recognition (OCR) technology is used on a limited basis; examples include the indexing of scanned documents and the digitizing of text documents. Intelligent character recognition (ICR) technology is being adopted slowly; examples include pen-based and handheld input devices. Radio frequency identification (RFID) is rapidly evolving; examples include the tracking of moveable patients, clinicians, medications, and equipment. Intelligent document recognition (IDR) has recently been developed; examples include document and form-type identification.

2. Electronic data interchange (EDI) was the health-care industry's first venture into direct electronic transmission of data between the computer system of one organization and the computer system of another organization (often called a business partner). By 2000, EDI as a term (not as a concept) had become dated and was replaced by e-commerce and e-health.

E-health now refers to the practice of e-commerce within the healthcare industry.

3. As discrete healthcare organizations come together to form integrated delivery networks (IDNs), the distribution of patient information among multiple databases and in multiple formats poses problems. The IDN wants to operate as a seamless delivery system for its customers and access longitudinal information about its business across the entire delivery network. As a result, healthcare providers are developing strategic enterprise master patient index (EMPI) initiatives because this technology, through an indexing scheme, ties a patient's information together across separate systems and databases, providing access to multiple repositories of information about overlapping patient populations.

4. An object-oriented database associated with a clinical data repository can contain several types of unstructured data (for example, streaming video, free text, real audio, or vector graphic data).

5. An ED/CM system is any electronic system that manages an organization's analog and digital documents or content to significantly improve business work processes.

Document imaging technology electronically captures, stores, identifies, retrieves, and distributes documents that are not generated digitally or are generated digitally but are stored on paper.

Workflow/business process management (BPM) technology allows computers to add and extract value from document content as the documents move throughout an organization. The documents can be automatically assigned, routed, activated, and managed through system-controlled rules that mirror business operations.

Computer output laser disk (COLD)/enterprise report management (ERM) technology electronically stores, manages, and distributes documents that are generated in a digital format and whose output data are report-formatted. These documents can be distributed through fax, e-mail, Web, and hard copy.

Automated forms processing technology allows users to electronically enter data into online forms and electronically extract the data from the online forms for data manipulation. The form document is stored in a form format, as the user sees it on the screen, for ease of interpretation.

Digital signature management technology offers both signer and document authentication for analog or digital documents. Signer authentication is the ability to identify the person who digitally signed the document. Document authentication ensures that the document and the signature cannot be altered.

6. Secure clinical messaging is not dependent upon time zones, it can be done in each clinical user's own timeframe, it gives clinical recipients time to think over and respond to issues appropriately, and it does not require all participants to be available at the same time.

7. Web browser-based systems are more complex than Web-enabled systems. Web browser-based systems use Web-based programming languages (such as HML, SGML, XML, or Java) as the system's code so that the Web browser acts as the primary desktop interface for accessing information directly from the organization's data repositories. Web-enabled systems do not use Web-based programming language. Instead, authorized users must access data in Web-enabled systems through a Web page from which the organization's applications (which may be written, for example, in Visual Basic) are then launched.

8. The clinical workstation (clinician/physician portal) provides the clinician with a single point of access with a common user interface (and a single log-on password) to launch and view information from disparate applications.

9. Web portals provided by providers/payers allow patients to schedule appointments, ask questions of their providers via secure messaging, request prescription renewals, securely view all or portions of their provider-based EHR, and pay bills online.

10. Web-based intranets are designed to enhance communication among an organization's internal employees and facilities. An employee handbook may be found on an organization's intranet. Web-based extranets are designed to enhance communication among an organization's business partners. A medical supply company might use an extranet to check an organization's inventory level to determine when to reorder.

11. Under an application service provider (ASP) model, a healthcare organization can gain quick access to functioning application software with the cost distributed over time and based on a set monthly or transaction-based fee structure. The organization is spared the burden of maintaining the system using internal technical staff because maintenance is the responsibility of the ASP. The drawbacks for the organization are that it must accept an off-the-shelf software application, it will lose control over the timing of upgrades, it remains responsible for firewalls and HIPAA compliance, and it must be prepared to transition its data from the ASP's control should the contract be dissolved.

Check Your Understanding 3.5

1. Data repositories are structured on relational and object-oriented database models that are well suited for online transaction processing (OLTP), and the data are updated in real time by current transactions. Data warehouses are structured on multidimensional database models that are well suited for online analytical processing (OLAP), and the data are historical in nature, subject-oriented, and nonvolatile.

2. Clinical decision support systems provide information that assists clinicians in making decisions related to patient care. Examples include reminders and alerts, clinical guideline advice, and benchmarking data. Expert decision support systems also provide information that assists clinicians. Expert decision support systems, however, first apply a set of rules or protocols to patient information, then provide a problem analysis, and finally offer advice similar to that which might be expected to be given by an expert serving as a consultant.

3. Artificial intelligence technology performs functions normally associated with humans, such as language, reasoning, learning, and problem solving.

Check Your Understanding 3.6

1. Distinct examples of diagnostic tests that involve physiological signal processing include electrocardiograms (EKGs), electroencephalograms (EEGs), electromyograms (EMGs), fetal tracings, digital blood pressure (BP) monitors, and digital thermometers.

2. Patient data that are typically collected and viewed (accessed) by care providers using point-of-care systems include order entry data, medication administration data, vital signs, input/output data, and lab test results.

3. Providers are recognizing the enormous variation in how they diagnose, treat, and care for patients. Therefore, they are looking to standardize care for both quality assurance and cost-containment purposes. Automation (computerization) of care plans, guidelines, pathways, and protocols promotes easier access to information by clinicians and easier ongoing maintenance.

4. Second- and third-generation telehealth applications rely on patient interaction and consultation, whereas first-generation applications relied on the transfer of patient information only. (The use of guided robotics is evident in third-generation telehealth applications. Telesurgeons in New York City, for example, can perform a gallbladder surgery on a patient in France via robots fed by high-speed signals sent across the Atlantic Ocean through fiber-optic cables.)

5. These IOM reports defined a computer-based patient record (CPR) as "an electronic patient record that resides in a system specifically designed to support users by providing accessibility to complete and accurate data, alerts, reminders, clinical decision support systems, links to medical knowledge and other aids." An electronic medical record (EMR) composed of digitized, bit-mapped images cannot provide the full functionality of the CPR as defined above. Alerts, reminders, links to medical knowledge, and so on are not functional components of a patient record that is primarily composed of digitized images of documents.

6. The EHR-S Functional Model and Standard laid the foundation for the first generation standards-based EHR and defined the EHR's components.

7. Examples of services using e-health technology that healthcare organizations offer include personal health records, patient appointment scheduling, patient registration, previsit health screening, postvisit patient education, and information on health conditions.

8. The e-health culture in a healthcare organization is characterized by quick response to communications from patients and customers and a high comfort level with working in partnership with a variety of other organizations.

9. The shared data record is a personal health record (PHR) supported by the provider and maintained by both the provider and the patient. In the EHR extension model, the provider allows access for an authorized patient to the record for review and extraction purposes only. PHRs built on the provider-sponsored information management model use communication vehicles between provider and patient so that reminders, appointment scheduling, prescription refills, and monitoring tools for disease management can be handled by the PHR system.

Check Your Understanding 3.7

1. Public key infrastructure (PKI) is a type of encryption technology. It involves a private key (known to one computer) and a public key that is given to a second computer. The second computer receives an incoming message from the first computer and decodes it with the public key and its own private key. PKI is becoming the standard encryption technology for securing data transfers and online authentication. Public key infrastructure is receiving much attention within the healthcare industry because secure data transfers and online authentication are vital in meeting the HIPAA security regulations.

2. In general, the major benefits of using biometrics to verify identity are that biometrics ensure unique positive identification without the fear of replication or duplication, and biometrics are very reliable personal identifiers. The major drawback of using biometrics is that, because biometric methods are so reliable, individuals might feel that their privacy is threatened or compromised when they are tracked by such devices.

   Fingerprints are the oldest and most popular type of biometric because they are accurate and easy to obtain. Fingerprint scanning requires the subject to pause and place a finger on a device while the imprint match is made. This is problematic for individuals with no or deformed fingers. Retinal and iris scanning are very accurate types of biometrics. However, they are not as popular as fingerprint scanning because of the close eye contact users must make with the scanning device. These scans are problematic for subjects who wear eyeglasses or contact lenses. Facial image recognition is the least obtrusive type of biometric. However, it requires the matching of dynamic images, which is more technologically difficult than the matching of static images such as fingerprints or retinal/iris scans.

3. Proxy services are special-purpose programs allowing network administrators to permit or deny user access to specific applications or features of applications. Filtering services allow routers to make permit/deny decisions for each piece of information that attempts to enter or leave a private network.

4. Delegating responsibility to users for examining their audit histories is one way to establish user trust. Another way to instill user trust is to frequently sample system usage by organizational managers and publish results of audit trails.

Check Your Understanding 3.8

1. As the patient record evolves into an EHR, the domains of HIM professional practice (clinical data quality, the legal and regulatory integrity of the record, and the privacy and security of the patient record) are transitioning from the paper-based environment into the electronic environment. Informatics is defined as information management applied in a computer-based environment, so HIM professionals functioning in an EHR environment are key players (along with IT professionals) within the informatics discipline.

Chapter 4

Check Your Understanding 4.1

1. The health information management (HIM) profession has been changed by government sponsorship and regulation of healthcare, the advent of computers, advances in medical practice, socioeconomic changes, and progress in higher education.

2. The information technology field is not specific to healthcare. It requires more in-depth knowledge of computer science, but less or no training in clinical processes, the healthcare industry, and other specifics of the HIM curriculum.

3. One of the HIM professional's principal roles is to develop systems that collect accurate and timely clinical information and make it available to decision makers. In contrast, other healthcare professionals collect and use these data in the direct provision of patient care.

4. Unlike the other forms of data for which health information managers are responsible, reference data are not derived from individual patient data.

Check Your Understanding 4.2

1. The benefits gained from HIM planning include making information available; ensuring appropriate access, security, and confidentiality; and making the process of accessing and retrieving information in clinical and administrative processes more efficient.

2. Data modeling defines the data that are required, whereas process or work-flow modeling identifies how and when the data will be captured.

3. A data dictionary defines all of the unique data elements in the data set and contains the definition, data attributes, edits, and authentication requirements.

4. In data modeling, understanding how data are used and their sources can help to identify what data are needed. For process and work-flow modeling, an understanding of the care process can assist in identifying what data can be collected and used by whom. Knowledge of the data meanings can help suggest data edits.

Check Your Understanding 4.3

1. The purpose of studying health services organization and delivery is to provide an understanding of the context in which health information is collected and used. This understanding is critical to effective data management and is one way that HIM is distinguished from other information management or informatics disciplines.

2. Accreditation standards are included in the healthcare information requirements and standards section of the curriculum.

3. The elements of healthcare data, content, and structure are:
   - structure and use of health information
   - health information media
   - type and content of health records
   - data quality assessment and integrity
   - secondary data sources
   - healthcare data sets
   - health information archival systems
   - National Healthcare Information Infrastructure
   - data collection tools

4. For performing research using health information, the following curriculum topics are useful:
   - biomedical sciences
   - healthcare statistics
   - biomedical research
   - quality management of healthcare statistics and research
   - quality management and performance improvement

Check Your Understanding 4.4

1. The American Health Information Management Association, the Association for American Transcription, the National Cancer Registrars Association, and the Health Information Management and Systems Society offer their members professional certification.

2. Membership in more than one professional association may be helpful if one's career involves more than one domain of practice.

3. Key services provided by professional associations include:
   - networking opportunities
   - continuing education
   - certification
   - advocacy

4. The International Medical Informatics Association (IMIA) and the International Federation of Health Record Associations (IFHRO) are both examples of international associations dealing with health information.

5. Individuals who hold AHIMA credentials are required to conduct themselves according to the AHIMA Code of Ethics. Violation of the code of ethics may result in disciplinary action, including revocation of credentials.

6. The code of ethics instructs all HIM professionals to advance health information management knowledge and practice through continuing education, research, publications, and presentations and to conduct themselves in the practice of the profession so as to bring honor to themselves, their peers, and the health information management profession.

7. The AHIMA code of ethics states that HIM professionals should perform honorably health information management association responsibilities, either appointed or elected, and preserve the confidentiality of any privileged information made known in any official capacity.

8. The benefits of certification include the following.
   - Certification demonstrates to colleagues and superiors a dedication to high-quality healthcare and to the highest standards of health information management.
   - Certification presents solid evidence to employers that an employee has been trained and tested to implement best practices and apply current technological solutions, abilities that, in turn, advance the organization.
   - Certification sets a person apart from uncredentialed job candidates. In recent AHIMA-sponsored research groups, healthcare executives and recruiters cited these reasons for preferring credentialed personnel: assurance of current knowledge through continued education, possession of field-tested experience, and verification of base-level competency.
   - Certification has value for employers because it supports a worker's commitment to upholding industry standards and regulations, thereby potentially saving organizations from fines and penalties due to errors or noncompliance.
   - Certification is a beneficial addition to a resume because it provides recognition of a candidate's capabilities. Because credentials appear after a person's name, they announce expertise with every signature.
   - Certification is maintained by abiding by the AHIMA Code of Ethics and completing the required continuing education activities.

9. RHIA applicants must pass AHIMA's RHIA examination and must hold one of the following educational requirements:
   - a baccalaureate degree from a CAHIIM-accredited health information administration (HIA) program
   - a baccalaureate degree from an accredited college or university and a certificate in HIA from a CAHIIM-accredited program
   - a degree from a foreign HIA baccalaureate program with which AHIMA has a reciprocal agreement (AHIMA currently has an agreement with the Health Information Management Association of Australia at the baccalaureate level)

10. Certification records are audited annually on a random sample of 2 percent of the reporting population.

11. Continuing education activities are reported to AHIMA through completion of a continuing education (CE) report form either in paper or via the Web site.

Chapter 5

Check Your Understanding 5.1

1. There are many possible answers to this question. An ICD-9-CM code is an example of data that would become information when aggregated into a report showing the top discharge diagnoses for the month.
2. Individuals within an organization need different levels of information. For example, a chief executive officer (CEO) might need a more advanced analysis of discharge statistics than a unit manager might need. A monthly report might already be information for the unit manager but might need to be inserted into a database for comparison with other facilities to become information for the CEO.

Check Your Understanding 5.2

1. The JCAHO IM plan begins with a needs assessment because each organization has unique information needs. No one information management plan would work for all.
2. Patient-specific, aggregate, comparative, and knowledge-based information go into the model. The JCAHO identifies five categories of information uses: clinical decision making, organizational decision making, research, performance improvement, and education (of patients, families, and healthcare providers).
3. The basic principles of information management are treating information as an essential organizational resource, obtaining top executive support for information systems (IS) planning and management, and developing an IS strategic plan and vision.
4. Healthcare organizations are information intensive. So much patient and ancillary information is created that it is imperative that it be managed effectively.

Check Your Understanding 5.3

1. These models have some characteristics in common, but their structures are different. The AHIMA model includes the dimensions of data quality and the MRI lists principles of documentation. The MRI model divides documentation into both information capture and report generation.
   a. Timeliness and accuracy
   b. AHIMA strives to include all healthcare data, but the MRI model limits the characteristics to clinical documentation. They are compatible.
2. The seven dimensions of data quality are relevancy, granularity, precision, timeliness, currency, consistency, and accuracy.
3. There are many possible answers to this question. Please refer to the examples provided in the chapter.

Check Your Understanding 5.4

1. Today, the most common type of database is the relational database.
2. Database design helps eliminate unnecessary redundancy and promotes data accuracy. Update, addition, and deletion errors are essentially eliminated in a well-designed relational database.
3. A data model is a "picture" or abstraction of real conditions. It shows how data are related within a database.
4. The conceptual data model has the highest level of abstraction; the physical model the lowest. The conceptual model is both software and hardware independent, the logical model is hardware independent, and the physical model is software specific. The physical model is essentially obsolete because most databases today are relational and do not require a physical-level model.
5. Entity relationship diagrams (ERDs) are used as communication tools among database developers and users at the conceptual level for any type of database and at the logical level for a relational database. Unified modeling language (UML) is a modeling language used to show a "picture" of an object-oriented database.
6. The components of an ERD are entity (relation), relationship, and attribute.
7. In an ERD, an entity is represented as a rectangle; a relationship is represented as a triangle.
8.

Check Your Understanding 5.5

1. A data dictionary contains detailed, agreed-upon database or enterprise-wide data element definitions. A data dictionary is very important for data consistency and in facilitating comparisons or aggregations of data across systems.
2. A list of terms and data elements would be housed in an enterprise-wide data dictionary. A system catalog would also include information about data tables, relationships, and other information pertinent to the development and maintenance of the database.

Check Your Understanding 5.6

1. The data administrator is responsible for managing the data that may be stored within a database. Database administrators manage the technical aspects of a database and focus on managing the data within the database. According to the AHIMA definition of data resource manager, the data resource manager also retrieves data and information from the database.
2. Health information managers would be excellent candidates for data administrators and data resource managers. There are multiple reasons that could be listed by learners.

Check Your Understanding 5.7

1. Data integrity is the assurance that data have been accessed or modified only by those authorized to do so and in a manner appropriate to the database. Data integrity is controlled by the database design. Numerous data integrity constraints or rules are built into databases.

2. Data security focuses on access authorization; that is, preventing unauthorized users from obtaining entry into the database. Data integrity includes access issues, but is also concerned with what happens to the data after they are accessed.

3. The authorization management features of the DBMS define users, assign passwords, define user groups, and assign access privileges.

Check Your Understanding 5.8

1. Graphs should:
   - show the data
   - induce the viewer to think about the substance rather than the methodology, graphic design, the technology or other things
   - avoid distorting what the data have to say
   - make large data sets coherent
   - encourage the eye to compare different pieces of data
   - reveal the data at several levels of detail
   - serve a reasonably clear purpose
   - be closely integrated with the statistical and verbal descriptions of the data set

2. The following are some basic guidelines for graphical excellence.
   - The well-designed presentation of interesting data is a matter of substance, statistics, and design.
   - Complex ideas should be communicated with clarity, precision, and efficiency
   - Excellent graphics give the viewer the greatest number of ideas in the shortest time with least ink in the smallest space.

3. Effective presentations should be:
   - *Big*—Make sure the font used is large enough to be seen from 2 meters away. Different fonts appear different, so it is best to test the font by moving away from the presentation. As a general rule, anything smaller than 24 points will be too small. When in doubt…go larger!
   - *Progressive*—Start with the main points of the presentation and then provide more detail for each point. Avoid giving the viewer all of the information at one time.
   - *Consistent*—Any differences should be planned. For example, if the viewer sees a different size, color, or font, they will interpret that as indicating importance. See figure 5.19.

- *Simple*—One of the most common mistakes with PowerPoint presentations is that the creator feels he or she must include lots of detail, color, fonts, pictures, sounds, animations, or slide transitions. Generally, follow the 6 × 7 rule when creating the text for slides: there should be no more than 6 lines per slide and no more than 7 words per line. See figure 5.20. Avoid too many colors and unnecessary pictures on a slide. Fonts should be consistent. Animations and transitions should be used sparingly and only for important emphasis.
- *Clear*—Avoid using italics or all capitals. Use San serif fonts. Use color for emphasis rather than underlining. Use contrasting and complementary colors.

Chapter 6

Check Your Understanding 6.1

1. Strategic information systems (IS) planning is important because it ensures that the IS plans are well aligned and integrated with the organization's overall strategic plans. Information systems generally require an enormous financial investment and require considerable resources (hardware, software, network, and personnel) to implement and maintain. Too often, they fail because of poor planning and inadequate involvement from key stakeholders, including clinicians and senior leadership. Most healthcare institutions have competing IS needs, and the strategic IS planning process enables leaders to set priorities and make informed decisions based on current and future needs.

   If the IS plan is not aligned with the organization's overall strategic plan, the organization may end up not having in place the information infrastructure or systems needed to support its strategic directions or initiatives. This can lead to cost overruns, the acquisition of ineffective or inadequate systems, low staff morale, and dissatisfied patients.

2. Senior-level managers and clinicians from key areas within the healthcare enterprise, including, but not limited to, information systems, medical staff, nursing, ancillary departments, and finance, should be involved in strategic IS planning. Senior-level input is critical. Different organizations might choose different individuals to lead the effort. In some cases, the chief information officer (CIO) is the best person. In other situations, a well-respected physician or senior administrator should be the leader. Whoever is selected should be well respected within the organization, have strong communication and project management skills, and have the power or clout to make things happen.

3. If an organization's overall strategic plan and the IS plan are not integrated or aligned, the healthcare organization runs the risk of not having in place the information infrastructure or systems needed to support its strategic directions or initiatives. This misalignment or lack of integration can lead to cost overruns, the acquisition of ineffective or inadequate systems, low staff morale, high staff turnover, and dissatisfied patients.

4. A healthcare organization should examine its current information systems before embarking on a new IS initiative. It should have a good handle on what systems are currently used, to what extent they meet the needs of end users, which ones will likely need to be replaced or upgraded, and which ones are likely to be obsolete. An organization also should examine how well existing systems support its strategic plans. If it moves forward without conducting this internal assessment of existing systems, it runs the risk of failing to identify needs or of acquiring new systems that are not needed.

5. A healthcare organization can prioritize its IS projects or needs in a number of ways. One way is to identify all proposed IS projects and hold an intensive retreat where key stakeholders rank and score each project in terms of its priority to the organization's mission and strategic goals. Another approach is to have senior leadership establish IS priorities as part of the strategic planning process.

Check Your Understanding 6.2

1. The systems development life cycle (SDLC) typically begins after the board of directors or senior administration has given the "go ahead" and approved funding for an IS project. Many institutions use the SDLC to select, implement, and evaluate healthcare information systems. IS priorities are generally established as part of the strategic IS planning process, after which the SDLC begins.

2. The four main phases of the SDLC are analysis, design, implementation, and maintenance and evaluation.

   • In the analysis phase, the organization further explores the need for a new IS, pinpoints problems with the existing system, identifies user needs, and establishes specifications. The primary focus is on the business problem, independent of any technology that might be used to implement a solution to the problem.

   • In the design phase, the organization considers how the new system will be designed or selected. Will it be built in-house, by an outside developer, or purchased from a vendor? Most organizations begin by exploring what products are currently available

from vendors through submission of a request for information (RFI). Responses to the RFI are used to narrow down the list to vendors who will be invited to respond to the subsequent request for proposal (RFP). Organizations may use a variety of other methods to assess vendors and their products, including contacting current users, attending user conferences, and hosting vendor demonstrations. Informal and formal mechanisms are used to obtain key stakeholder input on the various products. This phase ends with final contract negotiations for procurement of the system.

   • In the implementation phase, plans are made and executed to implement the new information system. This can be a lengthy process. Strong project management and leadership are required to coordinate the various activities. Key activities may include, but are not limited to, preparing the site, installing necessary hardware and software, preparing data tables, building interfaces, establishing a stable infrastructure, training staff, testing the new system, identifying and correcting errors, preparing documentation to support system use, implementing conversion plans, and testing backup and disaster recovery procedures.

   • In the maintenance and evaluation phase, problems in the new system are addressed. IT staff must be available to correct any problems and to identify new problems before they occur. For critical patient care systems, adequate technical staff and procedures must be in place for responding to system problems at all hours of the day, including weekends. Ongoing training must take place, and methods for monitoring data quality, integrity, and security should be established. It also is important to evaluate the new system on an ongoing basis to assess the degree to which it is contributing to the institution's goals and meeting user needs.

3. The RFI is generally sent to an extensive list of vendors and is used to assess the products available and to identify those vendors who offer products likely to meet the facility's needs. It typically outlines the facility's needs in general and broad terms. Responses from the RFI are used to narrow down the list of vendors to those who will be invited to respond to the RFP. In contrast to the RFI, the RFP includes detailed specifications and guidelines that the vendor should follow in submitting a bid.

4. The HIM professional can be an active participant throughout the SDLC. In the analysis phase, he or she may be able to assist in identifying problems with the current system, assessing user needs, and determining user specifications. In the design phase, he or she may be able to assist in evaluating vendors and their

products and also could provide valuable input when security and confidentiality issues are raised. Because the HIM professional has an understanding of both clinical and financial data, he or she could provide a broad perspective on how systems are integrated or how they interact with each other. In the implementation phase, the HIM professional could assume an active role in rolling out the new system through testing, training staff, and identifying problems.

Chapter 7

Check Your Understanding 7.1

1. Patient-specific data consist of data elements that describe characteristics about an individual patient, such as height, sex, principal diagnosis, and blood pressure. These data are contained in the health record of the specific patient and are identifiable as belonging to that patient.

   Aggregate data are data that have been extracted (or abstracted) from individual patient health records and collected into a database to describe characteristics about groups of patients. An example of aggregate data might be the number of men over age 50 who have had a myocardial infarction in the past year. Although identifying data may be kept in a database, aggregate data are generally presented and used without identifying individual patients.

2. The adage about "comparing apples to oranges" is applicable in healthcare data. To accurately collect, comb, compare, analyze, and interpret data, it is critical that data elements be defined in a common manner. For example, in studying the link between maternal risk factors and fetal death, it is very important that everyone use the same definition of fetal death and the same definitions of the risk factors. If data elements are not defined in a uniform way, conclusions drawn from the data may be erroneous.

3. Healthcare data sets provide standardized definitions (that have been determined by experts, usually through a process of negotiation and collaboration) of data elements. The data sets are then either mandated by a controlling agency, such as the federal government, or adopted by common consent in the healthcare industry. One example of a standardized definition is the one for principal diagnosis. The definition, as a result of a collaborative project in the 1960s, was adopted as part of the Uniform Hospital Discharge Data Set (UHDDS). It was subsequently adopted as part of a federal requirement under the prospective payment system (PPS) and is used across the United States to identify the principal diagnosis for all discharged hospital inpatients.

4. The National Center for Health Statistics (NCHS) sponsored the original conference on discharge data abstract systems that resulted in adoption of the UHDDS.

5. Before the widespread use of technology, data were collected and analyzed manually within hospitals and other healthcare facilities. The data were used internally but rarely reported or compared with the data of external organizations. As long as data definitions were applied consistently within an organization, there was no need to be concerned with external data definitions. The advent of computer systems allowed healthcare facilities to use data for clinical and administrative decision making and to develop comparative databases. Regulatory agencies such as federal and state agencies and the Joint Commission on Accreditation of Healthcare Organizations (JCAHO) began to demand sophisticated comparative data. Third-party payers and other external data organizations also developed reporting systems that required use of consistent and uniform data submission.

6. The MDS provides a structured way to organize resident information and to document problems identified in the assessment process. Documentation of a problem triggers a resident assessment protocol (RAP), which requires that the LTC facility evaluate the nature of the problem, the complications and risk factors associated with it, factors to consider in developing the care plan, and the need for referrals or further evaluation. LTC personnel use these data to outline a specific and personalized plan of care for the resident and to assess the resident's progress related to the indicated problems.

7. Data Elements for Emergency Department Systems (DEEDS) is a data set that supports the uniform collection of data in hospital-based emergency departments. The Essential Medical Data Set (EMDS) complements DEEDS and was designed to build a medical history of each individual emergency patient.

8. The common purpose for the use of data generated through the Health Plan Employer Data and Information Set (HEDIS) and ORYX is to evaluate outcomes of care by providing information about the effectiveness of interventions and treatments for specific diseases. Healthcare facilities can compare their success rates with those of other facilities to determine areas for performance improvement.

9. Clinical data provide the basis for evaluating patient progress and response to treatment. They also can provide information on the patient's long-term functional status following various treatment modalities. Because all these outcomes measurement systems focus on improving the quality of care for patients with specific disease conditions, it is critical to collect clinical data about the patient's disease, condition, treatment, functional status, survival, and so on in order to determine the efficacy and effectiveness of interventions.

10. A national health information network (NHIN) defines three dimensions of the infrastructure that provide a means for conceptualizing the capture, storage, communication, processing, and presentation of information for each group of information users:
   • Personal health dimension
   • Healthcare provider dimension
   • Population health dimension

Check Your Understanding 7.2

1. The transition from data sets to healthcare informatics standards has been evolutionary. The original data sets, such as the UHDDS and the UACDS, contained a list of data elements recommended or required for inclusion in a patient's record. They also contained definitions of the data elements, such as the UHDDS definition of principal diagnosis. In some cases, the data set also defined the manner in which data should be collected, such as using the postal zip code as a standard element in describing a patient's address.

   Healthcare informatics standards describe accepted methods for collecting, maintaining, and/or transferring healthcare data between computer systems. They are more inclusive than data sets in that they also specify hardware and/or software configurations, the mechanics of collecting and storing data, and the methods of transferring data. In addition, they are intended for computer-to-computer communication.

2. The computer revolution and the widespread use of technology have propelled the healthcare industry to develop standards that facilitate communication among providers, payers, regulators, researchers, and other users of healthcare data. Without healthcare informatics standards that set uniform definitions and link individualized platforms, data stored in specific computer systems could not be transmitted to other entities. The wealth of data stored in healthcare organization (HCO) systems would not be available for the variety of reimbursement, research, evaluation, and assessment purposes for which it is commonly used today.

3. The American Society for Testing and Materials (ASTM) Standard E1384 establishes structure and content standards for electronic health record systems. It describes data elements to be included in a CPR and gives clear definitions of these data elements. The Electronic Health Record System (EHR-S) Functional Model and Standards addresses the content and structure of an EHR.

4. The ASTM, Health Level Seven (HL7), the Accredited Standards Committee X12 (referred to as AST X12), and the creators of electronic data interchange (EDI) have been actively involved in developing healthcare informatics standards that are applicable to the EHR.

Check Your Understanding 7.3

1. ICD-9-CM and CPT/HCPCS codes represent clinical information and are used to communicate information about individual patients as well as to perform studies related to aggregate groups of patients. To generate high-quality data, coding systems must rely on data standards that set clear and concise definitions, conventions, and processes for coding. For coded data to be comparable across institutions, both data producers and data users must adhere to standard code sets and data standards.

2. Historically, healthcare consumers have received an identifier number called a medical record number at the time of admission or encounter with each healthcare provider. The result is that many consumers have health records at a variety of clinics, hospitals, emergency centers, nursing homes, and so on. These records are maintained in the facility and are not easily linked. Thus, healthcare can easily become fragmented because information about an individual is not coordinated. A unique healthcare identification number that would be used in every site of care would provide an effective means of linking the records of an individual consumer across disparate systems and would improve the quality of care.

3. Use of the Social Security number (SSN) as a unique identification number is considered inappropriate due to privacy, confidentiality, and security issues.

4. The extensible markup language (XML) was developed as a universal language to facilitate the storage and transmission of data published on the Internet. It allows each healthcare data item to be tagged with a descriptor that clearly defines and differentiates it from all other data items. Moreover, it allows data to be organized in a meaningful and searchable form and serves as an exchange standard for information transmitted over the Internet.

Chapter 8

Check Your Understanding 8.1

1. The primary purpose of patient health information is patient care and treatment.
2. Six other purposes or uses of patient health information are (1) support for clinical decision making and communication, (2) documentation or services, (3) evaluation of quality and efficacy of care, (4) research, (5) education, and (6) information for management as required by law and regulations.
3. The American College of Surgeons (ACS) developed the first standards for hospitals that included requirements for medical records.

   The Joint Commission on Accreditation of Healthcare Organizations (JCAHO) is the successor organization to the ACS and promotes voluntary accreditation. JCAHO develops and publishes standards to help improve the safety and quality of healthcare in the United States. A large portion of JCAHO's standards focus on information and documentation.

   The Centers for Medicare and Medicaid Services (CMS) includes requirements for records in its Conditions of Participation. The Conditions of Participation spell out requirements that facilities must meet to be part of CMS programs.

   State licensure has regulations for content of records and information that must be reported.

   The bylaws of individual facilities contain requirements and procedures that must be followed by the medical staff.
4. A longitudinal health record is a birth-to-death record that acts as an ongoing reference for and about the patient.
5. The provider is responsible for ensuring the quality of health record documentation.

Check Your Understanding 8.2

1. d   Orders
2. c   Physical examination
3. j   Ancillary notes
4. a   Care path
5. b   History
6. g   Advance directives
7. i   Discharge summary
8. f   Nursing notes
9. h   Emergency record
10. e   Consultations

Check Your Understanding 8.3

1. Source oriented
2. Universal chart order
3. Integrated
4. Problem oriented
5. Hospice

6. Ancillary
7. Long-term care
8. Shadow record

Check Your Understanding 8.4

1. The contract system, or outsourcing, of transcription saves money, provides for handling of overload, and can do all the work for the facility or partial work, as needed. Internal or in-house transcription provides internal control and protects confidentiality.
2. The formal education of medical transcriptionists at business schools or community colleges includes terminology, medical science, anatomy and physiology, English grammar, and other course work. Candidates for certification must also pass a certification examination.
3. Voice recognition technology will turn medical transcriptionists into editors and proofreaders.
4. The four benefits of an incentive pay plan would include the ability to reward productivity, motivate employees, reduce turnover, and provide a system for fair and equitable pay.
5. Factors to consider when determining the number of transcriptionists a facility needs include the kind and amount of information to be typed, specialties, whether the organization is a teaching facility, the presence of clinics, and additional nontranscription duties involved.

Check Your Understanding 8.5

1. Quantitative analysis is a review of the record for completeness and accuracy. For example, a quantitative analysis checks that the proper reports for the proper patient exist, that signatures are in order, and that the organization of the record is correct. Qualitative analysis is a more thorough review of the quality and accuracy of the documentation, ensuring that it meets standards and regulations.
2. Concurrent review, which may be qualitative or quantitative, is accomplished while patients are in the facility or under active treatment. Because the analysis is done in the location where the providers are, providers can easily be reminded of items that need to be accomplished to complete the chart, missing signatures that need to be obtained, and reports that need to be filed with the chart.

3. Universal chart order means leaving a paper record in the same order that compiled in the nurse's area. The order is the same while the patient is under treatment as it is for permanent filing. This method saves personnel time, and allows providers quick retrieval of needed materials because the order for the record is always the same.

4. Open-ended review is done concurrent with the patient's stay in the facility; closed-record review is done retrospectively, after the patient is discharged.

5. Incomplete records can hold up a facility's billing process and affect the timely reimbursement for patient care.

6. Incomplete records can be stored in an incomplete file area by either patient number or physician name. Some facilities do not have a separate incomplete file area but, instead, store incomplete records with all other records by patient number. If incomplete charts are filed by number in either a separate or permanent filing area, personnel must pull the records for the providers who wish to work on them.

7. Incomplete records are not finished; they become delinquent when they are not completed within a specified time frame, such as within 14 days after discharge. The definition of when a record becomes delinquent is set by the facility.

8. The HIM professional provides lists of what is needed to complete the record, conducts concurrent analysis, educates providers, flags or marks what needs to be signed, and does other tasks to make it easier for providers to complete records quickly.

9. Authentication proves authorship. Authentication in paper records is accomplished with a signature or initials handwritten in ink. Autoauthentication is a process by which providers can state, in advance, that dictated reports can be considered signed automatically if not corrected within a certain period of time. An electronic signature is a computer password used to authenticate a report or document.

10. Concurrent review processes often include notification of outstanding signatures. Facilities have discontinued retrospective notification because signing orders and notes after the patient has been discharged have no effect on the patient care process.

11. There must be control of the design and content of forms to ensure that the forms are compatible with the paper record and with imaging and microfilming systems.

12. The four parts of the forms control process are developing forms according to guidelines, controlling printing and the use of forms, educating providers about guidelines, and preventing duplication of unneeded forms.

13. Providers wanting a new form should go through the approval process to ensure control of forms, especially as the transition to imaging or computerized systems continues.

14. Bar codes and bar code labels are used to allow for indexing in imaging or computer systems.

Check Your Understanding 8.6

1. In a serial numbering system, each patient receives a new number at each visit. In a unit numbering system, the patient is assigned a number during the first encounter and keeps it permanently.

2. Terminal-digit filing allows for a more even distribution of files within the filing area and thus a more even distribution of work. In straight numerical filing, newer records are at the end of the file and most of the file work will be concentrated in the area with the new files.

3. The main factors in determining how long to maintain a health records are patient care needs, state laws, federal regulations, accreditation standards, and facility policies.

4. The major advantage of microfilming health records is that it saves space.

5. By using optical imaging in the chart completion process, images of the chart can be accessed and reviewed by simultaneous users.

6. The four primary steps in a good record retention program are conducting inventory, determining storage format and location, assigning retention periods, and destroying unnecessary records.

Check Your Understanding 8.7

1. The master patient index (MPI) is the key locator for records in a numerical filing system because it contains patient demographics and patient numbers.

2. Accurate information in an MPI ensures the correct identification of both the patient and the record.

3. Some of the reasons why incorrect patient information is obtained are that someone other than the patient provides the information, incorrect spelling, different names and/or initials are used for the same patient, clerical mistakes, and language differences.

4. The consequence of a patient having duplicate health record numbers is that providers will not have the proper information for patient care, resulting in duplicate testing and poor-quality healthcare.

Chapter 9

Check Your Understanding 9.1

1. A
2. B
3. G
4. H
5. E
6. D
7. F
8. C

Check Your Understanding 9.2

1. F
2. F
3. T
4. T
5. T
6. T
7. F
8. T
9. F
10. T

Check Your Understanding 9.3

1. *CDR*—clinical data repository
2. *CDS*—clinical decision support
3. *CDW*—clinical data warehouse
4. *COW*—computers on wheels
5. *COLD*—computer output to laser disk
6. *RAID*—redundant array of independent [or inexpensive] disks
7. *SAN*—storage area network
8. *Client/server architecture*—network where some computers house the applications and process data (servers), supporting local data capture and retrieval by other computers (clients)
9. *Full server redundancy*—contingency plan where duplicate servers process EHR transactions simultaneously so that if one crashes, processing falls over to the other
10. *Integration*—the ability to exchange data between systems without requiring an interface
11. *Interface*—a protocol that helps data to be passed from one disparate system to another
12. *Semantic interoperability*—information exchange where not only the format of the message is the same but the meaning of the content is the same because of using a standard vocabulary
13. *Source systems*—systems that supply data to the EHR (generally collected in a clinical data repository)
14. *Storage management*—the people, and now software, that keep track of where data are stored, making it accessible, and managing archival and retention processes.

Check Your Understanding 9.4

1. *Minimum necessary use requirement*—documentation of treatment relationships can support more granular access controls
2. *Individual right to request restriction*—discrete data can support specific restrictions if agreed upon by the covered entity
3. *Confidentiality of PHI when transmitted over the Internet*—data encryption can protect data transmitted in an open network
4. *Emergency operation procedures*—"break the glass" technology can support more granular access controls
5. *Authentication*—stronger forms of authentication can be applied and monitored
6. E
7. D
8. Z, E, and D
9. D
10. E

Check Your Understanding 9.5

1. Change, value, leadership, workflow, ownership, different systems between hospital and practice, security and privacy, patient acceptance, learning how to use system
2. Payback period calculates the number of years it will take to begin gaining positive financial results (sometimes described as how long it takes to pay for the system). IRR is a measure that considers the time value of money, or helps compare the percent of earnings a given investment will yield.
3. *ASP* is a model where the data and applications are housed (hosted) at a vendor site. The financial agreement is similar to a lease, where monthly payments are made for the duration of the time the application is being used by the organization. *An EHR acquisition model* is one in which the organization acquires a license to use the application and implements it internally and retains its own data. Usually there is a large upfront cost and then low, periodic maintenance fees.
4. Executives should provide the leadership necessary to achieve EHR benefits, by demonstrating their commitment and support, establishing appropriate expectations, and fostering a culture of quality and productivity improvement.
5. Most states require the accuracy and integrity of records in electronic form to be demonstrated.

Check Your Understanding 9.6

a. 6
b. 4
c. 5
d. 2
e. 3
f. 1
g. 12
h. 8
i. 11
j. 10
k. 7
l. 9

Chapter 10

Check Your Understanding 10.1

1. The four sources of law governing Americans are common law, statutory law, constitutional law, and administrative law.
2. Cases typically heard in federal courts include federal crimes such as racketeering and bank robbery, constitutional issues, and civil actions in which the parties do not live in the same state.
3. The court of last resort is the U.S. Supreme Court.
4. The two most common types of civil cases in healthcare are torts and contracts.
5. In a court, the trier of fact is the judge or the jury.
6. The result of a trial is called a verdict or a judgment.
7. Crimes that are wrongful acts against public health, safety, and welfare are covered by criminal laws.
8. The prosecutor in a criminal case is the attorney who, on behalf of the government, prosecutes an accused for a crime; the defendant is the person or group accused in a criminal or civil court action. The prosecutor has the burden of proving the charges against the defendant.
9. The defendant may plead guilty and be sentenced to probation or imprisonment and/or pay a fine or may plead not guilty, which results in a trial. The trial can result in a verdict of either guilty or not guilty. If found not guilty, the charges are dismissed. If found guilty, the defendant will be sentenced to probation or imprisonment and/or be required to pay a fine. In either case, the defendant has the right to appeal.
10. The three categories of torts are negligent torts, intentional torts, and product liability. Most healthcare cases arise from negligent torts.
11. Negligence results when a person does not act as a reasonably prudent person would act under the same circumstances. A negligent tort may result from a person committing an act or failing to act as a reasonably prudent person would or would not in the given circumstances. Typically, negligence is careless conduct that is outside the generally accepted standard of care.
12. The four elements of negligence are the duty to use due care, the breach of the duty to use due care, the injury (harm) that occurred, and the conduct that caused the injury/harm.
13. False imprisonment might occur in a hospital through the inappropriate use of restraints or the refusal to allow a patient to leave.
14. Truth and privilege are the available defenses to a defendant accused of defamation of character.
15. Healthcare providers may be held liable for a negligent disregard for patients' rights to privacy.
16. A contract is an agreement, whether written or oral, that, in most cases, is legally enforceable through the U.S. legal system.
17. A contract case arises when there is a breach of an agreement. This means that one party charges the other with failing to meet one or more of the obligations in the contract.

Check Your Understanding 10.2

1. The two sections of a health record are the demographic section and the clinical section. The demographic section includes, among other items, the patient's name, sex, age, insurance information, and the person to contact in case of emergency. The clinical section contains the patient's complaint, history of present illness, medical history, family history, social history, continuing documentation of ongoing medical care, report of diagnostic tests, x-ray reports, surgery and other procedure reports, consultant reports, nursing documentation, various graphs, and the final diagnoses.
2. Licensure is mandatory and government sponsored; accreditation is voluntary and not government sponsored.
3. National patient information confidentiality standards in the Health Insurance Portability and Accountability Act of 1996 (HIPAA) were promulgated in December 2000.
4. A plaintiff may make a claim of unauthorized disclosure of health information against a hospital (because of the breach of its duty to maintain confidentiality of information) on the basis of any job-related acts of the hospital's employees or agents and the consequences of any unauthorized disclosure, whether by employees, agents, or medical staff members.
5. The holding regarding privacy issued by the court in *Griswold v. Connecticut* was that the right to privacy limits governmental authority to regulate contraception, abortion, and other decisions affecting reproduction.
6. Federal/state laws; administrative policy; medical practice; varied purposes

7. Privacy, transactions and code sets, and security

8. Privacy Act of 1974, Freedom of Information Act, Controlled Substance Act, Medicare Conditions of Participation for Hospitals, Conditions of Participation for Clinics, Rehabilitation Agencies, and Public Health Agencies as Providers of Outpatient Physical Therapy and Speech-Language Pathology, Conditions of Participation for Home Health Agencies, Confidentiality of Alcohol and Drug Abuse Patient Records.

Check Your Understanding 10.3

1. Because they are the provider's business records, the healthcare provider (physician or hospital) that maintains the health records owns them.

2. The patient

3. The primary focus is how and for what purpose patient health information can be used.

4. Health plans, clearinghouses, and health care providers

5. No. The standard HIPAA rule is that it preempts state law if it is contrary to that state law except if one or more of the following conditions are met:
   • The Secretary of the Department of Health and Human Services determines that the provision of state law is necessary
   • To prevent fraud and abuse related to providing or paying for healthcare
   • To ensure appropriate state regulation of insurance and health plans
   • For state reporting on healthcare delivery or costs
   • For public health, safety, or welfare if the Secretary determines that the intrusion into privacy is warranted when balanced against this need
   • For the purpose of regulating the manufacture, registration, distribution, dispensing, or other control of controlled substances
   • The provision of state law relates to the privacy of individually identifiable health information and is more stringent that a provision in the HIPAA privacy rule
   • The provision of state law provides for reporting disease or injury, child abuse, birth, or death, or for the conduct of public health surveillance, investigation, or intervention
   • The provision of state law requires a health plan to report, or to provide access to, information for management audits, financial audits, program monitoring and evaluation, or licensure or certification of facilities or individuals

6. How covered entities may use and disclose PHI; the patient's rights regarding the covered entities' uses and disclosures; and the covered entities' obligations for protecting the patient's PHI

7. At the time of the first service delivery, including service delivered electronically. In emergency situations, covered entities providing care must provide the notice as soon as practicable after the emergency treatment situation is resolved. The covered entity is to make a good faith effort to obtain the patient's written acknowledgement of receipt of the notice. This requirement also is delayed until practicable in emergency treatment situations. If receipt is not obtained for any reason, including the patient refusing to provide the acknowledgement, the covered entity is required to document its good faith efforts and the reason why the acknowledgement was not obtained.

8. Oral, paper, and electronic

9. Oral information; psychotherapy notes; information compiled in anticipation of, or for use in, a civil, criminal, or administrative action or proceeding; PHI the covered entity maintains that is subject to or exempted from the Clinical Laboratory Improvements Amends (CLIA) of 1988

10. The most striking feature of the privacy rule is the individual's right to obtain an accounting of disclosures of his or her health information.

11. The types of disclosures that do not need to be included in an accounting are:
    • To carry out treatment, payment, and health care operations
    • To the patient who is the subject of the PHI
    • Those that are incidental
    • Those pursuant to patient authorization
    • For facility directory or to family or caregivers
    • For national security or intelligence purposes
    • To correctional institutions or law enforcement under specific circumstances
    • PHI included in a limited data set
    • Those made prior to the compliance date for the covered entity

12. The patient's request can be denied without giving the patient an opportunity to request review of the denial. In addition to the PHI types noted above to which the patient is not given access, access can be denied:

    If the covered entity is a correctional institution or a covered entity acting under the direction of the correctional institution and such access would jeopardize the health, safety, security, custody, or rehabilitation of the individual or others

    When PHI was created or obtained during research that includes treatment—the access is suspended while the research is in progress as long as the patient agreed to the access denial when consenting to participate in the research and the patient had to have been advised that the right would be reinstated upon completion of the research

    If the PHI is contained in records subject to the Privacy Act of 1974 and is also not available for access under the privacy act

13. According to HIPAA the patient or his or her legal representative may authorize the release of information.

14. The circumstances listed in the privacy rule under which a facility may deny a patient's request for access to his or her own health information without providing the patient the opportunity to have the denial reviewed are when the confidential medical information is excluded from the right of access and was obtained from someone other than a healthcare provider under a promise of confidentiality.

15.. Unless otherwise authorized by the patient, the organization may only release information to the news media that states the patient's general condition in terms of good, fair, or poor. No information may be released that reveals the patient's diagnosis. Furthermore, information may only be released on those patients that the news media identify by name.

16. The provider may release information to an employer when:
    - The care provider is a member of the employer's workforce or provides healthcare to the patient at the employer's request.
    - The care relates to a medical surveillance of the workplace or to a work-related illness or injury.
    - The information that is disclosed consists of findings concerning a work-related illness or injury or a workplace-related medical surveillance.
    - The employer needs the findings to comply with its obligations under federal and state laws.

17. Although the release of certain medical information is statutorily mandated under certain circumstances, a court may view the release to the wrong agency as a breach of confidentiality.

Check Your Understanding 10.4

1. No, the patient only must be given an opportunity to object (opt out) of the hospital's directory.

2. Only members of the clergy may receive this information. They may receive the information even if they do not ask for the patient by name.

3. When a patient is incapacitated or in an emergency situation and cannot object to being included in the facility's directory, the covered provider may disclose the information as noted if the disclosure is: In the patient's best interest as determined by the provider using professional judgment

4. Disclosure to family, friends, or other caregivers identified by the patient relevant to their involvement with the patient's care. The requirement for patient authorization typically extends to a request by a patient's family members, including the spouse. However, healthcare providers may discuss general information about the patient's condition with family members without authorization unless the patient

has instructed otherwise. If the patient is incapacitated, the physician and other caregivers may discuss health information and treatment plans with the next of kin or the patient's representative, however that is defined by a given state, to the extent necessary to make medical decisions on the incapacitated patient's behalf. The privacy rule permits the hospital to disclose to a family member, other relative, close personal friend, or any person identified by the patient health information directly relevant to that person's involvement in the patient's care or payment for healthcare [Section 164.510(b)(1)(i)].

Check Your Understanding 10.5

1. Yes. Except as permitted or required under the HIPAA Privacy rule, a valid patient authorization is required for the use or disclosure of PHI [45 CFR §164.508(a)(1)].

2. The authorization must include a specific description of the information to be used or disclosed. In addition, the name or other specific identification of the person(s) authorized to request and receive the requested information must be included. Further, the authorization must include the expiration date or event that relates to the individual or the purpose of the use or disclosure. The patient must be given the right to revoke the authorization in writing, the exceptions to this right, and a description of how he or she may revoke it. The authorization also must advise the patient that information released pursuant to the authorization may be subject to redisclosure by the recipient and may no longer be protected. Finally, the patient must sign and date the authorization.

   If a personal representative signs the authorization, a description of his or her authority to act for the patient must be included in the authorization form. Further, the form must be written in plain language. The patient must be advised that the hospital will not condition treatment, payment, enrollment in a health plan, or eligibility for benefits on his or her providing authorization for the requested information. The authorization must include a description of each purpose for the requested information. Further, the authorization must contain a statement to the effect that the patient may inspect or copy the information and may refuse to sign it. The hospital must disclose to the patient whether the release of the information will result in direct or indirect remuneration to the facility from a third party. If there is remuneration, the authorization must state that such remuneration will result. Also, the patient is entitled to a copy of the signed authorization.

3. Authorizations for uses and disclosures of health information created for research that includes treatment of the patient must contain additional elements.

For example, there must be a description of the extent to which the information will be used or disclosed to carry out treatment, payment, or healthcare operations. The authorization must further include a description of any health information that could be disclosed but will not be disclosed for facility directories or public health purposes. However, the facility may not include a limitation affecting its right to release information required by law.

4. For an unemancipated minor, the legal representative is the parent, guardian, or other person acting in loco parentis.

5. The two categories of uses and disclosures that the HIPAA Privacy rule specifically refers to as requiring patient authorization are psychotherapy notes and marketing.

Check Your Understanding 10.6

1. Treatment, payment and healthcare operations

2. No, patients and patient representatives have access to PHI without signing an authorization form (45 CFR §164.524).

3. Yes, because this is for continuation of care. The privacy rule, in sections 164.501 and 164.506(c)(1) and (2), permits the facility and healthcare providers to use or disclose confidential information for:
   - Providing, coordinating or managing healthcare and related services by one or more healthcare providers, including with a third party
   - Consulting between healthcare providers relating to a patient
   - Referring a patient for healthcare from one health care provider to another

4. Treatment, payment and healthcare operations; patient/patient representative; as required by law; public health activities; abuse, neglect, or domestic violence reporting; health oversight; judicial and administrative proceedings; Law enforcement; coroners, medical examiners, funeral directors; organ procurement organization; research; to avert a serious threat to health and safety; specialized governmental functions; fundraising; marketing exception

5. Common types of information reported for public health purposes include vital statistics (births and deaths); communicable diseases; child, adult, and elder abuse; wounds, such as from stabs and gunshots; and conditions affecting the ability to drive.

6. If the violation is committed with the intent to sell, transfer, or use PHI for commercial advantage, personal gain or malicious harm, the fine is not more than $250,000, imprisonment for not more than 10 years, or both.

Check Your Understanding 10.7

1. The physician–patient privilege may be created when a physician contracts to care for a particular group of people and a person from that group seeks care, when a physician enters into an express contract with a patient or his or her representative for care, and when a physician engages in conduct from which a patient can imply that a contract exists.

2. The care provider can be released from the privilege through words or actions. For example, a patient who places his or her treatment at issue in a trial cannot continue to claim a privilege to protect the information.

3. Both the Department of Health and Human Services (HHS) (for Medicare) and the state Medicaid agency may request information from the health record to support the healthcare provider's bill submitted for payment and for investigative purposes such as pursuant to the federal fraud and abuse statutes.

4. The custodian of records, typically the health information manager, may be called as a witness to identify the record as the one subpoenaed. He or she also may be called to testify as to policies and procedures relevant to the following:
   - Creation of the record
   - Maintenance of the record to prevent it from being altered
   - Maintenance of the record to prevent it from being accessed without proper authorization

Check Your Understanding 10.8

1. For QI purposes to ensure following policies and procedures; to measure employee performance; as a basis to request additional staff; as part of the annual evaluation process.

2. (1) Turnaround time for requests, (2) number of requests processed per employee per month, (3) number of subpoenas processed per employee per month.

3. Education that reinforces the organization's policies and the importance of following those policies. Staff also must be provided with and express an understanding of the expectations for them to follow ROI policies and procedures.

4. Yes, as the investigation relates to an alleged violation of HIPAA regulation by ROI staff. The ROI manager works with the Privacy Officer in such investigations pursuant to the organization's investigation policy. The investigation process may include the Human Resources Department to impose disciplinary action.

Check Your Understanding 10.9

1. The process of granting a physician membership in the hospital medical staff is called credentialing.
2. Typically, the documentation reviewed for the initial medical staff membership appointment includes medical education, including medical school, residencies, postdoctoral studies, and fellowships; license to practice; medical practice experience; and a search of the National Practitioner Data Bank (NPDB) regarding judgments and settlements above a specific amount in medical malpractice cases.
3. To grant specific privileges, the medical staff may require the physician to obtain a consultation before performing specific procedures; to have operative procedures proctored by an observing or assisting physician; or to have certification beyond a license, such as board certification in a particular medical specialty.
4. At reappointment, the medical staff may review, among other factors, the physician's blood usage patterns, lengths of stay, infection rates, complications and complication rates, health record documentation, closed malpractice claims, and the outcomes of focused studies. Physicians who have gained additional training since the last appointment may seek privileges not previously held. For any new privileges requested, the physician may be required to submit to consultation or proctoring.
5. Third parties such as the JCAHO and state and federal regulatory organizations may review credentialing files as part of their accrediting and licensing functions. Some states statutorily protect credentialing files from discovery in legal proceedings. However, when a plaintiff alleges negligent credentialing against a hospital, there is a question as to whether the protection will hold up.
6. Concurrent review consists of evaluating medical care as it is being given; retrospective review occurs after patient discharge.
7. Quality improvement and concurrent review files should be kept confidential because these review activities involve collecting outcomes and performance data on physician performance and may have an impact on continued medical staff membership.

Check Your Understanding 10.10

1. An incident is an occurrence that is inconsistent with the standard of care.
2. Incident reports may be protected by the following: certain state statutes that apply to quality improvement (QI) studies and activities, the attorney–client privilege doctrine, and the attorney work product doctrine.
3. Incident reports should be protected because they contain facts about occurrences.

4. The health information manager and the risk manager work as a team. The risk manager depends on the health information manager to alert him or her to potentially compensable events, and the health information manager also can advise the risk manager when an attorney requests a copy of a health record.

Chapter 11

Check Your Understanding 11.1

1. b   Employer
2. c   Public interest
3. a   Patients and the healthcare team
4. d   Oneself and one's peers and professional associations
5. d   Oneself and one's peers and professional associations
6. a   Patients and the healthcare team
7. d   Oneself and one's peers and professional associations
8. b   Employer
9. d   Oneself and one's peers and professional associations
10. b   Employer
11. a   Patients and the healthcare team
12. d   Oneself and one's peers and professional associations
13. a   Patients and the healthcare team
14. a   Patients and the healthcare team
15. d   Oneself and one's peers and professional associations
16. b   Employer
17. c   Public interest
18. c   Public interest
19. a   Patients and the healthcare team
20. d   Oneself and one's peers and professional associations
21. b   Employer
22. a   Patients and the healthcare team

Check Your Understanding 11.2

1. e
2. b
3. d
4. a
5. f
6. g
7. c

Check Your Understanding 11.3

1. e   Self-determination
2. d   Promote good
3. g   Do no harm
4. h   Fairness in applying rules

5. a   Right or wrong
6. b   Reasoned discourse
7. c   Right to be let alone
8. f   Healthcare communication
9. j   Electronic protection of information
10. i   Establishes privacy and security standards

Chapter 12

Check Your Understanding 12.1

1. A primary data source is created by the healthcare professionals providing the care. The medical record is considered a primary data source. A secondary data source is made up of data taken from a primary data source and put in a different format, such as a registry.

2. Patient-identifiable data are facts that can be connected with a particular patient, such as a single laboratory value. Aggregate data are data that have been grouped together, such as the number of discharges for a month. There is no way to determine information about a particular patient from these groups of data.

3. Secondary sources are created to put the information from the primary record into a format that is easier to query and manipulate. For example, it is difficult and time consuming for a cancer registrar to determine the number of patients with each type of cancer by looking at individual records. A database, which is a secondary record, can be queried to provide this information in a report from the secondary data that has been entered, thus speeding up the process.

4. An internal user is someone within the facility or enterprise, such as a cancer committee. An external user is someone or some agency outside of the facility or enterprise, such as the state vital records office.

Check Your Understanding 12.2

1. HIM departments use facility-specific indexes to locate data as requested by internal and external users. The operation index, for example, could be used to locate medical records for patients with a specific operation for a quality assessment study. It could also be used to provide information to external users. For example, residents often must provide data on the types of operations they have performed during their residency to the appropriate board for certification in their specialty.

2. The master population index allows users to locate patients by name and to find out their medical record number. It contains demographic information about the patient such as medical record number, name, address, dates of previous hospital admissions, name of attending physician, and date of birth.

3. Disease and operations indexes allow users to find medical records of patients with a particular diagnosis or operation. At minimum, they include the patient's health record number and disease/operation codes. They may also include other data such as physician or surgeon and date of discharge or operation as determined by the facility.

4. The purpose of the physician index is to locate medical records of patients that have been treated by a particular physician. It must, at a minimum, include the physician's name or a code number assigned and the patient's name and/or health record number.

Check Your Understanding 12.3

1. An index is a reference source that enables health records to be located by diagnosis, procedure, or physician. A registry contains more extensive data than an index does. Registries are collections of secondary data related to a patient's specific diagnosis, condition, or procedure.

2. Case definition refers to the process used by each registry to define the cases to be included in it. Case finding is a method used to identify patients who have been seen and/or treated in the facility for the particular disease or condition of interest to the registry.

3. A facility-based registry contains data used to provide information for the improved understanding of a specific disease or condition within a particular facility such as a hospital. A population-based registry contains data showing trends and changes in the incidence of the disease or condition within a geographic area covered by the registry, such as a city or state.

4. • **Cancer registry**
    – *Case definition:* the types of cancer to be included in the registry
    – *Case finding:* HIM discharge processing, disease index, review of cancer-related reports such as pathology, and lists of patients receiving cancer-related services such as radiation therapy
    • **Trauma Registry**
    – *Case definition:* trauma registries usually include cases with ICD-9-CM diagnosis codes in the range of 800–959
    – *Case finding:* disease index or deaths in services with frequent trauma diagnoses
    • **Birth Defects Registry**
    – *Case definition:* varies; may include cases found within the first year of life or cases within the first five years of life; may include stillborn
    – *Case finding:* disease index; labor and delivery logs; pathology and autopsy reports; ultrasound reports; cytogenetic reports; information from rehabilitation centers and children's hospitals; and birth, death, and fetal death certificates

- **Diabetes registry**
  - *Case definition:* may limit by type of diabetes or age of patient
  - *Case finding:* review of medical records, ICD-9-CM diagnosis codes, medication lists, identification by physician, and information from health plans
- **Implant registry**
  - *Case definition:* may include all implants or only certain types such as cochlear implants
  - *Case finding:* identifies patients who have been seen and/or treated in the facility for the particular disease or condition of interest to the registry
- **Transplant registry**
  - *Case definition/case finding:* physicians identify patients needing transplants
- **Immunization registry**
  - *Case definition:* all children in a population area or only those seen in public clinics are included; may include adults for immunization such as pneumonia and influenza vaccines
  - *Case finding:* electronic entry at birth from electronic vital records system or manual entry at birth from birth and death certificates

5.
- **Cancer registry:** For a facility-based registry, patient records are reviewed to collect demographic information, type and site of the cancer, diagnostic methodologies, and treatment methodologies. For a population-based registry, information is submitted by facilities within the population covered
- **Trauma registry:** Abstracting data from the medical record including demographic information, hospital care provided, status of patient at the time of admission, ICD-9-CM diagnosis and procedure codes, abbreviated injury scale, and injury severity score.
- **Birth defects registry:** Abstracting information from the sources used in case finding. Abstracted information includes demographic information, diagnosis codes, birth weight, status at birth, autopsy, cytogenetic reports, mother's and father's use of alcohol and drugs, and family history of birth defects.
- **Diabetes registry:** Abstracting information from physician office or clinic record including demographic information and laboratory values.
- **Implant registry:** Abstracting information from the health record including demographic data and data required by the FDA.
- **Transplant registry**
  - *Recipient information:* demographic data, patient diagnosis, medical urgency, functional status, life support status, and previous transplants
  - *Donor information/living donor:* relationship to recipient, clinical information, organ recovery information, and histocompatibility

  - *Donor information/deceased donor:* cause and circumstances of death, organ procurement and consent process, medications taken, and other donor history
- **Immunization registry:** Data is abstracted from vital records. The abstracted data includes core immunization data elements from the Centers for Disease Control and the National Vaccine Advisory Committee

6.
- **Cancer registry:** Annual report including aggregate data on the cancer cases for the year
- **Trauma registry:** Sometimes an annual report, or performance improvement reports such as delays in abdominal surgery
- **Birth defects registry:** No standard reports
- **Diabetes registry:** Laboratory monitoring, patient follow up, incidence of diabetes
- **Implant registry:** Reporting to the FDA and the manufacturer
- **Transplant registry:** Information on donors and recipients as well as survival rates, length of time on the waiting list for an organ, and death rates
- **Immunization registry:** Immunization rates are automatically reported to schools

7.
- **Cancer registry:** Review of medical records for treatment in the last year, contacting the patient's physician, contacting the patient, newspaper obituaries, and/or Internet sites
- **Trauma registry:** Follow up is done by some, but not all, registries; emphasis is on patient's quality of life
- **Birth defects registry:** Not routinely done
- **Diabetes registry:** Done to ensure appropriate continued care
- **Implant registry:** Follow up is done to assess performance of the implant over time
- **Transplant registry:** At intervals throughout the first year and then annually
  - *Living donor:* complications of the procedure, length of hospital stay
  - *Recipient:* status at time of follow up, functional status, graft status, treatment
- **Immunization registry:** Follow up reminders that immunizations are due, by postcard, telephone call, or autodialed call

8.
- **Cancer registry:** American College of Surgeons, North American Association of Central Cancer Registries, and Centers for Disease Control
- **Trauma registry:** American College of Surgeons
- **Birth defects registry:** None
- **Diabetes registry:** None
- **Implant registry:** None
- **Transplant registry:** None
- **Immunization registry:** Centers for Disease Control (CDC)

9. • **Cancer registry:** On-the-job training, seminars, and/or cancer registry program in a college; AHIMA's online Cancer Registry program
   • **Trauma registry:** Varies; may use RHITs, RHIAs, RNs, LPNs, EMTs or other health professionals or workshops and on-the-job training
   • **Birth defects registry:** None specified
   • **Diabetes registry:** None specified
   • **Implant registry:** None specified
   • **Transplant registry:** None specified
   • **Immunization registry:** None specified

10. • **Cancer registry:** Certified Cancer Registrar (CTR) is provided by the National Cancer Registrar's Association and requires passing an examination provided by the National Board for Certification of Registrars
   • **Trauma registry:** Certified Specialist Trauma Registry (CSTR) is provided through the American Trauma Society Registrar Certification Board. Certification requires passing an examination.
   • **Birth defects registry:** None
   • **Diabetes registry:** None
   • **Implant registry:** None
   • **Transplant registry:** None
   • **Immunization registry:** Proposed for Centers for Disease Control

Check Your Understanding 12.4

1. The MEDPAR file provides data on Medicare patients including demographic patient data, provider data, Medicare coverage, total charges, charges by service, ICD-9-CM diagnosis and procedure codes, and DRGs.

2. The limitation of MEDPAR data is that it only includes data on Medicare cases.

3. The National Practitioner Data Bank was developed to make information on malpractice claims, sanctions by Boards of Medical Examiners, and professional review actions available among all states. Before, physicians who had incurred such actions could move to another state and practice without anyone in the new state knowing his or her background. The Health Care Quality Improvement Act of 1986 mandated the creation of the NPDB.

    The Healthcare Integrity and Protection Data Bank was developed because there was no central repository for information on healthcare fraud and abuse. The Data Bank was mandated by the Health Insurance Portability and Accountability Act of 1996.

4. Information that must be reported to the National Practitioner Data Bank includes practitioner information, the reporting entity, and the judgment or settlement against the practitioner. Information that must be reported to the Healthcare Integrity and Protection Data Bank includes final adverse actions resulting in unnecessary costs to the program, improper payment, services that fail to meet professionally recognized standards of care or that are medically unnecessary, adverse patient outcomes, failure to provided covered or needed care in violation or contraction arrangements, and delays in diagnosis or treatment.

    There may be an overlap between the two data banks, so one report is made to both, and the information is then sorted to the appropriate data bank.

5. Healthcare organizations use the National Practitioner Data Bank in the credentialing process. They must query the data bank when the physician initially applies for medical staff privileges and every two years thereafter.

    Federal and state government agencies and health plans may access the Healthcare Integrity and Protection Data Bank. Practitioners, providers, and suppliers may only query about themselves.

6. Health information managers contribute to public health databases by providing information from the medical records of patients in their facilities.

7. The databases using data from health records include the National Discharge Survey, the National Ambulatory Medical Care Survey, the National Survey of Ambulatory Surgery, and the National Hospital Ambulatory Medical Care Survey.

8. A clinical trial is a research project in which new treatment and tests are investigated to see whether they are safe and effective.

    Clinical trial databases are developed to help physicians and patients find clinical trials.

    The Food and Drug Administration Modernization Act of 1997 mandated the development of a national clinical trials database.

9. The source of data for the Healthcare Cost and Utilization Project is data collected at the state level on claims data from the UB-92 or discharge abstracted data including the UHDDS reported by individual hospitals and, in some cases, ambulatory care centers.

10. The UMLS is of interest to health information managers because it includes data from the ICD-9-CM, CPT and HCPCS coding systems.

Check Your Understanding 12.5

1. The factors to be considered in determining the quality of data are its validity, reliability, completeness, and timeliness.
2. Errors in data that are used to make decisions concerning new treatment methods, healthcare policy, and physician credentialing and privileging may cause serious problems.
3. One method used to check validity in secondary data is the computer edit. Reliability may be checked through the interrater reliability method of having more than one person abstract data for the same case. Uniform terminology also improves reliability by ensuring that the same definitions are used for all concepts.
4. Security refers to controlling access to all health information. Confidentiality refers to efforts to guarantee the privacy of personal health information.
5. Methods used to control access to a health information system include the establishment of levels of access, audit trails, control of physical access to hardware and printouts, and encryption.
6. The best way to avoid potential loss of data is through regular backing up of data in the system. Anti-virus software also helps in preventing loss of data.
7. Factors to consider in developing a physical security program include placing computers in areas that are not available to unauthorized people, ensuring that reports and printouts are not left where they can be seen, and encrypting sensitive data.
8. Sensitive data, such as HIV status, should be encrypted.
9. Methods include employee training in confidentiality and the development of policies and procedures concerning who may access data.
10. Increased use of automated data entry is a current trend in the collection of secondary data. The development of the computer-based patient record will ensure that less data will have to be abstracted from the medical record into secondary records.

Chapter 13

Check Your Understanding 13.1

1. A classification system is a system for grouping similar diseases and procedures and organizing related information for easy retrieval, or a system for assigning numeric or alphanumeric code numbers to represent specific diseases and/or procedures.

   A terminology is a set of terms representing the system of concepts of a particular subject field; a clinical terminology provides the proper use of clinical words as names or symbols

2. One of the most significant problems in the field of healthcare terminology and vocabulary is that there are many definitions for vocabularies and terminologies. This is very important because a standardized terminology or vocabulary will be impossible to develop without consistent definitions.

Check Your Understanding 13.2

1. The original purpose of ICD-9-CM was to report morbidity data.
2. The four essential characteristics of ICD-10-PCS are:
   - *Completeness:* Content coverage is adequate for all known procedures
   - *Expandability:* The structure allows incorporation of new procedures as unique codes
   - *Standardized terminology:* Definitions for all the terms used in ICD-10-PCS are specific and consistent
   - *Multiaxial structure:* Each code character has the same meaning within the specific procedure section and across procedure sections to the extent possible
3. The primary function of CPT is to report physician services.
4. The topography code in ICD-O describes the site of origin of the neoplasm.

Check Your Understanding 13.3

1. The coder's primary responsibility is data accuracy.
2. The main factor in ensuring the quality of clinical coding is the quality of the clinical documentation.
3. It is important for organizations to establish and follow specific coding policies and procedures to ensure data consistency.
4. The quality assessment process for coding consists of:
   - Documenting the current coding process
   - Taking baseline measurements
   - Setting up benchmarks using comparative data
   - Continuing to evaluate coding in an ongoing manner

Check Your Understanding 13.4

1. Encoders use extensive user interaction. Computer-assisted coding uses natural language processing.
2. Speech recognition is one emerging technology that will affect classification and clinical terminologies because it can improve the accuracy of documenting the clinician's intent and it can make documentation easier. Other emerging technologies include handheld computers and personal digital assistants (PDAs), which will facilitate point-of-care data entry.

Check Your Understanding 13.5

1. Answers could include National Library of Medicine (NLM), Department of Veteran's Administration (VA), National Committee on Vital and Health Statistics (NCVHS), Department of Health and Human Services (HHS), Centers for Medicare and Medicaid Services (CMS), World Health Organization (WHO), National Center for Health Statistics (NCHS).
2. NGOs include Certification Commission for Health Information Technology (CCHIT), Health Level Seven (HL7), American Society for Testing and Materials (ASTM), American National Standards Institute (ANSI). See chapter text for description of each organization's activities.

3. Much like a dictionary defines a language, standards organizations are important for the EHR because they ensure transferability of information from one platform or system to another. SDOs also help to ensure the content of the EHR.

Check Your Understanding 13.6

1. Relationships are used to add meaning and context to a terminology. They can serve to identify anatomy, disease causes, broader groupings of terms, and so on.
2. The future goal of Digital Imaging and Communications in Medicine (DICOM) is to provide clinically relevant indexing for images.
3. The knowledge sources (identifier types) used in Unified Medical Language System (UMLS) are the UMLS Metathesaurus, the SPECIALIST Lexicon, and the UMLS Semantic Network.
4. Nosology is the branch of medical science that deals with classification issues.
5. The main advantage to using Logical Observation Identifier Names and Codes (LOINC) is that it enables the standardized communication of laboratory results. The main disadvantage to using the LOINC system is that it is a new standard that people have to learn about and incorporate into their existing system.
6. Universal Medical Device Nomenclature System (UMDNS) is a device classification system. Clinical situations in which it might be useful are identifying, processing, filing, storing, retrieving, transferring, and communicating data about medical devices; and hospital inventory and work-order controls to national agency medical device regulatory systems.
7. North American Nursing Diagnosis Association (NANDA II) is a nursing terminology used to develop and classify nursing diagnoses in a taxonomy.
   Nursing Interventions Classification (NIC) is a terminology that describes the treatments that nurses perform.
   Nursing Outcomes Classification (NOC) is a comprehensive standardized classification of patient/client outcomes developed to evaluate the effects of nursing interventions.
8. The National Library of Medicine (NLM) recently signed a contract to license and supply SNOMED-CT for use in healthcare information systems. This helps meet the clinical vocabulary needs of the U.S. healthcare industry by allowing any U.S. organization to freely acquire and use SNOMED-CT from NLM's UMLS Metathesaurus

Check Your Understanding 13.7

1. Permanence is important in clinical terminologies to preserve the longitudinal uniformity of a clinical terminology or classification.
2. Another name for *context representation* is grammar, which means that the meaning of a term is more than just the term because some terms have multiple meanings. To fully understand a term, all of the modifying words and terms related to the original term must be considered.

Chapter 14

Check Your Understanding 14.1

1. Until the late 1800s, Americans paid their own healthcare expenses or, if they did not have means to pay for care, they received charity care or no care at all. During the early part of the 20th century, both legislative and private efforts were initiated to cover the cost of healthcare. These efforts resulted in the development of private insurance systems for those who could afford it and public welfare for those who could not. Medicare and Medicaid, the first federal program developed specifically to provide funding for healthcare costs for specific populations, were instituted in 1965.
2. As a result of spiraling demand for healthcare services throughout the 1970s and early 1980s, the cost of funding Medicare and Medicaid services skyrocketed. The federal government developed the first prospective payment system for hospital inpatients in 1983 in order to control and manage the costs of the Medicare and Medicaid programs. Since that time prospective payment methodologies have been developed for other segments of healthcare such as long-term care, home health care, and ambulatory services.
3. According to table 14.1, percentage change in health insurance coverage status from 2002 to 2003 is −.4%.
4. The Centers for Medicare and Medicaid Services (CMS) administers the Medicare and Medicaid programs. This agency was known as the Health Care Financing Administration (HCFA) until 2001.
5. To counteract labor shortages during World War II, employers added health insurance coverage for hospital, surgical, and medical expenses to their accident and life insurance plans as a way of attracting workers.

Check Your Understanding 14.2

1. Fee-for-service reimbursement occurs when a patient pays cash for services on a retrospective basis (after the service has been rendered). Until the advent of managed care, capitation, and other prospective payment systems in the 1980s, most private insurance plans and government-sponsored programs also reimbursed providers on a retrospective fee-for-service basis. Fee-for-service is rarely used today because the government and most private insurers now compensate providers according to predetermined discounted rates rather than on a fee-for-service basis.
2. Private commercial insurance plans are financed through the payment of a pre-established monthly premium by each individual or family covered under the plan. The insurance company sets aside the premiums from all the people covered under the plan into a special fund, which is then used to pay claims for medical care.

3. When a claim for medical care is submitted to an insurance company, the company reviews the claim to determine whether the services described in the claim are covered by the patient's policy. The company also reviews the documentation provided with the claim to ensure that the services provided were medically necessary. If the claim is approved, payment is then made to either the provider or the policyholder.

4. Many employers have developed self-insurance programs to cover healthcare services for their workforce. Employer-based self-insurance programs often enter into administrative services only (ASO) contracts with private insurers. The employer funds the plan and the private insurer administers the self-insurance plan on behalf of the employer.

5. Medicaid pays for healthcare services for financially needy individuals.

6. TRICARE is a healthcare program for active-duty members of the military and other qualified family members, CHAMPUS-eligible retirees and their family members, and eligible survivors of members of the uniformed services. CHAMPVA is an acronym for the Civilian Health and Medical Program–Veterans Administration. It is a healthcare program for dependents and survivors of permanently and totally disabled veterans, survivors of veterans who died from service-related conditions, and survivors of military personnel who died in the line of duty.

7. Medicare Part B is a voluntary healthcare program in which a Medicare beneficiary pays a monthly premium in order to extend or supplement Medicare coverage for services not covered by Medicare Part A such as physician services, emergency and outpatient services, laboratory and x-ray services, physical and occupational therapy services, and durable medical equipment.

8. Medicare Advantage, often referred to as Medigap insurance, was established by the Balanced Budget Act of 1997 to expand the options for participation in private healthcare plans.

9. Medigap is private health insurance that pays, within limits, most of the healthcare service charges not covered by Medicare Part A. These policies, which must meet federal standards, are offered by Blue Cross and Blue Shield and various commercial health insurance companies.

10. Title XVIII of the Social Security Act, or Health Insurance for the Aged and Disabled, established the Medicare program, which became effective in July 1966. Title XIX of the Social Security Act established the Medicaid program, effective as of the same date. Medicare is a federally-funded health insurance program that covers most Americans over the age of 65. In 1973, several additional groups became eligible for Medicare benefits, including those entitled to Social Security or Railroad Retirement disability cash benefits, most persons with end-stage renal disease, and certain individuals over 65 who were not eligible for paid coverage but elected to pay for Medicare benefits. Medicaid was designed as a cost-sharing program between the federal and state governments. It pays for healthcare services provided to many low-income Americans and is administered by state governments.

11. Medicaid allows states to add health coverage to public assistance programs for low-income groups, families with dependent children, the aged, and the disabled. Eligibility criteria are determined within each state and the criteria vary from state to state. However, to be eligible for federal funds, states are required to provide Medicaid coverage to certain individuals defined by the federal government. Low income is only one test for Medicaid eligibility. Other financial resources are also compared against eligibility standards.

12. Preferred provider organizations (PPOs) represent contractual agreements between healthcare providers and a self-insured provider or a health insurance carrier. Beneficiaries of PPOs select providers from a list of participating providers who have agreed to furnish healthcare services to the covered population. Point-of-service (POS) plans are similar to HMOs in that subscribers select a primary care physician from a network of participating physicians. However, POSs are different in that subscribers are allowed to seek care from providers outside the network as long as they pay a greater share of the charges for out-of-network services.

13. The State Children's Health Insurance Program (SCHIP) is a program initiated by the Balanced Budget Act of 1997. It allows states to expand existing insurance programs by providing additional federal funds to states so that Medicaid eligibility can be expanded to include a greater number of uninsured children.

14. • Inpatient hospitalization: Medicare Part A
   • Prescription eyeglasses: No Medicare coverage
   • Emergency department visits: Medicare Part B
   • Dental care: No Medicare coverage
   • Ambulatory surgery center services: Medicare Part B
   • Hospice care: Medicare Part A

15. TRICARE offers three options to its beneficiaries: TRICARE Prime, TRICARE Extra, and TRICARE standard. TRICARE Prime provides the most comprehensive healthcare coverage at the lowest cost. TRICARE Extra is a cost-effective preferred provider network (PPO) option.

16. Federal workers are covered by the Federal Workers' Compensation program, while other nonfederal workers are generally covered by individual State Workers' Compensation coverage. In general, these programs cover healthcare costs and lost income associated with work-related injuries and illnesses.

17. A staff model health maintenance organization (HMO) directly employs physicians and other healthcare professionals to provide healthcare services to members.

18. In an independent practice association (IPA), the HMO enters into a contract with an organized group of physicians who join together for purposes of fulfilling the HMO contract but retain their individual practices. The IPA serves as an intermediary during contract negotiations. In a staff model HMO, physicians are directly employed by the HMO, are salaried, and are considered employees of the HMO. In general, the physician practice in a staff model HMO is limited to HMO clients.

19. Managed care is the generic term used to describe prepaid health plans that integrate the financial and delivery aspects of healthcare services. Managed care organizations work to control the cost of, and access to, healthcare services at the same time that they strive to meet high quality standards. Types of managed care plans available in the United States are:
    • Health maintenance organizations (HMOs)
    • Preferred provider organizations (PPOs)
    • Point-of-service (POS) plans
    • Exclusive provider organizations (EPOs)
    • Integrated delivery systems (IDSs)

20. Management services organizations (MSOs) provide practice management services, including administration and support, to individual physician practices. MSOs are usually owned by a group of physicians or a hospital.

Check Your Understanding 14.3

1. A prospective payment system is in place when the amount of payment is determined in advance.

2. A chargemaster lists the individual charges for every element of every service provided and serves as a provider's standard fee schedule. Chargemasters provide a reference so that fees billed to various payers are standardized. Chargemasters simplify the work of the billing department.

3. Usual, customary, and reasonable (UCR) charges represent the amount a third-party payer will reimburse a provider for a particular service or procedure based on the amount considered to represent reasonable compensation for those services in a specific geographic area.

4. The most typical cost share ratio is 80:20. This means that 80 percent of the costs are paid by the third-party payer and 20 percent of the costs are paid by the patient.

5. The most common utilization control associated with managed fee-for-service reimbursement is utilization review of the health services planned for, or provided to, patients. The review may be done on either a prospective (before admission) or retrospective (after discharge) basis. Prospective review is often referred to as precertification.

6. If a group of patients used more services than a managed care plan originally calculated in its contract, the plan would show a loss for the period. Conversely, if the group used fewer services than estimated, the plan would show a profit for the period.

7. Bundled payments are lump-sum payments to providers to compensate them for all of the healthcare services delivered to a patient for a specific illness and/or over a specified period of time. Bundled payments are also called episode-of-care (EOC) payments and include capitated payments, global payments, global surgery payments, Medicare ambulatory surgery center rates, and Medicare prospective payment systems.

8. Capitation is a payment methodology based on per-person premiums or membership fees rather than on itemized per-procedure or per-service charges. The capitated managed care organization (MCO) negotiates a contract with an employer or government agency representing a specific group of individuals. The MCO agrees to provide all of the contracted healthcare services that the covered individuals need over a specified period of time. Capitated premiums are calculated on the projected cost of providing covered services per patient or member per month.

9. Ambulatory surgery centers (ASCs) must accept assignment on Medicare claims, which means that the provider (the ASC) accepts as payment in full whatever Medicare reimburses. Because payments are subject to the Medicare Part B deductible and coinsurance requirements, reimbursement is 80 percent of the prospectively determined price for a specific surgical procedure.

10. The ASC is reimbursed at 100 percent for the procedure classified in the highest payment group, and any other procedure performed during the same session is reimbursed at 50 percent of the procedure's applicable group rate.

11. The inpatient prospective payment system using diagnosis-related groups (DRGs) was implemented by HCFA in 1983 as a method of controlling Medicare spending. It was effective in controlling inpatient costs. Medicare expenditures for inpatient care were significantly reduced as a result of the implementation of prospective payment.

12. Diagnosis-related groups are used in a payment methodology in which patient diagnoses are grouped into payment groups. DRGs are used to reimburse hospitals a predetermined amount for each Medicare inpatient stay.

DRGs were effective in reducing Medicare costs for inpatient treatment but, after their implementation, expenditures for Medicare post-acute care benefits escalated. This necessitated the development of prospective payment methodologies for nonacute care services. The Balanced Budget Act of 1997 mandated PPS implementation in nonacute segments of healthcare.

13. Coding is generally done by the facility's health information department. After the codes have been assigned, the billing department performs the following general steps to complete the billing process.
- Itemizes the services provided to the patient as represented by the procedural codes assigned to the case
- Assigns a fee to each service from the provider's standard fee schedule or chargemaster
- Applies the charges to the patient's account
- Transmits the detailed claim to the patient's third-party payer and sends an itemized account of the billed services to the patient

Check Your Understanding 14.4

1. Congress set the stage for prospective payment when it passed the Tax Equity and Fiscal Responsibility Act of 1982 (TEFRA) requiring implementation of the DRG-based prospective payment system in 1983. In 1983, Congress enacted legislation mandating the first Medicare PPS for Medicare Part A coverage.
2. Prior to the implementation of the DRG-based inpatient PPS, Medicare Part A payments to hospitals were based on traditional fee-for-service reimbursement. Reasonable cost and/or per-diem costs were used to determine payment.
3. The DRG prospective payment rate is based on the patient's principal diagnosis as well as complications, comorbidities, principal procedure, and other procedures.
4. The computer software program that assigns the appropriate DRG according to information provided for each episode of care is called a DRG grouper.
5. The Medicare acute care prospective payment system excludes the following types of hospitals:
- Psychiatric and rehabilitation hospitals and psychiatric and rehabilitation units within larger medical facilities
- Long-term care hospitals, defined as hospitals with an average length of stay of 25 days or more
- Children's hospitals
- Cancer hospitals
- Critical access hospitals

6. DRGs are organized within 25 Major Diagnostic Categories (MDCs). Most MDCs are based on a particular organ system of the body, although others are constructed to include multiple organ systems.
7. Case mix refers to the types or categories of patients treated by a hospital. The DRG system allows a hospital to relate its case mix to the costs incurred for inpatient care. This information supports administrative decisions about services to be offered to its patient population.
8. The Balanced Budget Act of 1997 mandated implementation of a skilled nursing facility prospective payment system (SNF PPS). The system was implemented on July 1, 1998.
9. Resident assessment data are standardized data collected about all residents of skilled nursing facilities (SNFs). They are collected from the Minimum Data Set, Version 2.0 (MDS 2.0). This is a data collection tool that includes the minimum core of defined and categorized patient assessment questions and serves as the basis for documentation and reimbursement in a SNF.
10. The resource-based relative value scale (RBRVS) was implemented by HCFA (now CMS) in 1992 as a reimbursement system for physician services covered under Medicare Part B. The system reimburses physicians according to a fee schedule based on predetermined values assigned to specific services.
11. The outpatient prospective payment system (OPPS) does not apply to critical access hospitals (CAHs) or hospitals in Maryland that are excluded because they qualify under the Social Security Act for payment under the state's payment plan. In addition, Indian Health Service hospitals and hospitals located outside the 50 states, the District of Columbia and Puerto Rico are excluded.
12. Discounting applies to the practice of multiple surgical procedures furnished during the same operative session. The full APC rate is paid for the surgical procedure with the highest weight, and other surgical procedures performed at the same time are reimbursed at 50 percent of the APC rate.
13. Home health agencies use the Outcome and Assessment Information Set (OASIS) to collect data elements that represent core items for the comprehensive assessment of adult home care patients.
14. The home health resource group (HHRG) is a classification system established for the prospective reimbursement of covered home care services to Medicare beneficiaries during a 60-day episode of care. Covered services include skilled nursing visits, home health aide visits, therapy services, medical social services, and nonroutine medical supplies.

15. An inpatient rehabilitation facility is required to complete a patient assessment instrument (PAI) on all patients upon both admission to and discharge from the facility.

16. CMS provides IRFs with IRVEN to collect the IRF-PAI in a database that can be transmitted electronically to a nationwide IRF database. This data is used in assessing clinical characteristics of patients in rehabilitation settings. Eventually it can be used to provide survey agencies with a means to objectively measure and compare facility performance and quality and to allow researchers to develop improved standards of care.

17. LTC hospitals are defined as having an average inpatient length of stay of more than 25 days.

18. A short-stay outlier is an adjustment to the payment rate for stays that are considerably shorter than the average length of stay for a particular LTC-DRG. A case would qualify for short-stay outlier status when the length of stay is between one day and up to and including 5/6 of the average length of stay for the LTC-DRG. Both the average length of stay and the 5/6 of the average length of stay periods are published in the Federal Register. Payment under the short-stay outlier is made using different payment methodologies.

19. The prospective systems for long-term care hospitals and inpatient psychiatric facilities both use the current DRGs for inpatient hospitals.

20. Patient-level or case-level adjustments are provided for age, specified DRGs, and certain comorbidity categories. Payment adjustments are made for eight age categories beginning with age 45 at which point costs are statistically increased as the patient ages.

   The IPF receives a DRG payment adjustment for a principal diagnosis that groups to 1 of 15 psychiatric DRGs. There is also a variable per diem adjustment to recognize higher costs in the early days of a psychiatric stay.

   The IPF prospective payment system also includes an outlier policy for those patients who require more expensive care than expected in an effort to minimize the financial risk to the IPF.

   The prospective payment system also includes regulations on payments when there is an interrupted stay, meaning the patient is discharged from an IPF and returns to the same or another facility before midnight on the third consecutive day.

Check Your Understanding 14.5

1. A coordination of benefits (COB) transaction is an electronic transmission from a healthcare provider to a healthcare plan. The purpose of a COB is to determine relative payment responsibilities for healthcare claims and/or payment information.

2. A remittance advice is sent by the third-party payer to the provider to explain payments made by the payer.

3. The CMS-1500 form is a standardized billing form used to bill third-party payers for reimbursement for provider services such as physician office visits. Though its precursor was the Attending Physician Statement (APS) (or COMB-1), the CMS-1500 currently has no alternate name.

4. The National Uniform Billing Committee (NUBC) is responsible for the data elements and design of the CMS-1450, which is also known as the UB-92 (Uniform Bill 92). This committee is made up of representatives from a wide variety of healthcare organizations.

5. The UB-92 is submitted by healthcare facilities in order to obtain reimbursement for patient services. Hospitals, ambulance companies, ambulatory surgery centers, home health agencies, hospice organizations, skilled nursing facilities, subacute facilities, stand-alone clinical laboratory facilities, and walk-in clinics use the UB-92. The revised UB-04 is targeted for implementation in 2007.

6. Revenue codes are reported using the CMS-1450 and are of particular importance since they identify services provided to patients.

7. Medicare carriers process Part B claims for services by physicians and medical suppliers and might include such agencies as a Blue Shield plan, a commercial insurance company, or another organization that contracts with Medicare. Carriers are responsible for performing the following functions:
   • Determining the charges allowed by Medicare
   • Maintaining the quality of performance records
   • Assisting in fraud and abuse investigations
   • Assisting both suppliers and beneficiaries as needed
   • Making payments to physicians and suppliers for Part B-covered services

   Medicare fiscal intermediaries (FIs) process Part A claims and hospital-based Part B claims for institutional services, including inpatient hospital claims, and claims from SNFs, home health agencies, and hospice services. They also process outpatient claims for supplemental medical insurance (Medicare Part B). The same types of organizations that serve as Medicare carriers might also contract as fiscal intermediaries. FIs are responsible for the following functions:
   • Determining costs and reimbursement amounts
   • Maintaining records
   • Establishing controls
   • Safeguarding against fraud and abuse or excess use
   • Conducting reviews and audits
   • Making payments to providers for covered services
   • Assisting both providers and beneficiaries, as needed

8. Electronic data interchange (EDI) allows a healthcare provider to transmit its claims data electronically to the third-party payer.

9. The HCFA (now known as the CMS) implemented the Correct Coding Initiative (CCI) in 1996 to develop correct coding methodologies to improve the appropriate payment of Medicare Part B claims. The CCI edits explain what procedures and services cannot be billed together on the same day of service for a patient.

10. The Correct Coding Initiative (CCI) policies are based on national and local policies and coding edits, coding guidelines developed by HCFA (now CMS), analysis of standard medical and surgical practices, and review of current coding practices.

Check Your Understanding 14.6

1. Generally, third-party payers update fee schedules on an annual basis.

2. A physician or other healthcare provider who participates in the Medicare program must agree to accept assignment for all covered services provided to Medicare patients. To accept assignment means that the provider or supplier accepts, as payment in full, the allowed charge from the Medicare fee schedule. The provider or supplier is prohibited from balance billing, which means the patient cannot be held responsible for charges in excess of the Medicare fee schedule.

3. Physicians, practitioners, and suppliers must notify Medicare by December 31 of each year whether they intend to participate in the Medicare program during the coming year. Medicare participation means that the provider or supplier agrees to accept assignment for all covered services provided to Medicare patients.

   Nonparticipating providers (NonPAR) do not sign a participation agreement with Medicare but may or may not accept assignment. If the nonPAR physician elects to accept assignment, he or she is paid 95 percent (5 percent less than participating physicians) of the Medicare Physician Fee Schedule or MFS. NonPAR providers who choose not to accept assignment are subject to Medicare's limiting charge policy.

4. The limiting charge policy states that a physician may not charge a patient more than 115 percent of the nonparticipating fee schedule. Under the limiting charge policy, the provider collects the full amount from the patient and Medicare reimburses the patient.

5. An inaccurate chargemaster can adversely affect facility reimbursement as well as compliance and data quality. Negative results that may occur because of an inaccurate chargemaster include overpayment, underpayment, undercharging for delivery of healthcare services, claims rejections, and fines or penalties.

6. • *Description of service:* Examples might be the evaluation and management visit, observation, or emergency room visit.
   • *CPT/HCPCS code:* Must correspond to the description of the service
   • *Revenue code:* Also called the UB-92 code, this is a three-digit code that describes a classification of a product or service provided to the patient. These revenue or UB-92 codes are required by CMS for reporting services.
   • *Charge amount:* The charge amount is the amount that the facility charges for the procedure or service. This does not necessarily equal what the facility will be reimbursed by the third-party payer.
   • *Charge or service code:* An internally assigned number that is unique to the facility. It identifies each procedure listed on the chargemaster and identifies the department or revenue center that initiated the charge. The charge code can be very useful for revenue tracking and budget analysis.
   • *General ledger key:* A two or three digit number that assigns a line item to a section of the general ledger in the hospital's accounting system.
   • *Activity/Status Date:* Indicates the most recent activity of an item

7. The chargemaster is generally maintained by representatives from health information management, clinical services, the business office, and compliance and information systems.

8. Revenue cycle management involves many different processes, and people all working to make sure that the healthcare facility is properly reimbursed for the services that are provided. Effective management of the revenue cycle is essential to improving the facility's revenues. Delays in payment, denied claims, and other lost revenues have a tremendous impact on the financial health of the facility. The major functions of revenue cycle management typically include admitting and access management, case management, charge capture, health information management, patient financial services and business office, finance, compliance, and information technology.

9. A good physician query form should:
   • Be clearly and concisely written
   • Contain precise language
   • Present the facts from the medical record and identify why clarification is needed
   • Present the scenario and ask the physician to make a clinical interpretation of a given diagnosis or condition based on treatment, evaluation, monitoring, and/or services provided. "Open-ended" questions that allow the physician to document the specific diagnosis are preferable to multiple-choice questions or questions requiring only a "yes" or "no" response. Queries that appear to lead the physician to provide a particular response could lead to allegations of inappropriate upcoding and should be avoided.

- Be phrased such that the physician is allowed to specify the correct diagnosis. The form should not indicate the financial impact of the response to the query. The form should not be designed so that only the physician signature is provided.
- Include patient name, admission date, medical record number, name and contact information (phone number and e-mail address) of the coding professional, specific question and rationale, place for the physician to document his or her response, and a place for the physician to sign and date his or her response

10. Coding compliance programs focus on preventing accusations of fraud and abuse. The Office of the Inspector General (OIG) of the Department of Health and Human Services (HHS) provides guidance for healthcare organizations in developing compliance programs.

11. Upcoding is the practice of assigning a reimbursement code specifically for the purpose of obtaining a higher level of payment. It is most often found when reimbursement-grouping systems are used. Unbundling is the practice of using multiple codes that describe individual components of a procedure rather than an appropriate single code that describes all steps of the procedure performed.

12. From Bowman, 2004:
- Inconsistent documentation
- Incomplete progress notes
- Undocumented care
- Test results not addressed in the physician documentation
- Historical diagnoses being documented as current diagnoses
- Long-standing, chronic conditions that are not documented
- Lack of documentation of postoperative complications
- Illegibility
- Documentation not completed on time

13.
- DRG Coding Accuracy
- Variations in case mix
- Discharge status (transfers vs discharges)
- Services provided under arrangement
- 72-hour window
- Medical necessity
- Evaluation and management services
- Chargemaster Description

14. Benefits of effective corporate compliance include a commitment to responsible conduct toward employees and the community, an accurate view of behavior related to fraud and abuse, identification and prevention of criminal and unethical conduct, and high-quality patient care improvements

Chapter 15

Check Your Understanding 15.1
1. Nominal
2. Ratio
3. Nominal/ordinal
4. Ratio
5. Nominal
6. Nominal
7. Ratio
8. Nominal
9. Ratio
10. Nominal/ordinal

Check Your Understanding 15.2
1. Ratio
2. Proportion
3. Rate

Check Your Understanding 15.3
1.
   a. 275 Inpatient census (268 + 16 − 9)
   b. 277 Daily inpatient census (275 + 2 patients admitted and discharged the same day)
   c. 277 Inpatient service days
   d. 547 Total inpatient service days for August 1 and 2 (277 + 270)
2.
   a. 10 Inpatient census (9 + 2 + 1 − 1 − 1)
   b. 12 Daily inpatient census (10 + 2 patients admitted and died the same day)

Check Your Understanding 15.4
1.

Inpatient Unit	Service Days	Bed Count	Occupancy Rate	
Medical	2,850	100	91.9%	[2,850/(100 × 31)]
Surgical	988	34	93.7%	[988/(34 × 31)]
Pediatric	422	15	90.8%	[422/(15 × 31)]
Orthopedic	502	18	90.0%	[502/(18 × 31)]
Obstetric	544	20	87.7%	[544/20 × 31)]
Newborn	524	18	93.9%	[524/(18 × 31)]
Total	5,830	6,355	97.7%	(5,830/6,355)

2.
   a. 183.9 (67,120/365)
   b. 13.3 (4,850/365)
   c. 83.6% (67,120/80,300)
   d. 60.4 (4,850/8,030)

Check Your Understanding 15.5
1.

Number of Patients Discharged	Total Length of Stay	Discharge Days
10	2	20
7	3	21
2	4	8
1	7	7
1	9	9
1	10	10
1	16	16

   a. Total length of stay 91
   b. Average length of stay 91/23 = 4.0

Check Your Understanding 15.6

1. <u>1.9%</u> $[(14 \times 100)/754]$
2. <u>1.1%</u> $[(14 - 6) \times 100/(754 - 6)]$
3. <u>2.1%</u> $[(3 \times 100)/(140 + 3)]$
4. <u>2.5%</u> $[(3 \times 100)/122]$
5. <u>1.9%</u> $[(14 + 3) \times 100/(754 + 122)]$
6. <u>1.5%</u> $(2 \times 100)/133$

Check Your Understanding 15.7

1. <u>50.0%</u> $[22 \times 100)/44]$
2. <u>52.4%</u> $[22 \times 100)/42]$

Check Your Understanding 15.8

1. $(5 \times 100)/20 = 26.0\%$
2. $(122 \times 100)/822 = 14.8\%$
3. The CMI for Dr. Green is 1.281 (26.4205/21).

DRG	DRG Title	RW	N	N*DRG
079	Respiratory Infections & Inflammations Age >17 w/ CC	1.6238	2	3.2476
085	Pleural Effusion w/ CC	1.2405	1	1.2405
087	Pulmonary Edema	1.3654	3	4.0962
089	Simple Pneumonia & Pleurisy Age >17 w/ CC	1.0320	1	1.0320
121	Circulatory Disorders w/ AMI & Major Complications, Discharged Alive	1.6136	1	1.6136
130	Peripheral Vascular Disorders w/ CC	0.9425	1	0.9425
143	Chest Pain	0.5659	1	0.5659
174	GI Hemorrhage w/ CC	1.0060	2	2.0120
182	Esophagitis, Gastroenteritis & Miscellaneous Digestive Disorders Age >17 w/ CC	0.8413	2	1.6826
240	Connective Tissue Disorder w/ CC	1.4051	1	1.4051
243	Medical Back Problems	0.7658	1	0.7658
316	Renal Failure	1.2692	1	1.2692
395	Red Blood Cell Disorders Age >17	0.8328	1	0.8328
416	Septicemia Age >17	1.6774	1	1.6774
450	Poisoning & Toxic Effects of Drugs Age >17 w/o CC	0.4282	1	0.4282
475	Respiratory System Diagnosis w/ Ventilator Support	3.6091	1	3.6091
Total			**21**	**27.4205**

Check Your Understanding 15.9

1. <u>84.5</u> $[(1{,}183{,}090 \times 10{,}000)/140{,}074{,}612]$
2. <u>84.9</u> $[(1{,}232{,}913 \times 10{,}000/145{,}238{,}309]$
3. <u>84.6</u> $[(1{,}183{,}090 + 1{,}232{,}913) \times 10{,}000]/$
         $(140{,}074{,}612 + 145{,}238{,}309)$
4. <u>26.9</u> $(58{,}184 \times 10{,}000)/22{,}464{,}182$
5. <u>14.8</u> $(33{,}510 \times 10{,}000)/22{,}675{,}474$

Check Your Understanding 15.10

1. *Incidence:* The number of new cases of a given disease in a population for a given period of time. *Prevalence:* The number of cases of a given disease in a population for a given period of time.
2. $(41{,}595 \times 100{,}000)/248{,}710{,}000 = 16.7$ per 100,000

Check Your Understanding 15.11

1. table
2. pie chart
3. line graph
4. bar chart
5. histogram
6. box plot

Check Your Understanding 15.12

1. The normal distribution is a family of distributions that are symmetrical and bell-shaped. Since it is symmetrical, 50 percent of the observations fall above the mean and 50 percent fall below the mean. In a normal distribution, the mean, median, and mode are equal.
2. When a distribution is asymmetrical it is said to be skewed. Skewness is the horizontal stretching of the distribution to one side so that one tail of the distribution is longer than the other.

Check Your Understanding 15.13

1. <u>2,418</u>   Mean
2. <u>2,540</u>   Median
3. <u>2,540</u>   Mode
4. <u>1,095</u>   Range
5. <u>139,617.1</u>   Variance
6. <u>373.7</u>   Standard deviation

Chapter 16

Check Your Understanding 16.1

1. Research is thoughtful, planned activity that expands or refines knowledge.
2. The research of health information professionals is considered applied research because it involves the use of research to improve practice.

3. Theories are made up of concepts that are abstract ideas generalized from particular instances, inter-relationships that are assumed to exist among these concepts, and consequences that are assumed to follow logically from the relationships proposed in the theory.

4. The "best" theories are often the simplest theories.

5. Health records are important to clinical research because clinical research, as opposed to epidemiology, focuses on the individual patient. Many protocols of clinical trials state that specific data will be obtained from health records.

6. An advantage of models is that they aid comprehension. Models include all known properties of theories and describe theories graphically or on a smaller scale.

7. Inductive reasoning involves creating conclusions based on a limited number of observations; deductive reasoning involves creating conclusions based on generalizations. Therefore, induction begins with the specific and deduction begins with the general.

8. Knowing their purpose is important to researchers because purpose determines research approach.

Check Your Understanding 16.2

1. The seven basic steps of research are defining the problem, reviewing the literature, determining the design and method, selecting the instrument, gathering the data, analyzing the data, and presenting the results.

2. A well-developed research question should be stated clearly and exactly; have theoretical significance, practical worth, or both; have obvious and explicit links to a larger body of knowledge; advance knowledge in a definable way; and be worthwhile.

3. The three rich sources of meaningful research questions are:
   • Research models
   • Recommendations of previous researchers
   • Gaps in the field's body of knowledge detected during the review of the literature

4. Conducting a literature review is important because it results in the researcher "owning" the body of knowledge. In other words, he or she knows the theories; the names of key researchers, theorists, and collaborators; the sources of data; the common research designs; and the gaps in the body of knowledge.

5. Five data sources, other than journal articles, that researchers should consider when doing a comprehensive search are videotapes, audiotapes, Web sites, government reports, and statistical data (such as census data, economic data, crime data, and Medicare data).

6. Journal articles from refereed journals should constitute the bulk of the literature review because articles in refereed journals have been evaluated for quality prior to publication.

7. A director of health information services might select the productivity standard recommended in a peer-reviewed journal rather than one recommended in a popular magazine because health information experts have evaluated the quality of the recommendations in the peer-reviewed journal.

8. Researchers use key terms (MeSH headings) to identify journal articles related to their topic.

9. A researcher might use bibliographic software because it saves time for the researcher by automatically converting the bibliographic information to the particular style required by a professor or journal.

10. Studies with contradictory results should be included in the review of the literature because readers could perceive the absence of contradictory studies as evidence of bias. Evidence of bias detracts from the credibility of the literature review.

11. In the review of the literature, readers should expect information about the study's design, time frame, method, sample, response rate, statistical techniques, and findings.

Check Your Understanding 16.3

1. The purpose of the study determines a researcher's choice of a research design.

2. A researcher would use correlational research to investigate the relationship between a supervisor's level of stress and the number of his or her subordinates.

3. An example of a direct relationship would be the higher the number of subordinates managed by the supervisor, the higher the level of the supervisor's stress.

4. The key characteristic of experimental research is control.

5. Quasi-experimental (for example, causal-comparative research) lacks random assignment to a group and manipulation of treatment.

6. The independent variable causes an effect in the dependent variable.

7. In a double-blind study, administrative assistants or researchers removed from the study know which subjects are in the study group. Neither the participants nor the researchers directly conducting the study knows which subjects are in the study control.

8. A longitudinal design is more credible than a cross-sectional study because it eliminates the possibility that the study occurred at some unrepresentative point in time. For an important topic, such as cancer, the investment of time is justifiable.

Check Your Understanding 16.4

1. A survey uses self-report data.
2. Question 1 is an unstructured question.
3. A researcher may choose a structured interview because it is easier to quantify, tabulate, and analyze than an unstructured interview. An interview guide provides the list of questions so all the researchers ask the same questions.
4. If researchers wanted to investigate the impact of the Hill-Burton Act on a region's healthcare, they would most likely choose to use the case study method.
5. Researchers would choose to conduct a questionnaire survey because it is efficient, it takes less time than other methods, and it generates great numbers of responses at a relatively low cost.
6. If researchers wanted to establish that a new drug causes a reduction in blood pressure, they would choose an experiment (randomized clinical trial or double-blind study), such as the pretest-posttest control group method, the Solomon four-group Method, or the posttest-only control group method.
7. Researchers might conduct a meta-analysis when many studies examined the same question, when the studies have common underlying characteristics, or when some of the studies' findings are contradictory.
8. The common characteristic that determined the researchers' choice of method in questions 3 through 7 was purpose (or definition of the question or problem).

Check Your Understanding 16.5

1. The alternative hypothesis states what the researcher believes.
2. If the researcher believes that the treatment increases output, the researcher would write a one-tailed hypothesis.
3. A type I error occurs when the researcher erroneously rejects the null hypothesis when it is true. A null hypothesis states that there is no difference between the groups. Rejecting the null implies that there is a difference in the groups. In the type I error, the researcher has said a difference exists when none does (that is, the drug really does not help the patient). A type II error occurs when the researcher erroneously fails to reject the null hypothesis when it is false. Failing to reject the null hypothesis implies that there is no difference in the groups. In a type II error, the researcher says no difference exists when a difference does exist (that is, the drug helps the patient but the researcher says it does not).
4. The p value represents the probability that the difference occurred by pure chance.
5. Internal validity ensures that the effect seen was caused by the independent variable. If internal validity is breached, the researcher cannot state that the independent variable caused a particular effect on the dependent variable. The issues involved in internal validity are history, maturation, testing, instrumentation, statistical regression, differential selection, experimental mortality, and diffusion of treatment.
6. Reliability is important because it represents the tests' dependability. Reliable tests result in the same or similar outcomes for multiple subjects in multiple situations. For example, scholastic aptitude tests or AHIMA's registration examination have the characteristic of reliability.

Check Your Understanding 16.6

1. A researcher would choose to use an instrument that someone else has created because the reliability and validity of the instrument are established. Construction of a reliable and valid measure is difficult. An established instrument can be matched to the purpose and theory of the researcher. In addition, it has the following characteristics: clarity of language, brevity and attractiveness, and a match between the levels of measurement.
2. An adequate sample depends upon the purpose of the study, the nature of the population, and the resources available to the researcher(s).
3. Directors of HIS departments would be considered a homogenous population (mostly female and white with similar educational backgrounds).
4. Institutional review boards (IRBs) are important because they help organizations comply with federal regulations and protect human subjects from abuses.
5. A pilot study is a "trial run." It shows that it is logistically feasible for the research study to be conducted on a larger scale.
6. Researchers are concerned about their response rates because low response rates could breach both internal and external validity of a study. A low response rate could represent bias, introduce inaccuracy, and/or make generalization to the population impossible.
7. Two common mistakes that researchers make in data collection are lack of planning and deviation from the original plan.

Check Your Understanding 16.7

1. Descriptive (summary) statistics describe the data through techniques such as means, frequency distributions, and variations. Inferential statistics allow the researchers to make inferences about the population characteristics (parameters) based on the characteristics of the sample.
2. Bivariate statistical techniques involve two variables.
3. Paired t test and analysis of variance (ANOVA) are inferential statistical techniques that emphasize differences in groups.
4. The two types of continuous data are interval data and ratio data.

5. Researchers must know the type of data that they are collecting because certain statistical techniques require data of a particular kind.

6. Researchers might use Epi-Info because it is especially designed for their type of study, epidemiological. It makes conducting the research easier by calculating the proper sample size and setting up the entry of data from questionnaires. In addition, Epi-Info is a dedicated statistical package. This means that Epi-Info requires less manipulation of the data and performs many statistical procedures. Finally, the software is free from the Centers for Disease Control and Prevention.

Check Your Understanding 16.8

1. The research findings and discussion sections differ in content and tone. The research findings section contains only the findings of the analysis of the data. No commentary about the findings is included. In the discussion section, researchers interpret and explain their findings and compare them to other researchers' findings. The researchers also comment on the significance of their study in terms of expanding the field's body of knowledge or of adding to a theory. The discussion section is more creative than the research findings section.

2. First, they should consider that they should present the element in only one mode (narrative, table, or figure). Second, they should consider which mode would be most meaningful and understandable to the reader.

3. A researcher should answer any three of the following questions when writing the discussion section:
   - What theoretical significance or practical worth do the findings have?
   - How do the findings link explicitly to the larger body of knowledge?
   - How have the findings improved the field's research model?
   - How have the findings expanded the body of knowledge?
   - What new definitions have the findings added to the field's area of practice?
   - How do the findings support practitioners in the workplace?
   - What problems do the findings solve?
   - What valid conclusions can the researchers and the readers draw from the findings?
   - How can other researchers expand or improve this research study?

4. When selecting a journal for manuscript submission, researchers should consider the journal's scope, content, and audience. A researcher should try to find a journal that matches their purpose, topic, and research design. They should apply the style to their manuscript and make revisions before submission.

Check Your Understanding 16.9

1. When using large databases for secondary analysis, researchers must know the underlying structure of the database.

2. Public databases are in the public domain (freely available), while proprietary databases are the property of an entity (access requires permission).

3. The discrepancy between the researcher's use of the term "anonymous" in the informed consent and the researcher's intent to track respondents. Anonymity demands that the researcher cannot link the response and the responder. The code would link the respondents to their data, so their data would no longer be anonymous.

4. The Common Rule is the set of regulations that stipulate the protection of human subjects in federally funded research under seventeen agencies.

5. Both HIPAA and the Common Rule apply to this researcher. Any state regulations that may be more stringent may also apply.

6. Research is important to an emerging profession, such as health information management, because the key characteristic of a profession is a body of knowledge. Research builds the body of knowledge.

Chapter 17

Check Your Understanding 17.1

1. The definition of quality will change based on the perspective of the individual. Products or services must meet the expectations of the individual(s) for whom they are provided. Failure to meet expectations means the product or service does not meet the basic standard of quality.

2. JCAHO has promoted quality of care since its inception. The organization's role has been to provide support and leadership for healthcare organizations in a variety of capacities and with the goal of improving quality.

3. The agencies involved in today's quality of care issues are JCAHO, state and federal agencies including the Food and Drug Administration [FDA]), the Centers for Disease Control (CDC), and the Centers for Medicare and Medicaid Services (CMS).

4. The Institute of Medicine (IOM) has identified six dimensions around which to frame the measurement of quality: safety, effectiveness, patient-centeredness, timeliness, efficiency, equity. These measures are helping HIM professionals devise ways to close the quality gap.

Check Your Understanding 17.2

1. The basic elements of a quality improvement (QI) program are:
   - Statement of mission
   - Supportive environment
   - Sufficient resources
   - Leaders with qualifications to provide direction
   - Sufficient staff
   - An organizational attitude that focuses on the importance of improvement
   - Coordinated and integrated effort
   - Continuous monitoring
2. The governing board/body is responsible for the overall care provided by a healthcare organization.
3. The HIM profession has a history of being involved in the evaluation of high-quality care and of having an understanding of QI. The backgrounds of HIM professionals in documentation, clinical data management, disease processes, and data analysis, as well as an understanding of the interdisciplinary responsibility for patient care quality add to the richness of the HIM vantage point.
4. HIM professionals can provide support to QI programs in the areas of research, data collection, use and development of spreadsheets and databases, data analysis (interpreting data in a meaningful way), data source evaluation, clinical process improvement, and documentation evaluation and improvement.
5. The goals of the Medicare Modernization Act (MMA) are to:
   - Improve patient safety
   - Enhance quality of care
   - Reduce scientific uncertainty and the unwarranted variation in medical practice that results in both lower quality and higher costs
6. Judicial decisions have influenced QI because they have provided the foundation for the hospital industry's responsibility for patient care. They have provided direction about what kinds of information to monitor regarding patient care, the work/services of physicians, and the processes necessary for selectin medical staff and granting of privileges.
7. The federal government and JCAHO have both set parameters regarding the quality of patient care. The federal government uses legislation to provide direction, and JCAHO develops and publishes accreditation standards to support quality of care initiatives.

Check Your Understanding 17.3

1. Performance measures are statements of expectation or performance. In QI processes, these indicators are tools that help measure the quality of care.
2. Structure, process, and outcome are part of an assessment model that provides a perspective of or orientation to the indicator statements used to measure the quality of care. For example, a statement may measure the qualifications of staff, which would be a statement developed around structure because it addresses the people who provide care.
3. Core measures, statements of outcomes, and clinical practice guidelines are all names of tools that can be used to measure the performance of an organization. They are all different in approach, definition, and process.
4. The four core measurement areas identified for hospitals by JCAHO and CMS are:
   - Acute myocardial infarction (AMI)
   - Heart failure (HF)
   - Pneumonia (PN)
   - Pregnancy and pregnancy-related conditions
   Data collection for surgical infection prevention (SIP) began in July 2004. Other topics that have been identified for the development of performance measures include pregnancy and related conditions, children's asthma care, and pain management.
5. Core performance measures require that healthcare facilities send data to JCAHO on a routine basis. Data from similar organizations will be compared, and areas for improvement will be identified that will be evaluated upon JCAHO accreditation review.
6. Students can visit the Web sites of these organizations to find specific items.
   - JCAHO
     - improve accuracy of patient identification
     - improve effectiveness of communication
     - improve safety of using high-alert medication
     - eliminate wrong-site, wrong-patient, wrong-procedure surgery
     - improve the safety of using infusion pumps
     - improve the effectiveness of clinical alarm systems
     - reduce the risk of healthcare-acquired infections
   - NQF
     - promote a culture of safety by reducing errors
     - match healthcare needs with service delivery capabilities to reduce healthcare errors
     - facilitate information transfer and clear communication to reduce healthcare errors
     - specific setting or processes of care targeted to reduce healthcare errors
     - increase the safe use of medications to reduce healthcare errors

- Leapfrog (4 quality/safety practices)
  - —use computer physician order entry (CPOE)
  - —use evidence-based hospital referral
  - —use ICU physician staffing
  - —use the Leapfrog practices score (the NQF's 27 safe practices)
- CMS
  - —use of best practice guidelines
  - —encourage use of shared decision making between providers and patients
  - —appropriate use of culturally and ethnically sensitive care
  - —provide incentives to improve safety, quality, and efficiency
  - —reduce scientific uncertainty through examination of service variation and outcomes measurement.

7. CMS, AHRQ, and the Food and Drug Administration (FDA) have been involved in developing safe practice protocols.

8. Managed care uses a system of checks and balances to ensure that patients receive the necessary care. The National Committee for Quality Assurance (NCQA) supports managed care organizations in evaluating their quality of care. The Health Plan Employer Data and Information Set (HEDIS) was developed to evaluate the quality of care provided by managed care plans.

9. The National Committee for Quality Assurance (NCQA) accredits health plans and develops performance standards.

10.
- HEDIS (Health Employers Data And Information Set)—Developed by the NCQA
- ICSI (Institute For Clinical Systems Improvement)—Sponsored by a variety of health plans in Minnesota
- CAHPS (Consumer Assessment Health Plan Survey)—Developed by the Agency For Healthcare Research And Quality

11. Severity indexing improves patient care because it provides information about the level of resource consumption. It allows those evaluating quality to determine whether a patient received sufficient resources and, therefore, adequate or high-quality care.

Check Your Understanding 17.4

1. It is important to include the licensed, independent medical staff in the healthcare organization's QI plan because the medical staff is a key player in providing healthcare in an organization, giving specific direction for virtually all patient care services.

2. The bylaws and rules and regulations of an organization provide the medical staff with structure, functions, and responsibilities. The bylaws set the parameters for how the medical staff functions in all capacities, including process improvement.

3. The credentialing process, when completed thoroughly and correctly, ensures that medical staff members are qualified and competent to provide the patient care services requested. Thus, it should eliminate unqualified or incompetent practitioners.

4. Reappointment/reappraisal ensures that the practice patterns of the medical staff are reviewed on a regular basis. The governing body is responsible for timely and appropriate reappointment/reappraisal.

Check Your Understanding 17.5

1. Utilization review (UR) and utilization management (UM) provide information about the appropriateness and necessity of patient care. UR helps ensure, in an efficient manner, that patients receive all needed services.

2. The different types of healthcare reviews (pre-admission, admission, continued stay, and discharge planning) provide information about appropriateness and medical necessity at different times during the patient's encounter. This time line begins before admission and continues to discharge and ensures effective and efficient use of resources and patient care.

3. A notice of noncoverage informs the patient, physician, family, and the organization that services are no longer covered and that the patient or family will have to assume responsibility for all remaining costs.

4. Risk management programs contribute to an organization's overall QI plan because they identify, reduce, or eliminate events that potentially jeopardize patients, staff, and visitors. Identifying and preventing these events contributes to the overall safety and quality of patient care.

5. Sentinel events are catastrophic events that require a system of intensive inquiry (called root-cause analysis) that leads to improvements in patient care systems.

Check Your Understanding 17.6

1. Clearly defined indicators, criteria, and/or data elements in data collection programs provide better information to use to address the system or process in question. Better, clearer information leads to more meaningful improvements.
2. The main data source of performance improvement data is the medical record.
3. Quality management is the foundation of providing high quality patient care. Risk management is a program designed to reduce injury or accidents to everyone who works in a healthcare organization. Reducing the likelihood of injuries to patients being treated in the organization or identifying likely PCEs is one aspect of providing a safer, higher quality environment. Utilization management assures the effective and efficient use of a healthcare organization resources so the patient gets the right services/treatment in a timely way. This assures that the patient is provided the necessary care in the most reasonable amount of time. Patient safety programs provide the patient with an environment that is as secure as possible. Keeping the patient from hazardous materials or unnecessary treatments and assuring appropriate medication use and administration equates to a higher quality of care for the patient.
4. QI data are sensitive information. They offer insight into an organization's inner workings and highlight what is most right and most wrong. Information is collected on the people who provide patient care and those who receive it. All information collected must be kept private and confidential. Laws, statutes, and professional organizations all encourage such safeguarding of this information.
5. • Provide decision support to the direct care providers such as allergic or interaction alerts (cross-check information).
   • Provide improved communication of test results by having all information available for better diagnosis.
   • Provide more accurate and complete information (large volumes of data) about all aspects of patient care.
   • Improve the quality of care by allowing quicker more complete analysis of data (benchmarking) involving practice patterns leading to a quicker understanding of what is best for patient care.
6. Communication is how an organization shares information. To be effective, information must flow freely from top to bottom and vice versa. Good communication increases clarity of understanding. Information is collected in many different areas for many different reasons. The results of QI efforts must be shared with all pertinent parties. There must be an openness to ensure that when areas for improvement are found, all appropriate staff and individuals work toward improvement. The challenge of collecting, analyzing, and improving does not just happen because of the efforts of one or two people. Effective communication can create an environment of sharing and caring, which then can lead to effective improvement of patient care services.

Chapter 18

Check Your Understanding 18.1

1. The Nuremberg Code outlines research ethics to guide the conduct of research involving human subjects. It was developed during the trials of Nazi war criminals following World War II. Its basic tenets are:
   • Informed consent is essential
   • Research should be based on prior animal work
   • The risks should be justified by the anticipated benefits
2. (1) Respect for persons, (2) beneficence, (3) justice
3. Respect for persons
4. Answer should include five of the following:
   • Lack of informed consent
   • Coercion or undue pressure on volunteers
   • Use of a vulnerable population
   • Withholding of information
   • Withholding available treatment
   • Withholding information about risks
   • Putting subjects at risk
   • Risks to subjects that outweigh the benefits
   • Deception
   • Violation of rights
5. The Public Health Service syphilis study

Check Your Understanding 18.2

1. False. The researcher, the research sponsor and/or organization in which the research is conduct are not exculpable for any harm caused to the human subject.
2. False. Only medical expenses related to the experimental portion of the research study are covered. Diagnositics such as x-ray, MRIs, etc., drugs and other treatments provided that are considered standard of care are the responsibility of the patient and/or the patient's insurance company.
3. False. Release of patient information is restricted to those identified in the informed consent. The subject must authorize the release of information to any other party.
4. True. A subject may withdraw from a research study at any time without penalty.

5. True. Individuals who have diminished autonomy are considered vulnerable. Autonomy means the ability to understand and process information (mental capacity) and the freedom from control or influence of other (voluntariness).

6. True

7. True

8.
   - A statement that the study involves research and its purpose
   - Expected duration of the subject's participation in the study
   - Description of the procedures to be followed
   - Indication that the procedures are experimental
   - Description of the risks and benefits
   - Description of alternative available treatments
   - Statement regarding confidentiality of collected information and how the privacy of the subject will be maintained
   - Fore research involving more than minimal risk, an explanation of whether compensation or medical care is available if injury occurs
   - Explanation of whom to contact for questions about the research
   - A statement that participation is voluntary and that refusal to participate will not result in loss of benefits to which the subject may otherwise be entitled

9. The HIPAA Privacy Rule protects medical records and other individually identifiable information from disclosure. It informs human subjects about how information about them will be used or disclosed. It also outlines their rights to access the information.

10. Office of Research Integrity (ORI) and Office of Human Research Protections

Check Your Understanding 18.3

1. The Privacy Rule provides individuals with certain rights about how their health information will be used and disclosed as well as how they can gain access to health records and information about when the PHI was released without their permission.

2.
   - Epidemiological studies
   - Case-control studies
   - Cohort studies
   - Cross-sectional study
   - Clinical trials

3.
   - Identify the cause of disease and associated risk factors
   - Determine the extent of disease in a given community
   - Study the natural history and prognosis of disease
   - Evaluate the preventive and therapeutic measures and new modes of healthcare delivery
   - Provide the foundation for public policy and regulatory decisions relating to environmental problems

4. Medical records may be used in case-control studies to retrospectively determine whether risk factors are present in exposed and unexposed groups. However, use of medical records may be problematic in that generalizability to a larger population is limited when only hospitalized patients are studied. In addition, medical records may be illegible, have poor documentation, or be unavailable.

5. In case-control studies, groups are defined on the basis of an outcome and then assessed on the basis of past exposure to possible risk factors. Case-control studies are quick and easy to conduct and inexpensive. However, because a case-control study is a retrospective study, recall bias may be a risk.

6. Randomized controlled clinical trials (RCCTs) are considered the gold standard for studying interventions. If properly designed, they can eliminate bias. In an RCCT, subjects are randomly assigned to either an experimental or control group. The experimental group receives the experimental treatment, and the control group receives a placebo or the standard method of treatment. If neither the subject nor the investigator is made aware of the treatment assignment until the conclusion of the study, it is called a double-blind study.

7. Relative risk is a ratio that compares the risk of disease between two groups; it is also referred to as risk ratio

8. Attributable risk is a measure of the public health impact of a causative factor on a population. It is assumed that the occurrence of a disease in an unexposed group is the baseline or expected risk for that disease. Any risk above that in the exposed group is the result of exposure to the risk factor. It is assumed that some individuals will acquire a disease whether or not they are exposed to the risk factor.

Check Your Understanding 18.4

1. The major objective of outcomes and effectiveness research is to understand the benefits, outcomes and end results of healthcare practices and interventions.

2.
   - Patient function
   - Quality of life
   - Patient satisfaction
   - Morbidity and mortality

3. The mission of the AHRQ is to support research designed to improve the outcomes and quality of healthcare, reduce its costs, address patient safety and medical errors, and broaden access to effective services. This information helps consumers make better decisions about healthcare.

4. The AHRQ is the sponsor of the HCUP. HCUP is a robust online query system that provides instant access to the largest set of all payer healthcare databases that are publicly available. It can be used to identify, track, analyze, and compare trends in hospital care at the national, regional and state levels.

5. • Prevention quality indicators—used to identify hospital admissions that could have been avoided
   • Inpatient quality indicators—used to assess quality of care including inpatient mortality and utilization
   • Patient safety quality indicators—indicators to evaluate potentially avoidable complications and iatrogenic events

6. • Structure—the setting in which healthcare is provided and the resources available to provide it
   • Process—the extent to which professionals perform to acceptable levels
   • Outcomes—changes in patient's condition, quality of life, and level of satisfaction

7. The purpose of the HEDIS measures is to:
   • Provide purchasers and consumers of healthcare with information to compare the performance of managed care programs
   • Develop a set of performance measures that serve as baseline measures
   • Standardize data reporting for comparative purposes
   • Provide accountability to the public
   • Build consensus among networks regarding data systems investment

8. HEDIS data are collected from healthcare claims and/ or health records.

9. The purpose of the ORYX core measures is to encourage organizations to examine their processes for providing care in order to improve the results (outcomes) of care. It allows healthcare organizations to benchmark their performance and outcomes with similar organizations.

10. • Acute Myocardial Infarction
    • Heart Failure
    • Pneumonia
    • Pregnancy and related conditions
    • Surgical Infection prevention

Chapter 19

Check Your Understanding 19.1

1. Because healthcare is a very information- and decision-intensive environment, with human lives as well as the financial soundness of organizations at stake, decision support systems are indispensable.

2. Some of the challenges facing healthcare that decision support can assist in addressing include locating and allocating financial resources, assisting health plan administrators in managing the medical care market and formulating appropriate payment plans, assisting hospital administrators in evaluating resource utilization, and preventing medical errors and adverse events.

3. A decision support system (DSS) is a computer-based system that gathers data from a variety of sources and assists in providing structure to this data by using various analytical models and visual tools. A decision support system facilitates and improves the outcomes of decision-making tasks associated with nonroutine and nonrepetitive problems.

4. Expert systems are designed to replace the expert. Decision support systems are designed to provide decision support for the decision maker, not to replace the decision maker.

5. The study and development of decision support systems evolved from the World War II discipline of operations research (also called management science).

6. The three phases in Simon's model of the decision making process are the intelligence phase, the design phase, and the choice phase.

7. The classical view of decision making involved postulating various decision alternatives and then selecting one from among them.

8. The key element in the DSS is the one that assists in "reasoning." The reasoning process considers the data and knowledge that has been provided and attempts to recognize and solve the problem. In expert systems, this key element is often called the inference engine.

9. The four classes of decision support systems are data-based, knowledge-based, model-based, and graphics-based.

10. An early medical DSS developed by Shortliffe and called MYCIN is an important medical decision support system that can be classified as a knowledge-based DSS. It used a knowledge base composed of rules (such as the one illustrated in figure 19.9 in the chapter), and an inference engine to "reason" from the rule base.

Check Your Understanding 19.2

1. A data warehouse serves as a neutral storage area for data extracted from an organization's transactional systems, is organized around specific business functions or requirements, and provides easy access to business data for analysis or data mining (decision support).

2. Normalization in a database seeks to eliminate redundancy in data storage.

3. Two well-known data models used for constructing a data warehouse are the star schema and the snowflake schema.

4. The architecture of a data warehouse and a clinical repository differ significantly. Because the clinical repository is integrated into the overall information systems, its architecture is best described by the systems with which it interacts. Though used in the design of a data warehouse, the star and snowflake schemas are typically not used in the design of the clinical repository. While nonclinical data warehouses will be static in nature (their data does not change except as specified on a periodic basis), the clinical repository will constantly be changing as new clinical data are available for patient care. The nonclinical data warehouse is focused on retrospective analyses of business data. The business analyst uses the nonclinical data warehouse to tap into corporate data to assist with future decisions. The clinical repository, however, is focused on assisting with patient care in a near real-time environment.

5. • OLAP: online analytical processing
   • ROLAP: relational online analytical processing
   • MOLAP: multidimensional online analytical processing
   • HOLAP: hybrid online analytical processing

6. In supervised learning, the algorithm learns the inherent patterns hidden in the data that predict a specified outcome or target variable. In supervised learning algorithms, this outcome or target variable must be present in the supplied data set in order for the algorithm to proceed. Unsupervised learning techniques seek to group together cases or data records that are similar or alike in certain respects. The goal of the analysis is to discover previously unknown groupings that exist in the data.

7. Important data-mining tools include artificial neural networks, decision trees, k-nearest neighbor clustering, and rule induction.

Check Your Understanding 19.3

1. The four types of decision support systems found in healthcare are clinical decision support systems (CDSSs), executive decision support systems, healthcare decision support systems, and nursing decision support systems.

2. A clinical decision support system (CDSS) is software that integrates information on the characteristics of individual patients with a computerized knowledge base for the purpose of generating patient-specific assessments or recommendations designed to aid clinicians and/or patients in making clinical decisions.

3. The name of one of the earliest CDSSs was MYCIN.

4. MYCIN used a knowledge base containing the production rules for the system, and an inference engine that "reasoned" based on the rules in the knowledge base.

5. Some of the difficulties in maintaining a CDSS include maintaining the rule base or the knowledge base to keep it current, eliciting the rules from medical experts (not all experts will agree on what is the most appropriate rule for a given situation), and ensuring that the knowledge base does not contain contradictory rules or rules that would lead to circular reasoning. All of these issues are part of what is often referred to as knowledge engineering in expert systems. Some have called it the Achilles' heel of expert systems.

6. The following are key characteristics of an EIS:
   • Generally, modeling and database capabilities are not as sophisticated as a DSS
   • Targets the top-level view and is not intended for the more in-depth analyses provided in a DSS
   • Is intended to allow executives to gain a "view" or "snapshot" of the organization as a whole, whereas a DSS often provides more detailed support in a particular area of the organization's operation
   • EISs typically incorporate external data into the information given to the user, while DSSs typically use internal data

7. The task of decision support for nursing is complex because the decisions faced by nurses are themselves broad and complex, making the development of nursing decision support systems very difficult.

Chapter 20

Check Your Understanding 20.1

1. Knowledge management can be applied to healthcare in the areas of determining cost effectiveness of treatment protocols, understanding cost structures of services, finding patterns and forecasting trends, and implementing process redesign initiatives for more enhanced customer service.

2. Knowledge is created from the translation of data and interpretation of information. Because people transform basic information and apply it as knowledge, knowledge in healthcare is found in individuals who make up the organization.

3. The five steps or components of a knowledge management program are:
    - Step 1: Categorize the organization's knowledge assets
    - Step 2: Analyze the cost and value of current knowledge assets
    - Step 3: Identify problems that current assets cannot solve
    - Step 4: Build a culture that encourages the capture of knowledge to help achieve the organization's objectives and goals
    - Step 5: Deploy and implement knowledge management and business intelligence applications
4. In the process of knowledge management, information comes before knowledge. Knowledge is only derived only after information is gathered, analyzed, and translated.
5. Knowledge management eventually creates wisdom, or business sense, for the organization. An organization can store and maintain knowledge, but wisdom is created only after knowledge is applied. In other words, wisdom is created when someone acts on acquired knowledge.
6. Explicit knowledge includes documents, databases, and other types of recorded and documented information. The actions, experiences, ideals, values, and emotions of individuals constitute tacit knowledge.

Check Your Understanding 20.2

1. A learning organization is one in which everyone within it progresses through a learning process in order to have sufficient knowledge of the business they are involved in. To allow staff to be fully engaged in their work and to reach their full potential, information is shared by everyone within the organization.
2. The four categories of healthcare data are patient-centric data, aggregate data, transformed base data, and comparative data.
3. A data warehouse contains all of an organization's data in one centralized place so that the organization can extract, maintain and send data to users. Data warehousing is a crucial element in the process of knowledge management because it is used to sort or convert large amounts of data into various arrangements and formats which help organizations solve problems and make good decisions.
4. Data mining discovers patterns and future trends in data. This, in turn, speeds up the process of knowledge management and information processing. Data mining also uncovers hidden patterns or trends, allowing organizations to maximize the full potential of their data. Data mining is an important tool because it converts data into information, creating business intelligence in the process.

5. Three basic forms of data mining include: decision trees, genetic algorithms, neural networks.
6. Customer relationship management involves finding solutions that enable products and services to meet customer needs. This strategic solution requires a thorough understanding of customer desires, business strategies, and organizational and technological issues.
7. Core communications in healthcare are the basic communications informing customers and others in the community about how they can maintain and improve their health. Branding communications include messages sent to a community to increase awareness of an organization's existence and to enhance an organization's image in the marketplace. Strategic communications are programs created to advance specific organizational goals.

Check Your Understanding 20.3

1. By applying knowledge management, healthcare organizations can allow their knowledge base to be updated and maintained by knowledge workers, thus closing the gap between the amount of information shared by the knowledge worker and the organization. If a sound knowledge management mechanism is in place, acquired knowledge can be shared among knowledge workers, which raises the strategic acumen of the organization as a whole. In order to discover trends and patterns, knowledge workers can navigate through the data and ask questions based on what they see at any given time. As knowledge workers share knowledge, they improve their performance and are able to make better decisions. Thus, the organization as a whole is able to strategically respond in a timely manner to changes in the marketplace.
2. The discovery phase of the decision-making process involves looking at comparisons and exceptions, and examining data from many different perspectives to identify trends and patterns. The analysis phase focuses on proving that the identified trends do exist, understanding them, forecasting the trends over time, and making solid predictions about the consequences of the trends. The presentation phase involves the creation of reports that are most appropriate for the identified goals and objectives of the organization.
3. OLAP offers fast access to multidimensional information from many different perspectives to help answer business queries and aid in strategic business decisions. OLAP also allows users to view large amounts of data while giving them the freedom to "slice and dice" through that data in order to answer questions users may have when making an informed decision.

4. A chief knowledge officer (CKO) oversees the entire knowledge management process in an organization, researches new knowledge management technologies that will benefit the organization, manages the sharing of knowledge between workers, and helps an organization successfully implement knowledge management applications.

Chapter 21

Check Your Understanding 21.1

1. The following are important management concepts that have persisted over the decades:
   - *Efficiency:* The early time and motion studies of Taylor, the Gilbreths, and others are still relevant to most organizations. The early studies are carried on in today's just-in-time inventory process, project management efforts, and emphasis on quality management.
   - *Management functions:* The four management functions of planning, organizing, leading, and controlling (plus Fayol's fifth function, coordination) have persisted in nearly all organizations and will likely continue to do so in the future.
   - *Fayol's 14 principles,* though modified in some cases, are still sound management concepts that are regularly practiced.

   These concepts have persisted because they enable managers to structure and monitor the functions of a business, regardless of size. They also create a common culture across organizations so that relocated or transferred staff encounter a shorter learning curve and require less time to adjust.
2. New management concepts, theories, and ideas have often been readily and quickly accepted because those who are in a position to adopt them have been ready to do so. These individuals see the need, understand the mechanism for implementing the idea, and understand that adoption of the idea presents obvious benefits. Because of limited or specialized applications at the time they were proposed, resistance to replacing established practices, and apprehension over uncertainty about new ideas, other ideas have required years to be accepted and adopted.
3. For example, the learner could time how long it typically takes to pack for a short trip and compare this time to packing time if a section of the closet is sectioned off with travel clothes already lightly folded, ready for placement in a suitcase. A travel kit of toiletries could be assembled and held ready for any trip. Socks, underwear, handkerchiefs, and so on, could be folded in stacks and placed in a special travel drawer for rapid packing. Another example might be to coordinate the several activities in making a dinner so that all of the dishes are done at the same time.

4. It appears that many of the executives in In Search of Excellence believed in Taylor's "one best way" of doing something and that the discovery of "that one way" in their own business led to their initial success. Some of the executives were so proud that they spent the next few years writing and giving workshops on how others could use the methods that made them successful. They ultimately failed because they stopped paying as much attention to their own businesses and how they made them successful in the first place. If they had recognized that success is a dynamic and ongoing process and continued reinventing new and successful ways to do business in a changing environment, they might have enjoyed longer success.

Check Your Understanding 21.2

1. Staff at different levels of the organization have different challenges and different responsibilities, and the required mix of the four management functions in any one employee often change to account for these differences. For example, while top executives certainly do provide a certain amount of leadership at the top levels of an organization, front-line supervisors and managers need to provide even more daily one-on-one and face-to-face leadership to their subordinates to accomplish goals.
2. An instructor in management, for example, must understand the purpose, principles, and concepts of management as described in this text. Interpersonal skills are used to encourage, challenge, coach, and motivate learners to do their best on assignments. Technically, the instructor must be able to design instructional materials, lecture, facilitate teamwork, and otherwise communicate instructional information.
3. For example, a manager of a museum store meets with staff to recognize best monthly sales performance (figurehead role), sends a memo on group tours planned for the next month (disseminator), coaches an employee who seems frequently late to work (disturbance handler), and so on.
4. See figure 21.4 (Sample Hospital Organizational Chart). The learner should create a chart similar to this.
5. For example, a student working part-time at a pizza store might define quality in terms of quickly attending to new customers, accurately getting the order from the customer, preparing the pizza quickly and in an attractive manner, serving the correct pizza slice to the correct person at each table, attending to other customer needs (for example, refills), and presenting the bill in a timely manner so the customers do not have to wait unnecessarily when they have finished. To get feedback on each key area of quality, a customer satisfaction card could be placed at each table.

Check Your Understanding 21.3

1. Cohesion refers to the interpersonal forces that influence a group to remain together and act with unity. There are several ways in which cohesion can be promoted, including: having a team name and identity, acquaintance and familiarity among members, shared goals, similarity of styles, team successes, smaller team size, and responding to a common "enemy" or competitor.

2. As much as cohesion is generally desirable, when it is excessive it can interfere with effective group functioning. Indicators of excessive cohesion include a lack of conflict, agreement in meetings but disagreeing privately, under-estimating the capability of competitors, believing that only the group holds the high ethical ground, making rapid decisions without considering alternatives or consequences, avoiding external opinions or evaluation, and not making contingency plans.

3. Groupthink can be reduced by encouraging members to voice disagreements and concerns, having leadership exert too much influence early in discussions, splitting the group into subgroups, having a devil's advocate argue for opposing points of view, inviting external observers to meetings, seeking external evaluation of group processes, and revisiting previous decisions to ensure soundness of arguments and decisions.

Chapter 22

Check Your Understanding 22.1

1. This list can be organized in several ways. For example, it could be interpreted as "good" and "bad" leaders as well as along effectiveness dimensions. Effectiveness refers to the extent to which their leadership served others and contributed to goal attainment. Effective leaders might include heads of state, business leaders, social leaders, and others (e.g., Franklin Roosevelt, Lee Iacoca of Chrysler, Congressional Representative Shirley Chisholm, etc.). Ineffective leaders—those whose performance did not serve their people or resulted in poor outcome—might include: Saddam Hussein, Kenneth Lay of Enron, Imelda Marcos of the Philippines, etc. Discuss how some leaders may attain temporary prominence (such as Hitler), but it does not serve others in the long run.

2. For example, assume you are very skilled and comfortable with providing structure and direction. This would be advantageous during the early stages of supervision or team formation, but as the supervisee or team gained experience and responsibility, such control would likely be perceived as restraining and inappropriate. As the supervisor, you might develop more flexibility in style, assess people's means of demonstrating responsibility, and empower them to perform more independently.

3. You might identify the range of behaviors that are associated with perceptions of effective or ineffective leadership, but emphasize that the person should not try to misrepresent or portray who he or she is not. Positive behaviors might include being a good listener, gatekeeping conversations, showing intelligence (but not too much), and taking a conventional ethical position. You might advise against speaking out too strongly, joking too much, or criticizing other leaders. The primary ethical issues is whether such behavioral practice can be viewed as manipulation.

4. The organization should examine what it most needs at the time and the direction it is developing, and select a leader who can best help them transition in that direction. The leader's ability to understand complex situations (for example, systems thinking), communication skills, experience in the field, stress management, and absence of dysfunctional behaviors (for example, alcohol abuse, anger problems, etc.) should be examined. Employees throughout the organization can be involved in reviewing applicants and background materials.

Check Your Understanding 22.2

1. For a specific decision you made, answer yes or no to each of the eight questions for the decision tree. When the questions have been answered, you will have identified the type of decision format recommended by the Normative Decision Tree (for example, autocratic, consultative, or group delegation). Compare the recommended decision with the procedure you used.

2. In general, leadership tends to be more directive, structured, and autocratic in the beginning and then more participative and delegative as people learn their roles, tasks become routine, skills become more developed, and they require less direct supervision. If knowledgeable and mature workers are overly supervised and controlled, they can become demoralized, resentful, and less productive.

3. Table may include the following:

Male Stereotypes	Female Stereotypes	Androgynous Characteristics
Competitive, aggressive, directive, logical	Collaborative, passive, permissive, emotional	Achieving, visionary, transformational, effective

Emphasize that any time stereotypes are used, the group stereotyped has important qualities overlooked. Also note that the gender dimension roughly corresponds to the task and social dimensions found in leadership and organizational studies, and that both are important to utilize.

Check Your Understanding 22.3

1. You might inform them of the disruptive nature of organizational change, and that the timing of it should be considered, given fluctuations in production or cash flows. You should also indicate that when new skills and perspectives are being learned, performance usually temporarily drops off—things get worse before they get better. Finally, during change people need a lot of reassurance and information, and clear communication is essential from top management.

2. You might start by reexamining what you want from your job and for your career, and whether job elimination might be an opportunity for change. Should you decide to stay, you would need to assess your skills related to the revised job, and decide how to present them as strengths. The stress of prospective unemployment can be high, and one should rely on a strong support group, be well rested, develop a plan and schedule for pursuing another job, talk with others to express your feelings, and identify your resources and resiliencies that will help you get through the transition.

3. People resist change for many reasons, among them: fear of losing what they value, they don't understand the reason for change, fear of failure, and lack of trust. Examples of measures to reduce these resistance include (respectively): showing people what they will continue doing that is important to them, providing clear rationale for the change, providing skills to help them succeed in the new organization, and building trust and respect before the change is introduced.

4. For example, you might notice that a few members of the group tend dominate the discussion, while others are very quiet. You might speculate and share with the group that you wonder if this reflects a split in the group, different levels of commitment, or lack of information by the low participators. A discussion of these possible meanings can help to decide what the group might want to do differently next meeting. For example, lack of information might be prevented by circulating the agenda and background information so all members can attend prepared to discuss the issue.

Chapter 23

Check Your Understanding 23.1

1. Temporary help should be secured for the weeks of 7/16 and 7/23 because the sole clerk is on a two-week vacation.

2. List the potential problem areas a work distribution analysis can reveal. Work distribution analysis can reveal the following:
   - If jobs being performed are developed enough so that qualifications and tasks complement each other
   - Findings related to the goals and objectives within the department, such as increases or decrease accounts receivable (AR) days
   - If employee qualifications are being used to the best of the employee's ability

3. Using the documentation that has been gathered by the employee in the position, that individual's supervisor or manager should write the job description.

4. An efficient work flow is best planned by creating a layout diagram or movement diagram to help visualize the functions and related tasks performed in a defined work area.

5. Light, color, sound, and temperature control considerations all contribute to the planning and creation of a good work environment.

Check Your Understanding 23.2

1. False: Input instead of conversion process.
2. True
3. True
4. False: Pilot tests should always be conducted because they can prevent unintended and unanticipated negative consequences.

Check Your Understanding 23.3

1. False: An organization has many customers and sometimes the expectations of one group of customers conflict with those of another group. Nevertheless, the goal of CQI is an admirable one and should be pursued because it can only serve to improve an organization's performance.
2. True
3. True
4. True
5. False: The main focus in reengineering is on reducing costs.

Chapter 24

Check Your Understanding 24.1
1. False
2. True
3. False
4. False

Check Your Understanding 24.2
1. False
2. False
3. True
4. False
5. True

Check Your Understanding 24.3
1. True
2. False
3. True
4. False
5. False

Check Your Understanding 24.4
1. True
2. True
3. False
4. True
5. False
6. True
7. True
8. False
9. False
10. True
11. False
12. True

Check Your Understanding 24.5
1. True
2. False
3. False
4. True
5. True
6. False
7. True
8. True
9. False
10. True
11. False
12. True
13. True
14. False
15. True

Chapter 25

Check Your Understanding 25.1
1. The purposes of the employee orientation program are to introduce the employee to the:
   - Organization's mission, policies, rules, and culture
   - Department or workgroup
   - Specific job he or she will be performing

   The orientation program also provides a period of socialization in which the employee learns the values, behavior patterns, and expectations of the organization.
2. The three levels of an orientation program and items reviewed, discussed, or accomplished at each level include the following:
   - Organizational level: Background and mission, policies and procedures, employee benefits, safety regulations, employee handbook, facility tour
   - Departmental level: Policies and procedures, introduction to other employees, tour of the department, work hours, time sheet, equipment operation, safety regulations
   - Individual level: Specific objectives for productivity and performance, instruction, and demonstration of specific job tasks
3. The orientation in large institutions may be conducted by the director of human resources or the director of education. In smaller organizations, the orientation is often conducted by the employee's supervisor. The departmental and individual portions of the orientation at both large and small organizations are typically performed by the employee's supervisor.
4. There are many things that can be done to make a new employee feel welcome in a new department. For example, the employee can be matched with a "buddy" on the first day who can escort him or her to lunch. On the first day, the new employee should also be introduced to coworkers, given a tour of the department, and shown his or her workstation.
5. Advantages of on-the-job training include its relatively low cost and the fact that work is still in progress while the employee is being trained. It also gives employee and supervisor opportunities to discuss specific problem areas and initiates socialization among employees and their coworkers. Disadvantages include distractions in the workplace and a feeling of pressure if employees do not accomplish work during the training period.
6. Skills that are often developed in on-the-job training include physical skills, academic knowledge, knowledge of institutional policies, and technical skills.
7. The most common technique used for on-the-job training is one-on-one training. For this to be successful, a trainer must be selected who is competent in the job content and capable of teaching and interacting

effectively with the trainee. Train-the-trainer workshops may be offered to develop skills in communication and instruction.

8. Job rotation is a useful training technique for employees who are supervisors and need to learn a variety of tasks performed by several subordinate employees.

9. The major steps in on-the-job training include:
   - Preparing the learner by putting him or her at ease and providing an overview of the job
   - Presenting the operation step by step
   - Having the learner demonstrate the steps
   - Following up with encouragement and correction, if necessary

10. In-service education is a continuous training process used to build on basic skills and to teach skills required to maintain job performance or retrain workers whose jobs have changed.

11. Events that suggest a need for in-service education include a restructuring of the department and/or organization, annual updates to coding or reimbursement requirements, implementation of new software or hardware, a decline in productivity or morale or an increase in absenteeism, a new organizational policy or procedure, or an external requirement imposed by accreditation or licensing organizations.

12. HIM in-service topics that might be of interest to other departments include ICD-9-CM or CPT annual updates, medical terminology, use of office productivity software for employee productivity measurement, and health record documentation.

13. Printed items that should be distributed at formal in-service programs include an agenda, a program schedule, materials or handouts to be used for instruction, and reference documents for posttraining reinforcement.

14. The effectiveness of an in-service program can be assessed by:
   - Completion of an evaluation form at the conclusion of the program
   - Formal or informal feedback from the employee's supervisor
   - Follow-up with the employee at a later time

15. The purpose of AHIMA's e-HIM initiative is to:
   - Promote the migration from paper to the electronic health record
   - Reinvent how institutional and personal health information and records are managed
   - Deliver measurable cost and quality results from improved information management.

16. Topics for training programs might include data analysis, data integration, privacy and security, encryption and deidentification methods, clinical vocabulary development and maintenance, and public health surveillance.

17. Diversity training programs might include topics such as review of other cultures from a social studies perspective, cultural norms such as communication styles, and perspectives or other cultures on privacy issues. Some employees may need training in English reading and writing skills, interpersonal communication skills, and customer service. Describe two skills that are desired as a result of customer service training.

   Skills to be developed in customer service training include communication and listening skills, as well as sensitivity training.

Check Your Understanding 25.2

1. The five models are:
   - Sensory: Does the learner prefer to listen, read, or practice in order to learn best?
   - Personality: One's personality traits affect how a person views the world
   - Information processing: People differ in how they receive and process information
   - Social interaction: Learning style differs by gender and social context
   - Instructional and environmental preference: The environment and its structure determine learning style.

2. Motivation plays a role in developing a training program because individual employee needs vary and even a single employee may have needs that differ at different points in his or her life or career. By calling attention to the relevance of training to specific needs and connecting the knowledge learned with a work goal, training can be facilitated for each employee.

3. Reinforcers other than monetary awards include a job schedule that allows more time with family or an opportunity for career advancement.

4. Performance standards should usually not be set higher than may reasonably be accomplished because they may reduce motivation and result in feelings of frustration, anxiety, and stress. Standards should be high enough to challenge employees, but not overwhelm them.

5. Adult learners typically like to control the speed of instruction and learn better when training is broken into manageable chunks. Training for adult learners should, therefore, be delivered in a modular fashion and over a longer period of time because adults learn better in smaller units and want to control the pace of their learning.

6. Trainers should accommodate diversity through acting in a culturally sensitive manner, such as encouraging females of non-Western cultures to participate more, and should adapt computer use to accommodate disabilities, such as using ADA compliant Web design or voice recognition.

Check Your Understanding 25.3

1. Factors that influence selection of a training method include:
   - Purpose of the training
   - Level of education and experience of the trainees
   - Amount of space, equipment, and media available for training
   - Number of trainees and their location
   - Cost of the method
   - Need for special accommodation due to disability or cultural differences

2. Computer-based training differs significantly from textbook learning. In computer-based training, the computer immediately responds to questions or reinforces answers. Textbooks, in this respect, are much less interactive than computer-based training programs. In addition, in computer-based learning, learners can repeat the interactive segments until they have fully mastered the material. The cost of developing computer-based training is higher than for a textbook, but the cost of delivery is less because the course can be used without an instructor and may be repeated as many times as necessary to gain mastery of the material.

3. Classroom training is appropriate when the goal is to train a large number of employees on largely factual knowledge within a short period of time, but it is not appropriate for developing problem-solving skills or improving interpersonal communication skills.

4. Distance learning removes training barriers associated with location and timing, both for individuals and groups. Learners can attend at a time and place of their choosing.

5. There are many ways that a healthcare organization can use an intranet to deliver training. Intranets are useful for distributing policies and procedures as well as for uploading educational courses for employee self-study. Material on CD-ROM can be installed and delivered to the employee's desktop, or customized for specific needs.

6. Topics appropriate for intensive study include cultural awareness, training on teamwork and empowerment, or management development.

Check Your Understanding 25.4

1. Organizations can reduce employee turnover by providing fair compensation, job flexibility, good communication, opportunities for mentoring and career growth, and good screening during the hiring process to seek employees with a high level of integrity.

2. An HIM department would benefit from a flextime arrangement when a workload has peaks and valleys, when equipment must be shared across employees and hours, and when employees need time to handle personal matters away from work.

3. An advantage for the employee of a compressed workweek is a reduction in commuting time and additional days off for personal time. An advantage to the department is increased productivity because of fewer start-and-stop periods.

4. One potential problem with flextime is that employees who work in positions that require interaction with others may be ineligible, which can produce feelings of favoritism or discrimination. This can be avoided with written policies that clearly state the positions that are open to flextime and those that are not. Another problem may be the increased fatigue of employees working long days in compressed workweeks. This can be avoided with an appropriate employee and supervisor orientation to explain appropriate work techniques and with extra break time.

5. In job sharing, two or more people share one full-time job and everyone sharing the job may perform parts of the same project. In traditional part-time employment, employees work less than full-time hours and perform their jobs independently of others.

6. A telecommuting agreement should include work schedule, communication frequency and methods, performance measures, confidentiality requirements, equipment maintenance responsibilities, and environmental safety requirements.

7. Functions that are commonly outsourced in an HIM department include transcription, release of information, and coding.

8. Factors that ensure the success of an outsourcing arrangement include:
   - Having assistance from someone skilled in negotiation when developing the contract
   - Engaging legal counsel to review the language of the contract
   - Requiring competitive bidding
   - Establishing expectations and performance standards for contractors
   - Monitoring compliance with performance standards
   - Performing periodic customer surveys to assess satisfaction with the service

9. Transcriptions jobs are suitable for offshoring as they do not require face-to-face customer service, they have high information content, low social networking requirements, and require very little interaction with managers or others in the organization.

10. Managers can empower employees by:
    - Getting others involved in selecting their work assignments and methods for accomplishing tasks
    - Creating an environment of cooperation, information sharing, discussion, and shared ownership of goals
    - Encouraging others to take initiative and make decisions
    - When problems arise, finding out what others think and letting them help design solutions
    - Giving others the freedom to put their ideas and solutions into practice
    - Recognizing successes and encouraging high performance

11. Managers may not empower employees because:
    - They feel that meetings take up too much time and take employees away from their "real work"
    - They may be afraid to share power with others

12. Delegation can provide employees the opportunity to try new tasks. Trying new tasks leads, in turn, to empowerment because employees can contribute ideas and fully use their skills.

13. Successful delegation includes assigning responsibility, granting authority, and creating accountability.

14. Employees may resist accepting delegated responsibilities if they feel unqualified to do the tasks or are being assigned too much work or unpopular work that has little value.

15. Effective coaches are dedicated leaders who display a high level of competence and can push or pull employees to their highest level of performance. They are role models, they provide praise or constructive feedback, and they are ready to help with routine work alongside the employee, if necessary. They defend and support their employees.

16. Mentors are senior employees who work with employees early in their careers. Mentoring is a form of coaching in that it helps employees become self-sufficient but is usually done on a one-on-one basis. Mentors share their knowledge of management styles and teach interpersonal skills, primarily for future job advancement. A coach, on the other hand, may work with several employees at the same time and is concerned more with helping them do the best job they can in their current job by removing obstacles and offering suggestions.

17. Promotion should be awarded on performance and competence, not on seniority, if it is to serve as a motivator. Promotion criteria should be published so that all employees have the opportunity to apply for consideration.

18. Incentive programs fail when there is an emphasis on quantity without a focus on quality, if the reward is not valued and not linked to the amount of effort displayed, or there is ineffective management of the reward program.

19. HIM professionals need continuing education to remain current in their knowledge of the field, which is changing rapidly, and so that they can provide high-quality skills to their organizations.

Check Your Understanding 25.5

1. The steps in a typical training and development plan include:
   - Performing a needs analysis
   - Setting training objectives
   - Designing the curriculum
   - Determining the location and method of delivery
   - Piloting the program
   - Implementing the program
   - Evaluating the effectiveness of the program
   - Making changes as needed
   - Providing feedback to interested groups

2. Outcomes of the needs analysis include:
   - An understanding of where training is needed in the organization
   - A list of the tasks to be learned at each level (entry, remedial, and management development)
   - An analysis of the deficiencies in employee knowledge and skills (accomplished by a comparison of desired and current levels of competence)

3. Objectives specify what employees should be able to accomplish upon completion of the training program. These should be set before starting the program so that results can be evaluated after completion.

4. Among the items to consider when designing a training program are the curriculum, the budget, who will teach the program, materials to be developed, location, and method of delivery.

5. Four outcomes to be measured in program evaluation include reaction of the trainees, what the trainees have learned, behavioral change, and results.

6. The Occupational Safety and Health Act of 1970 was passed to assure safe working conditions. Hospitals must train employees in safety measures, in the worker's native language.

   The Allied Health Reinvestment Act of 2005 encourages individuals to complete allied health education. It provides grants to healthcare organizations and scholarships to applicants.

   The Americans with Disabilities Act of 1990 requires employers to provide reasonable accommodations for physical or mental limitations regarding training, such as providing accessibility to computer-based training.

Chapter 26

Check Your Understanding 26.1

1. The HIM department is responsible for the coding of the records. While this is important in the billing process, the actual claims are filed by the patient accounts department. Therefore, the insurance company should be referred to the patient accounts department for resolution. If there is an individual who is specifically responsible for handling billing audits, that individual is an appropriate referral.

2. Revenue is recorded when known and earned. While the working DRG gives the "known" amount in an acute care situation, the revenue is technically not earned until discharge. Therefore, revenue is not recorded until after discharge. In longer term care situations, this is not the case. Interim payments are requested periodically and the associated revenue booked.

3. This is not a good strategy as it violates the Matching Principle. While the hospital should certainly make every effort to capture all of the associated expenses for THIS fiscal, next years expenses must be booked next year. If some of next year's expenses are actually paid this year, they would not be booked as expenses but rather as assets under the heading "prepaid expenses."

4. The federal government is the largest single payer of healthcare expenses in the United States. Although the CMS does not set accounting rules, it enforces the federal regulations regarding the reimbursement for Medicare and the federal portion of the Medicaid program and sets standards for the documentation and reporting of transactions related to such reimbursement.

5. Purely on the basis of the information in this chapter, yes the hospital can sell these services. The hospital would book nonoperating revenue. However, a not-for-profit hospital may have problems if the revenue is substantial, since the income is unrelated to its main business.

Check Your Understanding 26.2

1. *Examples of assets:* Cash, marketable securities, accounts receivable, inventory, building, equipment, land.
   Examples of liabilities: Accounts payable, notes payable, mortgage.

2. The excess of revenue over expenses increases the value of the organization. Conversely, the excess of expenses over revenue decreases the value of the organization. The net value of the organization (assets minus liabilities) is expressed in owner's equity (aka fund balance)

3. Anything that it sells as part of the services it provides. Typically, medications are inventory. Durable medical equipment may be considered inventory. In general, medical supplies may be considered inventory; however, for practical purposes they are more likely to be considered variable expenses in the provision of patient services.

4. In a double-entry bookkeeping system, all transactions have two sides, represented by an equal dollar amount of debits and credits. In a journal entry, the debits are listed on the left and the credits on the right. Assets and Expenses are increased by debits. Liabilities, Revenue, and Owners equity are increased by credits. In this manner, all transactions preserve the balance of the accounting equation: assets − liabilities = owners equity.

5. Nonfinancial managers are routinely asked to justify their activities in terms of their contribution to the financial well-being of the organization. Therefore, an understanding of accounting helps managers communicate with financial decision makers.

6. An organization's ability to pay current liabilities with current assets is very important to lenders. Current assets implicitly will be (or could be) converted to cash at some point within a year, either through collections, sales, or other business activity. The current ratio compares total current assets with total current liabilities.

Check Your Understanding 26.3

1. *Comparison:* Both branches of accounting deal with the recording, reporting, and analysis of transactions.
   Contrast: Financial accounting focuses on the financial statements and the needs of the users of those statements. Managerial accounting focuses on internal measurements of financial performance, such as budgets.

2. *Comparison:* Both types of budgets allocate the resources of the organization; both can originate at the department or administrative level; both can be analyzed and controlled at the departmental or administrative level.
   Contrast: Operational budgets are prepared annually. Capital budgets are prepared on an as-needed basis. Operational budgets last for one fiscal year. Capital budgets last for the life of the project. Operational budgets are measured and controlled by analyzing monthly and YTD variables from budget to actual amounts. Capital budgets are also measured in terms of return on investment.

3. In this particular situation, an activity-based budget may be more effective than a budget developed along organizational lines. With an activity-based budget, the financial effectiveness of the programs and services can be evaluated more easily. A zero-based budget may also be effective in ensuring that only effective programs and services are carried forward from one year to the next. Either a fixed or variable budget could be developed; however, it would be most effective on an activity basis rather than by department.

4. An organization whose activities do not follow a typical calendar year might find a noncalendar fiscal year more effective. For example, a not-for-profit organization that holds elections and an annual meeting in early summer might have trouble implementing a calendar year budget, since the fiscal accountability would be split between two administrations. Therefore, a fiscal year that ends as one administration leaves office would be more practical.

5. This is a favorable variance, since the payroll amount is actually less than budgeted. However, for a complete analysis, other line items, such as temporary employees and consulting expenses, must be analyzed. For example, a $2000 favorable payroll variance due to the resignation of a coder may be offset by a $3000 consulting fee for temporary coding services.

Chapter 27

Check Your Understanding 27.1

1. A project is undertaken because the organization has determined the need for some type of change. This need may be the result of a company's strategic agenda, such as the implementation of a new computer system, or may be due to the passage of a new government regulation.

   Some departments in an organization are primarily project oriented. For example, the information technology department is constantly in the process of implementing new or upgraded systems. Other departments, such as the registration department, can be thought of as primarily operation departments. These types of departments may undertake a project to improve a process.

2. Each project has an identified sponsor. The sponsor is the company employee with the most vested interest in the successful completion of the project. The project also has stakeholders. A stakeholder is anyone in the organization who is affected by the project product.

Both the sponsor and the stakeholders need to support the project to its successful conclusion. They need to ensure that issues are responded to, change factors are addressed, and that the appropriate resources are dedicated to the project. The main difference between the sponsor and the stakeholders is that the sponsor is the ultimate authority figure and has final say in any issue disputes. A stakeholder may be able to make budget decisions related to their area, but the sponsor usually approves the overall budget and any budget overruns that occur. The project manager generally has responsibility for the successful completion of the project objectives but usually does not have authority over the project team. The project manager must work with the sponsor and the stakeholders since they are typically the functional managers for the project team.

The stakeholders and sponsor often make up the oversight committee, sometimes named the steering committee.

3. A project differs from the day-to-day operations of an organization. Operations are concerned with the everyday jobs needed to run the business. The personnel involved in the operational aspects of the business perform the same functions on a routine basis. This work does not end. By contrast, a project has a precise, expected result produced by defined resources within a specific timeframe.

4. One of the reasons that many projects fail to meet the project objectives within the expected timeframe and budget is that the scope begins to grow as the project progresses. For example, new functions or features are added to a software implementation. This change is commonly known as "scope creep." The requester presents each change as a small revision with a low impact to the timeline or cost. Soon there are several minor changes that add up to a more significant modification to the original work or cost estimates. The project manager must be diligent to prevent scope creep. Examples:
   - Class assignment: What happens if your instructor asks for a 10-page document that is due in two weeks, but then two days prior to the due date, changes it to 25 pages? You'd want a new due date right? The scope changed, the resources stayed the same, so the timeline needs to be modified.
   - Building a house: If the foundation has been poured and you decide to have a den and additional bedroom added, this changes the scope. On the other hand, if you decide instead to upgrade to marble counters, you haven't created an impact on the schedule, but you have created an impact on the cost.

Check Your Understanding 27.2
Requires instructor guidance.

Check Your Understanding 27.3
The cost estimates will include personnel, equipment, and supplies. If an external company will be providing some project services, the answer should indicate if the engagement is based on time and materials or fixed fee pricing.

The skill set of the project team members will have an impact on the cost. It is a good idea to document the assumptions on which the cost estimates were based. If the project team members will receive raises during the project timeline, this should be reflected as well. Any costs associated with contingency plans should also be detailed.

Check Your Understanding 27.4
Requires instructor guidance.

Check Your Understanding 27.5
Requires instructor guidance.

Chapter 28

All of the Check Your Understanding exercises in this chapter require instructor guidance.

Glossary

Abbreviated Injury Scale (AIS): A set of numbers used in a trauma registry to indicate the nature and severity of injuries by body system

ABC Codes: A terminology created by Alternative Link that describes alternative medicine, nursing, and other integrative healthcare interventions

Ability (achievement) tests: Tests used to assess the skills an individual already possesses

Abstract: Brief summary of the major parts of a research study

Abstracting: 1. The process of extracting information from a document to create a brief summary of a patient's illness, treatment, and outcome   2. The process of extracting elements of data from a source document or database and entering them into an automated system

Accept assignment: A term used to refer to a provider's or a supplier's acceptance of the allowed charges (from a fee schedule) as payment in full for services or materials provided

Acceptance theory of authority: A management theory based on the principle that employees have the freedom to choose whether they will follow managerial directions

Access control: 1. A computer software program designed to prevent unauthorized use of an information resource   2. The process of designing, implementing, and monitoring a system for guaranteeing that only individuals who have a legitimate need are allowed to view or amend specific data sets

Accession number: A number assigned to each case as it is entered in a cancer registry

Accession registry: A list of cases in a cancer registry in the order in which they were entered

Accountability: Responsibility for a specific activity

Accounting: 1. The process of collecting, recording, and reporting an organization's financial data   2. A list of all disclosures made of a patient's health information

Accounting rate of return: The projected annual cash inflows, minus any applicable depreciation, divided by the initial investment

Accounts payable (A/P): Records of the payments owed by an organization to other entities

Accounts receivable (A/R): Records of the payments owed to the organization by outside entities such as third-party payers and patients

Accreditation: 1. A voluntary process of institutional or organizational review in which a quasi-independent body created for this purpose periodically evaluates the quality of the entity's work against preestablished written criteria   2. A determination by an accrediting body that an eligible organization, network, program, group, or individual complies with applicable standards

Accredited Standards Committee (ASC) X12N: A committee of the National Standards Institute that develops and maintains standards for the electronic exchange of business transactions, such as 837—Health Care Claim, 835—Health Care Claim Payment/Advice, and others

Accrue: The process of recording known transactions in the appropriate time period before cash payments/receipts are expected or due

Acid-test ratio: A ratio in which the sum of cash plus short-term investments plus net current receivables is divided by total current liabilities

Active listening: The application of effective verbal communications skills as evidenced by the listener's restatement of what the speaker said

Activities of daily living (ADL): The basic activities of self-care, including grooming, bathing, ambulating, toileting, and eating

Activity-based budget: A budget based on activities or projects rather than on functions or departments

Acute care: Medical care of a limited duration that is provided in an inpatient hospital setting to diagnose and/or treat an injury or a short-term illness

Acute care prospective payment system (PPS): The reimbursement system for inpatient hospital services provided to Medicare and Medicaid beneficiaries that is based on the use of diagnosis-related groups as a classification tool

Administrative information: Information used for administrative and healthcare operations purposes such as billing and quality oversight

Administrative information systems: A category of healthcare information systems that supports human resources management, financial management, executive decision support, and other business-related functions

Administrative law: A body of rules and regulations developed by various administrative entities empowered by Congress; falls under the umbrella of public law

Administrative management: A subdivision of classical management theory that emphasizes the total organization rather than the individual worker and delineates the major management functions

Administrative services only (ASO) contract: An agreement between an employer and an insurance organization to administer the employer's self-insured health plan

Adult learning: Self-directed inquiry aided by the resources of an instructor, colleagues/fellow students, and educational materials

Advance Beneficiary Notice (ABN): A statement signed by the patient when he or she is notified by the provider, prior to a service or procedure being done, that Medicare may not reimburse the provider for the service, wherein the patient indicates that he will be responsible for any charges

Advance directive: A legal, written document that describes the patient's preferences regarding future healthcare or stipulates the person authorized to make medical decisions in the event the patient is incapable of communicating his or her preferences

Affinity grouping: A technique for organizing similar ideas together in natural groupings

Age Discrimination in Employment Act (1967): Federal legislation that prohibits employment discrimination against persons between the ages of forty and seventy and restricts mandatory retirement requirements except where age is a bona fide occupational qualification

Agency for Healthcare Research and Quality (AHRQ): The branch of the U.S. Public Health Service that supports general health research and distributes research findings and treatment guidelines with the goal of improving the quality, appropriateness, and effectiveness of healthcare services

Agenda for Change: An initiative undertaken by the Joint Commission on Accreditation of Healthcare Organizations that focused on changing the emphasis of the accreditation process from structure to outcomes

Aggregate data: Data extracted from individual health records and combined to form de-identified information about groups of patients that can be compared and analyzed

All-patient diagnosis-related groups (AP-DRGs): A casemix system developed by 3M and used in a number of state reimbursement systems to classify non-Medicare discharges for reimbursement purposes

All-patient refined diagnosis-related groups (APR-DRGs): An expansion of the inpatient classification system that includes four distinct subclasses (minor, moderate, major, and extreme) based on the severity of the patient's illness

Alliance Standards Directory: Web site that includes 850 voluntary and mandatory standards and links to more than 200 standards development organizations (nahit.org/hitsdir/)

Alternative hypothesis: A hypothesis that states that there is an association between independent and dependent variables

Ambulatory care: Preventative or corrective healthcare services provided on a nonresident basis in a provider's office, clinic setting, or hospital outpatient setting

Ambulatory payment classification (APC) system: The prospective payment system used since 2000 for reimbursement of hospitals for outpatient services provided to Medicare and Medicaid beneficiaries

Ambulatory surgery center or ambulatory surgical center (ASC): Under Medicare, an outpatient surgical facility that has its own national identifier; is a separate entity with respect to its licensure, accreditation, governance, professional supervision, administrative functions, clinical services, record keeping, and financial and accounting systems; has as its sole purpose the provision of services in connection with surgical procedures that do not require inpatient hospitalization; and meets the conditions and requirements set forth in the Medicare Conditions of Participation

American Association for Medical Transcription (AAMT): The national professional association for medical transcriptionists

American Association of Medical Colleges (AAMC): The organization established in 1876 to standardize the curriculum for medical schools in the United States and to promote the licensure of physicians

American College of Healthcare Executives (ACHE): The national professional organization of healthcare administrators that provides certification services for its members and promotes excellence in the field

American College of Surgeons (ACS): The scientific and educational association of surgeons formed to improve the quality of surgical care by setting high standards for surgical education and practice

American Health Information Management Association (AHIMA): The professional membership organization for managers of health record services and healthcare information systems as well as coding services; provides accreditation, certification, and educational services

American Hospital Association (AHA): The national trade organization that provides education, conducts research, and represents the hospital industry's interests in national legislative matters; membership includes individual healthcare organizations as well as individual healthcare professionals working in specialized areas of hospitals, such as risk management

American Medical Association (AMA): The national professional membership organization for physicians that distributes scientific information to its members and the public, informs members of legislation related to health and medicine, and represents the medical profession's interests in national legislative matters

American Medical Informatics Association (AMIA): The membership organization composed of individuals, institutions, and corporations that develop and use information technologies in healthcare

American National Standards Institute (ANSI): The organization that accredits all U.S. standards development organizations to ensure that they are following due process in promulgating standards

American Nurses Association (ANA): The national professional membership association of nurses that works for the improvement of health standards and the availability of healthcare services, fosters high professional standards for the nursing profession, and advances the economic and general welfare of nurses

American Society for Testing and Materials (ASTM): A national organization whose purpose is to establish standards on materials, products, systems, and services

American Society for Testing and Materials Standard E1384 (ASTM E1384)—Standard Guide for Description of Content and Structure of an Automated Primary Record of Care: A standard that identifies the basic information to be included in electronic health records and requires the information to be organized into categories

Americans with Disabilities Act (ADA) (1990): Federal legislation that makes it illegal to discriminate against individuals with disabilities in employment, public accommodations, public services, transportation, and telecommunications

Analog: Data or information that is not represented in an encoded, computer-readable format

Analysis phase: The first phase of the systems development life cycle during which the scope of the project is defined, project goals are identified, current systems are evaluated, and user needs are identified

Analysis session: The process of mining a data segment

Ancillary systems: Electronic systems that generate clinical information (such as laboratory information systems, radiology information systems, pharmacy information systems, and so on)

Application programming interface (API): A set of definitions of the ways in which one piece of computer software communicates with another or a programmer makes requests of the operating system or another application; operates outside the realm of the direct user interface

Application service provider (ASP): A third-party service company that delivers, manages, and remotely hosts standardized applications software via a network through an outsourcing contract based on fixed, monthly usage or transaction-based pricing

Applied artificial intelligence: An area of computer science that deals with algorithms and computer systems that exhibit the characteristics commonly associated with human intelligence

Applied healthcare informatics: Automated information systems applied to healthcare delivery business and workflow processes, including the diagnosis, therapy, and systems of managing health data and information within the healthcare setting

Applied research: A type of research that focuses on the use of scientific theories to improve actual practice, as in medical research applied to the treatment of patients

Aptitude tests: Tests that assess an individual's general ability to learn a new skill

Architecture: The configuration, structure, and relationships of hardware (the machinery of the computer including input/output devices, storage devices, and so on) in an information system

Artificial intelligence (AI): High-level information technologies used in developing machines that imitate human qualities such as learning and reasoning

Artificial neural network (ANN): A computational technique based on artificial intelligence and machine learning in which the structure and operation are inspired by the properties and operation of the human brain

Assets: The human, financial, and physical resources of an organization

Association rule analysis (rule induction): The process of extracting useful if/then rules from data based on statistical significance; *See* **rule induction**

Assumptions: Undetermined aspects of a project that are considered to be true (for example, assuming that project team members have the right skill set to perform their duties)

Asynchronous: Occurring at different times

Attending Physician Statement (APS) (or COMB-1): The standardized insurance claim form created in 1958 by the Health Insurance Association of America and the American Medical Association

Attributable risk (AR): A measure of the impact of a disease on a population (for example, measuring additional risk of illness as a result of exposure to a risk factor)

Attributes: 1. Data elements within an entity that become the column or field names when the entity relationship diagram is implemented as a relational database   2. Properties or characteristics of concepts

Audioconferencing: A learning technique in which students in different locations can learn together via telephone lines while listening to a presenter and looking at handouts or books

Audit: A review process conducted by healthcare facilities (internally and/or externally) to identify variations from established baselines; *See* **external review**

Audit trail: A chronological set of computerized records that provides evidence of information system activity (log-ins and log-outs, file accesses) used to determine security violations

Authentication: 1. The process of identifying the source of health record entries by attaching a handwritten signature, the author's initials, or an electronic signature   2. Proof of authorship that ensures, as much as possible, that log-ins and messages from a user originate from an authorized source

Authority: The right to make decisions and take actions necessary to carry out assigned tasks

Authorization: The granting of permission to disclose confidential information; as defined in terms of the HIPAA privacy rule, an individual's formal, written permission to use or disclose his or her personally identifiable health information for purposes other than treatment, payment, or healthcare operations

Authorization management: The process of protecting the security and privacy of the confidential data in a database

Autoauthentication: A procedure that allows dictated reports to be considered automatically signed unless the health information management department is notified of needed revisions within a certain time limit

Autocoding: The process of extracting and translating dictated and then transcribed free-text data (or dictated and then computer-generated discrete data) into ICD-9-CM and CPT evaluation and management codes for billing and coding purposes

Autodialing system: A method used to automatically call and remind patients of upcoming appointments

Automated forms-processing (e-forms) technology: Technology that allows users to electronically enter data into online, digital forms and electronically extract data from online, digital forms for data collection or manipulation

Autonomy: A core ethical principle centered on the individual's right to self-determination that includes respect for the individual; in clinical applications, the patient's right to determine what does or does not happen to him or her in terms of healthcare

Average daily census: The mean number of hospital inpatients present in the hospital each day for a given period of time

Average length of stay (ALOS): The mean length of stay for hospital inpatients discharged during a given period of time

Balance billing: A reimbursement method that allows providers to bill patients for charges in excess of the amount paid by the patients' health plan or other third-party payer (not allowed under Medicare or Medicaid)

Balance sheet: A report that shows the total dollar amounts in accounts, expressed in accounting equation format, at a specific point in time

Balanced Budget Refinement Act (BBRA) of 1999: The amended version of the Balanced Budget Act of 1997 that authorizes implementation of a per-discharge prospective payment system for care provided to Medicare beneficiaries by inpatient rehabilitation facilities

Balanced scorecard (BSC): A strategic planning tool that identifies performance measures related to strategic goals

Baldridge Award: A congressional award that recognizes excellence in several areas of business

Bar chart: A graphic technique used to display frequency distributions of nominal or ordinal data that fall into categories

Bar-coding technology: A method of encoding data that consists of parallel arrangements of dark elements, referred to as bars, and light elements, referred to as spaces, and interpreting the data for automatic identification and data collection purposes

Baseline: The original estimates for a project's schedule, work, and cost

Basic research: A type of research that focuses on the development and refinement of theories

Bed count (complement): The number of inpatient beds set up and staffed for use on a given day

Bed count day: A unit of measure that denotes the presence of one inpatient bed (either occupied or vacant) set up and staffed for use in one twenty-four-hour period

Bed turnover rate: The average number of times a bed changes occupants during a given period of time

Behavioral description interview: An interview format that requires applicants to give specific examples of how they have performed a specific procedure or handled a specific problem in the past

Behavioral healthcare: A broad array of psychiatric services provided in acute, long-term, and ambulatory care settings; includes treatment of mental disorders, chemical dependency, mental retardation, and developmental disabilities, as well as cognitive rehabilitation services

Benchmarking: An analysis process based on comparison

Beneficence: A legal term that means promoting good for others or providing services that benefit others, such as releasing health information that will help a patient receive care or will ensure payment for services received

Benefit: Healthcare service for which the healthcare insurance company will pay

Bill hold period: The span of time during which a bill is suspended in the billing system awaiting late charges, diagnosis and/or procedure codes, insurance verification, or other required information

Bills of Mortality: Documents used in London during the seventeenth century to identify the most common causes of death

Bioethics: A field of study that applies ethical principles to decisions that affect the lives of humans, such as whether to approve or deny access to health information

Bit-mapped data: Data made up of pixels displayed on a horizontal and vertical grid or matrix

Bivariate: An adjective meaning the involvement of two variables

Blanket authorization: An authorization for the release of confidential information from a certain point in time and any time thereafter

Blended learning: A training strategy that uses a combination of techniques—such as lecture, Web-based training, or programmed text—to appeal to a variety of learning styles and maximize the advantages of each training method

Blood and blood component usage review: Evaluation of how blood and blood components are used using JCAHO guidelines

Blue Cross and Blue Shield (BC/BS): The first prepaid healthcare plans in the United States; Blue Shield plans traditionally cover hospital care and Blue Cross plans cover physicians' services

Blue Cross and Blue Shield Association: The national association of state and local Blue Cross and Blue Shield plans

Blue Cross and Blue Shield Federal Employee Program (FEP): A federal program that offers a fee-for-service plan with preferred provider organizations and a point-of-service product

Board of governors (board of trustees, board of directors): The elected or appointed group of officials who bear ultimate responsibility for the successful operation of a healthcare organization

Bounded rationality: The recognition that decision making is often based on limited time and information about a problem and that many situations are complex and rapidly changing

Boxplot: Tool in the form of a graph that displays five-number data summary

Brainstorming: A group problem-solving technique that involves the spontaneous contribution of ideas from all members of the group

Branding communications: Messages sent to increase awareness of, and to enhance the image of, a product in the marketplace

Break-even analysis: A financial analysis technique for determining the level of sales at which total revenues equal total costs beyond which revenues become profits

Breast Imaging Reporting and Data System Atlas (BI-RADS®): A comprehensive guide providing standardized breast imaging terminology and a report organization, assessment structure, and classification system for mammography, ultrasound, and MRI of the breast

Bridge technology: Technology such as document imaging and/or clinical messaging that provides some, but not all, the benefits of an EHR

Bubble chart: A type of scatter plot with circular symbols used to compare three variables; the area of the circle indicates the value of a third variable

Budget cycle: The complete process of financial planning, operations, and control for a fiscal year; overlaps multiple fiscal years

Buildings: A long-term (fixed) asset account that represents the physical structures owned by the organization

Bundled payments: A period of relatively continuous medical care performed by healthcare professionals in relation to a particular clinical problem or situation

Bureaucracy: A formal organizational structure based on a rigid hierarchy of decision making and inflexible rules and procedures

Business intelligence (BI): The end product or goal of knowledge management

Business process reengineering (BPR): The analysis and design of the work flow within and between organizations

Bylaws (rules and regulations): Operating documents that describe the rules and regulations under which a healthcare organization operates

Capital budget: The allocation of resources for long-term investments and projects

Capitation: A method of healthcare reimbursement in which an insurance carrier prepays a physician, hospital, or other healthcare provider a fixed amount for a given population without regard to the actual number or nature of healthcare services provided to the population

Care Map®: A proprietary care-planning tool similar to a clinical protocol that outlines the major aspects of treatment on the basis of diagnosis or other characteristics of the patient

Care path: A care-planning tool similar to a clinical practice guideline that has a multidisciplinary focus emphasizing the coordination of clinical services

Career development: The process of growing or progressing within one's profession or occupation

Case definition: A method of determining criteria for cases that should be included in a registry

Case fatality rate: The total number of deaths due to a specific illness during a given time period divided by the total number of cases during the same period

Case finding: A method of identifying patients who have been seen and/or treated in a healthcare facility for the particular disease or condition of interest to the registry

Case law: *See* **common law**

Case management: 1. The ongoing, concurrent review performed by clinical professionals to ensure the necessity and effectiveness of the clinical services being provided to a patient   2. A process that integrates and coordinates patient care over time and across multiple sites and providers, especially in complex and high-cost cases   3. The process of developing a specific care plan for a patient that serves as a communication tool to improve quality of care and reduce cost

Case manager: 1. A professional nurse who coordinates the daily progress of a patient population by assessing needs, developing goals, individualizing plans of care on an ongoing basis, and evaluating overall progress   2. A medical professional (usually a nurse or a social worker) who reviews cases to determine the necessity of care and to advise providers on payer's utilization restrictions

Case mix: A description of a patient population based on any number of specific characteristics, including age, gender, type of insurance, diagnosis, risk factors, treatment received, and resources used

Case study: A type of nonparticipant observation in which researchers investigate one person, one group, or one institution in depth

Case-control (retrospective) study: A study that investigates the development of disease by amassing volumes of data about factors in the lives of persons with the disease (cases) and persons without the disease

Case-mix group (CMG) relative weights: Factors that account for the variance in cost per discharge and resource utilization among case-mix groups

Case-mix index (CMI): The average relative weight of all cases treated at a given facility or by a given physician, which reflects the resource intensity or clinical severity of a specific group in relation to the other groups in the classification system; calculated by dividing the sum of the weights of diagnosis-related groups for patients discharged during a given period divided by the total number of patients discharged

Cash: The actual money that has been received and is readily available to pay debts; a short-term (current) asset account that represents currency and bank account balances

Categorical data: *See* **scales of measurement**

Categorically needy eligibility: Categories of individuals to whom states must provide coverage under the federal Medicaid program

Causal relationship: A type of relationship in which one factor results in a change in another factor (cause and effect)

Causal-comparative research: A research design that resembles experimental research but lacks random assignment to a group and manipulation of treatment

Cause-specific death rate: The total number of deaths due to a specific illness during a given time period divided by the estimated population for the same time period

Census: The number of inpatients present in a healthcare facility at any given time

Census survey: A survey that collects data from all the members of a population

Center for Drug Evaluation and Research (CDER) Data Standards Manual: A compilation of standardized nomenclature monographs for sharing information regarding manufactured drug dosage forms

Centers for Medicare and Medicaid Services (CMS): The division of the Department of Health and Human Services that is responsible for developing healthcare policy in the United States and for administering the Medicare program and the federal portion of the Medicaid program; called the Health Care Financing Administration (HCFA) prior to 2001

Certainty factor: The defined certainty percentage rate with which an occurrence must present itself to satisfy quality standards

Certification: 1. The process by which a duly authorized body evaluates and recognizes an individual, institution, or educational program as meeting predetermined requirements   2. An evaluation performed to establish the extent to which a particular computer system, network design, or application implementation meets a prespecified set of requirements

Certified coding associate (CCA): An AHIMA credential awarded to entry-level coders who have demonstrated skill in classifying medical data by passing a certification exam

Certified coding specialist (CCS): An AHIMA credential awarded to individuals who have demonstrated skill in classifying medical data from patient records, generally in the hospital setting, by passing a certification examination

Certified coding specialist—physician based (CCS-P): An AHIMA credential awarded to individuals who have demonstrated coding expertise in physician-based settings, such as group practices, by passing a certification examination

Certified in healthcare privacy (CHP): AHIMA credential denoting advanced competency in designing, implementing, and administering comprehensive privacy protection programs in all types of healthcare organizations; requires baccalaureate or master's degree, or healthcare information management credential plus experience

Certified in healthcare privacy and security (CHPS): Credential that recognizes advanced competency in designing, implementing, and administering comprehensive privacy and security protection programs in all types of healthcare organizations; requires successful completion of both the CHP and the CHS exams (jointly sponsored by AHIMA and HIMSS)

Certified in healthcare security (CHS): Credential (managed by HIMSS) that certifies advanced abilities in designing, implementing, and administering comprehensive security programs

Certified medical transcriptionist (CMT): A certification that is granted upon successful completion of an examination

Certified professional in health information management systems (CPHIMS): Credential (managed jointly by HIMSS, AHA Certification Center, and applied measurement professionals) that certifies knowledge of healthcare information and management systems and understanding of psychometrics (the science of measurement; requires baccalaureate or graduate degree plus associated experience

Chain of command: A hierarchical reporting structure within an organization

Change control: The process of performing an impact analysis and obtaining approval before modifications to the project scope are made

Change drivers: Forces in the external environment of organizations or industries that force organizations or industries to change the way they operate in order to survive

Charge description master (CDM): *See* **chargemaster**

Chargemaster: A financial management form that contains information about the organization's charges for the healthcare services it provides to patients; *See* **charge description master (CDM)**

Chart tracking: A system that identifies the current location of a record or information

Check sheet: A tool that permits the systematic recording of observations of a particular phenomenon so that trends or patterns can be identified

Chief executive officer (CEO): The senior manager appointed by a governing board to direct an organization's overall long-term strategic management

Chief financial officer (CFO): The senior manager responsible for the fiscal management of an organization

Chief information officer (CIO): The senior manager responsible for the overall management of information resources in an organization

Chief information security officer (CISO): IT leadership role responsible for ensuring that a healthcare organization's information systems are secure and safe from tampering or misuse; role has grown as a direct result of HIPAA security regulations

Chief information technology officer (CITO): IT leadership role that guides an organization's decisions related to technical architecture and evaluates latest technology developments and their applicability or potential use in the organization

Chief knowledge officer (CKO): A position that oversees the entire knowledge acquisition, storage, and dissemination process and that identifies subject matter experts to help capture and organize the organization's knowledge assets

Chief medical informatics officer (CMIO): An emerging position, typically a physician with medical informatics training, that provides physician leadership and direction in the deployment of clinical applications in healthcare organizations

Chief nursing officer (CNO): The senior manager (usually a registered nurse with advanced education and extensive experience) responsible for administering patient care services

Chief operating officer (COO): The role responsible for managing day-to-day activities of an organization

Circuit: The geographic area covered by a U.S. Court of Appeals

Civil law: The branch of law involving court actions among private parties, corporations, government bodies, or other organizations, typically for the recovery of private rights with compensation usually being monetary

Civil Rights Act (1991): The federal legislation that focuses on establishing an employer's responsibility for justifying hiring practices that seem to adversely affect people because of race, color, religion, sex, or national origin

Civil Rights Act, Title VII (1964): The federal legislation that prohibits discrimination in employment on the basis of race, religion, color, sex, or national origin

Civilian Health and Medical Program of the Uniformed Services (CHAMPUS): A federal program providing supplementary civilian-sector hospital and medical services beyond that which is available in military treatment facilities to military dependents, retirees and their dependents, and certain others

Civilian Health and Medical Program-Veterans Administration (CHAMPVA): The federal healthcare benefits program for dependents of veterans rated by the VA as having a total and permanent disability, for survivors of veterans who died from VA-rated service-connected conditions or who were rated permanently and totally disabled at the time of death from a VA-rated service-connected condition, and for survivors of persons who died in the line of duty

Claim: An itemized statement of healthcare services and their costs provided by a hospital, physician office, or other healthcare provider; submitted for reimbursement to the healthcare insurance plan by either the insured party or the provider

Claims processing: The process of accumulating claims for services, submitting claims for reimbursement, and ensuring that claims are satisfied

Classification: A clinical vocabulary, terminology, or nomenclature that lists words or phrases with their meanings, provides for the proper use of clinical words as names or symbols, and facilitates mapping standardized terms to broader classifications for administrative, regulatory, oversight, and fiscal requirements

Classification system: 1. A system for grouping similar diseases and procedures and organizing related information for easy retrieval   2. A system for assigning numeric or alphanumeric code numbers to represent specific diseases and/or procedures

Client/server architecture: A computer architecture in which multiple computers (clients) are connected to other computers (servers) that store and distribute large amounts of shared data

Clinical (or critical) pathway: A tool designed to coordinate multidisciplinary care planning for specific diagnoses and treatments; *See* **critical path and Care Map**

Clinical Care Classification (CCC): Two interrelated taxonomies, the CCC of Nursing Diagnoses and Outcomes and the CCC of Nursing Interventions and Actions, that provide a standardized framework for documenting patient care in hospitals, home health agencies, ambulatory care clinics, and other healthcare settings

Clinical care plans: Care guidelines created by healthcare providers for individual patients for a specified period of time

Clinical communication space: The context and range of electronic and interpersonal information exchanged among staff and patients

Clinical data: Data captured during the process of diagnosis and treatment

Clinical data repository (CDR): A central database that focuses on clinical information

Clinical data warehouse (CDW): *See* **data warehouse**

Clinical decision support system (CDSS): A special subcategory of clinical information systems that is designed to help healthcare providers make knowledge-based clinical decisions

Clinical Document Architecture (CDA): HL7 electronic exchange model for clinical documents (such as discharge summaries and progress notes)

Clinical informatics: A field of information science concerned with the management of data and information used to support the practice and delivery of patient care through the application of computers and computer technologies

Clinical information system (CIS): A category of a healthcare information system that includes systems that directly support patient care

Clinical messaging: The function of electronically delivering data and automating the work flow around the management of clinical data

Clinical practice guidelines: A detailed, step-by-step guide used by healthcare practitioners to make knowledge-based decisions related to patient care and issued by an authoritative organization such as a medical society or government agency

Clinical privileges: The authorization granted by a healthcare organization's governing board to a member of the medical staff that enables the physician to provide patient services in the organization within specific practice limits

Clinical repository: A frequently updated database that provides users with direct access to detailed patient-level data as well as the ability to drill down into historical views of administrative, clinical, and financial data; *See* **data warehouse**

Clinical Special Product Label (SPL): A LOINC standard that provides information found in the approved FDA drug label or package insert in a computer readable format for use in electronic prescribing and decision support

Clinical systems analyst: *See* **systems analyst**

Clinical trial: A controlled research study involving human subjects that is designed to evaluate prospectively the safety and effectiveness of new drugs, tests, devices, or interventions

Clinical value compass: Performance improvement approach that measures the association of quality and value

Clinical workstation: A single point of access that includes a common user interface to view information from disparate applications and to launch applications

Clinical/medical decision support system: A special subcategory of clinical information systems that is designed to help healthcare providers make knowledge-based clinical decisions

Clinician/physician Web portals: The media for providing physician/clinician access to the provider organization's multiple sources of data from any network-connected device

Closed records: The records of patients who have been discharged from the hospital or whose treatment has been terminated

Closed systems: Systems that operate in a self-contained environment

Closed-record review: A review of records after a patient has been discharged from the organization or treatment has been terminated

Cluster sampling: The process of selecting subjects for a sample from each cluster within a population (for example, a family, school, or community)

CMS-1500: A Medicare claim form used to bill third-party payers for provider services (for example, physician office visits)

Coaching: 1. A training method in which an experienced person gives advice to a less-experienced worker on a formal or informal basis   2. A disciplinary method used as the first step for employees who are not meeting performance expectations

Coalition building: A technique used to manage the political dimensions of change within an organization by building the support of groups for change

Coded data: Data that are translated into a standard nomenclature of classification so that they may be aggregated, analyzed, and compared

Coding: The process of assigning numeric representations to clinical documentation

Cohort study: A study, followed over time, in which a group of subjects is identified as having one or more characteristics in common

Coinsurance: Cost sharing in which the policy or certificate holder pays a preestablished percentage of eligible expenses after the deductible has been met

Collaborative Stage Data Set: A new standardized neoplasm-staging system developed by the American Joint Commission on Cancer

College of Healthcare Information Management Executives (CHIME): A membership association serving chief information officers through professional development and advocacy

Commission on Accreditation of Health Informatics and Information Management Education (CAHIIM): The accrediting organization for educational programs in health informatics and information management

Commission on Accreditation of Rehabilitation Facilities (CARF): A private, not-for-profit organization that develops customer-focused standards for behavioral healthcare and medical rehabilitation programs and accredits such programs on the basis of its standards

Common cause variation: The source of variation in a process that is inherent within the process

Common law: Unwritten law originating from court decisions where no applicable statute exists; *See* **case law**

Communication plan: A documented approach to identifying the media and schedule for sharing information with affected parties

Comorbidity: A medical condition that coexists with the primary cause for hospitalization and affects the patient's treatment and length of stay

Compensable factor: Characteristic used to compare the worth of jobs (for example, skill, effort, responsibility, and working conditions)

Compensation and benefits: The payment package offered to employees in return for work

Competencies: Demonstrated skills that a worker should perform at a high level

Compliance: 1. The process of establishing an organizational culture that promotes the prevention, detection, and resolution of instances of conduct that do not conform to federal, state, or private payer healthcare program requirements or the healthcare organization's ethical and business policies   2. The act of adhering to official requirements

Compliance program guidance: The information provided by the Office of the Inspector General of the Department of Health and Human Services to help healthcare organizations develop internal controls that promote adherence to applicable federal and state guidelines

Complication: A medical condition that arises during an inpatient hospitalization (for example, a postoperative wound infection)

Compressed workweek: A work schedule that permits a full-time job to be completed in less than the standard five days of eight-hour shifts

Compromise: A mutual agreement

Computer Output Laser Disk/Enterprise Report Management (COLD/ERM) technology: Technology that electronically stores the documents and distributes them with fax, email, Web, and traditional hard-copy print processes

Computer virus: A software program that attacks computer systems and sometimes damages or destroys files

Computer-assisted coding: The process of extracting and translating dictated and then transcribed free-text data (or dictated and then computer-generated discrete data) into ICD-9-CM and CPT evaluation and management codes for billing and coding purposes

Computer-based training: A type of training that is delivered partially or completely using a computer

Computerized provider order entry (CPOE): Systems that allow physicians to enter medication or other orders and receive clinical advice about drug dosages, contraindications, or other clinical decision support

Concept: A unit of knowledge or thought created by a unique combination of characteristics

Conceptual data model: The highest level of data model, representing the highest level of abstraction, independent of hardware and software

Conceptual framework of accounting: The concept that the benefits of financial data should exceed the cost of obtaining them and that the data must be understandable, relevant, reliable, and comparable

Conceptual skills: One of the three managerial skill categories that includes intellectual tasks and abilities such as planning, deciding, and problem solving

Concurrent analysis: A review of the health record while the patient is still hospitalized or under treatment

Conditions of Participation: The administrative and operational guidelines and regulations under which facilities are allowed to take part in the Medicare and Medicaid programs; published by the Centers for Medicare and Medicaid Services, a federal agency under the Department of Health and Human Services

Confidentiality: A legal and ethical concept that establishes the healthcare provider's responsibility for protecting health records and other personal and private information from unauthorized use or disclosure

Conflict management: The process of working with individuals to find a mutually acceptable solution to a problem that has arisen between them

Confounding (extraneous, secondary) variable: An event or a factor that is outside a study but occurs concurrently with the study

Connecting For Health: A public-private collaborative designed to address the barriers to development of an interconnected health information infrastructure

Connectivity: The ability of one computer system to exchange meaningful data with another computer system

Consent: A means for residents to convey to healthcare providers their implied or expressed permission to administer care or treatment or to perform surgery or other medical procedures

Conservatism: The concept that resources must not be overstated and liabilities not understated

Consistency: The idea that all time periods must reflect the same accounting

Consolidated Health Informatics (CHI): The notion of adopting existing health information interoperability standards throughout all federal agencies

Consolidated Health Informatics (CHI) initiative: The effort to achieve CHI through federal agencies spearheaded by the Office of National Coordinator for Health Information Technology

Construct validity: The ability of an instrument to measure hypothetical, nonobservable traits

Constructive confrontation: A method of approaching conflict in which both parties meet with an objective third party to explore perceptions and feelings

Consultation: The response by one healthcare professional to another healthcare professional's request to provide recommendations and/or opinions regarding the care of a particular patient/resident

Consultation rate: The total number of hospital inpatients receiving consultations for a given period divided by the total number of discharges and deaths for the same period

Consumer informatics: The field of information science concerned with the management of data and information used to support consumers by consumers (the general public) through the application of computers and computer technologies

Content: The substantive or meaningful components of a document or collection of documents

Content analysis: A method of research that provides a systematic and objective analysis of communication effectiveness, such as the analysis performed on tests

Content validity: The extent to which an instrument's items represent the content that the instrument is intended to measure

Context: The text that illustrates a concept or the use of a designation

Contingency: A plan of action to be taken when circumstances affect project performance

Continuing education: A type of training that enables employees to remain current in the knowledge base of their profession

Continuity of care record (CCR): Documentation of care delivery from one healthcare experience to another

Continuous data: Data that represent measurable quantities but are not restricted to certain specified values

Continuous quality improvement (CQI): 1. A management philosophy that emphasizes the importance of knowing and meeting customer expectations, reducing variation within processes, and relying on data to build knowledge for process improvement   2. A continuous cycle of planning, measuring, and monitoring performance and making knowledge-based improvements

Continuous record review: *See* **open-record review**

Continuous speech input: The quality of speech/voice recognition technology that does not require users to pause between words to allow the computer to distinguish between the beginnings and endings of words

Continuous variables: Discrete variables measured with sufficient precision

Continuum of care: The range of healthcare services provided to patients, from routine ambulatory care to intensive acute care

Contra-account: Any account set up to adjust the historical value of a balance sheet account (for example, cumulative depreciation is a contra-account to an equipment [fixed-asset] account)

Contract law: A branch of law based on common law that deals with written or oral agreements that are enforceable through the legal system

Contract service: An entity that provides certain agreed-upon services for the facility, such as transcription, coding, or copying

Control: One of the four management functions in which performance is monitored in accordance with organizational policies and procedures

Control group: A comparison study group whose members do not undergo the treatment under study

Controlled Substances Act: The legislation that controls the use of narcotics, depressants, stimulants, and hallucinogens

Controlling: The monitoring and maintenance of a project's structure

Convenience sample: A type of nonrandom sampling in which researchers use any unit at hand

Coordination of benefits (COB) transaction: The electronic transmission of claims and/or payment information from a healthcare provider to a health plan for the purpose of determining relative payment responsibilities

Core communications: A series of triggered, event-specific communications based on need and data such as age, sex, and health profile that gives providers an appropriate time and personalized reason to communicate with recipients

Core data elements/core content: A small set of data elements with standardized definitions often considered to be the core of data collection efforts

Core measure/core measure set: Standardized performance measures developed to improve the safety and quality of healthcare (for example, core measures are used in the Joint Commission on Accreditation's ORYX initiative)

Corporation: An organization that may have one or many owners in which profits may be held or distributed as dividends (income paid to the owners)

Corrective controls: Internal controls designed to fix problems that have been discovered, frequently as a result of detective controls

Correlational research: A design of research that determines the existence and degree of relationships among factors

Cost accounting: The specialty branch of accounting that deals with quantifying the resources expended to provide the goods and/or services offered by the organization to its customer/client/patients

Cost justification: A rationale developed to support competing requests for limited resources

Cost outlier: Exceptionally high costs associated with inpatient care when compared with other cases in the same diagnosis-related group

Cost outlier adjustment: Additional reimbursement for certain high-cost home care cases based on the loss-sharing ratio of costs in excess of a threshold amount for each home health resource group

Cost report: A report that analyzes the direct and indirect costs of providing care to Medicare patients

Court of Appeals: A branch of the federal court system that has the power to hear appeals on the final judgments of district courts

CPT (Current Procedural Terminology): A comprehensive, descriptive list of terms and numeric codes used for reporting diagnostic and therapeutic procedures and other medical services performed by physicians; published and updated annually by the American Medical Association

Credentialing: The process of reviewing and validating the qualifications (degrees, licenses, and other credentials), of physicians and other licensed independent practitioners, for granting medical staff membership to provide patient care services

Credits: The amounts on the right side of a journal entry

Criminal law: A branch of law that addresses crimes that are wrongful acts against public health, safety, and welfare, usually punishable by imprisonment and/or fine

Critical path/critical path method: The sequence of tasks that determine the project finish date; *See* **clinical pathway and Care Map**

Cross-sectional study: A biomedical research study in which both the exposure and the disease outcome are determined at the same time in each subject; *See* **prevalence study**

Cross-training: The training to learn a job other than the employee's primary responsibility

Crude birth rate: The number of live births divided by the population at risk

Crude death rate: The total number of deaths in a given population for a given period of time divided by the estimated population for the same period of time

Cultural competence: Skilled in awareness, understanding, and acceptance of beliefs and values of the people of groups other than one's own

Current Dental Terminology (CDT): A medical code set of dental procedures, maintained and copyrighted by the American Dental Association (ADA), referred to as the

Uniform Code on Dental Procedures and Nomenclatures until 1990

Current ratio: The total current assets divided by total current liabilities

Customer relationship management (CRM): A management system whereby organizational structure and culture and customer information and technology are aligned with business strategy so that all customer interactions can be conducted to the long-term satisfaction of the customer and to the benefit and profit of the organization

Customer service training: Training that focuses on creating a true customer orientation within the work environment

Cybernetic systems: Systems that have standards, controls, and feedback mechanisms built in to them

Cyclical staffing: A transitional staffing solution wherein workers are brought in for specific projects or to cover in busy times

Daily inpatient census: The number of inpatients present at census-taking time each day, plus any inpatients who were both admitted and discharged after the census-taking time the previous day

Data: The dates, numbers, images, symbols, letters, and words that represent basic facts and observations about people, processes, measurements, and conditions

Data administrator: An emerging role responsible for managing the less technical aspects of data, including data quality and security

Data capture: The process of recording healthcare-related data in a health record system or clinical database

Data confidentiality: The extent to which personal health information is kept private

Data cube: A collection of one or more tables of data, assembled in a fashion that allows for dynamic analysis to be conducted on the joins, intersections, and overall integration of these predefined tables

Data definition language (DDL): A special type of software used to create the tables within a relational database, the most common of which is structured query language

Data dictionary: A descriptive list of the data elements to be collected in an information system or database whose purpose is to ensure consistency of terminology

Data display: A method for presenting or viewing data

Data element: An individual fact or measurement that is the smallest unique subset of a database

Data Elements for Emergency Department Systems (DEEDS): A data set designed to support the uniform collection of information in hospital-based emergency departments

Data exchange standards: Protocols that help ensure that data transmitted from one system to another remain comparable

Data integrity: 1. The extent to which healthcare data are complete, accurate, consistent, and timely 2. A security principle that keeps information from being modified or otherwise corrupted either maliciously or accidentally

Data manipulation language (DML): A special type of software used to retrieve, update, and edit data in a relational database, of which the most common is structured query language

Data mart: A well-organized, user-centered, searchable database system that usually draws information from a data warehouse to meet the specific needs of users

Data miners: Those individuals who extract data from a database with the intention of quantifying and filtering them

Data mining: The process of extracting information from a database and then quantifying and filtering discrete, structured data

Data model: A picture or abstraction of real conditions used to design the definitions of fields and records and their relationships in a database

Data modeling: The process of determining the users' information needs and identifying relationships among the data

Data quality management: A managerial process that ensures the integrity (accuracy and completeness) of an organization's data during data collection, application, warehousing, and analysis

Data quality model: A managerial process that ensures the integrity (accuracy and completeness) of an organization's data during data collection, application, warehousing, and analysis; also called data management model

Data repository: An open-structure database that is not dedicated to the software of any particular vendor or data supplier, in which data from diverse sources are stored so that an integrated, multidisciplinary view of the data can be achieved; also called a central data repository or, when related specifically to healthcare data, a clinical data repository

Data resource manager: A role that ensures that the organization's information systems meet the needs of people who provide and manage patient services

Data security: The process of keeping data safe from unauthorized alteration or destruction

Data set: A list of recommended data elements with uniform definitions that are relevant for a particular use

Data types: A technical category of data (text, numbers, currency, date, memo, and link data) that a field in a database can contain

Data warehouse: A database that makes it possible to access data from multiple databases and combine the results into a single query and reporting interface; *See* **clinical repository**

Database: An organized collection of data, text, references, or pictures in a standardized format, typically stored in a computer system for multiple applications

Database administrator: The individual responsible for the technical aspects of designing and managing databases

Database life cycle (DBLC): A system consisting of several phases that represent the useful life of a database, including initial study, design, implementation, testing and evaluation, operation, and maintenance and evaluation

Database management system (DBMS): Computer software that enables the user to create, modify, delete, and view the data in a database

Data-based DSS: Decision support system that focuses on providing access to the various data sources within the organization through one system

Debit: The amount on the left side of an account entry that represents an increase in an expense or liability account or a decrease in a revenue or asset account

Debt ratio: The total liabilities divided by the total assets

Debt service: The current obligations of an organization to repay loans

Decentralization: The shift of decision-making authority and responsibility to lower levels of the organization

Decision support system (DSS): A computer-based system that gathers data from a variety of sources and assists in providing structure to the data by using various analytical models and visual tools in order to facilitate and improve the ultimate outcome in decision-making tasks associated with nonroutine and nonrepetitive problems

Decision tree: A structured data-mining technique based on a set of rules useful for predicting and classifying information and making decisions

Deductive reasoning: The process of developing conclusions based on generalizations

Deemed status: An official designation indicating that a healthcare facility is in compliance with the Medicare Conditions of Participation; to qualify for deemed status, facilities must be accredited by the Joint Commission on Accreditation of Healthcare Organizations or the American Osteopathic Association

Default judgment: A court ruling against a defendant in a lawsuit who fails to answer a summons for a court appearance

Defendant: In civil cases, an individual or entity against whom a civil complaint has been filed; in criminal cases, an individual who has been accused of a crime

Delegation: The process by which managers distribute work to others along with the authority to make decisions and take action

Delegation of authority: The act of assigning responsibility

Delinquent health record: An incomplete record not finished or made complete within the time frame determined by the medical staff of the facility

Demographic data: *See* **demographic information**

Demographic information: Information used to identify an individual, such as name, address, gender, age, and other information linked to a specific person

Dental informatics: A field of information science concerned with the management of data and information used to support the practice and delivery of dental healthcare through the application of computers and computer technologies

Department of Health and Human Services (HHS): The cabinet-level federal agency that oversees all the health- and human-services–related activities of the federal government and administers federal regulations

Dependency: The relationship between two tasks in a project plan

Dependent variable: A measurable variable in a research study that depends on an independent variable

Depreciation: The allocation of the dollar cost of a capital asset over its expected life

Derived attribute: An attribute whose value is based on the value of other attributes (for example, current date minus date of birth yields the derived attribute age)

Descriptive research: A type of research that determines and reports the current status of topics and subjects

Descriptive statistics: A set of statistical techniques used to describe data such as means, frequency distributions, and standard deviations; statistical information that describes the characteristics of a specific group or a population

Design phase: The second phase of the systems development life cycle during which all options in selecting a new information system are considered

Designated record set: A group of records maintained by or for a covered entity that may include patient medical and billing records; the enrollment, payment, claims adjudication, and cases or medical management record systems maintained by or for a health plan; or information used, in whole or in part, to make patient care-related decisions

Detective control: An internal control designed to find errors that have already been made

Development: The process of growing or progressing in one's level of skill, knowledge, or ability

Diagnosis-related group (DRG): A unit of case-mix classification adopted by the federal government and some other payers as a prospective payment mechanism for hospital inpatients in which diseases are placed into groups because related diseases and treatments tend to consume similar amounts of healthcare resources and incur similar amounts of cost; in the Medicare and Medicaid programs, one of more than 500 diagnostic classifications in which cases demonstrate similar resource consumption and length-of-stay patterns

Diagnostic image data: Bit-mapped images used for medical or diagnostic purposes (for example, chest x-rays or computed tomography scans)

Digital: 1. A data transmission type based on data that have been binary encoded   2. A term that refers to the data or information represented in an encoded, computer-readable format

Digital dictation: A process in which vocal sounds are converted to bits and stored on computer for random access

Digital Imaging and Communication in Medicine (DICOM): A standard that promotes a digital image communications format and picture archive and communications systems for use with digital images

Digital signature management technology: The practice of validating the identity of an individual sending data through the use of an electronic signature

Direct costs: Resources expended that can be identified as pertaining to specific goods and/or services (for example, medications pertain to specific patients)

Direct method of cost allocation: A budgeting concept in which the cost of overhead departments is distributed solely to the revenue-producing areas

Discharge analysis: An analysis of the health record at or following discharge

Discharge planning: The process of coordinating the activities related to the release of a patient when inpatient hospital care is no longer needed

Discharge summary: A summary of the resident's stay at the long-term care facility that is used along with the post-discharge plan of care to provide continuity of care for the resident upon discharge from the facility

Discharged, no final bill (DNFB) report: A report that includes all patients who have been discharged from the facility but for whom, for one reason or another, the billing process is not complete Disciplinary action

Discipline: A field of study characterized by a knowledge base and perspective that is different from other fields of study

Disclosure: The act of making information known; in the health information management context, the release of confidential health information about an identifiable person to another person or entity

Discounting: The application of lower rates of payment to multiple surgical procedures performed during the same operative session under the outpatient prospective payment system; the application of adjusted rates of payment by preferred provider organizations

Discrete data: Data that represent separate and distinct values or observations; that is, data that contain only finite numbers and have only specified values

Discrete variables: A dichotomous or nominal variable whose values are placed into categories

Discrimination: The act of treating one entity differently from another

Disease index: A list of diseases and conditions of patients sequenced according to the code numbers of the classification system in use

Disease registry: A centralized collection of data used to improve the quality of care and measure the effectiveness of a particular aspect of healthcare delivery

Disposition: For outpatients, the healthcare practitioner's description of the patient's status at discharge (no follow-up planned; follow-up planned or scheduled; referred elsewhere; expired); for inpatients, a core health data element that identifies the circumstances under which the patient left the hospital (discharged alive; discharged to home or self-care; discharged and transferred to another short-term general hospital for inpatient care; discharged and transferred to a skilled nursing facility; discharged and transferred to an intermediate care facility; discharged and transferred to another type of institution for inpatient care or referred for outpatient services to another institution; discharged and transferred to home under care of organized home health services organization; discharged and transferred to home under care of a home intravenous therapy provider; left against medical advice or discontinued care; expired; status not stated)

Distance learning: A learning delivery mode in which the instructor, the classroom, and the students are not all present in the same location and at the same time

Diversity training: A type of training that facilitates an environment that fosters tolerance and appreciation of individual differences within the organization's workforce and strives to create a more harmonious working environment

Do not resuscitate (DNR) order: An order written by the treating physician stating that in the event the patient suffers cardiac or pulmonary arrest, cardiopulmonary resuscitation should not be attempted

Document: Any analog or digital, formatted, and preserved "container" of data or information

Document image data: Bit-mapped images based on data created and/or stored on analog paper or photographic film

Document imaging: The practice of electronically scanning written or printed paper documents into an optical or electronic system for later retrieval of the document or parts of the document if parts have been indexed

Document management technology: Technology that organizes/assembles, secures, and shares documents, and includes such functions as document version control, check in-check out control, document access control, and text/word searches

Double distribution: A budgeting concept in which overhead costs are allocated twice, taking into consideration that some overhead departments provide services to each other

Double-blind study: A type of clinical trial conducted with strict procedures for randomization in which neither researcher nor subject knows whether the subject is in the control group or the experimental group

Downsizing: A reengineering strategy to reduce the cost of labor and streamline the organization by laying off portions of the workforce

DRG grouper: A computer program that assigns inpatient cases to diagnosis-related groups and determines the Medicare reimbursement rate

Duration: The amount of time, usually measured in days, for a task to be completed

e-commerce: The use of the Internet and its derived technologies to integrate all aspects of business-to-business and business-to-consumer activities, processes, and communications

Edit: A condition that must be satisfied before a computer system can accept data

Effectiveness: The degree to which stated outcomes are attained

Efficiency: The degree to which a minimum of resources is used to obtain outcomes

Effort: The mental and physical exertion required to perform job-related tasks

e-health: The application of e-commerce to the healthcare industry, including electronic data interchange and links among healthcare entities

e-HIM: The application of technology to managing health information

EHR collaborative: A group of healthcare professional and trade associations formed to support Health Level Seven, a healthcare standards development organization, in the development of a functional model for electronic health record systems

Eighty-five/fifteen (85/15) rule: The total quality management assumption that 85 percent of the problems that occur are related to faults in the system rather than to worker performance

e-learning: The use of the Internet and its derived technologies to deliver training and education

Electronic data interchange (EDI): A standard transmission format using strings of data for business information communicated among the computer systems of independent organizations

Electronic document management system (EDM): A storage solution based on digital scanning technology in which source documents are scanned to create digital images of the documents that can be stored electronically on optical disks

Electronic health record (EHR): A computerized record of health information and associated processes

Electronic medical record (EMR): A form of computer-based health record in which information is stored in whole files instead of by individual data elements

Electronic medication administration record (EMAR): System designed to prevent medication errors by checking a patient's medication information against his or her bar-coded wristband

Electronic performance support system (EPSS): Sets of computerized tools and displays that automate training, documentation, and phone support; that integrate this automation into applications; and that provide support that is faster, cheaper, and more effective than traditional methods

Electronic records management technology: Systems that create and preserve electronic records

Electronic remittance advice (ERA): A classification of payment information from third-party payers that is communicated electronically

Electronic signature: 1. Any representation of a signature in digital form, including an image of a handwritten signature   2. The authentication of a computer entry in a health record made by the individual making the entry

Emergency Maternal and Infant Care Program (EMIC): The federal medical program that provides obstetrical and infant care to dependents of active-duty military personnel in the four lowest pay grades

Emergency preparedness: A state of readiness to react to an emergency situation

Emotional intelligence (EI): The sensitivity and ability to monitor and revise one's behavior based on the needs of and responses by others

Empiricism: The quality of being based on observed and validated evidence

Employee record: The document in which an employee's information relating to job performance and so on is kept

Employer-based self-insurance: An umbrella term used to describe health plans that are funded directly by employers to provide coverage for their employees exclusively in which employers establish accounts to cover their employees' medical expenses and retain control over the funds but bear the risk of paying claims greater than their estimates

Employment contract: A legal and binding agreement of terms related to an individual's work, such as hours, pay, or benefits

Employment-at-will: Concept that employees can be fired at any time and for almost any reason based on the idea that employees can quit at any time and for any reason

Empowerment: The condition of having the environment and resources to perform a job independently

Encoder: Specialty software used to facilitate the assignment of diagnostic and procedural codes according to the rules of the coding system

Encounter: The direct personal contact between a patient and a physician or other person who is authorized by state licensure law and, if applicable, by medical staff bylaws to order or furnish healthcare services for the diagnosis or treatment of the patient

Encryption: The process of transforming text into an unintelligible string of characters that can be transmitted via communications media with a high degree of security and then decrypted when it reaches a secure destination

Enterprise master patient index (EMPI): An index that provides access to multiple repositories of information from overlapping patient populations that are maintained in separate systems and databases

Entity: An individual person, group, or organization

Entity relationship diagram (ERD): A specific type of data modeling used in conceptual data modeling and the logical-level modeling of relational databases

Environmental Protection Agency (EPA) Substance Registry System (SRS): Interoperability standard for chemicals that provides a common basis for identification of chemicals, biological organisms, and other substances listed in EPA regulations and data systems

Environmental scanning: A systematic and continuous effort to search for important cues about how the world is changing outside and inside the organization

Epidemiological data: Data used to reveal disease trends within a specific population

Epidemiological studies: Studies that are concerned with finding the causes and effects of diseases and conditions

Episode-of-care (EOC) reimbursement: A category of payments made as lump sums to providers for all healthcare services delivered to a patient for a specific illness and/or over a specified time period; also called bundled payments because they include multiple services and may include multiple providers of care

Equal Employment Opportunity Act (1972): Federal legislation prohibiting discrimination in the workplace based on gender, race, religion, or national origin

Equal Pay Act of 1963 (EPA): The federal legislation that requires equal pay for men and women who perform substantially the same work

Equipment: A long-term (fixed) asset account representing depreciable items owned by the organization that have value over multiple fiscal years (for example, the historical cost of a CT scanner is recorded in an equipment account)

Ergonomics: A discipline of functional design associated with the employee in relationship to his or her work environment, including equipment, workstation, and office furniture adaptation to accommodate the employee's unique physical requirements so as to facilitate efficacy of work functions

Esprit de corps: Enthusiasm among the members of a group supporting the group's existence

Essential Medical Data Set (EMDS): A recommended data set designed to create a health history for an individual patient treated in an emergency service

Established Name for Active Ingredients and FDA Unique Ingredient Identifier (UNII) Codes: Interoperability standard for active ingredients in medications

Ethical agent: An individual who promotes and supports ethical behavior

Ethical decision making: The process of requiring everyone to consider the perspectives of others, even when they do not agree with them

Ethicist: An individual trained in the application of ethical theories and principles to problems that cannot be easily solved because of conflicting values, perspectives, and options for action

Ethics: A field of study that deals with moral principles, theories, and values; in healthcare, a formal decision-making process for dealing with the competing perspectives and obligations of the people who have an interest in a common problem

Ethics training: The act of teaching others about moral principles, theories, and values

Ethnography: A method of observational research that investigates culture in naturalistic settings using both qualitative and quantitative approaches

Evaluation research: A design of research that examines the effectiveness of policies, programs, or organizations

Evidence: Something that provides proof

Evidence-based management: A management system in which practices based on research evidence will be effective and produce the outcomes they claim

Evidence-based medicine: Healthcare services based on clinical methods that have been thoroughly tested through controlled, peer-reviewed biomedical studies

Exclusive provider organization (EPO): Hybrid managed care organization that provides benefits to subscribers only when healthcare services are performed by network providers; sponsored by self-insured (self-funded) employers or associations and exhibits characteristics of both health maintenance organizations and preferred provider organizations

Executive dashboard: An information management system providing decision makers with regularly updated information on an organization's key strategic measures

Executive information system (EIS): An information system designed to combine financial and clinical information for use in the management of business affairs of a healthcare organization

Executive manager: A senior manager who oversees a broad functional area or group of departments or services, sets the organization's future direction, and monitors the organization's operations

Exempt employees: Specific groups of employees who are identified as not being covered by some or all of the provisions of the Fair Labor Standards Act

Exit interview: The final meeting an employee has with his or her employer before leaving the organization

Expenses: Amounts that are charged as costs by an organization to the current year's activities of operation

Experimental (study) group: A group of participants in which the exposure status of each participant is determined and the individuals followed forward to determine the effects of the exposure

Experimental research: 1. A research design used to establish cause and effect   2. A controlled investigation in which subjects are assigned randomly to groups that experience carefully controlled interventions that are manipulated by the experimenter according to a strict protocol; *See* **experimental study**

Experimental study: *See* **experimental research**

Expert decision support system: A decision support system that uses a set of rules or encoded concepts to construct a reasoning process

Expert system (ES): A type of information system that supports the work of professionals engaged in the development or evaluation of complex activities that require high-level knowledge in a well-defined and usually limited area

Explanation of Benefits (EOB): A statement issued to the insured and the healthcare provider by an insurer to explain the services provided, amounts billed, and payments made by a health plan

Explicit knowledge: Documents, databases, and other types of recorded and documented information

Extended care facility: A healthcare facility licensed by applicable state or local law to offer room and board, skilled nursing by a full-time registered nurse, intermediate care, or a combination of levels on a twenty-four-hour basis over a long period of time

Extensible markup language (XML): A standardized computer language that allows the interchange of data as structured text

External review (audit): A performance or quality review conducted by a third-party payer or consultant hired for the purpose

External validity: An attribute of a study's design that allows its findings to be applied to other groups

Extranet: A system of connections of private Internet networks outside an organization's firewall that uses Internet technology to enable collaborative applications among enterprises

Facility-based registry: A registry that includes only cases from a particular type of healthcare facility, such as a hospital or clinic

Facility-specific system: A computer information system developed exclusively to meet the needs of one healthcare organization

Factor comparison method: A complex quantitative method of job evaluation that combines elements of both the ranking and point methods

Fair Labor Standards Act of 1938 (FLSA): The federal legislation that sets the minimum wage and overtime payment regulations

Family and Medical Leave Act of 1993 (FMLA): The federal legislation that allows employees time off from work (up to twelve weeks) to care for themselves or their family members with the assurance of an equivalent position upon return to work

Family numbering: A filing system, sometimes used in clinic settings, in which an entire family is assigned one number

Favorable variance: The positive difference between the budgeted amount and the actual amount of a line item, that is, when actual revenue exceeds budget or actual expenses are less than budget

Federal Employees' Compensation Act (FECA): The legislation enacted in 1916 to mandate workers' compensation for civilian federal employees, whose coverage includes lost wages, medical expenses, and survivors' benefits

Federal Register: The daily publication of the U.S. Government Printing Office that reports all changes in regulations and federally mandated standards, including HCPCS and ICD-9-CM codes

Fee schedule: A list of healthcare services and procedures (usually CPT/HCPCS codes) and the charges associated with them developed by a third-party payer to represent the approved payment levels for a given insurance plan; also called table of allowances

Fee-for-service basis: See **fee-for-service (FFS) reimbursement**

Felony: A serious crime such as murder, larceny, rape, or assault for which punishment is usually severe

Fetal autopsy rate: The number of autopsies performed on intermediate and late fetal deaths for a given time period divided by the total number of intermediate and late fetal deaths for the same time period

Fetal death (stillborn): The death of a product of human conception before its complete expulsion or extraction from the mother regardless of the duration of the pregnancy

Fetal death rate: A proportion that compares the number of intermediate and/or late fetal deaths to the total number of live births and intermediate or late fetal deaths during the same period of time

Financial Accounting Standards Board (FASB): An independent organization that sets accounting standards for businesses in the private sector

Financial data: The data collected for the purpose of managing the assets of a business (for example, a healthcare organization, a product line); in healthcare, data derived from

the charge generation documentation associated with the activities of care and then aggregated by specific customer grouping for financial analysis

Financial transaction: The exchange of goods or services for payment or the promise of payment

Fiscal intermediary (FI): An organization that contracts with the Centers for Medicare and Medicaid Services to serve as the financial agent between providers and the federal government in the local administration of Medicare Part B claims

Fiscal year: One business cycle or tax year, which may or may not coincide with the calendar year

Fishbone diagram: A performance improvement tool used to identify or classify the root causes of a problem or condition and to display the root causes graphically

Fixed budget: A type of budget based on expected capacity

Fixed costs: Resources expended that do not vary with the activity of the organization (for example, mortgage expenses do not vary with patient volume)

Flex years: A work arrangement in which employees can choose, at specific intervals, the number of hours they want to work each month over the next year

Flexible budget: A type of budget that is based on multiple levels of projected productivity (actual productivity triggers the levels to be used as the year progresses)

Flexible work schedule: See **flextime**

Flextime: A work schedule that gives employees some choice in the pattern of their work hours, usually around a core of midday hours

Float employee: An employee who is not assigned to a particular shift or function and who may fill in as needed in cases of standard employee absence or vacation

Flow process chart: See **flowchart**

Flowchart: A graphic tool that uses standard symbols to visually display detailed information, including time and distance, of the sequential flow of work of an individual or a product as it progresses through a process

Focused studies: Studies in which a researcher orally questions and conducts discussions with members of a group

Food and Drug Administration (FDA): The federal agency responsible for controlling the sale and use of pharmaceuticals, biological products, medical devices, food, cosmetics, and products that emit radiation, including the licensing of medications for human use

Force-field analysis: A performance improvement tool used to identify specific drivers of, and barriers to, an organizational change so that positive factors can be reinforced and negative factors reduced

Forecasting: To calculate or predict some future event or condition through study and analysis of available pertinent data

Foreign key: A key attribute used to link one entity/table to another

For-profit organizations: The tax status assigned to business entities that are owned by one or more individuals or organizations and that earn revenues in excess of expenditures that are subsequently paid out to the owners or stockholders

Fourteen principles of management: Henri Fayol's key points in the formulation of the administrative approach to management

Fraud and abuse: The intentional and mistaken misrepresentation of reimbursement claims submitted to government-sponsored health programs

Freedom of Information Act (FOIA): The federal law, applicable only to federal agencies, through which individuals can seek access to information without the authorization of the person to whom the information applies

Free-text data: Data that are narrative in nature

Frequency distribution: A table or graph that displays the number of times (frequency) a particular observation occurs

Frequency polygon: A type of line graph that represents a frequency distribution

Full-time equivalent (FTE): A statistic representing the number of full-time employees as calculated by the reported number of hours worked by all employees, including part-time and temporary, during a specific time period

Fund balance: In a not-for-profit setting, the entity's net assets or resources remaining after subtracting liabilities that are owed; in a for-profit organization, the owner's equity

Fuzzy logic: An analytic technique used in data mining to handle imprecise concepts

Galen Common Reference Model (CRM): A computer-based clinical terminology developed in Europe for representing medical concepts

Gantt chart: A graphic tool used to plot tasks in project management that shows the duration of project tasks and overlapping tasks

General ledger: A master list of individual revenue and expense accounts maintained by an organization

Generalizability: The ability to apply research results, data, or observations to groups not originally under study

Generally accepted accounting principles (GAAP): Refers to the way organizations record and report financial transactions so that financial information is consistent between organizations

Generally accepted auditing standards (GAAS): Refers to the way organizations record and report financial transactions so that financial information is consistent between organizations

Genetic algorithms: Optimization techniques that can be used to improve other data-mining algorithms so that they derive the best model for a given set of data

Geographic information system (GIS): A decision support system that is capable of assembling, storing, manipulating, and displaying geographically referenced data and information

Geographic practice cost index (GPCI): An index developed by the Centers for Medicare and Medicaid Services to measure the differences in resource costs among fee schedule areas compared to the national average in the three com-

ponents of the relative value unit: physician work, practice expenses, and malpractice coverage

Geographical information system (GIS): A decision support system that is capable of assembling, storing, manipulating, and displaying geographically referenced data and information

Gesture recognition technology: A method of encoding handwritten, print, or cursive characters and of interpreting the characters as words or the intent of the writer

Global Medical Device Nomenclature (GMDN): A collection of internationally recognized terms used to accurately describe and catalog medical devices, in particular, the products used in the diagnosis, prevention, monitoring, treatment or alleviation of disease or injury in humans

Global payment: A form of reimbursement used for radiological and other procedures that combines the professional and technical components of the procedures and disperses payments as lump sums to be distributed between the physician and the healthcare facility

Global surgery payment: A form of reimbursement used for radiological and other procedures that combines the professional and technical components of the procedures and disperses payments as lump sums to be distributed between the physician and the healthcare facility

Goal: A specific description of the services or deliverable goods to be provided as the result of a business process

Going concern: An organization that can be assumed to continue indefinitely unless otherwise stated

Government Accounting Standards Board (GASB): The federal agency that sets the accounting standards to be followed by government entities

Graphical user interface (GUI): A style of computer interface in which typed commands are replaced by images that represent tasks (for example, small pictures [icons] that represent the tasks, functions, and programs performed by a software program)

Graphics-based decision support system: A decision support system in which the knowledge base consists primarily of graphical data and the user interface exploits the use of graphical display

Grievance: A formal, written description of a complaint or disagreement

Grievance procedures: The steps employees may follow to seek resolution of disagreements with management on job-related issues

Gross autopsy rate: The number of inpatient autopsies conducted during a given time period divided by the total number of inpatient deaths for the same time period

Gross death rate: The number of inpatient deaths that occurred during a given time period divided by the total number of inpatient discharges, including deaths, for the same time period

Group health insurance: A prepaid medical plan that covers the healthcare expenses of an organization's full-time employees

Group model health maintenance organization: Type of health plan in which an HMO contracts with an independent multispecialty physician group to provide medical services to members of the plan

Group practice without walls (GPWW): A type of managed care contract that allows physicians to maintain their own offices and share administrative services

Grouper: A computer software program that automatically assigns prospective payment groups on the basis of clinical codes

Groupthink: An implicit form of group consensus in which openness and effective decision making are sacrificed to conformity

Habit: An activity repeated so often that it becomes automatic

Harassment: The act of bothering or annoying someone repeatedly

Hard-coding: The process of attaching a CPT/HCPCS code to a procedure located on the facility's chargemaster so that the code will automatically be included on the patient's bill

Hawthorne effect: A research study that found that novelty, attention, and interpersonal relations have a motivating effect on performance

Hay method of job evaluation: A modification of the point method of job evaluation that numerically measures the levels of three major compensable factors: know-how, problem-solving ability, and accountability

Health care provider dimension (HCPD): One of three dimensions of the National Health Information Infrastructure privacy concept that addresses the needs of providers for complete and accurate patient data

Health information exchange (HIE): The exchange of health information electronically between providers and others with the same level of interoperability, such as labs and pharmacies

Health information management (HIM): An allied health profession that is responsible for ensuring the availability, accuracy, and protection of the clinical information that is needed to deliver healthcare services and to make appropriate healthcare-related decisions

Health Information Management and Systems Society (HIMSS): A national membership association that provides leadership in healthcare for the management of technology, information, and change

Health Information Standards Board (HISB): A subgroup of the American National Standards Institute that acts as an umbrella organization for groups interested in developing healthcare computer messaging standards

Health Insurance Portability and Accountability Act (HIPAA) of 1996: The federal legislation enacted to provide continuity of health coverage, control fraud and abuse in healthcare, reduce healthcare costs, and guarantee the security and privacy of health information

Health Level Seven (HL7): A standards development organization accredited by the American National Standards Institute that addresses issues at the seventh, or application, level of healthcare systems interconnections

Health maintenance organization (HMO): Entity that combines the provision of healthcare insurance and the delivery of healthcare services, characterized by: (1) organized healthcare delivery system to a geographic area, (2) set of basic and supplemental health maintenance and treatment services, (3) voluntarily enrolled members, and (4) predetermined fixed, periodic prepayments for members' coverage

Health management information system (HMIS): An information system whose purpose is to provide reports on routine operations and processing (for example, a pharmacy inventory system, radiological system, or patient-tracking system)

Health or healthcare information technology (HIT): A term that encompasses the technical roles that process health data and records, such as classification, abstracting, retrieval, and so on

Health Plan Employer Data and Information Set (HEDIS): A set of performance measures developed by the National Commission for Quality Assurance that are designed to provide purchasers and consumers of healthcare with the information they need to compare the performance of managed care plans

Health record review: A concurrent or ongoing review of health record content performed by caregivers or HIM professionals while the patient is still receiving inpatient services to ensure the quality of the services being provided and the completeness of the documentation being maintained; also called health record analysis

Health Research Extension Act (1985): Federal legislation that established guidelines for the proper care of animals used in biomedical and behavioral research

Health savings accounts: Savings accounts designed to help people save for future medical and retiree health costs on a tax-fee basis, part of the 2003 Medicare bill

Health science librarian: A professional librarian who manages a medical library

Health services research: Research conducted on the subject of healthcare delivery that examines organizational structures and systems as well as the effectiveness and efficiency of healthcare services

Health systems agency: An agency that promotes and provides community-based health planning services

Healthcare Common Procedure Coding System (HCPCS): A classification system that identifies healthcare procedures, equipment, and supplies for claim submission purposes; the three levels are as follows: I, Current Procedural Terminology codes, developed by the AMA; II, codes for equipment, supplies, and services not covered by Current Procedural Terminology codes as well as modifiers that can be used with all levels of codes, developed by CMS; and III (eliminated December 31, 2003 to comply with HIPAA), local codes developed by regional Medicare Part B carriers and used to report physicians' services and supplies to Medicare for reimbursement

Healthcare Cost and Utilization Project (HCUP): A group of healthcare databases and related software tools developed through collaboration by the federal government, state governments, and industry to create a national information resource for patient-level healthcare data

Healthcare informatics: The field of information science concerned with the management of all aspects of health data and information through the application of computers and computer technologies

Healthcare information standards: Guidelines developed to standardize data throughout the healthcare industry (for example, developing uniform terminologies and vocabularies)

Healthcare information systems steering committee: An interdisciplinary team of healthcare professionals generally responsible for developing a strategic information system plan, prioritizing information system projects, and coordinating IS-related projects across the enterprise

Healthcare Integrity and Protection Data Bank (HIPDB): A national database that collects information on cases of healthcare fraud and abuse

Healthcare provider: A provider of diagnostic, medical, and surgical care as well as the services or supplies related to the health of an individual and any other person or organization that issues reimbursement claims or is paid for healthcare in the normal course of business

Heterogeneity: The state or fact of containing various components

Heuristic thought: Exploratory thinking that helps in solving certain types of problems but offers no guarantees

Hierarchy: An authoritarian organizational structure in which each member is assigned a specific rank that reflects his or her level of decision-making authority within the organization

Hierarchy of needs: Maslow's theory that suggested that human needs are organized hierarchically from basic physiological requirements to creative motivations; *See* **Maslow's hierarchy of needs**

Hill-Burton Act: The federal legislation enacted in 1946 as the Hospital Survey and Construction Act to authorize grants for states to construct new hospitals and, later, to modernize old ones

Hiring: Engaging the services of an individual in return for compensation

Histocompatibility: The immunologic similarity between an organ donor and a transplant recipient

Histogram: A graphic technique used to display the frequency distribution of continuous data (interval or ratio data) as either numbers or percentages in a series of bars

Historical cost: The resources expended by an organization to acquire an asset

Historical research: A research design used to investigate past events

History: The pertinent information about a patient, including chief complaint, past and present illnesses, family history, social history, and review of body systems

Home Assessment Validation and Entry (HAVEN): A type of data-entry software used to collect Outcome and Assessment Information Set (OASIS) data and then transmit them to state databases; imports and exports data in standard OASIS record format, maintains agency/patient/employee information, enforces data integrity through rigorous edit checks, and provides comprehensive online help

Home health agency (HHA): A program or organization that provides a blend of home-based medical and social services to homebound patients and their families for the purpose of promoting, maintaining, or restoring health or of minimizing the effects of illness, injury, or disability

Home health prospective payment system (HH PPS): The reimbursement system developed by the Centers for Medicare and Medicaid Services to cover home health services provided to Medicare beneficiaries

Home health resource group (HHRG): A classification system with eighty home health episode rates established to support the prospective reimbursement of covered home care and rehabilitation services provided to Medicare beneficiaries during sixty-day episodes of care

Home healthcare: The medical and/or personal care provided to individuals and families in their place of residence with the goal of promoting, maintaining, or restoring health or minimizing the effects of disabilities and illnesses, including terminal illnesses

Honesty (integrity) tests: Tests designed to evaluate an individual's honesty using a series of hypothetical questions

Hospice: An interdisciplinary program of palliative care and supportive services that addresses the physical, spiritual, social, and economic needs of terminally ill patients and their families

Hospice care: The medical care provided to persons with life expectancies of six months or less who elect to forgo standard treatment of their illness and to receive only palliative care

Hospital autopsy: A postmortem (after death) examination performed on the body of a person who has at some time been a hospital patient by a hospital pathologist or a physician of the medical staff who has been delegated the responsibility

Hospital autopsy rate: The total number of autopsies performed by a hospital pathologist for a given time period divided by the number of deaths of hospital patients (inpatients and outpatients) whose bodies were available for autopsy for the same time period

Hospital death rate: The number of inpatient deaths for a given period of time divided by the total number of live discharges and deaths for the same time period

Hospital discharge abstract system: A group of databases compiled from aggregate data on all patients discharged from a hospital

Hospital information system (HIS): The comprehensive database containing all the clinical, administrative, financial, and demographic information about each patient served by a hospital

Hospital inpatient autopsy: A postmortem (after death) examination performed on the body of a patient who died during an inpatient hospitalization by a hospital pathologist or a physician of the medical staff who has been delegated the responsibility

Hospital newborn inpatient: A patient born in the hospital at the beginning of the current inpatient hospitalization

Hospital-acquired infection rate: The number of hospital-acquired infections for a given time period divided by the total number of inpatient discharges for the same time period

Hospitalization insurance (HI) (Medicare Part A): A federal program that covers the costs associated with inpatient hospitalization as well as other healthcare services provided to Medicare beneficiaries

Human Genome Nomenclature (HUGN): Interoperability standard for exchanging information regarding the role of genes in biomedical research and healthcare

Human relations movement: A management philosophy emphasizing the shift from a mechanistic view of workers to concern for their satisfaction at work

Human subjects: Individuals whose physiologic or behavioral characteristics and responses are the object of study in a research program

Human–computer interface: The device used by humans to access and enter data into a computer system, such as a keyboard on a PC, personal digital assistant, voice recognition system, and so on

Hybrid online analytical processing (HOLAP): A data access methodology that is coupled tightly with the architecture of the database management system to allow the user to perform business analyses

Hybrid record: A health record that is includes both paper and electronic elements

HyperText Markup Language (HTML): A standardized computer language that allows the electronic transfer of information and communications among many different information systems

Hypothesis: A statement that describes a research question in measurable terms

ICD-9-CM (International Classification of Diseases, Ninth Revision, Clinical Modification): A classification system used in the United States to report morbidity and mortality information

Identifier standards: Recommended methods for assigning unique identifiers to individuals (patients and clinical providers), corporate providers, and healthcare vendors and suppliers

Identity management: In the master patient index, policies and procedures that manage patient identity, such as prohibiting the same record number for duplicate patients or duplicate records for one patient

Implementation phase: The third phase of the systems development life cycle during which a comprehensive plan is developed and instituted to ensure that the new information system is effectively implemented within the organization

Incentive: Something that stimulates or encourages an individual to work harder

Incentive pay: A system of bonuses and rewards based on employee productivity; often used in transcription areas of healthcare facilities

Incidence: The number of new cases of a specific disease

Incidence rate: A computation that compares the number of new cases of a specific disease for a given time period to the population at risk for the disease during the same time period

Incident: An occurrence in a medical facility that is inconsistent with accepted standards of care

Incident report review: An analysis of incident reports or an evaluation of descriptions of adverse events

Income statement: A statement that summarizes an organization's revenue and expense accounts using totals accumulated during the fiscal year

Indemnity plans: Health insurance coverage provided in the form of cash payments to patients or providers

Independent practice organization (IPO) or association (IPA): An open-panel health maintenance organization that provides contract healthcare services to subscribers through independent physicians who treat patients in their own offices; the HMO reimburses the IPA on a capitated basis; the IPA may reimburse the physicians on a fee-for-service or a capitated basis

Independent practitioners: Individuals working as employees of an organization, in private practice, or through a physician group who provide healthcare services without supervision or direction

Independent variable: An antecedent factor that researchers manipulate directly

Index: An organized (usually alphabetical) list of specific data that serves to guide, indicate, or otherwise facilitate reference to the data

Indian Health Service (IHS): The federal agency within the Department of Health and Human Services that is responsible for providing federal healthcare services to American Indians and Alaska natives

Indirect costs: Resources expended that cannot be identified as pertaining to specific goods and/or services (for example, electricity is not allocable to a specific patient)

Individually identifiable health information: Personal information that can be linked to a specific patient, such as age, gender, date of birth, and address

Inductive reasoning: A process of creating conclusions based on a limited number of observations

Infant mortality rate: The number of deaths of individuals under one year of age during a given time period divided by the number of live births reported for the same time period

Infection review: Evaluation of the risk of infection among patients and healthcare providers, looking for, preventing, and controlling the risk

Inference engine: Specialized computer software that tries to match conditions in rules to data elements in a repository (when a match is found, the engine executes the rule, which results in the occurrence of a specified action)

Inferential statistics: A set of statistical techniques that allows researchers to make generalizations about a population's characteristics (parameters) on the basis of a sample's characteristics

Informatics: A field of study that focuses on the use of technology to improve access to, and utilization of, information

Information: Factual data that have been collected, combined, analyzed, interpreted, and/or converted into a form that can be used for a specific purpose

Information assets: Information that has value for an organization

Information capture: The process of recording representations of human thought, perceptions, or actions in documenting patient care, as well as device-generated information that is gathered and/or computed about a patient as part of health care

Information management: The acquisition, organization, analysis, storage, retrieval, and dissemination of information to support decision-making activities

Information science: The study of the nature and principles of information

Information system (IS): An automated system that uses computer hardware and software to record, manipulate, store, recover, and disseminate data (that is, a system that receives and processes input and provides output); often used interchangeably with information technology (IT)

Information technology (IT): Computer technology (hardware and software) combined with telecommunications technology (data, image, and voice networks); often used interchangeably with information system (IS)

Information technology professional: An individual who works with computer technology in the process of managing health information

Informed consent: 1. A legal term referring to a patient's right to make his or her own treatment decisions based on the knowledge of the treatment to be administered or the procedure to be performed 2. An individual's voluntary agreement to participate in research or to undergo a diagnostic, therapeutic, or preventive medical procedure

Injury Severity Score (ISS): An overall severity measurement maintained in the trauma registry and calculated from the abbreviated injury scores for the three most severe injuries of each patient

Inpatient: A patient who is provided with room, board, and continuous general nursing services in an area of an acute care facility where patients generally stay at least overnight

Inpatient bed occupancy rate (percentage of occupancy): The total number of inpatient service days for a given time period divided by the total number of inpatient bed count days for the same time period

Inpatient psychiatric facility (IPF): A healthcare facility that offers psychiatric medical care on an inpatient basis; CMS established a prospective payment system for reimbursing these types of facilities using the current DRGs for inpatient hospitals

Inpatient rehabilitation facility (IRF): A healthcare facility that specializes in providing services to patients who have suffered a disabling illness or injury in an effort to help them achieve or maintain their optimal level of functioning, self-care, and independence

Inpatient Rehabilitation Validation and Entry (IRVEN): A computerized data-entry system used by inpatient rehabilitation facilities

Inpatient service day (IPSD): A unit of measure equivalent to the services received by one inpatient during one twenty-four-hour period

In-service education: Training that teaches employees specific skills required to maintain or improve performance, usually internal to an organization

Institute for Clinical Systems Improvement (ICSI): A collaboration of healthcare organizations that provides an objective voice dedicated to supporting healthcare quality and helping its members identify and achieve implementation of best practices for their patients

Institute of Electrical and Electronics Engineers (IEEE): A national organization that develops standards for hospital system interface transactions, including links between critical care bedside instruments and clinical information systems

Institute of Electrical and Electronics Engineers (IEEE) 1073: Interoperability standard for electronic data exchange

Institute of Medicine (IOM): A branch of the National Academy of Sciences whose goal is to advance and distribute scientific knowledge with the mission of improving human health

Institutional review board (IRB): An administrative body that provides oversight for the research studies conducted within a healthcare institution

Instrument: A standardized and uniform way to collect data

Insured: A holder of a health insurance policy

Insurer: An organization that pays healthcare expenses on behalf of its enrollees

Integrated delivery network (IDN): *See* **integrated delivery system**

Integrated delivery system (IDS): A system that combines the financial and clinical aspects of healthcare and uses a group of healthcare providers, selected on the basis of quality and cost management criteria, to furnish comprehensive health services across the continuum of care

Integrated health record: A system of health record organization in which all of the paper forms are arranged in strict chronological order and mixed with forms created by different departments

Integrated provider organization (IPO): An organization that manages the delivery of healthcare services provided by hospitals, physicians (employees of the IPO), and other healthcare organizations (for example, nursing facilities)

Integration: The complex task of ensuring that all elements and platforms in an information system communicate and act as a uniform entity; or the combination of two or more benefit plans to prevent duplication of benefit payment

Integrity: The state of being whole or unimpaired

Integrity constraints: Limits placed on the data that may be entered into a database

Intellectual capital: The combined knowledge of an organization's employees with respect to operations, processes, history, and culture

Intelligent character recognition (ICR) technology: A method of encoding handwritten, print, or cursive characters and of interpreting the characters as words or the intent of the writer

Intelligent document recognition (IDR) technology: Technology that automatically recognizes analog items, such as tangible materials or documents, or recognizes characters or symbols from analog items, enabling the identified data to be quickly, accurately, and automatically entered into digital systems

Interface: The zone between different computer systems across which users want to pass information (for example, a computer program written to exchange information between systems or the graphic display of an application program designed to make the program easier to use)

Interim period: Any period that represents less than an entire fiscal year

Internal controls: Policies and procedures designed to protect an organization's assets and to reduce the exposure to the risk of loss due to error or malfeasance

Internal rate of return (IRR): An interest rate that makes the net present value calculation equal zero

Internal validity: An attribute of a study's design that contributes to the accuracy of its findings

International Classification for Nursing Practice (ICNP®): Unified nursing language system into which existing terminologies can be cross-mapped

International Classification of Diseases for Oncology (ICD-O): A classification system used for reporting incidences of malignant disease

International Classification of Primary Care (ICPC-2): Classification used for coding the reasons of encounter, diagnoses, and interventions in an episode-of-care structure

International Classification on Functioning, Disability and Health (ICF): Classification of health and health-related domains that describe body functions and structures, activities, and participation

International Federation of Health Record Organizations (IFHRO): Organization that supports national associations and health record professionals to implement and improve health records and the systems that support them

International Medical Informatics Association (IMIA): Worldwide not-for-profit organization that promotes medical informatics in healthcare and biomedical research

Interoperability: The ability, generally by adoption of standards, of systems to work together

Interoperable: Adjective form of interoperability

Interoperate: Verb form of interoperability

Interpersonal skills: One of the three managerial skill categories that includes skills in communicating and relating effectively to others

Interrater reliability: A measure of a research instrument's consistency in data collection when used by different abstractors

Interrogatories: Discovery devices consisting of a set of written questions given to a party, witness, or other person who has information needed in a legal case

Interval data: A type of data that represents observations that can be measured on an evenly distributed scale beginning at a point other than true zero

Interval scale: Situation where the intervals between adjacent scale values are equal with respect to the attributes being measured

Intervention: 1. A clinical manipulation, treatment, or therapy 2. A generic term used by researchers to mean an act of some kind

Interview: A formal meeting, often between a job applicant and a potential employer

Interview guide: A list of written questions to be asked during an interview

Interview survey: A type of research instrument with which the members of the population being studied are asked questions and respond orally

Intranet: A private information network that is similar to the Internet and whose servers are located inside a firewall or security barrier so that the general public cannot gain access to information housed within the network

Intrarater reliability: A measure of a research instrument's reliability in which the same person repeating the test will get reasonably similar findings

Intuition: Unconscious decision making based on extensive experience in similar situations

Inventory: Goods on hand and available to sell, presumably within a year (a business cycle)

Investor-owned hospital chain: Group of for-profit healthcare facilities owned by stockholders

ISO 9000: An internationally agreed-upon set of generic standards for quality management established by the International Standards Organization

Issue log: A form of documentation that describes the questions, concerns, and problems that must be solved in order for a task to be completed

Job classification method: 1. A method of job evaluation that compares a written position description with the written descriptions of various classification grades 2. A method used by the federal government to grade jobs

Job description: A list of a job's duties, reporting relationships, working conditions, and responsibilities

Job evaluation: The process of applying predefined compensable factors to jobs to determine their relative worth

Job procedure: A structured, action-oriented list of sequential steps involved in carrying out a specific job or solving a problem

Job ranking: A method of job evaluation that arranges jobs in a hierarchy on the basis of each job's importance to the organization, with the most important jobs listed at the top of the hierarchy and the least important jobs listed at the bottom

Job rotation: A work design in which workers are shifted periodically among different tasks

Job sharing: A work schedule in which two or more individuals share the tasks of one full-time or one full-time-equivalent position

Job specifications: A list of a job's required education, skills, knowledge, abilities, personal qualifications, and physical requirements

Joint Commission on Accreditation of Healthcare Organizations (JCAHO): A private, not-for-profit organization that evaluates and accredits hospitals and other healthcare organizations on the basis of predefined performance standards

Journal entry: An accounting representation of a financial transaction or transfer of amounts between accounts that contains at least one debit and one credit and in which the dollar value of the debits and the credits is the same

Judge-made law: Unwritten law originating from court decisions where no applicable statute exists; *See* **common law or case law**

Jurisdiction: The power and authority of a court to hear and decide specific types of cases

Justice: The impartial administration of policies or laws that takes into consideration the competing interests and limited resources of the individuals or groups involved

Just-in-time training: Training provided anytime, anyplace, and just when it is needed

Key attributes: Common fields (attributes) within a relational database that are used to link tables to one another

Key indicator: A quantifiable measure used over time to determine whether some structure, process, or outcome in the provision of care to a patient supports high-quality performance measured against best practice criteria

K-nearest neighbor (K-NN): A classic technique used to discover associations and sequences when the data attributes are numeric

Knowledge: The information, understanding, and experience that give individuals the power to make informed decisions

Knowledge assets: Assets that are the sources of knowledge for an organization (for example, printed documents, unwritten rules, work flows, customer knowledge, data in databases and spreadsheets, and the human expertise, know-how, and tacit knowledge within the minds of the organization's workforce)

Knowledge base: A database that not only manages raw data but also integrates them with information from various reference works

Knowledge management: 1. The process by which data are acquired and transformed into information through the application of context, which in turn provides understanding

2. A management philosophy that promotes an integrated and collaborative approach to the process of information asset creation, capture, organization, access, and use

Knowledge production: Involves the creation of knowledge through collection, generation, synthesis, and identification and organization of knowledge through codification, storage, packaging, and coordination

Knowledge refinement: Consists of evaluation, reflection, adaptation, and sustainability of knowledge

Knowledge use: Consists of distribution, sharing, application, and integration of knowledge

Knowledge worker: An employee who improves his or her performance by sharing his or her experience and expertise with other employees

Knowledge-based data: The sources of knowledge for an organization (for example, printed documents; unwritten rules; work flows; customer knowledge; data in databases and spreadsheets; and the human expertise, know-how, and tacit knowledge within the minds of the organization's workforce); also called knowledge-based assets

Knowledge-based DSS: Decision support system in which the key element is the knowledge base; often referred to as a rule-based system because the knowledge is stored in the form of rules (for example, the IF, THEN, ELSE format)

Kolb's "Learning Loop": A theory of experiential learning involving four interrelated steps: concrete experiences, observation and reflection, formation of abstract concepts and theories, and testing new implications of theory in new situations

Labor relations: Human resources management activities associated with unions and collective bargaining

Labor-Management Relations Act (Taft-Hartley Act): Federal legislation passed in 1947 that imposed certain restrictions on unions while upholding their right to organize and bargain collectively

Labor-Management Reporting and Disclosure Act (Landrum-Griffin Act): Federal legislation passed in 1959 to ensure that union members' interests were properly represented by union leadership; created, among other things, a bill of rights for union members

Layoff: A suspension of work, usually termporary

Leading: One of the four management functions in which people are directed and motivated to achieve goals

Leapfrog Group: Organization that promotes healthcare safety by giving consumers the information they need to make better-informed choices about the hospitals they choose

Learning content management system: Training software development tools that assist with management, sharing, and reuse of course content

Learning curve: The time required to acquire and apply certain skills so that new levels of productivity and/or performance exceed prelearning levels (productivity often is inversely related to the learning curve)

Learning management system: A software application that assists with managing and tracking learners and learning events and collating data on learner progress

Learning organization: An organization in which the emphasis is on acquiring and sharing business knowledge along with delivering information quickly, clearly, and visually to everyone within the organization

Lecture: A one-way method of delivering education through speaking in which the teacher delivers the speech and the student listens

Legacy system: A type of computer system that uses older technology but may still perform optimally

Length of stay (LOS): The total number of patient days for an inpatient episode, calculated by subtracting the date of admission from the date of discharge

Level of significance: 1. The relative intensity of services given when a physician provides one-on-one services for a patient (such as minimal, brief, limited, or intermediate) 2. The relative intensity of services provided by a healthcare facility (for example, tertiary care); also called level of service

Lexicon: 1. the vocabulary used in a language or a subject area or by a particular speaker or group of speakers 2. A collection of words or terms and their meanings for a particular domain, used in healthcare for drug terms

Liability: 1. A legal obligation or responsibility that may have financial repercussions if not fulfilled 2. An amount owed by an individual or organization to another individual or organization

Licensure: The legal authority or formal permission from authorities to carry on certain activities that by law or regulation require such permission (applicable to institutions as well as individuals)

Likert scale: An ordinal scaling and summated rating technique for measuring the attitudes of respondents; a measure that records level of agreement or disagreement along a progression of categories, usually five (five-point scale), often administered in the form of a questionnaire

Line authority: The authority to manage subordinates and to have them report back, based on relationships illustrated in an organizational chart

Line graph: A graphic technique used to illustrate the relationship between continuous measurements; consists of a line drawn to connect a series of points on an arithmetic scale; often used to display time trends

Linear programming: An operational management technique that uses mathematical formulas to determine the optimal way to allocate resources for a project

Linkage analysis: A technique used to explore and examine relationships among a large number of variables of different types

Liquidity: The degree to which assets can be quickly and efficiently turned into cash, for example, marketable securities are generally very liquid, the assumption being that they can be sold for their full value in a matter of days, whereas buildings are not very liquid, because they cannot usually be sold quickly

Literature review: A systematic and critical investigation of the important information about a topic; may include books, journal articles, theses, dissertations, periodicals, technical and research reports, proceedings of conferences, audiovisual media, and electronic media

Litigation: A civil lawsuit or contest in court

Logical (or conceptual) repository: The compilation of multiple physical repositories

Logical data model: The second level of data model that is drawn according to the type of database to be developed

Logical Observation Identifier Names and Codes (LOINC): A database protocol developed by the Regenstrief Institute for Health Care aimed at standardizing laboratory and clinical codes for use in clinical care, outcomes management, and research

Longitudinal: A type of time frame for research studies during which data are collected from the same participants at multiple points in time

Longitudinal health record: A permanent, coordinated patient record of significant information listed in chronological order and maintained across time, ideally from birth to death

Long-term assets: Assets whose value to the organization extends beyond one fiscal year, for example, buildings, land, and equipment are long-term assets

Long-term care: Healthcare services provided in a nonacute care setting to chronically ill, aged, disabled, or mentally handicapped individuals

Long-term care hospital (LTCH): A healthcare organization that provides medical, nursing, rehabilitation, and sub–acute care services to residents who need continual

Loss prevention: A risk management strategy that includes developing and revising policies and procedures that are both facilitywide and department specific

Loss reduction: A component of a risk management program that encompasses techniques used to manage events or claims that already have taken place

Low-utilization payment adjustment (LUPA): An alternative (reduced) payment made to home health agencies instead of the home health resource group reimbursement rate when a patient receives fewer than four home care visits during a sixty-day episode

Machine learning: An area of computer science that studies algorithms and computer programs that improve employee performance on some task by exposure to a training or learning experience

Maintenance and evaluation phase: The fourth and final phase of the systems development life cycle that helps to ensure that adequate technical support staff and resources are available to maintain or support the new system

Major diagnostic category (MDC): Under diagnosis-related groups (DRGs), one of twenty-five categories based on single or multiple organ systems into which all diseases and disorders relating to that system are classified

Major medical insurance (catastrophic coverage): Prepaid healthcare benefits that include a high limit for most types of medical expenses and usually require a large deductible and sometimes place limits on coverage and charges (for example, room and board)

Malpractice: The improper or negligent treatment of a patient, as by a physician, resulting in injury, damage, or loss

Managed care: 1. Payment method in which the third-party payer has implemented some provisions to control the costs of healthcare while maintaining quality care   2. Systematic merger of clinical, financial, and administrative processes to manage access, cost, and quality of healthcare

Managed care organization (MCO): A type of health-care organization that delivers medical care and manages all aspects of the care or the payment for care by limiting providers of care, discounting payment to providers of care, and/or limiting access to care

Management by objectives (MBO): A management approach that defines target objectives for organizing work and comparing performance against those objectives

Management functions: Traditionally, the tasks of planning, organizing, directing, coordinating, and controlling

Management information system (MIS): A computer-based system that provides information to a healthcare organization's managers for use in making decisions that affect a variety of day-to-day activities

Management service organization (MSO): An organization, usually owned by a group of physicians or a hospital, that provides administrative and support services to one or more physician group practices or small hospitals

Managerial accounting: The development, implementation, and analysis of systems that track financial transactions for management control purposes, including both budget systems and cost analysis systems

Many-to-many relationship: The concept (occurring only in a conceptual model) that multiple instances of an entity may be associated with multiple instances of another entity

Mark sense technology: Technology that detects the presence or absence of hand-marked characters on analog documents; used for processing questionnaires, surveys, and tests, such as filled-in circles by Number 2 pencils on exam forms

Maslow's Hierarchy of Needs: A theory developed by Abraham Maslow suggesting that a hierarchy of needs might help explain behavior and guide managers on how to motivate employees; *See* **hierarchy of needs**

Massed training: An educational technique that requires learning a large amount of material at one time

Master patient index (MPI): A list or database created and maintained by a healthcare facility to record the name and identification number of every patient who has ever been admitted or treated in the facility

Master population index: *See* **master patient index**

Matching: A concept that enables decision makers to look at expenses and revenues in the same period to measure the organization's income performance

Materiality: The significance of a dollar amount based on predetermined criteria

Maternal death rate (hospital based): For a hospital, the total number of maternal deaths directly related to pregnancy for a given time period divided by the total number of obstetrical discharges for the same time period; for a community, the total number of deaths attributed to maternal conditions during a given time period in a specific geographic area divided by the total number of live births for the same time period in the same area

Maternal mortality rate (community based): A rate that measures the deaths associated with pregnancy for a specific community for a specific period of time

Mean: A measure of central tendency that is determined by calculating the arithmetic average of the observations in a frequency distribution

Measures of central tendency: The typical or average numbers that are descriptive of the entire collection of data for a specific population

Median: A measure of central tendency that shows the midpoint of a frequency distribution when the observations have been arranged in order from lowest to highest

Medicaid: An entitlement program that oversees medical assistance for individuals and families with low incomes and limited resources; jointly funded between state and federal governments

Medical care evaluation studies (medical audits): Audits required by the Medicare Conditions of Participation that dictate the use of screening criteria with evaluation by diagnosis and/or procedure

Medical foundation: Multipurpose, nonprofit service organization for physicians and other healthcare providers at the local and county level; as managed care organizations, medical foundations have established preferred provider organization, exclusive provider organizations, and management service organizations, with emphases on freedom of choice and preservation of the physician-patient relationship

Medical Group Management Association (MGMA): A national organization composed of individuals actively engaged in the business management of medical groups consisting of three or more physicians in medical practice

Medical informatics: A field of information science concerned with the management of data and information used to diagnose, treat, cure, and prevent disease through the application of computers and computer technologies

Medical informatics professionals: Individuals who work in the field of medical informatics

Medical Literature, Analysis, and Retrieval System Online (MEDLINE): A computerized, online database in the bibliographic Medical Literature Analysis and Retrieval System (MEDLARS) of the National Library of Medicine

Medical staff bylaws: A collection of guidelines adopted by a hospital's medical staff to govern its business conduct and the rights and responsibilities of its members

Medical staff classifications: Categories of clinical practice privileges assigned to individual practitioners on the basis of their qualifications

Medical Subject Headings database (MeSH): The National Library of Medicine's (NLM's) controlled vocabulary for indexing journal articles

Medical transcriptionist: A medical language specialist who types or word-processes information dictated by providers

Medically needy option (Medicaid): An option in the Medicaid program that allows states to extend eligibility to persons who would be eligible for Medicaid under one of the mandatory or optional groups but whose income and/or resources fall above the eligibility level set by their state

Medicare: A federally funded health program established in 1965 to assist with the medical care costs of Americans sixty-five years of age and older as well as other individuals entitled to Social Security benefits owing to their disabilities

Medicare Advantage (Medicare Part C): Optional managed care plan for Medicare beneficiaries who are entitled to Part A, enrolled in Part B, and live in an area with a plan; types include health maintenance organization, point-of-service plan, preferred provider organization, and provider-sponsored organization

Medicare carrier: A health plan that processes Part B claims for services by physicians and medical suppliers (for example, the Blue Shield plan in a state)

Medicare fee schedule (MFS): A feature of the resource-based relative value system that includes a complete list of the payments Medicare makes to physicians and other providers

Medicare prospective payment system: The reimbursement system for inpatient hospital services provided to Medicare and Medicaid beneficiaries that is based on the use of diagnosis-related groups as a classification tool

Medicare Provider Analysis and Review (MEDPAR) database system: A database containing information submitted by fiscal intermediaries that is used by the Office of the Inspector General to identify suspicious billing and charge practices

Medicare Summary Notice (MSN): A summary sent to the patient from Medicare that summarizes all services provided over a period of time with an explanation of benefits provided

Medication usage review: An evaluation of medication use and medication processes

Medigap: A private insurance policy that supplements Medicare coverage

Mental ability (cognitive) tests: Tests that assess the reasoning capabilities of individuals

Mentor: An advisor; an experienced individual who coaches another individual who is at the beginning stages of his or her career

Message format standards: Protocols that help ensure that data transmitted from one system to another remain comparable

Meta-analysis: A specialized form of systematic literature review that involves the statistical analysis of a large collection of results from individual studies for the purpose of integrating the studies' findings

Metadata: Descriptive data that characterize other data to create a clearer understanding of their meaning and to achieve greater reliability and quality of information

Microfilming: A photographic process that reduces an original paper document into a small image on film to save storage space

Middle managers: The individuals in an organization who oversee the operation of a broad scope of functions at the departmental level or who oversee defined product or service lines

Migration path: A series of steps required to move from one situation to another

Minimum Data Set 2.0 (MDS): The instrument specified by the Centers for Medicare and Medicaid Services that requires nursing facilities (both Medicare certified and/or Medicaid certified) to conduct a comprehensive, accurate, standardized, reproducible assessment of each resident's functional capacity

Minimum Data Set for Long-Term Care-Version 2.0 (MDS 2.0): A federally mandated standard assessment form that Medicare- and/or Medicaid-certified nursing facilities must use to collect demographic and clinical data on nursing home residents

Misdemeanor: A crime that is less serious than a felony

Mission statement: A short description of an organization or group's general purpose for existing

m-learning: Mobile learning; the application of e-learning to mobile computing devices and wireless networks

Mode: A measure of central tendency that consists of the most frequent observation in a frequency distribution

Model: The representation of a t heory in a visual format, on a smaller scale, or with objects

Model-based DDS: Decision support system that attempts to include as many different models as can be accommodated to provide the user the greatest flexibility in framing the decision situation

Moral values: A system of principles by which one guides one's life, usually with regard to right or wrong

Morality: A composite of the personal values concerning what is considered right or wrong in a specific cultural group

Mortality (attrition): 1. A term referring to the incidence of death in a specific population 2. The loss of subjects during the course of a clinical research study

Mortality review: A review of deaths as part of an analysis of ongoing outcome and performance improvement

Mortgage: A loan that is secured by a long-term asset, usually a building

Motion for summary judgment: A request made by the defendant in a civil case to have the case ruled in his or he favor based on the assertion that the plaintiff has no genuine issue to be tried

Motion (or streaming) video/frame data: A medium for storing, manipulating, and displaying moving images in a format, such as frames, that can be presented on a computer monitor

Motivation: The drive to accomplish a task

Movement diagram: A chart depicting the location of furniture and equipment in a work area and showing the usual flow of individuals or materials as they progress through the work area

Multidimensional analysis: Simultaneous analysis of data from multiple dimensions using different data elements

Multidimensional data structure: A structure whereby data are organized according to the dimensions associated with them

Multidimensional database management system (MDDBMS): A database management system specifically designed to handle data organized into a data structure with numerous dimensions

Multidimensional online analytical processing (MOLAP): A data access methodology that is coupled tightly with a multidimensional database management system to allow the user to perform business analyses

Multimedia: The combination of free-text, raster or vector graphics, sound, and/or motion video/frame data

Multivariate: A term used in reference to research studies indicating that many variables were involved

Multivoting technique: A decision-making method for determining group consensus on the prioritization of issues or solutions

National Alliance for Health Information Technology (NAHIT): A partnership of government and private-sector leaders from various healthcare organizations working to use technology to achieve improvements in patient safety, quality of care and operating performance; founded in 2002

National Association of Healthcare Quality (NAHQ): An organization devoted to advancing the profession of healthcare quality improvement through its accreditation program

National Cancer Institute (NCI) Thesaurus: Interoperability standard that describes anatomical locations for clinical, surgical, pathological and research purposes

National Cancer Registrars Association (NCRA): An organization of cancer registry professionals that promotes research and education in cancer registry administration and practice

National Centers for Health Statistics (NCHS): The federal agency responsible for collecting and disseminating information on health services utilization and the health status of the population in the United States

National Committee for Quality Assurance (NCQA): A private not-for-profit accreditation organization whose mission is to evaluate and report on the quality of managed care organizations in the United States

National Committee on Vital and Health Statistics (NCVHS): A public policy advisory board that recommends policy to the National Center for Health Statistics and other health-related federal programs

National conversion factor (CF): A mathematical factor used to convert relative value units into monetary payments for services provided to Medicare beneficiaries

National Correct Coding Initiative (NCCI): A series of code edits on Medicare Part B claims

National Council for Prescription Drug Programs (NCPDP): An organization that develops standards for exchanging prescription and payment information

National Drug Code (NDC) Directory: A list of all drugs manufactured, prepared, propagated, compounded, or processed by a drug establishment registered under the Federal Food, Drug, and Cosmetic Act

National Drug Codes (NDC): Codes that serve as product identifiers for human drugs, currently limited to prescription drugs and a few selected over-the-counter products

National Drug File—Reference Terminology (NDF-RT): File of drug products centrally maintained and developed by the Department of Veterans Affairs that can be locally modified and deployed

National Health Care Survey: A national public health survey that contains data abstracted manually from a sample of acute care hospitals or from discharged inpatient records or that are obtained from state or other discharge databases

National health information network (NHIN): System that links various healthcare information systems together, allowing patients, physicians, healthcare institutions, and other entities nationwide to share clinical information privately and securely

National Information Infrastructure-Health Information Network Program (NII-HIN): A national quasi-governmental organization that provides oversight of all healthcare information standards in the United States

National Institutes of Health (NIH): Federal agency of the Department of Health and Human Services comprising a number of institutes that carry out research and programs related to certain types of diseases, such as cancer

National Labor Relations Act (Wagner Act): Federal pro-union legislation passed in 1935, later amended by the Taft-Hartley Act

National Library of Medicine (NLM): The world's largest medical library and a branch of the National Institutes of Health

National Practitioner Data Bank (NPBD): A data bank established by the federal government through the 1986 Health Care Quality Improvement Act that contains information on professional review actions taken against physicians and other licensed healthcare practitioners, which healthcare organizations are required to check as part of the credentialing process

National provider file (NPF): A file developed by the Centers for Medicare and Medicaid Services that includes all healthcare providers, including nonphysicians, and sites of care

National provider identifier (NPI): An eight-character alphanumeric identifier used to identify individual healthcare providers for Medicare billing purposes

National Quality Forum: A private, not-for-profit membership organization created to develop and implement a strategy nationwide to improve the measurement and reporting of healthcare quality

National Uniform Billing Committee (NUBC): The national group responsible for identifying data elements and designing the CMS-1500

National Uniform Claim Committee (NUCC): The national group that replaced the Uniform Claim Form Task Force in 1995 and developed a standard data set to be used in the transmission of noninstitutional provider claims to and from third-party payers

National Vaccine Advisory Committee (NVAC): A national advisory group that supports the director of the National Vaccine Program

National Vital Statistics System (NVSS): A federal agency responsible for the collection of official vital statistics for the United States

Natural language processing (NLP): *See* **natural language processing technology**

Natural language processing technology: The extraction of unstructured or structured medical word data, which are then translated into diagnostic or procedural codes for clinical and administrative applications

Naturalism: A philosophy of research that assumes that multiple contextual truths exist and bias is always present

Naturalistic observation: A type of nonparticipant observation in which researchers observe certain behaviors and events as they occur naturally

Needs assessment: A procedure performed to determine what is required, lacking, or desired by an employee, a group, or an organization

Need-to-know principle: The release-of-information principle based on the minimum necessary standard that means that only the information needed by a specific individual to perform a specific task should be released

Negative (inverse) relationship: A relationship in which the effects move in opposite directions

Negligence: A legal term that refers to the result of an action by an individual who does not act the way a reasonably prudent person would act under the same circumstances

Neonatal mortality rate: The number of deaths of infants under twenty-eight days of age during a given time period divided by the total number of births for the same time period

Net autopsy rate: The ratio of inpatient autopsies compared to inpatient deaths calculated by dividing the total number of inpatient autopsies performed by the hospital pathologist for a given time period by the total number of inpatient deaths minus unautopsied coroners' or medical examiners' cases for the same time period

Net death rate: The total number of inpatient deaths minus the number of deaths that occurred less than forty-eight hours after admission for a given time period divided by the total number of inpatient discharges minus the number of deaths that occurred less than forty-eight hours after admission for the same time period

Net income: The difference between total revenues and total expenses

Net loss: The condition when total expenses exceed total revenue

Net present value: A formula used to assess the current value of a project when the monies used were invested in the organization's investment vehicles rather than expended for the project; this value is then compared to the allocation of the monies and the cash inflows of the project, both of which are adjusted to current time

Network administrators: The individuals involved in installing, configuring, managing, monitoring, and maintaining network computer applications and responsible for supporting the network infrastructure and controlling user access

Network model health maintenance program: Program in which participating HMOs contract for services with one or more multispecialty group practices

Network provider: A physician or another healthcare professional who is a member of a managed care network

Neural networks: Nonlinear predictive models that, using a set of data that describe what a person wants to find, detect a pattern to match a particular profile through a training process that involves interactive learning

Newborn (NB): An inpatient who was born in a hospital at the beginning of the current inpatient hospitalization

Newborn autopsy rate: The number of autopsies performed on newborns who died during a given time period divided by the total number of newborns who died during the same time period

Newborn death rate: The number of newborns who died divided by the total number of newborns, both alive and dead

Nomenclature: A recognized system of terms used in a science or art that follows preestablished naming conventions; a disease nomenclature is a listing of the proper name for each disease entity with its specific code number

Nominal data: *See* **nominal-level data**

Nominal group technique: A group process technique that involves the steps of silent listing, recording each participant's list, discussing, and rank ordering the priority or importance of items

Nominal-level data: Data that fall into groups or categories that are mutually exclusive and with no specific order (for example patient demographics such as third party payer, race, and sex)

Nonexempt employees: All groups of employees covered by the provisions of the Fair Labor Standards Act

Nonmaleficence: A legal principle that means "do no harm"

Nonparametric (distribution-free) technique: A type of statistical procedure used for variables that are not normally distributed in a population

Nonparticipant observation: A method of research in which researchers act as neutral observers who do not intentionally interact or affect the actions of the population being observed

Nonparticipating provider: A healthcare provider who did not sign a participation agreement with Medicare and so is not obligated to accept assignment on Medicare claims

Nonprogrammed decision: A decision that involves careful and deliberate thought and discussion because of a unique, complex, or changing situation

Nonrandom sampling: A type of convenience or purposive sampling in which all members of the target population do not have an equal or independent chance of being selected for a research study

Normal distribution: A theoretical family of continuous frequency distributions characterized by a symmetric bell-shaped curve, with an equal mean, median, and mode, any standard deviation, and with half of the observations above the mean and half below it

Normalization: 1. A formal process applied to relational database design to determine which variables should be grouped together in a table in order to reduce data redundancy across and within the table   2. Conversion of various representational forms to standard expressions so that those that have the same meaning will be recognized by computer software as synonymous in a data search

North American Nursing Diagnosis Association (NANDA II): Nursing terminology used to develop and classify nursing diagnoses in a taxonomy

Nosocomial (hospital-acquired) infection: An infection acquired by a patient while receiving care or services in a healthcare organization

Nosology: The branch of medical science that deals with classification systems

Not-for-profit organizations: An organization that is not owned by individuals, where profits may be held for a specific purpose or reinvested in the organization for the benefit of the community it serves

Notice of Privacy Practices: A statement (mandated by the HIPAA Privacy Rule) issued by a healthcare organization that informs individuals of the uses and disclosures of patient-identifiable health information that may be made by the organization, as well as the individual's rights and the organization's legal duties with respect to that information

Notifiable disease: A disease that must be reported to a government agency so that regular, frequent, and timely information on individual cases can be used to prevent and control future cases of the disease

Null hypothesis: A hypothesis that states there is no association between the independent and dependent variables in a research study

Nursing informatics: The field of information science concerned with the management of data and information used to support the practice and delivery of nursing care through the application of computers and computer technologies

Nursing Information and Data Set Evaluation Center (NIDSEC): The Nursing Information & Data Set Evaluation Center was established by the American Nurses Association (ANA) to review, evaluate against defined criteria, and recognize information systems from developers and manufacturers that support documentation of nursing care within automated Nursing Information Systems (NIS) or within computer-based patient record systems (CPR)

Nursing Interventions Classification (NIC): A terminology that describes the treatments that nurses perform

Nursing Management Minimum Data Set (NMMDS): A data set that supports description, analysis, and comparisons of nursing care and nursing resources in the context of complex healthcare outcomes; designed to complement the clinical patient oriented data designated in the nursing minimum data set (NMDS)

Nursing Minimum Data Set (NMDS): A data set that provides uniform definitions and categories of nursing care; built on the uniform minimum health data sets (UMHDS)

Nursing Outcomes Classification (NOC): A classification of patient/client outcomes developed to evaluate the effects of nursing interventions

Object: The basic component in an object-oriented database that includes both data and their relationships within a single structure

Objective: A statement of the end result expected, stated in measurable terms, usually with a time limitation (deadline date) and often with a cost estimate or limitation

Object-oriented database (OODB): A type of database that uses commands that act as small, self-contained instructional units (objects) that may be combined in various ways

Object-oriented database management system (OODBMS): A specific set of software programs used to implement an object-oriented database

Observational research: A method of research in which researchers obtain data by watching research participants rather than by asking questions

Observational study: An epidemiological study in which the exposure and outcome for each individual in the study is observed

Occasion of service: A specified identifiable service involved in the care of a patient that is not an encounter (for example, a lab test ordered during an encounter)

Occupational Safety and Health Act of 1970 (OSHA): The federal legislation that established comprehensive safety and health guidelines for employers

Occurrence/generic screening: A risk management technique in which the risk manager reviews the health records of current and discharged hospital inpatients with the goal of identifying potentially compensable events

Odds ratio: A relative measure of occurrence of an illness; the odds of exposure in a diseased group divided by the odds of exposure in a nondiseased group

Office for Human Research Protections (OHRP): The department with the Department of Health and Human Services that monitors compliance with federal regulations governing the conduct of biomedical research

Office of Research Integrity (ORI): Organization that provides integrity in biomedical and behavioral research, monitoring incidents of research misconduct and facilitating responsible research conduct through educational, preventive, and regulatory activities

Office of the National Coordinator of Health Information Technology (ONC): Office that provides leadership for the development and implementation of an interoperable health information technology infrastructure nationwide to improve healthcare quality and delivery

Offshoring: Outsourcing jobs to countries overseas, wherein local employees abroad perform jobs that domestic employees previously performed

Omaha System: A research-based taxonomy designed to generate data following routine client care

Omnibus Budget Reconciliation Act (OBRA) of 1989: Federal legislation that mandated important changes in the payment rules for Medicare physicians; specifically, the legislation that requires nursing facilities to conduct regular patient assessments for Medicare and Medicaid beneficiaries

One-tailed hypothesis: An alternative hypothesis in which the researcher makes a prediction in one direction

One-to-many relationship: A relationship that exists when one instance of an entity is associated with multiple instances of another entity

One-to-one relationship: A relationship that exists when an instance of an entity is associated with only one instance of another entity, and vice versa

Ongoing records review: *See* **open-record review**

Online analytical processing (OLAP): A data access architecture that allows the user to retrieve specific information from a large volume of data

Online analytical processing (OLAP) engine: An optimized query generator that can retrieve the correct information from the warehouse to accommodate what-if queries

Online/real-time analytical processing (OLAP): *See* **online analytical processing**

Online/real-time transaction processing (OLTP): The real-time processing of day-to-day business transactions from a database

On-the-job training: A method of training in which an employee learns necessary skills and processes by performing the functions of his or her position

Open-record review: A review of the health records of patients currently in the hospital or under active treatment; part of the Joint Commission on Accreditation of Healthcare Organizations (JCAHO) survey process

Open systems: Processes that are affected by what is going on around them and must adjust as the environment changes

Operation index: A list of the operations and surgical procedures performed in a healthcare facility that is sequenced according to the code numbers of the classification system in use

Operational budget: A type of budget that allocates and controls resources to meet an organization's goals and objectives for the fiscal year

Operational plan: The short-term objectives set by an organization to improve its methods of doing business and achieve its planned outcomes

Operations management: The application of mathematical and statistical techniques to production and distribution efficiency

Operations research (OR): A scientific discipline primarily begun during the Second World War that seeks to apply the scientific method and mathematical models to the solution of a variety of management decision problems

Operations support system (OSS): An information system that facilitates the operational management of a healthcare organization

Optical character recognition (OCR) technology: A method of encoding text from analog paper into bit-mapped images and translating the images into a form that is computer readable

Optical imaging technology: The process by which information is scanned onto optical disks

Ordinal data: Data with inherent order and with higher numbers usually associated with higher values; also referred to as ordinal-level data

Ordinal scale of measurement: Measurement scale that consists of separate categories with separate names ranked in terms of magnitude

Organization: The planned coordination of the activities of more than one person for the achievement of a common purpose or goal

Organizational chart: A graphic representation of an organization's formal structure

Organizing: The process of coordinating something, such as activities

Orientation: A set of activities designed to familiarize new employees with their jobs, the organization, and its work culture

Orion project: A Joint Commission on Accreditation of Healthcare Organizations initiative designed to assess accreditation models, develop a continuous accreditation process, and test alternative processes for reporting survey findings to hospitals

ORYX: *See* **ORYX initiative**

ORYX initiative: A Joint Commission on Accreditation of Healthcare Organizations initiative that supports the integration of outcomes data and other performance measurement data into the accreditation process; often referred to as ORYX

Outcome and Assessment Information Set (OASIS): A standard core assessment data tool developed to measure the outcomes of adult patients receiving home health services under the Medicare and Medicaid programs

Outcome measures: The process of systematically tracking a patient's clinical treatment and responses to that treatment, including measures of morbidity and functional status, for the purpose of improving care

Outcomes and effectiveness research (OER): A type of research performed to explain the end results of specific healthcare practices and interventions

Outcomes management: The process of systematically tracking a patient's clinical treatment and responses to that treatment, including measures of morbidity and functional status, for the purpose of improving care

Out-of-pocket expenses: Healthcare costs paid by the insured (for example, deductibles, copayments, and coinsurance) after which the insurer pays a percentage (often 80 or 100 percent) of covered expenses

Outpatient: A patient who receives ambulatory care services in a hospital-based clinic or department

Outpatient code editor (OCE): A software program linked to the Correct Coding Initiative that applies a set of logical rules to determine whether various combinations of codes are correct and appropriately represent the services provided

Outpatient prospective payment system (OPPS): The Medicare prospective payment system used for hospital-based outpatient services and procedures that is predicated on the assignment of ambulatory payment classifications

Outpatient visit: A patient's visit to one or more units located in the ambulatory services area (clinic or physician's office) of an acute care hospital

Outsourcing: The hiring of an individual or a company external to an organization to perform a function either on site or off site

Overhead costs: The expenses associated with supporting but not providing patient care services

Owner's equity: The value of the investment in an organization by its owners

Packaging: A payment under the Medicare outpatient prospective payment system that includes items such as anesthesia, supplies, certain drugs, and the use of recovery and observation rooms

Panel interview: An interview format in which the applicant is interviewed by several interviewers at the same time

Par level: The accepted, standard inventory level for all supplies and equipment in an organization

Paradigm: A philosophical or theoretical framework within which a discipline formulates its theories and makes generalizations

Parallel work division: A type of concurrent work design in which one employee does several tasks and takes the job from beginning to end

Parametric technique: A type of statistical procedure that is based on the assumption that a variable is normally distributed in a population

Pareto chart: A bar graph that includes bars arranged in order of descending size to show decisions on the prioritization of issues, problems, or solutions

Partial hospitalization: A term that refers to limited patients stays in the hospital setting, typically as part of a transitional program to a less intense level of service; for example, psychiatric and drug and alcohol treatment facilities that offer services to help patients reenter the community, return to work, and assume family responsibilities

Participant observation: A research method in which researchers also participate in the observed actions

Partnership: The business venture of two or more owners for whom the profits represent the owners' personal income

Part-time employee: An employee who works less than the full-time standard of forty hours per week, eighty hours per two-week period, or eight hours per day

Patient care charting system: A system in which caregivers enter data into health records

Patient Care Data Set (PCDS): A terminology of patient problems, patient care goals, and patient care orders that represents and captures clinical data for inclusion in patient care information systems

Patient/member Web portals: The media for providing patient/member access to the provider organization's multiple sources of data from any network-connected device

Patient-specific data: *See* **patent-specific/identifiable data**

Patient-specific/identifiable data: Data in the health record that relates to a particular patient identified by name

Pay for performance: The Integrated Healthcare Association initiative in California based on the concept that physician groups would be paid for documented performance

Payback period: A financial method used to evaluate the value of a capital expenditure by calculating the time frame that must pass before inflow of cash from a project equals or exceeds outflow of cash

Payer of last resort (Medicaid): A Medicaid term that means that Medicare pays for the services provided to individuals enrolled in both Medicare and Medicaid until Medicare benefits are exhausted and Medicaid benefits begin

Payment status indicator (PSI): An alphabetic code assigned to CPT/HCPCS codes to indicate whether a service or procedure is to be reimbursed under the Medicare outpatient prospective payment system

PDSA cycle (Plan-do-study-act): A performance improvement model designed specifically for healthcare organizations

Peer review: A service that provides diagnostic and therapeutic services for patients under the age of fourteen years

Peer review organization (PRO): Until 2002, a medical organization that performs a professional review of medical necessity, quality, and appropriateness of healthcare services provided to Medicare beneficiaries; now called quality improvement organization (QIO)

Peer-reviewed (refereed) journal: A type of professional or scientific journal for which content experts evaluate articles prior to publication

Per member per month (PMPM): *See* **per patient per month**

Per patient per month (PPPM): A type of managed care arrangement by which providers are paid a fixed fee in exchange for supplying all of the healthcare services an enrollee needs for a specified period of time (usually one month but sometimes one year)

Performance counseling: Guidance provided to an individual in an attempt to improve his or her work performance

Performance improvement (PI): The continuous study and adaptation of a healthcare organization's functions and processes to increase the likelihood of achieving desired outcomes

Performance measure: A quantitative tool used to assess the clinical, financial, and utilization aspects of a healthcare provider's outcomes or processes

Performance measure/measurement system: System designed to improve performance by providing feedback on whether goals have been met

Performance measurement: The process of comparing the outcomes of an organization, work unit, or employee against preestablished performance plans and standards

Performance review: An evaluation of an employee's job performance

Performance standards: The stated expectations for acceptable quality and productivity associated with a job function

Permanent budget variance: A financial term the refers to the difference between the budgeted amount and the actual amount of a line item that is not expected to reverse itself during a subsequent period

Personal digital assistant (PDA): A hand-held microcomputer, without a hard drive, that is capable of running applications such as e-mail and providing access to data and information, such as notes, phone lists, schedules, and laboratory results, primarily through a pen device

Personal health dimension (PHD): One of three dimensions of the National Health Information Infrastructure privacy concept that supports individuals in managing their own wellness and healthcare decision making

Personal health record (PHR): An electronic or paper health record maintained and updated by an individual for himself or herself

Physical data model: The lowest level of data model with the lowest level of abstraction

Physical data repository: A repository organized into data fields, data records, and data files, storing structured, discrete, clinical, administrative, and financial data as well as unstructured, patient free-text, bit-mapped, real audio, streaming video, or vector graphic data

Physician assistant (PA): A healthcare professional licensed to practice medicine with physician supervision

Physician index: A list of patients and their physicians that is usually arranged according to the physician code numbers assigned by the healthcare facility

Physician-hospital organization (PHO): An integrated delivery system formed by hospitals and physicians (usually through managed care contracts) that allows for cooperative activity but permits participants to retain some level of independence

Physiological signal processing systems: Systems that store vector graphic data based on the human body's signals and create output based on the lines plotted between the signals' points

Pie chart: A graphic technique in which the proportions of a category are displayed as portions of a circle (like pieces of a pie)

Piece-rate incentive: An adjustment of the compensation paid to a worker based on exceeding a certain level of output

Pilot study: A trial run on a smaller scale

Pixel: An abbreviation for the term picture element, which is defined by many tiny bits of data or points

Placebo: A medication with no active ingredients

Plaintiff: The group or person who initiates a civil lawsuit

Planning: An examination of the future and preparation of action plans to attain goals; one of the four traditional management functions

Point method: A method of job evaluation that places weight (points) on each of the compensable factors in a job whereby the total points associated with a job establish its relative worth and jobs that fall within a specific range of points fall into a pay grade with an associated wage

Point-of-care information system: A computer system that captures data at the location (for example, bedside, exam room, or home) where the healthcare service is performed

Point-of-care review: *See* **open-record review**

Point-of-service (POS) plan: A type of managed care plan in which enrollees are encouraged to select healthcare providers from a network of providers under contract with the plan but are also allowed to select providers outside the network and pay a larger share of the cost

Policy: 1. A governing principle that describes how a department or an organization is supposed to handle a specific situation 2. Binding contract issued by a healthcare insurance company to an individual or group in which the company promises to pay for healthcare to treat illness or injury

Policyholder: An individual or entity that purchases healthcare insurance coverage

Population health dimension (PHD): One of three dimensions of the National Health Information Infrastructure privacy concept that addresses protecting and promoting the health of the community

Population-based registry: A type of registry that includes information from more than one facility in a specific geopolitical area, such as a state or region

Population-based statistics: Statistics based on a defined population rather than on a sample drawn from the same population

Position (job) description: A document that outlines the work responsibilities associated with a job

Positive (direct) relationship: A relationship in which the effect moves in the same direction

Positivism: A philosophy of research that assumes that there is a single truth across time and place and that researchers are able to adopt a neutral, unbiased stance and establish causation; *See* **quantitative approach**

Post–acute care: Care provided to patients who have been released from an acute care facility to recuperate at home

Postneonatal mortality rate: The number of deaths of persons aged twenty-eight days up to, but not including, one year during a given time period divided by the number of live births for the same time period

Postoperative infection rate: The number of infections that occur in clean surgical cases for a given time period divided by the total number of operations within the same time period

Potentially compensable event (PCE): An event (for example, an injury, accident, or medical error) that may result in financial liability for a healthcare organization

Practice guidelines: Protocols of care that guide the clinical care process

Practice management system (PMS): Software designed to help medical practices run more smoothly and efficiently

Precision factor: The definitive tolerable error rate to be considered in calculations of productivity standards

Predecessor: A task that affects the scheduling of a successor task in a dependency relationship

Predictive modeling: A process used to identify patterns that can be used to predict the odds of a particular outcome based on the observed data

Preemption: In law, the principle that a statute at one level supercedes or is applied over the same or similar statute at a lower level (for example, the federal HIPAA privacy provisions trump the same or similar state law with certain exceptions)

Preferred provider organization (PPO): A managed care arrangement based on a contractual agreement between healthcare providers (professional and/or institutional) and employers, insurance carriers, or third-party administrators to provide healthcare services to a defined population of enrollees at established fees that may or may not be a discount from usual and customary or reasonable charges

Pregnancy Discrimination Act (1978): The federal legislation that prohibits discrimination against women affected by pregnancy, childbirth, or related medical conditions by requiring that affected women be treated the same as all other employees for employment-related purposes, including benefits

Premium: Amount of money that a policyholder or certificate holder must periodically pay an insurer in return for healthcare coverage

President's E-Gov Initiative: An initiative introduced in the 2002 budget submission to eliminate redundant systems and improve the government's quality of customer service for citizens and businesses

President's Information Technology Advisory Committee (PITAC): A committee that advises the federal administration on information technology, including EHR interoperability issues

Prevalence rate: The proportion of people in a population who have a particular disease at a specific point in time or over a specified period of time

Preventive controls: Internal controls implemented prior to an activity and designed to stop an error from happening

Primary analysis: The analysis of original research data by the researchers who collected them

Primary care manager (PCM): The healthcare provider assigned to a TRICARE enrollee

Primary care physician (PCP): 1. Physician who provides, supervises, and coordinates the healthcare of a member and who manages referrals to other healthcare providers and utilization of healthcare services both inside and outside a managed care plan   2. The physician who makes the initial diagnosis of a patient's medical condition

Primary data source: A record developed by healthcare professionals in the process of providing patient care

Primary key: An explanatory notation that uniquely identifies each row in a database table

Primary source: An original work of a researcher who conducted an investigation

Principal diagnosis: The disease or condition that was present on admission, was the principal reason for admission, and received treatment or evaluation during the hospital stay or visit

Principal investigator: The individual with primary responsibility for the design and conduct of a research project

Principal procedure: The procedure performed for the definitive treatment of a condition (as opposed to a procedure performed for diagnostic or exploratory purposes) or for care of a complication

Priority focus process (PFP): A process used by the JCAHO to collect, analyze, and create information about a specific organization being accredited in order to customize the accreditation process

Privacy: The quality or state of being hidden from, or undisturbed by, the observation or activities of other persons or freedom from unauthorized intrusion; in healthcare-related contexts, the right of a patient to control disclosure of personal information

Privacy Act of 1974: The legislation that gave individuals some control over information collected about them by the federal government

Privacy Rule: The federal regulations created to implement the privacy requirements of the simplification subtitle of the Health Insurance Portability and Accountability Act of 1996

Privacy standards: Rules, conditions, or requirements developed to ensure the privacy of patient information

Privilege: The professional relationship between patients and specific groups of caregivers that affects the patient's health record and its contents as evidence; the services or procedures, based on training and experience, that an individual physician is qualified to perform; a right granted to a user, program, or process that allows access to certain files or data in a system

Privileging process: The process of evaluating a physician's or other licensed independent practitioner's quality of medical practice and determining the services or procedures he or she is qualified to perform

Problem-oriented medical record (POMR): A way of organizing information in a health record in which clinical problems are defined and documented individually; also called problem-oriented health record

Procedure: A document that describes the steps involved in performing a specific function

Process and work-flow modeling: The process of creating a representation of the actions and information required to perform a function, including decomposition diagrams, dependency diagrams, and data flow diagrams

Process measures: Specific measures that enable the assessment of the steps taken in rendering a service; also called process indicators

Productivity: A unit of performance defined by management in quantitative standards

Professional component (PC): 1. The portion of a healthcare procedure performed by a physician   2. A term generally used in reference to the elements of radiological procedures performed by a physician

Profitability index: An index used to prioritize investment opportunities, where the present value of the cash inflows is divided by the present value of the cash outflows for each investment and the results are compared

Program evaluation and review technique (PERT) chart: A project management tool that diagrams a project's time lines and tasks as well as their interdependencies

Programmed decisions: An automated decision made by people or computers based on a situation being so stable and recurrent that decision rules can be applied to it

Programmers: Individuals primarily responsible for writing program codes and developing applications, typically performing the function of systems development and working closely with system analysts

Programs of All-Inclusive Care for the Elderly (PACE): A state option legislated by the Balanced Budget Act of 1997 that provides an alternative to institutional care for individuals fifty-five years old or older who require the level of care provided by nursing facilities

Progress notes: The documentation of a patient's care, treatment, and therapeutic response that is entered into the health record by each of the clinical professionals involved in a patient's care, including nurses, physicians, therapists, and social workers

Progressive discipline: A four-step process for shaping employee behavior to conform to the requirements of the employee's job position that begins with a verbal caution and progresses to written reprimand, suspension, and dismissal upon subsequent offenses

Project charter: A document that defines the scope and goals of a specific project

Project components: Related parameters of scope, resources, and scheduling with regard to a project

Project definition: First step in the project management life cycle that sets expectations for the what, when, and how of a project he organization wants to undertake

Project deliverables: The tangible end results of a project

Project management life cycle: The period in which the processes involved in carrying out a project are completed, including project definition, project planning and organization, project tracking and analysis, project revisions, change control, and communication

Project management software: A type of application software that provides the tools to track a project

Project network: The relationship between tasks in a project that determines the overall finish date

Project office: A support function for project management best practices

Project plan: A plan consisting of a list of the tasks to be performed in a project, a defined order in which they will occur, task start and finish dates, and the resource effort needed to complete each task

Project schedule: The portion of the project plan that deals specifically with task start and finish dates

Project scope: 1. The intention of a project   2. The range of a project's activities or influence

Project team: A collection of individuals assigned to work on a project

Promotion: The act of being raised in position or rank

Proportion: A type of ratio in which the elements included in the numerator also must be included in the denominator

Proportionate mortality ratio (PMR): The total number of deaths due to a specific cause during a given time period divided by the total number of deaths due to all causes

Prosecutor: An attorney who prosecutes a defendant accused for a crime on behalf of a local, state, or federal government

Prospective payment system (PPS): A type of reimbursement system that is based on preset payment levels rather than actual charges billed after the service has been provided; specifically, one of several Medicare reimbursement systems based on predetermined payment rates or periods and linked to the anticipated intensity of services delivered as well as the beneficiary's condition

Prospective studies: Studies designed to observe outcomes or events that occur after the identification of a group of subjects to be studied

Protected health information (PHI): Under HIPAA, all individually identifiable information, whether oral or recorded in any form or medium, that is created or received by a healthcare provider or any other entity subject to HIPAA requirements

Protocol: In healthcare, a detailed plan of care for a specific medical condition based on investigative studies; in medical research, a rule or procedure to be followed in a clinical trial; in a computer network, a protocol used to address and ensure delivery of data

Public assistance: A monetary subsidy provided to financially needy individuals

Public Company Accounting Oversight Board (PCAOB): A not-for-profit organization that oversees the work of auditors of public companies

Public health: An area of healthcare that deals with the health of populations in geopolitical areas, such as states and counties

Public Health Informatics Institute (PHII): A cooperative of public health, health information systems, and informatics experts established to develop health information systems for public and population health purposes

Public Health Service (PHS): Services concerned primarily with the health of entire communities and population groups

Public key infrastructure (PKI): A system of digital certificates and other registration authorities that verify and authenticate the validity of each party involved in a secure transaction

Purchase order: A paper document or electronic screen on which all details of an intended purchase are reported, including authorizations

Purposive sampling: A strategy of qualitative research in which researchers use their expertise to select representative units and unrepresentative units to capture a wide array of perspectives

Qualitative analysis: A review of the health record to ensure that standards are met and to determine the adequacy of entries documenting the quality of care

Qualitative approach: *See* **naturalism**

Qualitative standards: Service standards in the context of setting expectations for how well or how soon work or a service will be performed

Quality: The degree or grade of excellence of goods or services, including, in healthcare, meeting expectations for outcomes of care

Quality assurance (QA): A set of activities designed to measure the quality of a service, product, or process with remedial action, as needed, to maintain a desired standard

Quality gap: The difference between approved standards, criteria, or expectations in any type of process and actual results

Quality improvement (QI): A set of activities that measures the quality of a service or product through systems or process evaluation and then implements revised processes that result in better healthcare outcomes for patients, based on standards of care

Quality improvement organization (QIO): An organization that performs medical peer review of Medicare and Medicaid claims, including review of validity of hospital diagnosis and procedure coding information; completeness, adequacy, and quality of care; and appropriateness of prospective payments for outlier cases and nonemergent use of the emergency room; until 2002, called peer review organization

Quality indicator (QI): A standard against which actual care may be measured to identify a level of performance for that standard

Quality management: Evaluation of the quality of healthcare services and delivery using standards and guidelines developed by various entities, including the government and independent accreditation organizations

Quantitative analysis: A review of the health record to determine its completeness and accuracy

Quantitative approach: *See* **positivism**

Quantitative standards: Measures of productivity in the context of setting expectations for how efficiently or effectively work will be performed

Questionnaire survey: A type of survey in which the members of the population are questioned through the use of electronic or paper forms

Queuing theory: An operations management technique for examining customer flow and designing ideal wait or scheduling times

Radio frequency identification (RFID): An automatic recognition technology that uses a device attached to an object to transmit data to a receiver and does not require direct contact

Random sampling: An unbiased selection of subjects that includes methods such as simple random sampling, stratified random sampling, systematic sampling, and cluster sampling

Randomization: The assignment of subjects to experimental or control groups based on chance

Randomized clinical trial (RCT): A special type of clinical trial in which the researchers follow strict rules to randomly assign patients to groups

Range: A measure of variability between the smallest and largest observations in a frequency distribution

Raster image: A digital image or digital data made up of pixels in a horizontal and vertical grid or a matrix instead of lines plotted between a series of points

Rate: A measure used to compare an event over time; a comparison of the number of times an event did happen (numerator) with the number of times an event could have happened (denominator)

Ratio: 1. A calculation found by dividing one quantity by another   2. A general term that can include a number of specific measures such as proportion, percentage, and rate

Ratio analysis: Mathematical computations that compare elements of an organization's financial statements

Ratio data: Data with a defined unit of measure, a real zero point, and with equal intervals between successive values; also called ratio-level data

Ratio scale: Continuous data having both equal intervals and an absolute zero point

Real audio (or sound) data: The storing, manipulating, and displaying of sound in a computer-readable format

Recruitment: The process of finding, soliciting, and attracting employees

Redundant array of independent (or inexpensive) disks (RAID): A method of ensuring data security

Reengineering: Fundamental rethinking and radical redesign of business processes to achieve significant performance improvements

Reference check: Contact made with an individual that a prospective employee has listed to provide a favorable account of his or her work performance or personal attributes

Reference data: Information that interacts with the care of the individual or with the healthcare delivery system, such as a formulary, protocol, care plan, clinical alert, or reminder

Reference terminology: A set of concepts and relationships that provide a common consultation point for the comparison and aggregation of data about the entire healthcare process, recorded by multiple individuals, systems, or institutions

Referred outpatient: An outpatient who is provided special diagnostic or therapeutic services by a hospital on an ambulatory basis but whose medical care remains the responsibility of the referring physician

Regional health information network (RHIN): System that links various healthcare information systems in a region together so that patients, healthcare institutions, and other entities can share clinical information

Regional health information organization (RHIO): An organization that manages the local deployment of systems promoting and facilitating the exchange of healthcare data within a national health information network

Registered health information administrator (RHIA): A type of certification granted after completion of an AHIMA-accredited four-year program in health information management and a credentialing examination

Registered health information technician (RHIT): A type of certification granted after completion of an AHIMA-accredited two-year program in health information management and a credentialing examination

Rehabilitation services: Health services provided to assist patients in achieving and maintaining their optimal level of function, self-care, and independence after some type of disability

Reinforcement: The process of increasing the probability of a desired response through reward

Relational database: A type of database that stores data in predefined tables made up of rows and columns

Relational database management system (RDBMS): A database management system in which data are organized and managed as a collection of tables

Relational online analytical processing (ROLAP): A data access methodology that provides users with various drill-down and business analysis capabilities similar to online analytical processing

Relationship: A type of connection between two terms

Relative risk (RR): A ratio that compares the risk of disease between two groups

Relative value unit (RVU): A measurement that represents the value of the work involved in providing a specific professional medical service in relation to the value of the work involved in providing other medical services

Reliability: A measure of consistency of data items based on their reproducibility and an estimation of their error of measurement

Remittance advice (RA): An explanation of payments (for example, claim denials) made by third-party payers

Report cards: A method used by managed care organizations (and other healthcare sectors) to report cost and quality of care provided

Report generation: The process of analyzing, organizing, and presenting recorded patient information for authentication and inclusion in the patient's healthcare record; the formatting and/or structuring of captured information

Request for information (RFI): A written communication often sent to a comprehensive list of vendors during the design phase of the systems development life cycle to ask for general product information

Request for production: A discovery device used to compel another party to produce documents and other items or evidence important to a lawsuit

Request for proposal (RFP): A type of business correspondence asking for very specific product and contract information that is often sent to a narrow list of vendors that have been preselected after a review of requests for information during the design phase of the systems development life cycle

Research: An inquiry process aimed at discovering new information about a subject or revising old information

Research data: Data used for the purpose of answering a proposed question or testing a hypothesis

Research method: The particular strategy used by a researcher to collect, analyze, and present data

Research methodology: A set of procedures or strategies used by researchers to collect, analyze, and present data

Resident Assessment Instrument (RAI): A uniform assessment instrument developed by the Centers for Medicare and Medicaid Services to standardize the collection of skilled nursing facility patient data; includes the Minimum Data Set 2.0, triggers, and resident assessment protocols

Resident assessment protocols (RAPs): A summary of a long-term care resident's medical condition and care requirements

Resident Assessment Validation and Entry (RAVEN): A type of data-entry software developed by the Centers for Medicare and Medicaid Services for long-term care facilities and used to collect Minimum Data Set assessments and to transmit data to state databases

Resource Utilization Groups, Version III (RUG-III): A case-mix–adjusted classification system based on Minimum Data Set assessments and used by skilled nursing facilities

Resource-based relative value scale (RBRVS): A Medicare reimbursement system implemented in 1992 to compensate physicians according to a fee schedule predicated on weights assigned on the basis of the resources required to provide the services

Resources: The labor, equipment, or materials needed to complete a project

Respect for Persons: The principle that all people are presumed to be free and responsible and should be treated accordingly

Respite care: A type of short-term care provided during the day or overnight to individuals in the home or institution to temporarily relieve the family home caregiver

Responsibility: The accountability required as part of a job, such as supervising work performed by others or managing assets or funds

Restitution: The act of returning something to its rightful owner, of making good or giving something equivalent for any loss, damage, or injury

Resume: A document that describes a job candidate's educational background, work experience, and professional achievements

Retained earnings: Undistributed profits from a for-profit organization that stay in the business

Retention: 1. The process whereby inactive health records are stored and made available for future use in compliance with state and federal requirements 2. The ability to keep valuable employees from seeking employment elsewhere

Retention schedules: Timetables specifying how long various records are to be maintained according to rules, regulations, standards, and laws

Retrospective: A type of time frame that looks back in time

Retrospective payment system: Type of fee-for-service reimbursement in which providers receive recompense after health services have been rendered; also called retrospective payment method

Retrospective study: A type of research conducted by reviewing records from the past (for example, birth and death certificates and/or health records) or by obtaining information about past events through surveys or interviews

Return on equity (ROE): A more comprehensive measurement of profitability that takes into consideration the organization's net value

Return on investment (ROI): The financial analysis of the extent of value a major purchase will provide

Revenge effects: Unintended and typically negative consequences of a change in technology

Revenue: The charges generated from providing healthcare services; earned and measurable income

Revenue codes: A three- or four-digit number in the chargemaster that totals all items and their charges for printing on the form used for Medicare billing

Reverse mentoring: The opposite of the usual coaching process where the younger goes to the older instructor

Risk: 1. The possibility of injury or loss 2. The probable amount of loss foreseen by an insurer in issuing a contract

Risk analysis: An assessment of possible security threats to the organization's data

Risk prevention: One component of a successful risk management program

Role playing: A training method in which participants are required to respond to specific problems they may actually encounter in their jobs

Role theory: Thinking that attempts to explain how people adopt specific roles, including leadership roles

Roles and responsibilities: The definition of who does what on a project and the hierarchy for decision making

Root-cause analysis: A technique used in performance improvement initiatives to discover the underlying causes of a problem

Rule induction: *See* **association rule analysis**

Run chart: A type of graph that shows data points collected over time and identifies emerging trends or patterns

RxNorm: A clinical drug nomenclature developed by the Food and Drug Administration, the Department of Veterans Affairs, and HL7 to provide standard names for clinical drugs and administered dose forms

Safe practices: Behaviors undertaken to reduce or prevent adverse effects and medical errors

Sample: A set of units selected for study that represents a population

Sample size: The number of subjects needed in a study to represent a population

Sample size calculation: The qualitative and quantitative procedures to determine an appropriate sample size

Sample survey: A type of survey that collects data from representative members of a population

Satisficing: A decision-making process in which the decision maker accepts a solution to a problem that is satisfactory rather than optimal

Scalar chain: A theory in the chain of command in which everyone is included and authority and responsibility flow downward from the top of the organization

Scale: Measure with progressive categories, such as size, amount, importance, rank, or agreement

Scales of measurement: A reference standard for data collection and classification; *See* **categorical data**

Scanning: The process by which a document is read into an optical imaging system

Scatter chart: *See* **scatter diagram**

Scatter diagram: A graph that visually displays the linear relationships among factors

Scenarios: Stories describing the current and feasible future states of the business environment

Scheduling engine: A specific functionality in project management software that automates the assignment of task start-and-finish dates and, as a result, the expected project finish date

Scientific inquiry: A process that comprises making predictions, collecting and analyzing evidence, testing alternative theories, and choosing the best theory

Scientific management: A principle that states that the best management is a science based on laws and rules and that secures maximum prosperity for both employer and employee

Scope creep: A process in which the scope of a project grows while the project is in process, virtually guaranteeing that it will be over budget and behind schedule

Scope of command: The number and type of employees who report to a specific management position in a defined organizational structure

Scope of work: The time period an organization is under contract to perform as a quality improvement organization

Secondary analysis: A method of research involving analysis of the original work of another person or organization

Secondary data source: Data derived from the primary patient record, such as an index or a database

Secondary release of information: A type of information release in which the initial requester forwards confidential information to others without obtaining required patient authorization

Secondary source: A summary of an original work, such as an encyclopedia

Secure messaging systems: A system that eliminates the security concerns that surround e-mail, but retains the benefits of proactive, traceable, and personalized messaging

Securities and Exchange Commission (SEC): The federal agency that regulates all public and some private transactions involving the ownership and debt of organizations

Security: 1. The means to control access and protect information from accidental or intentional disclosure to unauthorized persons and from unauthorized alteration, destruction, or loss 2. The physical protection of facilities and equipment from theft, damage, or unauthorized access; collectively, the policies, procedures, and safeguards designed to protect the confidentiality of information, maintain the integrity and availability of information systems, and control access to the content of these systems

Security standards: Statements that describe the processes and procedures meant to ensure that patient-identifiable health information remains confidential and protected from unauthorized disclosure, alteration, and destruction

Selection: The act or process of choosing

Self-directed learning: An instructional method that allows students to control their learning and progress at their own pace

Self-monitoring: The act of observing the reactions of others to one's behavior and making the necessary behavioral adjustments to improve the reactions of others in the future

Semantic clinical drug (SCD): Standardized names created in RxNorm for every clinical drug; consists of components and a dose form

Semantic Clinical Drug (SCD) of RxNorm: *See* **semantic clinical drug**

Semantic differential scale: A measure that records a group's perception of a product, organization, or program through bipolar adjectives on a seven-point continuum, resulting in a profile

Semantics: The meaning of a word or term; sometimes refers to comparable meaning, usually achieved through a standard vocabulary

Semistructured question: A type of question that begins with a structured question and follows with an unstructured question to clarify

Sentinel event: According to the JCAHO, an unexpected occurrence involving death or serious physical or psychological injury, or the risk thereof

Serial filing system: A health record identification system in which a patient receives sequential unique numerical identifiers for each encounter with, or admission to, a healthcare facility

Serial numbering system: A type of health record identification and filing system in which patients are assigned a different but unique numerical identifier for every admission

Serial work division: A system of work organization where each task is performed by one person in sequence

Serial-unit numbering system: A health record identification system in which patient numbers are assigned in a serial manner but records are brought forward and filed under the last number assigned

Server redundancy: Situation where two servers are duplicating effort

Service: An act performed by a person on behalf of another person

Seven dimensions of data quality: The seven characteristics—relevancy, granularity, precision, timeliness, currency, consistency, and accuracy—used to evaluate the quality of data

Severity indexing: 1. The process of using clinical evidence to identify the level of resource consumption 2. A method for determining degrees of illness

Shift differential: An increased wage paid to employees who work less desirable shifts, such as evenings, nights, or weekends

Shift rotation: The assignment of employees to different periods of service to provide coverage, as needed

Simon's decision-making model: A model proposing that the decision-making process moves through three phases: intelligence, design, and choice

Simple random sampling: The process of selecting units from a population so that each one has exactly the same chance of being included in the sample

Simulation: A training technique for experimenting with real-world situation by means of a computerized model that represents the actual situation

Simulation and inventory modeling: The key components of a plan that are computer simulated for testing and experimentation so that optimal operational procedures can be found

Simulation observation: A type of nonparticipant observation in which researchers stage events rather than allowing them to happen naturally

Simultaneous equations method: A budgeting concept that distributes overhead costs through multiple iterations, allowing maximum distribution of interdepartmental costs among overhead departments

Single-blinded study: A study design in which (typically) the investigator but not the subject, knows the identity of the treatment and control groups

Six Sigma: Disciplined and data-driven methodology for getting rid of defects in any process

Skill: The ability, education, experience, and training required to perform a job task

Skilled nursing facility (SNF): A long-term care facility with an organized professional staff and permanent facilities (including inpatient beds) that provides continuous nursing and other health-related, psychosocial, and personal services to patients who are not in an acute phase of illness but who primarily require continued care on an inpatient basis

Skilled nursing facility prospective payment system (SNF PPS): A per-diem reimbursement system implemented in July 1998 for costs (routine, ancillary, and capital) associated with covered skilled nursing facility services furnished to Medicare Part A beneficiaries

Snowflake schema: A modification of the star schema in which the dimension tables are further divided to reduce data redundancy

Social Security Act 1935: The federal legislation that originally established the Social Security program as well as unemployment compensation, and support for mothers and children; amended in 1965 to create the Medicare and Medicaid programs

Social Security number (SSN): A unique numerical identifier assigned to every U.S. citizen

Socialization: The process of influencing the behavior and attitudes of a new employee to adapt positively to the work environment

Sole proprietorship: A venture with one owner in which all profits are considered the owner's personal income

Source systems: An information system that operates independently of a CPR system but provides data to it

Source-oriented health record: A system of health record organization in which information is arranged according to the patient care department that provided the care

Spaced training: The process of learning a task in sections separated by time

Span of control: The number of subordinates reporting to a supervisor

Special cause variation: An unusual source of variation that occurs outside a process but affects it

Speech recognition technology: Technology that translates speech to text

Sponsor: A person or an entity that initiates a clinical investigation of a drug (usually the drug manufacturer or research institution that developed the drug) by distributing it to investigators for clinical trials; a person in an organization that supports, protects, and promotes an idea within the organization; the company position with the ultimate responsibility for a project's success

Stable monetary unit: The currency used as the measurement of financial transactions

Staff authority: The lines of reporting in the organizational chart in which the position advises or makes recommendations

Staff model health maintenance organization: A type of health maintenance that employs physicians to provide healthcare services to subscribers

Staffing structure: The arrangement of staff positions within an organization

Staging system: A method used in cancer registers to identify specific and separate different stages or aspects of the disease

Stakeholder: An individual within the company who has an interest in, or is affected by, the results of a project

Standard: 1. A scientifically based statement of expected behavior against which structures, processes, and outcomes can be measured   2. A model or example established by authority, custom, or general consent or a rule established by an authority as a measure of quantity, weight, extent, value, or quality

Standard deviation: A measure of variability that describes the deviation from the mean of a frequency distribution in the original units of measurement; the square root of the variance

Standard of care: An established set of clinical decisions and actions taken by clinicians and other representatives of healthcare organizations in accordance with state and federal laws, regulations, and guidelines; codes of ethics published by professional associations or societies; regulations for accreditation published by accreditation agencies; usual and common practice of equivalent clinicians or organizations in a geographical regions

Standards development organization (SDO): A private or government agency involved in the development of healthcare informatics standards at a national or international level

Star schema: A visual method of expressing a multidimensional data structure in a relational database

State Children's Health Insurance Program (SCHIP): The children's healthcare program implemented as part of the Balanced Budget Act of 1997; sometimes referred to as the Children's Health Insurance Program, or CHIP

State workers' compensation insurance funds: Funds that provide a stable source of insurance coverage for work-related illnesses and injuries and serve to protect employers from underwriting uncertainties by making it possible to have continuing availability of workers' compensation coverage

Statement: A list of unpaid invoices; sometimes a cumulative list of all transactions between purchaser and vendor during a specific time period

Statement of cash flow: A statement detailing the reasons why cash amounts changed from one balance sheet period to another

Statement of retained earnings: A statement expressing the change in retained earnings from the beginning of the balance sheet period to the end

Statement of stockholder's equity: A statement detailing the reasons for changes in each stockholder's equity accounts

Statement of work: A document that defines the scope and goals of a specific project

Statistical process control chart: A type of run chart that includes both upper and lower control limits and indicates whether a process is stable or unstable

Statute of limitations: A specific time frame allowed by a statute or law for bringing litigation

Statutory law: Written law established by federal and state legislatures

Stem and leaf plots: A visual display that organizes data to show its shape and distribution, using two columns with the stem in the left-hand column and all leaves associated with that stem in the right-hand column; the "leaf" is the ones digit of the number, and the other digits form the "stem"

Step-down allocation: A budgeting concept in which overhead costs are distributed once, beginning with the area that provides the least amount of non-revenue-producing services

Storytelling: A group process technique in which group members create stories describing the plausible future state of the business environment

Strategic communications: Programs created to advance specific organizational goals such as promoting a new center or service, establishing a new program, or positioning the organization as a center of excellence in a specific discipline such as cardiology or oncology

Strategic IS planning: A process for setting IS priorities within an organization; the process of identifying and prioritizing IS needs based on the organization's strategic goals with the intent of ensuring that all IS technology initiatives are integrated and aligned with the organization's overall strategic plan

Strategic management: The art and science of formulating, implementing, and evaluating cross-functional decisions that enable an organization to achieve its objectives

Strategic plan: A broad organization-wide plan by which the facility accomplishes its strategic goals

Strategic planning: A disciplined effort to produce fundamental decisions that shape and guide what an organization is, what it does, and why it does it

Strategy: A course of action designed to produce a desired (business) outcome

Strategy map: A visual representation of the cause-and-effect relationships among the components of an organization's strategy

Stratified random sampling: The process of selecting the same percentages of subjects for a study sample as they exist in the subgroups (strata) of the population

Structure: A term from Donabedian's model of quality assessment that assesses an organization's ability to provide services in terms of both the physical building and equipment and the people providing the healthcare services

Structure and content standards: Common data elements and definitions of the data elements to be included in an electronic patient record

Structure measures: Indicators that measure the attributes of the healthcare setting (for example, adequacy of equipment and supplies)

Structured analysis: A pattern identification analysis performed for a specific task

Structured (close-ended) question: A type of question that limits possible responses

Structured data: Binary, computer-readable data

Structured decision: A decision made by following a formula or a step-by-step process

Structured interview: An interview format that uses a set of standardized questions that are asked of all applicants

Structured query language (SQL): A fourth-generation computer language that includes both DDL and DML components and is used to create and manipulate relational databases

Sub–acute care: A type of step-down care provided after a patient is released from an acute care hospital (including nursing homes and other facilities that provide medical care, but not surgical or emergency care)

Subprojects: Smaller components of a larger project

Successor: A task in a dependency relationship between two tasks that is dependent on the predecessor task

Supervised learning: Any learning technique that has as its purpose to classify or predict attributes of objects or individuals

Supervisory managers: Managers who oversee small (two- to ten-person) functional workgroups or teams and often perform hands-on functions in addition to supervisory functions

Supplemental medical insurance (SMI) (Medicare Part B): A voluntary medical insurance program that helps pay for physicians' services, medical services, and supplies not covered by Medicare Part A

Surgical review: Evaluation of operative and other procedures, invasive and noninvasive, using JCAHO guidelines

Survey: A method of self-report research in which the individuals themselves are the source of the data

Synchronous: Occurring at the same time

Syntax: A term that refers to the comparable structure or format of data, usually as they are being transmitted from one system to another

System: A set of related and highly interdependent components that are operating for a particular purpose

System catalog: An integrated data dictionary (which is a component of a database management system) that generally contains information on data tables and relationships in addition to data definitions

Systematic literature review: Methodical approach to literature review the reduces the possibility of bias; characterized by explicit search criteria to identify literature, inclusion and exclusion criteria to select articles and information sources, and evaluation against consistent methodological standards

Systematic sampling: The process of selecting a sample of subjects for a study by drawing every nth unit on a list

Systemized Nomenclature of Medicine (SNOMED): A comprehensive clinical vocabulary developed by the College of American Pathologists that is the most promising set of clinical terms available for a controlled vocabulary for healthcare

Systemized Nomenclature of Medicine Clinical Terminology (SNOMED CT): A comprehensive, controlled clinical vocabulary developed by the College of American Pathologists

Systemized Nomenclature of Medicine Reference Terminology (SNOMED RT): A concept-based terminology consisting of more than 110,000 concepts with linkages to more than 180,000 terms with unique computer-readable codes

Systems analysis and design: A performance improvement methodology that can be applied to any type of system

Systems analyst: An individual who investigates, analyzes, designs, develops, installs, evaluates, and maintains an organization's healthcare information systems; is typically involved in all aspects of the systems development life cycle; and serves as a liaison among end users and programmers, database administrators, and other technical personnel

Systems development life cycle (SDLC): A model used to represent the ongoing process of developing (or purchasing) information systems

Systems thinking: An objective way of looking at work-related ideas and processes with the goal of allowing people to uncover ineffective patterns of behavior and thinking and then finding ways to make lasting improvements

Tacit knowledge: The actions, experiences, ideals, values, and emotions of an individual that tend to be highly personal and difficult to communicate (for example, corporate culture, organizational politics, and professional experience)

Tactic: A method for accomplishing an end

Tactical plan: A strategic plan at the level of divisions and departments

Target population: A large group of individuals who are the focus of a study

Task: The step to be performed in order to complete a project or part of a project

Task analysis: A procedure for determining the specific duties and skills required of a job

Tax Equity and Fiscal Responsibility Act of 1982 (TEFRA): The federal legislation that modified Medicare's retrospective reimbursement system for inpatient hospital stays by requiring implementation of diagnosis-related groups and the acute care prospective payment system

Taxonomy: The principles of a classification system, such as data classification, and the study of the general principles of scientific classification

Team building: The process of organizing and acquainting a team, and building skills for dealing with later team processes

Technical component (TC): The portion of radiological and other procedures that is facility based or nonphysician based (for example, radiology films, equipment, overhead, endoscopic suites, and so on)

Technical skills: One of the three managerial skill categories, related to knowledge of the technical aspects of the business

Telecommuting: A work arrangement (often used by coding and transcription personnel) in which at least a portion of the employee's work hours is spent outside the office (usually in the home) and the work is transmitted back to the employer via electronic means; *See* **telestaffing**

Telehealth: A telecommunications system that links healthcare organizations and patients from diverse geographic locations and transmits text and images for (medical) consultation and treatment; also called telemedicine

Telestaffing: *See* **telecommuting**

Temporary Assistance for Needy Families (TANF): A federal program that provides states with grants to be spent on time-limited cash assistance for low-income families, generally limiting a family's lifetime cash welfare benefits to a maximum of five years and permitting states to impose other requirements

Temporary budget variance: The difference between the budgeted and actual amounts of a line item that is expected to reverse itself in a subsequent period; the timing difference between the budget and the actual event

Temporary privileges: Privileges granted for a limited time period to a licensed, independent practitioner on the basis of recommendations made by the appropriate clinical department or the president of the medical staff

Ten-step monitoring and evaluation process: The systematic and ongoing collection, organization, and evaluation of data related to indicator development promoted by the Joint Commission on Accreditation of Healthcare Organizations in the mid-1980s

Terminal-digit filing system: A system of health record identification and filing in which the last digit or group of digits (terminal digits) in the health record number determines file placement

Termination: The act of ending something (for example, a job)

Terminology: A set of terms representing the system of concepts of a particular subject field; a clinical terminology provides the proper use of clinical words as names or symbols

Terminology standard: A terminology adopted by the appropriate standards-setting organizations for use in healthcare

Test statistics: A set of statistical techniques that examines the psychometric properties of measurement instruments

Testing: The act of performing an examination or evaluation

Text mining: The process of extracting and then quantifying and filtering free-text data

Theory: A systematic organization of knowledge that predicts or explains the behavior or events

Theory X and Y: A management theory developed by McGregor that describes pessimistic and optimistic assumptions about people and their work potential

Third-party payer: An insurance company (for example, Blue Cross/Blue Shield) or healthcare program (for example, Medicare) that reimburses healthcare providers (second party) and/or patients (first party) for the delivery of medical services

360-degree evaluation: A method of performance evaluation in which the supervisors, peers, and other staff who interact with the employee contribute information

Time and motion studies: Studies in which complex tasks are broken down into their component motions to determine inefficiencies and to develop improvements

Time ladder: A form used by employees to document time spent on various tasks

Time period: A specific span of dates to which data apply

Tort: An action brought when one party believes that another party caused harm through wrongful conduct and seeks compensation for that harm

Total length of stay (discharge days): The sum of the days of stay of any group of inpatients discharged during a specific period of time

Total quality management (TQM): A management philosophy that includes all activities in which the needs of the customer and the organization are satisfied in the most efficient manner by using employee potentials and continuous improvement

Traditional fee-for-service (FFS) reimbursement: A reimbursement method involving third-party payers who compensate providers after the healthcare services have been delivered; payment is based on specific services provided to subscribers

Train the trainer: A method of training certain individuals who, in turn, will be responsible for training others on a task or skill

Trainee: A person who is learning a task or skill

Trainer: A person who gives instruction on a task or skill

Training: A set of activities and materials that provide the opportunity to acquire job-related skills, knowledge, and abilities

Training and development model: A nine-step plan designed to help the health information manager or human resources department identify the training needs of an employee group

Transaction standards: Standards that support the uniform format and sequence of data during transmission from one healthcare entity to another

Transactional system: A computer-based information system that keeps track of an organization's business transactions through inputs (for example, transaction data such as admissions, discharges, and transfers in a hospital) and outputs (for example, census reports and bills); also called transaction-processing system

Transcription: The process of deciphering and typing medical dictation

Traumatic injury: A wound or injury included in a trauma registry

Treatment: The manipulation, intervention, or therapy; a broad term used by researchers to generically mean some act, such as a physical conditioning program, a computer training program, a particular laboratory medium, or the timing of prophylactic medications

TRICARE: The federal healthcare program that provides coverage for the dependents of armed forces personnel and for retirees receiving care outside military treatment facilities in which the federal government pays a percentage of the cost; formerly known as Civilian Health and Medical Program of the Uniformed Services

TRICARE Extra: A cost-effective preferred provider network TRICARE option in which costs for healthcare are lower than for the standard TRICARE program because a physician or medical specialist is selected from a network of civilian healthcare professionals who participate in TRICARE Extra

TRICARE Prime: A TRICARE program that provides the most comprehensive healthcare benefits at the lowest cost of the three TRICARE options, in which military treatment facilities serve as the principal source of healthcare and a primary care manager is assigned to each enrollee

TRICARE Prime Remote: A program that provides active-duty service members in the United States with a specialized version of TRICARE Prime while they are assigned to duty stations in areas not served by the traditional military healthcare system

TRICARE Senior Prime: A managed care demonstration TRICARE program designed to better serve the medical needs of military retirees, dependents, and survivors who are sixty-five years old and over

TRICARE Standard: A TRICARE program that allows eligible beneficiaries to choose any physician or healthcare provider, which permits the most flexibility but may be the most expensive

Trier of fact: The judge or jury hearing a civil or criminal trial

Two-tailed hypothesis: A type of alternative hypothesis in which the researcher makes no prediction about the direction of the results

Type I error: A type of error in which the researcher erroneously rejects the null hypothesis when it is true

Type II error: A type of error in which the researcher erroneously fails to reject the null hypothesis when it is false

UB-04 (Uniform Bill-04): The single standardized Medicare form for standardized uniform billing, scheduled for implementation in 2007 for hospital inpatients and outpatients; this form will also be used by the major third-party payers and most hospitals

UB-92 (Uniform Bill-92/ CMS-1450): A Medicare form used for standardized uniform billing

Unallocated reserves: Monies that have not been assigned a specific use

Unified Medical Language System (UMLS): A program initiated by the National Library of Medicine to build an intelligent, automated system that can understand biomedical concepts, words, and expressions and their interrelationships

Unified Medical Language System (UMLS) Metathesaurus: A list containing information on biomedical concepts and terms from more than 100 healthcare vocabularies and classifications, administrative health data, bibliographic and full-text databases, and expert systems

Unified Medical Language System (UMLS) Semantic Network: A categorization of all concepts UMDNS in the UMLS Metathesaurus

Unified Medical Language System (UMLS) SPECIALIST Lexicon: An English-language lexicon containing biomedical terms

Unbundling: The practice of using multiple codes to bill for the various individual steps in a single procedure rather than using a single code that includes all of the steps of the comprehensive procedure

Unfavorable variance: The negative difference between the budgeted amount and the actual amount of a line item, where actual revenue is less than budget or where actual expenses exceed budget

Unified modeling language (UML): A common data-modeling notation used in conjunction with object-oriented database design

Uniform Ambulatory Care Data Set (UACDS): A data set developed by the National Committee on Vital and Health Statistics consisting of a minimum set of patient/client-specific data elements to be collected in ambulatory care settings

Uniform Hospital Discharge Data Set (UHDDS): A core set of data elements adopted by the U.S. Department of Health, Education, and Welfare in 1974 that are collected by hospitals on all discharges and all discharge abstract systems

Uniformed Services Employment and Reemployment Rights Act (1994): Federal legislation that prohibits discrimination against individuals because of their service in the Armed Forces Reserves, National Guard, or other uniformed services

Union: A collective bargaining unit that represents groups of employees and is authorized to negotiate with employers on the employees' behalf in matters related to compensation, health, and safety

Unique identification number: A combination of numbers or alphanumeric characters assigned to a particular patient

Unique identifier: A type of information that refers to only one individual or organization

Unique physician identification number (UPIN): A unique numerical identifier created by the Health Care Financing Administration (now called the Centers for Medicare and Medicaid Services) for use by physicians who bill for services provided to Medicare patients

Unit filing system: A health record filing system in which all inpatient and outpatient visits and procedures are arranged together under a permanent unit number

Unit numbering system: A health record identification system in which the patient receives a unique medical record number at the time of the first encounter that is used for all subsequent encounters

Unit work division: A method of work organization where each task is performed by one person at the same time that another person is doing a task, but one does not have to wait for the other

United Nations International Standards Organization (ISO): An international standards organization that coordinates all international standards development

Unity of command: A human resources principle that assumes that each employee reports to only one specific management position

Univariate: A term referring to the involvement of one variable

Universal chart order: A system in which the health record is maintained in the same format while the patient is in the facility and after discharge

Universal Medical Device Nomenclature System (UMDNS): A standard international nomenclature and computer coding system for medical devices, developed by ECRI

Universal protocol: A written checklist developed by the JCAHO to prevent errors that can occur when physicians perform the wrong procedure, for example

Unstructured analysis: A pattern identification analysis performed through a database without the specific goal of discovering interesting patterns that were not conceived previously

Unstructured data: Nonbinary, human-readable data

Unstructured decision: A decision that is made without following a prescribed method, formula, or pattern

Unstructured (open-ended) question: A type of question that allows free-form responses

Unsupervised learning: Any learning technique that has as its purpose to group or cluster items, objects, or individuals

Upcoding: The practice of assigning diagnostic or procedural codes that represent higher payment rates than the codes that actually reflect the services provided to patients

User groups: Groups composed of users of a particular computer system

Usual, customary, and reasonable (UCR) charges: Method of evaluating providers' fees in which the third-party payer pays for fees that are "usual" in that provider's practice, "customary" in the community, and "reasonable" for the situation

Utilization management: 1. The planned, systematic review of the patients in a healthcare facility against care criteria for admission, continued stay, and discharge   2. A collection of systems and processes to ensure that facilities and resources, both human and nonhuman, are used maximally and are consistent with patient care needs

Utilization review (UR): The process of determining whether the medical care provided to a specific patient is necessary according to preestablished objective screening criteria at time frames specified in the organization's utilization management plan

Utilization Review Act: The federal legislation that requires hospitals to conduct continued-stay reviews for Medicare and Medicaid patients

Validity: 1. The extent to which data correspond to the actual state of affairs or that an instrument measures what it purports to measure   2. A term referring to a test's ability to accurately and consistently measure what it purports to measure

Values statement: A short description that communicates an organization's social and cultural belief system

Variability: The dispersion of a set of measures around the population mean

Variable: A factor

Variable costs: Resources expended that vary with the activity of the organization, for example, medication expenses vary with patient volume

Variance: A measure of variability that gives the average of the squared deviations from the mean; in financial management, the difference between the budgeted amount and the actual amount of a line item; in project management, the difference between the original project plan and current estimates

Variance analysis: An assessment of a department's financial transactions to identify differences between the budget amount and the actual amount of a line item

Vector graphic (or signal tracing) data: Digital data that have been captured as points and are connected by lines (a series of point coordinates) or areas (shapes bounded by lines)

Vendor system: A computer system developed by a commercial company not affiliated with the healthcare organization

Verification service: An outside service that provides a primary source check on information that a physician makes available on an application to the medical staff

Vertical structure: The levels and relationships among positions in an organizational hierarchy

Virtual reality (VR): An artificial form of reality experienced through sensory stimuli and in which the participant's actions partly affect what happens

Vision: A picture of the desired future that sets a direction and rationale for change

Vision statement: A short description of an organization's ideal future state

Vital statistics: Data related to births, deaths, marriages, and fetal deaths

Vocabulary: A list or collection of clinical words or phrases and their meanings

Vocabulary standard: A common definition for medical terms to encourage consistent descriptions of an individual's condition in the health record

Voice recognition technology: A method of encoding speech signals that do not require speaker pauses (but uses pauses when they are present) and of interpreting at least some of the signals' content as words or the intent of the speaker

Volume logs: Forms used (sometimes in conjunction with time ladders) to obtain information about the volume of work units received and processed in a day

Voluntary Disclosure Program: A program unveiled in 1998 by the OIG that encourages healthcare providers to voluntarily report fraudulent conduct affecting Medicare, Medicaid, and other federal healthcare programs

Vulnerable subjects:

Web browser–based (or Web native) architectures: Systems and applications written in one or more Web programming languages; also called Web browser-based systems

Web content management systems: Systems in which information placed in a Web site can be labeled and tracked so that it can be easily located, modified, and reused

Web portal: A Web site entryway through which to access, find, and deliver information

Web services: an open, standardized way of integrating disparate, Web browser-based and other applications

Web-based systems and applications: Systems and applications that use Internet technology

Web-based training: Instruction via the Internet that enables learners to work when, where, and at a pace suited to them and offers interaction with other students and the instructor via the listserv

Webmasters: Individuals who support Web applications and the healthcare organization's intranet and Internet operations

Wireless technology: A type of technology that uses wireless networks and wireless devices to access and transmit data in real time

Wisdom: The intelligence that gives individuals the empowerment and courage to act

Word-processing services: Companies outside the healthcare facility that specialize in the deciphering and typing of medical dictation

Work: The effort, usually described in hours, needed to complete a task

Work breakdown structure: A hierarchical structure that decomposes project activities into levels of detail

Work distribution analysis: An analysis used to determine whether a department's current work assignments and job content are appropriate

Work distribution chart: A matrix that depicts the work being done in a particular workgroup in terms of specific tasks and activities, time spent on tasks, and the employees performing the tasks

Work division: The way in which tasks are handled within an organization

Work flow: Any work process that must be handled by more than one person

Work measurement: The process of studying the amount of work accomplished and how long it takes to accomplish work in order to define and monitor productivity

Work products: Documents produced during the completion of a task that may be a component of, or contribute to, a project deliverable

Work sampling: A work measurement technique that uses random sample measurements to characterize the performance of the whole

Workers' Adjustment and Retraining Notification (WARN) Act: Federal legislation that requires employers to give employees a sixty-day notice in advance of covered plant closings and covered mass layoffs

Workers' compensation: The medical and income insurance coverage for certain employees in unusually hazardous jobs

Work-flow technology: Technology that allows computers to add and extract value from document content as the documents move throughout an organization

Workforce trends: Referring to changes that will likely take place in the workforce in the future

Working conditions: The environment in which work is performed (surroundings) and the physical dangers or risks involved in performing the job (hazards)

X12N: Referring to standards adopted for electronic data interchange

Zero-based budget: Types of budgets in which each budget cycle poses the opportunity to continue or discontinue services based on available resources so that every department or activity must be justified and prioritized annually to effectively allocate resources

Index

(continued)

Ensure Career Success with an AHIMA Certification

Registered Health Information Administrator (RHIA)

AHIMA's Registered Health Information Administrator (RHIA) credential helps you stand out from the crowd, showing employers a commitment to working in HIM and a higher competency level.

RHIAs are skilled in the collection, interpretation, and analysis of patient data. RHIAs interact with all levels of a healthcare organization, including clinical, financial, and administrative, to ensure quality information in patient data.

RHIAs enjoy job placements in a variety of settings, including hospitals, physician practices, nursing homes, home health agencies, and public agencies. RHIAs are key team members and leaders in the delivery of successful health information management content and delivery.

> *"The credential is a recognizable symbol of professionalism. I believe it opens doors for higher-level, better-paying, and more interesting jobs."*
>
> Marilyn Davidian, RHIA
> Chair
> Department of Health Information Management
> Loma Linda University
> Loma Linda, CA

Make the right move…pair your degree and experience with AHIMA certification to maximize your career possibilities.

AHIMA is the premier organization for HIM professionals, with more than 50,000 members. AHIMA certification carries a strong reputation for quality and for mastering rigorous certification requirements.

For more information on AHIMA credentials, you can:
Visit our Web site at **www.ahima.org/certification**
E-mail AHIMA at **info@ahima.org**
Call **(800) 335-5535**

Look for These **Quality AHIMA Publications** at **Bookstores, Libraries,** and **Online**

- *Applying Inpatient Coding Skills under Prospective Payment*
- *Basic CPT/HCPCS Coding*
- *Basic ICD-9-CM Coding*
- *The Best of In Confidence*
- *Calculating and Reporting Healthcare Statistics*
- *Clinical Coding Workout: Practice Exercises for Skill Development*
- *Coding and Reimbursement for Hospital Inpatient Services*
- *Coding and Reimbursement for Hospital Outpatient Services*
- *CPT/HCPCS Coding and Reimbursement for Physician Services*
- *Documentation for Acute Care* (Book and CD)
- *Documentation for Ambulatory Care*
- *Documentation and Reimbursement for Behavioral Healthcare Services*
- *Documentation and Reimbursement for Long-Term Care* (Book and CD)
- *Documentation and Reimbursement for Home Care and Hospice Programs*

- *Effective Management of Coding Services*
- *Electronic Health Record*
- *Essentials of Healthcare Finance* (Workbook)
- *Health Information Management*
- *Health Information Management Technology*
- *Health Information Management Compliance* (Book and CD)
- *HIPAA in Practice*
- *ICD-9-CM Diagnostic Coding and Reimbursement for Physician Services*
- *ICD-9-CM Diagnostic Coding for Long-Term Care and Home Care*
- *ICD-10-CM and ICD-10-PCS Preview* (Book and CD)
- *Pocket Glossary of Health Information Management and Technology*
- *Principles of Healthcare Reimbursement*
- *Quality and Performance Improvement in Healthcare*
- *Statistical Applications for Health Information Management*

More Information

For details and easy ordering, visit **www.ahima.org/store.**

For textbook content questions, contact **publications@ahima.org** or **(800) 335-5535.**

American Health Information Management Association®

© 2006 AHIMA

P086

Play a Key Role in the Migration to an Electronic Health Record

AHIMA Helps You Take Center Stage in Advancing Healthcare

AHIMA Offers These Free Practice Standards

- Core Data Sets
- Delving into Computer-assisted Coding
- The Complete Medical Record in a Hybrid EHR Environment
- The Strategic Importance of Electronic Health Records Management
- Implementing e-Signatures
- E-mail as Provider-Patient Electronic Communication Medium and Its Impact on the EHR
- Electronic Document Management as a Component of the EHR
- Core Data Sets for the Physician Practice EHR
- Speech Recognition in the EHR
- HIM Practice Transformation

- The Role of the Personal Health Record in the EHR
- The Legal Process and EHR
- Guidelines for Defining the Legal Health Record
- Update: Maintaining a Legally Sound Health Record—Paper and Electronic
- Surveying the RHIO Landscape
- Guidelines for Developing a Data Dictionary
- Interpretation of Emerging Federal Guidelines for EHR as Legal Evidence and the Impact on Providers
- Standards for Minimum Content for the Legal EHR

And much more.
Go to www.ahima.org and click on "HIM Resources."

The e-HIM® work groups are supported in part by grants to the Foundation of Research and Education (FORE) from Dictaphone Corporation, McKesson, MedQuist, Meta Health Technology Inc., 3M Healthcare Services, Initiate Systems, Inc, and Precyse Solutions, Inc.

AHIMA provides its industry-leading e-HIM® education and advocacy programs to support the effective use of information technology to manage patient information and healthcare data.

American Health Information Management Association®

AHIMA is the premier association of health information management (HIM) professionals. AHIMA's 50,000 members are dedicated to the effective management of personal health information needed to deliver quality healthcare to the public. Founded in 1928 to improve the quality of medical records, AHIMA is committed to advancing the HIM profession in an increasingly electronic and global environment through leadership in advocacy, education, certification, and lifelong learning. For information about the Association, go to www.ahima.org.